ANIMAL MODELS IN TOXICOLOGY

DRUG AND CHEMICAL TOXICOLOGY

1. Toxicity Screening Procedures Using Bacterial Systems, *edited by Dickson Liu and Bernard J. Dutka*
2. Chemically Induced Birth Defects, *James L. Schardein*
3. Neurotpxicology, *edited by Kenneth Blum and Luigi Manzo*
4. Statistics for Toxicologists, *David S. Salsburg*
5. Photobiology of the Skin and Eye, *edited by Edward M. Jackson*
6. Product Safety Evaluation Handbook, *edited by Shayne Cox Gad*
7. Safer Insecticides: Development and Use, *edited by Ernest Hodgson and Ronald J. Kuhr*
8. Animal Models in Toxicology, *edited by Shayne Cox Gad and Christopher P. Chengelis*

ADDITIONAL VOLUMES IN PREPARATION

ANIMAL MODELS IN TOXICOLOGY

EDITED BY

SHAYNE COX GAD

Becton Dickinson and Company
Research Triangle Park, North Carolina

CHRISTOPHER P. CHENGELIS

WIL Research Laboratories, Inc.
Ashland, Ohio

Marcel Dekker, Inc.   New York • Basel • Hong Kong

Library of Congress Cataloging-in-Publication Data

Animal models in toxicology / edited by Shayne Cox Gad, Christopher P.
  Chengelis.
    p.   cm.
  Includes bibliographical references and index.
  ISBN 0-8247-8456-1 (acid-free paper)
    1. Toxicology--Animal models.   2. Toxicity testing.   I. Gad,
Shayne C.   II. Chengelis, Christopher P.
  RA1199.4.A54A52   1992
  615.9'00724--dc20   92-12643
                                           CIP

This book is printed on acid-free paper.

MARCEL DEKKER, INC.
270 Madison Avenue, New York, New York 10016

Current printing (last digit):
10 9 8 7 6 5 4 3 2 1

PRINTED IN THE UNITED STATES OF AMERICA

To my beloved babies (Samantha, Katina, and Jake),
forever in Daddy's heart,
and to Suzann, whom I'll always love.

—S. C. G.

To my wife, MaryAnne.

—C. P. C.

About the Series

Toxicology has come a long way since the ancient use of botanical fluids to eliminate personal and political enemies. While such means are still employed (often with more potent and subtle materials), toxicology has left the boiling-pots-and-vapors atmosphere of the "old days" and evolved into a discipline that is at the forefront of science. In this process, present-day toxicologists adopted a variety of techniques from other scientific areas and developed new skills unique to the questions asked and the studies being pursued. More often than not, the questions asked have never been thought about before, and only through the advances made in other disciplines (for example, in analytical chemistry) were the needs for answers raised. The compounding concerns of society for public safety, the maintenance of environmental health, and the improvement of the welfare of research animals have expanded the boundaries in which toxicologists work. At the same time, society has spotlighted toxicology as the science that will offer the hope of safety guarantees, or at least minimal and acceptable risks, in our everyday chemical encounters.

This *Drug and Chemical Toxicology* series was established to provide a means by which leading scientists may document and communicate important information in the rapidly growing arena of toxicology. Providing relevant and forward-looking subjects with diverse and flexible themes in an expedited and prompt publication format will be our goal. We will strive in this vehicle to provide fellow toxicologists and other knowledgeable and interested parties with appropriate new information that can be promptly applied to help answer current questions.

The present volume systematically explains how animals are best employed in testing and research to improve human health and safety. Clearly, these efforts are indispensable for much-needed, and often long-awaited, progress.

Frederick J. Di Carlo
Frederick W. Oehme

Preface

The use of animals as predictive models in experimental biology in general, and in toxicology and pharmacology in particular, continues to cause more than a little controversy. On one hand, animal models have provided the essential building blocks that have permitted the explosive growth of understanding in these fields, with the multitude of benefits to both humans and other animal species. At the same time, the benefits of such use, balanced against costs, in terms of animal lives and potential suffering and discomfort, have been subject to an increasing level of questioning.

How many animals are used in research, of what species, and from what sources are not clear cut. The best estimates come from the U.S. Department of Agriculture (APHIS) annual reports, as shown in Table 1. These do not include rats and mice, but Table 2 presents a logical extrapolation to estimate total annual animal use in all biomedical research and education (approximately 7,910,000 in 1989). About one-quarter of these animals (i.e., no more than 2,000,000 a year) (Gad, 1990a) are consistently used in toxicology and product-safety evaluation. While great strides have been made in the development of alternative in vitro methods for specific narrow endpoint, there can be little doubt that the use of animals in testing will continue into the foreseeable future.

Scientists have used animal models for so long that the case can be made that many are used purely out of habit, with little or no thought as to "is this the best way?" Although there is an element of this failing that is real, by and large, animals have worked exceptionally well as predictive models for humans—when properly used (Gad, 1990b and Chapters 12 and 13 in this volume).

Regulations governing the purchase, husbandry, and use of animals in research received a great deal of attention during the late 1980s and early 1990s. Table 3 illustrates the degree of this attention by summarizing one aspect (current specifications for housing of species in the laboratory).

The problems behind the failure of animal models lie largely in selecting the wrong model, in not using an animal model correctly, or in extrapolating results to humans poorly. In addition, most graduate degree programs do not currently address these issues well (if at all) in their curricula. Indeed, broad training in animal model selection and use, and the techniques involved in such research, is currently available. This test was developed to address these needs. Indeed, it is essential to the performance of good science that the correct species be used as a model, and that data be analyzed appropriately.

Chapter 1 presents a historical review of the use of animal models and an overview of broad considerations of metabolism and relevance to use in toxicology. The core of the book, however, is in Chapters 2 through 9. Each of these chapters represents the joint efforts of experts in toxicology (addressing techniques for animal use and husbandry and peculiarities of the species as a toxicological model), toxicological pathology, and metabolism. For an investigator who is not well versed in the use of a particular species, each of these chapters provides an excellent introductory "course," along with guidance to the literature for more detailed understanding. All the major species used (and strains or breeds within these species) are addressed in these core chapters.

Chapter 10 presents the case for a range of species (fish, pigs, earthworms, etc.) not commonly used for safety assessment studies but which may provide useful alternative models for some specfic endpoints.

In Chapter 11, Robert Hall presents and discusses the special considerations regarding the evaluation and interpretation of clinical pathology of the eight major model species.

Chapters 12 and 13 address in detail the general case of how to select a model species and how to extrapolate the results to humans. Chapter 13 details the pitfalls in the process—the situations that cause either human or model to be significantly more sensitive than the other or totally irrelevant to each other in specific cases.

Chapter 14 presents an overview of the regulations that govern how laboratory animals are obtained, maintained, and utilized. Such laws have become increasingly complex, and an understanding of what can (and cannot) be done is essential for the modern researcher.

The Appendix provides a quick guide to the major commercial sources of laboratory animals, whether common (rats and mice) or harder to come by (Chinese hamsters and primates). Information on the selection and use of common anesthetics, drugs, and pharmacological agents for use in laboratory animals is available in Borchards' *Drug Dosage In Laboratory Animals: A Handbook* (Telford Press).

Our aim in this volume is to provide a single source reference for the use of animal models in toxicology.

Shayne Cox Gad
Christopher P. Chengelis

REFERENCES

Gad, S. C. (1990a) Recent developments in replacing, reducing, and refining animal use in toxicologic research and testing. *Fund Appl. Toxicol.* 15, 8–16.

Gad, S. C. (1990b) Model selection in toxicology: Principles and practice. *J. Am. Coll. Toxicol.* 9, 291–302.

Table 1   U.S. Experimental Animal Usage

	APHIS 1983	APHIS 1986	APHIS 1987	APHIS 1988	APHIS 1989
Rabbits	509,052	521,773	554,385	459,254	471,037
Guinea pigs	521,237	462,699	538,998	431,457	481,712
Hamsters	454,479	370,655	461,001	331,945	389,042
Dogs	182,425	176,141	180,169	140,471	156,443
Wild animals	Not reported	144,470	168,032	178,249	153,722
Cats	55,346	54,125	50,145	42,271	50,812
Primates	59,336	48,540	61,392	51,641	51,688
Total[a]	NA[b]	1,778,403	1,969,122	1,635,288	1,754,456

[a]Does not include rats and mice.
[b]But would appear (from species reported) to be more than in 1986, 1988, or 1989.
Source: Gad (1990a).

Table 2   Estimating U.S. Rat, Mouse, and Total Animal Use 1986–1989

	U.K. rat and mouse use				
	1985	1986	1987	1988	X
Total #	3,213,673	3,042,633	3,588,838	3,437,571	
Rat #	884,343	830,159	866,349	860,284	
% of total #	27.5	27.3	24.1	25.0	25.97
Mouse #	1,724,616	1,622,138	2,017,289	1,850,463	
% of total #	53.7	53.3	56.2	53.8	54.25

Therefore the average % of total that is rats and mice, and therefore not included in U.S. totals, is 80.2%. If one accepts that patterns of use in the U.S. and U.K. are similar, this means the U.S. total usage should be multiplied by

$$\frac{80.2}{100 - 80.2} = \frac{80.2}{19.8} = 4.05.$$

Applying this to the existing APHIS figures, we get the figures below. 1982 APHIS figures showed mice to be 60.5% of total and rats 23.9%.

	U.S. total animal, rat and mouse use[a]			
	1986	1987	1988	1989
Total #	8,980,935	9,944,066	8,258,204	7,910,157
Mouse	3,907,373	4,326,407	3,592,932	3,854,759
Rat	1,870,497	2,071,092	1,719,971	2,300,943

[a]Extrapolated based on U.K. figures.

Table 3   Laboratory Animal Husbandry

Animals	Weight (g)	Type of housing	Floor area/animal[a] in.²	Floor area/animal[a] cm²	Cage height in.	Cage height cm	Ambient temperature °C	Ambient temperature °F	Relative humidity (%)
Mice	<10	Cage	6.0	38.71	5	12.70	18–26	64.4–78.8	40–70
	10–15	Cage	8.0	51.62	5	12.70	18–26	64.4–78.8	40–70
	15–25	Cage	12.0	77.42	5	12.70	18–26	64.4–78.8	40–70
	>25	Cage	15.0	96.78	5	12.70	18–26	64.4–78.8	40–70
Rats	<100	Cage	17.0	109.68	7	17.78	18–26	64.4–78.8	40–70
	100–200	Cage	23.0	148.40	7	17.78	18–26	64.4–78.8	40–70
	200–300	Cage	29.0	187.11	7	17.78	18–26	64.4–78.8	40–70
	300–400	Cage	40.0	258.08	7	17.78	18–26	64.4–78.8	40–70
	400–500	Cage	60.0	387.12	7	17.78	18–26	64.4–78.8	40–70
	>500	Cage	70.0	451.64	7	17.78	18–26	64.4–78.8	40–70
Hamsters	<60	Cage	10.0	64.52	6	15.24	18–26	64.4–78.8	40–70
	60–80	Cage	13.0	83.88	6	15.24	18–26	64.4–78.8	40–70
	80–100	Cage	16.0	103.23	6	15.24	18–26	64.4–78.8	40–70
	>100	Cage	19.0	122.59	6	15.24	18–26	64.4–78.8	40–70
Guinea pigs	<350	Cage	60.0	387.12	7	17.78	18–26	64.4–78.8	40–70
	>350	Cage	101.0	651.65	7	17.78	18–26	64.4–78.8	40–70
	kg		ft²	m²					
Rabbits	<2	Cage	1.5	0.14	14	35.56	16–21	60.8–69.8	40–60
	2–4	Cage	3.0	0.28	14	35.56	16–21	60.8–69.8	40–60
	4–5.4	Cage	4.0	0.37	14	35.56	16–21	60.8–69.8	40–60
	>5.4	Cage	5.0	0.46	14	35.56	16–21	60.8–69.8	40–60
Cats	<4	Cage	3.0	0.28	24	60.96	18–29	64.4–84.2	30–70
	>4	Cage	4.0	0.37	24	60.96	18–29	64.4–84.2	30–70
Dogs	<15	Pen/run	8.0	0.74	—	—	18–29	64.4–84.2	30–70
	15–30	Pen/run	12.1	1.12	—	—	18–29	64.4–84.2	30–70
	>30	Pen/run	24.0	2.23	—	—	18–29	64.4–84.2	30–70
	<15	Cage	8.0	0.74	32	81.28	18–29	64.4–84.2	30–70
	15–30	Cage	12.1	1.12	36	91.44	18–29	64.4–84.2	30–70
	>30	Cage	[b]	[b]	[b]	[b]	18–29	64.4–84.2	30–70

Table 3 *(continued)*

Animals	Weight (kg)	Type of housing	Floor area/animal[a]		Cage height		Ambient temperature		Relative humidity (%)
			ft²	m²	in.	cm	°C	°F	
Nonhuman primates[c]									
Group 1	<1	Cage	1.6	0.15	20	50.80	18–29	64.4–84.2	30–70
Group 2	1–3	Cage	3.0	0.28	30	76.20	18–29	64.4–84.2	30–70
Group 3	3–10	Cage	4.3	0.40	30	76.20	18–29	64.4–84.2	30–70
Group 4	10–15	Cage	6.0	0.56	32	81.28	18–29	64.4–84.2	30–70
Group 5	15–25	Cage	8.0	0.74	36	91.44	18–29	64.4–84.2	30–70
Group 6	>25	Cage	25.1	2.33	84	213.36	18–29	64.4–84.2	30–70

[a]Space recommendations comparable to the regulations of the Animal Welfare Act (CFR, 1984). Mothers with litters require more space.

[b]Some dogs, especially those near the upper limit of each weight range, may require additional floor space or cage height to ensure compliance with the regulations of the Animal Welfare Act. The height of each cage must be sufficient to allow the occupant to stand in a "comfortable position," and the minimum square footage of floor space must be equal to the "mathematical square of the sum of the length of the dog in inches, as measured from the tip of its nose to the base of its tail, plus 6 inches, expressed in square feet." If dogs are housed in group pens/runs, only compatible animals should be housed together.

[c]The designated groups are based on approximate sizes of various nonhuman primate species used in biomedical research. Examples of species included in each group are: Group 1—marmosets, tamarins, and infants of various species; Group 2—capuchins, squirrel monkeys, and similar species; Group 3—macaques and African species; Group 4—male macaques and large African species; Group 5—baboons and nonbrachiating species larger than 15 kg; Group 6—great apes and brachiating species.

Institutions are encouraged to provide alternatives to individual caging. If adults are to be housed in groups, it is essential that only compatible animals be kept together. The minimum height of pens and runs for nonhuman primates should be 6 ft (1.8 m). For chimpanzees and brachiating species, the minimum cage height should be such that the animals can, when fully extended, swing from the cage ceiling without having their feet touch the floor.

N.B. Definitive housing requirements for ferrets have not been addressed by the U.S. Department of Agriculture or other regulatory bodies. See text for further information.

Table assembled by Christine L. Merrill, D.V.M.

Contents

About the Series   iv

Preface   v

Contributors   xiii

1. **Introduction**   **1**
   Christopher P. Chengelis and Shayne Cox Gad

2. **The Rat**   **21**
   Toxicology   David E. Semler   21
   Pathology   Shayne Cox Gad   76
   Metabolism   Christopher P. Chengelis   103

3. **The Mouse**   **165**
   Toxicology   James M. Andress   165
   Pathology   Charles H. Frith, Dawn G. Goodman, and
            Byron G. Boysen   233
   Metabolism   Chyung S. Cook   272

4. **The Hamster**   **295**
   Toxicology   Anne C. Costello   295
   Pathology   Frederick G. Hess   324
   Metabolism   Christopher P. Chengelis   331

5. **The Guinea Pig**   **351**
   Toxicology   Shayne Cox Gad   351
   Pathology   John C. Peckham   394
   Metabolism   Christopher P. Chengelis   418

6. **The Rabbit**   **441**
   Toxicology   Clare M. Salamon and Karen M. MacKenzie   441
   Pathology   Robert R. Dahlgren   471
   Metabolism   Chyung S. Cook   479

7. **The Ferret** **497**
   Toxicology Daniel E. McLain and Richard M. Hoar 497
   Pathology Glen K. Miller 551
   Metabolism Christopher P. Chengelis 555

8. **The Dog** **567**
   Toxicology Gillian C. Haggerty 567
   Pathology Robert W. Thomassen 600
   Metabolism Christopher P. Chengelis 657

9. **Nonhuman Primates** **675**
   Toxicology Gene B. Fuller, William C. Hobson, and
   David M. Renquist 675
   Pathology Curtis D. Port 710
   Metabolism Christopher P. Chengelis 721

10. **Alternative Species** **737**
    Christopher P. Chengelis

11. **Clinical Pathology of Laboratory Animals** **765**
    Robert L. Hall

12. **Model Selection and Scaling** **813**
    Shayne Cox Gad

13. **Susceptibility Factors** **841**
    Shayne Cox Gad

14. **Laws and Regulations Governing Animal Care and Use in Research** **861**
    Curtis D. Port

Appendix: Commercial Sources of Laboratory Animals **877**
    Shayne Cox Gad

Index 881

Contributors

James M. Andress   G. D. Searle and Company, Skokie, Illinois

Byron G. Boysen   Hazleton Wisconsin, Inc., Madison, Wisconsin

Christopher P. Chengelis   WIL Research Laboratories, Inc., Ashland, Ohio

Chyung S. Cook   G. D. Searle and Company, Skokie, Illinois

Anne C. Costello   S. C. Johnson & Son, Inc., Racine, Wisconsin

Robert R. Dahlgren   WIL Research Laboratories, Inc., Ashland, Ohio

Charles H. Frith   Toxicology Pathology Associates, Little Rock, Arkansas

Gene B. Fuller   New Mexico Regional Primate Research Laboratory (PRL), New Mexico State University, Holloman Air Force Base, New Mexico

Shayne Cox Gad   Becton Dickinson and Company, Research Triangle Park, North Carolina

Dawn G. Goodman   PATHCO, Inc., Ijamsville, Maryland

Gillian C. Haggerty   G. D. Searle and Company, Skokie, Illinois

Robert L. Hall   Hazleton Wisconsin, Inc., Madison, Wisconsin

Frederick G. Hess   Agricultural Research Division, American Cyanamid Company, Princeton, New Jersey

Richard M. Hoar   Argus International, Inc., Horsham, Pennsylvania

William C. Hobson   New Mexico Regional Primate Research Laboratory (PRL), New Mexico State University, Holloman Air Force Base, New Mexico

Karen M. MacKenzie   RMT, Inc., Madison, Wisconsin

Daniel E. McLain   Searle European Development Centre, Mont-Saint-Guibert, Belgium

Glen K. Miller   G. D. Searle and Company, Skokie, Illinois

John C. Peckham   Experimental Pathology Laboratories, Inc., Research Triangle Park, North Carolina

Curtis D. Port   G. D. Searle and Company, Skokie, Illinois

David M. Renquist   University of Tennessee, Memphis, Memphis, Tennessee

Clare M. Salamon   Hazleton Wisconsin, Inc., Madison, Wisconsin

David E. Semler   G. D. Searle and Company, Skokie, Illinois

Robert W. Thomassen   G. D. Searle and Company, Skokie, Illinois

ANIMAL MODELS IN TOXICOLOGY

1

Introduction

Christopher P. Chengelis
WIL Research Laboratories, Inc.
Ashland, Ohio

Shayne Cox Gad
Becton Dickinson and Company
Research Triangle Park, North Carolina

BACKGROUND

The use of animals in experimental medicine, pharmacological study, and toxicological assessment has become a well-established and essential practice. Whether serving as a source of isolated cells or tissues, a disease model, or as a prediction for drug or other xenobiotic action in man, experiments in animals have provided the necessary building blocks that permitted the explosive growth of medical and biological knowledge in the later half of the twentieth century (Meier and Stocker, 1989). Animal experiments also have served rather successfully as identifiers of potential hazards to and toxicity in humans for synthetic chemicals with many intended uses.

Animals have been used as models for centuries to predict what chemicals and environmental factors would do to humans. The earliest uses of experimental animals are lost in prehistory, and much of what is recorded in early history about toxicology testing indicates that humans were the test subjects. The earliest clear description of the use of animals in the scientific study of the effects of environmental agents appears to be by Priestley (1792) in his study of gases. The first systematic use of animals for the screening of a wide variety of agents was published by Orfila (1814), and was described by Dubois and Geiling (1959) in their historical review. This work consisted of dosing test animals with known quantities of agents (poisons or drugs), and included the careful recording of the resulting clinical signs and gross necropsy observations. The use of animals as predictors of potential ill effects has grown since that time.

CURRENT ANIMAL STUDIES

The current regulatorily required use of animal models in acute testing began by using them as a form of instrument to detect undesired contaminants. For example, canaries were used by miners to detect the presence of carbon monoxide—a case in which an animal model is more sensitive than humans (Burrell, 1912). In 1907, the U.S. Food and Drug Administration (FDA) started to protect the public by the use of a voluntary testing program for new coal tar colors in foods. This was replaced by a mandatory program of testing in 1938, and such regulatorily required animal testing programs have continued to expand until recently.

The knowledge gained by experimentation on animals has undoubtedly increased the quality of our lives, an observation that most reasonable people would find difficult to dispute, but in (as reviewed by Ewald and Gregg, 1983) has also benefited animals as well. As is the case with many tools, animals have sometimes been used inappropriately. These unfortunate instances have helped fuel an increasingly vituperative animal "rights" movement. This movement has encouraged a measure of critical self-appraisal on the part of scientists concerning the issues of the care and usage of animals. The Society of Toxicology, for example, has established Animals in Research Committees, and has published guidelines for the use of animals in research and testing. In general, the purpose of these committees is to foster thinking on the four "Rs" of animal-based research: Reduction, Refinement, research into Replacements, and Responsible use. This book is, in part, a response to these concerns.

The media commonly carry reports which state that most (if not at all) animal testing and research is not predictive of what will happen in people, and therefore such testing is unwarranted. Many of the animal rights groups also present this argument at every opportunity, and reinforce it with examples which entail seemingly great suffering in animals but which add nothing to the health, safety, and welfare of society. This is held to be especially the case for safety testing and research in toxicology. Animal rights activists try to "prove" this point by presenting examples of failure (such as thalidomide*). In light of the essential nature of animal research and testing in toxicology, this is equivalent to seeking to functionally disarm us as scientists. Our primary responsibility (the fourth "R") is to provide the information to protect people and the environment, and without animal models we cannot discharge this responsibility.

When confronted with this argument, all too many toxicologists cannot respond with examples to the contrary. Indeed, many may not even fully understand the argument at all. And very few are familiar enough with some of the history of toxicity testing to be able to counter with examples where it has not only accurately predicted a potential hazard to humans, but where research has directly benefited both people and animals. There are, however, many such examples. Demonstrating the actual benefit of toxicology testing and research with examples which directly relate to the everyday lives of most people and not esoteric, basic research findings (which are the most exciting and interesting products to most scientists) is not an easy task. Examples that can be seen to affect neighbors, relatives, and selves on a daily basis would be the most effective. The problem is that toxicology is, in a sense, a negative science. The things we find and discover are usually adverse. And if the applied end of our science works correctly, then the results are things that do not happen (and therefore are not seen).

If we correctly identify toxic agents (using animals and other predictive model systems) in advance of a product or agent being introduced into the market place or environment, then generally it will not be introduced (or it will be removed) and society will not see death, rashes, renal and hepatic diseases, cancer, or birth defects (for example). And as these things already occur at some level in the population, it would

---

*Where the lack of adequate testing (or of interpretation of existing test results) prior to marketing is not pointed out.

seem that seeing less of them would be hard to firmly tie to the results of toxicity testing that rely on animals. In addition, the fact that animals are predictive models for man is controversial.

ORIGINS OF PREDICTIVE ANIMAL TESTING

The actual record of evidence for the predictive value of animal studies and how they have benefited man and domestic animals will be reviewed in the following two sections. However, the negative image needs to be rebutted. First, it must be remembered that predictive animal testing in toxicology, as we now know it, arose largely out of three historical events.

The "Lash Lure" Case

Early in the 1930s, an untested eyelash dye containing p-phenylenediamine (Lash Lure) was brought onto the market in the United States. This product (as well as a number of similar products) rapidly demonstrated that it could sensitize the external ocular structures, leading to corneal ulceration with loss of vision and at least one fatality (McCalley et al., 1933).

The Elixir of Sulfanilamide Case

In 1937, an elixir of sulfanilamide dissolved in ethylene glycol was introduced into the marketplace. One hundred and seven people died as a result of ethylene glycol toxicity. The public response to these two tragedies helped prompt Congress to pass the Federal Food, Drug, and Cosmetic Act of 1938 (Pendergrast, 1984). It was this law that mandated the premarket testing of drugs for safety in experimental animals. The most compelling evidence that should be considered is "negative"—It is the fact that since the imposition of animal testing as a result of these two cases, no similar occurrence has happened. Even though society uses many more consumer products and pharmaceuticals today than during the 1930s.

Thalidomide

The use of thalidomide, a sedative-hypnotic agent, lead to some 10,000 deformed children being born in Europe. This which in turn led directly to the 1962 revision of the Food, Drug and Cosmetic Act, requiring more stringent testing. Current testing procedures (or even those at the time in the United States, where the drug was never approved for human use) would have identified the hazard and prevented this tragedy. And, in fact, it has not occurred in Europe or the United States except when the results of animal tests have been ignored. Table 1 presents an overview of cases where animal data predicted adverse effects in humans.

For example, birth defects have occurred with isotretinoin (Accutane) where developmental toxicity had been clearly established in animals and presented on labeling, but the drug has continued to be used by potentially pregnant women.

Research into replacements such as cellular cultures, organs harvested from slaughter houses, computer modeling, and physical/chemical systems has been extensive (Frazier, 1990). While each of these have their utility (Gad, 1989), they will not replace animals for the foreseeable future. Some degree of animal use will continue. We hope that this book

Table 1 Animal Models Which Predicted Adverse Effects of Xenobiotics on Humans

Agent	Effect	Animal species	In man
Thalidomide	Phocomelia	Rat	N/Y
Accutane	Developmental toxicity of CNS (neural tube defects)	Rat, rabbit, dog, primate	Y
AZT	Bone marrow depression	Dog, rat, monkey	Y
Valproic acid	Cleft palate	Rat, mouse, rabbit	Y
Cyclosporine	Nephropathy	Rat, dog	Y
	Reversible immune response suppression (essential aid to organ transplantation)	Rat, monkey	
Benoxaprofen (Oraflex)	Hepatotoxicity,	No	Y
	photosensitivity	Guinea pig	Y
Zomepirac (Zomax)	Anaphylactic shock	No	Y
MPTP	Parkinsonism	Monkey	Y
Cyclophosphamide	Hemorrhagic cystitis	Rat, dog	Y
Mercury	Encephalopathy	Rat, monkey	Y
Diethylene glycol	Nephropathy	Rat, dog	Y
Razoxin	Myelomonocytic leukemia	Mouse	Y

will assist the responsible investigator in designing and interpreting appropriate experiments (refinement) that will require fewer animals (reduction) in which the animals are appropriately husbanded and utilized (responsibility).

CHOOSING AN ANIMAL MODEL

Choosing the appropriate animal model for a given problem is sometimes guess work and often a matter of convenience. One often uses a species with which one is most familiar, with little consideration as to whether the chosen species is actually the most appropriate for the problem at hand. For example, the rat is probably a poor model for studying the chronic toxicity of any new nonsteroidal anti-inflammatory drug (NSAID) because the acute gastrointestinal toxicity will probably mask any other toxic effects. The guinea pig is less sensitive to most NSAIDs than the rat, and would therefore be a more appropriate species for investigating the chronic (nongastrointestinal) toxicity of an NSAID. This practice of not rationally choosing an appropriate species for an experiment undoubtedly results in questionable science. This alone should be considered a waste of animals and resources. It results also in additional, and sometimes duplicative, experiments. We hope that this book will contribute to the reduction and refinement of the use of animals by helping to alleviate this practice. What the editors consider to be the core chapters (Chaps. 2–10) include discussions of the strengths and weaknesses of each of the common laboratory species, and recommendations for potential appropriate uses. Chapter 12 directly addresses the issue of how to select the best practical model.

HUSBANDRY AND CARE

The quality of an experiment often hinges on the details of animal husbandry and care. At one extreme, inappropriate handling could result in unhealthy animals, and an experiment yielding variable and irreproducible results. All animals have optimal temperature, humidity, light cycle, light intensity, cage size and bedding, and dietary requirements. Rabbits, for example, have a different optimal temperature range than rats. Rats and ferrets have completely different dietary requirements. Albino rodents have very sensitive eyes, and lights of too high a candle power can cause incidental ocular damage, especially in those animals on the top row of a cage rack. Infrequent changing of indirect bedding materials can result in exposure of rodents to a high airborne concentration of ammonia, which can cause ocular damage. Recently, it has become clear that ad lib feeding of rodents in chronic or carcinogenicity studies both shortens their lives and alters the patterns of spontaneous tumors that occur. These are all examples of how inattention to the details of animal care can compromise an experiment, particularly a long-term one. A refined and responsibly designed experiment accommodates these details. It is hoped that this book will provide a convenient source of husbandry procedures for the more common animal species used in toxicological and pharmacological research.

Caging

Caging deserves special mention for two reasons. First, not all animals can be group housed. Hamsters, for example, are notoriously antisocial. Even breeding pairs cannot be left in the same small cage together for protracted periods. Guinea pigs, on the other hand, thrive when group housed. Obviously these factors need to be considered when designing an experiment. In modern toxicology practice, animals are seldom group housed during chronic studies in order to maintain identification, facilitate clinical observations, and ensure necropsy of moribund or dead animals (mice, in particular, are very cannibalistic). With short-term experiments, however, group housing of certain animals may not compromise a study and may decrease the amount of housing space needed. This book will discuss appropriate housing, including instances when animals should or should not be group housed.

Second, cage size is of importance because the animal rights movement has made it important. While most investigators (and cage manufacturers) have long recognized that cages have optimal sizes, the 1989 proposed Animal Welfare Codes (which became law in 1991) attempted to specify somewhat larger cages with several size cutoffs mediating cage changes. For example, there are three to four different cage specifications for guinea pigs depending on their age and/or weight. Many caging systems currently in use would no longer be permitted and their replacement would be very expensive. There is no scientific basis for believing that these changes will improve animal husbandry or quality of life. This is just an example of how the animal rights movement, and the resultant animal care laws, could effect the conduct of pharmacologists and toxicologists. This book contains in-depth discussion on current animal welfare laws. The investigator needs to be aware of not only the four "Rs," but also of the relevant laws and regulations governing animal experimentation. These are discussed in greater detail in Chapter 14.

CHOOSING SPECIES AND STRAINS

Not only is it important to pick the correct species for an experiment, but sometimes the correct strain. For most of the species discussed in this book there are a handful of commonly used strains. In some cases, an inbred strain may provide qualitative and specific characteristics that make it a good disease model such as the spontaneously hypertensive rat. There are other more quantitative strain-related differences such as size, color, temperament, and background disease. For example, the Fischer 344 rat is smaller than the Sprague-Dawley rat. The CD-1 mouse is shorter lived than the C57B6/F$_1$ hybrid. These differences may make a particular strain more appropriate for one experiment than others. For example, the Fischer 344 rat has a high rate of spontaneous Leydig cell tumors as compared to the Sprague-Dawley rat, which would make the latter less appropriate for determining if a chemical is a testicular carcinogen. For these reasons, this book includes discussions of strain-related differences. Rats and mice provide the greatest array of strains from which to choose, including outbred and some inbreed. There are literally hundreds to choose from, but the majority are specialized-use animals, such as the athymic nude mouse. For the majority of generalized pharmacology and toxicology testing, a relatively small handful of rat and mouse strains are used and the emphasis in those chapters will be on those more commonly used strains. Many chapters will include some mention of strain; however, the situation with dogs is somewhat different.

All domestic dogs belong to the same family, which is subdivided by breed. Only the beagle breed is purposely raised for biomedical medical research; otherwise one uses mongrel or random-source dogs (obtained from pounds and used without regard to breed). Hence, the chapter on the dog will focus on the beagle. There may be supplier-related differences in beagles, but these have not been systemically studied.

DOSING

In order to study the effects of a drug or other chemical in an animal, the two have to be brought together; i.e., the animal has to be dosed. Dosing is the act of introducing a drug or chemical into a living organism. It requires active interaction between man and animal. There are, however, passive dosing techniques that are also used frequently in which the chemical is placed in the animals air, water, or feed, and the animal doses itself by breathing, drinking, or eating. Hence, administering an antibiotic intravenously is active dosing; giving it in the feed is passive dosing. In the former case, dosimetry (i.e., calculating milligrams per kilograms of exposure) is generally intuitively simple (an exception being for the dermal route). In the latter case, other measurements must be taken (e.g., feed consumption) and a variety of formulas are used in dosimetry. The main routes used for active dosing are oral, intravenous, intraperitoneal, dermal, and sub-cutaneous. Other routes are sometimes used, and these will be mentioned where appropriate (for a complete discussion of different routes, see Gad and Chengelis, 1988, Chap. 10). For oral dosing, for example, one may have a choice of using capsules or gavaging. However, capsules are rarely used with rats and gavage seldom used with dogs. When necessary, a dog can be gavaged, but the technique is different from that used with rats. Intravenous dosing of ferrets is especially difficult, but can be done. It is hoped that this book will present the appropriate techniques, "tricks of the trade," so that animals can be appropriately and humanely dosed.

Second, some of the information (e.g., average feed consumption) and formulas needed to calculate or estimate dosimetry in passive dosing procedures are presented and discussed. With regard to dosing and dosimetry, it should be kept in mind that the terms *dose* and *dosage* are not synonymous. The dose is the total amount of test article given, e.g., 1000 mg. The dosage is a rate term and is the dose divided by the weight of the test animal, i.e. 1000 mg/10 kg (for a dog) = 100 mg/kg. In most instances, when one speaks of a dose-response curve, a dosage-response curve is being described.

ANIMAL PHYSIOLOGY

All animal species and strains have their own distinctive physiology. As a result, values pertaining to blood pressure, breathing rates, ECGs, rectal temperatures, and normal clinical laboratory parameters often vary between species. Clearly, appropriate interpretation of an in vivo experiment requires one to have a firm understanding of these baseline data. For example, there are well-established differences between species with regard to red blood cell size. What is normal for a dog would be high for a rat. The converse is true for breathing rates. This book provides a convenient source for this important background data.

Background Incidence of Disease

All animals also have their own baseline, or natural incidence, or diseases that complicates the conduct and interpretation of chronic toxicity experiments. The background incidence of liver tumors in C57B6/F$_1$ mice is quite high. It would, perhaps, be prudent to investigate a suspect hepatocarcinogen in a species with a lower spontaneous incidence than these. Ferrets in the United States are currently contaminated by the Aleutian mink virus, which could make this species inappropriate for chronic experiments. The background incidence of these diseases and pathological lesions are discussed to aid the investigator in choosing the more appropriate species for an experiment and in the interpretation of the results.

Responses to Biologically Active Agents

An animal's responses to drugs or other biologically active agents may be just as important as the background incidence of disease, and species-related differences in sensitivity are important for two reasons. First, animals will often have to be anesthetized or receive other treatment such as antibiotics during an experiment. Appropriate dosages vary between species. Thus, this book presents the appropriate dosages of common anesthetics for the model species discussed here.

Second, the other reason species-related differences are important is that in toxicity testing, these differences are the major hurdle in applying toxicity data to human hazard assessment. This is perhaps too broad a topic for a single book, but mention is made so that an investigator is aware of such differences. Cats, for example, are far more sensitive to digitoxin (LD$_{50}$ $\simeq$ 180 μg/kg po), than other species, such as the rat (LD$_{50}$ $\simeq$ 56 mg/kg po, as reported in RTECS, 1979).

There can also be qualitative differences between species. Morphine, for example, is infamous for causing different clinical signs in different species: straub tail in mice, catatonia in rats, and extreme reactivity in cats. Some of the more frequent examples of these distinctions will be mentioned in the core chapters. The salient message is that species often differ both quantitatively and qualitatively in their responses to drugs and/or chemicals. These differences must be investigated and considered in choosing a species for an experiment, and in interpreting the results. Incidentally, cats (with the exception of veterinary products intended for use in cats) are seldom used in toxicity testing and are used in pharmacology mainly for acute, terminal neurophysiological experiments. For these reasons, an in-depth discussion of cats is not included in this book.

Absorption, Distribution, Metabolism, and Excretion of Chemicals

When studying the effects of drugs and other chemicals on intact animals, it is also vitally important to investigate the processes of absorption, distribution, metabolism, and excretion (ADME). These have been intensely studied widely. Space does not permit a review of this large body of work. Some basic degree of knowledge must be presumed. We have compiled a list of references to which the reader can refer if additional information is needed (Table 2). For the remainder of this chapter, we will touch upon some basic principles that apply across all species. In each individual core chapter (Chaps. 2–9) of this book, some basic information on ADME will be presented on a species-specific basis. The emphasis will be on providing the information necessary to assist one in (1) the appropriate selection of an animal model, (2) the design of the experiment, (3) the interpretation of resultant data, and (4) the applicability of the results to humans.

The principles that govern absorption and distribution apply fairly equally across all species (Goldstein et al., 1974), and therefore will not be discussed to any great extent on an animal-by-animal basis. It is most difficult to predict species differences in bioavailability (absorption across gastrointestinal tract into the blood) or systemic bioavailability (bioavailability + first-pass metabolism) of a specific chemical. Species differences in gastric or intestinal pH, for example, may dictate species differences in GI permeability to specific chemicals, but will not account for differences in GI transit time or hepatic metabolism. Assumptions based solely on phylogenetic grounds can be quite

Table 2 Summary of Review Material for General Reviews of Xenobiotic Metabolism

Topic	Source
General reviews on process of drug metabolism and disposition	LaDu et al., 1972
	Goldstein et al., 1974
	Klaassen, 1986
	Sipes and Gandolfi, 1986
	deBethizy and Hayes, 1988
	Rozman, 1988
Cytochrome P-450	Gonzales, 1988
	Black and Coon, 1986
	Kadlubar and Hammons, 1987
Flavin-dependent microsomal mixed function oixdase	Ziegler, 1988
	Tynes and Hodgson, 1985
Epoxide hydrolase	Seidegard and DePierre, 1983
	Oesch, 1972
Glutathione S-transferase	Jarina and Bend, 1977
	Pickett and Lu, 1989
UDP-glucuronosyl transferase/glucronidation	Boutin, 1987
	Mulder, 1986
	Siest et al., 1989
PAPS-Sulfotransferase/sulfate formation	Singer, 1985
	Jacoby et al., 1984
Amino acid conjugations	Hirom et al., 1977
Acetylations	Lower and Bryan, 1973
Esterases	Leinweber, 1987
Alcohol metabolism	Hawkins and Kalant, 1972
	Crabb et al., 1987
Billiary excretion	Klaassen and Watkins, 1984
	Levin, 1978

misleading. We had recent experience with a drug found to be bioavailable in the rat and dog, but not at all absorbed in the monkey. In fact, the dog was the species most similar to the human. One needs to strive to ascertain test article bioavailibility experimentally for any specific chemical, as general principles always come encumbered with exceptions.

Absorption

After dosing, a chemical must be absorbed in order to cause an effect. Absorption is the process of the chemical passing through a barrier to gain access to the general systemic circulation. The most common dosage routes are oral, inhalation, topical, intraperitoneal, intravenous, subcutaneous, and intramuscular. Absorption is not generally a problem by the latter three routes as the test substance is introduced directly to the body. It is normally a foregone conclusion that drugs so administered will reach the systemic circulation. Plasma concentrations will depend on rates of delivery (iv), or rates of diffusion (im/sc). While there are some technical concerns, the principles are either independent of species, or the species difference are obvious. For example, because of relative small muscle mass and rapid circulation time, drugs given intramuscularly will more rapidly equilibrate in rats than in monkeys. Via the intraperitoneal route, systemic availability will depend not only on the rates of diffusion, but also on the first-pass metabolism effect. There are no known species differences with regard to intraperitoneal absorption, but there are species differences with regard to rates of hepatic metabolism which may dictate the degree of first-pass metabolism. Interestingly, first-pass effects are generally of greater concern in smaller species, rat and mice, where the intraperitoneal route is more commonly used.

With regard to the oral, dermal, and inhalation routes there are very real species differences. For example, thickness and length of the small intestine, size of cecum (if, indeed there is one), and gut transit time will all play a role in gastrointestinal absorption.

Species differences in facilitated or active transport may also play a role in absorption. Whether an animal is an obligate nose breather or not, the structure of the nasal turbinates, respiration rate, and minute volume will all influence the size and number of the particles reaching the alveoli by the inhalation route. The rat is a poor model for inhalation pharmacokinetic studies in extrapolating the results to humans for these reasons. There are well-described differences in skin structure that control dermal absorption and result in species differences. Such species differences will vary with chemical class.

This book may help one sort through this maze, but there are few scientifically sound generalizations. Our best recommendation is that investigators substantiate their assumptions on dermal or inhalation absorption before rendering any conclusion on studies conducted using these routes of administration.

Distribution

After gaining access to the systemic circulation, the toxin/drug is distributed among the organs. Distribution will depend on:

Blood flow to the organ
Extent and avidity of binding to plasma proteins*
The "natural" affinity a particular organ may have
The degree and extent to which the chemical crosses barriers such as the blood/brain
    barrier, the placenta.
The extent to which metabolism and/or excretion competes with these processes.

---

*Interestingly, it has recently become clear that even proteins (such as some of the biotechnologically generated pharmaceutical agents) can be bound to plasma proteins.

There are probably species differences with regard to all these processes. Not all have been vigorously explored, however. For example, there are few comparative studies on the blood/testes barrier, or comparisons on plasma protein binding of different chemicals in the monkey, so the database in this area is surprisingly small. A few transspecies comparisons of plasma protein binding have been done. As a broad generalization, binding is most extensive in humans and least extensive in mouse. Such information is presented and discussed in the core chapters, but the reader should be aware of the holes in the available knowledge.

Metabolism

In the area of ADME, the processes of metabolism or bioconversion are of greatest concern with regard to species-specific differences. Indeed, species differences in metabolism are a leading cause for species differences in toxicity. First, very few administered xenobiotics are excreted unchanged. Therefore, rates of metabolism often dictate the time length of a pharmacodynamic response. Second, metabolism of a xenobiotic may result in metabolites of similar potency and/or produce metabolites that are responsible for toxicity. For example, most genotoxic carcinogens require metabolic activation. Finally, because the metabolism of xenobiotics is an enzyme-based phenomenon, it shows a great deal of species differences. For example, Williams (1972) examined the metabolism of phenol, a relatively simple chemical, in 13 different species and found that no two species provided the same spectrum of metabolites. Species differences can be either quantitative (differing amounts of the same metabolites) or qualitative (different metabolites). Because of the importance of metabolism in toxicity testing, each individual animal chapter contains in-depth discussion of xenobiotic metabolism.

Xenobiotic Metabolism.   The area of species differences in xenobiotic metabolism is not new. Some of the efforts in this area are summarized in Tables 1–3. It is not the objective of this book to provide yet another interspecies comparison, but rather to present information on a species-specific basis. For example, what type of regimen is required to induce increases in microsomal multifunction oxidase (MMFO) activity in the dog? The metabolism of xenobiotics by mammals is a phenomenon that has been recognized since 1842 when Keller (Mandel, 1972) identified that benzoic acid was excreted in the urine as the glycine conjugate (hippuric acid). As a modern science, drug (or xenobiotic) metabolism was formalized in the late 1940s when Williams (1947) published the first text on the subject. Williams (see references for 1972 and 1974 for reviews) has been particularly instrumental in the area of species differences in metabolism. Early works in this area tended to concentrate on isolating and identifying various conjugations of simple chemicals given to intact animals. Miller and Mueller published on the importance of liver microsomes in xenobiotic metabolism in their studies on the oxidative metabolism of aminazodyes (Mannerig, 1972; Miller and Mueller, 1949). The field has grown explosively since the mid 1950s, catalyzed by the studies of Brodie and colleagues in the United States (Brodie et al., 1955; Quinn et al., 1958) and Remmer in Germany (Remmer and Menker, 1963; Mannering, 1972). Their works confirmed the quantitative importance of the liver in xenobiotic metabolism, and that the major underlying enzymes were located in the microsomal fraction. It was during this period that the practice of naming an enzyme by its activity, such as aminopyrine demethylase or aniline hydroxylase, was adopted. It was only later that it was recognized that all these activities are catalyzed by the same enzymes (or family thereof); i.e., the cytochrome P-450–dependent microsomal

Table 3 Compilation of Selected Papers that Compare Xenobiotic Metabolism in Different Species

Species compared	Parameters examined	Comments	References
Dog, guinea pig, rat, rabbit, monkey, human, mouse	Gastrointestinal differences which affect absorption. Plasma and tissue binding. Drug metabolism in liver and intestine	Rhesus monkey best predictor for ADME in man Excellent Bibliography	Rozman, K., 1988
Rat, mouse, guinea pig	GSH-T	With CDNB total activity mouse>guinea pig>rat. Parallel to AFT sensitivity. Quantitative differences in isozymes	Neal et al., 1987
Rat, hamster, mouse, guinea pig	Induction of P-450 and MMFO activities (AP demethyl, BP-OH, EC-deethyl) by 2-AAF and 3-MC	In general, MMFO activity, rat had lowest, but BP activity most inducible. In some species, induction had no effect or decreased some activities	Anstrom et al., 1986
Mouse, guinea pig, rabbit, hamster	GSH-T (1-chloro-2,4-dinitrobenzene)	Hamster>rabbit=gp>mouse>rat. S-sepharose elution patterns different	Igarashi et al., 1986
Rat, rabbit, dog, mouse	Chlorfenvinphos deethylation (in vitro)	Dog>rabbit=mouse>rat with same order to LD_{50}	Hutson and Logan, 1986
Rat, dog, monkey	Metabolism and kinetics of Tolrestat	Highest bioavailability in rats. More unchanged drug in dogs and monkeys	Cayen et al., 1985
Rat, mouse, guinea pig	Induction of MMFO, GSH-T, EH	EH-M gp>rat>mouse, but gp is less inducible. For GSH-T; mouse>rat>gp and gp not induced. For, MMFO, gp>mouse>rat.	Thabrew and Emerole, 1983
Rat, dog, monkey	Inducing effect of hexahydroindazole (P-450, AP-demeth, AN-OH)	Increases in relative liver weights in all species. For P-450, monkey>rat>dog; for AP, monkey>rat=dog; for AN, rat=monkey>dog (gram basis, different if on protein). Best induction in dog	Lan et al., 1983

Table 3   *(continued)*

Species compared	Parameters examined	Comments	References
Rat, mouse, guinea pig, dog, monkey	Conjugation reactions	A review	Caldwell, 1982
Rats, rabbits, hamster, guinea pig, ferret	Metabolism of glyceryl trinitrite	Species differences in plasma half-life a function of body weight	Ioannides et al., 1982
Various: emephasis on dog, mouse, rat, rabbit, monkey	Various aspects of metabolism covered: spectrum of metabolites, plasma half-lifes, developmental differences, inhibitors, inducers	Excellent comprehensive review with emphasis on mixed function oxidase activity	Kato, 1979
Rat, mouse, rabbit, hamster, guinea pig	Changes in iron "spin-state" as determined by EPR induced by different binding spectra.	Proportion of high spin P-450 in vivo: rabbit> gp=hamster=mouse> rat	Kumaki et al., 1978
Rat, rabbit, guinea pig	Different inducing agents. Glucuronide vs sulfate in conjugation of 4-hydroxy-3-methoxy-phenylethanol	Glucuronide formed only by liver, other organ involved in sulfation. Both produced in liver of rat rabbit and gp, only sulfate formed by mouse	Wong, 1976
Rat, mouse, rabbit, hamster, guinea pig	Protein, P-450 content, reductase concentrations, model substrates, GSH and UDPG transferase activities, lung, liver, kidney	For all species, liver most active with lung and kidney 15–40% of liver. No species superior in all activities, but hamster tended to have greatest activities	Litterst et al., 1975
Rat, mouse, guinea pig, rabbit	Microsomal protein, BP-OH, UDPG transferase, small intestine vs liver	No real differences in microsomal protein (30–35 mg/g). For BP, liver> >gut for all species. For liver gp =mouse> rat>rabbit; for gut, gp>rabbit> rat=mouse; for UDPG liver, gp> rabbit= mouse> rat; for UDPG-gut, rabbit>rat> mouse=gp	Hietanen and Vanio, 1973

Rat, mouse, guinea pig, hamster, rabbit, dog, pig, monkey	Metabolism of [^{3}H]styrene oxide: EH and GSH-T in liver, lung, and kidney	For EH, liver>kidney> lung. In general, mouse is lowest and primate is highest. For GSHT, liver>kidney> lung. gp is highest and primate is lowest. Includes lit comp. of EH activities	Pacific et al., 1981
Rat, mouse, guinea pig, rabbit, pig, monkey	P-450, b5, cytochrome c reduct, K_m and V_{max} of various substrates	Not big differences in micro: P-450 ranged 0.38 (pig) to 0.75 nmol/mg (gp). b5 ranged 0.20 (mouse) to 0.49 nmol/ mg (gp). Cytochrome c red ranged 115 (rabbit) to 136 (gp) nmol/min/ mg	Amri et al., 1986
Rat, mouse, guinea pig, hamster	Induction of EH UDPG transferase, and GSH-T by 2-AAF or 3-MC	Large species variation (3- to 12-fold) in control activities. Except for EH in guinea pig, enzymes induced only in rat by 2-AAF. Except for GSH-T in hamster, enzymes induced only in rat by 3-MC. Rats not representative of activities or inducibility of other species	Astrom et al., 1987
Rat, mouse, guinea pig, hamster	Effects of DDT on AHH activity and cytochrome P450	Induction in hamsters, decreases in other species. Acute toxic effects depend on route and species	Haietanen and Vainio, 1976
Rat, mouse, guinea pig, hamster	Total GSH, γ-GTP, GSH synthetases, peroxidease, and reductase	GSH lowest in guinea pig, highest in mouse. Synthesis lowest in hamster highest in rat. γ-GT much higher in gp. GSH-T highest in gp, lowest in rat and not affected by fasting. GR lowest in rat= mouse, highest in hamster, fasting affects species dependent. Px highest in mouse= hamster, lowest in rat and mouse, depend on substrate and fasting state	Igarashi et al., 1983

Table 3 *(continued)*

Species compared	Parameters examined	Comments	References
Rat, mouse, rabbit, guinea pig	GSH-T activity with different substrates, different age animals, and with different inducing agents	Wide range of activities, depending on species and substrate. Age-related changes evident in all species, peak (up to 120 days) varies with species. Activity inducible in all species, but extent depends on inducer and substrate. Rat and mouse most inducible	Gregus et al., 1985
Rat, mouse, hamster, guinea pig, monkey	Review on role of intestinal microflora in drug metabolism. Excellent bibliography with references to primary articles and other reviews	Gut flora (β-glucosidase and β-glucuronidase; nitro, nitrite, and azo reductases) have large species difference, guinea pigs tend to have lowest amounts, mice the highest.	Rowland, 1988
Rat, mouse, hamster, rabbit, guinea pig, dog, primate others	Excellent review. Qualitative differences (lack of specific enzymes) and quantitative differences. Emphasis on in vivo data. Species differences in the metabolism of [1-14c-acetyl]phenacetin	Examples: Only in the rat is aromatic hydroxylation the major route of amphetamine metabolism. Dogs and guinea pigs have a deffect in N-acetylation. Guinea pigs do not make mercapturic acids	Williams, 1972, 1979
Rat, rabbit, guinea pig, ferret	Case reviews on how species differences in drug metabolism lead to differences in toxicity	Deacetylation highest in rat and ferret, aromatic hydroxylation high in ferret, low in others. Glucuronide formation dominant in rabbit, guinea pig, ferret: sulfation is dominant in rat.	Smith and Timbrell, 1974
Rat, mouse, guinea pig, hamster, rabbits, dogs, primates	Review chapter in monograph. Species differences in biotransformation, plasma protein binding, biliary excretion, and pharmacokinteics	Example: Dog has increased risk of bladder cancer (in response to) aromatic amines because of ability to N-hydroxylate but limited capacity to acetylate	Calabrese, 1988
Rat, mouse, guinea pig, hamster, rabbits, dogs, primates		Example: In general, protein binding is highest in primate, and lowest in mouse	Cayen, 1987

Rat, mouse, rabbit, guinea pig, dog	A citation classic. Species and other factors, in the metabolism of four different chemical explored.	In general, most rapid half-life in mice, longest in dog. Correlates with rates of microsomal demethylation	Quinn et al., 1958
Rat, mouse, guinea pig, rabbit, rat, dog, quail, trout	Cytochrome P-450, MMFO, EH UDPG transferase, PAPS-sulfotransferase, N-acetyl transferase	A good basic comparison. Convenient source for species comparison	Gregus et al., 1983
Rat, mouse, guinea pig, rabbit, dog	Drug metabolism by nasal tissue in vitro	Highest activities in hamster, lowest in dog	Hadley and Dahl, 1983

Abbreviations:

AP—demeti-aminopyrine demethylase, BP-OH—benzo(a)pyrene hydroxylase, EC—deethyl-7-ethoxycoumain deethylase

2-AAF—2-acetylaminofluorene, 3-MC—3-methylcholanthrene

EH—epoxide hydrolase, AN-OH—aniline hydroxylase

GSH—glutathione, UDPG—UDP-glucuronic acid

γ-GTP—γ-glutamyltranspeptidase, gp—guinea pig

GSH-T—glutathione s-transferase

mixed function oxidase system (Gonzales, 1988; Guengerich, 1988). Cytochrome P-450 was discovered almost a decade after Miller and Mueller described microsomal metabolism requiring NADPH (Coon, 1978; Kingenberg, 1958; Mannering, 1972). The importance of the identification and characterization of the cytochrome P-450–dependent MMFO system to the fields of biochemistry, pharmacology, and toxicology could not be understated. The reader is referred to any one of several reviews of the system (see Tables 1 and 2).

The process of xenobiotic metabolism has traditionally been divided in phase I (oxidative) and phase II steps. In general (as reviewed more extensively by de Bethizy and Hayes [1988]), all mammalian processes are designed to convert lipophilic chemicals to more polar and more easily excreted metabolites. In reality, the process can be more complicated than two steps because the products of phase I oxidation can be (1) further hydroxylated at different sites, (2) further oxidized at the same site (by a different enzyme such as alcohol dehydrogenase), or (3) Conjugated with glutathione or glucuronic acid, sulfate, or one of several amino acids. This process is discussed in greater detail elsewhere (see Tables 1 and 2). The result is that any one xenobiotic may have an astonishing spectrum of metabolites. For example, benzene is a relatively simple chemical, yet over 15 different metabolites have been described.

Enzymes Involved in Xenobiotic Metabolism: The main enzymes involved in xenobiotic metabolism are fairly uniform across species. In all mammalian species, the liver is quantitatively the most important site of xenobiotic metabolism, and the MMFO system is the most important enzyme. While this system is ubiquitous, there are species differences in isozymic characteristics, substrate specificity, activity, and inducibility. More recently, flavin-dependent microsomal multifunction oxidase, which is distinct from the MMFO, has been identified (Ziegler, 1988), and has been shown to play a role in the metabolism of many chemicals. There are also differences in phase II enzyme activities and cosubstrate availability (Gregus et al., 1983). Seldom do two species dispose of the same chemical that way. Each species produces a spectrum of metabolite or chomatographic "fingerprints" that are often distinct. The characteristics of the MMFO for each of the most highly used species will be discussed in this book some detail. Other enzyme systems such as the flavin-dependent (non–cytochrome P-450) monoxygenase may also be involved in xenobiotic oxidative metabolism, and are discussed where available information permits. The species characteristics of other important enzymes such as epoxide hydrolase and UDP-glucuronosyl transferase are also discussed. Some enzymes are ubiquitous, such as the alcohol dehydrogenase and carboxylesterase. All species metabolize primary alcohols to aldehyde, and subsequently to carboxylic acids. This will only be discussed, therefore, when there is some species-specific characteristic. This is also true for esterases, as all species rapidly hydrolyze esters.

Excretion

The processes of elimination will not be dealt with in great detail in the core chapter. This is not to say, however, that excretion is not important. Like absorption, elimination can be both active and passive, and most xenobiotics are passively excreted. In most cases, conjugated metabolites are actively excreted. The process of xenobiotic metabolism can be viewed, to a certain extent, as packaging for the excretory process. Across species, the active excretion of a metabolite by the liver into the bile is probably (quantitatively) the most important active excretory process concerning xenobiotic disposition. Glucuronide conjugates (as reviewed by Levine, 1978; Klassen and Watkins, 1984; and Williams, 1972) are actively excreted by the liver into the bile ultimately into the feces. Amino acid conjugates, in contrast, tend to be excreted by the kidney into the urine. These are definite species-related differences in the molecular weight cut-off between 300 and 500 for the biliary transport of the metabolite which dictate whether a metabolite will end up in either the feces or the urine.

Species differences do not follow any particular phylogenetic lines. For example, rats and dogs effectively excrete phenolphthalein glucuronide (50% in bile), whereas guinea pigs and monkeys do not (<10%) (Williams, 1972). While there are species differences in excretions, these tend to be overshadowed by the species differences in metabolism. That is, a particular species may not need an efficient biliary excretory process because with a particular chemical, it may produce glucuronides sparingly or not at all. This information may be of interest to the pharmacokinist in determining where to look for a metabolite. Generally, however, such information is of academic interest to the pharmacologist or toxicologist in interpreting an experiment because glucuronides are generally inactive endproducts, and it does not really matter whether they end up in the urine or feces. (As with any rule, these are exceptions: Mualder [1986] sites several examples of glucuronides being active metabolites; i.e. causing toxicity.) There are several instances, however, where biliary excretion actually influences the toxicity of a chemical, such as with some of the cardiac glycosides or heavy metals where biliary excretion occurs without metabolism and biliary excretion is the "detoxification" mechanism (Klossen and Watkins, 1984). Cayen (1987) has pointed out that species-related differences in indomethacin-induced intestinal damage directly correlates to the degree of exposure of the mucosa owing to biliary excretion and resultant enterohepatic circulation. Such instances are discussed on a species-specific basis where such data permit.

SUMMARY

We have attempted to assemble a source book of basic information on laboratory animals. We trust that this book will provide a convenient source of information for either the skilled or novice investigator to aid in the design and interpretation of in vivo pharmacological or toxicological studies.

REFERENCES

Amri, H., Batt, A., and Siest, G. (1986) Comparison of cytochrome P-450 content and activities in liver microsomes of seven species including man. *Xenobiotica* 16, 351–358.

Anon. (1980) *1979 Registry of Toxic Effects of Chemical Substances*, National Institute of Occupational Safety and Health, Washington, D.C., Publication number 80–111.

Astrom, A., Maner, S., and DePierre, J. (1987) Induction of liver microsomal epoxide hydrolase, UDP-glucuronosyl transferase and cytosolic glutathione transferase in different rodent species by 2-acetylaminofluroene or 3-methylcholanthrene. *Xenobiotica* 17, 155–163.

Astrom, A., Maner, S., and DePierre, J. (1986) Induction of cytochrome P-450 and related drug-metabolizing activities in the livers of different rodent species by 2-acetylaminofluorene or by 3-metylcholanthrene. *Biochem. Pharmacol.* 35, 2703–2713.

Black, S., and Coon, M. (1986) Comparative structure of P-450 cytochromes, in *Cytochrome P450: Structure, Mechanisms and Biochemistry*, Oriz de Montellano, P., ed. Plenum, New York, pp. 161–216.

Boutin, J., Antoine, B., Batt, A., and Siest, G. (1984) Heterogeneity of hepatic microsomal UDP-glucuronyltransferase activities: Comparison between human and mammalian species activities. *Chem.-Biol. Int.* 52, 173–184.

Boutin, J. (1987). Indirect evidence of UDP-glucuronosyl-transferase heterogeneity: How can it help purification? *Drug Metab. Revs.* 18, 517–553.

Brodie, B., Axelrod, J., Cooper, J., Gaudette, L., LaDu, B., Mitoma, C., and Udenfriend, S. (1955) Detoxification of drug and other foreign compounds by liver microsomes. *Science* 148, 1547–1554.

Burrell, G. A. (1912). *The Use of Mice and Birds for Detecting Carbon Monoxide After Mine Fire and Explosions*. Technical Paper 11, Department of Interior, Bureau of Mines, Washington, D.C., pp. 3–16.

Calabrese, E. (1988) Comparative biology of test species. *Environ. Health Perspec.* 77, 55–62.

Caldwell, J. (1981) The current status of attempts to predict species differences in drug metabolism. *Drug Metab. Rev.* 12, 22–237.

Caldwell, J. (1982) Conjugation reactions in foreign-compound metabolism: Definition, consequences, and species variations. *Drug Metab. Revs.* 13, 745–777.

Cayen, M. (1987) Retrospective evaluation of appropriate animal models based on metabolism studies in man, in *Human Risk Assessment—The Role of Animal Selection and Extrapolation*, Roloff, M., Wilson, A., Ribelin, W., Ridley, W., and Ruecker, F., eds., Taylor & Francis, New York, pp. 99–112.

Cayen, M. Hicks, D., Ferdinandi, E., Kraml, M., Greselin, E., and Dvornik, D. (1985) Metabolic disposition and pharmacokinetics of aldose reductase inhibitor tolrestat in rats, dogs and monkeys. *Drug Metab. Dispos.* 13, 412–419.

Coon, M. (1978) Oxygen activation in the metabolism of lipids, drugs and carcinogens. *Nutr. Rev.* 36, 319–328.

Coon, M., and Vaz, A. (1987) Mechanism of microsomal electron transfereactions. *Chem. Scripta* 27A, 17–19.

Crabb, D., Borson, W., and Li, T.-K. (1987) Ethanol metabolism. *Pharmacol. Ther.* 34, 59–73.

deBethizy, J., and Hayes, J. (1989) Metabolism: A determinent of toxicity, in *Principles and Methods of Toxicology*, Hayes, A., ed., Raven Press, New York, pp. 29–66.

Dubois, K. P., and Geiling, E.M.K. (1959) *Textbook of Toxicology*, Oxford University Press, New York, pp. 11–12.

Ewald, B., and Gregg, D. (1983) Animal research for animals. *Annl. N.Y. Acad. Sci.* 406, 48–58.

Frazier, J. M. (1990) *In Vitro Toxicology*, Marcel Dekker, New York.

Gad, S., and Chengelis C. (1989). *Acute Toxicity Testing*; *Perspectives and Horizons*, Telford Press, Caldwell, N.J..

Gad, S. C. (1989) *A Tier Testing Strategy Incorporating In Vitro Testing Methods for Pharmaceutical Safety Assessment, Humane Innovations and Alternatives in Animal Experimentation* 3:75–79.

Goldstein, A., Aranow, L., and Kalman, S. (1974) *Principles of Drug Action: The Basis of Pharmacology*, Wiley Biomedical, New York, pp. 129–217, 227–300.

Gonzales, F. (1988) The molecular biology of cytochrome P-450s. *Pharmacol. Rev.* 40, 243–288.

Gregus, Z., Watkins, J., Thompson, T., Harvey, M., Rozman, K., and Klaassen, C. (1983) Hepatic phase I and phase II biotransformations in quail and trout: Comparison to other species commonly used in toxicity testing. *Toxicol. Appl. Pharmacol.* 67, 430–441.

Gregus, Z., Varga, F., and Schmelas, A. (1985). Age-development and inducibility of hepatic glutathione S-transfersase activities in mice, rats, rabbits and guinea-pigs. *Comp. Biochem. Physiol.* 80C, 85–90.

Guengerich, F., Minireview; cytochromes P-450 (1988) *Comp. Biochem. Physiol.* 89C, 1–4.

Hadley, W., and Dahl, A. (1983) Cytochrome P-450 dependent monooxygenase activity in nasal membranes. *Drug Metab. Dispos.* 11, 275–276.

Haietanen, E., and Vainio, H. (1973) Interspecies variations in small intestinal and hepatic drug hydroxylation and Glucuronidation. *Acta Pharmacol. Toxicol.* 33, 57–64.

Haietanen, E., Vainio, H. (1976) Effect of administration route on DDT acute toxicity and on drug biotransformation in various rodents. *Arch. Environ. Contam. Toxicol.* 4, 201–16.

Hawkins, R., and Kalant, H. (1972) The metabolism of ethanol and its metabolic effects. *Pharmacol. Rev.* 24, 67–157.

Hirom, P., Idle, J., and Millburn, P. (1977) Comparative aspects of the biosynthesis and excretion of xenobiotic conjugates by non-primate mammals, in *Drug Metabolism: From Microbes to Man*, Park, D., and Smith, R., eds., Taylor & Francis, Philadelphia, pp. 299–329.

Hutson, D., and Logan, C. (1986). Detoxification of the organophosphorus insectiside chlorfenvinphos by rat, rabbit and human liver enzymes. *Xenobiotica* 16, 87–93.

Igarashi, T., Satoh, T., and Ueno, K., and Kitagawa, H. (1983) Species difference in Glutathione level and glutathione related enzyme activities in rats, mice, guinea pigs and hamsters. *J. Pharm. Dyn.* 6, 941–949.

Igarashi, T., Tomihari, N., and Ohmori, S. (1986) Comparison of glutathione S-transferase in mouse, guinea pig, rabbit, and hamster liver cytosol to those in rat liver. *Biochem. Int.* 13, 641–648.

Ioannides, C., Parke, D., and Taylor, I. (1982) Elimination of glyceryl trinitrate: Effects of sex age, species and route of administration, *Br. J. Pharmacol.* 77, 83–88.

Jacoby, W., Duffel, M., Lyon, E., and Ramasway, S. (1984) Sulfotransferases active with xenobiotics—Comments on mechanism, in *Progress in Drug Metabolism*, Vol 8., Bridges, J., and Chasseaud, L., eds., Taylor & Francis, London, pp. 11–33.

Jarina, D., and Bend, J. (1977) Glutathione S-transferases, in *Biological Reactive Intermediates*: *Formation, Toxicity and Inactivation*, Jallow, D., Kocsis, J., Snyder, R., and Vanio, H., eds., Plenum Press, New York, pp. 207–236.

Kadlubar, F., and Hammons, G. (1987) The role of cytochrome P-450 in the metabolism of chemical carcinogens, in *Mammalian Cytochrome P-450*, Vol 1, Guengerich, F., ed. CRC Press, Boca Raton, Florida, pp. 1–54.

Kato, R. (1979) Characteristics and differences in the hepatic mixed function oxidases of different species *Pharmacol. Ther.* 6, 41–98.

Kumaki, K., Sato, M., Kon, H. and Nebert, D. (1978) Correlation of type I, type II, and reverse type I, difference spectra with absolute changes in spin state of hepatic microsomal cytochrome P-450 iron from five mammalian species *J. Biol. Chem.* 253, 1048–1058.

Klaassen, C., and Watkins, J. (1984) Mechanisms of bile formation, hepatic uptake, and biliary excretion. *Pharmacol. Rev.* 36, 1–67.

Klaassen, C. (1986) Distribution, excretion and absorption of toxicants, in *Casarett and Doull's Toxicology; the Basic Sciences of Poisons*. Klaassen, C., Amdur, M., and Doull, J., eds., Macmillan, New York, pp. 33–63.

Klingenberg, M. (1958) Pigments of rat liver microsomes. *Arch. Biochem. Biophys.* 75, 376–386.

Klinger, W. (1982) Biotransformation of drugs and other xenobiotics during postnatal development *Pharmacol. Ther.* 16, 377–429.

LaDu, B., Mandel, H., and Way, E. (eds.) (1972) *Fundamentals of Drug Metabolism and Drug Disposition*, Williams & Wilkins, Baltimore.

Lan, S., Weinstein, G., and Keim, G., and Migdalof (1983) Induction of hepatic drug-metabolizing enzymes in rats, dogs, and monkeys after repeated administration of an anti-inflammatory hexahydroindazole. *Xenobiotica* 13, 329–335.

Leinweber, F. (1987) Possible Physiological roles of carboxylic ester hydrolases. *Drug Metab. Revs.* 18, 379–440.

Levin, W. (1978) Biliary excretion of drugs and other xenobiotics. *Ann. Rev. Pharmacol. Toxicol.* 18, 81–96.

Lower, G., and Bryan, G. (1973) Enzymatic N-acetylation of carcinogenic aromatic amines by liver cytosol of species displaying different oran susceptibilities. *Biochem. Pharmacol.* 22, 1581–1588.

Litterst, C., Mimnaugh, E., Reagan, R., and Gram, T. (1975) Comparison of in vitro drug metabolism by lung, liver, and kidney of several common laboratory species. *Drug Metab. Dispos.* 3, 259–265.

Mandell, H. (1972) Pathways of Drug Biotransformation: Biochemical conjugation, in *Fundamentals of Drug Metabolism and Drug Disposition*, LaDu, B., Mandel, H., and Way, E. eds., Williams & Wilkins, Baltimore, pp. 149–186.

Mannering, G. (1972) Microsomal Enzyme systems which catalyze drugs, in *Fundamentals of Drug Metabolism and Drug Disposition*, LaDu, B., Mandel, H., and Way, E., eds. Williams & Wilkins, Baltimore, pp. 206–252.

McCally, A. W., Farmer, A. G., and Loomis, E. C. (1933). Corneal ulceration following use of lash lure. *J.A.M.A.* 101, 10560–1561.

Meier, J., and Stocker, K. (1989) Review article: On the significance of animal experiments in toxinology. *Toxicon* 27, 91–104.

Miura, T., Shimada, H., Ohi, H., Komori, M., Kodama, T., and Kamataki, T. (1989) Interspecies homology of cytochrome P-450: Inhibition by anti-P-450-male antibodies of testosterone hydroxylases in liver microsomes from various animal species including man. *Jpn. J. Pharmacol.* 49, 365–374.

Mueller, G., and Miller, J. (1949). The reductive cleavage of 4-dimethylaminoazobenzene by rat liver; the intracellular distribution of the enzyme system and its requirement for triphosphoropyridine nucleotide. *J. Biol. Chem.* 180, 1125–1136.

Mulder, G., Meerman, J., and van den Goorbergh, J. (1986) Bioactivation of xenobiotic by conjugation, in *Advances in Xenobiotic Conjugation Chemistry*, American Chemical Society Symposium Series, A.C.S., Washington, D.C., pp. 282–200.

Mulder, G. (1986) Sex differences in drug conjugation and their consequences for drug toxicity, sulfation, glucuronidation, and glutathione conjugation. *Chem.-Biol. Int.* 57, 1–15.

Neal, G., Nielsch, U., Judah, D., and Hulbert, P. (1987) Conjugation of model substrates or mocrosomally-activated aflatoxin b1 with reduced glutathione, catalyzed by cytosolic glutathione-S-transferase in livers of rats, mice and guinea pigs. *Biochem. Pharmacol.* 36, 4269–4276.

Oesch, F. (1972) Mammalian epoxide hydrases: Inducible enzymes catalysing the inactivation of carcinogenic and cytotoxic metabolites derived from aromatic and olefinic compounds. *Xenobiotica* 3, 305–340.

Orfila, M.J.B. (1814) *Traite de toxicologie*.

Pacifici, G., Boobis, A., Brodie, M., McManus, M., and Davies, D. (1981) Tissue and species differences in enzymes of epoxide metabolism. *Xenobiotica* 11, 73–79.

Pendergrast, W. (1984). *Biological Drug Regulation in the Seventy-fifth Anniversary Commemorative Volume of Food and Drug Law*. Edited and Published by the Food and Drug Law Institute, Washington, D.C., pp. 293–305.

Pickett, C., and Lu, A. (1989) Glutathione S-transferases: Gene structure, regulation, and biological function. *Annu. Rev. Biochem.* 58, 743–64.

Priestley, J. (1792). *On Different Kinds of Air, Philosophical Transactions*.

Quinn, G., Axelrod, J., and Brodie, B. (1958) Species, strain and sex differences in metabolism of hexobarbitoane, amidopyrine, antipyrine, and aniline. *Biochem. Pharmacol.* 1, 152–159.

Remmer, H., and Merker, H. (1963) Drug-induced changes in liver endoplasmic reticulum: Association with drug-metabolizing enzymes. *Science* 142, 1567–1568.

Rowland, I., Mallett, A., and Bearne, C. (1986) Enzyme activities of the hindgut of microflora of laboratory animals and man. *Xenobiotica* 16, 519–523.

Rowland, I. (1988) *Role of the Gut Flora in Toxicity and Cancer*, Academic Press, New York.

Rozman, K. (1988) Disposition of Xenobiotics: Species differences. *Toxicol. Pathol.* 16, 123–129.

Siest, G., Magdalou, J., and Burchell, B. eds. (1989) *Cellular and Molecular Aspects of Glucuronidation*, Colloque Inserm, Vol. 173, John Libbey Eurotext, London.

Seidegard, J., and DePierre, J. (1983) Microsomal epoxide hydrolase: Properties, regulation, and function. *Biochim. Biophys. Acta.* 695, 251–270.

Sipes, I., and Gandolfi, A. (1986) Biotransformation of toxicants, in *Casarett and Doull's Toxicology; the Basic Sciences of Poisons*. Klaassen, C., Amdur, M., and Doull, J., eds., Macmillan, New York, pp. 64–98.

Singer, S. (1985) Preparation and characterization of the different kinds of sulfotransferases, in *Biochemical Pharmacology and Toxicology*, Vol I, Zakim, D., and Vessay, D., eds., Wiley Interscience, New York, pp. 95–159.

Smith, R., Timbrell, J. (1974) Factors affecting the metabolism of phenacetin I. Influence of dose, chronic dosage, route of administration and species on the metabolism of [1-14C-acetyl]phenacetin. *Xenobiotica* 8, 489–501.

Thabrew, M., and Emerole, G. (1983) Variation in induction of drug metabolizing enzymes by trans-stilbene oxide in rodent species. *Biochem. Biophys. Acta* 756, 242–246.

Tynes, R., and Hodgson, E. (1985) Catalytic activity and substrate specificity of the flavin-containing monooxygenase in microsomal systems: Characterization of the hepatic, pulmonary and renal enzymes of the mouse, rabbit, and rat. *Arch Biochem. Biophys.* 240, 77–93.

Wong, K. (1976) Species differences in the conjugation of 4-hydroxy-3-methoxypheylethanol. *Biochem. J.* 158, 33–37.

Williams, R. T. (1947) *Detoxification Mechanisms. The Metabolism of Drugs and Allied Organic Compounds*, Wiley, New York.

Williams, R. T. (1972) Species variation in drug biotransfromations, in *Fundamentals of Drug Metabolism and Drug Disposition*, LaDu, b., Mandel, H., and Way, E., eds., Williams & Wilkins, Baltimore, pp. 187–205.

Williams, R. T. (1974) Inter-species variations in the metabolism of xenobiotics. *Biochem. Soc. Transat.* 2, 359–377.

Ziegler, D. M. (1988) Flavin-containing monooxygenase: Catalytic mechanism and specificities. *Drug Metab. Rev.* 19, 1–32.

2

The Rat

Toxicology: **David E. Semler**

G. D. Searle and Company
Skokie, Illinois

Pathology: **Shayne Cox Gad**

Becton Dickinson and Company
Research Triangle Park, North Carolina

Metabolism: **Christopher P. Chengelis**

WIL Research Laboratories, Inc.
Ashland, Ohio

Toxicology   **David E. Semler**

HISTORY

The Norway Rat (*Rattus norvegicus*) is believed to have originated in Asia and spread throughout the world with modern civilization as an economic pest. The rat was first used experimentally in France in the study of adrenal gland function (Philipeaux, 1856, as cited in Lindsey, 1979), and it is considered to be the first animal to be domesticated for strictly scientific purposes (Richter, 1959). Use of the rat as a research tool in North America began shortly before 1900 (Lindsey, 1979). Early research with the rat in the areas of nutrition, endocrinology, physiology, and behavior led to the discoveries such as the nutritional quality of various amino acids in mammals, the existence of vitamins, the characterization of the hormones of the anterior pituitary, and the existence of biological clocks. The advantages of the rat as an experimental tool were recognized quickly and the use of the rat spread to almost every field of biological and medical research.

To minimize the variability in their experiments and emphasize specific desirable characteristics, early researchers established breeding programs. Henry Donaldson and his colleagues at the Wistar Institute (Philadelphia, Pennsylvania) were prominent in this effort. Many of the rat strains commonly used in toxicology today, including the Wistar, Sprague-Dawley, and Long Evans, can be traced to the Wistar lineage. The Fischer 344 rat, used commonly in carcinogenicity studies, was developed for use in cancer research at the Crocker Research Institute of Columbia University, New York City. Lindsey (1979) presents a history of commonly used strains.

Use of the rat in toxicology has paralleled its use in other fields. With the exception of topical irritation studies and studies dealing with immunology, the rat is a species of choice in most toxicology studies.

CHOICE OF THE RAT IN TOXICOLOGICAL RESEARCH

Theoretically, the choice of an appropriate species for use in toxicology studies should be made based on a comparison of pharmacokinetics and metabolism of the test compound in various laboratory species vs man. In many instances, this comparison is not possible, and the choice is based on more economic or practical reasons. The subject of model selection is discussed in detail in Chapter 10. In addition, to many metabolic similarities between the rat and human, some of the reasons that the rat has been used in toxicology studies are their small size, relatively docile nature, short life span, and short gestation period. Since the rat has been so widely used in research, a large database has been developed about their nutrition, diseases, and general biology. This section summarizes some basic physiological data about the rat and discusses some species and strain differences that may be useful in making a decision to use the rat or in the interpretation of toxicological data from rat studies.

Normal Physiological Values

Some general values for selected physical parameters are given in Tables 1 and 2. Normal values will vary with the strain of animal, supplier, food, and conditions under which the animals are housed and the data are taken; the data given should be used only as a point of reference.

Species Differences

While rats, other laboratory animals, and humans share many physiological and anatomical characteristics, there are some anatomical or physiological peculiarities which affect compound absorption, pharmacokinetics, and metabolism or cause an unexpected reaction to a test compound. The investigator should be aware of these (some of which are mentioned in this section) when selecting the rat as a model or interpreting data from toxicology studies in rats. Rats are obligate nose breathers and inhaled material is more subject to nasal filtration or absorption, whereas humans are much more likely to breathe through their mouth (Page, 1977). Owing to differences in structure, the placenta is considerably more porous in the rat than in the human. This difference may increase chances of prenatal exposure to xenobiotics (Oser, 1981). Owing to differences in their distribution within the gut, intestinal microflora are much more likely to metabolize an orally administered compound, possibly into a toxic or active metabolite, in the rat than in the human (Williams, 1972). Rats are much more susceptible to zinc phosphide, a rodenticide, because their stomach acid secretion is continuous, whereas in the dog the mechanism for secretion is complex, requiring stimuli (Johnson and Voss, 1952). The mechanism of action of this rodenticide is that it reacts with hydrochloric acid in the stomach to produce phosphine, which is lethal. The species-specific nephrotoxicity observed in male rats as a result of volatile hydrocarbon exposure appears to be a consequence of a predisposition to spontaneous hyaline droplet formation in the aged rat (Alden, 1985). Uterine tumors appearing in the rat, but not in the mouse, dog, or human after chronic bromocriptine administration appear to be due to an effect on various sex

Table 1 Selected Normative Data

General	
lifespan	2.5–3.0 years
surface area	0.03–0.06 cm^2
chromosome number (diploid)	42
water consumption	80–110 ml/kg/day
food consumption	100 g/kg/day
body temperature	37.5°C
basal metabolism	35 kcal/24 hr (400-g rat)
Reproduction	
puberty	50 ± 10 days
breeding season	All year
type of estrous cycle	Polyestrous
length of estrous cycle	4–5 days
duration of estrous	10–20 hr
mechanism of ovulation	Spontaneous
time of ovulation	8–11 hr after onset of estrous
time of implantation	Late day 5[a]
length of gestation	21–23 days
litter size	8–14 pups
birth weight	5–6 g
eyes open	10–12 days
weaning age	21 days
weaning weight	40–50 g
Cardiovascular	
arterial blood pressure	
systolic	84–184 mmHg
diastolic	58–145 mmHg
heart rate	330–480 beats/min
cardiac output	10–80 ml/min
blood volume	
plasma	40.4 (36.3–45.3) ml/kg
whole blood	64.1 (57.5–69.9) ml/kg
Respiratory	
respiration frequency	85.5 (66–114)/min
tidal volume	0.86 (0.60–1.25) ml
alveolar surface area	7.5 m^2 (400-g rat)
pattern	Obligate nasal
Renal	
urine volume	55 ml/kg/24 hr
Na$^+$ excretion	16.3 mEq/kg/24 hr
K$^+$ excretion	8.3 mEq/kg/24 hr
urine osmolarity	1659 mOsm/kg of H$_2$O
urine pH	7.3–8.5
urine specific gravity	1.04–1.07

Source: Data from Baker et al. (1979), Bivin et al. (1979), and Peplow et al. (1974).

[a]Day 1 is the day on which sperm is found in the vagina.

Table 2 Growth Rates in Selected Rat Strains

Weight (g)	Age (days)							
	Crl:CD(SD)BR		Crl:(WI)BR		Crl:(LE)BR		CDF(F-344)/ CrlBR	
	M	F	M	F	M	F	M	F
Up to 50	21	21	21	21–22	21–22	21	21–23	21–23
51–75	22–28	22–27	22–28	23–31	23–28	22–28	24–28	24–28
76–100	29–32	28–32	29–33	32–37	29–32	29–35	29–33	29–35
101–125	33–37	33–36	34–39	38–45	33–37	36–40	34–36	36–42
126–150	38–41	37–41	40–43	46–51	38–41	41–49	37–42	43–57
151–175	42–44	42–46	44–49	52–63	42–46	50–56	43–48	58–63
176–200	45–48	47–54	50–53	64–69	47–49	57–66	49–54	
201–225	49–52	55–63	54–58	70–89	50–53	67–92	55–57	
226–250	53–56	64–74	59–63	90 plus	54–63	93 plus		
251–275	57–61		64–67		64–68			
276–300	62–66		68–75		69–78			
301–325	67–72		76–85		79–87			
326–350	73–80		86–96		88–96			
351–375	81–88		97–105		97–110			
376 plus	89 plus		106 plus		111 plus			

Source: Adapted from Charles River (1988).

hormones superimposed on the endocrine system of the aging female (Richardson et al., 1984). Several other differences are known; comprehensive examinations of these differences and their impact can be found in reviews by Oser (1981), Calabrese (1984), Hart and Fishbein (1985), and Roe (1987a).

Strain Differences

Breeding rats for specific characteristics has understandably produced some physiological differences between strains of rats. Some of these differences are known to affect how the various strains react to toxicants. Among others, strain-specific differences have been found in sensitivity to thiourea (Dieke and Richter, 1945), sensitivity to acetaminophen nephrotoxicity (Newton et al., 1985), the incidence of spontaneous glomerular sclerosis (Bolton et al., 1976), sensitivity to the carcinogenic actions of 7,12-dimethylbenz(a)anthracene (Boyland and Sydnor, 1962), the ability to metabolize phenobarbital (Shefer et al., 1972), the sensitivity to the renal toxicity of caprolactam (Powers et al., 1984), and differences in the levels of drug-metabolizing enzymes (Page and Vesell, 1969).

Of importance for carcinogenicity studies, strain differences have been found in the incidence of spontaneous tumors. Table 3 gives the incidence of common spontaneous tumors found in Sprague-Dawley and Fischer 344 rats, the two strains most commonly used in carcinogenicity studies. The background tumor incidence is important because a high spontaneous rate may mask a small test compound–related increase in tumor incidence.

HUSBANDRY

As will be discussed in this section, the environment to which a rat is exposed can have a profound affect on the results of a toxicology study. Even subtle or short-term changes in

Table 3 Incidence of Common Spontaneous Tumors in Fischer 344 and Sprague-Dawley Rats

| | % Tumors in untreated rats | | | |
| | Fischer 344[a] | | Sprague Dawley[b] | |
Tumor type	males	females	males	females
Testicular interstitial cell	85	—	6	—
Pituitary tumors	24	36	42	64
Mammary tumors	23	41	4	49

[a]From Sass et al. (1975).
[b]From Charles River.

environment can alter a response to a test compound. Good animal husbandry is essential to maintain the health of the animals being studied, increase the reproducibility of the results, and eliminate potential variables that may confound the interpretation of the results of a study.

Facilities

Temperature and Relative Humidity

Current specifications for temperature and humidity are 18–26°C and 40–70% relative humidity (ILAR, 1985). These ranges are designed to allow rats to maintain a minimum metabolic rate or to be within their thermoneutral zone (Bligh and Johnson, 1973). Exposed to temperatures outside of the thermoneutral zone, rats will adapt metabolically (by increasing or decreasing the metabolic rate) or behaviorally (by actively controlling heat production and loss, modifying food and water uptake, nest building with bedding material, or huddling) to maintain their core temperature (Weihe, 1973). The degree to which they are able to adapt will depend upon the conditions under which the animals are housed; i.e., number of animals per cage, type of caging, and type of bedding.

The process of adaptation may affect basic growth parameters. Rats exposed to a room temperature of 32°C for just 1 day had markedly decreased food consumption and body weights (Hamilton, 1967). Male rats exposed to temperatures of 26.7–31.7°C for 48 hr developed testicular atrophy consistent with degeneration of the seminiferous epithelium and failure of spermatocyte maturation (Pucak et al., 1977). Groups of rats raised for two generations at room temperatures from 12 to 32°C had statistically significant differences in body weights, feed intakes, hematological and serum biochemical parameters, and reproductive parameters (Yamauchi et al., 1981).

The influence of temperature on the toxic response has been well reviewed (Fuhrman and Fuhrman, 1961; Weihe, 1973; Clough, 1982). Fuhrman and Fuhrman (1961) discuss three patterns by which toxicity may vary with temperature: toxicity may increase at temperature extremes; toxicity may increase linearly with temperature; or toxicity may remain constant with increasing temperature to some threshold, then increase with increasing temperature. Examples of these patterns are evident in the work of Keplinger et al. (1959) where groups of animals were exposed to temperatures of 8, 26, and 36°C and administered various drugs intraperitoneally (Table 4).

Table 4 Effects of Room Temperature on Approximate Lethal Dose (mg/kg) of Compounds Administered Intraperitoneally to Rats

Compound	Room temperature		
	8°C	26°C	36°C
Toxicity increased at temperature extremes			
acetylsalicytic acid	80	420	55
atropine	280	420	55
benzene	500	1150	225
carbon tetrachloride	1400	7100	940
kerosene	2100	10,700	940
pentobarbital	55	80	10
chlorpromazine	12	210	62
strychnine	0.25	1.5	0.25
Toxicity increased with increasing temperature			
diphenhydramine	180	80	16
ephedrine	420	180	120
pentachlorophenol	620	420	120
quinidine sulphate	210	140	94
Toxicity increased at some threshold			
caffeine	280	280	55
DDT	940	940	120
procaine	280	280	120
promethazine	140	140	42

Source: Keplinger et al. (1959), used with permission.

The magnitude of temperature fluctuation or time of exposure can be small, yet still cause an effect. The toxicity of caffeine and dextroamphetamine was increased in mice that were exposed to temperatures of 30 or 15°C for 1 hr compared to those at 22°C (Muller and Varnikos-Danellis, 1970). In pregnant rats, a lowering of the core body temperature 4°C for 5 min or 2.5°C for 1 h during critical periods of gestation caused teratogenic changes such as microphthalmia, encephalocele, facial clefting, and maxillary hypoplasia (Germain et al., 1985).

Relative humidity (RH) is of importance for the heat balance of an animal, but variations from recommended ranges will also have other affects on animals. In 1961, Weihe et al. (as cited by Clough, 1982) found that at a constant temperature of 21°C rats housed at 35% RH consumed 5% more food than rats housed at 75% RH. Ringtail, a lesion observed in young animals and characterized by annular constrictions of the tail, is thought to be associated with relative humidities below 40% (Njaa et al., 1957; Flynn, 1959). Mice were more susceptible to the PR8 strain of influenza virus when maintained at 35.6°C, 22% RH than at 35.6°C, 90% RH (Baetjer, 1968). Pathological changes in the respiratory tract can result from high ammonia levels (Gamble and Clough, 1976), which can be encouraged in rodent cages by high RH (Clough, 1976).

Lighting

Light and light cycles play a key role in many physiological processes and circadian rhythms (Axelrod, 1974; Moore et al., 1967; Wurtman, 1975). Animal facility lighting can be an important environmental variable in toxicology studies. The activity of some drug-metabolizing enzymes and sensitivity to certain drugs such as ouabain, steroids, alcohol, and barbituates can vary with circadian periodicity (Radzialowski and Bousquet, 1968; Nair and Caspar, 1969; Pauly and Scheving, 1969). Constant light for as few as 3 days may induce persistent estrus, hyperestrogenism, polycystic ovaries, and endometrial hypertrophy or metaplasia (Baker et al., 1979).

Lighting recommendations are governed by the need to provide sufficient lighting for animal care activities and healthy living conditions for the animals. The current guideline for laboratory rats is that levels be at 323 lux approximately 1 m above the floor (ILAR, 1985). These levels are considered sufficient for performance of routine animal care (Bellhorn, 1980), yet take into account that rats are susceptible to retinal damage if exposed to too high a light intensity (Noell et al., 1977). Where specific animal room activities require a higher light intensity, it has been suggested that variable-intensity controls be used which would increase illumination to 525–800 lux (Rao, 1986).

Variations in light intensity should be considered when arranging animals on cage racks for toxicology studies. There can be as much as an 80-fold increase in light intensity inside transparent plastic cages on the tops of racks compared to those on the bottom (Weihe et al., 1969). This difference in illumination can be important in long-term studies. Weisse et al. (1974) found that occurence of retinal lesions in a 3-year study appeared to be directly related to light exposure and position of the cages: there was retinal damage in 79% of the males and 96% of the females in the top row of cage racks (exposed to 223 lux), whereas 38% of the males and 50% of the females were affected in the bottom row (exposed to 30 lux).

Most facilities operate their lights on a 12-h light/12-h dark cycle. It is important that monitoring procedures are in place to assure that the lighting cycle is operating correctly. Retinal photoreceptors undergo a continual renewal process (Young, 1973) and this process is influenced by environmental light-dark cycles (Basinger et al., 1976; LaVail, 1976). The lack of a dark cycle can be a causative factor in retinal degeneration in rats. As few as 4 days of continuous light at 194 lux will cause retinal degeneration in rats (O'Steen, 1970) and a level of 65 lux for the same period can also show some evidence of damage (Anderson et al., 1972). It is possible that failure of the light controls over a weekend could cause retinal degeneration in susceptible strains.

In addition to retinal damage, exposure to continuous lighting could have an effect on the pharmacokinetics of test compounds. Continuous lighting tends to equalize day and night food consumption and speed gastrointestinal transit rate in rats (Siegel, 1961; Zucker, 1971; Wong and Oace, 1981). Since gastric emptying can be affected by the amount of food in the stomach, the speed of absorption, and hence blood levels, can be changed especially in a study where test compound is being administered in the diet.

Ventilation

An adequate ventilation system will control temperature and humidity, and provide a sufficient airflow to dilute chemical pollutants and control transmission of infectious agents. Current guidelines recommend a ventilation rate of 0.815 ft^3/min/250 g rat (Runkle, 1964) or 10–15 air changes per hour (ILAR, 1985). When placing racks within a room, consideration should be given to their spacial arrangement to avoid cross-contamination and possible convection currents (Clough, 1976). Teelman and Weihe (1974) recommend racks be placed at least 2 m apart to minimize the between-rack spread of airborne microorganisms. Racks should be placed such that they do not block the airstream or subject specific cages to drafts (Nevins, 1971). There may be a difference in airflow in upper cages compared to lower cages within a rack (McGarrity et al., 1969). This fact should be considered when positioning treatment groups within a rack.

To minimize the spread of disease or contaminants within a facility, animals should be maintained in rooms with a slightly positive static pressure compared with possibly contaminated areas such as halls, quarantine areas, or cage washing facilities. An exception to this might be in rooms with studies in which animals are receiving test compound in their diet. In this case, thought should be given to keeping animal rooms at negative pressure with respect to the hallway to minimize the possibility of facility contamination (Sansone and Fox, 1977). In clean/dirty corridor systems, air should flow from the access corridor, through the animal room, to the dirty corridor (Sontag et al., 1976).

Noise

Gamble (1982) has reviewed the effects of noise on laboratory rats. Exposed to various levels of noise for a variety of durations, rats have shown audiogenic seizures in susceptible strains (D'Amour and Shaklee, 1955); changes in uterus and adrenal weights (Sackler et al., 1959; Nayfield and Besch, 1981); reproductive disturbances, including total litter resorptions and developmental abnormalities (Geber, 1966; Geber, 1973); increases in eosinophils in peripheral blood, serum cholesterol concentrations, and adrenal ascorbic acid levels (Geber et al., 1966); and increased serum lipid concentrations (Friedman et al., 1967). Barrett and Stockham (1963) found that the noise associated with feeding and changing cage pans produced marked increases in plasma corticosterone levels. While noise from cage changing or dosing activities is unavoidable in an animal facility, personnel should be trained to minimize the noise. Noisy animals, such as dogs or nonhuman primates, should be housed in areas separate from those housing rats.

Caging

The environmental conditions which rats experience within their cages (the microenvironment) may be markedly different from the conditions within the animal room, the macroenvironment (Clough, 1976). Cage design may significantly affect temperature, humidity, ventilation, and exposure of animals to microorganisms and contaminants. As discussed, these factors may alter an animal's response to the test compound and should be taken into consideration when choosing a caging system for a study.

Shoebox Caging

Shoebox cages are rectangular boxes with solid bottoms, sides, and walls (Fig. 1). They can be made of metal (preferably stainless steel), but molded plastic boxes of polycarbonate (clear) or polypropylene (translucent) are popular. Lids for those cages are made of wire, metal with ventilation holes, or filter tops. Cages may also be suspended from shelves in a rack; in this case, the shelf covers the cage.

Filter tops provide some protection against airborne spread of disease (Kraft, 1958; Brick, et al., 1969; Simmons and Brick, 1970). Serrano (1971) found that filter covers reduce the intercage transfer of vectors for infectious organisms—feces, soiled bedding, and hair. However, Sansone, et al. (1977) demonstrated that fine particulates could penetrate the filter cover. A disadvantage in using filters is that ventilation of the cage is reduced; air exchange rates can be decreased by as much as 50% compared to rodent cages with open tops (Woods, 1978). This reduction in ventilation results in increased humidity, temperature, and levels of carbon dioxide and ammonia (Simmons et al., 1968; Serrano,

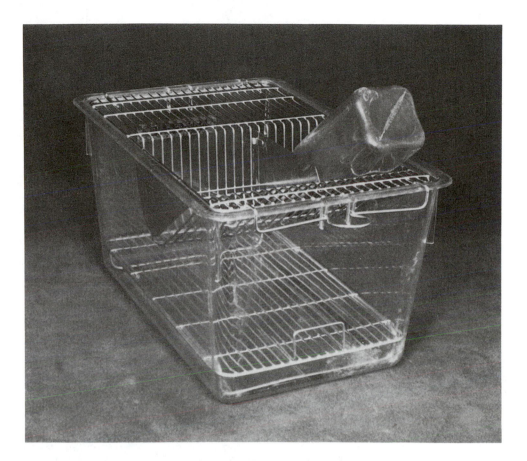

Figure 1 Shoebox cage with wire lid for food pellets and water bottle, and raised wire floor.

1971) Broderson et al. (1976) found that ammonia plays an important role in the pathogenesis of murine respiratory mycoplasmosis.

The bottoms of shoebox cages are usually filled with an absorbant bedding. The choice of bedding should be made with care. The use of cedar or soft-wood bedding has been associated with increases in hepatic microsomal enzyme levels (Ferguson, 1966; Wade et al., 1968; Hasimoto, 1972); increased pup mortality (Burkhart and Robinson, 1978; Smith et al., 1968); and an increase in the rate of spontaneous tumors in mice (Sabine et al., Heston, 1975). Bedding may also be a source of toxicity as a result of contamination with organophosphates (Gibson et al., 1987). Solid-bottom shoebox caging can allow rats to consume fecal pellets which can contain potentially toxic or carcinogenic metabolites (Laqueur, 1970). Some cage designs have raised wire floors to minimize direct contact with excreta and bedding. These can significantly reduce the amount of airborne bedding particles within the cage that can be inhaled or ingested by the rats (Raynor et al., 1983).

Shoebox cage designs may have other affects on study results. DePass et al. (1986) found that mice treated topically with benzo(a)pyrene and housed in polycarbonate cages with wood-chip bedding developed dermal neoplasms at an earlier time and with a greater incidence than those housed in stainless steel wire mesh cages without bedding. Winter and Flataker (1962), working with respiratory-depressant drugs, were able to demonstrate a more than 10-fold increase in LD_{50} by placing animals after injection in cages with wire mesh bottoms compared to animals in cages with solid bottoms. It was observed that under depressant-induced anesthesia the animal's nose would be pressed against the junction between the cage wall and bottom and the animal would suffocate.

Suspended Caging

Suspended wire-bottom cages (Figs. 2 and 3) are usually made entirely of metal, although some cages with plastic sides and wire mesh bottoms are available. The wire mesh floors in this design of cage allow excrement to fall to absorbant papers underneath the cages. This minimizes the need to disturb the cage occupants while changing papers. Gartner et al. (1980) found that heart rate, hemoglobin, plasma protein content, and serum glucose, pyruvate, and lactate concentrations in rats were elevated after cage movement to a table; the presence of a familiar animal care person working in the room without moving cages did not cause marked changes.

This cage design allows more ventilation within the cage than shoebox cages. This is an advantage in that ammonia concentrations will be lower. However, it is also a disadvantage in that these cages offer little protection against the airborne transmission of disease or contaminants such as test compound in diet admixture studies (Sansone et al.,

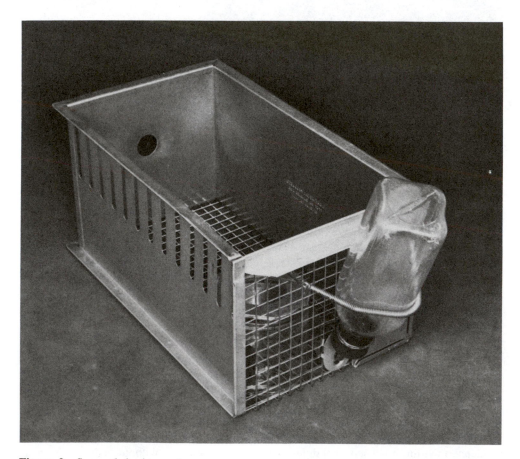

Figure 2 Suspended wire mesh cage.

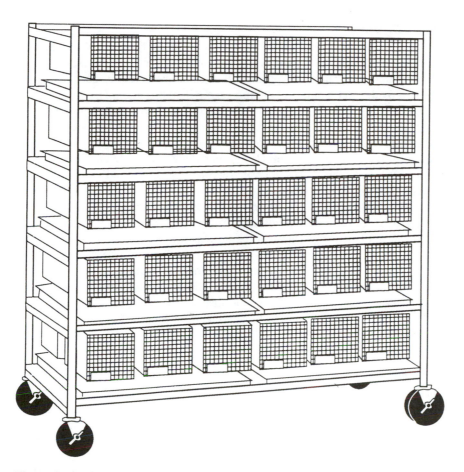

Figure 3   Rack of suspended wire mesh cages.

1977). There are other disadvantages that may be linked to the flooring itself. Decubital
ulcers on the plantar surface of the hindfeet are common in rats housed chronically in
wire-bottomed cages. Some biological differences have been noted between rats housed
on wire mesh floors compared to rats reared on solid floors. Mundy and Porter (1969)
found that rats housed for 12 weeks on wire floors weighed less, yet had heavier adrenal
weights than littermates housed on solid floor cages. Rats housed in cages where the floor
grating was widely spaced had increased serum creatine phosphokinase concentrations
compared to those housed on solid floors or more closely spaced grating (Frolich et al.,
1981); the creatine increase was ascribed to increased muscle tonus or muscle damage.

Laminar Airflow Systems

Laminar airflow systems have been developed to minimize the airborne spread of bacterial
infections. Studies have shown significantly lowered viral infection of mice housed in
cages with laminar airflow compared to mice housed in conventional caging (McGarrity
and Coriell, 1973). Respiratory tract infections were significantly reduced in hamsters
housed in laminar flow housing compared to conventionally housed hamsters (Smith et
al., 1975).

Minimum Space Recommendations

Current minimum space recommendations for rats are given in Table 5. When deciding how many rats to house per cage it must be remembered that the population density can have an effect on microenvironmental parameters such as the levels of heat, moisture, oxygen, carbon dioxide, and ammonia within a cage (Clough, 1976). These parameters will have effects on the animals, as previously discussed. Density may also have an impact on reproductive success (Christian and Lemunyan, 1958) and behavior (Stern et al., 1960). Several studies have been done comparing the effects of group versus individual housing. Barrett and Stockham (1963) found that animals housed in groups of 20 per cage for 18 h had higher plasma corticosterone levels than individually housed animals. Individual housing for 3 weeks results in a decreased sleep time in response to barbiturates (Wiberg and Grice, 1965); however, this decrease in response time does not appear to be due to an induction of microsomal drug-metabolizing enzymes (Balazs and Dairman, 1967). It has been suggested that the decreases in sleep time could be due to alterations in central nervous system (CNS) activity resulting in decreased barbiturate sensitivity or a change in the pharmacokinetic parameters in the CNS (Dairman and Balazs, 1970). Rats housed individually for 3 months develop larger adrenal and thyroid glands, smaller spleens and thymus glands, and display an increased sensitivity to the cardiotoxicity of isoprenaline (Balazs et al., Diarman and Balazs, 1970).

Food

Physical Form and Presentation

Food is usually supplied to rats in a pelleted or a meal form. Pellets, which are usually presented to rats in wire or perforated metal hoppers attached to the side of the cage, are considered a more efficient form in that they are less easily scattered by the animal and more easily handled by caretakers. Pelleted diets are available from commercial manufacturers but may be formulated in the laboratory, if necessary (Green and Turner, 1974). Making relatively hard pellets from finely ground materials will reduce wastage (Ford, 1977). The meal form of diet is useful when test compounds must be mixed with the diet. Food in this form is usually presented to animals in wide-mouthed jars with lids

Table 5 Minimum Cage Sizes for Rats

Weight of rat (g)	Floor area/ Animal[a]	
	in^2	cm^2
Up to 100	17	109.68
100–200	23	148.40
200–300	29	187.11
300–400	40	258.08
400–500	60	387.12
Over 500	70	451.64

[a]Cage height should be at least 7 in (17.78 cm).
Source: NIH (1985).

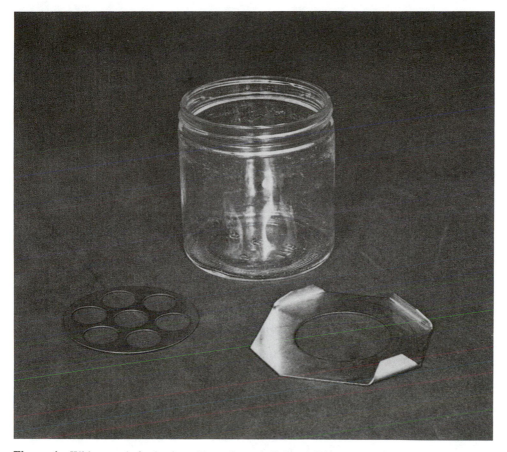

Figure 4 Wide mouth feeder jar with perforated disc and lid to reduce food spillage.

which minimize spillage (Fig. 4). Devices, such as perforated discs which sit on the feed below the lid or boxes which restrict full access to the feed jar, have been developed to further reduce spillage and contamination by excreta (Joy, et al., 1967; Fukushima et al., 1979; Thomsen, 1981). Devices have also been developed for pair-feeding studies or for studies where feed aliquots must be presented to animals throughout the day (Quarterman et al., 1970; Loveless et al., 1972). For specific applications, semimoist diets made with powdered ingredients mixed with water (50% v/v) and agar (0.1%) or liquid diets have been used (Navia, 1977; Pleasants, 1984).

Nutrition

Nutrient Requirements.   Nutrient requirements for the laboratory rat have been reviewed by Rogers (1979). Recommendations for dietary nutrient contents are given in Table 6.

Common Diets and the Effect of Nutrient Variability.   Several complete rat diets which are adequate for normal growth, reproduction, and maintenance are available from commercial sources. These diets are available in natural-ingredient and purified forms. Natural-ingredient diets use unrefined or minimally processed ingredients such as cereals, cereal biproducts, fish meals, soya-bean meals, skimmed milk, meat and bone-meals, and molasses (Clarke et al., 1977). The sources, proportions, and nutrient content of natural

Table 6   Recommended Dietary Content of Nutrients
for Rats

Nutrient	Amount in diet (90% dry matter)
Protein (%)	12.0[a]
Fat (%)[b]	5.0
Digestible energy (kcal/kg)	3800
L-Amino acids	
arginine (%)	0.6
asparagine (%)	0.4
glutamic acid (%)	4.0
histidine (%)	0.3
isoleucine (%)	0.5
leucine (%)	0.75
lysine (%)	0.7
methionine[c] (%)	0.6
phenylalanine[d] (%) (and tyrosine)	0.8
proline (%)	0.4
threonine (%)	0.5
tryptophan (%)	0.15
valine (%)	0.6
nonessential[e] (%)	0.59
Minerals	
calcium (%)	0.5
chloride (%)	0.05
chromium (mg/kg)	0.3
copper (mg/kg)	5.0
fluoride (mg/kg)	1.0
iodine (mg/kg)	0.15
iron (mg/kg)	35.0
magnesium (mg/kg)	400.0
manganese (mg/kg)	50.0
phosphorous (%)	0.4
potassium (%)	0.36
selenium (mg/kg)	0.10
sodium (%)	0.05
sulfur (%)	0.03
zinc (mg/kg)	12.0
Vitamins	
A (IU/kg)	4000.0
D (IU/kg)	1000.0
E (IU/kg)	30.0
K_1 (IU/kg)	50.0
choline (mg/kg)	1000
folic acid (mg/kg)	1.0
niacin (mg/kg)	20.0
pantothenate (calcium) (mg/kg)	8.0
riboflavin (mg/kg)	3.0
thiamin (mg/kg)	4.0

vitamin B_6 (mg/kg)	6.0
vitamin B_{12} (μg/kg)	50.0

[a]Ideal protein adequate to support growth, gestation, and lactation.
[b]Linoleic acid is required at 0.3%.
[c]One-third to one-half can be supplied by L-cystine.
[d]One-third to one-half can be supplied by L-tyrosine.
[e]Mixture of glycine, L-alanine, and L-serine.
Source: Rogers (1979), used with permission.

diet ingredients will vary depending upon cost, availability, and growing conditions (Newberne, 1975; Greenman et al., 1980; Wise and Gilburt, 1980; Wise, 1981; Wise and Gilburt, 1981). Purified diets use refined ingredients such as casein, vegetable oil, starch, and sucrose. Cellulose is used as a nonnutritive filler in purified diets.

Natural-ingredient diets are more economical and more widely used; however, the variability of the nutrient content of natural-ingredient diets may make interpretation of toxicology study results difficult. In a review of drug-nutrient interactions, Conner and Newberne (1984) discuss the implications of choice of diet in toxicology studies. Rats fed a diet deficient in lipotropes were resistent to a single high dose of aflatoxin B_1, but not to repeated small doses of aflatoxin B_1 compared to controls fed a complete diet (Rogers and Newberne, 1971). A higher incidence of colon carcinomas was associated with rats exposed to aflatoxin B_1 and a fed diet deficient in or with marginal levels of vitamin A (Newberne and Rogers, 1973).

Natural-ingredient diets tend to have a higher fiber content. Dietary fiber has been shown to counteract the toxicity of a number of compounds. Chadwick et al. (1978) found that the dietary fiber found in a natural-ingredient diet significantly altered the bacterial metabolism of lindane and suggested that this might be the source of the fiber's protective effect. Conner and Newberne (1984) make the point that purified diets (low in fiber) may increase the sensitivity of the bioassay such that it exceeds that required to assess the risk of human exposure.

Commercially available diets (natural-ingredient and purified) typically contain 20.0–23.5% protein (Table 7), whereas the National Research Council (1978) has defined a dietary protein content of 12% as adequate for rats (see Table 6). High-protein diets may increase microsomal enzyme activity and decrease the toxic effects of pesticides and aflatoxin (Campbell and Hayes, 1974). Butler and Dauterman (1988) found that animals fed diets with 22% protein produced increased rates of xenobiotic metabolism as compared to animals receiving 12% diet. The authors suggested that this increase in metabolism may affect the interpretation of biological responses and their significance to man.

Contaminants

Chemical contaminants may occur in diets as constituents of the raw materials or be introduced accidentally during manufacture. In analyses of commercial laboratory diets selenium, DDT, dieldrin, cadmium, lead, and nitrosamine have been found at concentrations near those shown to have biological effects (Edwards et al., 1979; Greenman et al., 1980). Fox et al. (1976) and Fox and Boylen (1978) found that 39% of the diets they analyzed had greater than 1 ppm of lead. Current toxicology study regulations and guidelines require or recommended analysis of diets for contaminants known to be capable of influencing the results of toxicology studies (ILAR, 1976; Food and Drug

Table 7   Protein Content of Commonly Used Rodent Diets

Diet	Protein (%)
Purina rodent lab chow 5002	20.0[a]
NIH-07 open formula mouse and rat diet	23.5[a]
AIN-76 purified rodent diet	20.0[b]

[a]As crude protein.
[b]As casein.
Source: Data from Ralston Purina Co., Rao and Knapka (1987), and Bieri *et al*. (1977).

Administration, 1978; National Academy of Sciences, 1978; Environmental Protection Agency, 1979; Oller et al., 1980). Additionally, recommendations for tolerance levels of dietary contaminants have been set (Pal et al., 1984).

Food Restriction in Chronic Studies

Food restriction in chronic studies has been found to increase life expectancy and decrease the incidence of some types of tumors. Tucker (1979) found that a 20% restriction in food consumption resulted in decreased tumor incidence (Table 8). Overfeeding has been found to influence hormonal status and increase the incidence of hormonally mediated neoplasia (Roe, 1987b). Conybeare (1980) found that mice fed at 75% of their ad libitum level had higher survival rates and significant decreases in the incidence of neoplasms of all types. Berg (1960) found that male rats on restricted diets (33–46% less than ad libitum controls) had a survival rate of 81–87% at 800 days of age compared to 48% for males on unrestricted diets. In addition, the animals on restricted diets had significantly fewer lesions and a lower tumor incidence than unrestricted males. Food restriction may be a way to decrease spontaneous tumor rates and increase the sensitivity of carcinogenity studies.

Sterilization

Sterilization of diets for gnotobiotic animals is manidtory or is recommended for diets used by specific pathogen-free animals (Wostman, 1975; Coates, 1984). Common means of sterilization are heat, ionizing radiation, and fumigation. Heat may affect the nutrient

Table 8   Effect of Food Restriction on Incidence of Pituitary and Mammary Tumors

Tumor	% of rats with tumors			
	males		females	
	ad lib	restricted	ad lib	restricted
Pituitary	32	0[a]	66	39[b]
Mammary	0	0	34	6[b]

[a]$p < 0.001$.
[b]$p < 0.005$.
Source: Data from Tucker (1979).

value of diets and affect the physical nature of the diet by causing pellets to disintegrate or become hard or increase the tendency for mold growth (Ford, 1976; Clarke et al., 1977). Heat-labile nutrients may need to be replaced following sterilization. Fumigation with ethylene oxide may affect the nutrient value of diets somewhat (Ford, 1976); care must be taken to remove all traces of ethylene oxide following treatment. The use of ionizing radiation is an effective means of sterilizing diets (Ley et al., 1969); Clarke et al., (1977) found that cereal-based diets survive gamma radiation with little harm to their nutrient value. Coates (1987) reviews additional points to consider in choosing a sterilization method.

Water

Bottles or automatic watering systems are used to supply water to rats. Where bottles are used, they are capped with rubber stoppers fitted with stainless steel tubes. The tubes have constricted apertures or ball valves. When the bottles are inverted and attached to the cages, rats can lick the aperture or valve and a drop of water will be delivered. Water bottle systems are useful where water consumption is to be measured or test compound is to be given in the water. They are inexpensive to set up, but incur increased labor costs due to the bottle washing, sterilization, and replacement required; bottles are commonly changed every 2–3 days. Animals may contaminate the water supply when drinking from bottles, but infection is limited to the specific cage. Tober-Meyer et al. (1981) used acidified water in an attempt to minimize bacterial growth and allow replacement of bottles less frequently. The acidified water had no effect on growth rates, or on the hematology or serum biochemical parameters measured. Automatic watering systems connect the cage and rack to the laboratory water supply by a series of pipes and tubes. Animals activate the system by licking a valve attached to their cage. This system requires less maintenance, but can malfunction if air becomes trapped in the rack, laboratory water pressure fails, or the rack is incorrectly attached to the laboratory plumbing. Since cages and racks are connected by plumbing, there is an increased risk of pathogen spread. Microorganism build-up in the plumbing is minimized by daily flushing of the system. In both systems, a malfunction could result in flooding of shoebox cages.

Since the water supply can be an important source of environmental contamination, including known or suspected carcinogens, such as carbon tetrachloride, polychlorinated biphenyls, and benzene (National Academy of Sciences, 1977), current toxicology guidelines or regulations require periodic analyses of water for contaminants which may be capable of affecting the outcome of the study.

Prevention of Infectious Diseases

Obviously, a disease outbreak which results in the death or severe clinical illness of test animals will affect the results of a toxicology study. Less pathogenic agents causing subclinical or less severe signs may also affect study results by surpressing or modifying the immune response, affecting fetal viability or organogenesis, or causing specific histological changes (Hsu et al., 1980; Jacoby and Barthold, 1981). By suppressing immune responses, a mycoplasma infection can result in an increase in the incidence of lung tumors in rats treated with N-nitrosoheptamine, a respiratory carcinogen (Schreiber et al., 1972). Keratoconjunctivitis, which can result from a sialodacryoadenitis viral infection, will make rats unsuitable for opthalmoscopic studies. If only a portion of the animals are affected in a study, this could lead to misleading or uninterpretable results. Common diseases which can affect the laboratory rat are discussed by Weisbroth (1979),

Cassell et al. (1979), Jacoby et al. (1979), and Kohn and Barthold (1984). The use of specific pathogen-free animals and good animal husbandry will minimize major disease outbreaks.

Microbial Status

Because study results may well be affected by infectious disease, researchers have shown increasing interest in using animals of known or stated health status. The range of different levels of microbic association goes from *axenic* (or *germ-free*) animals, which are produced by hysterectomy and reared behind germ-free barriers, to *conventional* rats from which microbes have not been excluded. *Specific pathogen–free* (SPF) or *barrier-reared* (BR) rats are animals derived from axenic animals, reared in barrier-protected colonies, and shown to be free of certain specific pathogens. The SPF animals are preferred by researchers, especially for longer-term studies, for their health and relative longevity compared to conventional animals (Baker et al., 1979).

Disease Prevention

The challenge facing the toxicologist and laboratory management is to maintain the microbial status of the rats once they arrive at the facility.

Suppliers should be asked to ship animals in boxes with polyester fiber filters to avoid contamination of the animals in transit. Animals face stress in transit from the supplier (Slanetz et al., 1956; Bantin et al., 1984). To minimize the stress, suppliers should provide sufficient feed and water (Foster et al., 1967; Weisbroth et al., 1977) and, if possible, ship the animals in environmentally controlled vehicles. To avoid potential contamination from the outside of the shipping containers, these should not be brought into the room where animals will be quarantined.

Once at the facility, animals should be quarantined to allow them to recover from the stresses of transit, resume normal weight gain, and allow existing disease to express itself. Periods recommended for this quarantine have varied from 48 hr to 4 weeks (Dymsza et al., 1963; Grant et al, 1971; Sontag et al., 1976); however, a period of 2 weeks appears to be common. Animals can be quarantined in a specially designed room or in the room to be used for the study. Baseline values for a disease-surveillance program can be established during this period: groups of excess animals ordered specifically for this purpose can be killed upon receipt and at preselected intervals during the course of the study for various serological, clinical laboratory, and histological examinations. Fox et al. (1979) discusses surveillance programs.

Elements in barriers against disease introduction include (1) treatment of materials, including equipment, feed, and bedding entering the room; (2) personnel entry procedures; and (3) environmental systems. ILAR (1976) discusses procedures to be used for various classifications of barrier areas. Specific procedures will be determined by research objectives and the cost of possibly repeating a compromised study. The health status of other animals within the facility will greatly influence the chances of disease introduction (Baker et al., 1979). The use of conventional and SPF animals in the same facility will increase the risk of exposure.

Jacoby and Barthold (1981) discuss various options available to the investigator if an outbreak occurs. These include ignoring the infection, quarantine of specific animals or the colony, purposeful exposure of animals to generalize the infection, culling, and termination of the study or population. The selection of an option will be dependent on the type of infection and chances for control, research objectives, husbandry practices, and facility design.

STUDY DESIGN

The length and design of toxicology studies used to predict human risk are, to a large part, determined by guidelines issued by regulatory bodies such as the FDA, the Environmental Protection Agency (EPA), and their counterparts worldwide (Alder and Zbinden, 1988). The length of dosing varies, depending on the purpose, from single-dose (acute) studies to studies of 1–2 years in length. Acute toxicity studies assess adverse effects from a single dose of a test compound (Table 9). Regulatory agencies no longer require the determination of an LD_{50} value as a result of an acute study. Short-term or subchronic studies (Table 10), which are usually 14–90 days in duration, assess the effects of a test compound at dosages which do not cause immediate toxic effects. Chronic studies (Table 10), which are 6 months or longer in duration, assess the test compound effect following prolonged periods of exposure. The highest dosage level in each of these studies should produce a toxic effect such that target organs may be defined. The lowest dosage should exceed the estimated human exposure and, ideally, should define a no observable effects level. Some

Table 9 Typical Protocol for an Acute Study with Rats

Animals	Male and female; young adults; acclimated for at least 5 days prior to test; weight variation should not exceed ±20% of the mean weight.
Dose levels	At least 3; or just 1 at 5000 mg/kg if this dosage is not lethal
No. of animals/dose	10: 5 male and 5 female
Dosing specifications	
fasting	Overnight prior to dosing
dosing volume (for gavage studies)	1 ml/100 g body weight; if the vehicle is an aqueous solution, 2 ml/100 g
duration	Dose should be delivered in single administration if possible; if multiple administrations required, dose should be given over a period not exceeding 24 hr
Observations	
duration	At least 14 days
frequency	At least once per day
content	Observations should include changes in the skin and fur, eyes, and mucous membranes, the respiratory, circulatory, autonomic, and central nervous systems, and in somatomotor activity and behavior pattern. Observe particularly for tremors, convulsions, salivation, diarrhea, lethargy, sleep, and coma. The time of death should be recorded as precisely as possible
Body weights	Shortly before test substance administration, then weekly and at death
Necropsy	On all animals found dead or killed, when indicated by the nature of the toxic effects observed
Microscopic examination	Should be considered for organs showing evidence of gross pathology in animals surviving 24 hr or more

Table 10 Typical Protocol for a Subchronic or Chronic Toxicity Study with Rats

Duration	90 days (subchronic) or 6 months to 2 years (chronic)
Age at start (weeks)	<6
No. of treatment groups	3
No. of control groups	1
No. of animals/sex/group	15–20 (additional animals for interim sacrifices, reversal, and pharmacokinetics groups)
Body weights	Weekly for 13 weeks then monthly
Food consumption	Weekly for 13 weeks then monthly
Daily observations	2 times daily (minimum)
Physical exams	Weekly
Ophthalmic exams	Prestudy, at an intermediate point, and at termination
Blood collections	
frequency	1–2 interim points and at termination
parameters	
hematology	HGB, HCT, RBC, WBC, MCH, MCHC, MCV, differential smear evaluation, platelet count, prothrombin time
blood chemistry	AST, ALT, ALP, glucose, urea, total protein, albumin, globulin, total bilirubin, cholesterol, creatinine, electrolytes
Urinalysis	
frequency	Same as blood collections
parameters	pH, specific gravity, glucose, bilirubin, ketones, protein, occult blood, urobilinogen, 24-hr volume, microscopic exam on spun sediment
Necropsy	
organs weighed	Adrenals, brain, epididymis, heart, kidneys, liver, ovaries, pituitaries, prostate, salivary gland, spleen, testes, thymus, thyroids, uterus
Tissues taken for microscopy	Above plus aorta, bone, bone marrow, esophagus, eye with lacrimal gland, doudendum, jejunem, ileum, cecum, colon, rectum, lung, lymph node, mammary gland, pancreas, peripheral nerve, skeletal muscle, seminal vesicle, skin, spinal cord, tongue, trachea, urinary bladder, vagina

researchers have questioned the value of toxicity studies longer than 6 months in duration (Lumley and Walker, 1985, 1986).

Additional studies are performed to assess the potential of a test compound to cause specific types of toxicity. The carcinogenicity study (Table 11), typically 18 months to 2 years in length, is designed to assess the potential of the test compound to induce neoplastic lesions. The highest dosage in a carcinogenicity study should cause minimal toxic effects; i.e., the maximum tolerated dose. Reproduction studies are performed to assess the potential to affect general fertility and reproductive performance (Segment I), cause developmental toxicity (Segment II), or affect perinatal and postnatal development (Segment III). The highest dose in the reproductive studies should be chosen so that it causes some minimal toxic effect. Typical protocols for reproductive studies are in Tables

Table 11 Typical Protocol for a Carcinogenicity Study with Rats

Duration	2 years to lifetime
Age at start (weeks)	<6
No. of treatment groups	3
No. of control groups	1 or 2
No. of animals/sex/group	50 minimum
Body weights	Weekly for 13 weeks then monthly
Food consumption	Weekly for 13 weeks then monthly
Daily observations	2 times daily (minimum)
Physical exams and mass palpations	Weekly
Blood collections	
frequency	12 and 18 months, and at termination
parameters	Differential smear at interim collections plus RBC and WBC at termination
Necropsy	
Tissues taken for microscopy	Adrenal, aorta, bone, bone marrow, brain, epididymis, esophagus, eye with lacrimal gland, heart, duodenum, jejunum, ileum, cecum, colon, rectum, kidney, liver, lung, lymph node (submaxillary and mesenteric), mammary gland, ovary, pancreas, peripheral nerve, pituitary, prostate, salivary gland, skeletal muscle, seminal vesicle, skin, spinal cord, spleen, stomach, testis, thymus, thyroid, tongue, trachea, urinary bladder, uterus, vagina

12, 13, and 14. These represent typical studies to meet United States guidelines and would need to be modified to meet the additional European and Japanese requirements.

DOSING TECHNIQUES

With the extensive use of the laboratory rat in biological sciences, a wide range of dosing routes and techniques have been published (Kraus, 1979; Petty, 1982; Flecknell, 1987). In toxicology studies where results are to extrapolated to human risk, convention and guidelines dictate that rats should be dosed by a route closely approximating that of human exposure. For mechanistic studies, where specific organs may be targeted, the route of administration will be dictated by research objectives.

Oral Route

Rodents have some unique characteristics to be considered regarding the oral administration of test compounds. One characteristic is the lack of an emetic response. The fact that rodents lack an emetic response allows a higher dose of an otherwise emetic compound to be given to rats. Many compounds cause dogs and other species with emetic responses to vomit when orally dosed; this results in problems determining the actual dose received and leads to erratic blood levels. The lack of an emetic response has been useful in designing rodenticides (Lisella et al., 1971). A second factor to consider is that rodents are nocturnal and eat most of their food at night. When maintained on 12-h light and dark periods, rats

Table 12   General Fertility and Reproductive Performance (Segment I)

Age at start of dosing	
males	40 days (minimum)
females	Adult or at least sexually mature
No. of treatment groups	2 minimum
No. of control groups	1
No. of animals/dose	10 males and 20 females
Dosing duration	
males	60–80 days prior to mating
females	14 days prior to mating and throughout pregnancy and lactation
Mating	One male is mated with two females; day 0 is the day evidence of copulation is found (sperm or sperm plug)
Examinations	
day 13 of pregnancy	Half the females are killed and examined for pre- or postimplantation embryo lethality
Postweaning	The remaining females are allowed to deliver and wean their offspring; weanlings are sacrificed and subjected to gross and visceral examinations for malformations.
Parameters determined	
preimplant. deaths	No. corpora lutea in ovaries/no. implantation sites in uterine horns
postimplant. deaths	No. resorption sites in uterus/no. implantation sites $\times$ 100.
fertility index	No. pregnancies/no. matings $\times$ 100
gestation index	No. live fetuses/litter
sex ratio[a]	No. of each sex/total no. offspring
viability index[a]	No. pups alive/no. pups born alive (or remaining after cull) $\times$ 100
weaning index	No. pups alive at 21 days/no. pups maintained at 4 days $\times$ 100
growth index[a]	Average male and female pup weights

[a]Determined at birth (except viability) and at days 4, 7, 14, and 21 after birth.

consume 75% of their 24-hr food intake during the 12 dark hours (Wong and Oace, 1981). This pattern of consumption will affect blood levels in studies where test compound is administered in the diet. The rat stomach appears to act as a reservoir for energy supply during the first half of the light period (Armstrong et al., 1978). The stomach shows a variation in content over a 24-hr period with the maximum content occurring at the end of the dark and early light hours, whereas the proximal part of the small intestine holds a relatively constant amount over 24-hr periods. These factors will have some affect on gastric emptying and the speed of absorption of test compounds. Chasseaud and Taylor (1974) and Smyth and Hottendorf (1980) discuss other considerations regarding oral administration and absorption of test compounds.

Techniques for orally administering test compounds include mixing in the diet, by gavage or stomach tube, by capsule, or with drinking water. The dietary and gavage techniques are much more widely used than the others.

Dietary vs Gavage Methods

The choice between dietary and gavage dosing techniques is by no means straightforward and the choice is often a matter of convenience or manpower considerations. A scientific decision can only be made with a knowledge about pharmacokinetics of the test com-

Table 13 Teratology Study (Segment II)

Age at start of dosing	Adult or at least sexually mature
No. of treatment groups	2 minimum
No. of control groups	1
No. of animals/dose	20 females
Dosing duration	Day 6 through day 15 of pregnancy; day 0 is the day evidence of copulation is found (sperm or sperm plug)
Examination	On day 21 of pregnancy, females are sacrificed and fetuses are delivered by hysterectomy, weighed, sexed, and examined for gross, visceral, and skeletal abnormalities. See Manson and Kang (1989) for a description of examinations.

pound administered by both methods. Other considerations which might be used in making the decision are given below.

The dietary method can be used if a compound (1) can be mixed in the diet, (2) is stable under storage conditions and in the cage, and (3) is palatable to the rat. A major advantage of the dietary method is that it requires less manpower to perform the study. The diet mixing process can be performed weekly or, if stability allows, even less frequently. The mixing and feeding process is much less labor intensive than gavaging rats on a daily basis. A disadvantage is that to prove homogeneity and stability analytical procedures must be developed and validated; this can be a difficult and time-consuming process. In addition, since the concentration of compound mixed in the feed is based on predicted feed consumption and body weights, the dietary method of dosing can be less exact than the gavage method. Contamination of the facility or control animals by the spread of

Table 14 Perinatal and Postnatal Study (Segment III)

Age at start of dosing	Adult or at least sexually mature
No. of treatment groups	2 minimum
No. of control groups	1
No. of animals/dose	20 females
Dosing duration	Day 15 of pregnancy and throughout pregnancy and lactation; day 0 is the day evidence of copulation is found (sperm or sperm plug)
Examinations	Weanlings are autopsied and subjected to gross and visceral examinations for malformations
Parameters determined	
fertility index	No. pregnancies/no. matings × 100
gestation index	No. live fetuses/litter
sex ratio[a]	No. of each sex/total no. offspring
viability index[a]	No. pups alive/no. pups born alive (or remaining after cull) × 100
weaning index	No. pups alive at 21 days/no. pups maintained at 4 days × 100
growth index[a]	Average male and female pup weights

[a]Determined at birth (except viability) and at days 4, 7, 14, and 21 after birth.

compound dust or vapor must be addressed in dietary studies (Sansone et al., 1977; Sansone and Losikoff, 1978).

The gavage method can be used where the test compound is not stable in the diet or is not palatable. If the test compound is not a solution and has to be mixed with a vehicle prior to administration, an analysis must be developed to confirm concentration, homogeneity, and stability of the mixture; however, this analysis is usually easier to develop than in the diet. With the gavage method of dosing, a more precise amount of compound can be delivered. A disadvantage of the gavage method is that it involves handling rats on a daily basis; handling rats has been shown to increase plasma corticosterone levels (Barrett and Stockham, 1963) and may affect study results. Additionally, daily intubation may lead to deaths due to esophageal punctures or inhalation pneumonia.

A common assumption is that higher peak plasma levels will be achieved in gavage studies than in dietary studies because test compound is given as a bolus in gavage studies and over a prolonged period in dietary studies. This is not necessarily the case. Van Harken and Hottendorf (1978) found 23% higher peak plasma levels and 44% greater 24-hr area under the curve values in groups where cefatrizine was administered for 5 days in the diet compared to groups receiving the drug by single daily gavage. They suggested that the drug might be absorbed in the upper small intestine and that gavage dosing resulted in a drug bolus that passed beyond the site of absorption before absorption was completed. A method for comparing availability of drugs given by gavage vs by diet is given in Smyth et al. (1979).

Dietary

Utilizing the dietary method, test compound is mixed with the diet and administered to animals ad libitum. The dosage received by an animal is regulated by varying the concentration of compound in the diet based on predicted food consumption and body weight. Food consumption and body weight predictions are based upon historical laboratory data for early time points in a study. After growth and food consumption curves can be established for groups during the study, group mean data can be used for predictions. Different concentrations are made for each sex.

Test compound and diet are mixed in two steps: (1) the compound and about 10% of the total amount of diet are blended in a premix, then (2) the premix and rest of the diet are mixed. The total amount of diet to be mixed is first weighed out, then 10% of this amount is separated for the premix. To make a premix, all the test compound and an aliquot of diet (from the 10%) are put into a mortar. These ingredients are ground with a pestle until the mixture appears homogeneous. This mixture and the remainder of the 10% are layered in a small-capacity mixer and mixed for 5–10 mins. The time for this mixing process can be varied if analysis shows the total mixture is not homogeneous. For the final mix, the premix and the remainder of the diet are layered in a large-capacity mixer. The mixing time will vary with type of blender and can be varied if analysis shows the total mixture is not homogeneous.

Several types of blenders are available for the mixing process, including open-bowl "kitchen" mixers, V or PK blenders, and Turbula mixers. Metal parts should be grounded to eliminate electrostatic forces. A complete discussion of concentration calculations and diet mixing is given in Stevens and Gallo (1989). Food jars and other equipment for presentation of compound-diet mixtures have been discussed in the section on food.

Alternative methods of mixing test compound with diet have been published. Microencapsulation has been used as a means of incorporating volatile, reactive, or unpalatable chemicals into animals food in toxicology studies (Melnick et al., 1987a, b). Shimamura and Shimamura (1986) present an alternative method for delivering oil-soluble compounds in the diet. In a limited study, they dissolved the test compound in olive oil and placed a small amount in a hole made in the center of a food pellet. They found that rats will preferentially eat this pellet if it is placed on the floor of the cage.

Gavage

In the gavage procedure, test article is introduced into the eosphagus through a stomach tube or needle attached to a graduated syringe.

Test Article Preparation. If not already a liquid, the test compound is prepared for administration by adding it to the appropriate vehicle. The choice of vehicle will depend on the characteristics of the compound; however, consideration must be given to the effect of the vehicle on the rat (Gad and Chengelis, 1988). Common vehicles used are water or food-grade oil. Suspensions are made when aqueous vehicles are desired and the test compound is not soluble. Suspending agents such as methylcellulose are added to increase the viscosity and hold the compound in suspension. A wetting agent such as polysorbate 80 can also used. Pekas (1974) used ingesta or semiliquefied meals to overcome problems he was having formulating microgram quantities of lipophilic substances.

Equipment. Soft catheters made of rubber (Shay and Gruenstein, 1946) or polyethylene, e.g., size 8 French infant feeding tubes, or stainless steel gavage needles with smooth, ball-shaped tips (Ferrill, 1943; Clark and Harland, 1969) are commonly used in gavage dosing (Fig. 5); all are commercially available. Soft catheters minimize the chances of

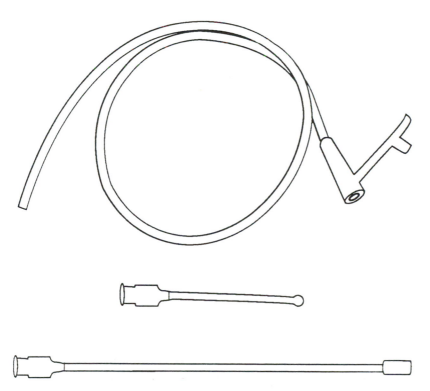

Figure 5 Gavage needle, size 8: French infant feeding tube, and capsule needle.

esophageal trauma. The ball-shaped tips of gavage needles reduce the chances of tracheal injections, however, if an animal struggles while a gavage needle is in the esophagus, the rigid needle increases the chances of esophageal punctures. A disadvantage of the soft catheter is that it can allow small amounts of fluid to leak past the catheter, out of the esophagus, and be aspirated. Even a small amount of solution can cause inhalation pneumonia. Conybeare and Leslie (1988) observed deaths in gavage studies as a result of the aspiration of small amounts of irritant solutions or acidic, hypertonic solutions. They found that the use of a ball-tip 4 mm in diameter would eliminate these deaths. With gentle handling, rats will become used to the dosing technique. Gags should not be necessary to aid in dosing rats under normal conditions. Where necessary, various aids made of wire or dowels have been described (Lehr, 1945; Woodnott, 1962; Kesel, 1964; Pekas, 1974).

Technique. The description below is appropriate for either a gavage needle or catheter; for simplicity, only the needle will be mentioned in the description. The method for holding a needle and syringe combination while dosing is illustrated in Figure 6; the method for the catheter and syringe combination is shown in Figure 7.

Prior to picking up the animal, the syringe should be filled with the amount of test liquid to be delivered and the needle attached. Any air bubbles should be eliminated. It is a good practice to wipe off the needle prior to dosing the animal; if the dosing liquid is distasteful, the rat may begin to struggle after repeated dosings and increase the chances of being injured.

To position the animal for gavage, it should be grasped by the skin of the back and neck (see Fig. 6) ensuring that the head, neck, and back are in a straight line. Alternatively, the animal can be grasped about the shoulders, with the index finger and thumb on either side of the head (see Fig. 7). The objective is to firmly hold the animal and to be able to control any struggling if it occurs. For even more control, the animal may be placed on a table or brought up against the operator's chest.

Once the animal is positioned, the needle can be inserted into the mouth of the animal, moved over the tongue, and down into the esophagus. The full length of the needle should be able to be inserted into the animal. A slight rotary movement of the needle may help insertion into the esophagus. If the needle is inserted into the trachea, the animal may struggle. The syringe should be grasped lightly such that, if the animal does struggle, chances of an esophageal tear are minimized. If the animal continues to struggle, the needle should be withdrawn to allow the animal to settle down, then the placement can be attempted once again.

With the needle in place, the test compound should be slowly expelled into the animal. Too rapid an administration may cause a reflux of the liquid back up the esophagus, resulting in an inaccurate dose being given and possible aspiration of the test compound. Once the dose is delivered, the needle should be withdrawn and the animal observed for any signs of distress or respiratory difficulty. An experienced technician should be able to dose 250–350 animals per hour without causing discomfort to the animals and with minimal (1 per 80,000 dosings) dosing-related deaths (Conybeare and Leslie, 1988).

Gavage liquids are commonly administered at a volume of 5–10 ml/kg body weight. The volume should be enough to be delivered accurately, but not so much that it will adversely affect the animal. The maximum volume should be no more than 20 ml/kg. The volume chosen can have an effect on the results. Ferguson (1962) found that a change in

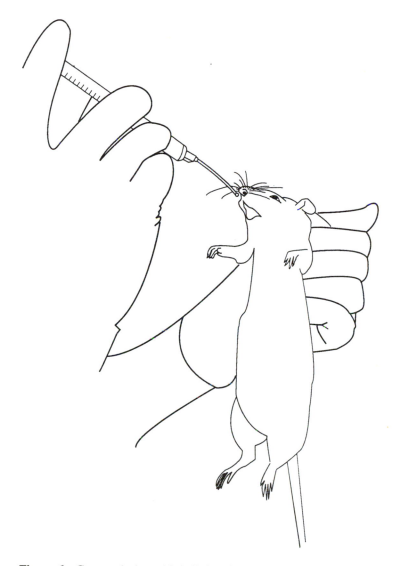

Figure 6   Gavage dosing with ball-tipped needle. Note method of restraint.

dose volume of from 5 to 1% of body weight could change mortality rate from approximately 95% to approximately 5%, respectively, at equivalent doses.

Intragastric Infusion.   To allow continuous intragastric infusions, rats can be fitted with chronic gastric tubes (Fig. 8) running from a spot between their ears, subcutaneously to their nostrils, then through the nasopharynx and esophagus to the stomach (Epstein and Teitelbaum, 1962a). The tube running from the ears is connected to a water-tight swivel joint (Epstein and Teitelbaum, 1962b) through which test solutions are pumped. Animals will move, eat, and drink freely for months and without developing infection or respiratory difficulties. Additionally, Waynforth et al. (1977) have developed a device which

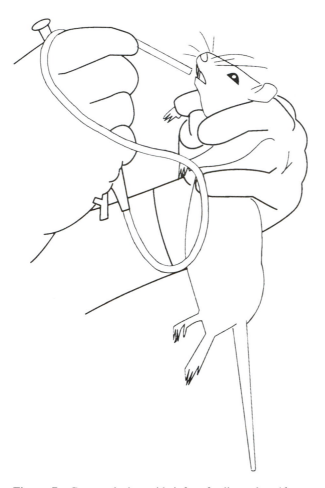

Figure 7 Gavage dosing with infant feeding tube. Alternate method of restraint.

allows short-term, continuous infusion; however, the animals have to be restrained during infusions and cannot eat or drink.

Neonatal Administration.   Neonatal intragastric injections can be made orally with thin silicone tubing (Gibson and Becker, 1967; Smith and Kelleher, 1973) or by intragastric injection with a 27-gauge needle through the abdominal wall (Worth et al., 1963; Bader and Klinger, 1974).

Capsule

To eliminate the possibility of dosing errors and to deal with compounds which can not be delivered through conventional means, methods have been developed for the administration of capsules into the esophagus of rats (Nelson and Hoar, 1969; Shani et al., 1970; and Lax et al., 1983). In these methods, a small capsule is inserted into the esophagus in the tip of a tube or in a stainless steel cap attached to a gavage needle (see Fig. 5). By injecting air or pushing a rod, the capsule is forced out and into the esophagus. The capsules move into the stomach by peristaltic action and are dissolved within 10

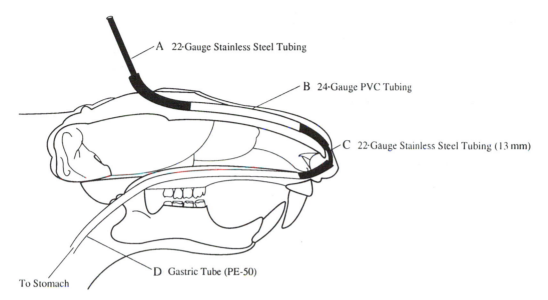

Figure 8   Intragastric cannula placement. (Redrawn from Epstein and Teitlebaum [1962a].)

min (Lax et al., 1983). Up to 150 mg of test compound can be administered at one time using this method (Shani et al., 1970).

Water

As an alternative to dietary administration, compounds that are water soluble, palatable to the rat, and stable in water may be administered to rats in their drinking water. This method offers similar advantages as adding a test compound to the diet. Additionally, compounds will be more easily mixed and analyses will be more easily developed than when a compound is in the diet. However, spillage of water makes measurement of the actual dose received difficult.

Intravenous Route

Veins which have been used for intravenous injections are the lateral tail (caudal), jugular, femoral, saphenous, lateral marginal, dorsal metatarsal, sublingual, and dorsal penile vein. While most are superficial and available for injection, several require the use of anesthesia or an assistant and may be of limited usefulness in repeated dose studies. While anesthesia may be acceptable for acute studies or for surgery, its repeated use may have an affect on toxic responses. Ether exposure is known to increase plasma cholinesterase levels, whereas barbiturates can induce drug-metabolizing enzymes.

Lateral Tail Vein

The lateral tail veins are currently the most widely used for intravenous injections in the rat. The veins are visible, especially in young animals, and injections can be performed by one person without the use of anesthesia.

Bolus Injection Technique.   A 23-gauge needle attached to an appropriately sized syringe should be used. After putting the animal into a suitable restrainer, the vein should be dilated with heat. This can be accomplished by placing the tail in warm water (40–45°C) or under a heat lamp. Alternatively, the area of the tail to be injected can be wrapped with a gauze pad which has been dipped in warm water. Care must be taken to avoid using excessive heat. Minsaian (1980) describes a tourniquet made from a plastic syringe and thread which may be of use.

The tip of the tail should be held taunt with the thumb and index finger of one hand (Fig. 9). With the other hand, the needle should be held bevel up and at a shallow angle parallel to the vein. The skin of the tail should then be pierced and the needle advanced until resistance is no longer felt. The thumb and forefinger holding the tail can then be moved to hold the hub of the needle as well, while the other hand is free to pull back slightly on the plunger of the syringe. The use of a needle with a clear or transparent hub will facilitate confirmation of correct placement. Blood backflow into the needle chamber confirms entry into the vein.

If repeated dosings are to be performed, initial venipunctures should be performed as close to the tip of the tail as possible. During the injection, a small bleb will occur if the needle has come out of the vein. The needle should be immediately repositioned to prevent infiltration of solution around the vein. Infiltration of an irritating solution can cause necrosis and make future injections difficult or impossible. Injection of 2 ml/100 g body weight can be accomplished without stress to the rat. Barrow (1968) found that injections of volumes over this amount produced respiratory difficulty and pulmonary edema.

Tail Vein Infusions.   The tail is convenient for infusions because catheter placement can

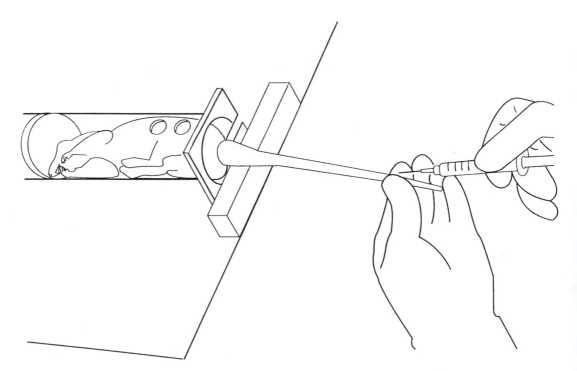

Figure 9   Tail vein injection.

be done with no anesthesia (Cotlove, 1961). A 23-gauge needle connected with polyethylene tubing to a pump is inserted into the tail. The needle and polyethylene tubing are secured to the tail with waterproof plastic tape and test solutions can then be infused. The tail may be taped to a wooden stick or tongue depressor to further protect the needle from being dislodged (Fig. 10). Commercially available over-the-needle catheters (Nachtmann et al., 1988) offer an advantage to resident needles in that they are less likely to damage or penetrate the vein wall. The advantages of this tail vein infusion technique over techniques using indwelling catheters are that it can be repeated daily, there is no permanent cannula to become clogged, and it does not require anesthesia. A disadvantage is that restraint is required during infusions. This may cause the animals stress, so infusions should be limited in duration.

In alternative techniques (Born and Moller, 1974; Rhodes and Patterson, 1979), a cannula is inserted into the lateral vein and protected with electrical shielding. The advantage of this technique is that the animal is unrestrained and, therefore, can be

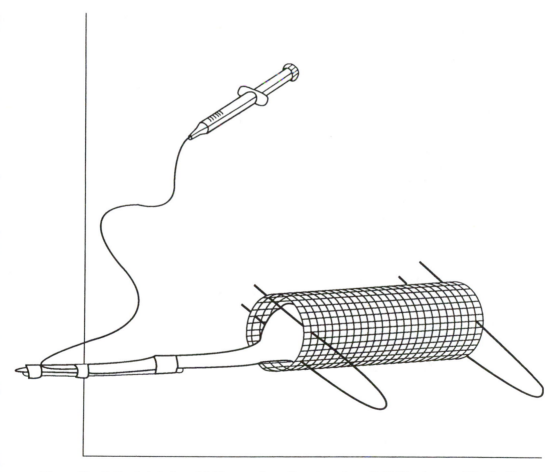

Figure 10 Tail vein infusion with 23-gauge butterfly set taped to tail. Tail has been stabilized with a splint.

infused for longer periods of time; Born and Moller (1974) suggest the infusion can be maintained for several weeks.

Jugular Vein

Although this route has been used for bolus injections, it is most widely used as a site for cannulation for indwelling catheters. The use of anesthesia is required for bolus injections and for the cannulation procedure.

Bolus Injection Technique. Although injections can be made by exposing the jugular vein by incision (see the jugular vein blood collection method), this method is not acceptable for repeated dosings. Phillips et al. (1973) describe a method performed without incision. The animal is anesthetized and placed on its back. The head should be positioned to the left or right for entrance into the respective jugular vein. A 23-gauge, 0.75-inch needle fitted to an appropriately sized syringe bevel up is inserted in a cephalocaudal direction into the angle made by the neck and shoulder. The needle should enter the vein anterior to the point at which it disappears between the pectoralis muscle and the clavicle. When about one-half the length of the needle has penetrated the skin, the bevel should be in the lumen of the vessel. Insertion of the needle through the muscle stabilizes the needle and minimizes bleeding.

Infusion. To perform the surgical procedure (Popovic and Popovic, 1960), the anesthetized animal is placed on a board with its head and forelegs secured; the forelegs should be in an outstretched position. A 3-cm incision should be made in the median neck vein skin and the body of the jugular vein cleaned for a length of 1 cm just before it enters the chest. Manipulation of the vein should be minimized to prevent collapse. A cephalic ligature is then tied and the jugular is lifted slightly. After making a small incision at the anterior part of the jugular, a cannula is pushed into the body of the jugular. When correctly positioned, the tip of the cannula will be at the junction of both venae cavae. The cannula should then be secured with ligatures. Pope (1968) and Rezek and Havlicek (1976) have cannulation devices to facilitate the cannula insertion. Harms and Ojeda (1974) describe an alternative procedure using a catheter attached to a needle to feed the cannula through the vein and anchor the cannula to the pectoralis muscle (Fig. 11). This technique avoids closing off the venous flow with ligations and may increase the life of the cannula.

The useful lifetime for jugular cannulas is quite variable; the lumen of the cannula is eventually obstructed by a blood clot or fibrous mass. The position of the cannula end is

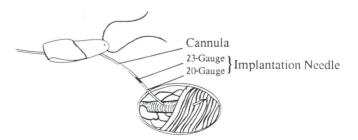

Cannula
23-Gauge
20-Gauge } Implantation Needle

Figure 11 Jugular vein cannula and insertion technique. (From Harm and Ojeda [1974], used with permission.)

important. There will be less coagulation and the cannula will last longer if the tip is in the venous stream rather than in the jugular (Popovic and Popovic, 1960). Cannulas have been constructed of several materials to prolong their life or for specific purposes (Stewart and Sanislow, 1961; Weeks and Davis, 1964; Herd and Barger, 1964; Smith and Davis, 1975; Brandstaetter and Terkel, 1977). If the test compound and objectives of the study permit, the cannula can be tested for patency by injecting 3–6 mg of pentobarbital solution (0.05–0.10 ml of a 60mg/ml solution) into the cannula (Weeks, 1972). If the cannula is functional, the rat will lose its righting reflex and become ataxic in 10–15 sec. The rat will recover in approximately 10–15 mins.

Since rats will destroy unprotected cannulas and animals used for long-term infusions need to be relatively free to move about their cages, cannulas are generally brought subcutaneously to the back of the neck or head and externalized. At this point, the cannula can be treated in several ways. The free end of the cannula can be plugged with a wire so that it can be accessed for daily injections. The cannula can be connected to a subcutaneously implanted port which serves as a daily injection site (Novin et al., 1974). Various forms of osmotic pumps which can be connected to cannulas and implanted subcutaneously have been developed (Rose and Nelson, 1955; Rose and Rabinov, 1967; Nielsen, 1981). Finally, the cannula can be attached by way of a harness support apparatus to a swivel and pump. Eve and Robinson (1963), Dalton et al. Wilson (1969), Evans (1970), Weeks (1972), Steiger et al. (1972), Cox and Beazley (1975), and Brown et al. (1976) describe swivel and harness systems for jugular infusions. When performing long-term infusion studies, the effects of the cannula and harness should be considered. Infections, septicemia, a variety of visceral lesions, endothelial lesions, and increased platelet consumption have been observed in cannulated animals (Hysell and Abrams, 1967; Meuleman et al., 1980; Vilageliu et al., 1981). Birkhahn et al. (1976) saw decreased or erratic weight gains and decreased liver weights in harnassed animals compared to animals without harnesses. These changes were attributed to the stress involved from harnessing rats for chronic intravenous infusion. Even light restraint can cause depressed growth, adrenal histological changes, and slight thymic involution (Pfeiffer, 1967).

Femoral Vein

A skin incision is necessary to expose the femoral vein. Owing to its placement, this vein has been used predominantly for terminal procedures or procedures involving catheterization. The catheterization technique is similar to that used for the jugular vein. The animal is anesthetized, a 2- to 3-cm incision is made over the vein, and a 1- to 2-cm length of vein is exposed by blunt dissection. Suture material is placed posterior and anterior to where the vein incision is to be made, keeping opposing tension on both to cut off the blood flow once the incision has been made. As with the jugular vein, a small hole should be made in the vein and the cannula inserted. The cannula should be advanced until the tip is in the inferior vena cava (3.5–4.5 cm in 100 to 200-g rats). The cannula should then be secured in the vein with sutures.

Jones and Hynd (1981) and Slack and Jones (1987) discuss the use of the femoral vein in long-term infusions. In each, the cannula is run subcutaneously through the groin and tail where it is exteriorized and passed through a protective spring to a infusion pump. Rats have been continuously infused for 3 weeks using this method (Slack and Jones, 1987).

Saphenous, Lateral Marginal, and Metatarsal Veins

These veins in the leg and foot of the rat are easily visualized and can be injected without anesthesia; however, an assistant is required. Shaving the area over the saphenous or lateral marginal vein will make it easier to see. For the injection, the assistant restrains the rat and occludes the vein to cause it to dilate. Wiping the skin over the vein with 70% alcohol will increase the dilation. The opearator is then free to inject the animal. A 26- to 27-gauge needle is appropriate for these veins (Everett and Sawyer, 1956; Pearce, 1957; Nobunaga et al., 1966).

Dorsal Penis Vein

It is not clear whether anesthesia is required for injection into the dorsal penis vein. In the original description (Salem et al., 1963), the use of anesthesia was not mentioned; however, Nightingale and Mouravieff (1973) lightly anesthetized their animals. To perform the procedure, an assistant holds the animal by the skin on its back with one hand and by either the feet or tail with the other hand. The vertebral column should be hyperextended. The operator grasps the tip of the penis between the thumb and forefinger, and injects test solution into the dorsal vein using a 26- to 30-gauge needle. Nightingale and Mouravieff (1973) compared the metabolism of 4-aminoantipyrine injected intracardially and by dorsal penis vein. The results suggested that injection of the drug through the penis vein lead directly to the general circulation and that a first-pass effect on drug metabolism is not to be expected.

Sublingual Vein

While the method of sublingual vein injection has the disadvantage of requiring anesthesia, it can be performed by one person (Anderson, 1963; Waynforth and Parkin, 1969). The animal should be placed on its back with the head facing the operator. Holding the tongue between the thumb and forefinger and, using a 26- to 30-gauge needle, the vein should be entered at a very shallow angle and the test solution injected. After the injection, the bleeding can be stopped using direct pressure with the thumb. Once bleeding has stopped, a small cotton-wool pledget should be placed over the vein and the tongue and pledget put back into the animal's mouth. When the animal regains consciousness, it will spit out the cotton.

Neonatal Administration

Intravenous injections in neonatal rats using 30-gauge needles have been made into the tail vein (Gibson and Becker, 1967) and into the subcutaneous vein at the junction of the superior and inferior palpebral veins (Anderson et al., 1959). Volumes of 0.1 ml were injected. Grazer (1958) delivered the same volume with a 30-guage needle in an intracardiac injection.

Intraperitoneal Route

Test compound injected into the peritoneal cavity will be absorbed into the portal circulation and transported to the liver. As a result, the compound will be subjected to the metabolic activity of the liver before gaining access to the general circulation and possibly excreted in the bile before gaining access to the remainder of the animal. Owing to the amount of blood flow and circulatory surface area in the region, compounds injected intraperitoneally (ip) will be absorbed relatively quickly into the circulation.

One person can perform the injection, but an assistant holding the animal's legs may minimize the chances of the operator being scratched and permit the operator to have more control of the injection process. The needle (< 21 gauge) should be inserted anteriorly into the lower part of the abdomen, just lateral to the ventral midline (Fig. 12). Aspiration of the syringe prior to injection will help the operator determine if the needle is positioned in an organ. Lewis et al. (1966) studied errors occurring as a result of intraperitoneal dosing. In 127 injections with a radiopaque dye, the authors found that 19.6% had been injected into a site other than the peritoneal cavity (GI tract, subcutaneously, retroperitioneally, or urinary bladder). It was suggested that fasting, 0.25- to 0.50-in needles, and maintaining steady restraint be used as means to minimize the errors. Fifteen to 25 ml of solution can be injected into the peritoneal space.

In choosing the intraperitoneal route of injection, the researcher should be aware that multiple injections can be stressful to the animal and that injection of some substances into the peritoneal cavity can lead to irritation or inflammation. Golba et al. (1974) found that dosing rats with 1 ml of an aqueous solution of sodium chloride intraperitoneally for several days resulted in a decrease in the white blood cell count. The authors attributed the decrease to the stress of the multiple intraperitoneal injections. Teoh (1961) found that the injection of methylcellulose intraperitoneally lead to splenomegaly and the presence of foam cells throughout major organs in the body.

Intramuscular Route

Intramuscular injection of compounds will result in rapid absorption into the general circulation owing to the abundant supply of blood vessels. However, the speed of

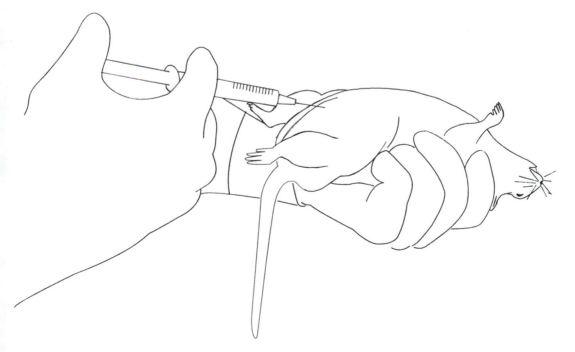

Figure 12   Intraperitoneal injection technique.

absorption will not be as fast as with an interperitoneal injection. Acceptable sites in the rat are the quadriceps, the thigh, and the triceps. An assistant will be required to hold the rat (Fig. 13). The selected muscle mass should be stabilized with the thumb and forefinger of one hand and the needle ($<$ 21 gauge) guided into the muscle with the other. The syringe should be aspirated to ensure that the injection will not be accidentally done intravenously, then the solution slowly injected. A slow injection will minimize the pain. Approximately 0.3 ml of solution can be injected.

Subcutaneous Route

Absorption after subcutaneous injection will usually be slower than after intramuscular injection; however, this may be an advantage if a relatively sustained period of absorption is desired. Suitable sites for injection are the ventral body, flank, or shoulders. To perform the injection, the skin is grasped between the thumb and forefinger and raised to make a tent (Fig. 14). The needle ($<$ 20 gauge) is inserted through the skin to make the injection. Injection sites can be varied for multiple-dose studies where the solution is a potential irritant. Five to 10 ml can be injected.

To minimize the stress of manipulation and to provide a means for continuous infusion, perforated cannulas have been implanted in the dorsal subcutis. Wittgenstein and Rowe (1965) secured the cannula with a harness, attached it to pumps in a manner similar to that described for jugular infusions, and infused rats for up to 10 days. Mucha (1980) injected sodium pentobarbital directly into the cannula and showed it was absorbed much more rapidly following injection through the cannula than following hypodermic injection. Hock and Beyhl (1984) have described the use of an osmotic minipump for continuous

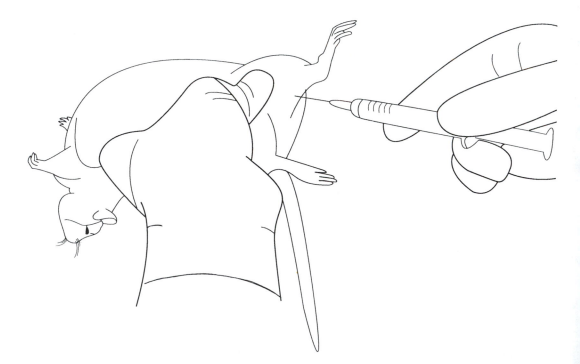

Figure 13 Intramuscular injection technique.

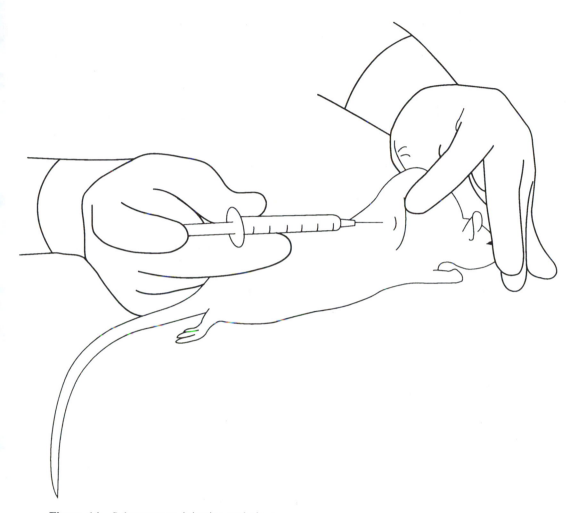

Figure 14 Subcutaneous injection technique.

subcutaneous infusion. This method offers several advantages in that it is continuous, constant, and animals are not encumbered with the infusion apparatus. To utilize the minipump, however, solutions to be infused must be stable at the rat's body temperatures for the duration of the infusion period. Additionally, pellets of test compound have been implanted subcutaneously for chronic delivery (Borbely et al., 1979).

Topical Route

The rat has not traditionally been used as a model in skin irritation or sensitization studies. However, it has been used in systemic toxicity studies where skin was used as a portal of entry for whole body exposure and in skin painting studies where carcinogenic potential is being accessed. In a comparison of absolute absorption rates of several compounds, Bartek et al. (1972) found dermal absorption rates in the rat tended to be slightly lower than in the rabbit, and higher than in the monkey, swine, and human.

Exposure in dermal studies is usually to the anterior dorsal portion of the back. Skin is shaved weekly or 24 hr prior to skin painting. Test area of application should be clearly marked; for repeated dose studies the area of this site is often 10% of the body area. Usually 0.25–1.0 ml of test solution is applied in skin painting studies; the amounts of creams or ointments applied will vary with the test compound. Dosing is usually performed every day; however, 5-day/week regimens have been used.

Since the actual dose in dermal toxicity studies is the amount of compound absorbed (Chaube et al., 1982), factors which influence absorption should be considered. Several design features in the topical study may affect absorption: abraded skin will tend to absorb faster than intact skin; test compound may adhere or build up at the site of exposure, and this may impede absorption (and test compound may be chemically changed owing to exposure to air or light); the test compound may be licked or scratched from the site; and test compound may be ingested by the animals, particularly if they are group housed.

Several techniques have been developed to avoid removal or ingestion of test compound, since this is a particularly confounding factor in topical studies. For acute studies, Rice and Ketterer (1977) describe a cable-type restrainer attached to a stainless steel plate. Loops just behind the front legs and just in front of the hind legs hold the animal immobile. To allow the animal mobility, "Elizabethan" collars have been used (Barnett, 1958; Einheber et al., 1967; Lykke and Cummings, 1969); these are 4- to 5-cm wide strips of polyethylene or metal that fit around the animal's neck and restrict access to the back. Harness and collar devices (Bartek et al., 1972) and acrylic chambers (Nixon and Reer, 1973; Swan, 1975) have also been used.

Rectal Route

The rectal route is not a routinely used method of administration in toxicology. However, administration by this route is sometimes required to support drugs given rectally by suppository. For dosing, the animal is held up by the base of its tail and a stainless steel, ball-tipped gavage needle (5 cm) or vinyl tube (6 cm) attached to a syringe is inserted into the rectum. Care must be taken not to damage the rectum when inserting the needle. The syringe should be held lightly; the weight of the needle and syringe will propel the needle. The animal can either be awake or anesthetized. If animals are awake, excretion of the unabsorbed test compound may be a problem. Methods to control excretion have included ligation of the rectum (Nishihata et al., 1984), or various types of septums which are tied or glued in place (DeBoer et al., 1980; Iwamoto and Watanabe, 1985). Anesthetized animals can be placed on an inclined board to retard expulsion.

An important factor in rectally dosing the rat is that the depth of deposition of test material will affect the rate of absorption and should be standardized. Drugs subject to extensive first-pass metabolism, such as propranolol and lidocaine, have been found to be much more bioavailable when injected close to the anus rather than in the upper areas of the rectum (DeBoer et al., 1980; Iwamoto and Watanabe, 1985). DeLeede et al. (1983) found that the systemic availability of lidocaine given by the oral route was 16%. Lidocaine systemic availability was 16% when given rectally, 4 cm from the anus, 21% at 2 cm, 45% at 1 cm, and 72% when delivered as close to the anus as possible. The reason for this difference is that drug in the upper rectal area is absorbed into the upper rectal veins which go via the portal circulation to the liver; the lower hemorrhoidal veins are not connected to the portal system, but go directly to the inferior vena cava (Iwamoto and Watanabe, 1985).

Intranasal Route

With the increasing number of drugs being delivered nasally, methods have been developed to support this route. A rather crude method of exposing unanesthetized animals to test liquids is to allow small drops to fall from a syringe onto their nares. These drops will be inhaled into the nasal cavity. This technique will work more successfully in an anesthetized animal. More sophisticated methods using nebulizers or aerosolizer pumps are available. For acute, quantitative studies, Hussain et al. (1980) describe a surgical cannulation of the nasal cavity.

Inhalation Route

Owing to the complexities and equipment involved in generating, maintaining, and measuring appropriate atmospheres, the inhalation study is one of the most technically difficult to perform. A complete discussion of the skills necessary to perform an inhalation study is outside of the scope of this chapter and the reader is directed to reviews by Gad and Chengelis (1988) and Kennedy (1989). This section will deal with general considerations about the three major steps in exposing rats by the inhalation route: generation of the test atmosphere, exposure of the test animals, and measurement and characterization of the test atmosphere.

Generation of Test Atmospheres

Atmospheres that are commonly generated are those which include test material in the form of gases, vapors, aerosols, and/or dusts. Gases are the easiest atmospheres to generate, since they can be metered into an air stream, mixed to some appropriate concentration, then introduced into the test chamber. Vapors are the gas phase of a liquid or solid that has been heated. These can be passed at an appropriate concentration to the exposure chamber in nitrogen or compressed air. Considerations with vapors involve avoiding chemical modification during the heating process and avoiding condensation. Aerosols (stable suspensions of fine solid or liquid particles) and dusts (solid particles in air, but not necessarily in a stable suspension) are more difficult to generate. A variety of generators have been developed to nebulize or disperse the particles into the air. Once generated, aerosols and dusts are mixed to appropriate concentrations and introduced into the exposure chamber. Considerations involved in aerosol and dust generation include particle size, size distribution, and particle shape, as these parameters will primarily determine where in the respiratory tract the particles will be deposited and the rate at which they will be absorbed. As discussed earlier, rats are obligate nasal breathers. As a result of this characteristic and their smaller nasal passages, particulates above 1 μm are essentially excluded from rodent lungs.

Exposure of Test Animals

The three major chamber designs, whole body, nose-only, and head-only, are pictured in Figure 15. Design features common to these chambers include: they are made of nonreactive material and have provisions for easy access to and viewing of the animals; they are designed to ensure a uniform flow of test material to the animals; and they have a number of ports for monitoring test compound concentrations, and chamber temperature, humidity, and pressure. The advantages of head- and nose-only chambers are that they require much less compound, compound exposure is limited to the nose or to the head, and animals are more accessible for physiological measures. A major disadvantage is that animals must be restrained in tubes and, therefore, exposure limits must be limited to

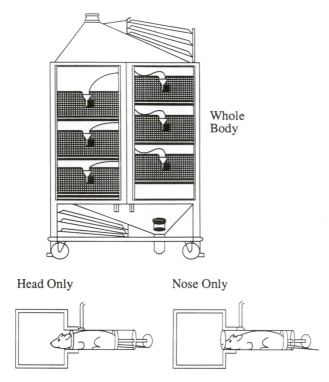

Whole
Body

Head Only   Nose Only

Figure 15 Major inhalation chamber designs including whole body, head-only, and nose-only exposure chambers.

minimize stress and possible overheating. Advantages of the whole body chambers are that loading and unloading are much less labor intensive than other designs and the animals are maintained in cages, allowing longer exposure times. A disadvantage of whole body chambers is that aerosols and dusts are deposited on the fur and may be eaten or absorbed dermally.

In the exposure process, animals are placed into the chambers and exposed for a predetermined amount of time to the test atmosphere. Generally, exposures in head- and nose-only chambers are limited to hours, whereas whole body exposures can be longer, even chronic or lifetime. Dosages in inhalation studies are generally stated on the basis of the period of time at a stated atmosphere concentration. Estimations of actual dosage received are complex and are based on the physiology and anatomy of the rat and upon several characteristics of the atmosphere (Gad and Chengelis, 1988; and Kennedy, 1989).

Measurement and Characterization of Test Atmosphere
An important part of the exposure process is documenting the atmosphere to which the animals were exposed. Measurements are made to determine characteristics, including the concentration of the atmosphere, homogeneity of distribution, and, in aerosol or dust studies, the size of particles generated. Samples should be drawn from a number of sites within the chamber to determine homogeneity. Gases and vapors can be analyzed using chromatography or spectrophotometry. Aerosols and dusts are collected and then measured using methods such as sedimentation, filtration, centrifugation, impaction, thermal or electrostatic precipitation, or by optics (Kennedy, 1989).

Intratracheal Administration

To avoid the expenses of maintaining an inhalation facility or in cases where test compound supply is limited, techniques have been developed to instill compound directly into the trachea. Instillation allows a more accurate and quantifiable method of lung exposure to test compounds. Murrow (1975) inserted a speculum into the trachea of anesthetized rats and instilled radionuclides with a syringe and needle to which a 5 cm piece of tubing was attached. He found that with a 2-ml injection volume radionuclide was distributed approximately evenly between the right and left lungs. The author found less variability in the amount of radionuclide in the lungs of rats after instillation than after inhalation. A nebulizer has been described for this technique (Sabaitis et al., 1989) that more closely approximates the behavior of an inhaled dose.

Miscellaneous Routes

While not widely used in toxicology, techniques have been developed to deliver test compounds to specific target vessels or organs. These include techniques for injection of test compounds into the vitreous chamber (Rose and Glow, 1965), uterine lumen (Chwalisz et al., 1983), vas deferens (Wadsworth and Ratnasooriya, 1981), portal vein (Gallo-Torres and Ludorf, 1974; Smadja et al., 1988), superior sagittal sinus (Lipton, 1972), renal artery (Beuzeville, 1968), and several sites in the central nervous system (Popick, 1976; Pass and Ondo, 1977; Sloane-Stanley and Chase, 1981; and Caulfield et al., 1983).

DATA COLLECTION TECHNIQUES

Observations and Physical Examinations

Rats are routinely monitored during toxicology studies as an assessment of their general health and to define the effects of the test article. In acute and subchronic studies, animals may be observed frequently in an effort to define short-term pharmacological changes induced by the test compound which may become apparent at peak blood levels. In chronic studies, these observations are critical in tracking tumor development and for determining animals in extremis which should be euthanized to minimize suffering, autolysis, and tissue loss. Arnold et al. (1977) contains a useful description of a clinical assessment program for chronic studies.

Daily observations are performed first thing in the morning and last thing before leaving in the afternoon to assess the health of the animals. In this observation, behavioral status, respiratory signs, skin, eyes, and excretory products are noted. Care should be taken to disturb the animal as little as possible, since this will be a source of stress. The animal should be picked up and examined more closely if abnormalities are detected. Special attention should be paid to the amount of feces present, since a decrease in fecal output may be the first sign of a watering system malfunction. In acute studies or where pharmacological effects are expected, animals may be examined continuously or at peak plasma levels.

A more thorough physical examination should be done weekly. Each animal is taken from its cage and placed on an examination table where respiration, behavior, general appearance, and locomotion are observed. The technician should then pick up the animal, examine its body orifices, skin, and coat, and perform a palpation of the trunk and limbs to check for tumors. The detection and tracking of the size and fate of masses (potential tumors) is essential for carcinogenicity studies.

Animals which have experienced severe weight loss over the previous week, a progressive decline in weight over several weeks, or other severe clinical signs should be marked for more frequent examination and possible euthanasia.

Body and feeder weights can be measured as part of the physical examination or as a separate function. Performance of these operations as a part of physical examinations will minimize animal handling and potential stress. If the operations are combined, it is important that the physical examination be done completely and not rushed.

Neurobehavioral Examination

Neurobehavioral examinations are included in toxicology studies to assess the behavioral and neurological effects of test chemicals. These examinations, which may be done as part of acute or repeated dose studies, typically involve screens consisting of a functional observational battery and some measure of locomotor activity. The Environmental Protection Agency (EPA) has written guidelines on the design and conduct of these studies (EPA, 1985). The screen is performed prior to the start of treatment, then periodically during the course of treatment. It may be performed as a separate study, on satellite groups of animals in conjunction with the main study, or on animals in the main portion of the toxicology study. Where initial screens indicate the possibility of a test compound–related change, more specialized series of tests are performed to assess the nature of the effect and the extent of central nervous system involvement. These secondary tests evaluate motor and sensory function as well as cognitive ability. Examples of secondary tests include sensory-evoked potential experiments and schedule-controlled behavior studies. Descriptions of these secondary tests can be found in Annau (1986).

Functional Observational Battery
The typical functional observation battery (FOB) includes observations of home-cage and open-field activity as well as measurements of reflexive, physiological, and neuromuscular function. Observations and measurements which have been suggested for an FOB (Haggerty, 1989; Moser, 1989) are in Table 15. The order of measurement should be

Table 15 Functional Observation Battery

Home cage and open field	Manipulative	Physiological and Neuromuscular
Posture	Ease of removal from cage	Body weight
Convulsions	Ease of handling rat	Body temperature
Biting	Lacrimation	Hindlimb extensor strength
Palpebral closure	Salivation	Grip strength
Time to first step	Piloerection	Rotarod performance
Number of rears	Fur appearance	Hindfoot splay
Number of defecations	Approach response	
Number of pools of urine	Touch response	
Mobility	Click response	
Gait	Tail pinch	
Convulsions	Pupil response	
Ataxic gait	Eye blink response	
Tremors	Forelimb extension	
Arousal	Hindlimb extension	
Stereotyped behavior	Righting reflex	
Bizarre behavior		

Source: From Haggerty (1989) and Moser (1989).

consistent, progressing from the least interactive to the most interactive measurements. Home-cage observations are made first. The animals are then transferred to the open field. During the transfer, certain physical observations such as how the animal responds to handling, the animal's appearance, and notations of any exudations are made. Animals are observed for 2 min in the open-field apparatus; during this period behavior and locomotor activity are observed. When the open-field period is completed, reflexive, physiological and neuromuscular measurements are performed.

Procedures used during the performance of an FOB must be standardized because some observations made have a subjective component. If at all possible, a single observer should be used throughout a single study. The EPA guidelines (EPA, 1985) recommend that observers be blind with respect to the animal's treatment group.

Locomotor Activity

Methods used for recording motor activity include direct observation and automated techniques such as photocell devices and mechanical measurements (Reiter and MacPhail, 1979; Macphail et al., 1989). In direct observations, the observer can make quantitative measurements of the frequency, duration, or sequencing of various motor components of behavior or qualitative records on the presence or absence of certain components of activity. Photocell devices record the number of times an animal interrupts a beam in specially designed chambers. In mechanical chambers, the animal's movements result in a vertical or horizontal displacement of the chamber; records are kept of the chamber's movements. The EPA guidelines (EPA, 1985) specify the use of automated techniques for recording locomotor activity.

To make activity determinations, an animal or group of animals is put into an observation or recording chamber and activity is recorded for a specific period of time. Since activity will normally decline over the course of the session, the length of the observation period is important. The EPA guidelines (EPA, 1985) specify that activity should approach asymptotic levels by the last 20% of the session. Haggerty (1989) uses a 15-min recording session, accumulating data over three 5-min test intervals. Since a large number of environmental conditions can affect motor activity, e.g., sound level, cage design, lighting, temperature and humidity, or odors, it is important to minimize variations in the test environment.

Cardiovascular Parameters

Examinations of the cardiovascular system may be scheduled routinely into toxicology studies or performed only when the cardiovascular system is a suspected target of the test compound. Measurement of cardiovascular system function as a routine part of toxicology studies is more common in Europe than in the United States. Examinations of the cardiovascular system function should be performed prior to the start of treatment to set baseline values and periodically during the course of the study.

Electrocardiography

Although the dog has traditionally been the species of choice in toxicology studies of effects on ECG, research with the rat has progressed and increased over the years. Detweiler (1981) provides an excellent review of the use of electrocardiography in toxicology studies with rat. This section will present a general discussion on the aspects of the recording methods and interpretation of the ECG in the rat. For a more complete discussion, the reader is referred to Budden et al. (1981b).

Recording Methods

Restraint: One of the disadvantages of studying ECGs in rats is that it is difficult to keep the animals still while recording. It is important that the animal remain in a constant position during the procedure to avoid muscular artifact in the ECG. Hundley et al. (1945) manually restrained rats in a supine position using rubber gloves to prevent short circuiting. The authors reported that rats become accustomed to the procedure and tracings were relatively free of muscular interference. Various forms of anesthesia have also been used, including pentobarbital (Lombard, 1952), light ether anesthesia (Sambhi and White, 1960), and urethane (Zbinden et al., 1980). Restraint devices developed to allow ECG recording without anesthesia have included cork boards to which the rats were pinned (Ensor, 1946), boards with clamps (Hill et al., 1960), and plastic tubes with slits on either side which allow electrodes to be positioned (Osborne, 1973; Zbinden et al., 1980).

No conclusion has been reached about the best method of restraint, though Osborne (1974) and Driscoll (1981) have discussed the issue. The basic concerns are that manual methods and physical restraint often require training periods before the animal becomes accustomed to the procedure and tracings can be reasonably free of muscular artifact. Also, varying pressures of clamps or hands during restraint may change the results. Opponents of anesthetic use argue that the use of anesthesia has been shown to produce changes in the ECG and there may be a possibility of synergism between the anesthetic and the compound being tested.

Position: The most common positions are the prone (on the stomach) position when animals are awake and the supine (on the back) position when animals are anesthetized. Beinfield and Lehr (1956) compared the positions and felt the prone position gave advantages in that several recordings were stabilized, the R wave was increased, and it avoided unfavorable cardiac rotation and an undesirable variation in the projection of the spacial QRS loop.

Robineau (1988) has developed an electrode system which can be implanted subcutaneously a few days before the recording is to take place. The device has a quick-disconnect plug which is exteriorized near the back of the head. The advantage of this system is that a cable can be connected to the plug and the ECG can be taken in unrestrained rats. While the signal quality is sufficient for the detection of arrhythmias, it still has room for improvement.

Leads: For the most part, investigators have used Einthoven's bipolar limb lead system, lead I (right and left foreleg), lead II (right foreleg and left hindleg), and lead III (left foreleg and left hindleg), with and without the augmented unipolar limb leads aVR (right foreleg), aVL (left foreleg), and aVF (one of the hindlegs). Since foreleg position can alter the scalar ECG wave amplitudes, investigators must standardize foreleg positions during recording.

Various types of electrodes have been used to connect the ECG wires. Hill et al. (1960) and Fraser et al. (1967) used hypodermic needles inserted under the skin in the appropriate limbs. Sambi and White (1960) used a small-gauge insulated copper wire which was wrapped around the shaved distal portion of the limbs. Currently, alligator clips are commonly used (Osborne, 1974).

ECG Waveform.   A diagrammatic example of a normal rat ECG is illustrated in Figure 16. The major points to notice about the rat ECG are that the conventional waves of the mammalian ECG (P, QRS, and T) are all identifiable in the rat ECG, there is no isoelectric line during the electrocardiographic complex, and there is no ST segment.

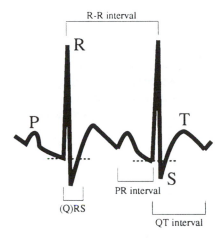

R-R interval

R

P T

S

(Q)RS

PR interval

QT interval

Figure 16 Diagrammatic representation of rat ECG waveform with intervals indicated. (From Driscoll [1981], used with permission.)

Normal time ranges for unanesthetized rats are: P, 10–20; PR, 35–50; QRS, 12–25; and QT, 38–80 (Detweiler, 1981). These intervals may be prolonged under deep anesthesia. Two good discussions about the analysis of waveforms are available: Spear (1981) discusses the relationships between the waveforms and the electrophysiology of the heart; and Detweiler (1981) discusses characteristic waveforms and their variation. Several efforts have been made to computerize the analysis process (Caprino et al., 1978; MacFarlane et al., 1981; Schumacher et al., 1981; and Watkinson et al., 1985).

Spontaneous Abnormalities. Various authors have addressed abnormalities and age-related changes in the rat ECG. Zbinden (1981) found that spontaneous arrhythmias were rather rare in his laboratory (1 in 200 recorded ECGs). Budden et al. (1981a) compared rats from 1 to 24 months of age. The study found an age-related decrease in heart rate and increases in PR and QT intervals and ECG abnormalities, including sinus arrhythmia, bradycardia, ectopic beats, and partial AV block in the 24-month-old animals. Detweiler et al. (1981) observed a high incidence of atrial and ventricular arrhythmias associated with an outbreak of sialodacryoadenitis (SDA) virus. The arrhythmias persisted long after physical evidence of the disease subsided and were associated with myocardial lesions. The author speculated that the SDA virus might produce myocarditis, causing arrhythmias.

Drug Effects on the Rat ECG. To establish background data on the effects of drugs on the rat ECG, Budden et al. (1981a) tested a wide variety of drugs affecting the central nervous system, autonomic nervous system, and cardiovascular system. Their conclusion was that the ECG changes observed were generally comparable to those seen in man. Detweiler (1981), in a review of the literature, came to a similar conclusion. The one known exception is the rat's resistence to the toxic effects of cardiac glycosides; the acute lethal dose of digitoxin for the rat is over 20 times that for the dog, cat, or rabbit (Detweiler, 1967). Although species differences in metabolism are known, the reason for this resistence appears to lie within the myocardium.

Heart Rate

Heart rates can be calculated from standard limb lead ECGs; the distance between two peaks of a prominent waveform (such as the R wave) is measured and this distance is divided by the paper speed. However, manipulating animals to obtain an ECG that is free of muscular artifact has an effect on the heart rate. Detweiler (1981), in a review of the literature, found that published heart rates for rats varied between 250 and 750 beats/min. Awake, restrained adult rats had heart rates from 330 to 600 beats/min; trained, quieted animals had heart rates from 250 to 350 beats/min; and in anesthetized animals heart rates were from 300 to 400 beats/min. The higher rates in restrained animals are probably due to the fact that the heart rate is increased more by emotional stimuli than by movement (Moses, 1946).

Where effects of restraint or anesthesia need to be avoided, the heart rate can be measured in relatively unrestrained animals using just two electrodes. Eisenstein and Woskow (1958) placed two metal suture electrodes on the back, about 2.5 cm from the doral midline, and just above the scapula. The sutures were connected to a monitor by wires that were suspended over the cage. Other investigators have placed the electrodes on the skull and sacral region (Eisman, 1965) or on either side of the rib cage (Barnard et al., 1974). Telemetry methods have been used to eliminate the connecting wires (Longo and Pellegrino, 1967; Burns et al., 1971; and Buttner and Wollnik, 1982). Vetterlein et al. (1984) designed a specialized cage with metal plates built into the floor in which the heart rate is recorded through the paws.

Blood Pressure

Indirect Measurement.   Indirect methods of blood pressure measurement detect systolic blood pressures by the occlusion of arterial inflow to the tail and subsequent detection of the pressure at which the first arterial pulsation occurs. The two places where indirect measurements have been made in the rat are the tail and hindpaw.

Tail Cuff Method: The tail cuff method monitors pressures in the ventral caudal artery. In this method, the animal is put into a suitable restrainer that allows the tail to be accessible and a tail cuff is put around the base of the tail (Fig. 17). Pressure in the cuff is increased until blood flow stops, then pressure is slowly released. The cuff pressure at the time when blood flow resumes is the systolic blood pressure. Various methods have been used to determine the point at which blood flow returns. These include plethysmography (Williams et al., 1939), ultrasonic doppler flowmeter (Rowberg et al., 1969), microphonic manometer (Friedman and Freed, 1949), photoelectric sensors (Ablondi et al., 1947; Hermansen, 1970), electrical impedance monitors (Wen et al., 1988), and visual observation (Alexander, 1957).

Because the caudal pulse is rather weak, several of the above methods require preheating of the animals in boxes at temperatures of 30–42°C for periods of up to 10 min

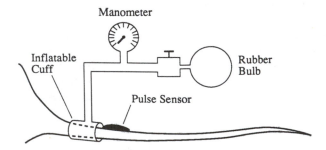

Figure 17   Indirect blood pressure measurement. (Adapted from Bivin et al. [1979]).

to dilate the caudal artery. As discussed earlier in this chapter, changes in body temperature can have widespread effects on the animal. With respect to blood pressures, preheating will increase the systolic blood pressure (Proskauer et al., 1945; Borg and Viberg, 1980). Kersten et al, (1947) and Ablondi et al. (1947) found that responses to the same heating conditions will vary with different rats and even in the same rat on different days. Sobin (1946) suggested the use of local rather than general warming and used a double coil of tubing wrapped around the plethysmograph chamber to heat (43°C) just the tail. The photoelectric sensor method does not require preheating, but becomes unreliable if the room temperature falls below 27°C. For this reason, preincubation of the animals at 27–30°C is recommended. The electrical impedance method is useful at ambient temperatures of 21–24°C and, therefore, is probably the most appropriate one for toxicology studies.

The placement and width of the tail cuff is important. There is a gradient in pressure along the caudal artery which amounts to 4.5 mmHg/cm. For this reason, the cuff should be placed close to the base of the tail and this placement should be standardized. Variation in the width of the rubber tubing can be a major source of error. Bunag (1973) found that the most accurate readings were given by 15-mm cuffs; shorter cuffs gave falsely elevated readings, whereas longer ones gave erroneously low readings.

Hindpaw Method: Measurement of blood pressure in the hindpaw does not measure the pressure in a specific vessel. In this method, the animal is placed in a restrainer, as in the tail cuff technique. A pressure cuff is placed around the ankle to occlude blood flow and blood pressure is measured as the cuff pressure is released and blood flow returns. As in the tail cuff method, several techniques have been used to determine the return of blood flow: visual observation (Griffith, 1934–1935), photoelectric cell (Kersten et al., 1947), and oximeter (Korol and McShane, 1963). The advantage of the photoelectric and oximeter methods is that they do not require preheating to dilate the vessels in the hindpaw. The oximeter technique measures mean arterial pressure rather than systolic pressure.

Direct Measurement.   The direct measurement techniques involve the cannulation of an artery with the blood pressure being determined with a manometer or transducer connected to the free end of the cannula. Surgery and cannula placement for the techniques are generally similar to those discussed previously for venous cannula placement. Where chronic use is desired, cannulas are usually run subcutaneously and exteriorized at the back of the head. The arteries which have generally been used are the carotid (Popovic and Popovic, 1960) or the abdominal aorta (Weeks and Jones, 1960). The carotid artery cannulas can be expected to remain patent for 24–30 days (Ross, 1977; Andrews, Jones and Simpson, 1978). Weeks and Jones (1960) reported that abdominal aorta cannulas could be used for up to 6 months. The femoral artery has been used in acute experiments (Ablondi et al., 1947; Kudo et al., 1981).

Blood Collection Techniques

Blood samples are routinely collected in safety studies to determine (1) direct test article effects on the blood or bone marrow, (2) effect on other organs as indicated by the contents of the blood, for instance, leakage enzymes like aspartate aminotransferase, and (3) blood levels of the test compound or its metabolites. A variety of techniques have been described for blood collection in the rat. Choice of a specific technique will depend upon factors such as (1) the volume to be collected, (2) whether the animal is to survive the procedure, (3) the frequency with which samples will need to be collected, (4) whether anesthetics can be used, (5) impact on the study if the animal does not survive the procedure, and (6) impact of organ damage resulting from the procedure. The rat has a blood volume of about 50 ml/kg; approximately 10% of the total blood volume can be collected from a rat without endangering its survival and physiological stability.

Technique and anesthetic used for blood drawing should be standardized throughout a study if repeated samples are being taken. Several studies have shown that the technique, anesthetic, or stress involved with the technique may have an effect on the blood parameters to be examined (Table 16). Activities or conditions occurring prior to the blood collection may also have an effect. Overnight fasting and subsequent decreases in water consumption have been shown to cause changes in hematology values (Apostolou et al., 1976). Glucose residues from diabetic urine on the tail of rats resulted in erroneous blood sugar values in blood collected from tail veins (Schreiber and Schmidt, 1979). Consideration should be given to the effect of blood sampling on the animal's response to the test compound; repeated handling, anesthesia, and blood sampling can create sufficient stress to alter the binding characteristics of a highly bound drug (Hulse et al., 1981).

Retroorbital Plexus

The retro-orbital plexus is a convenient site for periodic sampling during the course of a study. Sorg and Buckner (1964) reported that exsanguination of a 115- to 130-g rat will yield 4–6 ml of blood, and in large rats more than 8 ml can be obtained without sacrifice. Collection can be done with or without anesthesia; however, light anesthesia will minimize struggling. Since the plexus cannot be visualized, some degree of expertise is necessary to perform this technique well.

Blood is collected with a microcapillary tube (Riley, 1960; Sorg and Buckner, 1964), the fine end of a Pasteur pipet, or with polyethylene tubing (Cate, 1969). To collect blood, the animal is held immobile on its side against a table top by a firm grip (Fig. 18). The head should be pressed down with the thumb and forefinger. The pipet or tubing is then inserted into the orbit of the eye at the anterior angle formed by the lids and the nictitating membrane (Fig. 19). A short thrust past the eyeball will make the tube enter the slightly resistent horny membrane of the sinus. It may help to slightly rotate the tube as it is

Table 16 Factors in Blood Collection Techniques Which May Influence Results

Factor	References
Site or method of collection	Doell and Hegarty (1970), Upton and Morgan (1975), Dohler et al. (1977, 1978), Neptun et al. (1985), Suber and Kodell (1985), Smith et al. (1986)
Stress of handling or sampling conditions	Neill (1970), Besch and Chou (1971), Carney and Walker (1973), Brown and Martin (1974), Bellinger and Mendel (1975), Hulse et al. (1981), Boehm et al. (1982), Iversen and Andersen (1983), Sadjak et al. (1983), Conahan et al. (1985)
Choice of anesthesia	McAllister (1938), Wuttke and Meites (1970), Chi and Shin (1978), Meltzer et al. (1978), Fowler et al. (1980).

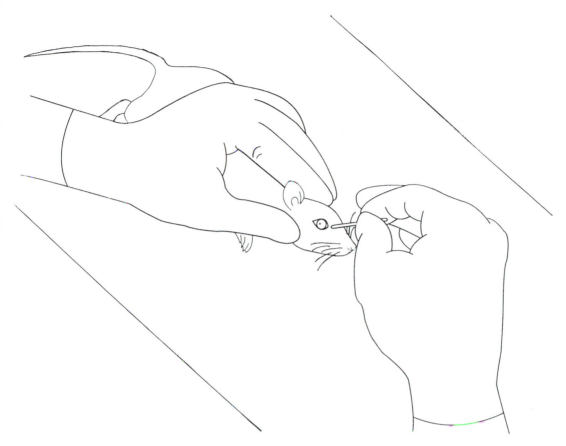

Figure 18 Retro-orbital venous plexus blood collection.

advanced. As soon as the sinus is punctured, blood enters the tubing by its own pressure. If flow stops, pull our the tube slightly and flow will restart.

In the hands of an experienced technician, there is minimal risk to the animal. Puncture of the bone behind the eye, epistaxsis, loss of an eye, or death are possible complications. McGee and Maronpot (1979) reported localized necrotizing inflammation of the Harderian gland as a sequela to retro-orbital blood collection.

Tail

A tail vein bleed offers a visible target and is of minimal risk to the animal. Blood will flow faster if the tail has been dipped in warm (40–45°C) water or warmed with a lamp. If anesthesia is used, select one that does not alter blood pressure; pentobartibal, chloralose, and urethane have all been found unacceptable. Minasian (1980) describes a tourniquet made from a syringe to aid in venipuncture.

Tail Clip.   The animal should be lightly anesthetized. To collect blood, 2–3 mm of the distal part of the tail should be amputated with sharp scissors. Three to 4 ml of blood can be collected in 20–30 sec from 200- to 250-g rats (Enta et al., 1968). When finished, the cut surface can be cauterized with a hot spatula or glass rod. Wright (1970) found collection faster and with less hemolysis when a Unopette Macro Sampler was used.

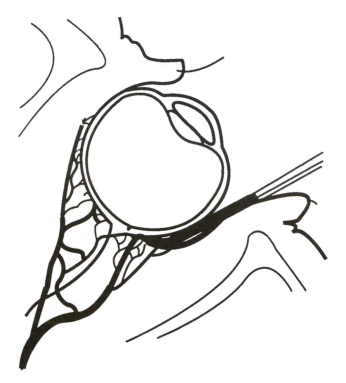

Figure 19 Diagrammatic indication of venous plexus location and pipette insertion. (Redrawn from Riley [1960].)

Several devices have been described to aid the collection of blood by the use of vacuum (Sandiford, 1965; Stuhlman et al., 1972; Levine et al., 1973; Nerenberg and Zedler, 1975).

Vein Incision.   Animals should be restrained in a holder that allows complete access to the tail. The transitional area between the body and the tail should be shaved then the lateral vein dilated near the base of the tail using a tourniquet. The vein should be punctured with a 21-gauge needle then the needle should be immediately withdrawn. Blood will run freely from the site of the puncture into a collecting tube. Pressure can be applied with a finger to stop bleeding. Two to 4 ml of blood can be collected (Videm, 1980).

Puncture of the Artery.   With the use of an appropriate restrainer, this technique can be done without anesthesia (Omaye et al., 1987). A 21-gauge needle should be inserted into the artery in the midventral surface of the tail, close to the tip. As a result of arterial pressure, the blood will flow immediately. Several needle assemblies have been reported. Hurwitz (1971) used a Caraway-type microblood collecting tube inserted into the clear hub of a 21-gauge needle. Furuhama and Onodera (1983) used a 22-gauge needle with the hub cut off. Omaye et al. (1987) found a needle with a clear polyethylene hub was useful to let the operator observe the blood flow into the collection tube. The authors found that blood clotting was frequent unless the needle was heparinized.

Cardiac Puncture

The technique of cardiac punctures offers a rapid way to remove a large amount of blood from the rat; Burhoe (1940) found that although it was possible to remove 5 ml of blood in 20 sec, it usually took 40–60 sec to remove that quantity. It is possible to exsanguinate the animal with this technique. Because repeated puncture of the myocardium can lead to damage, hemorrhage, and death, this technique is of high risk to the animal and may not be appropriate for interim bleeds.

To collect blood, the animal should be anesthetized and placed it on its back. The heart can be located by placing the index finger over the 4th and 5th left ribs with the thumb on the right side of the thorax. The area over the heart should then be shaved and an appropriate antiseptic applied. The collection needle (25–26 gauge, 1–2 cm long; a large-gauge needle can be used if the animal will not be retained) should be inserted at a 45-degree angle into the heart. Once the needle is introduced, the plunger of the syringe should be drawn back slightly to produce a slight vacuum then the needle can be slowly advanced until blood is obtained. Falabella (1967) attached polyethylene tubing directly to a needle without a hub and eliminated the need for a syringe.

Abdominal Aorta and Vena Cava

Collection from the abdominal aorta offers a convenient way to exsanguinate an animal and obtain a maximal amount of blood. To perform the procedure, the animal should be anesthetized and the aorta exposed by dissection (Lushbough and Moline, 1961). A 2- to 3-cm length of aorta just ventral to the diaphram should be exposed and clamped off with hemostats. The aorta should then be severed approximately 0.5 cm below the point of clamping and the open end of the aorta placed into a collection tube. If the hemostat pressure is carefully released, blood will run into the collection tube. An alternate technique, rather than clamping and severing the aorta, is to use a butterfly needle attached to a piece of tubing. The free end of the tubing should be placed into a collection tube and the needle inserted directly into the vein.

Winsett et al. (1985) describe a method of repeated sampling from the vena cava of conscious rats. An assistant holds the animal while the operator grasps the rat with the left hand so that the thumb and index finger are just beneath the last rib. The needle (25 gauge) is inserted 1 cm to the right of the spinous process of the first lumbar vertebra at an angle of 45 degrees until contact is felt. At that point, the needle is partially withdrawn and reinserted at a slightly more acute angle to miss the bone and enter the vena cava (Fig. 20). The manuver of first identifying the bone is essential to the procedure. The authors of this reference have performed 350 venipunctures and have had three deaths.

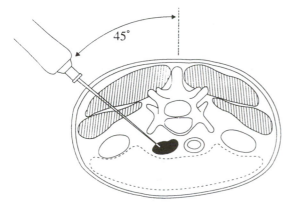

Figure 20 Blood collection from the vena cava. Coronal plane at level of first lumbar vertebrae. (Redrawn from Winsett et al. [1985].)

Jugular Vein

The jugular vein provides a means of chronic blood sampling that is of relatively low risk to the animal's health. Although the technique described is invasive, the venipuncture can be achieved through the skin if necessary.

To perform the collection (Mouzas and Weiss, 1960; Renaud, 1969), the head and front limbs of an anesthetized animal should be secured to an operating board. The area over the vein should be shaved and an antiseptic applied. One jugular vein should be exposed by incision of the skin and rapid dissection of the subcutaneous tissue. A needle (20 gauge, 2.5 cm) can be inserted bevel up into the vein by passing it through the pectoral muscle and directing it toward the animal's head. Inserting the needle through the muscle will minimize bleeding and stabilize the needle in the vein. Blood should flow freely with a minimum of aspiration. Once the collection is complete, the incision can be closed with a wound clip. Ten to 20 animals can be bled per hour. Archer and Riley (1981) suggested the use of a 23-gauge needle bent at an angle of 135 degrees to keep the attached syringe away from the thoracic cavity.

Proximal Saphenous and Metatarsal Veins

A small amount of blood can be collected from animals at minimal risk to their health utilizing the proximal saphenous and metatarsal veins. No anesthesia is required.

Proximal Saphenous Vein.   The inner aspect of the thigh of the hind limb should be shaved. While an assistant holds the rat and compresses the inguinal area to dilate the vein, a longitudinal nick should be made in the vein with a 20-gauge needle or a hematocrit lancet. Blood can be collected into heparinized capillary tubes. Rusher and Birch (1975) found that they could collect 0.1–0.2 ml of blood in approximately 45 sec using this method.

Metatarsal Vein.   This procedure can be done with or without an assistant. The animal is restrained and a nick is made in the vessel with a needle. Blood (0.1–0.2 ml) is collected with a capillary tube or through a needle into a syringe (Nobunaga et al., 1966).

Sublingual Vein

When using the sublingual vein for blood sampling, the animal should be cradled in the palm of the hand. By holding the animal's head between the thumb and index fingers, the head can be stretched back and the skin of the face pulled backward. This will force the mouth open and the tongue against the palate. The right or left vein should be cut with iris scissors and the animal held such that blood drips into the collection tube. Bleeding is stopped with a gauze pad held against the vein. Angelov et al. (1984) found that bleeding animals in this way did not affect their weight gain or food consumption, and that hematology and serum chemistry values from blood collected in this manner were comparable to those derived from retro-orbital plexus blood.

Decapitation

Decapitation should be performed only by trained technicians with the appropriate equipment. An easily fabricated decapitation device is described by Bush and Bush (1971). Immediately after decapitation, mixed venous and arterial blood is collected by suspending the carcass over a funnel placed into a collecting tube.

Cannulation

While the blood collection methods described above will give sufficient volumes and quality of sample for the majority of toxicology studies, specific protocols may require blood sampled from animals which have been subjected to a minimum of handling. Cannulation is one method researchers have tried to meet this requirement. A variety of veins and arteries have been cannulated for the purpose of blood collection. Yoburn et al. (1984) compared jugular, carotid, and femoral cannulas for long-term sampling of blood. They found the femoral artery cannula preferable in terms of patency and postsurgical weight loss. Giner et al. (1987) expressed the opinion that none of the current methods are totally reliable. Although some investigators have used blood from cannulated rats as an indicator of normal values in unstressed animals (Milakofsky et al., 1984), it should be remembered that the values derived may have been altered by the stress of cannulation itself (Laasko et al., 1984).

Jugular Vein. The cannulation procedure is the same as that described for infusion techniques. The cannulas are patent for variable periods of time: Upton (1975) found that cannulas with tips trimmed to an arrowhead then cut with a transverse cut would allow blood sampling for 5 weeks or longer; Tsukamoto et al. (1984) in a study with 18 rats found 94% patent after 6 weeks and 75% after 11 weeks. Various methods of anchoring the cannula to the rat's back or head have been developed for ease of sampling or as a connection point for continuous infusion apparatus (Steffens, 1969; Brown and Breckenridge, 1975; Carruba et al., 1981).

Inferior Vena Cava. The inferior vena cava appears to provide a site for long-lived cannulas. Kaufman (1980) placed a Silastic cannula in the inferior vena cava in the area of the renal vein and advanced it to the area of the xiphisternum. The cannula was held in place by the elasticity of the musculature of the vena cava and ligatures placed around the right psoas muscle and exteriorized at a point between the ears. The cannula remained patent for months. Koeslag et al. (1984) used a similar technique; 100% of the cannulas implanted were functional after 30 days and 59% were functional after 120 days. Hall et al. (1984) exteriorized a cannula at the caudalmost part of the scrotum. When the cannula was not used for blood sampling, it was stored in a pouch made in the scrotum. The authors of this reference found this technique acceptable for experiments of several days' duration.

Abdominal Aorta. Still and Whitcomb (1956) described a technique in which a polyethylene cannula is implanted in the aorta, 2.5–3.0 cm above the bifurcation. The free end of the cannula is brought subcutaneously to the dorsal base of the neck. The cannula was used for blood sampling up to 2 weeks. A problem with aneurysms was traced to the clamps used to occlude the aorta during cannula placement. When softer clamps and older animals were used, the problem was minimized.

Subcutaneous Ports. Exteriorized cannulas are sources of contamination and are subject to destruction if several animals are housed together. To avoid exteriorizing the cannulas, Bodziony and Schwille (1985), Aguiar et al. (1987), and Paulose and Dakshinamurti (1987) have connected venous cannulas to subcutaneously placed silicone ports (Fig. 21). Paulose and Dakshinamurti (1987) compared plasma catacholamine levels of blood collected from the port with those obtained from blood collected from decapitation and found there was minimal stress when blood was collected from the port.

Urine Collection

Urine is generally collected in toxicology studies to assess kidney function. While several varieties of metabolism cages have been described in the literature (Howells et al., Harrison, 1964; Cruickshanks and Wood, 1970; Hansen and Holm, 1971; Blass, 1972;

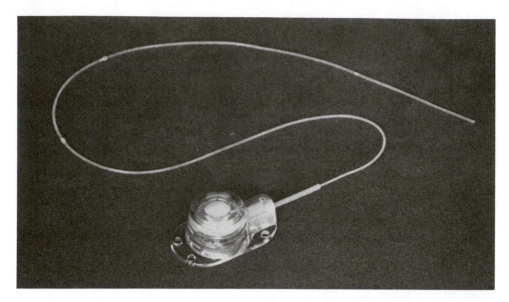

Figure 21   Venous port for infusions and blood collection (Access Technologies, Skokie, Illinois).

Black and Claxton, 1979; and Tomkins and O'Donovan, 1986), the most common method of collection is a stainless steel, commercially available unit (Fig. 22). In this unit, urine and feces are separated by a cone-shaped device; urine drains off the collecting walls into a tube and the feces fall into an inverted cone. Food and water are made available in such a way that the urine will not be contaminated. While this unit produces urine of acceptable quality for the normal urinalysis, some hair and fecal contamination of the urine can occur. Descriptions of collection methods using capillary tubes (Hayashi and Sakaguchi, 1975), catheters (White, 1971), beakers (Khosho et al., 1985), or anal cups (Frape et al., 1970; Ryer and Walker, 1971) have been described to solve this problem.

Necropsy

The necropsy is the link between antemortem findings and histological observations. It is an essential portion of the toxicology study and, since a necropsy will involve the processing of a large number of animals, it is important that the procedure be well planned (Black, 1986). At a prenecropsy meeting involving the pathologist, prosectors, and the study director, necropsy responsibilities can be discussed. Additionally, the study director can summarize clinical observations and discuss potential target organs. Prosectors should be familiarized with the protocol and amendments for the study involving the animals being necropsied. During the necropsy, devices such as check lists or prelabeled compartmentalized trays should be present to ensure that all required organs are taken and weighed. Copies of the last clinical observations should be present at the necropsy so the prosecters are alerted to lesions which might require special attention. Palpation records are particularly important at carcinogenicity study necropsies to ensure that all masses detected at the last examination are confirmed and collected.

The necropsy itself will involve a check of animal identification and sex, an external

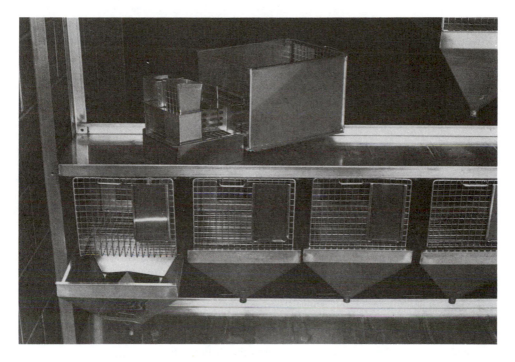

Figure 22 Rack of stainless steel metabolism cages.

examination of the animal, an in situ examination of all tissues and organs (prior to dissection), and the collection and weighing of the required tissues. A step-by-step guide to the necropsy process is outside of the scope of this chapter; the reader is referred to Feldman and Seely (1988).

SUMMARY

In summary, there are several advantages to the use of the rat in toxicology studies. Because of its widespread use in many fields of biology, there is a large base of information about the anatomy and needs of the species. This knowledge, along with information about the species' metabolism and response to toxicants, has shown the rat, to be generally a good model for the prediction of the human's response to toxicants. Rats have a lifespan of 24–30 months, which is convenient for chronic toxicity and carcinogenicity studies where animals need to be exposed for the majority of their lifetime. The short gestation time and large litter size make the rat a good model for reproduction studies. The development of specific pathogen–free rats and improved husbandry have eliminated most of the disease outbreaks that may have introduced variability into studies. The lack of an emetic response allows the testing of higher dosages of compounds that might cause vomiting in other species. The small size of the rat is useful in that large numbers can be housed relatively economically. The size is also useful where test compounds are in short supply or are expensive.

The relatively small size of the rat is also one of its major disadvantages. The amount of blood that can be taken from the animal limits the number of parameters that can be investigated in any one animal, especially when the animals are young. This problem can be overcome by adding additional animals in interim sacrifice groups or satellite groups. However, increased numbers of animals mean increased work in the conduct of the study. The small size and relatively active nature of the rat makes some procedures, such as intravenous dosing or taking electrocardiograms, more difficult. These have been overcome with the use of suitable restrainers or, in some cases, anesthesia.

Pathology   **Shayne Cox Gad**

There is an enormous amount of literature available on the pathology of the laboratory rat. It is not the intention of this section to reproduce that literature here. Rather, the desire is to provide an overview of those elements which most commonly influence the design, conduct, and interpretation of toxicity studies and then to give access to the relevant literature for those who need more information or detail.

Before the initiation of any study there are three inputs from the laboratory animal professional and pathologist which are essential to the success of the study. First, the source of test animals must be carefully selected and all individual shipments carefully screened to ensure that only healthy rats with the desired characteristics (e.g., age, sex, strain) are used. This screening process should include a period of acclimation/health surveillance after the rats have been received to the facility (though 2 weeks is generally desirable, 7 days is adequate).

Second, the objective of the study and the degree of variability in the pathology of the animals must be considered in the design of the study, as should any factors such as the known time course of a response. Sufficient animals need to be used so that an effect may reasonably be detected (if present) as an increase above the existing background levels of morphological variation. In other words, the study design must be adequate to allow development of a pathological response and yet also include "sampling" (collection of blood and tissues) at appropriate time points so that the effects of age or other confounding processes do not obscure results.

Finally, the necropsy must be designed to be both efficient and effective, and the involved personnel must have adequate training and experience with the type of animals being utilized.

NECROPSY

Except for dose-ranging studies, unexpected mortalities in rodent toxicity studies should be limited to rare accidental deaths associated with procedures (dosing mistakes in intubation studies, for example) and deaths due to unexpected toxicity. Otherwise animals should live to the time of scheduled termination, providing for optimal tissue collection and fixation and proper correlation of clinical signs and pathology. Because moribund or dead animals frequently have treatment-induced or important spontaneous lesions, they must receive complete necropsies. Rats should be observed a minimum of twice daily to identify moribund individuals. If there is a significant chance that death may occur before the next observation, the animal should be sacrificed. Little is gained by attempting to have the animal live a few days longer, considering the risk of loss of data due to premature death and autolysis.

Dead animals should be refrigerated immediately on discovery and necropsied as soon as possible thereafter. Refrigeration will significantly delay autolysis (for up to 8 hr [Kupp and Strolle, 1977]). Dead animals should not be frozen, as ice crystals created during the freezing and thawing process will damage or destroy cellular integrity and severely limit or impair any interpretation of histopathology. For scheduled necropsies, animals should generally be fasted overnight to provide for the natural emptying of the gastrointestinal tract and for a standard physiological baseline for evaluation of clinical pathology parameters.

Clinical observation records of the animal should be available at the time of necropsy, enabling the prosector to focus on target sites of disease and decreasing the chance of missing important lesions. The necropsy technique may have to be modified to suit the clinical signs. For example, the standard necropsy calls for collecting a piece of lumbar spinal cord. If paralysis or paresis was noted clinically, the entire spinal cord and possibly the brachial or lumbar plexuses would need to be examined.

A standard necropsy procedure should be followed. After reviewing the clinical records, one should palpate the animal thoroughly and examine all external orifices, eyes, and skin. Essentially, a physical examination is performed before the necropsy. The actual necropsy should follow a standardized format. This provides increased efficiency, optimal tissue accountability, and improved fixation. A thorough necropsy is probably the first essential step to assure eventual quality in pathology. General methods for rat necropsies and guides to gross anatomy have been published (NCI, 1976; Reuber, 1977; Bohensky, 1986; Chiasson, 1988; and Feldman and Seely, 1988).

Table 17 provides a list of the tissues which whould be collected from a rat at necropsy, along with an indication of which should normally be weighed to provide an indication of potential morphological indications of treatment related effects.

Table 17 Tissues Collected and Weighed at Necropsy

Skin	Liver[a]
Mammary gland	Pancreas
Lymph node(s)	Spleen[a]
Salivary gland	Kidneys[a]
Sternum/costochondral junction	Adrenal gland[a]
Femur (including bone barrow)	Urinary bladder
Muscle (PSOAS)	Seminal vesicle
Thymus[a]	Prostate[a]
Trachea	Testes[a]
Lung[a]	Ovary[a]
Heart[a]	Uterus[a]
Thyroid gland (with parathyroid)[a]	Vagina
Tongue	Brain[a]
Esophagus	Pituitary gland[a]
Stomach	Spinal cord
Duodenum	Eyes
Jejunum	Lacrimal gland
Ileum	Any additional tissues or organs with "abnormal findings"
Colon	or deemed appropriate

[a]Tissues to be weighed at necropsy.

Organ weights can be extremely useful if accurately determined and when considered in the proper context. They can help to identify subcellular changes (such as enzyme induction in the liver), target organs (though they are more useful for some organs than others—see Gad et al., 1985), and they can assist in identifying hormonal influences in some target organs. The downside is that improper tissue handling by the prosector can lead to artifactual tissue damage and organ weights may not correlate with other findings (in which case a weight of evidence and nature of the data warrant consideration).

If tissues, lesions, or observations are missed at necropsy, they will never be recovered.

Accurate observations must be recorded and descriptions should include the location, size, color, and consistency of the lesion. Whenever possible, lesions should be collected and fixed with some adjacent normal tissue. Facilities for gross photography should be available to document significant study findings. Not all gross lesions must be photographed: however, representative toxic lesions should be recorded on film.

Routine tissues should be fixed in approximately 10 volumes of neutral buffered formalin. Excellent fixation of lungs can be obtained by inserting a 14- to 18-gauge blunt needle into the lower trachea and inflating the lungs to their original size with formalin. The stomach should be opened and examined carefully for ulcers, erosions, etc. The small intestine of rodents can be opened and examined or flushed with formalin and examined by transillumination. If the latter is done, the gut should be opened and examined at the time of tissue trimming. The bladder should also be inflated with formalin and examined by transillumination, followed by an open examination when trimmed for embedding. The pituitary is one tissue most often lost in rodent necropsies. This can be minimized by leaving the organ attached to the basisphenoid bone. The bone and attached pituitary can be placed in a special tissue capsule until embedding. After removal of the eyes, brain, pituitary, tongue, and mandible, the nasal turbinates can be fixed by flushing from the nasopharynx to the nares with formalin followed by immersion in formalin. Tissue sections should have a maximum thickness of 0.5 cm for good fixation, and should be fixed for a minimum of 48 hr before trimming and processing.

CLINICAL PATHOLOGY

Clinical pathology comprises both hematology and clinical chemistry. These are extremely powerful tools for both assessing specific target organ toxicities during the in-life phase and providing correlative information for understanding both disease processes and the relevance of anatomical findings.

Laboratory determination of various clinical chemistry parameters in the rat is not particularly difficult, especially with the recent development of many automated analyzers. Most of these instruments require from 1.5 to 50.0 μl of serum or plasma and are preprogrammed to perform up to 20 different clinical chemical tests. The primary challenge of the clinical pathology laboratory is to validate equipment or procedures designed for use with human serum, or blood, and modify these into reliable methodology for the evaluation of organ function and toxicity in rats.

Toxicologists must be aware of a seemingly infinite number of variables which impact upon the interpretation of clinical pathology. Controllable sources of variation can be divided into at least three general categories: (1) variation related to the physiological status of the animal and its environmental condition, (2) variation related to sampling, and (3) variation related to analytical instrumentation and methodology.

Several authors have addressed the effect of these factors on many of the common clinical chemistry procedures. Variations related to the physiological status of the rat and its environment include disease status (Deb and Hart, 1956; Cotchin and Roe, 1967), age (Kozma et al., 1969; Vondruska and Greco, 1973; and Weisse et al. 1974), sex (Kozma, 1967; Weisse et al., 1974), husbandry, nutritional condition, and degree of hydration. Variations related to sampling collection include method of collection, anesthetic used, the time of day the sample is collected, restraint technique, anticoagulant used, hemolysis, sample processing and storage, and site of sampling. Blood sampling techniques are described and discussed elsewhere in this chapter.

In the rat as in other species, prompt separation of serum from cells is critical. Hemolyzed or transparent serum that has remained in contact with erythrocytes can have falsely elevated values for potassium, lactic dehydrogenase, and total protein, less consistently and to a lesser degree for phosphorus, and sometimes for bilirubin. Prolonged contact of serum with erythrocytes reduces serum glucose. Centrifugation and prompt removal of the serum from the clot should occur at intervals not exceeding 30 min after collection in order to yield reliable data.

Tables 18 and 19 summarize literature values for clinical chemistries and hematological values of common laboratory rats. One notable variation in hematologies for different strains of rats is the life span of red blood cells (Derelanko, 1987), which suggests that other functional aspects of the hematological system may vary between strains to the point that they can influence interpretation. All such tabular summaries of normal or control values (such as Mitruka and Rawnsley, 1977; Leonard and Ruben, 1986; and Loeb and Quimby, 1989), however, should be considered critically and used only as general guidance.

COMMON DISEASES

Common diseases which occur in modern caesarian-derived (CD), specific pathogen–free (SPF) rats used in toxicology laboratories can be viral, bacterial, parasitic, or rickettsial. Outbreaks of infectious disease are becoming less common in well-managed laboratory animal facilities but sporadic outbreaks and subclinical infections do occur. It behooves the laboratory animal professional to maintain high operating standards to minimize the impact of infectious diseases in toxicity studies. Infectious diseases can produce lesions and functional defects which may be difficult to distinguish from those of target organ toxicity. Infectious agents may produce lesions at the site of entry equivalent to local toxicity, and lesions equivalent to systemic toxicity. Either local or systemic effects can predominate, or the disease may be expressed as a combination of both. Infectious skin diseases are uncommon in most laboratory animals, and the two most frequently affected portals of entry are the respiratory and digestive tracts. In rats, infections of the respiratory tract are more frequent.

Viral Pneumonitis

Viral pneumonitis is a subclinical respiratory infection producing a lung lesion that is a focal alveolitis, which may be observed in any phase of the inflammatory process from acute to chronic and is accompanied by prominent perivascular leukocyte foci, usually lymphoid, with occasional eosinophils. The alveolitis is generally of little clinical significance, but its presence can seriously confound the interpretation of inhalation toxicity

Table 18 Clinical Chemistry Values

	Male		Female		
	Mean	SD	Mean	SD	Range
Bilirubin (mg/dl)	0.35	0.02	0.24	0.07	0.00–0.55
Cholesterol (mg/dl)	28.3	10.2	24.7	9.62	10–54
Creatinine (mg/dl)	0.46	0.13	0.49	0.12	0.20–0.80
Glucose (mg/dl)	78.0	14	71	16	50–135
Urea nitrogen (mg/dl)	15.5	4.44	13.8	4.15	5–29
Uric acid (mg/dl)	1.99	0.25	1.79	0.24	1.20–7.5
Sodium (mEq/I)	147	2.65	146	2.50	143–156
Potassium (mEq/I)	5.82	0.11	6.70	0.12	5.40–7
Chloride (mEq/I)	102	0.85	101	0.90	100–110
Bicarbonate (mEq/I)	24	3.80	20.8	3.60	12.6–32
Phosphorous (mg/dl)	7.56	1.51	8.26	1.14	3.11–11
Calcium (mg/dl)	12.2	0.75	10.6	0.89	7.2–13.9
Magnesium (mg/dl)	3.12	0.41	2.60	0.21	16–4.44
Amylase (Somogyi units/dl)	245	32	196	34	128–313
Alkaline phosphatase (IU/I)	81.4	14.8	93.9	17.3	56.8–128
Acid phosphatase (IU/I)	39	4.30	37.5	3.70	28.9–47.6
Alanine transaminase(SGPT) (IU/I)	25.2	2.05	22.5	2.50	17.5–30.2
Aspartate transaminase (SGOT) (IU/I)	62.5	8.40	64.0	6.50	45.7–80.8
Creatine phosphokinase (CPK) (IU/I)	5.60	1.30	6.80	2.40	0.80–11.6
Lactic dehydrogenase (LDH) (IU/I)	92.5	13.9	90	14.5	61.0–121
Serum total protein (g/dl)	7.61	0.50	7.52	0.32	4.70–8.15
Albumin (g/dl)	3.73	0.53	3.62	0.52	2.70–5.10
(%)	49	7.10	48.1	7.40	33.3–63.8
α_1-Globulin (g/dl)	1.03	0.22	0.89	0.25	0.39–1.60
(%)	13.5	2.20	11.9	3.80	4.30–21.1
α_2-Globulin (g/dl)	0.71	0.14	1.40	0.32	0.20–2.10
(%)	9.3	1.80	8.60	2.70	3.20–14.7
β-Globulin (g/dl)	1.07	0.35	1.31	0.26	0.35–2.00
(%)	14.1	4.70	17.4	3.60	5.70–26.8
γ-Globulin (g/dl)	1.05	0.21	1.18	0.21	0.62–1.60
(%)	13.8	2.70	14	2.80	10–19.8
Albumin/globulin	0.96	0.24	0.93	0.25	0.72–1.21

studies, particularly of some of the low-grade focal dust-induced lesions. Hyperplasia of the mandibular lymph node is also common in infected rats, and probably represents an immune reaction to viral infection. The causal organism may be the pneumonia virus of mice (PVM).

Sialodacryoadenitis

Sialodacryoadenitis (SDA) is a frequent epizootic disease in rat colonies with a high morbidity and negligible mortality. It was first recognized in rats in 1961 (Innes and Stanton, 1961). Sialodacryoadenitis is a generic term for infection with several serotypes of a coronavirus. These serotypes have a spectrum of virulence, primarily infecting the upper respiratory tract with variable infection of the glands around the head and neck.

Table 19 Hematology Values of Common Rat Strains

Test	Unit	Long-Evans (Blu:(LE)	Wistar/Lewis Albino	Osborne-Mendel	Fischer inbred strain 344/Cr
Erythrocytes (RBC)	($\times 10^6$/mm^3)	5.98–8.30	7.20–9.60	36.26–8.96	6.68–9.15
Hemoglobin	(g/dl)	13.1–16.7	12–17.5	14.30–17.7	13.4–17.2
MCV	(v^3)	52–69	57–65	52–66	54–67.5
MCH	(vvg)	18.5–23.5	14.6–21.3	18.8–23.3	17–21.8
MCHC	(%)	32–38.5	26–38	32–42	26–35.5
Hematocrit (PCV)	(ml%)	39–48	42.5–49.4	39.4–46.2	46–52.5
Leukocyte (WBC)	($\times 10^3$/mm^3)	3.30–7.90	5–8.96	6.23–12.6	5.35–11.2
neutrophils	(%)	5.50–35.5	9–34	4.50–23.5	11.5–41.6
basophils	(%)	0	0–1.50	0	0
lymphocytes	(%)	60–93.5	65–84.5	72–94	43–79.5
monocytes	(%)	0–5.50	0–5	0.50–3.50	0–2
eosinophils	(%)	0–1.50	0–2.50	0–1	0–4
Platelets	($\times 10^3$/mm^3)	140–460	160–470	145–450	150–450

Respiratory tract lesions include rhinitis and focal interstitial pneumonitis, but this is generally subclinical. In contrast, infection of the glands often produces striking clinical symptoms. The most striking clinical features are red staining around the eyes due to infection of the Harderian gland, and swelling of the ventral neck region associated with infection of the submaxillary salivary gland. The swollen neck ("rat mumps") rapidly subsides and the rats appear normal within about a week. Thus, SDA is a disease dominated by acute local effects.

The main finding at necropsy, depending on the stage of the disease, is either a swollen or shrunken salivary gland. Histologically, the gland progressively shows various combinations of degeneration, inflammation, and regeneration, but it is quickly restored to normal. The Harderian gland shows a similar cycle of disease, but squamous metaplasia is very prominent in the proliferative repair phase. In some animals, there are ophthalmic lesions, including reddish discharge, cloudy cornea, and corneal ulceration. Microscopically, the changes in the harderian and submaxillary salivary glands can be dramatic: there is necrosis, intense inflammation, and often marked squamous metaplasia of the ductal epithelium.

Lesions in the eye associated with SDA consist of keratoconjunctivitis, corneal ulcers, and synechiae of the iris and ciliary body, and are largely resolved by 10 weeks; however, megaloglobus persisted in 6% of the rats in one study (Lai et al., 1976). Such severe alterations of ocular structures make infected rats unsuitable for research in which the eye is the target organ. Apparently, this disease is widespread in rat colonies, invading the ear canal, and usually has both sebaceous and squamous differentiation.

Sendai Virus Infection

The Sendai virus is a paramyxovirus which is enzootic in many modern rat colonies. Enzootic infections generally affect weanlings as maternal milk-transmitted immunity wanes. The pups develop a respiratory disease that is generally subclinical. At necropsy, many rats appear normal, but some have small red foci scattered over the surface of the lung. Histologically, there are acute necrotizing inflammatory lesions in the mucosal epithelium of the nose, trachea, and pulmonary airways, the last of these often extending into the alveoli. Most of the airway mucosal lesions repair rapidly and completely, but focal fibrosis and scarring may occur in terminal airways and associated alveoli. In general, however, Sendai infection can be considered an acute transient infection of the rat respiratory tract with little or no residual effects.

Although it is widely recognized that Sendai virus is a respiratory pathogen of mice that produces pneumonia and death, its role in naturally occurring respiratory diseases of rats is much less clear. In one report, a Sendai virus epidemic occurred in an aging rat colony paralleling an outbreak in a mouse colony at the same institute (Burek et al., 1977). The epidemic was characterized by seroconversion, but increased mortality and clinical signs were not observed. During this period, however, rats coming to necropsy had distinct microscopic pulmonary lesions not found before the outbreak. Three types of lesions were found: perivascular cuffing of pulmonary vessels by plasma cells and lymphocytes; multifocal interstitial pulmonary infiltrates of macrophages, lymphocytes, and neutrophils; and hyperplasia of peribronchial lympholid tissue.

Corynebacterium kutscheri Infection

Corynebacterium kutscheri is an example of a bacterial disease dominated mainly by acute local effects in the respiratory tract. The infection is usually latent or inapparent, but may become activated to produce acute suppurative pulmonary lesions which are either fatal or resolve by fibrosis and the formation of granulomas. Activation of this disease is usually associated with factors that lower host resistance. Administration of chemicals could be such a factor, either through immunosuppression or the general stress of toxicity. As a result, a pathologist could be presented with a pattern of minor lesions in controls and a dose-related increase in lung lesions in treated groups. This apparent "pulmonary toxicity" is another example of the complex interaction between different causal agents that may occur in animal models.

Pinworms

Pinworms are parasitic nematodes which may be very common and are visible living free in the lumen of the large intestine without producing any obvious lesions. They are common in many species and are a good example of an asymptomatic local infection.

Mycoplasmosis

Mycoplasmosis tends to be tissue and host specific, and in the rat the disease primarily affects the respiratory tract and to a lesser extent the female reproductive tract. The respiratory disease begins in early life, and progresses as a chronic condition; therefore respiratory mycoplasmosis in the rat is commonly termed chronic respiratory disease. Chronic respiratory disease (CRD) has been the major health problem affecting the laboratory rat. When endemic in a colony, it is generally the life-limiting factor. This disease has been eliminated from most modern colonies, but is still occasionally encountered as a highly contagious, chronic enzootic disease of the respiratory tract.

Mycoplasmosis often begins with inner ear involvement, and only later is pulmonary involvement seen (Kohn, 1971). The most characteristic clinical sign in the young rat is snuffling and wheezing during the first 3 months of life. This snuffing is associated with inflammation in the upper respiratory tract, notably rhinitis, and with increasing severity or age progressively affects the larynx, trachea, and lungs to produce the bronchiectatic abscess characteristic of the older rat. After mycoplasmal colonization small amounts of purulent exudate appear in the airway lumen. This is followed by hyperplasia and increased mucus production in the respiratory epithelium and by lymphoid infiltration and proliferation. The hallmarks of chronic infection are thus exudate, epithelial hyperplasia, squamous metaplasia, and lymphoid cell accumulation. The infection may also affect the middle ear, and subsequent labyrinthitis may produce clinical symptoms such as circling.

Like *C. kutscheri* infection, the disease pattern may be altered by extraneous factors such as ammonia levels in the animal room as well as by interaction with other infectious agents such as the Sendai virus, and of course by effects related to test article administration. Any stress such as crowding or experimental procedure will cause increased mortality and decreased life span.

Gross pathological findings include areas of red to gray consolidation of the lung, often containing abscesses. In a majority of rats, the bullae of the ears contain a green-yellow exudate. The most spectacular pathological changes are seen in the old rat, and in protracted cases, the lung may be converted to a mass of bronchiectatic tissue and abscesses. Microscopically, there is a severe chronic purulent bronchopneumonia with bronchiectasis and marked peribronchial lymphoid hyperplasia. The histopathological findings in advance stages are fairly typical or chronic disease, consisting of a combination of chronic inflammation and reparative processes.

While numerous agents have been proposed as the cause of CRD, *Mycoplasma pulmonis* appears to be the main, and in many cases the sole, agent responsible. The organism can continue to be isolated from the pneumonic lung, and rats with more severe respiratory involvement are more infectious for other rats. Although high complement fixation antibody titers are present and may serve as an aid in diagnosis, there is no correlation between circulating antibody and the presence of the organism. This suggests that circulating antibody does not play a role in protection against the mycoplasma infection. Occasionally, *Mycoplasma arthritidis* can be a secondary invader in CRD of rats. Common nonneoplastic lesions are summarized in Table 20.

HISTOPATHOLOGY OF THE RAT

Though there are several ways that one might organize an overview of the microscopic pathology of the laboratory rat, a good (and fairly common) approach is to compare the patterns commonly found in both young and aged animals, as these form very different backgrounds to evaluate (or detect) any toxicological response against secondary patterns of concern which may complicate or confound determinations of causality, such as a response to generalized stress which is not uncommonly seen at high doses, may then also be considered. In all cases, reference to some standard glossary for use in the description of findings (such as that of Greaves and Faccini, 1984).

PATHOLOGY OF YOUNG RATS

Strain-to-strain variations for patterns of age-related lesions are recognized in rats. Though the patterns associated with old animals are generally of more interest, there are also common spontaneous lesions in young animals.

Control rats rarely die in short-term studies and neoplasia is also rare. The observed

Table 20 Example of a Pattern of Pathology in Young Rats

Organ	Diagnosis	% incidence male	% incidence female
Skin	Alopecia/fur loss	5	9
	Dermatitis/sore	4	4
Tail	Dermatitis/sore	5	3
	Other lesions	3	3
Esophagus	Myositis	2	6
Eye	Periorbititis	10	11
	Other lesions	6	8
Heart	Leukocyte foci	7	2
Kidney	Leucocyte foci	12	7
	Hyaline droplets	15	0
	Tubular regeneration	32	4
	Mineralization	0	6
	Hydronephrosis	10	10
Liver	Leukocyte foci	80	80
Lung	Leukocyte foci	52	56
	Pneumonitis	20	18
	Foamy histiocytes	20	16
	Mandibular lymph node hyperplasia	40	26
	Large intestine nematodes	8	3
Pituitary	Cyst	3	3
Stomach	Erosions and ulcerations	10	10[a]
Thyroid	Ectopic thymus	2	3
Prostate	Leukocyte foci	14	—
Testis	Atrophy	2	—[b]
Thymus	Atrophy	—	—[b]
Uterus	Distension	—	14

[a]Seems to be increasing in recent years (1988 onward).
[b]Commonly found associated with nonspecific stress at higher dose levels.
Source: Adapted from Glaister, 1986.

pattern of pathology is, therefore, of nonneoplastic lesions and is usually presented in tabular form, such as in Table 20. Only lesions occurring with an incidence greater than 1% are listed. A toxicologist presented with such a table should try to understand what the diagnoses and their frequencies mean in terms of the general background of pathology in control animals. Among the 40 organs commonly evaluated, only a minority have lesions, and relatively few lesions have incidence rates greater than 10%. Thus, the majority of organs of a young rat are either normal or rarely show histopathological changes. There are numerous subpatterns within this general overall pattern of infrequent lesions. The observations presented in incidence summary tables, such as Table 20, are usually listed on an organ-by-organ basis, but lesions within any particular organ may represent degenerations, inflammations, or proliferations; they may be trivial or severe; and they

Table 21 Incidence (%) of Morbidity and Mortality in Sprague-Dawley Rats Due to the Major Groups of Nonneoplastic and Neoplastic Causes

| | Study internal (weeks) | | | | | |
| | male | | | female | | |
Cause	52–78	79–104	>104	52–78	79–104	>104
Nonneoplasia						
degenerations	8	8	12	2	1	0
inflammations	8	8	8	2	2	2
other conditions	2	2	8	1	1	5
Uncertain/multifactorial	14	19	8	2	2	0
Neoplasia						
pituitary	40	30	21	45	41	45
subcutis	19	13	16	1	2	2
mammary	0	0	0	33	43	32
other tumors	9	20	27	14	8	14

Coleman et al. (1977) has extensive incidence tables on male Fischer 344 rats.
Source: Adapted from Glaister, 1986.

may be related to a variety of causes. It is the association between cause and effect that is the main interest in toxicological pathology and, in young animals, it is convenient to describe the pathology in terms of causation rather than in terms of lesions within any one organ.

Rats are commonly housed in small groups, often in metal cages with wire mesh floors. A variety of minor external inflammatory lesions are encountered owing to attrition between rats and between rats and their cages. Fur loss and dermatitis are typical changes seen on the skin and on the tail in group-housed rats. Lesions on the feet and ears may also be seen. These lesions are usually dismissed as insignificant, but differences between control and treated groups may occur in certain circumstances, such as a decrease in the incidence of fight wounds in rats given tranquilizers.

Some lesions are associated with the method of administration of the chemical or with the removal of blood samples for analysis. Rats may struggle when gavaged and the esophagus can be traumatized by the cannula. This bruising appears histologically as a focal myositis with evidence of acute inflammation and/or with healing and repair. The usual appearance is one of basophilic regenerating myofibers accompanied by a few leukocytes. Although the oral route is the most common method of test article administration, equivalent inflammatory lesions such as phlebitis or myositis may be common following intravenous and intramuscular administration.

Hair Fragments in the Lung

Another lesion sometimes associated with intravenous injections is hair fragments in the lung. These fragments lodge in pulmonary vessels as hair emboli after their introduction into a peripheral vein during venipuncture. Blood sampling by orbital sinus puncture is another common procedure, and this may cause a variety of inflammatory changes around the eye and orbit, designated by the general term periorbitis. Repeated sampling or poor technique may produce other lesions such as degeneration of the optic nerve (optic neuropathy). The severity and incidence of these procedure-related lesions are variable depending on the nature and frequency of the procedure and on the skill of the technician. Lesions may be uncommon and minor in short-term, well-conducted studies, or at the other extreme may be fatal if the esophagus or eyeball is accidentally punctured.

Congenital or Developmental Defects

The thymus has the same embryological origin as the parathyroid and during its migration toward the base of the heart, small nests of tissue descending from the third and fourth branchial pouch may remain adjacent to or be embedded in the parathyroid/thyroid. These may be quite striking histologically, but they are of trivial significance. Similarly, pituitary cysts are usually trivial. They are derived from remnants of the upgrowth of the craniopharyngeal (Rathke's) pouch, which develops into the adenohypophysis. They vary in site and appearance, but they are usually seen in the pars distalis as small colloid-filled cysts lined by ciliated epithelium. Hydronephrosis (dilation of the renal pelvis) may be caused by urinary tract obstruction, but more commonly is usually due to developmental or congenital defects. It tends to be unilateral, of little significance, and is associated with normal renal function. Severe bilateral and fatal cases may occasionally occur, but care must be taken to exclude obstruction of the lower urinary tract in these instances.

Background Changes

A variety of minor inflammations, degenerations, and proliferations of diverse or un-certain cause may be encountered in the young rat. They are grouped together as miscellaneous "background" changes and include (see Table 20) hyaline droplets, tubular regeneration and mineralization in the kidney, foamy histiocytes in the lung, testicular atrophy, and uterine distension. One also sees leukocyte foci in the liver and lung.

Renal Hyaline Droplets
Renal hyaline droplets are common findings in the kidneys of the male rat. These appear as bright eosinophilic globules of various sizes in the cytoplasm of the proximal tubular epithelium. The glomerulus of the male rat is "leaky" to low molecular weight proteins, and these droplets represent protein resorbed by the proximal tubule cells and sequestered in lysosomes prior to recycling into the blood. Although these droplets are common and are generally considered trivial, like many other background observations, the severity of the change occasionally increases in a dose-related manner. The cause of such an increase in hyaline droplets is related to the interaction of the test article or a metabolite with a protein, α_2 microglobulin, and interference with the recycling of the globulin by renal tubules. In some cases, the increase in hyaline droplets is accompanied by focal tubular degeneration, and/or tubular necrosis (Swenberg et al., 1989). Thus, a common change may be accentuated to a sufficient extent in treated animals to be variably interpreted as evidence of nephrotoxicity. The kidneys of females are usually normal.

Renal Tubular Regeneration
Renal tubular regeneration is another common but minor finding in male rat kidneys. Synonyms are "blue tubules," tubular atrophy, and tubular basophilia. The affected tubules stand out against the generally eosinophilic cortex because of their basophilia. On closer inspection, they appear as slightly shrunken tubules with cuboidal basophilic epithelium and sometimes a thickened basement membrane. The response of tissues to

injury is limited, and tubular regeneration is one sequel to nephrotoxicity. This otherwise trivial lesion may therefore assume importance if it confounds the interpretation of no-effect levels in studies of nephrotoxic chemicals.

Renal Tubular Mineralization

Renal mineralization, also termed nephrocalcinosis, is a common minor renal lesion, but is seen mainly in females. The mineral may be found under or in the pelvic epithelium, or more commonly in the tubules at the corticomedullary junction. The corticomedullary mineralization usually appears between weaning and sexual maturity, and the etiology appears to be multifactorial, involving dietary and endocrine factors. Manipulation of dietary components in nutritional studies on certain food or protein substitutes may increase the incidence and severity of mineralization. This is another example of synergism between the specific substance of interest and background factors, and it may be difficult to establish no-effect levels if there is a high incidence of mineralization in controls.

Foamy Histiocytes

In the lung, the main observation of interest is foamy histiocytes. These are also called foam cells or termed lipidosis. The condition is characterized by accumulations of plump pale cells in the alveolar lumen, often located subpleurally so that they appear at necropsy as pinpoint gray spots on the surface of the lung. The foamy appearance of these alveolar macrophages is due to the uptake of surfactant released from type II alveolar cells. This condition may be considered an uptake, storage, and recycling process analogous to the hyaline droplets seen in the male rat kidney and, similarly, may become enhanced in response to certain treatments. This enhancement is seen most commonly in response to inhaled particles such as silica and in association with phospholipidosis-inducing compounds such as cationic amphiphilic drugs. A high control incidence of foam cells may interfere with the assessment of no-effect levels with these compounds.

Testicular Atrophy

Testicular atrophy is usually minor, unilateral, and affects the subcapsular tubules. Occasionally, it may be severe and diffuse, and appear at necropsy as a small, watery, blue testis. Histologically, the affected tubules are small and show partial or complete lack of germ cells, leaving only Sertoli cells. This condition can have many causes, including congenital origin, obstructive lesions, and physical restraint as in nose-only inhalation studies. It may also result from treatment with chemicals and hormones, and a high background incidence in controls may hinder the evaluation of these substances. It is not uncommon to see significant incidences of testicular and thymic atrophy in high-dose group animals attibutable to nonspecific stress rather than any specific target organ toxicity. In these cases, however, the animals also generally have reduced food consumption and reduced absolute body weight.

Leukocyte Inflammatory Cell Foci in the Liver and Lung

Leukocyte inflammatory cell foci are frequently encountered in certain tissues, especially the liver and lung and to a lesser extent the prostate. They may be related to enzootic viral infections such as PVM or Sendai, but the relationship is difficult to establish. The foci are usually minor and multifocal, and usually comprise mononuclear leukocytes in various admixtures, but mainly lymphoid. These foci appear histologically as small basophilic cellular aggregates scattered across the plane of section. Other terms used are round cell foci, lymphoid foci, inflammatory foci, and similar nonspecific terms. This tendency to use nonspecific terms is quite common among toxicological pathologists because of the frequent misunderstanding of the more specific terms when crossing species' lines or scientific disciplines. Thus, leukocytes in the liver may occasionally surround a necrotic liver cell and could justify the term hepatitis. However, such a diagnosis may be interpreted as a serious condition by a medical pathologist or a toxicologist unfamiliar with laboratory animal pathology.

In terms of the two basic scales for assession lesions—incidence and severity—pathology findings in the young rat can be considered to be generally infrequent, and when present, of minor biological significance. Their main importance is in the two ways in which they can complicate the interpretation of treatment-related responses. In the first place, they may mimic the effect of treatment. For example, renal tubular regeneration may complicate the assessment of no-effect levels of nephrotoxins. Second, the incidence or severity of background pathology may be enhanced in a dose-related manner. The enhancement may be of endogenous processes such as the lysosomal cycling of pulmonary surfactant and renal protein, or it may be of processes initiated by exogenous agents such as infections. In either case, the precise causal relationship of treatment to the observed response may be difficult to unravel.

PATHOLOGY OF OLD RATS

The pathology of the aged rat is an important confounding factor in long-term bioassays for chronic toxicity and carcinogenicity. In contrast to the pattern of infrequent and generally minor lesions seen in young rats, the pattern seen in aging animals during chronic studies is one of an increasing incidence and severity of lesions culminating in death. Although lesions related to husbandry, procedures, development, and infections still occur, these are relatively minor compared with the main age-associated lesions and, therefore, the pattern of pathology will be classified in a different way. The three main items of interest in chronic rodent studies are morbidity/mortality, nonneoplastic lesions, and neoplasms. These will vary from strain-to-strain (more so than the patterns associated with very young animals), but a basic pattern is still present. The two main parameters of interest in analysis of morbidity (illness) and mortality (death) are the rate at which they occur and the causation. These data give the toxicologist an excellent opportunity to overview some of the major background characteristics of the rat strain. One or both of these parameters may be affected by treatment, but must also always be considered in study design and conduct. The status of changes in body weight (Are the animals gaining, losing, or stable?) is an important indicator of general health status for a group of rats.

Age at Which to Terminate Animals

A key issue in rodent carcinogenicity studies is the age at which to terminate the animals. As such a study progresses, the rise in the background level of tumors makes it more and more difficult to clearly partition treatment-effect tumors from age-effect tumors. Swenberg (Solleveld et al., 1984; Swenberg, 1985) has made the point that the incidence of many tumor types has increased from 100 to 500% when control rat results from 2-year studies (rats 110–116 weeks of age) were compared to those from life-span studies (140–146 weeks of age). If such an increase in age (25%) can result in such extreme increases in spontaneous tumors, what is the effect on interpretation of incidence rates seen in concurrent treatment groups? This is especially the case if, as Salsburg (1980) has suggested, any biologically active treatment will result in a shift in the patterns of neoplastic lesions occurring in aging animals. The current practice is to interpret tumor incidence on an independent site-by-site basis (on the assumption that what happens at each tissue site is independent of what happens elsewhere), and no allowance or factoring is made for the fact that what may be occurring in animals over their life span (as expressed by tumor incidence levels at an advanced age) is merely a shifting of patterns from one tumor site to another. In other words, commonly the "significantly" increased incidence of liver tumors is focused on, whereas the just as statistically significant decrease in kidney tumors compared to controls is ignored. Clearly, we should not be trying to analyze tumor data from rats that are advancing into senescence in the same manner that we do the data from those which lack these confounding factors. Where should a cut-off point be? This is a problem, but clearly Cameron's data (Cameron et al., 1985) suggest that the growth curves of 9385 B6C3F1 mice and 10,023 F344 rats from control groups in NCI/NTP studies show consistent patterns of decline in body weights from these animals starting at the following ages (in weeks).

	Males	Females
B6C3F1 mice	96	101
Fischer 344 rats	91	106
Sprague-Dawley rats	112	104

The existence of similar data for tumor incidences (unfortunately not available from NCI/NTP studies) would certainly improve our confidence in selecting cutoff points for age, but the above ages merit consideration as termination points.

Patterns of Lesions

The patterns of lesions are equally as important as the rates and incidences at which they occur, as these can also be altered by treatment and may provide essential insight into the causal relationship. Such patterns can be altered without any change in survival rates.

In rats, the patterns of neoplasia associated with deaths on carcinogenicity studies are sex specific. Approximately 80% of unscheduled deaths in females are attributable to tumors in two organs, the pituitary and mammary gland, and this pattern is constant throughout the aging period. Other lethal tumors considered on an individual organ basis account for less than 5% of morbidity and mortality, and a similar case holds for various types of nonneoplastic lesions. Pituitary tumors cause illness and death because of their critical position at the base of the brain, and relatively small tumors may be fatal. Mammary tumors are not critically located. These subcutaneous tumors may exceed 100 g without causing any apparent ill health unless they ulcerate or impede the animal's movement.

The patterns of mortality associated with neoplastic lesions in males are more diverse. Two main tumor types, pituitary tumors and fibrous tumors of the subcutis, account for many losses, but the pattern is not as prevalent in females, in which several other tumor types occur. The incidence of these other lethal tumors tends to increase with time, but rarely exceeds 5% if they are considered on an individual tissue basis. Two tumors predominate, liver tumors and various endocrine tumors, and are accompanied with time by a slowly increasing range of low-frequency tumor types such as bone tumors.

About one-third of unscheduled necropsies in males are not associated with any large, ulcerated, or critically situated neoplasms, and morbidity and mortality in these cases has to be attributed to nonneoplastic causes. In many cases, there may be no major morphological lesion to account for illness, or there may be two or more conditions of equivalent biological impact and the cause has to be stated as uncertain or multifactorial. In other cases, there may be major degenerative lesions in the kidney, nervous system, or heart or inflammation in the skin, appendages, or genitourinary tract, and these together with other obvious lesions can be attributed unequivocally as the cause of the animal's demise. The pattern of these nonneoplastic causes of death has a reasonable constancy with time, except that the uncertainty tends to decrease as the major degenerations associated with old age become more prominent. In some strains, particularly those fed high-protein diets ad libitum, kidney disease can be the major cause of morbidity and mortality in males.

Analysis of the incidence and causes of morbidity and mortality is not a common practice in long-term studies, but has much to commend it in assessing the biological significance of lesions. Changes in mortality rate or in the major patterns of causation are easily detected and are more likely to be relevant in risk assessment than any minor increases in the incidence of microscopic or small tumors found in groups of animals dying from other causes. The survival pattern in most strains of rat also suggests that assay sensitivity is unlikely to be increased by extending a study beyond 2 years. As already pointed out, 2 years is approximately the 50% survival point and the patterns of causation after this point are relatively constant. These patterns are dominated by three or four major entities, and the sudden appearance of a biologically and statistically significant increase in other lesions in the remaining rats could be difficult to detect. Similar considerations apply to many other strains of rat. The majority of morbidity and mortality is usually dominated by a small number of nonneoplastic and neoplastic conditions throughout the aging period.

The common morphological lesions can be grouped into degenerative, inflammatory, and proliferative lesions, the later overlapping to some extent with neoplasms (Table 22). Most other lesions reported in aging control rats are of low incidence and of minor biological significance, and are not discussed. The biological significance of a lesion is equally as important as frequency and the common lesions in Table 22 can be divided into two main groups on this basis. For example, degenerations of the kidney and nervous system can be lethal, whereas those in the liver and reproductive organs are usually incidental findings at necropsy. The main emphasis in this section will be on the clinically significant lesions and on lesions that cause problems in data analysis.

Nonneoplastic Lesions

Nonneoplastic proliferations are a particular problem in analysis. The main use of long-term studies in rats is as a model bioassay for carcinogenicity. Nonneoplastic proliferations are seldom of clinical significance, but are extremely important because of the diagnostic difficulties they create in differentiation from preneoplastic lesions and from neoplasms. For example, spontaneous liver tumors are rare, but the liver is a common target organ of carcinogens and, therefore, spontaneous proliferations are important because they mimic preneoplastic changes. However, the presence or absence of preneoplastic proliferative lesions associated with tumors in the same organ can be important in evaluating the carcinogenic potential of xenobiotics. In contrast, endocrine proliferations and tumors are common in rats, and the choice of criteria to differentiate nonneoplastic and neoplastic proliferations can profoundly alter the reported incidence of endocrine tumors in various laboratories.

Table 22 Common Nonneoplastic Lesions in Aging Sprague-Dawley Rats

Morphotogical Lesion	Clinical Condition
Degeneration	
kidney	Glomerulonephropathy
nerve	Radiculoneuropathy
testis	Atrophy
ovary	Atrophy/cyst
liver	Steatosis
	Microcystic degeneration
	Telangiectasis
Inflammation	
foot	Pododermatitis/arthritis
tail	Dermatitis/folliculitis
pancreas	Pancreatitis
Proliferation	
liver	Biliary proliferation
	Altered cell foci/nodules
adrenal	Altered cell foci/nodules
mammary	Hyperplasia

Kidney

Glomerulonephropathy. Of the degenerations, glomerulonephropathy is probably the major nonneoplastic condition in the aging rat of all strains (Gray, 1977), in that it accounts for a significant proportion of morbidity and mortality. The inbred Lewis rat appears to be less susceptible and the inbred Fischer 344 rat more susceptible to the development of chronic nephrosis than many random-bred rat strains (Bolton et al., 1976). Males are more susceptible than females. The severity of renal disease can be profoundly influenced by factors such as genotype and diet, and its presence hinders evaluation of chronic nephrotoxicity.

Glomerulonephropathy has numerous synonyms, including nephropathy, nephrosis, and glomerulonephrosis; theories regarding its pathogenesis are equally numerous. The incidence and severity of disease are greater in males than in females. In advanced cases, the kidneys are enlarged, tan, and irregular in shape at necropsy and the cut surface in severe cases may be grossly cystic. Histologically, both glomerular and tubular changes are present, but the latter are dominant. Some tubules are shrunken with thickened basement membranes accompanied by variable degrees of interstitial fibrosis. Other tubules contain hyaline casts or form large cysts filled with proteinaceous material. Glomerular changes are relatively inconspicuous and are characterized mainly by varying degrees of sclerosis and cystic dilation of Bowman's space. Such severe cases are unusual in 2-year-old rats, and in most instances 50% or more of the kidney may appear reasonably normal.

The kidneys play a major role in fluid and electrolyte homeostasis and are important in the excretion of waste products. However, there is considerable reserve capacity and a rat may survive for an extended period with severely damaged kidneys before dying of renal failure. Because the kidneys play a central role in fluid and electrolyte balance, advanced cases may lead to secondary patterns of pathology (syndromes) in other organs. The two main syndromes affect the cardiovascular system and calcium/phosphorus homeostasis.

Cardiovascular Disease: The kidney receives 25% of the cardiac output and is intimately concerned with blood pressure regulation through the renin-angiotensin system. It is not surprising, therefore, that severe renal disease sometimes results in secondary cardiovascular disease. Myocardial fibrosis, especially in the left ventricle, is a common complication of severe renal disease, while the more advanced cases may show left atrial thrombosis or arteritis. Arteritis may be seen in one or more vessels, including renal vessels, but is not commonly recorded in the pancreatic, mesenteric, and testicular arteries. Advanced involvement of mesenteric vessels can be seen at necropsy as blue tortuous or nodular vessels in the mesentery around the duodenum and pancreas. Histologically the affected vessels show varying degrees of thrombosis, aneurysmal dilatation, fibrinoid necrosis, and leukocyte infiltration.

Mineralization Syndrome: The mineralization syndrome is related to the kidney's role in calcium and phosphorus homeostasis via control of tubular resorption, and also via synthesis of the 1,25-dihydroxy derivative of vitamin D_3. The pathogenesis of the syndrome is incompletely understood, but renal impairment results in hyperphosphatemia and acidosis. Calicum phosphorus imbalance stimulates parathyroid hyperplasia and there is increased bone resorption in an attempt to correct the hypocalcemia. Severe cases can be identified at necropsy. The parathyroids are grossly enlarged, the bones are thin and brittle, and the aorta is dilated and rigid owing to mineral deposited in the media. This mineralization affects many tissues histologically, and is known as metastatic mineralization in contrast to the focal dystrophic mineralization (nephrocalcinosis) that is a common finding in the young rat.

Nerve

Radiculoneuropathy. Another major degenerative lesion in the aging rat is radiculoneuropathy. This disease may appear clinically as minor ataxia or as hind limb paralysis with urinary incontinence in severe cases. The lesion is predominant in males. Histologically, degeneration is seen in the posterior spinal cord (myelopathy), posterior nerve roots (radiculoneuropathy), and sciatic nerve (peripheral neuropathy) and results in secondary changes in the hind limb muscles (atrophy). Paralysis and urinary incontinence may predispose to infection of the urogenital tract, resulting in inflammation of the prostate (prostatitis), bladder (cystitis), or kidney (pyelonephritis). Inflammation in these organs can be severe and fatal in contrast to the minor lesions in young animals, and illustrate the importance of qualifying terms in diagnoses.

Histological evidence of degeneration of myelin sheaths include vacuoles and avoids within the sheaths, associated with foamy macrophages or in severe cases, cholesterol deposits (clefts) and astrocytic, Schwann cell, or proliferation of fibroblasts.

Radiculoneuropathy is very common in aging males, but it is usually asymptomatic. In contrast, there is a less frequent degeneration of the central nervous system, which may produce obvious neurological symptoms and the animal has to be removed from the study. This condition, termed encephalopathy, or more descriptively spongiform encephalopathy, consists of a maultifocal vacuolation of the gray and white matter, most notable histologically in the cerebral cortex. Minor cases can be easily masked by artifacts, but the brain of old rats showing acute neurological symptoms in the absence of pituitary or brain tumors should be examined carefully for this condition.

Inflammations of biological significance are uncommon in aging rats unless they suffer from enzootic diseases such as mycoplasmosis. Prostatitis and other urogenital tract lesions are occasionally seen in animals with hind limb paralysis, but apart from these, lesions of the hind feet are the only common inflammations likely to make a significant impact on the health of the rat. Foot lesions are basically husbandry-related and comprise of two entities, pododermatitis and arthritis. Rats are commonly housed on grid or mesh floors and males may reach 1 kg body weight on ad libitum feeding. It is not surprising, therefore, that this combination of high body weight and mesh floors occasionally results in lesions of the feet, particularly in the heavier males. Up to 5% of aging males may be removed from a study because of these foot lesions.

Foot

Pododermatitis. Pododermatitis is a local inflammation of the skin of the foot. It begins initially as a wartlike growth or callus on the foot pad due to constant pressure, and subsequent proliferation of the skin. However, infection, ulceration, and bleeding may subsequently occur. Histologically, the lesion consists of inflamed granulation tissue variably covered by a hyperplastic squamous epithelium.

Arthritis. Arthritis is inflammation of the joint and surrounding tissues. Severe cases appear clinically as grossly swollen, firm, blue feet and hocks and may significantly impair the animal's mobility. The initial lesion is a periarthritis or tenosynovitis, resulting in marked periarticular edema with fibrosis and mononuclear leukocyte infiltration. The metatarsal joint ultimately becomes affected, and in some cases the persistent chronic inflammation may incite a dramatic reactive bony proliferation which results in ankylosis of the involved joint.

Liver

The liver is such a frequent target organ in toxicity studies (in fact, the most common) that a discussion of some of the more common lesions that occur with aging in the rat seems warranted. More than half of aging male Fischer and Sprague-Dawley rats have nonneoplastic hepatic lesions such as bile ductule hyperplasia and focal chronic hepatitis (Cohen et al., 1978). The National Toxicology program has its own systemic nomenclature specifically for rat hepatoproliferative lesions (Maronpot et al., 1986).

Steatosis. Steatosis in the liver is a very general term unless qualified further, and includes both focal and diffuse change, the latter being either centrilobular or periportal. The appearance of fat droplets is equally variable and may be either macrocytic or microcytic. The pathogenesis of steatosis may be equally diverse and includes dysfunction in the hepatocyte or imbalance in general lipid homeostatis. The latter is probably more common in aging rats either because of obesity due to ad libitum feeding or due to lipid mobilization in debilitated or clinically ill animals secondary to pituitary tumors or other debilitating lesions. In these cases, diffuse periportal steatosis is common.

Microcystic Degeneration. Microcystic degeneration occurs in the liver, and is also known as spongiosa hepatica. It may be visible at necropsy, but is usually a histological finding characterized by groups of thin-walled cysts containing pale-pink proteinaceous material and occasionally a few erythrocytes. The microcysts are thought to be derived from the fat-storing (Ito) cell in the liver. They are found mainly in males.

Telangiectasis. Telangiectasis is another common liver lesion. It is a vascular lesion, but is probably secondary to or associated with atrophy of the hepatic cords. It is most obvious at necropsy as depressed red foci on the surface of the liver and is particularly conspicuous when the liver is slightly yellow due to steatosis. Histologically, these foci are groups of dilated sinusoids usually located below the liver capsule. Telangiectasis is also very common in the adrenal cortex.

Biliary Proliferations.   Focal proliferations of the bile ducts are common in the liver. They are generally minor histological observations. Biliary proliferation (bile duct hyperplasia) consists of clusters or chains of bile duct–like formations lined by cuboidal or flattened epithelium. The proliferations are generally in the vicinity of the portal triad and may show varying degrees of basement membrane thickening or fibrosis. These structures do not progress to neoplasia, but the more basophilic cellular lesions could possibly mimic early-phase oval cell (ductular) hyperplasia, which is a response sometimes observed in the liver of rats fed carcinogens.

Foci of Cellular Alteration.   Foci of cellular alteration, a controversial entity (from an interpretive view point), is not uncommon in the liver of aging rats. It remains unclear whether foci of cellular alteration are preneoplastic or "progress" to adenomas. The focal proliferations consist of groups of hepatocytes which stand out from the normal liver parenchyma because of their arrangement, size, or tinctorial properties. They also demonstrate a variety of biochemical and functional properties such as the inability to store iron and increased γ-glutamyl-transpeptidase activity, which can be utilized to distinguish foci of alteration from normal hepatocytes. However, not all foci of cellular alteration demonstrate consistent biochemical or functional properties in a given animal.

In routine H&E sections, foci are usually classified into vacuolated (clear), acidophilic, basophilic, or mixed cell foci. Clear cell foci are characterized by "empty" cytoplasm representing the space occupied by glycogen or occasionally fat. The cells are usually larger than the surrounding hepatocytes. An increased amount of acidophilic cytoplasm is the characteristic feature of acidophilic foci, and the hepatocytes may also have an enlarged nucleus with a prominent nucleolus. In contrast, the hepatocytes forming basophilic foci are smaller than normal and the cytoplasm contains prominent clumps of basophilic granules. Mixed foci, as the name suggests, contain hepatocytes of two or more of the previous types. Foci exceeding the size of a hepatic lobule are sometimes called areas of cellular alteration, and ones larger still that compress the surrounding parenchyma may be referred to as nodules. Basophilic foci are the most common and are encountered mainly in aging females while most in males tend to be acidophilic foci. Overall, these altered cell foci and areas are uncommon in most strains of rat and do not significantly mask the interpretation of hepatocarcinogenic effects (Maronpot et al., 1986).

Hepatic cysts are, however, a common aging change in many rat strains. The lesion consists of cysts of different sizes that are lined by cuboidal or flat, endothelial-like cells. A moderate amount of connective tissue often surrounds the cysts. In the brown Norway rat these lesions are especially common where large multilocular cysts often bulge from the hepatic surface (Squire and Levitt, 1975). Occasionally, large foci of endothelial-lined spaces containing eosinophilic amorphous material are found. The pathogenesis of these lesions is not clear, but they may represent a sequela to hepatic necrosis.

Adrenals

Altered Cell Foci.   In contrast to the liver, altered cell foci areas and nodules are very common in the adrenal cortex, particularly in females. As in the liver, the lesions can be classified on the basis of staining characteristics into vacuolated, acidophilic, basophilic, etc., although there are subclasses of each type.

Finely vacuolated foci are found in both sexes and usually affect the zona glomerulosa and other zona fasciculata. Coarsely vacuolated foci are most common in males and usually lie in the central zona fasciculata. The small acidophilic cell focus (sometimes called hyperplastic focus) is often multiple and in the outer zona fasciculata. The lesion of most concern is the large acidophilic cell focus. These proliferations are common in aging females and may grow to grossly visible nodules of debatable diagnostic classification.

The proliferation of hyperbasophilic pheochromocytes in the adrenal medulla is an example of classification in the other direction. In this case, there is a reasonable continuity in both cytology and incidence to suggest progression from small basophilic foci to large metastasing proliferations in rats nearing the end of their life span. Similar continuities are seen in the anterior pituitary and in the C-cell population of the thyroid. In all these cases, foci may be considered adenomas even though they are small, noncompressing, and with infrequent mitoses. There is no easy answer to these diagnostic problems, but they are often at the center of debate regarding the conclusions from carcinogenicity studies. It cannot be stressed too frequently that toxicologists and statisticians should appreciate the level of uncertainty that surrounds the classification of microscopic proliferations as hyperplasias or as neoplasias and evaluate the data accordingly.

Heart

Loss and degeneration of myocardial fibers with fibrosis is a common lesion of older rats. It occurs most frequently in the wall of the left ventricle or intraventricular septum and is characterized by areas of fibrosis surrounding myocardial fibers showing loss of striation, fragmentation, and vacuolization. The lesions vary from small foci involving only a few myocardial fibers to extensive areas of fibrosis. The lesion becomes progressively more severe with age (Squire and Levitt, 1975). Cartilaginous foci at the base of the aortic valve are quite common in some Sprague-Dawley strains and were once attributed to aging. However, similar cartilaginous foci have been observed in young rats (Hollander, 1968).

An unusual, but not uncommon, endomyocardial lesion has been described in several strains of rats. The lesion is characterized by proliferation of undifferentiated mesenchymal cells in the subendocardium and usually involves the left ventricle. The lesion is usually sharply demarcated from the myocardium but in places extends along muscle bundles or vessels. A few lymphocytes and occasional cell debris are found in the lesion. An occasional sarcoma is associated with endomyocardial disease, but it is not known whether it represents a progression of the lesion. The lesion is definitely age associated. It is most common in rats over 30 months of age and is rarely observed in rats less than 27 months of age (Squire and Levitt, 1975). Myxomatous degenerative change of heart valves occurs in a majority of old rats.

Testes

Testicular atrophy may appear as a primary condition in aging rats, but it is also secondary to large pituitary tumors and to testicular arteritis. This is an example of a condition which may appear as a single entry on an incidence summary table, but its occurrence may be due to a variety of causes. Toxicologists and statisticians should be aware of the conditions in which pooling data due to different causes is commonly done. Atrophy of the seminiferous tubules ranges from focal unilateral to diffuse bilateral, and severe cases appear grossly as small, blue or brown, sometimes flaccid and watery gonads. Histologically, the tubules are shrunken and the seminiferous epithelium is lost, leaving only Sertoli cells. Interstitial edema is also frequent, and Leydig cell hyperplasia may occur.

Eye

Because the eye can be the target organ of toxicological studies, it is important to be aware of spontaneous lesions in order to avoid misinterpretation. In a study involving 400 rats up to 3 years of age, retinal lesions were found in more than one-third of the animals (Weisse et al., 1974). The lesions consisted of the loss of nuclei in the outer and inner nuclear layer of the retina, neuronal atrophy, and degeneration and thickening plus increased tortuosity of retinal capillaries. The lesions were both age and light dependent. The authors stated that while the lighting was not unlike that in other animal facilities, 12-hr light-dark exposures to less than 200 lux m/m^2 of light resulted in retinal lesions that appeared to be directly related to the amount of light exposure. There was retinal damage in 79% of the males and 96% of the females in the top rows of cage racks; 38% of the males and 50% of the females were affected in the bottom row. In a study involving Fischer 344 rats that were exposed to less than 10–320 lux m/m^2 of light, there was similar light-related retinal degeneration (Lai et al., 1978). In addition, the gradual loss of photoreceptor cells in rats that were exposed to less than 10 lux m/m^2 suggested to the authors that some cell loss in an age-related change. Peripheral retinal degeneration was unrelated to light intensity or severity of photoreceptor cell loss in other parts of the retina. Both studies indicate that age-related and light-associated retinal lesions are common and must be considered in long-term toxicological studies.

Skin and Appendages

The most common inflammatory lesions of the skin and appendages is inflammation of the hair follicle (folliculitis) in the tail. Nodules or postules are frequent along the tail and are primarily a logistic problem related to good laboratory practice (GLP) rather than a clinical problem. Theoretically, a tail nodule could be a tumor, and occasionally this is the case, but the vast majority are various stages of suppurative folliculitis. Many long-term study protocols state that all gross lesions will be examined histologically and a histopathologist will rapidly become an expert on rat tails (and ears or feet) if this requirement is adhered to strictly. These appendigeal lesions could reasonably be treated in the same way as erect fur or fur loss in the skin, or as roundworms and tapeworms in the intestine. Mechanical abrasion from feeders is another possible cause. The clinical and necropsy data can be regarded as a definitive diagnosis in the vast majority of cases without the need to resort to histopathology.

Two other lesions of the integument pose similar problems. These are small nodules in the subcutis of the preputial region or on the back of males. These may be faithfully recorded week after week during the in-life phase of the study as palpable masses which grow slowly if at all, and some may regress. These two entities are preputial abscesses and squamous (epidermoid inclusion) cysts, respectively. Repeated palpation may aggravate and rupture the lesions and necessitate removal of the animal from the study.

Pancreas

Another minor inflammatory lesion affects the pancreas. The histological appearance of this lesion is quite characteristic, but its status as a degenerative lesion (atrophy, micro-ductular change) or postinflammatory lesion (adenitis, pancreatitis) is ill defined. There is focal loss of acinar epithelial cells, producing a ductular structure often accompanied by a mild interstitial inflammatory response. The lesion may be multifocal, but most of the exocrine pancreas is normal.

NEOPLASIA

Rats, like mice, develop a wide variety of tumors. Some of the factors known to affect tumor incidence include age at time of necropsy, strain of rat, sex, diet, and diligence with which tumors are sought. Careful macroscopic examination of the animal at necropsy plus multiple histological sections will result in a higher tumor incidence, especially of the smaller tumors. In this review, only some of the more common or controversial tumors are discussed.

Interpretation and Classification of Tumors

The two main criteria used in the classification of proliferations as tumors are morphology and the probability of progression. Morphological criteria include atypical cytology and organization. Nuclear:cytoplasmic ratio, tinctorial properties, anaplasia, and mitotic rate are the main cytological characteristics that distinguish neoplastic cells from normal cells. Organizational atypia includes abnormal growth patterns, compression, or invasion, and abnormal relationships between proliferating cells and blood vessels or other mesenchymal elements. These patterns serve to differentiate neoplasms from nonneoplastic proliferations.

Probability criteria (which incorporate both severity and incidence data) are mathematical assessments of the degree of association between small lesions of debatable classification and large clear-cut neoplasms. Crudely stated, if large, lethal masses are common in an organ, then common microscopic lesions are probably microscopic tumors or at least precursor lesions with a high probability of neoplastic transformation. On the other hand, if microscopic foci are common and gross tumors are rare in old animals, there is a low probability of any biologically significant degree of progression suggestive of neoplastic transformation. Pathologists use all of these criteria in assessing proliferations, but with different degrees of emphasis. This results in highly variable incidence data for certain types of proliferative lesions. The reviewing toxicologist must become familiar with the main problem areas in a given study and evaluate the data in the perspective that application of diagnostic criteria may influence the incidence rates.

If the above criteria are applied to the large acidophil proliferations in the adrenal cortex, then on a morphological basis large compressing nodules of cytologically distinct cells, sometimes with frequent mitoses, are common in the female adrenal. On this basis, there could be a 40% or more incidence of cortical tumors in some rat strains. Alternatively, the probable fate of many of these proliferations is to undergo vacuolar degeneration, resulting in a large blood-filled cyst which may thrombose. Further evidence against a neoplastic diagnosis is that large undoubted cortical neoplasms are often composed of small acidophilic cells cytologically distinct from the hypertrophied acidophilic cell of the commonly occurring nodules. Thus, if diagnosis is based on this cytological discontinuity and the high incidence of degeneration, these nodules would be regarded as hyperplastic rather than neoplastic.

The incidence and types of neoplasia are usually the patterns of pathology of most concern in long-term studies. The pattern of common tumors in the Fischer 344 was presented in detail in Table 23, and this is reasonably representative of other strains (except that more mammary tumors—up to a 55% incidence—are seen in Sprague-Dawleys). The pattern is dominated by subcutaneous connective tissue tumors, mammary proliferations, and by endocrine tumors. Other tumor types occur at incidence rates of less than 10% and in most cases rarely exceed 3%.

Table 23 Reported Background Tumor Incidences in Fischer 344 Rats

Organ/Tissue	Chu (1977)		Fears et al. (1977); Page (1977), Gart et al. (1979)		Goodman et al.[a] (1979)		Chu et al. (1981)		Tarone et al. (1981)	
	M	F	M	F	M	F	M	F	M	F
Brain	0.9	0.6	1.3	<0	8.1	0.55	.8	0.6		
Skin/subcutaneous	6.6	3.2	5.7	2.5	6.4	3	7.8	3.2		
Mammary gland	1.4	17.9	0	18.8	1.54	8.5	1.5	20.9		
Circulatory system	0.4	0.5	<1	<1	3.8	0.27	0.7	0.4		
Lung/trachea	3.1	1.8	2.4	<1	2.9	2	3.0	1.9		
Heart	0.3	0.1	<1	<1	0.2	0.05				
Liver	1.8	3.1	1.2	1.3	1.74	3.9	2.2	1.9	0.7–3.4	0.5–2.9
Pancreas	0.2	—	<1	<0	0.16	0	0.2	—		
Stomach	0.3	0.2	<1	<1	0.32	0.2	0.3	0.2		
Intestines	0.3	0.5	<1	<1	0.31	0.36	0.6	0.3		
Kidney	0.4	0.2	<1	<1	0.38	0.16	0.5	0.2		
Urinary/bladder	0.1	0.2	<1	<1	0.1	0.22	0.1	0.3		
Preputial gland	1.4	1.2	—	—	1.4	1.2	2.4	1.8		
Testis	80.6	NA	76.2	NA	80.1	NA	2.3	NA		
Ovary	NA	0.3	NA	<1	NA	0.33	NA	0.4		
Uterus	NA	15.6	NA	16.8	NA	5.55	NA	17		
Pituitary	11.5	30.5	10.2	29.5	11.4	0.3	4.7	34.9	7.5–31.2	32.0–58.6
Adrenal	10	4.6	8.7	4	9.95	4.58	2.4	5.2		
Thyroid	7.1	6.5	5.1	5.6	7.16	6.65	8.2	6.8	3.6–	4.7–
Pancreatic islets	0.8	1	3.2	1.3	3.89	1.05	3.9	0.8		
Body cavities	1.1	0.3	<1	<1	2.51	0.38	2.6	0.4	2.8–9	1–1.9
Leukemia/lymphoma	11.7	9.1	6.5	5.4	12.3	9.9	9.9	13.4	9.1–23.6	7.5–15.4
N	1806	1765	846	840	1794	1754	b	b		

[a]Gives detailed breakdown of neoplastic and nonneoplastic lesions in aged animals.
[b]Range of averages, 6 different laboratories.

The rat represents the most commonly employed animal model in toxicological research and testing. As all other animal species, it has certain background incidences of lesions (particularly of neoplastic lesions) which are characteristic of it and which may confound interpretation of results. These vary from strain-to-strain, but there are general patterns for the species. Table 23 presents a summary of findings of tumor incidences in large groups of control Fischer 344 rats. These incidences show, in some cases, great degrees of variability. Haseman et al. (1989) discusses the major reasons behind such variability.

Pituitary

In several strains, one of the most prevalent spontaneous neoplastic alterations is the pituitary adenoma. Female Fischer 344 rats have been found to develop such tumors at a 30% rate by the time they were 110 weeks old in an investigation involving a total of 1754 females (Goodman et al., 1979), and most of the pituitary tumors were described as chromophobe adenomas. Carcinomas, on the other hand, consist of cells with anaplastic features and/or show invasion. Pituitary adenomas have also been observed frequently in other strains such as the Crl:CD(SD)BR strain (Cohen et al., 1978). Females appear to develop pituitary adenomas more often than males, although the incidence of such tumors in male F344 rats has been reported to be 14.7% (Coleman et al., 1977). In Wistar-derived SAG/Rij female rats, adenomas of the pituitary gland were found in 69% out of a total of 290 animals which had an average life span of 31 months (Boorman and Hollander, 1973). The incidences of spontaneous pituitary tumors in various rat strains have been reviewed by Carlton and Gries (1984).

Mammary Gland

Another frequently observed spontaneous neoplasm in the rat is the mammary tumor, the incidence of which varies from 10 to 40% depending on the strain and the age of the animals. While in WAG/Rij rats, pituitary tumors appeared to be the most usual cause of death in animals over 1 year of age, mammary tumors tended to develop later in life and were most often seen in animals which had survived for 2 years (Boorman and Hollander, 1973). Moreover, 68% of such rats with mammary tumors simultaneously revealed adenomas of the pituitary gland. Histologically, fibroadenomas and adenocarcinomas represent the most common varieties of benign and malignant mammary tumors.

Lymphoreticular System

Spontaneous tumors of the lymphoreticular system are fairly rare in rats, although a 25% incidence has been reported in Wistar-Furth and Fischer strains (Moloney et al., 1969, 1970). In contrast to mice, such neoplasms have not been studied widely and are, therefore, not well classified. They usually progress with secondary involvement of the spleen, liver, lung, and often of renal adipose tissue. Generally, tumors of the lymphoid system are not common, but a 25% incidence has been reported in Wistar and Fischer rats (Squire and Goodman, 1978). Lymphoreticular cell tumors have not been widely studied and are not well classified. They usually involve the spleen with secondary involvement of liver, lung, and often the renal adipose tissue. Large granular lymphocyte leukemia (previously called mononuclear cell leukemia) is the most common "natural" cause of death in Fischer-344 rats used in chronic toxicity and carcinogenicity studies. From 30 to

50% of aging Fischer-344 rats in "control" populations die from the primary and secondary effects of this leukemia between 14 and 30 months of age (Losco and Ward, 1984).

Thyroid

After many strains have reached 2 years of age, neoplasms of the thyroid gland occur spontaneously at high frequencies. Again in WAG/Rij females, such tumors were found in 40% of 290 examined animals (Boorman and Hollander, 1973). In this study, electron microscopy revealed the cells of origin to be parafollicular.

Testes

Spontaneous testicular tumors are not common in the majority of rat strains (Sertoli cell tumors are especially rare in rats). However, a 100% incidence of interstitial (Leydig cell) tumors occurs in male Fischer rats by the time they are 30 months of age. Table 17 presents a summary of neoplastic lesions incidences in this strain (the most commonly used in long-term toxicology studies) as reported by various investigators.

Skin/Subcutaneous Tissues

Large subcutaneous masses are common finding in aging rats and may exceed 100 g in weight. In males, a variety of connective tissue tumors occurs, but they are usually fatty or fibrous, the latter predominating.

Fatty tumors (lipomas) are seen at necropsy as large, smooth, soft, glistening masses and are most easily defined in debilitated animals when the normal subcutaneous adipose tissue is depleted. In obese males, the distinction between small lipomas and large fat depots is not clear cut. Histologically, the lipoma consists of mature lipocytes sometimes with small bands of fibrosis.

Large Fibroma

Large, well-differentiated fibromas are the predominant subcutaneous connective tissue in males. Large tumors may impede movement or become ulcerated and the animal has to be removed from the study. They appear grossly as well circumscribed, firm, multinodular masses with a variable appearance on cut surface ranging from uniform white to a mosaic of white, cream-pink, and red areas. The histological appearance may vary widely within different areas of the same tumor. Fibroblasts are elongated cells producing collagen and ground substance and the histological appearance of tumors depends on the arrangement of the cells and the relative proportion of cells and extracellular material. Most tumors contain abundant collagen, but in some areas ground substance may predominate, producing a myxomatous appearance. The more cellular areas may suggest malignant transformation, but the fate of these cells appears to be differentiation rather than progression to fibrosarcoma, since cellular areas are common and metastases from these large subcutaneous masses are virtually nonexistent. Fibrosarcomas do occur, but are not common. Their characteristic histological feature is basophilia due to uniform hypercellularity in contrast to the largely eosinophilic fibroma. Mitotic figures are frequent and some tumors contain bizarre giant cells and multinucleate cells.

Dermal Fibroma

Another frequently encountered, but generally small mass, is the dermal fibroma. This is a distinct entity composed of an irregular mass of coarse collagen fibers similar to those of the normal dermis. Larger nodules extend into the subcutis. Both small and large nodules may contain sufficient adipose tissue to justify the combined diagnosis fibrolipoma. The relationship of this tumor to the large subcutaneous fibroma is uncertain, but it is more likely a separate entity rather than a precursor lesion.

Subcutaneous masses are more common in females than in males. Tthey are frequently multiple and usually mammary in origin. The gross and histological appearance of these tumors is highly variable, but the majority are variants of a single entity; i.e., mammary fibroadenoma. The rat has six pairs of mammary glands consisting of milk-secreting epithelium and supporting or contractile stroma. Both epithelial and stromal elements proliferate, hence the diagnosis fibroadenoma. The degree of proliferation often varies in different parts of the same tumor, resulting in areas that are predominantly fibrous, predominantly epithelial, or mixed fibroepithelial. Diagnostic terms such as adenofibroma or fibroadenoma may be used to reflect the relative proportions of each component, but this division is probably unnecessary. Purely fibrous tumors may be impossible to distinguish from subcutaneous fibromas on one single section, but glandular formations may be found if multiple samples of the mass are examined. For statistical classification it is reasonable to consider fibrous tumors in females as a variant of mammary fibroadenoma. Subcutaneous masses are the tumors most frequently seen as "palpable masses" in the in-life phase of long-term studies, but endocrine tumors are just as frequent in the final pathology phase. This group is dominated by the pituitary adenoma both in incidence and biological significance. Pituitary tumors are frequently visible at necropsy and are a common cause of morbidity and mortality. Thyroid C-cell tumors and adrenal pheochromocytomas are less common and frequently microscopic entities.

Endocrine System

Pituitary Adenoma

The anterior pituitary secretes several hormones and pituicytes fall into three main groups, acidophilic, basophilic, and chromophobe depending on the tinctorial properties of the cytoplasm. In the past, attempts were made to use tinctorial classifications in the diagnosis of pituitary tumors, but this has largely been abandoned in favor of the nonspecific diagnosis pituitary adenoma or pituitary tumor. More sophisticated investigational techniques such as ultrastructure, immunocytochemistry, and hormone assay suggest that the majority of tumors secrete prolactin and the term prolactinoma is sometimes used. However, in routine H&E sections it is impossible to delineate functional properties and it is inappropriate to use specific terms without any evidence for the functional status of the tumor. Pituitary adenomas are the most common tumors in several strains of laboratory rats (Boorman and Hollander, 1973; Squire and Levitt, 1975; Cohen et al., 1978). Pituitary tumors range in size from microscopic to macroscopic, raising the question of hyperplasia vs neoplasia. Since large lethal tumors 10 mm or more in diameter are common in this strain, the equally common microscopic lesions of similar cytology but just smaller in terms of size can reasonably be considered in the spectrum of adenomas. The microscopic appearance varies. In females, the cells are generally small to medium in size with relatively little cytoplasm (chromophobes). Dilated vascular channels are frequent and hemosiderin pigment is sometimes found. In males the cytology is much more diverse and bizarre pale eosinophilic cells are often seen. Microscopic tumors may be multicentric, and the larger tumors are nodular masses compressing the brain, often causing hydrocephalus. Most tumors are considered benign even though the cytology may be bizarre. Invasion of the meninges and along vascular channels into the brain is occasionally seen, but metastases are extremely rare.

The large tumors are space occupying and often functional, and frequently result in other histological lesions. In females, acinar hyperplasia of the mammary gland and ovarian atrophy are commonly associated with pituitary neoplasms. Testicular atrophy may occur in males. Other components of the pituitary syndrome are splenic atrophy with hemosiderosis, squamous hyperplasia of the forestomach, and steatosis in the liver. The clinical syndrome of a thin, neurologically abnormal rat with red tear stains around the eyes is almost pathognomonic of large pituitary tumors.

Thyroid Tumors

Naturally occurring thyroid neoplasms occur with high frequency in many strains of rats, particularly after 2 years of age. These tumors have been shown to originate from C or parafollicular cells and to produce calcitonin (Boorman et al., 1972; Deftos et al., 1976; DeLellis et al., 1979). The lesions begin as diffuse or nodular hyperplasia of C cells. When the cells extend through the basement membrane or have distant metastases, they are called medullary thyroid carcinomas because they are similar to this tumor in humans. Unless one is aware of these tumors they are easily missed because they are often microscopic. They tend to metastasize first to the deep cervical lymph nodes. Their malignant nature is more easily assessed if the lymph nodes are examined microscopically.

The thyroid C-cell proliferations are slightly more of a diagnostic problem than those in the pituitary. A minor degree of diffuse proliferation is common and is usually termed hyperplasia. Focal proliferations range from single perifollicular aggregates to grossly visible masses. Terminology varies, but proliferations occupying large areas of the thyroid are common and the smaller foci could reasonably be considered part of the adenoma spectrum. However, other diagnoses used range from nodular hyperplasia to microscopic carcinoma depending on the diagnostic criteria applied by different pathologists. The cells usually form large pale acidophilic nests of round cells, compressing adjacent thyroid follicles. The larger tumors tend to incite fibrous encapsulation and occasionally show focal invasion of the capsule, surrounding tissues, or metastasis to the cervical nodes. These large masses are designated carcinomas, although the cytology and mitotic rate may not markedly differ from the smaller proliferations. Hence, the tendency for some pathologists to refer to all proliferations as carcinoma.

A variety of chemical carcinogens can also induce zymbal gland tumors in the rat (Ward, 1975).

Metabolism   **Christopher P. Chengelis**

GENERAL BACKGROUND

The processes of xenobiotic transformation have been well characterized in the rat. It has been largely the species of choice for the study of hepatic microsomal enzymes. As such, the literature on xenobiotic metabolism in the rat is huge and no attempt will be made here to summarize it exhaustively. We will attempt to cite in a snapshot fashion the necessary information on xenobiotic metabolism to aid the investigator in the design and interpretation of studies of drug action in the rat.

In considering xenobiotic metabolism, one should keep in mind that there can be quantitative as well as qualitative differences between species. For example, at a low dosage (0.16 μg/kg), of benzo(a)pyrene, 1.7% will accumulate in the lungs of rats, whereas 7.9% accumulates in hamster lungs. At a high dosage, these percentages become 9.01 and 8.04% for rat and hamster, respectively (Weyland and Bergman, 1987). This is an example of a quantitative species-related difference. At the low dose of benzo(a)pyrene, the predominant metabolites in all species were thioether (glutathione) conjugates. In contrast, thioethers remained dominant at a high dose of benzo(a)pyrene in guinea pigs, but there was a considerable shift toward glucuronide formation in rats. This is an example of a more qualitative species related difference. Studying metabolism in different species does not always mean that an investigator has to sort through a morass of species related differences. Frequently, more similarities in metabolism exist between species than differences. For example, Berman et al. (1984) studied the in vitro microsomal metabolism of α-naphthaflavone (ANF) by various species. For the most part, all species produced ANF-5, 6 oxide and ANF-dihydrodiol as the predominant metabolites. In addition, total hydrophobic (solvent extractable) metabolite formation was amazingly close between species, ranging from 2.7 to 3.2 nmol/15 min/mg microsomal protein.

As in all species, the liver in the rat is the main site of xenobiotic metabolism. In general, the liver to body weight ratio in the rat is about 2.5–3.2% in fasted rats and about 3.3–4.0% in (ad libitum) fed rats owing to the differences in glycogen content. Many of the characteristics of hepatic xenobiotic metabolism of the rat are summarized in Table 24.

MICROSOMAL MIXED FUNCTION OXIDASE (MMFO)

Native concentration of cytochrome P-450 range from 0.20 to 1.0 nmol/mg microsomal protein, depending on age, sex, and strain of rat examined. The rat was one of the first animals in which cytochrome P-450 was isolated and studied. And it was one of the first animals for which it was realized that cytochrome P-450 exists as a family of isozymes. As the literature in this field is extensive and complex, the reader is referred to reviews by Luand West (1980), Nebert (1981), Gonzales (1989), and Okey (1990), or the compilation assembled by Ortiz de Montellano (1986) for more details. Perhaps as many as 14 different isozymes of cytochrome P-450 have been isolated and characterized with regard to molecular weight, substrate specificity, inducing agent sensitivity, site specificity (the same molecule, testosterone, for example, can be hydroxylated at several different positions by the MMFO, and each site preferentially involves a specific cytochrome P-450 isozyme, as shown by Wood and colleagues in 1983), and Soret visible wavelength absorption (447–452 nm). The isozymic nature of cytochrome P-450 serves as a fundamental explanation for many of the characteristics of the rat MMFO. For example,

Table 24 Summary of Hepatic Xenobiotic Metabolizing Enzymes in Rats

Enzyme	Conentration or activity	Comments and references
Cytochrome P-450 (microsomal)	0.20–1.00 nmol/mg-m 10 to 40 nmol/g (est.)	Variability due to differences in sex, age, and strain of rats used. When these variables are controlled, there is generally good agreement between animals (<10% difference). Astrom et al. (1986), Galinsky et al. (1986), Kiai et al. (1986), Souhaili-el Amri et al. (1986), Chengelis (1988).
Cytochrome b_5 (microsomal)	0.10–0.40 nmole/mg-m 6–17 nmol/g (est.)	Differences with regard to strain, sex, and age are not as prominent as with cytochrome P-450. Astrom et al. (1986), Kiai et al. (1986), Souhaili-el Amri et al. (1986), Chengelis (1988).
NADPH : cytochrome P-450 reductase (microsomal)	75–200 nmol/min/mg-m	For the more common strains. Fuller et al. (1972), Litterest et al. (1975), Souhali-el Amri et al. (1986), Chengelis (1988).
MMFO activities aminopyrene demethyl. aniline hydroxyl. p-nitroanisole demethyl. aryl hydrocar. hydroxyl.	2.3–10.0 nmol/min/ mg-m 0.3–1.6 nmol/min/mg-m 0.3–1.25 nmol/min/ mg-m 0.1–0.4 nmol/min/mg-m	Determined under staturating conditions. Variations with age, sex, and strain. Page and Vessel (1969), Litterest et al. (1975), Astrom et al. (1986), Chengelis (1988), Kai et al. (1988), Koster et al. (1989).
Epoxide hydrolase (with styrene oxide) microsomal cytosolic	2–12 nmol/min/mg-m 30–46 nmol/min/mg-c	Sex-, strain-, and age-related differences. Birnbaum and Baird (1979), Astrom et al. (1983), Chengelis (1988), Kizer et al. (1985), Oesch et al. (1988).
UDP-glucuronosyl transferase 1-naphthol 4-nitrophenol	5–40 nmol/min/mg-m 15–30 nmol/min/mg-m	Boutin et al. (1984), Galainsky et al. (1986), Atrom et al. (1987), Chengelis (1988).
Glutathione S-transferase CDNB 4-nitrobenzyl chloride	360–1400 nmol/min/ mg-c 110–380 nmol/min/ mg-c	James et al. (1977), Gregus et al. (1985), Galinsky (1986), Neal et al. (1987), Chengelis (1988).

Abbreviations: mg-m = mg microsomal protein
mg-c = mg cytosolic protein
g = grams liver
CONB = 1-chloro-2,4,-dinitrobenzene

aromatic hydrocarbon metabolism is high, induced by 3-methylcholanthrene (3-MC) because this agent induces an isozyme (once called cytochrome P-448 in the rat; now known as cytochrome P-450c by most investigators) with high affinity for aromatic hydrocarbons. Also, the well-described differences in MMFO between male and female rats is apparently due to different isozymes of cytochrome P-450 (Kamataki et al., 1985). Hence, we will continually refer to the isozymic nature of rat cytochrome P-450 in the ensuing discussions on age, sex, and hormonal effects on MMFO.

The enzyme NADPH:cytochrome C reductase (also known as NADPH:cytochrome P-450 reductase) is the other main enzymic component of the MMFO. It has also been isolated, purified, and well characterized in the rat. Unlike cytochrome P-450, it does not exist as a family of isozymes. Only one enzyme exists and different isozymes are not induced by different agents. In fact, in the rat, phenobarbital and pregnenolone-16α-carbonitrile (PCN)–type inducing agents induce increases in both cytochrome P-450 and the reductase, whereas 3-MC–type agenst induce cytochrome P-450, but not the reductase in rats (Lu et al., 1972). The more effective inducer of the reductase than of cytochrome P-450 is PCN, whereas phenobarbital is the better inducer of cytochrome P-450. There has been recurring debate as to whether the reductases of cytochrome P-450 are the rate-limiting step in MMFO activity, but it is generally believed in the activity of the reductase is the rate-limiting step in MMFO activity (Mannering, 1971). Miwa et al. (1978) reported that incorporation of previously isolated reductase into freshly prepared micromal preparations resulted in rate enhancements which depended on the substrate examined and whether the micromes were isolated from induced animals.

The concentrations of cytochrome b_5 range from 0.1 to 0.4, and remain remarkably constant across age, sex, and strain of rats. Inducing agents generally have little effect on cytochrome b_5 concentrations in the rat. The role of cytochrome b_5 in MMFO oxidation was once the center of some controversy (see Jansson and Schenkman, 1973) and has been most highly investigated in rats. The nub of the controversy was whether or not cytochrome b_5 played a facilitative role in the electron transfer in the "oxygen reduction" phase of the MMFO cycle. Tamburini et al. (1985) demonstrated that cytochrome b_5 tightly binds to cytochrome P-450, and this binding results in enhanced affinity of cytochrome P-450 for MMFO substrates. In rabbits, cytochrome b_5 has also been shown to play a facilitative or inhibitory role depending on the substrate (Pompon and Coon, 1984). Janssen and collegueges (1985) subsequently established that cytochrome b_5 interacts differently with different rat cytochrome P-450 isozymes, and thus plays a facilitative role in the oxidation of some substrates, and an inhibitory role in others, depending on the cytochrome P-450 isozyme involved. Given that the isozymic character of cytochrome P-450 is under a variety of controls, the involvement of cytochrome b_5 in xenobiotic metabolism is the rat can also be expected to shift accordingly.

The activities of the MMFO with several model substrates are also summarized on Table 24. Across rodent species, the rat does not have either the highest concentrations of cytochrome P-450 or levels of MMFO activity. This was highlighted by Kato in his review in 1979. Souhaili-el Amri et al. (1986) also noted that the male rat had less cytochrome P-450 than either the guinea pig or the male rabbit. In addition, when maximal velocities where examined, the rat had the highest activities with only one substrate, benzo(a)pyrene. The guinea pig had the highest activities with four of the substrates (aminopyrine, benzphetamine, p-nitroanisole, and 7-ethoxycoumarin). This can have obvious toxocological consequences. For example, Hutson and Logan (1986) attributed the higher sensitivity of rats as opposed to other rodents to chlorofenvinphos (an organophosphate insecticide) to a lower rate of metabolism in the rat. One should not assume, therefore, that the rat has the highest rates of metabolism for the chemical under study. In fact, there are several instances where a nonrodent, such as the dog (Duignan et al., 1987) have higher rates of oxidation for a substrate than the rat.

The previous paragraph stressed quantitative differences between the rat MMFO and those of other species. There are also qualitative differences. The rat has a high tendency to hydroxylate aromatic structures (e.g., benzene to phenol). The rat has a considerable ability to produce "phenolic" metabolites from chemicals like benzo(a)pyrene and aniline. Take the often sited example of the metabolism of amphetamine. The major pathway in the rat is the formation of 4-hydroxyamphetamine, whereas in other species the major pathway is through oxidative deamination to benzoic acid derivatives. There are exceptions. The rat, for example, lacks the ability to metabolize warfarin to 7-hydroxy-warfarin as other species do. Also, unlike many other species, the rat lacks the ability to oxidize the terminal nitrogen in aliphatic amines (Caldwell, 1981). N-Octylamine is, in fact, a very good inhibitor of cytochrome P-450–dependent MMFO activity in the rat. Similarly, the rat produces relatively few deaminated metabolites in the metabolism of amphetamine.

Not all reactions catalyzed by the MMFO (in the rat as well as other species) are oxidative in nature. Several reductive pathways of toxocological importance are also catalyzed by this system. For example, the carcinogenic activation of azo dyes by rat liver preparations has been extensively explored, with p-dimethylaminoazobenzene (DAB) being the prototypical agent. As reviewed by Zbaida (1989), N-demethylation and N-oxidation reactions are inovlved in the activation of DAB to ultimate carcinogens, whreas detoxification is associated with C-oxidation and reductive cleavage of the azo bond. Their work clearly demonstrates the MMFO is involved in the reductive as well as the oxidative reactions. The rat is obviously a good model for the study of these reactions. Interestingly, azoreductase activity is highly inducible by β-naphthaflavone (a "3-MC–type" inducing agent that is commonly used because, unlike 3-MC, it is not carcinogenic). In the case of azo dyes, induction of "carcinogen-specific cytochrome P-450," leads to decreases in carcinogenic activation.

The MMFO of the rat has been shown to have definite stereospecificity. Traiger and collegueges (Bush and Traiger, 1985; Heinmark and Traiger, 1985) have published a very elegant series of studies on the metabolism of warfarin, demonstrating stereospecificity, both in terms of preferred substrate (R over S) and major metabolite formed (8-hydroxy vs 6-hydroxy) in rats. Cook et al. (1982) examined the stereospecificity of disopyramide metabolism and observed in vivo that the (S)-enatiomer was more extensively metabolized. In addition, the major metabolite with the (S)-enatiomer was the 3-methoxyphenol metabolite, whereas none of this was produced from the (R)-enantionmer (which was largely excreted unchanged) where the predominant metabolite was mono-N-dealkylated disopyramide. Hence, in the rat, optical activity can govern both the rate and the pattern of metabolism. As one can judge on the basis of these two examples, it is difficult to determine a priori which enantiomer will be preferred and may vary with substrate. In addition, there may well be species differences; the preferred isomer in rats may not be preferred isomer in human subjects.

Inhibition (of the MMFO)

The MMFO of the rat is inhibited by a wide variety of chemicals. We will limit ourselves to a discussion of the of four different major classes of inhibition: (1) direct competitive agents, (2) suicide substrates, (3) synthesis inhibitors, and (4) antibodies.

Direct Competitive Agents

The classic competitive inhibitors of the MMFO are represented by agents such as SKF 525-A, metyrapone, and 2,4'-dichloro-6-phenyl-phenoxyethylamine (HCl) which avidly bind the catalytic site on cytochrome P-450 (Soliman et al., 1974). SKF 525-A has been widely used by many investigators to block the metabolic activation of many indirect hepatotoxins. Generally, the dose administered is 75 mg/kg (intraperitoneally in saline) 30–60 min prior to the administration of the chemical under study. Murray (1989) reviewed these mechanisms of reversible inhibition associated with the imidazole or quinoline drugs. Ketoconazole, for example, is the prototypical imidazole antifungal agent that inhibits cytochrome P-450–mediated reactions in both the liver and the adrenal gland. Piperonyl butoxide (Freidman and Couch, 1974) was used as an adjunct with various insectisides to inhibit their metabolism and detoxification in the target species. It is also an inhibitor in rats and is most commonly given 500 mg/kg ip in corn oil. In theory, any substrate for the MMFO can competitively inhibit the metabolism of any other substrate, depending on the affinity constants, dosages, and isozymes of cytochrome P-450 involved. Such interactions are, in fact, a major concern in polypharmacy and the rat provides an excellent model for the study of these types of interactions.

Suicide Substrates

In contrast to the reversible inhibitors just discussed, the suicide substrates are irreversible substrates that are not necessarily distinctive on the basis of affinity or low turnover number. Upon oxidation by the MMFO, they form reactive metabolites that subsequently irreversibly bind to and denature cytochrome P-450. Substrate specificity can be used to selectively inhibit specific cytochrome P-450 isozymes. Halpert et al. (1985), for example, have reported that chloramphenicol (300 mg/kg ip given in 0.5 ml propylene glycol) can lead to the destruction of only three of eight of the major cytochrome P-450 isozymes as determined by their methodology. These included the major phenobarbitol-inducible isozymes, whereas the isozymes induced by β-NF, PCN, or clofibrate were unaffected by chloramphenicol treatment. Dekker et al. (1986, 1989) have reported that 7α-thiosteroids specifically deactivate the rat cytochrome P-450 induced by dexamethasone. It is probably only a matter of time before highly specific suicide substrates are available for all known rat cytochrome P-450 species.

Synthesis Inhibitors

Chemicals that inhibit cytochrome P-450 synthesis or stimulate its breakdown will also have an inhibitory effect on MMFO activity. Agents that generally block protein synthesis have been used to study mechanisms of induction, but lack specificity to be used as MMFO inhibitors. Generally, agents that inhibit the synthesis of hemoprotein or stimulate hemoprotein deactivation (by increasing the activity of heme oxygenase) are more acceptable MMFO inhibitors. Cobalt (as the chloride salt) inhibits heme syntheses and has long been used as a tool to inhibit the MMFO-mediated activation of indirect hepatotoxins. The typical treatment regimen is 250 μmol/kg sc given 48, 36, 24, and 12 hr prior to hepatotoxic challenge (Chengelis, 1988a). As discussed by Spaethe and Jallow (1989); however, the use of $CoCl_2$ as an MMFO inhibitor has several disadvantages in that its effect on cytochrome P-450 is relatively brief and that other enzyme systems are affected as well. They discovered that cobaltic protoporphyrin IX can profoundly depress cytochrome P-450 from 3 to 5 weeks. In rats, a single dose (90 μg/kg sc) led to approximately 90% depletion in cytochrome P-450 1 week posttreatment. This resulted in large decreases in the V_{max} of the MMFO toward all typical model substrates but had no effect on FMFO, UDP-glucuronosyl transferase, PAPS-sulfotransferase, or glutathione S-transferase activities. Hence, Co-protoporphyrin would made an excellent inhibitor to use as a tool for studying the involvement of the MMFO in the metabolism and/or toxicity of a drug or chemical in the rat.

Antibodies

Antibodies to cytochrome P-450 represent a fourth class of cytochrome P-450 inhibitor. They have the disadvantage of being useful only for in vitro broken cell studies. The specificity of antibodies can be used to discern or confirm the specific isozyme of cytochrome P-450 involved in a reaction. For example, Thomas et al. (1977) compared antibody inhibition patterns against various substrates to demonstrate the marked differences in the spectrum of cytochrome P-450 isozymes induced in control vs phenobarbital-, 3-MC–, and PCN-treated rats. As discussed elsewhere, antibodies to NADPH:cytochrome c reductase can be used to discriminate between MMFO- and FMFO-catalyzed metabolic transformations.

There are a variety of miscellaneous other agents that inhibit the MMFO by mechanisms that do not involve direct interaction with cytochrome P-450. These include agents such as menadione, which is a substrate for, and therefore competes with cytochrome P-450 for, NADPH:cytochrome c reductase (Utley and Mehendale, 1989). In fact, it is the reduction of menadione by NADPH:cytochrome c reductase that is believed to be responsible for menadione cytotoxicity (Utley and Mehendale, 1989). Ethanol has also been repeatedly shown to inhibit MMFO activity, but the mechanism is the subject of debate. There is little doubt, however, that at high concentrations (80–100 mM) ethanol inhibits the MMFO. Both menadione and ethanol have pharmacological and toxicological properties that limit their usefulness as in vivo as MMFO inhibitors. For example, ethanol is not a MMFO-potent inhibitor and, regardless of the underlying mechanism, would be a poor choice to use as an in vivo MMFO inhibitor because of the CNS depression that would be caused at the dosages required.

Induction (of the MMFO)

The fact that the activity of the MMFO with different substrates respond differently to various inducing agent played a key role in the elucidation of the molecular biology of cytochrome P-450. Induction (or hepatic enzyme induction) refers to the process whereby treatment of an animal with a chemical results in an increased amount of endoplasmic reticulum, accompanied by an increased activity of the MMFO. Induction will almost always result in an increased amount of microsomal protein, and this alone will cause increased MMFO activity. In the strictest sense of the word, however, induction will also result in increased specific activity (i.e., increased V_{max} on a milligram protein basis). The term *induction* had come to be applied loosely to both situations. In the rat, enzyme induction is almost always accompanied by increases in liver weight. In fact, the rat is a highly inducible species, and subchronic treatment with almost any organic chemical may well cause increases in liver weight. There are generally three classes of inducing agents, each class named for the prototypical agent: phenobarbital, 3-methylcholanthrene (3-MC), and pregnenalone-16-carbonitrile (PCN). They are differentiable on the basis of the classes of cytochrome P-450 isozymes they induce as well as the exact mechanisms of induction (as reviewed by Gonzlaes, 1989). Some agents are more specific than others. Mixtures of polychlorinated hydrocarbons (e.g., Aroclor 1254) induces both phenobarbital and 3-MC-type activities. It is for this reason that hepatic preparations used in the Ames Salmonella assay for mutagenicity are taken from rats treated with Arocolor 1254. Other enyzmes could also be affected. Phenobarbital, for example, will also induce increases in UDP-glucuronosyl and glutathione S-transferases in the rat. With phenobarbital, good induction (approximate doubling of cytochrome P-450 with about 30% increases in liver weight) is obtained with three dosages of 80 mg/kg (intraperitoneally in saline with the pH corrected by HCl) over a 3-day period. For 3-MC–type induction, current practice is to use one dose of 100 mg/kg (intraperitoneally in corn oil) β-naphthaflavone (β-NF, which is not carcinogenic) followed by a 3-day rest period. Induction with PCN is usually affected by giving 25–50 mg/kg ip for 3–4 days. Induction can provide a convenient tool for studying metabolism of a specific chemical in the rat. For example, Decker et al. (1989) reported that spironolactone caused slight losses of cytochrome P-450 in naive rats, but will cause much more profound losses in rats pretreated with dexamethasone (a PCN-type agent that causes increases in cytochrome P-450p). This allowed for more thorough study of this phenomenon: the "suicide substrate" destruction of hepatic cytochrome P-450 by spironolactone.

What are the implications of microsomal enzyme induction? The rat is a highly inducible species, and teleologically, this may explain why it tends to have lower baseline activity than other less inducible rodent species, such as the hamster. It is a rare chemical that (if given in a high enough dosage for a long enough period of time) will not have some inductive effect in the rat. Increases in liver weight with centrilobular hepatocyte hypertrophy (due to proliferation of the smooth endoplasmic reticulum) is a common finding in toxicity studies using the rat. This is a reversible, adaptive response and should not be considered (of and by itself) evidence of toxicity.

Alterations of intrinsic hormone metabolism can be another implication of induction. In the rat, a frequent example of this is increased metabolism and clearance of thyroid hormones (T3 and T4). While not cytochrome P-450 mediated (rather these reactions are primarily catalyzed by UDP-glucuronosyl transferase, discussed below), they are still inducible. The increased clearance of thyroid hormones, a primary effect of microsomal enzyme induction, results in increased synthesis and release of the pituitary hormone TSH. Hence, an increased size and weight, and sometimes a frank increase in thyroid tumors in long-term studies, may be a secondary effect of hepatic microsomal enzyme induction.

Induction may be accompanied by other physiological changes that may have little to do with increases in xenobiotic metabolism. Induction of MMFO in the rat often causes concomitant changes in plasma proteins. Typical clinical chemical panels in toxicity studies can result in the increased production of various microglobulins by the liver (Makvananda et al., 1987). Hence, MMFO induction in the rat may be accompanied by slight increases in serum proteins associated with an increase in the globulin fraction. Such changes are of little, if any, toxicological importance. As discussed by Makaranaada (1987), however, chemical-induced liver damage will also cause changes in the components of the globulin fraction, albeit different ones than those changed by induction. One should not, therefore, jump to a conclusion concerning an increase in the globulin fraction without examining the liver histologically and/or examining plasma proteins by electrophoresis.

An other implication with regard to induction is that the rat is more inducible than most species. For example, Astrom et al. (1986) compared the effects of 3-MC induction in the rat, hamster, guinea pig, and two strains of mice. In rats, 3-MC produced a threefold increase in cytochrome P-450 and a 100-fold increase in 7-ethoxyresorufin deethylation activity. In hamsters and guinea pigs, the same treatment induced only 1.5- to 2.5-fold increases in cytochrome P-450 and five- to sevenfold increases in 7-ethoxyresorufin deethylation activity, respectively. In mice, the responses were strain dependent: 3-MC did not induce increases in DBA/2 mice, but did induce increases in cytochrome P-450 and MMFO activity in C57bl/6 mice. Hence, one can not always extrapolate from the results obtained in rats to other species. In fact, it is likely that a weak inducer in rats will have little inductive effect in other species.

Another implication of induction in the rat is that increases in cytochrome P-450 are not always accompanied by increases in MMFO activity. The inducing agent may cause a change in the isozymic spectrum of cytochrome P-450 such that the activity of the MMFO toward some substrates may actually decrease. For example, Astrom et al. (1986) have reported that 3-MC induction resulted in decreases in the rate of aminopyrine metabolism in vitro. Rhodes and Houstan (1983) have reported that phenobarbital caused a slight decrease in the formation of $14C-CO_2$ from 14C-antipyrene in vivo in rats, whereas β-NF caused a 50% increase. Ioannides et al. (1981) demonstrated 3-MC induction in rats enhanced subsequent benzo(a)pyrene mutagenicity in the Ames assay, whereas phenobarbital decreased it. The opposite occurred with 2-AAF induction. Thus, the type of induction (i.e., the isozyme of cytochrome P-450) can have important implications with regard to the toxicity of other agents in the rat. For example, as discussed by Lesca (1984), different mutagenic agents are preferentially activated by different cytochrome P-450 isozymes: Ethidium bromide is preferentially activated by 3-MC–inducible MMFO activity. A single 80 mg/kg treatment of rats with 3-MC caused over a 100-fold increase in the number of revertant colonies in the Ames assay vs the response obtained with liver enzyme preparations obtained from control rats. Phenobarbital and PCN, in contrast, caused only modest (2.5–3.5%) increases. Phenobarbital, however, did induce 100-fold increases in response in the Ames assay to cyclophosphamide, whereas 3-MC caused no increase in this response. Aroclor caused increases in the mutagenic activity of both ethidium bromide and cyclophosphamide, indicative of the broad spectrum of isozymes induced by this agent. Lesca (1984) recommended using changes in responses in the Ames assay to known mutagens to determine the nature of cytochrome P-450 induced by new chemical entities in the rat.

Rats are common species used for carcinogenicity testing. What are the potential implications of chronic exposure of rats to an inducing agent? Kurata et al. (1989) studied the long-term effects of phenobarbital on the liver and the MMFO. The greatest degree of induction was achieved with 7 weeks of treatment. MMFO activity and cytochrome P-450 concentrations fell off slightly thereafter, but remained at a plateau 2.5- to 3.5-fold greater than control levels for the remainder of the study. Hence, induction has a finite effect: The liver cannot hypertrophy indefinitely. In pharmacological terms, rats accommodate to induction but do not become tachyphylactic. Many chemicals induce increases in their own metabolism. In a chronic toxicity study, plasma levels of the parent test article often decrease, whereas levels of metabolites increase during the test period. This can result in changes in toxicity depending on whether the parent or the metabolite is most responsible for toxicity.

Other than expected pharmacokinetic consequences does induction have any other implications? Lubet et al. (1989) explored the relationship between induction and hepatocellular tumor promotion. They suggested that potent inducing agents of cytochrome P-450b (e.g., phenobarbital, DDT) are all potent liver tumor promoters. Structural analogs (e.g., hexobarbital) which are not potent inducing agents are also poor liver tumor promoters. In addition, hamsters, where cytochrome P-450 is not inducible, are resistant to hepatocellular tumor promotion. Hence, in chronic toxicity studies in the rat with inducing agents, promotion of naturally occurring "background" hepatic neoplasias is a real possibility such that an nongenotoxic chemical could appear to be an hepatic carcinogen.

Most of the implication of induction in the rat have to do with the specific isozymes of cytochrome P-450 induced. Therefore, if in the testing of a chemical, one has reason to believe that it is an inducing agent (gross increases in liver weight, centrilobular hypertrophy, increases in the grossly measurable cytochrome P-450), then identification of the specific isozyme of cytochrome P-450 induced would aid in determining the implications of such findings. This can be accomplished without isolating and characterizing microsomal proteins by immunoelectrophoresis (Thomas et al., 1983, 1984) by simply looking at shifts in metabolic patterns in crude microsomal preparations. Wood et al. (1983) used changes in in vitro testosterone metabolism to discriminate or categorize types of induction. For example, a shift in in vitro metabolize spectrum that includes a large increase in 16β-testosterone formation would be indicative of cytochrome P-450a, or phenobarbital-type induction in the rat. 7-Ethoxyresorufin is a specific substrate for 3-MC–inducible cytochrome P-450b and e. Iwasaki et al. (1986) reported that 3-MC treatment (50 mg/kg ip for 3 days) increased 7-ethoxyresorufin deethylation 32-fold (from 0.05 to 1.6 nmol/min/nmol. These increases will appear even larger when corrected for increases in microsomal protein. Thus, the estimation of changes in the metabolic rate and/or metabolite profile for a handful of well-studied model MMFO substrates can provide useful metabolic and toxicological information.

In summary, the phenomenon of microsomal enzyme induction rat has been well studied in the rat. Different chemical classes have somewhat different specific effects but, in general, most of the implications of microsomal induction are due to the increases in specific isozymes of cytochrome P-450. The rat is a highly inducible species, but there are age-, sex-, and strain-related quantitative differences. Given that, and also given the implications induction may have for the metabolism and toxicity of a chemical in the rat, the careful investigator should consider inspection of the type of induction related to a specific chemical under study. The technology for doing so is available and easily adaptable.

Microsomal induction studies generally involve biochemical analyses conducted at a single time point following treatment with the suspect inducing agent. One needs to be cautious in the design and interpretation of such studies, however, as different isozymes have time courses of response to different inducing agents. For example, Parkinson et al. (1983a) examined the time course of the response of Long-Evans rats to a single dose of Aroclor 1254 (500 mg/kg ip). Cytochrome P-450c was maximally induced 2 days after treatment and remained constant. In contrast, cytochrome P-450a was not maximally induced until 9 days after treatment. Other isozymes had yet different patterns. All isozymes started to decline 15 days following treatment. Hence, if one is concerned about the nature of the hepatic induction affected by a poorly characterized chemical in the rat, several time points should be examined.

Sex-Related Differences

The hepatic MMFO is under a variety of hormonal controls that are responsible for the well-reported differences in male and female rats. In fact, sex-related differences have been most frequently and convincingly demonstrated in the rat as opposed to other species. Hormonal control of drug oxidation is very complex but has been most well characterized in the rat. This effort dates back to the late 1950s and early 1960s, when it was first noticed that there was a sex difference in drug metabolism, with males generally having higher activity than females. For example, Kato et al. (1964) demonstrated that male Wistar rats had consistently higher in vitro rates of microsomal aniline, aminopyrine, and strychnine metabolism. Furner et al. (1969) reported that regardless of the strain of rats examined, male rats generally had higher rates of microsomal metabolism with aniline, aminopyrine, ethylmorphine, and other model substrates. The extent of this difference varied depending on age, strain, and substrate examined. These earlier works were among the first to also note that the sex-related difference were less apparent in sexually immature rats. This has also been confirmed repeatedly and will be discussed in greater detail below (under Age-Related Changes).

Ariyoshi et al. (1981) demonstrated in Wistar rats that there was no difference in cytochrome P-450 content between males and females at 30 days of age, but there were large differences at 300 days. Tht fact that the sex-related differences in xenobiotic metabolism were less apparent in sexually immature rats led to many experiments exploring the hormonal control of MMFO activity. The work in this area has been reviewed in detail by Skett (1988).

In general, there are substantial data suggesting that the androgenic and estrogenic hormones exert different and competing modulating effects on MMFO activity. For example, early work demonstrated that castration reduced activity in males to female levels and testosterone supplementation "remasculinzed" drug metabolism in rats. The differences are due to differences in the total amount of as well as the spectrum of cytochrome P-450 isozymes induced. Kato and coworkers (Kamataki et al., 1985) have identified two distinct (by immunological methods and by electrophoretic mobility) forms of cytochrome P-450 (termed cytochrome P-450–male and P-450–female) that are specific to the respective sexes in Fischer 344 rats. Cytochrome P-450–male is associated with a higher rate of MMFO activity with several model substrates (e.g., 7-propoxycoumarin, aniline, and benzphetamine) than cytochrome P-450–female. High levels of cytochrome P-450–male are induced by testosterone: Castration leads to decreases in this isozyme. In contrast, cytochrome P-450–female is present only in female rats and the levels are attenuated after oophorectomy and exogenous testosterone administration. Other hormonal effects on MMFO activity have been reported. Growth hormone (a pituitary hormone) has been shown to have a feminizing effect on xenobiotic metabolism in the rat (Skett, 1988), also presumably due to differences in expression of cytochrome P-450 isozymes. Waxman et al. (1985), example, have described a distinct isozyme of cytochrome P-450 (termed P450 2c($\male$)/UT-A) which is responsible for testosterone 16α-hydroxylation activity in liver microsomes from male rats. Castration of male rats at birth led to diminished amounts (to levels found in female rats) of both this cytochrome P-450 isozyme and 16α-hydroxylation activity.

While hormonal effects on MMFO activity are generally attributed to control and expression of specific cytochrome P-450 isozymes, other actions are also involved. Waxman et al. (1989) demonstrated that hypothesectomy resulted in elevated amounts of several cytochrome P-450 isozymes and decreases in others, but there was little correlation between the changes in cytochrome P-450 with changes in MMFO activity. They demonstrated that this was due to decreases (26–30% of control) in NADPH:cytochrome P-450 reductase activity and was restored by exogenous T_4 treatment, but not by other hormones. They concluded that the reductase is subject to hormonal controls that are distinct from those for cytochrome P-450. This observation is also consistent with the observation that reductase activity is also the rate-limiting step in MMFO reactions.

In summary, the well-described sex-related differences in MMFO activity (toward xenobiotics and endogenous steroid hormones) in the rat (with males generally having higher activity than females) are due to the implicit hormonal differences that result in the expression of different isozymes of cytochrome P-450 and total NADPH:reductase activity. Hence, it is not at all uncommon for a chemical to have different pharmacokinetic behavior in male vs female rats, or for there to be quantitative differences in chemical toxicity between the two sexes of this species. In addition, as the use of surgically altered rats in pharmacological experiments is not uncommon, these potential effects that the resulting hormone changes may have on drug metabolism should be kept in mind.

Strain-Related Differences

Strain-related differences in MMFO activity and inducibility have long been recognized, as Conney (1967) mentioned in an early review on the subject of microsomal drug metabolism. In their classic 1969 article, Page and Vessel compared native and induced rates of in vitro (with S-9 fractions) oxidation of ethylmorphine and aniline in 10 different strains of rat. They noted several strain-related differences. For example, baseline aniline hydroxylation activity in males varied from 6.9 (Wistar) to 20.2 nmol/min/mg (Long-Evans). Interestingly, there were these baseline differences in activity despite the fact that cytochrome P-450 content did not differ substantially between strains. Following induction by phenobarbital, activity tripled in Wistar rats but increased only 50% in Long-Evans rats. More recently, Koster et al. (1989) examined strain-related differences in the MMFO of 14 highly inbred strains which had originated from four different European facilities, and identified considerable strain-related variations. Kai et al. (1988) determined that Sprague-Dawley rats had lower amounts of cytochrome P-450 as well as lower MMFO activity with the model substrates aniline and aminopyrine than Wistar rats. The Sprague-Dawley rat, however, was more inducible with malotilate than the Wistar rat. Augustine and Zemaitis (1989) also demonstrated that there were significant differences in MMFO activity between Wistar, Sprague-Dawley, and Fischer 344 rats. Jackson et al. (1987) reported that citral was a more potent inducer in Long-Evans than in Wistar rats.

There are also strain-related differences in the metabolism of endogenous substrates. Shefer (1972), for example, compared testosterone 7α-hydroxylation activity in Charles River Sprague-Dawley (CD-1) and Wistar rats. Activity was 3.59 and 2.36 nmol/min/mg (approximately 50% difference), respectively. Following phenobarbital treatment, there was essentially no change in this enzyme activity in Sprague-Dawley rats, but a sixfold increase in Wistar rats. While there are exceptions, three generalizations tend to emerge from the literature with regard to strain-related differences in MMFO activity in rats: (1) In all strains, males have higher activity than females. Quantitatively, this difference is greater in the Fischer 344 and Long-Evans strains than the Sprague-Dawley and Wistar strains. (2) Baseline (native) activities in Wistar rats tend to be lower than those of the Fischer 344 and Long-Evans strains, and the Sprague-Dawley strain tends to be intermediate. (3) The Wistar strain tends to show the greater inductive response to phenobarbital-type inducers.

Strain-related differences are an important consideration in the design and interpretation of toxicity studies, but they can also be used as specific experimental tools. The Lewis and DA rats are closely related strains that differ in that the DA rat has poor hepatic debrisoquine 4-hydroxylation activity (Kahn et al., 1985). Hietanen et al., (1986) demonstrated that S-9–mediated mutagenicity of aflatoxin B_1 in the Ames assay (as well as the metabolism toward ochratoxin) were also much lower in DA rats. Tucker et al. (1981)

made interesting use of strain-related differences in rats to study the metabolism and toxicity of carbon disulfide. In their hands, the extent of CS_2-mediated hepatic hydropic degeneration varied considerably in four different inbred strains of rats, and was accompanied by hepatic necrosis in the most susceptible strain. There was also a good correlation between the extent of hepatic damage and the CS_2-mediated loss of cytochrome P-450 (CS_2 being a suicide substrate). Hence, while the exact mechanism is unclear, these results demonstrate the loss of cytochrome P-450 is involved in the mechanism of CS_2-mediated hepatotoxicity. These examples demonstrate the utility of using strain-related differences for studying the relationship between metabolism and toxicity of a drug or chemical.

Celier et al. (1989) have recently described an interesting strain-related phenomenon involving the Gunn rat. As discussed elsewhere (see under Conjugation Reactions) this strain has a well-characterized lack of UDP-glucuronosyl transferase activity. Celier and colleagues further demonstrated that the Gunn rat also does not respond to 3-MC induction with increases in total cytochrome P-450, but does develop increases in MMFO activity with substrates such as 7-ethoxyresorufin, generally associated with this type of induction. Immunoquantification methods demonstrated that 3-MC–treated male (a different pattern was seen in females) Gunn rats had increases in cytochrome P-450c and P-450d, but with a equivalent decrease in other isozymes. A more usual inductive pattern would have been an increase in specific isozymes while the levels of others remained constant. Interestingly, while 3-MC has been shown to induce UDP-glucuronosyl transferase (as well as cytochrome P-450) in other rat strains, it does not induce increases in Gunn rats. The example of the Gunn rat provides an interesting example of a sex difference nested within a strain difference in inductive response. This highlights the need to be very cautious in interpreting the implication of microsomal induction in the rat.

The Zucker rat is a strain with a marked tendency to develop obesity and is frequently used as a model to study the physiological consequences of this condition. This strain is not commonly used to study toxicological problems, but does provide an interesting example of strain-related differences which can be tied to phenotypic expression. Brouwer et al. (1984) compared the inductive response of lean vs obese Zucker rats to Sprague-Dawley rats and found that phenobarbital treatment caused similar increases in Sprague-Dawley and lean Zucker rats; that is, increases in antipyrine clearance, liver weight, microsomal protein, and cytochrome P-450 content. The obese Zucker rat, however, failed to respond to phenobarbital treatment with increases in any of these parameters.

Another implication in considering strain-related differences is illustrated by the case of pregnenolone-16α-carbonitrile. There has been some debate on whether or not pregnenolone-16α-carbonitrile induced increases in benzo(a)pyrene metabolism in the rat. This disagreement resulted from strain-, age-, and sex-related differences, as reported by Gorski et al. (1985). They demonstrated that PCN did induce increases in benzo(a)pyrene metabolism in 1-month-old rats regardless of strain (Long-Evans, Sprague-Dawley, Wistar, or Holtzman). Differences began to develop as the rats matured. In male (but not female) Long-Evans rats, for example, inducibility of benzo(a)pyrene metabolism with PCN decreased with age. Hence, the age, sex, and strain of rat used as well as the model substrate and assay techniques can all influence the apparent inductive response in the rat. It is not unusual to see this type of disagreement in the literature. This example also underscores the need to pay close attention to experimental details, such as the sex, strain, and age of rats used when one needs to replicate the work of another investigator.

While strain-related differences in metabolism may often be the basis for the differences in toxicity, this is not always the case. For example, acetaminophen is nephrotoxic in Fischer 344 rats but not in Sprague-Dawley rats. Tarloff et al. (1989) extensively explored the metabolism and pharmacokinetics of acetaminophen in age- and sex-matched rats for these two strains and could not identify any differences to account for the strain-related differences in toxicity. Further, Newton et al. (1983) were unable to identify any specific differences in renal xenobiotic metabolism that could provide an explanation for the difference in acetaminophen nephrotoxicity in these two strains of rat. Elsewhere, Plummer et al. (1987) were unable to identify any metabolic differences between Fisher 344 and DA rats that could account for the strain-related differences in sensitivity to aflatoxin. In other studies (Kahn et al., 1987), this group was also unable to demonstrate differences between DA and Fischer 344 rats with regard to phenacetin metabolism.

Age-Related

Age-related changes in xenobiotic metabolism, particularly that affected by the MMFO, has been studied in the rat for quite some time. In general, these studies fall into two categories: those on postnatal or perinatal changes, and those on senescent changes. Perinatal changes will be discussed first.

In 1964, Kato et al. claimed (quoting earlier works by Fouts and Jondorf) that "It is a well known fact that in new born animals there is a deficiency in certain drug metabolizing enzymes." They demonstrated (using female Sprague-Dawley rats) that the in vitro microsomal metabolism of five different model substrates was quite low in neonatal rats (approximately 5% of the activities observed in 30-day-old rats), but these activities increased gradually and steadily to a peak in 30-day-old rats and declined thereafter. They also demonstrated that there were age-related changes in NADPH:cytochrome P-450 reductase that paralleled the changes in MMFO activity.

Nearly 10 years after the publication by Kato et al. (1964), Muller et al. (1973) published on age-related changes in cytochrome P-450 in male Wistar rats; the concentrations in 10-day-old rats were less than half of those observed in adult (30- to 60-day-old) rats. Barbital was a poor inducer in young rats. This paper also noted that changes in MMFO with age did not correlate well with the amount of cytochrome P-450, but did not mention the earlier work by Kato. The additional literature in this area through 1980 is summarized by Klinger (1982). While he questioned whether the activity of NADPH:cytochrome P-450 reductase is the rate-limiting step in all MMFO activities, his review clearly indicates that neonatal rats have low MMFO activity which may be due to a combination of factors: low amounts of cytochrome P-450 (not always seen by all investigators), the low activity of NADPH:cytochrome P-450 reductase, and the isozymic character of the cytochrome P-450 present.

Depending on the model substrate, there are different time courses of MMFO development and responsiveness to inducing agents. Devasagayam et al. (1983), for example, reported that female Wistar rats at 1 day of age have 25% of the cytochrome P-450 and 20% of the NADPH:cytochrome P-450 reductase as those at 75 days of age. While there are exceptions, in general, the sex-dependent differences in MMFO activity are not apparent in neonatal rats and tend to develop concurrently with sexual maturity. Waxman and collegeuges (1985) demonstrated that this was because different gonadal hormones control the levels of different cytochrome P-450 isozymes. For example, both males and females are born with very low testosterone 16α-hydroxylating ability. This increases rapidly in males, but remains low in females even after sexual maturation (4–6 weeks of age).

The quantitative and qualitative responsiveness of neonatal and perinatal rats to inducing agents is still a matter of some debate. In contrast to the aforementioned results with barbital, Pyykko (1983) reported that perinatal (3-day-old) rats are as responsive to the inducing effects of toluene as adults. In toxicological research, experiments which require the treatment of neonatal rats are probably quite rare. The inducibility of 2-day-old rats may be of intellectual interest, but the implications in developmental/reproductive toxicity are not clear. In contrast to inducibility, the fact that neonatal rats have a low metabolic capacity has definite toxicological implications. Depending on the toxicological mechanism of action of chemical, neonatal rats will respond differently than adult rats. For example, CC14 requires metabolic activation for hepatotoxicity, and neonatal rats are refractory to CC14-induced hepatic damage.

The activity of MMFO in rats has also been shown to change with advancing age. Kato et al. (1964) also discussed changes in senescence. In general, MMFO activity appears to decrease as rats age. For example, Kato (1964) noted that cardosopil metabolism peaked at 30 days of age and declined progressively thereafter. The rates of plasma clearance were equivalent in 15- vs 250-day-old rats. Baird et al. (1974) reported that there were age-related (30- to 900-day-old) changes in CFN male rats in that while the concentrations of cytochrome P-450 did not decline appreciably, in vitro microsomal metabolism of zoxazolamine did, and this decline seemed to reflect an age-related decline in NADPH:cytochrome P-450 activity. Rikens and Notley (1981, 1982a,b) examined age-related changes in male Fischer 344 rats, and found that microsomal cytochrome P-450, cytochrome b_5, and NADPH:cytochrome c reductase decreased in middle-aged (14–15 month) and old (24–25 months) rats compared to young rats (3–5 months). Changes in MMFO activity were variable (sometimes increasing, sometimes decreasing with age) depending on substrate. Schmucker and Wang (1980) reported the levels of cytochrome P-450 and NADPH:cytochrome c reductase was highest in middle-aged (16 months) rats, with marked decreases in older rats (27 months). The MMFO activities tended to be lowest in older rats (Schmucker and Wang, 1980). Additionally, they reported that the microsomal cholesterol/phospholipid ratio increased in senescent rats. The resulting change in membrane fluidity was thought to change the interaction between the reductase and cytochrome P-450 (Schmucker et al., 1984).

While age-related changes in MMFO activity in Fischer 344 rats has been extensively studied, relatively few reports on age-related changes in Sprague-Dawley rats have been published. Chengelis (1988a) reported a rather extensive investigation of age-related changes in MMFO activity in male and female Sprague-Dawley rats. In a pattern similar to that observed in Fischer 344 rats, cytochrome P-450 peaked (on a gram liver basis) in rats at 39 weeks of age. NADPH:Cytochrome P-450 reductase activity also peaked at 39 months of age and declined thereafter. In senescent rats (greater than 78 weeks of age), there were apparent differences between sexes with regard to the levels of the components of the MMFO and MMFO activity. Interestingly, there was little correlation between MMFO activity and the amounts of cytochrome P-450. For example, the activity toward p-nitroanisole was lowest in 39-week-old rats (when cytochrome P-450 was highest). Aniline hydroxylase was lowest in 104-week-old rats. These results suggest that there are not only age-related changes in total cytochrome P-450, but also age-related changes in the isozymic spectrum. This would be consistent with the earlier findings by Kamataki et al. (1985), who reported that there were definite age-related changes in male Fischer 344 rats. Benzo(a)pyrene hydroxylation and 7-propoxycoumarin dealkylation activities peaked at 6 months of age in males, but not in females where activities remained constant throughout adult life. In males, there was a drop in MMFO activities after 24 months of age to female levels. For benzo(a)pyrene hydroxylation, for example, peak in vitro activity was approximately 350 pmol/min/mg microsomal protein in 6-month-old male rats and approximately 90 pmol/min/mg in both sexes at 24 months of age. These changes directly reflected the amounts of cytochrome P-450–male, as well as the appearance of cytochrome P-450–female in senescent male rats. Hence, while there are quantitative and qualitative exceptions, depending on strain, sex, and age of the rats as well as the substrate of interest MMFO activity in rats tends to be highest in middle-aged rats (9–14 months) and lowest in senescent rats (24 months). Age-related changes are due to a combination of changes in total cytochrome P-450, the spectrum of cytochrome P-450 isozymes, NADPH:cytochrome P-450 reductase, and microsomal lipid content. A further complication is that microsomal protein will also change with age (Chengelis, 1988c). Because of this variability, one should not base too many conclusions on these generalizations with out specific examination.

Given there are age-related changes in cytochrome P-450 in rats, can there also be age-related changes in response to inducing agents? Age-related changes in the sensitivity of rats to inducing agents has been discussed since the late 1960s. The literature in this field is mixed. For example, Kato and Takanaka reported that phenobarbital (60 mg/kg ip for 3 days) caused much larger increases in 40-day-old than 300-day-old rats; 23 vs 8% in microsomal protein, 249 vs 52% in NADPH:cytochrome c reductase, 259 vs 60% in cytochrome P-450, and 713 vs 173% in aminopyrine N-demethylation activity. Kao and Hudson (1979) compared and contrasted the inducing effect of phenobarbital (80 mg/kg ip for 4 days) vs β-naphthaflavone ((80 mg/kg ip for 4 days) in young (10 weeks) vs old (100 weeks) male Fischer 344 rats. As expected, the baseline amount of MMFO components as well as the MMFO activities examined were higher in young adult rats than senescent rats, but both agents caused comparable degrees of increase in both age groups. They concluded that young and old rats responded to inducing agents in relatively the same quantitative fashion. In contrast, Rikans and Notley (1988) reported that age affected the response to different inducing agents differently. They concluded that phenobarbital induced increases to approximately the same extent in old vs young rats, whereas β-naphthaflavone induced larger increases in older rats. They further suggested that age-related differences in sensitivity to induction are due to differences in the inducibility of specific cytochrome P-450 isozymes. This latter conclusion is consistent with the work of Sun et al. (1986), who examined the levels of six different forms of cytochrome P-450 as a function of both age and inducing agents using immunochemical techniques. They noted that phenobarbital induced a different pattern of isozymes in 2- vs 52-week-old rats. Sitar and Desai (1983) reported that male Sprague-Dawley rats lost responsiveness with age to phenobarbital but not β-naphthaflavone. McMartin et al. (1980) observed the same pattern in Sprague-Dawley rats. In contrast, Baird et al. (1975) reported no decline in responsiveness of male CFN rats to phenobarbital. Birnbaum and Baird (1978) examined the effectiveness of three different inducing agents (phenobarbital, 3-MC, and PCN) in Fischer 344 rats. They observed that inducibility of microsomal benzphetamine demethylation and aniline hydroxylation decreased with age, whereas inducibility of p-nitroanisole demethylation increased with age.

Thus, despite the lack of uniformity in the literature, age clearly plays a role in the response of rats to inducing agents. The extent that age plays depends on the stain and sex of the rats used, the class of inducing agent, and the specific MMFO parameter examined. As a broad generality, most rats loose responsiveness to phenobarbital induction as they age.

What are the implications of age-related changes in MMFO activity? One should expect changes in pharmacokinetic behavior of a given drug or chemical in rats. Kapetanovic et al. (1983), for example, reported that the plasma half-life was longer and plasma clearance rate lower in old (32–34 months) rats than in young (3–4 months) rats. If toxicity of a chemical depends on metabolic activation (e.g., an indirect hepatotoxin) there may well be age-related changes in sensitivity. Rikans (1984) examined age-related changes in response to various hepatotoxins and reported that old (24–25 months) rats were more sensitive to allyl alcohol but more sensitive to bromobenzene that middle age (14–15 months) rats. The sensitivity of rats in acute toxicity testing varies considerably with age, and this may be due in part to age-related differences in metabolism. Hence, one should always consider the age of the rats in attempting to reproduce an experimental result.

Other Influences of MMFO Activity

Age, sex, and the strain of rats used all have play modulating roles in xenobiotic metabolism. Husbandary and other external events have also been shown to influence xenobiotic metabolism. The feeding regimen is a good example: Gram et al. (1970) reported almost 20 years ago that 72 hr of starvation elicited increases in cytochrome P-450 and MMFO activity. This is consistent with the authors' experience that fasting increases the sensitivity of the rat to many indirect hepatotoxins. Radzialowski and Bousquet (1968) reported that MMFO activity followed a diurnal cycle that tended to mirror the diurnal cycles in plasma corticosterone levels. Hence, the time of day a rat is dosed can affect the subsequent metabolism and pharmacokinetic behavior of the drug or chemical under investigation. In another classic work, Fuller et al. (1972) demonstrated that cold exposure (4°C for 4 days) stimulated hepatic drug metabolism in the rat. Hence, environmental conditions can also influence MMFO activity in the rat. Room conditions in a toxicity study should be carefully controlled and monitored to avoid temperature extremes that could alter rates of test article metabolism.

PEROXISOMAL PROLIFERATION

There is a class of chemicals that induce not only increases in cytochrome P-450, but other changes as well; namely, those that induce peroxisomal proliferation (Hawkins et al., 1987). In general, these fall into two classes: hypolipidimic drugs related in structure to clofibrate and plasticizers related in structure to di(2-ethylhexeyl)phthalate. These agents cause hepatomegaly, proliferation of smooth endoplasmic reticulum with increases in MMFO activity, increases in peroxisomal number with associated enzyme level changes, and changes in mitochondrial number and function with increases in certain enzyme levels. This phenomenon has been most extensively studied by Reddy and colleagues (1983) in rats and mice. The phenomenon is diagnosed microscopically by increased content of peroxisomes, or biochemically by measuring the activity of peroxisomal-specific enzymes, such as catalase or carnatine-acetyl transferase. They also, as reported by Oesch et al. (1988), cause large increases in cytosolic epoxide hydrolase. For example, these investigators have reported 1 week of treatment with clofibrate (200 mg/kg/r day, dietary admix) will cause a 50% increase in liver relative organ weights (from 4.1 to 6.3%), and eightfold increase in both palmatyol-CoA transferase activity (from 11.4 to 90.0 nmol/min/mg) and c-EH activity (38–312 pmol/min/mg protein) in rats.

Bezofibrate is a hyperlipidemic drug that is a potent peroxisomal-proliferating agent. Halvorson (1983) reported that administration of bezofibrate (by dietary admix, 12.4

μmol/g feed for 9 days) caused 60% increases in liver weight and total hepatic protein, and a 2.4-fold increase in carnitine palmatoyl transferase activity in male Wistar rats. Watanabe et al. (1989) demonstrated that a longer dosing period (100 mg/kg for 13 weeks) can have even more dramatic effects; e.g., a 35.8-fold increase in carnatine acyltransferase. Increases were seen in other species, but (except for mice) nowhere near the increases seen in rats.

The safety of peroxisomal-proliferating agents is an of issue because these agents are also liver carcinogens in rats and mice. Rats and mice are the most inducible and other species are less responsive. It would appear that rats are good models to determine if an agent causes peroxisomal proliferation, but poor models to determine if such agents are genotoxic carcinogens. These agents will almost always uniformly (100% response) cause hepatocellular tumors at the maximally tolerated dose (MTD) in rats. As these tumors are probably a result of the peroxisomal proliferation, the relevance of these findings to nonresponsive species is questionable. The potential carcinogenicity of peroxisomal-proliferating agents may be better assessed in a species such as the guinea pig, which Oesch et al. (1988) have shown to respond poorly to peroxisomal-proliferating agents.

The mechanism by which peroxisomal-proliferating agents cause hepatic carcinomas in rodents is a subject of some debate. One theory holds that the increase in peroxisomal number leads to an increase in the generation of reactive oxygen species that can damage DNA. The oxidative stress hypothesis has come under some question because there is little evidence to suggest that oxidative injury in and of itself is sufficient to cause genotoxic changes. An alternative explanation is that peroxisomal-proliferating agents also have promoting activity. Cattley and Popp (1989) have studied this hypothesis using WY-14643 as a model peroxisomal-proliferating agent and compared its promoting activity with that of phenobarbital. Both agents were very effective (100% response in 4–5 weeks) in promoting altered hepatic foci in diethylnitrosamine-initiated rats, but with qualitative differences. In contrast to phenobarbital, WY-14643 promoted foci were larger, did not stain for γ-glutamyl transpeptidase, and were highly ATPase deficient. The authors concluded that these differences were evidence that WY-14643 is a tumor promoter (as well as a peroxisomal-proliferating agent), but the mechanism of promotion differs from that of phenobarbital. In fact, the mechanisms of WY-14643 promotion and peroxisomal proliferation may be distinct. Whether these findings can be generalized to all peroxisomal-proliferating agents remains to be established and the role of peroxisomal proliferation in carcinogenicity needs to be more thoroughly examined. The rat is probably the species of choice for such investigations.

FLAVINE-DEPENDENT MIXED FUNCTION OXIDASE (FMFO)

Not all the microsomal mixed function oxidase activity is cytochrome P-450 dependent. There is a separate flavin-dependent mixed function oxidase (FMFO) which is different and distinct from the cytochrome P-450–dependent MMFO. Dannan and Guengerich (1982) clearly identified with immunochemical techniques the presence of this enzyme in various rat tissues, including the rat liver. The literature on this enzyme has been extensively reviewed by Ziegler (1988). There are species- and organ-related isozymes, but the presence of more than one different isozyme in the same organ has not yet been demonstrated. There is currently no data to suggest that this enzyme in inducible in the strictest sense of the word (i.e., causes increases in specific activity). The literature is inconsistent with regard to sex-related differences. Ziegler reported that, as with cytochrome P-450–dependent activity, there is a greater activity in males than in female rats (approximately 5:1), while Dannan and Guengerich (1982) reported nearly equivalent activity in male and female rats. Also in rats, the highest amounts of activity are found in the liver, although in female rats nearly equivalent amounts (on a gram tissue basis) are found in the liver and kidney (Dannan and Guengerich, 1982).

N-Octylamine (an inhibitor of cytochrome P-450–dependent MMFO) is an allosteric activator of the hog liver FMFO (the preparation traditionally used to study this enzyme), but not of the rat hepatic FMFO. The FMFO metabolizes chemicals containing thiol, sulfide, thioamide, (secondary and tertiary) amine, hydrazine, and phosphine substituents. This enzyme requires NADPH as a cofactor and is inhibited by both carbon monoxide and SKF 525A. With these similarities to the MMFO, it can be difficult to distinguish between them and determine which enzyme system is actually playing the predominant role in the metabolism of a specific chemical, especially in vivo. In in vitro preparations, however, enzyme-specific antibodies can be used to determine the relative contributions of each system. For example, Tynes and Hodgson (1985) used antibodies to the NADPH:cytochrome c reductase to demonstrate that 100% of the thiobenzamide S-oxidation is due to the FMFO.

The implication of such findings is that for the aforementioned classes of chemicals, there may be two competing pathways of oxidative metabolism (in addition to the competing isozymic cytochrome P-450 pathways). For example, Cashman (1989) reported that verapamil is oxidiazed by both systems in rats; via the FMFO the main metabolite is 3,4-dimethoxystyrene and via the MMFO the main metabolite is N-desmethylverapamil. As 3,4-dimethoxystyrene is the predominant metabolite, the FMFO is the major enzyme involved in verapamil metabolism in the rat. Interestingly, the FMFO is stereoselective for the S(+)-enantiomer of verapamil, which results in steroeoselective first-pass metabolism of verapamil with shifts in the S(+)/R(-) ratio. In general, the FMFO is probably stereoselective in the metabolism of many chemicals. In studying the metabolism of racemic mixtures of potential FMFO substrates, one should be aware of the possibility of stereoselective first-pass metabolism. As pharmacological properties of optical isomers are frequently different, stereoselective metabolism may cause changes in pharmacological actions that do not follow changes in plasma concentrations of a drug.

EPOXIDE HYDROLASE

Epoxide hydrolase (EH) is an important microsomal enzyme in the study of xenobiotic metabolism and toxicity in the rat. The products of MMFO metabolism of many aromatic and olefinic chemicals are highly reactive arene and alkene oxides. These are, in turn, substrates for EH, which converts them to inactive dihydrodiols. Epoxide hydrolase is thusly truly protective, as many of the endogenous substrates of the MMFO are oxidized to epoxides. It has been the subject of many reviews (see also the introductory chapter) such as those by Oesch (1972), and Seidegard and DePierre (1982). The enzyme has been found in every avian and mammalian species examined, including the rat. Highest activity is present in the liver, testis, kidney, ovary, and lung. Microsomal EH activity is induced in the rat by phenobarbital treatment, but only sparingly induced by 3-MC–type inducing agents. Microsomal EH is not affected by the more common MMFO inhibitors, such as SKF-525A. In fact, some of the more common MMFO inhibitors, such as metyrapone, are allosteric activators of microsomal EH. Specific inhibitors of microsomal EH include 1,1,1-trichloropropane-2,3-oxide, and cyclohexane oxide. This enzyme also has some interesting substrate conformational specificity. For example, *cis*-stilbene oxide is hydrated 700 times more rapidly than the *trans* isomer. Treatment of rats with poor substrates like *trans*-stilbene oxide (400 mg/kg ip in corn oil) was once thought to specifically induce EH. This is true only in a relative sense, as transstilbene will cause slight increases in MMFO activity. It, however, causes much larger increases in EH. Few, if any, chemicals induce EH without also increasing MMFO activity to some extent.

If one plans on using inducing agents to study EH, they need to be aware that the time course of the response of cytochrome P-450 and EH are different. For example, Parkinson et al. (1983b) demonstrated that following treatment of 4-week-old male Long-Evans rats with Arochlor 1254 (single intraperitoneal injection, 500 mg/kg), peak total cytochrome P-450 increases occurred in 4 days, whereas maximal EH activity increase did not occur until about 10 days. The implications of this finding is that longer pretreatment periods may well be required than normally used in experiments with inducing agents (e.g., 3 days of treatment with phenobarbital tends to be common practice) if one wants assurance that maximal induction of both cytochrome P-450 and EH has occurred.

As might be expected, EH follows a similar pattern of distribution as cytochrome P-450. Thus, the centrilobular hepatocytes contain higher amounts than those of the periportal region (Seidegard and DePierre, 1983). Whether or not microsomal EH has more than one isomeric form has been the subject of some debate. It was once held that the enzyme existed as a single form with a molecular weight of 50,000 but the presence of multiple forms can not be ruled out. Guengerich and co-workers (1979) demonstrated that there were at least two and possibly three isozyme of EH in rat liver microsomes that could be distinguished on quantitative differences in amino acid content, activities toward different substrates, sensitivities toward different substrates and inducers, and the effectiveness of different different allosteric activators. Walz et al. (1983) have also identified two hepatic microsomal froms of EH. Despite such evidence, the concept of the multiplicity of EH isozymes has not been as easily digested as the same concept applied to cytochrome P-450. For example, Parkison et al. (1983a) examined the turnover time of various microsomal proteins. Isozymes of cytochrome P-450 were examined individually, but epoxide hydrolase was described in terms of a single enzyme. No mention was made of the aforementioned article by Guengerich et al. (1979) which appeared 4 years previously. Given the broad substrate specificity and the fact that the differences between the isozymes reported by Guengerich et al. (1979) were largely more quantitative than qualitative in nature, the implications of isozymic forms of EH are of more theoretical than of practical concern in toxicological and pharmacological testing.

Some strained-related differences in rat hepatic EH have been identified. Oesch et al. (1983) examined microsomal EH activity with styrene 7,8-oxide (a common model substrate) in 22 different rat strains. They found that the activity was highest in Sprague-Dawley and lowest in Fischer 344 rats (4.3 vs 12.7 nmol/min/mg protein). No qualitative differences were identified to account for these differences; they were due entirely to strain-related differences in the amounts of enzyme synthesized.

The effects of age and sex on microsomal EH have been examined to some extent in the rat. Birnbaum and Baird (1979) studied EH in male CFN rats, and reported that there were age-related increases in young (3 months), middle age (12 months), and old (27 months) rats. They also noted that induction of EH with phenobarbital also increased with age. Chengelis (1988d) reported on the age-related changes in epoxide hydrolase in Sprague-Dawley (Charles River) male and female rats. At 4 weeks of age, rats of both sexes had about the same activity (about 90 nmol/min/gm tissue) but it increases dramatically in males thereafter, peaking (at 340 nmol/min/g) at 78 weeks of age. In females, activity remained relatively constant throughout their lifetime. This could result in age-related shifts in the metabolite profile for a chemical in male but not in female rats. One should be aware, therefore, that the extent of EH activity, and gender-related differences, may depend upon the age of the rats studied.

EH was once thought to be solely considered to be a microsomal protein, but recently, a distinct cytosolic isozyme has been identified. The activity of this enzyme (with the same model substrates) is an order of magnitude less than that of the microsomal enzyme, so its biological and toxicological significance is obscure. Levels of this enzyme, however, increases markedly in rats treated with peroxisomal-proliferating agents (Oesch et al., 1988) and may have some utility as a marker for this effect. In contrast, microsomal EH is greatly increased in hepatic hyperplastic nodules and hepatomas (Seidegard and DePierre, 1982). Kizer et al. (1984) examined the induction of microsomal epoxide hydrolase by known carcinogens, such as 2-acetylaminofluorene, thioacetamide, and aflatoxin. They noted that 3 weeks of feeding with various carcinogens which require metabolic activation resulted in four- to 10-fold increases in EH activity in Holtzman rats. They recommended that the induction of EH (direct measurement of the enzyme by ELISA techniques) could be used as part of a preliminary screen for determining the carcinogenic potential of new chemical entities. In our opinion, such data are useful, but only as part of an overall package of short-term tests (including but not limited to genetic toxicology testing).

CONJUGATION REACTIONS

Conjugation, or biosynthetic pathways, are those that take the products of MMFO, FMFO, or epoxide hydrolase and add an additional functionality to form a new chemical moiety. In the past, these were frequently called phase II reactions, whereas the MMFO reaction were called phase I reaction. The oxidation of benzene to phenol is phase I, whereas the formation of phenol sulfate in a phase II reaction. The rat has a complete set of conjugative reactions, including (in ascending order of importance) N-acetylation, amino acid (almost always either glycine or glutamate) conjugation, sulfate conjugation, glutathione conjugation (thio-ether formation), and glucuronic acid conjugation. The reader is refered to Caldwell (1982) for a more complete descriptions of these processes. The preference for a specific conjugation reaction is very much substrate specific. For example, Huckle et al. (1981) examined the in vivo metabolism of 3-phenoxybenzoic acid, and found that the 5-hydroxy-3-phenoxbenzoic acid sulfate to be the major metabolite (accounting for > 60% of the radioactivity in the urine). In contrast, Weyland and Bevan (1987) reported that the predominant conjugate metabolites of benzo(a)pyrene were thio-ethers (glutathione conjugates), whereas sulfates accounted for only 10% of the excreted metabolites. Both quantitative and qualitative differences in species also lead to further complications. In contrast to the rat, for example, the major metabolite of 3-phenoxybenzoic acid in the guinea pig is 3-phenoxybenzoic acid glucuronide (Huckle 1987). The basic apects of the classic conjugation reactions as they apply to the rat are as follows.

Amino Acid Conjugates

In general, amino acid conjugation is more highly developed in larger species, and amino acid conjugates are seldom major metabolites in rats. Amino acid conjugates are also usually quite stable and not involved in further activation reactions.

Acetylation

While O-acetylation of hydroxyl groups (ester formation) is theoretically possible, in the rat this is apparently very rare; whereas acetylation of free amines to amides is a common reaction in rats. It is catalyzed by the cytosolic enzyme N-acetyl transferase, using acetyl-CoA as the cosubstrate. N-Acetyl transferase has gathered most attention with regard to the metabolism (and activation) of carcinogenic aromatic amines and hydrazides. The acetylation of 2-aminofluorine is the first step in the activation of this chemical to an ultimate carcinogen. Interestingly, in comparison to other rodent species, the rat is a relatively poor acetylator. As reported by Lower and Byran (1973) the hamster, guinea pig, and mouse have approximately 16, 10.5, and 9 times greater (in vitro) activity as the rat with 2-aminofluorene as the substrate. Lotlikar et al. (1967) reported the rat has relatively low aromatic amide hydroxylation capabilities; it is not detectable in uninduced rats. Highest activity (both baseline and induced) is found in the hamster. Hence, in the study of aromatic amine metabolism and toxicity, the hamster (not the rat) is the preferred species.

Depending on substituents, hydrazines can have a number of effects. Of most concern, however, are carcinogenicity and hepatotoxicity. Many hydrazines, hydrazones, and hydrazides have caused cancer in laboratory animals (Toth, 1979). McKennis et al. (1959) first demonstrated (in rabbits) that acetylhydrazine is the final common reactive metabolite in the hepatotoxicity of both hydrazine and isoniazid. This work was further developed using the rat as a model by Timbrell et al. (1980). Single doses of acetylhydrazine (30 mg/kg) or acetylisoniazid (200 mg/kg) produced liver necrosis in rats. Isoniazid itself, however, is poorly hepatotoxic in the rat, an observation which is consistent with the observation that rats have relatively poor N-acetyltransferase activity. Rats must be pretreated with phenobarbital and then aggressively treated with (100 mg/kg every hour for 6 hrs) isoniazid to develop hepatic damage. Thus, rats are apparently poor models to study hydrazine toxicity, but are good models for the study of the metabolism and toxicity of these chemicals once they are acetylated.

Sulfate Conjugates

Sulfate ester formation (e.g., phenol sulfate formation from phenol) is catalyzed by the cytosolic enzyme PAPS-sulfotransferase using 3'-phospho-adenosine-5'-phosphosulfate (PAPS) as the cosubstrate. The reaction has important toxicological involvements. For example, N-sulfo-acetyl-2-aminofluorene is the ultimate carcinogen formed from 2-acetyl-aminoflurorene involving a reaction catalyzed by phenolic-specific sulfotransferase. Generally, the availability of sulfate to be activated (PAPS formulation) is the rate-limiting step (Weinshilboum, 1990). Agents that depress PAPS formation also depress sulfate formation (Hjelle et al., 1985) in the rat. Chemicals with free phenolic hydroxyl groups are the most common substrates. Hence, PAPS-sulfotransferase and UDP-glucuronosyl transferase usually compete for the same substrate, and both conjugates are frequently found together. The one that predominates will depend on the specific chemical, dose of parent chemical, and metabolic state of the rat. As a broad generalization, because of K_m differences between PAPS-sulfotransferase and UDP-glucuronosyl transferases, sulfates tend to predominate at lower dosages, whereas the percentage of glucuronides increases with increases in dosage (Mulder, 1986).

PAPS-Sulfotransferases exist as a collection of enzymes; some with broad and some with narrow substrate specificity (Mulder et al., 1986). Steroid hormones are the natural endogenous substrates for a specific class of sulfotransferases. As there are sex-related differences in steroidal hormones, it is not surprising that the rat displays considerable sex-related variation in sulfotransferases involved in steroid metabolism (as reviewed by Mulder, 1986). Common aryl sulfotransferase (p-nitrophenol) activity is 2–3 times higher in the male than female rat (Matsui and Watanabe, 1982). As a matter of course, sulfotransferases now tend to be classified as phenol sulfotransferase and steroid sulfotransferases (STs). Sekura and Jakoby (1979) isolated from rats two closely related phenol STs with activity toward a wide variety of xenobiotic phenolic chemicals, such as phenol, β-naphthol, and p-nitrophenol. Maas et al. (1982) studied phenol sulfotransferase using 3-methoxy-4-hydroxyphenol glycol as the substrate. While there are measurable amounts of activity in the brain and kidney, the activity in the liver is two orders of magnitude greater, and would by far make the greatest contribution to sulfate formation from xenobiotics. Hepatic activity peaks at about 10 weeks of age and is somewhat induced by dexamethasone (1 μmol/kg for 2 days). There are some slight strain-related differences in activity, but generally it falls between 25 and 50 Units/mg cytosolic protein. Chengelis (1988d) examined age- and sex-related differences in Sprague-Dawley rats using β-naphthol as a substrate. No consistent sex-related differences were identified; however, males did have greater activity at 12 and 26 weeks of age, and at no point did females have statistically significant greater activity than males. Activity in both sexes peaked at 78 weeks of age. As UDP-glucuronosyl transferase peaks at an earlier time point, the ratio of sulfate to glucuronide conjugates may also change as a function of age. In contrast to Sprague-Dawley rats, 5 months of age Fischer 344 male rats had twice the in vitro activity with acetaminophen (phenol transferase) then females, whereas with glycol lithocholic acid, females had 5 times the activity than males (Galinski et al., 1986a). Using a relatively small dose (30 mg/kg, which is not hepatotoxic), these authors observed an age-related decrease in the sulfate to glucuronide ratio in male rats. This was confirmed with a higher dose (Galinsky 1986b). The reasons for the lack of consistent reportedly sex-related differences for the phenol sulfotransferase are unclear, but are likely due to strain, age, and methodology (e.g., model substrate).

As mentioned, there are clear sex-related differences in the steroid sulfotransferases. Female rat liver cytosol contains at least three sulfotransferases that transform a variety of hydroxymethyl polyaromatics (e.g., 5-hydroxy-methylchrysene) to sulfates that are potent mutagens (Ogura, et al. 1990). This is an interesting exception to the "rule" that conjugates are inactive endproducts. The dominant isozyme in this class had no activity with p-nitrophenol, but was competitively inhibited by dehydroepiandrosterone, but not 2,6-dichloro-4-nitrophenol. Interestingly, according to Ogura et al. (1990), neither hydroxymethylarenes nor the methylarenes are heptocarcinogens in rats because of the high activity of hepatic glutathione S-transferase.

In summary, the rat has an appreciable capability to form organic (ethereal) sulfates. As the rat has a high tendency to form phenolic chemicals when given aromatic-fused ring structures, one can almost always expect sulfate (and glucuronide)–containing metabolites to be formed in the rat. Activity is classified (by isozymic specificity) as either phenolic or steroid sulfotransferases. Both, however, are capable of activity toward xenobiotics and the products can sometimes be toxic "activated metabolites."

Glucuronide Conjugates

UDP-Glucuronosyl transferases are microsomal enzymes that catalyzes the formation of glucuronide conjugates using uridine-diphosphoglucuronic acid (UDP-glucuronosyl) as the cosubstrate. In general, glucuronides are usually inactive endproducts, but this is not always the case. Smith et al. (1986) have demonstrated that glucuronidation of zomepirac results in a reactive chemical moiety that binds to macromolecules. Generally, the generation of glucuronic acid is considered the rate-limiting step in rate limiting. Gregus et al. (1988) have demonstrated that treatments that decrease UDP-glucuronate also decrease glucuronide formation. Large numbers of functional groups are capable of being glucuronidated, including hydroxyls carboxyls, primary amines, and thiols (Burchell and Coughtrie, 1989; Caldwell, 1982). Substrates containing phenolic hydroxyl groups are the most commonly studied substrates. As with the sulfotransferases, different types of phenolic substrates are used to type or characterize the different isozymes. UDP-Glucuronosyl transferase (UDPGT) of the rat has been extensively studied. At least eight different isozymes have been isolated and characterized from rat liver (Boutin, 1987; Burchell and Coughtrie, 1989; Tephly et al., 1988). Known molecular weights vary from 52,000–56,000. Isozymes are divided between those that have primary activity against xenobiotics (4-nitrophenol, morphine, phenol, and 4-hychroxyphenol UDPGT) and those that have primary activity against endogenous substrates (17β-hydroxysteroids, 3α-hydroxysteroids, bilirubin, and estrone UDPGT). In general, isozymes that prefer xenobiotic substrates have broader substrate specificity than those that prefer endogenous substrates (Chowdhury et al., Tephly et al. 1988). The activity of this system is particularly important in the rat. Glucuronides are actively transported and excreted in the bile, and the rat has an extremely efficient biliary excretion system. Enterohepatic circulation of xenobiotics and metabolites is always a factor to consider in rats. For example, indomethacin is so highly ulcerogenic in the rat as opposed to the guinea pig (Mariani and Bonanomi, 1978) because the enterohepatic circulation of indomethacin results in greater exposure of the intestinal mucosa. Despite the efficiency of this species in biliary excretion, UDPGT activity in the rat is not distinctively high. Astrom et al. (1987) examined the activity of microsomal preparations against 1-naphthol for various species (rat, mouse guinea pig, and hamster). There were not large differences between species; mean activity from 5.9 to 12 nmol/mg/min. Guinea pigs had the highest activity. Boutin et al. (1984) examined a much larger number of substrates in five different species. Again, there was nothing either quantitatively or qualitatively distinctive about the activity in rats, and activity in guinea pigs tended to have the highest activity.

In the rat liver, UDPGT is also a highly inducible enzyme, particularly those with isozyme activity toward exogenous substrates. It has been conclusively known since the early 1970s that phenobarbital and polycyclic aromatic hydrocarbons induce not only P-450, but UDPGT as well (Vanio et al., 1974). Mulder (1970) reported that phenobarbital increased p-nitrophenol UDPGT activity nearly 90%. Bock et al. (1988) have isolated and characterized the 3-MC–inducible form of (phenol) UDPGT, and found that 3-MC (40 mg/kg ip in olive oil; single treatment) increased microsomal UDPGT activity with 1-naphthol almost 4 times, whereas having no effect with testosterone as the substrate. As with the MMFO, different types of inducers induce different enzymes. For a complete review of the inducible characteristics of UDPGT, the reader is referred to Burchell and Coughtrie (1990). The induction of UDPGT, however, is not a common mammalian characteristic, and may be distinctive to the rat. Astrom et al. (1987) reported that 3-MC caused a 6 times increase in microsomal UDPGT activity (with 1-naphthol) in male rats, had at best modest effects in guinea pigs and C57BL/6 mice (17 and 20% increase, respectively, and caused actual decreases in hamsters and DBA/2 mice (27 and 21%, respectively). The different isozymes also have different lobular distribution in the rat liver. As could be expected, those that prefer xenobiotic substrates (p-nitrophenol) have a distribution similar to the MMFO, with the largest amount in the centrilobular region. 3α- and 17β-Hydroxysteroid UDPGTs were uniformly spread across the lobule, with equal amounts in the centrilobular, midzonal, and periportal regions (Knapp et al., 1987).

As reviewed by Mulder (1986), male rats generally have higher heaptic UDPGT activity than female rats. There are exceptions, particularly with endogenous substrates; females, for example, have higher 17β-steroid UDPGT activity than males. Mulder suggests that differences between sexes were quite variable; and dependent on assay conditions. This was confirmed by Astrom et al. (1987), who demonstrated that there was no difference in the microsomal activity toward 1-naphthol unless the preparations were treated with a detergent. This situation may also be complicated because there are sex-related differences in age-related changes. Chengelis (1988d) reported that microsomal p-nitrophenol UDPGT in Sprague-Dawley rats peaked in both sexes at 39 weeks of age, but males had significantly higher activity at 12, 26, and 39 weeks of age. There were no sex-related differences after 52 weeks of age, and activity fell off precipitously in senescent rats. In contrast, while Galinsky et al. (1986) identified no age-related changes in UDPGT activity with variety of substrates, males (also 5-month-old) had consistently higher activity than females (also 5-month-old). Borghoff et al. (1988) also reported decreases in UDPGT activity in male Fischer 344 rats. Using 4,4'-thio-bis(6-t-butyl-m-cresol) as a model, they detected a decrease in the amount of glucuronide formed, decreased microsomal activity in vivo, and age-related decreases in UDPGT as substrate. Thus, gender as well as age-related changes could play a role in glucuronide formation.

Developmental changes in UDPGT have been characterized in the rat, as reviewed by Burchell and Coughtrie (1988). For the isozymes most involved in xenobiotic metabolism, there are two developmental clusters. Activities toward planar phenolic structures (e.g., 4-nitrophenol) develop prior to birth and reach a perinatal maximum 2 days postpartum. Activity toward more bulky molecules (morphine, chloramphenicol) does not appear until after birth and reaches a perinatal maximum 25–30 days postpartum. These changes should be kept in mind when one is examining the metabolism or toxicity of xenobiotics in neonatal animals.

Considerable strain variation is demonstrated by UDPGT. The Gunn rat, for example, is an inbred substrain of the wistar rat that has life-long hyperbilirubinemia because of low UDPGT activity with bilirubin. The Gunn rat has very low activity with a variety of planar phenolic substrates, and activity is not inducible by 3-MC (Buschell and Coughtrie, 1989), but almost the expected level of activity with testosterone and similar substrates. Boutin et al. (1984) reported that the microsomal activity of Wistar rats with 1-naphthol was 34 nmol/min/mg and with testosterone was 6.4 nmol/min/mg. In Gunn rats, these activities were 11.3 and 4.3 nmol/min/mg. Other genetic variations have been described in Wistar rats; approximately 50–60% have high (whereas 40–50% have low) 3-hydroxysteroid UDPGT (Knapp et al., 1988). While such differences obviously will alter the metabolism of some endogenous chemicals, the implications for the metabolism of xenobiotics is unclear. One should be aware, however, that different Wistar rats may produce unpredictably different metabolic profiles with some chemicals.

Glutathione and the Glutathione S-Transferase(s)

This system is probably the most important conjugation system in the rat liver with regard to "inactivation" of activated metabolites. Glutathione is a tripeptide (γ-glutamyl-cystinyl-glycine) that accounts for over 90% of nonprotein thiols in the liver (Levine, 1983). From a xenobiotic viewpoint, the cystinyl group is the most important. Glutathione readily reacts (nucleophilic attack) with arene-oxides, epoxides, and aryl and alkyl halides to form thio-ethers. The oxidation of reduced glutathione (GSH) to the dithiol (GSSG) also plays an important role in protection against oxidative stress (Boyd, 1980). As reviewed by Koplowitz et al. (1985), the transport, synthesis, and activity of the glutathione redox cycle (glutathione reductase, glutathione peroxidase) acts to keep glutathione at a fairly constant level. The concentration of (reduced) glutathione in rat liver tends to range between 4 and 8 μmol/g liver (e.g., see Chengelis, 1988b, 1989d; Igarashi et al., 1983; Moron, 1979), and is present in much larger amounts than the oxidized disulfide form by an approximately a 20 :1 ratio (Igarashi et al., 1983). No consistent sex-related differences in glutathione content have been reported. The effects of different inducing agents on hepatic glutathione levels have not been thoroughly explored, but at least one author has reported that treating rats with phenobarbital results in increases in glutathione (Utley and Mehendale, 1989). Within the hepatocyte, glutathione exists in different distinct pools (Levine, 1983). Reed (1990) recently reviewed the toxicological implication of mitochondrial, as opposed to cytosolic, glutathione. About 10–15% of hepatic glutathione in the rat is in the mitochondrial fraction. For example, the cytotoxic effect of erthacrynic acid in isolated hepatocytes correlated with depletion of mitochondrial not cytosolic glutathione.

While glutathione is generally considered a cosubstrate in a synthetic reaction (for every mole of conjugate, 1 mole of xenobiotic and 1 mole of glutathione are consumed), glutathione can also play a catalytic role. In the rat (and probably other species as well), glutathione is involved in the metabolism of formaldehyde (Levine, 1983) and dihalomethanes (Ahmed and Anders, 1978). In both cases, the first step is the formation of a conjugate which is then the substrate for a final enzyme. For example, bromoethane is first conjugated (with release of one halide ion) to a s-halomethyl-glutathione intermediate; this is further metabolized by a cytosolic enzyme to form formaldehyde, another bromide ion and intact glutathione.

Additionally, while glutathione conjugates are generally inactive endproducts, there are numerous examples of glutathione conjugates that are toxic or "activated metabolites in and of themselves" (Caldwell, 1982; Picket and Lu, 1989). Booguard et al. (1989) clearly demonstrated that the cysteine-s conjugates of tetrachloroethylene (TFE), chlorotrifluorethylene, and other chlorofluorocarbons are potent nephrotoxins in rats. Marik et al. (1990) demonstrated in vitro that glutathione conjugates of ethylene dibromide lead to the formation of an active metabolite (as measured by DNA adduct formation). The same results were obtained using both purified enzymes and isolated hepatocytes (human and rat), suggesting that the rat is a good predictive model for these types of activation reactions.

Glutathione conjugates are both actively further metabolized and excreted (Levine, 1983) in the rat and most species. As reviewed by Picket and Lu (1989), GSH conjugates undergo stepwise cleavage (first by γ-glutamyltranspeptidase, then by cysteinylglycine dipeptidase) of two amino acid residues to a cysteine conjugates. This is a breakpoint; the cysteinyl conjugate is either acetylated (by N-acetyl transferase) to a mercapturic acid or cleaved to a free thiol (by the enzyme cysteine conjugate β-lyase). This latter reaction has been shown to have important toxicological implications in the rat in that the free thiols formed, for example, are responsible for the nephrotoxicity discussed in the previous paragraph.

The reactions between glutathione and activated xenobiotics are catalyzed by the enzyme glutathione S-transferase (GSHT). The structure and molecular biology of this enzyme has been thoroughly explored, especially in the rat (Boyer, 1989; Keen and Jacoby, 1989; Picket and Lu, 1989). In general, roughly eight different isozymes of the rat cytosolic enzyme have been identified. They represent different heterodimeric combinations of different monomeric structures. This organization contributes to the very broad substrate specificity displayed by the rat cytosolic GSHT (Keen and Jacoby, 1978). A brief survey of the literature indicates that the most common model substrates used for examining total activity are 1-chloro-2,4-dinitrobenzene (CDNB), p-nitrobenzyl chloride, and 1,2-dichloro-4-nitrobenzene (DCNB). This have been used probably because they are a good substrate for the widest spectrum of isozymes.

The total activity of cytosolic GSHT is high in the rat; as much as 5% of the cytosolic protein in the rat may be GSHT. As reviewed elsewhere (Boyer, 1989; Picket and Lu 1989), these macromolecules also have binding and transport rules distinct from the role they play in xenobiotic metabolism. They are extremely stable; rat cytosolic preparations can be left at refrigerator temperatures for several days with no change in GSHT activity. Rarely is GSHT activity the rate limiting step in glutathione conjugation. Generally, the amount of glutathione is rate limiting and glutathione depletion has important metabolic and toxicological consequences. For a variety of metabolically activated hepatotoxins, cell damage does not occur until the metabolism results in glutathione depletion. In comparison to other species, the activity of GSHT in the rat is by no means the highest. Astrom et al. (1987) reported that the hamster, mouse, and guinea pig all had greater activity then the rat with CDNB as the substrate. Gregus et al. (1985) have reported that species-related differences in glutathione S-transferase can be highly substrate dependent. Perhaps the best way to summarize GSHT activity in the rat in comparison to other species is that the rat may not always have the highest activity, but it generally has good activity with a wider range of substrates than most species. Rodents, in general, tend to have higher activity than nonrodent. Down and Chasseaud (1979), for example, compared GSHT activity in cytosolic preparations in the rat, baboon, and rhesus monkey with four different substrates; the rat had from 5 to 20 times the activity depending on substrate. As discussed elsewhere (see Chapt. 9), primates have higher amounts of epoxide hydratase than rats. As GSHT and EH serve the same "deactivating" role in the metabolism of potential toxins, this difference does not necessarily result in phylogenetic differences in toxicity, but can result in predictable differences in metabolites formed.

Hepatic GSHT in the rat is influenced by a variety of factors such as age, sex, strain, and diet. As reviewed by Mulder (1986), data on sex-related differences have been highly complex, and often dependent on the substrate examined and the age of the rat. Chengelis (1988d) examined age- and sex-related changes in hepatic GSHT in Sprague-Dawley rats with two substrates (p-nitrobenzyl chloride and CDNB). Activity was greater with both in males than females only in rats 26 through 78 weeks of age; there were no significant differences in young (4–12 weeks) or senescent rats (104 weeks of age). In both sexes, activity peaked at 52 weeks of age. This is consistent with the earlier findings of Igarashi et al. (1983), who also demonstrated that there were no sex-related differences in GSHT activity in young adult rats. The different monomeric subunits are evidently under different controlling influences that complicate generalizations about sex-related differences in the rat. For example, Hale et al. (1981) reported that orchidectomy resulted in decreased activity toward three substrates, but an increase toward a fourth. James and Pheasant (1978) reported that GSHT activity is very low in neonatal rats. Given the complex tapestry of such controls, it is sometimes difficult to predict the extent glutathione conjugation will play in the metabolism of a specific chemical in the rat, and the presence or (absence) thereof will always have to be confirmed experimentally.

In the rat, GSHT is also an inducible enzyme, although (as could be expected) the different monomers are differentially effected by different agents. Baars et al. (1978) examined the effect of phenobarbital, 3-MC, and TCDD treatment of rats on cytosolic GSHT activity with three different substrates (styrene oxide, 1,2-butylene oxide, and CDNB). In general, while all three treatments caused increases in activity with all three substrates, 3-MC appeared to be the best inducing agents. Down and Chasseaud (1979) reported that DDT was a better inducing agent than phenobarbital, and that neither agent increased GSHT activity in nonhuman primates. Astrom et al. (1987) compared the inducing effect of 3-MC on GSHT activity (with CDNB) in four different rodent species; increases were induced in the rat and hamster, but not the mouse or guinea pig. In general, induction of GSHT activity is a trait seen in relatively few species, including the rat, where only 3-MC and DDT appear to induce at best relatively modest increases in this type of activity.

Inhibition of GSHT can occur; for example, Aitio and Bend (1979) reported on the inhibitory effect of various common solvents (e.g., ethanol). Dierickx (1982) reported on the inhibitory effect of divalent metal ions (such as Hg^{2+}). Jakobson et al. (1979) reported that oxidized glutathione (GSSG) and S-octylglutathione are effective inhibitors of GSHT. As a tool in the study of xenobiotic metabolism, inhibition of GSHT in the rat has not been widely used. This is probably because the enzyme has such high activity that partial inhibition has little effect on actual conjugate formation. As mentioned, glutathione availability tends to be the limiting factor in glutathione adduct formation. Most investigators have relied on glutathione depletion not GSHT inhibition to study the involvement of this system in metabolism and toxicity. Dielthylmalonate is a substrate for GSHT (Early and Schnell, 1972) that rapidly depletes hepatic glutathione, and, therefore, is frequently used in studies that require glutathione depletion. For example, Chengelis (1988b), reports that diethylmalonate (640 mg/kg ip, neat) resulted in an 86% decrease in hepatic glutathione content in 60 min.

Not all the GSHT isozymes are present in the rat liver under all circumstances. Ito and colleagues (1989) have identified a placental form which is expressed in altered hepatic or preneoplastic foci in rat liver. They have demonstrated that this is an excellent marker for these types of changes, and has the advantages of being detectable (by immunohistochemical staining) in formalin-fixed tissues.

There is also ample evidence that there is a distinct microsomal GSHT in the rat (Boyer et al., 1982; Morganstern et al., 1982). While Boyer has suggested that this enzyme plays an important role in xenobiotic metabolism, the full implications of this enzyme in metabolism and toxicity in the rat remain to be clarified.

OTHER ENZYMES

As mentioned in the introduction to this section, all species have a wide variety of esterases. For example, 15 different isozymes have been described for the rat brain and five for the rat liver (Lienweber, 1987). Any ester given to a rat will be rapidly hydrolyzed. Like all other species, the rat possesses alcohol dehydrogenase (ADH). Unlike the situation in other species, however, methanol is not a substrate for rat ADH, being oxidized to formate by the catalase/hydrogen peroxide system (Tephly et al., 1964).

EXTRAHEPATIC XENOBIOTIC METABOLISM

That various tissues other than liver possess xenobiotic-metabolizing ability has been recognized for quite some time (Litterst et al., 1975). In general, given the relatively small size of these organs and the relatively low activity of the salient enzymes (compared to the liver), extrahepatic metabolism rarely plays a major role in the overall disposition of xenobiotics. For example, Litterst et al. (1975) noted that the lungs had only 7% of the cytochrome P-450 as the liver on a microsomal basis and only 35% of the microsomal protein as the liver in the rat. A possible exception to this generalization is the intestine. The presence of the gut flora give this organ considerable hydrolytic and reductive capability which plays a major role in enterophepatic circulation. This is especially true in the rat, as it has a very effective biliary excretory capacity. The organs most frequently examined are the lung, liver, kidney, adrenal, and gastrointestinal tract. While the metabolic capabilities of these organs may not necessarily play a major role in xenobiotic disposition, they can play major roles in target organ toxicity. This short review will highlight some examples of this phenomenon in the rat.

Adrenal Cortex

The adrenal cortex is a steroidogenic organ and, therefore, actually quite rich in cytochrome P-450–dependent MMFO. (The testis and ovary are also quite rich in these enzymes, but will not be discussed here.) There are two different systems: microsomal and mitochondrial. The latter system is distinctive because of the presence of an additional protein, adrenodoxin, in the MMFO system, which serves as the electron carrier between NADPH:cytochrome P-450 reductase and the hemoprotein. These systems are primarily involved in the production of glucocorticoid and mineralocorticoid by this organ. As a generality, the toxicity associated with the MMFO in the adrenal gland is not the production of toxic reactive intermediates but is secondary to the effects of xenobiotics on adrenal hormone production. For example, 7α-thiosteroids, such as spironolactone, are suicide substrates and cause the destruction of adrenal cytochrome P-450 (Menard et al., 1979; Sherry et al., 1988). Ketoconazole also blocks adrenal steroidogenesis by inhibiting cytochrome P-450–dependent activities (Loose, et al., 1983). Veltman and Maines (1986a) reported that relatively small doses of mercury can cause major alterations in adrenal MMFO activity. A single dose of $HgCl_2$ (30 nmol/kg sc) in male rats caused (24 hr) increases in adrenal mitochondrial cytochrome P-450 accompanied by increases in 11β-steroid hydroxylase and side-chain cleavage activities. In contrast, adrenal microsomal cytochrome P-450 was decreased, accompanied by decreases in 21α-steroid hydroxylase activity. These effects would result in decreased corticosterone production and increased progesterone production. In a continuation on their investigations on heavy metals and adrenal hormone formation, Veltman and Maines (1986b) also reported that 7 days of treatment with cupric chloride significantly decreased 11β-hydroxylase activity, which resulted in a decreased plasma level of corticosterone. The metabolic concerns associated with TCDD are normally focused on the liver, but Mebus and Piper (1986) have demonstrated that TCDD can cause decreases in adrenal 21α-hydroxylase activity. Brownie et al. (1988) reported that methylandrostenediol treatment decreased 11β-hydroxylase activity and that, therefore, the resulting accumulation of 11β-deoxycorticosterone may play a major role in androgen-induced hypertension in rats.

Hence, there are numerous examples of xenobiotics exerting potential toxic effects by disrupting adrenal steroid hormone production in the rat. It is important to note that such effects are not always accompanied by morphological evidence of adrenal damage. Unless one specifically examines for effects on adrenal steroidogenesis, these inhibitory effects on adrenal MMFO are difficult to asses in the context of a routine toxicity study.

Gastrointestinal Tract

The gastrointestinal tract (GI) has two separate identifiable sources of xenobiotic-metabolizing capability: that associated with the gut flora and that associated with the mucosa. As review by Rowland (1988), the reactions catalyzed by the gut bacteria are largely hyydrolytic and reductive in nature. In comparison to other species, rats tend to have the highest activity in β-glucuronidase, but also have high nitrate, nitrite, and azo-reductase activities. The high β-glucuronidase activity doubtlessly contributes to the high tendency of rats toward the enterohepatic circulation of xenobiotic metabolites. The metabolism of metronidazole by the rat provides an example of the important role that the gut flora can play in the metabolism of a synthetic chemical. N-(2-Hydroxyethyl) oxamic acid is formed from metronidazole via the reductive action of intestinal bacteria. When metronidazole is given to routinely maintained laboratory rats N-(2-hdroxyethyl), oxamic acid is excreted in the urine, whereas none is detected in the urine of germ-free (gnotobiotic) rats (Koch and Goldman, 1979; Yeung et al., 1983).

The GI mucosa itself has low but detectable cytochrome P-450–dependent MMFO activity in the rat. The relationship between intestinal MMFO activity and chemical carcinogenesis has attracted considerable attention. Stobel and coworkers (1980, 1987) and Tamura et al. (1987) reported that isolated gut mucosal microsomes are capable of the metabolism of many of the same model substrates (e.g., ethylmorphine, p-nitroanisole) as the liver, including the carcinogen benzo(a)pyrene. The system was induced by both β-naphthaflavone and phenobarbital, and inhibited by both SKF 525A and 7,8-benzoflavone. The system produced positive results against known mutagens which required metabolic activation in the Ames assay. In fact, MMFO activity has been found along the entire intestinal tract in the rat; Bankovosky et al. (1985) and Lindeskog et al. (1986) characterized small but measurable amounts of phenobarbital-inducible cytochrome P-450 in the small intestine. Pascoe and Correia (1985) demonstrated that intestinal cytochrome P-450 is regulated by both dietary selenium and iron concentrations; deprivation of either or both can lead to decreases in cytochrome P-450. Hence, it is clear that the GI tract of the rat possesses the ability to activate chemical carcinogens. Intestinal MMFO can be manipulated in the same manner (with regard to inducers and inhibitors) as the liver MMFO to study the activation of suspected GI carcinogens in vivo or in vitro.

Kidney

Litterst et al. (1975) was among the first to publish on the MMFO of the kidney. On a microsomal protein basis, the rat kidney has about 13% of the cytochrome P-450 as the liver, but only about 6% of the activity with aminopyrine, and scantly detectable activity with aniline. Endou (1983) examined the distribution of cytochrome P-450 along the nephron in rats, and found that it was localized only in the proximal tubule. Within the proximal tubule, the straight segment possesses higher amounts than the convoluted tubules. This was confirmed by Sugita et al. (1988); they also demonstrated that starvation induced cytochrome P-450 in the convoluted tubule, whereas 3-MC induced preferentially in the straight portion. Cojocel et al. (1988) demonstrated that cephladoxin rather specifically causes the depletion of cytochrome P-450 in the rat kidney cortex. Babany et al. (1985) and Barry et al. (1987) explored the relationship between renal and hepatic MMFO activity, and noted that procedures (e.g., inhibition of the hepatic MMFO, partial hepatectomy, cholestasis, and biliary cirrhosis) which decrease MMFO activity resulted in increased renal MMFO. These reports suggest that there is an inverse relationship between activities of the hepatic and renal MMFO.

In an interesting similarity to the liver, the kidney also develops preneoplastic lesions that have different enzyme concentrations and staining characteristics than the surrounding normal tissue. Tsuda et al. (1987) demonstrated that the preneoplastic lesions induced by N-ethyl-N-hydroxyethylnitrosamine in the kidney and liver differed in that in the liver these foci contained decreases in all forms of cytochrome P-450 examined and increased in epoxide hydratase, whereas in the kidney the altered foci contained increased levels of the cytochrome P-450 isozyme PB3a and decreases in epoxide hydratase. This observation also demonstrates that the rat kidney also has considerable epoxide hydrolase activity. Knoll et al. (1988) have demonstrated that nephrotoxic doses of $HgCl_2$ induce large increases in renal epoxide hydrolase activity. Greater increases were observed in Sprague-Dawley than in Fischer 344 rats. Whether this indicates a role for epoxide hydrolase in $HgCl_2$ nephrotoxicity, or whether this is a generalized response to nephrotoxicity remains to be established.

Not only is the renal cytochrome P-450 localized in the proximal tubule, but also anatomically located in the renal cortex of the rat and probably other species as well. Thus, agents that require metabolic activation via the MMFO tend to produce renal damage that is restricted to the renal cortex. Acetaminophen, for example, causes renal cortical necrosis in rats (Newton et al., 1985). In addition, Fischer 344 rats are more susceptible, whereas Sprague-Dawley rats are resistant. Newton et al. (1985) reported that when rats were treated with radiolabeled acetaminophen, the extent of covalently bound radioactivity in the renal cortex was much higher in Fischer 344 than in Sprague-Dawley rats. These results clearly suggest that acetaminophen nephrotoxicity in the rat is due to metabolic activation, and that strain-related differences are due to strain-related differences in renal MMFO activity. Beierschmitt et al. (1986) reported that there were also age-related differences in the sensitivity of Fischer 344 rats to acetaminophen toxicity. At 600 mg/kg (ip), acetaminophen caused severe renal lesions in old (22–25 months of age) rats, but no evidence of damage in 2- to 4-month-old rats and only intermediate damage in middle aged (12–15 months) rats. Tarloff et al. (1988) confirmed this and further demonstrated that the aforementioned strain-related differences between Sprague-Dawley and Fischer 344 rats became less noticeable as the animals aged. At 12 months of age, rats of both strains have equivalent sensitivity to acetaminophen nephrotoxicity, a finding not necessarily due to age-related differences in renal MMFO activity.

Lungs

Relative the rat liver, the rat lung has even less MMFO activity that the kidneys. According to Litterst et al. (1975), the lung has only about 7% of the cytochrome P-450 as the liver (on a microsomal protein basis) and also only 35% of the microsomal protein. As reviewed by Mitchell and Boyd (1983), however, there is ample evidence that the lung has sufficient MMFO activity to generate toxic reactive intermediate. In fact, for a few chemicals, such as 4-ipomeanol, the enzyme kinetic constants are such that MMFO metabolism in the lung is favored over metabolism in the liver, so that toxicity is restricted to the lung (Mitchell and Boyd, 1983). Garst et al. (1983) demonstrated a positive correlation between pulmonary cytochrome P-450 content and species differences in the pulmonary toxicity of 4-ipomeanol; the rat tends to be among the most sensitive of species.

Also as reviewed by Mitchell and Boyd (1983) and Guengerich (1990), the lung is extremely heterogeneous with regard to cell type. The Clara cells tend to be relatively rich, whereas type I epithelial cells are devoid of MMFO activity. Keith et al. (1987) have demonstrated the presence of specific cytochrome P-450 isozymes in both Clara and type II epithelial cells. Hence, toxins that required activation tend to have these two cell types as targets. The molecular biology and enzymology of pulmonary cytochrome P-450 has been most thoroughly explored in the rabbit, but some work has been completed in the rat (Guengerich, 1990). Rat pulmonary cytochrome P-450 exists as several different isozymes (some of which are indistinguishable from the corresponding isozymes of the liver). Pulmonary cytochrome P-450 in the rat is induced by chemicals such as phenobarbital and 3-MC, and different isozymes are induced by different classes of inducers. For example, Robinson et al. (1986) reported that 3-MC induction increases the levels of a pulmonary cytochrome P-450 that is identical to 3-MC–induced hepatic cytochrome P-450. Rampersaud and Walz (1986) demonstrated that rat lung contains at least six different cytochrome P-450s, one of which is cytochrome P-450b, whereas cytochrome P-450e (which is coinduced in the liver with cytochrome P-450b) was not induced under any circumstances in the lung. Hence, despite the similarities, the genetic controls over pulmonary cytochrome P-450 differ somewhat from those of the liver.

In a fashion similar to the liver, however, different isozymes show different sensitivities to different inhibitors. For example, Rabovsky and Judy (1989) reported that rat pulmonary MMFO activity towrd benzyloxyphenoxazone was exquisitely sensitive in vitro to 1-octanol inhibition (IC50 $\simeq$ –3.8 μM), whereas activity toward ethoxyphenoxazone was completely unaffected by 1-octanol (at the limits of solubility). Naslund and Halpert (1984) reported that chloramphenicol (100 mg/kg ip or iv) is a selective suicide substrate for the pulmonary cytochrome P-450 isozyme involved in the 2-hydroxylation of n-hexane. Elovaara et al. (1987) reported that inhalation of m-xylene (300 ppm) resulted in the selective destruction of pulmonary cytochrome P-450 in rats with no effects on any other enzyme system and visible morphological changes. Pyykko et al. (1987) reported that various substituted benzenes also caused decreases in pulmonary cytochrome P-450 and 7-ethoxycoumarin deethylation activity, but increases in 7-ethoxyresorufin deethylation activity. Rietjens et al. (1988) reported that prolonged (7 days) exposure of rats to ozone (by inhalation: 1.6 mg/M^3) results in increases in cytochrome P-450 owing to proliferation of Clara cells. There was, however, a shift in cytochrome P-450 isozymes such that activity toward 7-ethoxycoumarin decreases, whereas activity toward 7-pentoxyresorufin increased. Thus, the MMFO of the rat lung is localized to two main cells types, and (like that of the liver) is controlled by different cytochrome P-450 isozymes. These different isozymes can be induced or inhibited by a variety of different chemical treatments.

Most of this discussion has focused on the pulmonary MMFO. The rat lung, however, also has appreciable flavin-dependent MFO activity (Tynes and Hodgeson, 1983; Ziegler, 1988). This system has been shown to play an important role in the species selectivity of different rodenticides. For example, α-naphthylthiurea (ANTU) causes pulmonary edema in the rat, but not in larger species. Evidently, this difference is due to species differences in activity toward ANTU (and the formation of reactive metabolites), as reviewed by Mitchell and Boyd (1983).

Xenobiotic metabolism by the lung has important implications in toxicology and (based on the preceding paragraph) the rat is an appropriate model for the study of this system. The first concern has to do with localized (pulmonary) toxicity due to the formation of reactive metabolites. Inhalation can result in direct exposure of the lung to relatively high (enzyme-saturating) amounts of potential toxins (although inhalation is not required for a chemical to be a pulmonary toxin, e.g., 4-ipomeanol). For example, 2-nitrofluorene is a potent carcinogen that is rapidly converted in vitro to the potent mutagen (and presumed ultimate carcinogen) 9-hydroxy-2-nitrofluorene by rat lung microsomes (Tornquist, 1988). Agents that induce pulmonary MMFO activity will result in increased pulmonary sensitivity to procarcinogens. The second concern with regard to pulmonary MMFO activity has to do with pulmonary first-pass metabolism of chemicals administered by inhalation. Metabolism by the lung can influence toxicity at more distal sites. Hexane, for example, is metabolized to a neurotoxic chemical, 2,5-hexanediol. Toftgard et al. (1986) reported that the lungs can facilitate the formation of this metabolite by catalyzing the formation of 2-hexanol, which is then transported to the liver for further metabolism to 2,5-hexanediol. These implications are of concern because for the majority of the general human population, inhalation is one of the major routes of incidental exposure to environmental and occupational chemical hazards. Thus, chemicals that influence pulmonary MMFO activity may have potentially serious human health implications. As noted, pulmonary MMFO activity can be altered under circumstances where no other noticeable effects occur, and this is the type of effect that would be easily missed in a traditional toxicology study. The rat would provide a good model for the study of the toxicological implications of pulmonary MMFO induction or inhibition in a tier 2 or single endpoint type of study.

REFERENCES

Ablondi, F., Subbaow, Y., Lipchuck, L., and Personeus, G. (1947) Comparison of blood pressure measurements in the rat as obtained by use of the tail and foot methods and by direct femoral puncture. *J. Lab. Clin. Med.* 32, 1099–1101.

Ahmed, A., and Anders, M. (1978) Metabolism of dihalomethanes to formaldehyde and inorganic halide II. Studies on the mechanism of the reaction. *Biochem. Pharmacol.* 27, 2021–2025.

Alden, C. L. (1985) Species, sex, and tissue specificity in toxicologic and proliferative responses. *Toxicol. Pathol.* 13, 135–140.

Alder, S., and Zbinden, G. (1988) *National and International Drug Safety Guidelines.* M. T. C. Verlag Zollikon, Zollikon, Switzerland.

Alexander, C. S. (1957) A new simple method for indirect determination of blood pressure in the rat. *Proc. Soc. Exp. Biol. Med.* 94, 368–372.

Anderson, J. M. (1963) Lingual vein injection in the rat. *Science* 140, 195.

Anderson, K. V., Coyle, F. P., and O'Steen, W. K. (1972) Retinal degeneration produced by low-intensity colored light. *Exp. Neurol.* 35, 233–238.

Anderson, N. F., Delorme, E. J., Woodruff, M. F. A., and Simpson, D. C. (1959) An improved technique for intravenous injection of newborn rats and mice. *Nature* 184, 1952–1953.

Andrews, D. I., Jones, D. R., and Simpson, F. O. (1978) Direct recording of arterial blood pressure and heart rate in the conscious rat. *J. Pharm. Pharmacol.* 30,524–525.

Angelov, O., Schroer, R. A., Heft, S., James, V. C., and Noble, J. (1984) A comparison of two methods of bleeding rats: the venous plexus of the eye versus the vena sublingualis. *J. Appl. Toxicol.* 4, 258–260.

Annau, Z. (1986) *Neurobehavioral Toxicology.* The Johns Hopkins University Press, Baltimore.

Apostolou, A., Saidt, L., and Brown, W. R. (1976) Effect of overnight fasting of young rats on water consumption, body weight, blood sampling, and blood composition. *Lab. Anim. Sci.* 26, 959–960.

Aquiar, J. L., Bartkowski, R., Berger, M. R., Petru, E., Schlag, P., and Schmahl, D. (1987) Feasible model for locoregional and systemic longterm administration of drugs and concomitant blood sampling in Sprague-Dawley rats. *J. Cancer Res. Clin. Oncol.* 113, 27–30.

Archer, R. K., and Riley, J. (1981) Standardized method for bleeding rats. *Lab. Anim.* 15, 25–28.

Ariyoshi, T., Kazumitsu, T., and Hamasaki, K. (1981) Effects of age and sex on microsomal heme oxygenase and cytochrome P-450 content in liver of rats. *J. Pharm. Dyn.* 4, 664–669.

Armstrong, S., Clarke, J., and Coleman, G. (1978) Light-dark variation in laboratory rat stomach and small intestine content. *Physiol. Behav.* 21, 785–788.

Arnold, D. L., Charbonneau, S. M., Zawidzka, Z. Z., and Grice, H. C. (1977) Monitoring animal health during chronic toxicity studies. *J. Environ. Pathol. Toxicol.* 1, 227–239.

Astrom, A., Maner, S., and DePierre, J. (1986) Induction cytochrome P-450 and related drug-metabolizing activities in the livers of different rodent species by 2-acetylaminofluorene and 3-methylcholanthrene. *Biochemical. Pharmacol.* 35, 2703–2713.

Astrom, A., Maner, S., and DePierre, J. (1987) Induction of liver microsomal epoxide hydrolase, UDP-glucuronyl transferase and cytosolic glutathione transferase in different rodent species by 2-acetylaminofluorene and 3-methylcholanthrene. *Xenobiotica* 17, 155–163.

Atio, A., and Bend, J. (1979) Inhibition of rat liver glutathione S-transferase activity by aprotic solvents. *F.E.B.S. Lett.* 101, 187–190.

Augustine, J. A., and Zemaitis, M. A. (1989) A comparison of the effects of cyclosporine (CsA) on hepatic microsomal drug metabolism in three different strains of rat. *Gen. Pharmacol.* 20(2), 137–141.

Axelrod, J. (1974) The pineal gland: A neurochemical transducer. *Science* 184, 1341–1348.

Baars, A., Jansen, M., and Breimer, D. (1978) The influence of phenobarbital. 3-methylcholanthrene, and 2,3,7,8-tetrachlorodibenzo-p-dioxin on glutathione S-transferase activity of rat liver cytosol. *Biochem. J.* 27, 2487–2494.

Babany, G., Descatoire, V., Corbic, M., Gendre, S., Degott, C., Larrey, D., Letteron, P., Wandscheer, N. C., Funck-Brentano, C., and Pessayre, D. (1985) Regulation of renal cytochrome P-450. Effects of two-thirds hepatectomy, cholestasis, biliary cirrhosis and post-necrotic cirrhosis on hepatic and renal microsomal enzymes. *Biochem. Pharmacol.* 34, 311–320.

Bader, M., and Klinger, W. (1974) Intragastric and intracardial injections in newborn rats. Methodical investigation. *Z. Versuchstierk.* 16, 40–42.

Baetjer, A. M. (1968) Role of environmental temperature and humidity in susceptibility to disease. *Arch. Environ. Health* 16, 565–570.

Baird, M., Nicolosi, R., Massie, H., and Samis, H. (1975) Microsomal mixed function oxidase activity and senescence—I. Hexobarbital sleep time and induction of components of the hepatic microsomal enzyme system in rats of different ages. *Exp. Gerontol.* 10, 89–99.

Baker, H. J., Lindsey, J. R., and Weisbroth, S. H. (1979) Housing to control research variables, in *The Laboratory Rat*, Vol. I, Baker, H. J., Lindsey, J. R., and Weisbroth, S. H., eds. Academic Press, New York, pp. 169–192.

Balazs, T., and Dairman, W. (1967) Comparison of microsomal drug-metabolizing enzyme systems in grouped and individually caged rats. *Toxicol. Appl. Pharmacol.* 10, 409–410.

Balazs, T., Murphy, J. B., and Grice, H. C. (1962) The influence of environmental changes on the cardiotoxicity of isoprenaline in rats. *J. Pharm. Pharmacol.* 14, 750–755.

Bantin, G. C., Deeny, A. A., Gregory, D. J., and Hewitt, R. A. (1984) Animals in transit. *Anim. Technol.* 35, 113–122.

Barnard, R. J., Duncan, H. W., and Thorstensson, A. T. (1974) Heart rate responses of young and old rats to various levels of exercise. *J. Appl. Physiol.* 36, 472–474.

Barnett, M. (1958) The use of polythene for "Elizabethan" collars. *J. Anim. Tech. Assoc.* 9, 50–52.

Barrett, A. M., and Stockham, M. A. (1963) The effect of housing conditions and simple experimental procedures upon the corticosterone level in the plasma of rats. *J. Endocrinol.* 26, 97–105.

Barrow, M. V. (1968). Modified intravenous injection technique in rats. *Lab. Anim. Care* 18, 570–571.

Barry, M., Duenas-Laita, A., Mathuan, P. M., and Feely, J. (1987) Increse in renal cytochrome P-450 and NADPH cytochrome c reductase activity following drug inhibition of hepatic monooxygenase activity. *Biochem. Pharmacol.* 36, 768–769.

Bartek, M. J., LaBudde, J. A., and Maibach, H. I. (1972) Skin permeability in vivo: Comparison in rat, rabbit, pig, and man. *J. Invest. Dermatol.* 58, 114–123.

Basinger, S., Hoffman, R., and Matthes, M. (1976) Photoreceptor shedding is initiated by light in the frog retina. *Science* 194, 1074–1076.

Beierschmitt, W., Keenan, K., and Weiner, M. (1986) The development of acetaminiphen-induced nephrotoxicity in male Fischer 344 rats of different ages. *Arch. Toxicol.* 59, 206–210.

Beinfield, W. H., and Lehr, D. (1956) Advantages of ventral position in recording electrocardiogram of the rat. *J. Appl. Physiol.* 9, 153–156.

Bellhorn, R. W. (1980) Lighting in the animal environment. *Lab. Anim. Sci.* 30, 440–450.

Bellinger, L. L., and Mendel, V. E. (1975) Hormone and glucose responses to serial cardiac puncture in rats. *Proc. Soc. Exp. Biol. Med.* 148, 5–8.

Benson, J., Royer, R., Galvin, J., and Shimizu, R. (1983) Metabolism of Phenathridine to Phenathridone by rat lung and liver microsomes after induction with benzo(a)pyrene and Aroclor. *Toxicol. Appl. Pharmacol.* 68, 36–42.

Berg, B. N. (1960) Nutrition and longevity in the rat. *J. Nutrition* 71, 242–263.

Berman, H., Bryant, B., and Nesnow, S. (1984) Metabolism of α-naphthaflavone by rat, mouse, rabbit and hamster liver microsomes. *Toxicol. Appl. Pharmacol.* 72, 469–470.

Besch, E. L., and Chou, B. J. (1971) Physiological responses to blood collection methods in rats. *Proc. Soc. Exp. Biol. Med.* 138, 1019–1021.

Beuzeville, C. (1968) Catheterization of renal artery in rats. *Proc. Soc. Exp. Biol. Med.* 129, 932–936.

Bieri, J. G., Stoewsand, G. S., Briggs, G. M., Phillips, R. W., Woodard, J. C., and Knapka, J. J. (1977) Report of the American Institute of Nutrition ad hoc committee on standards for nutritional studies. *J. Nutr.* 107, 1340–1348.

Birkhahn, R. H., Bellinger, L. L., Bernardis, L., and Border, J. R. (1976) The stress response in the rat from harnessing for chronic intravenous infusions. *J. Surg. Res.* 21, 185–190.

Birnbaum, L., and Baird, M. (1978) Induction of hepatic mixed function oxidases in senescent rodents. *Exp. Gerant.* 13, 299–303.

Birnbaum, L., and Baird, M. (1979). Senescent changes in rodent hepatic epoxide hydrolase. *Chem.-Biol. Interact.* 26, 245–256.

Bivin, W. S., Crawford, M. P., and Brewer, N. R. (1979) Morphophysiology, in *The Laboratory Rat*, Vol. I, Baker, H. J., Lindsey, J. R., and Weisbroth, S. H., eds. Academic Press, New York, pp. 73–103.

Black, H. E. (1986) A manager's view of the "musts" in a quality necropsy, in *Managing Conduct and Data Quality of Toxicology Studies*, Hoover, B. K., Baldwin, J. K., Uelner, A. F., Whitmire, C. E., Davies, C. L., and Bristol, D. W., eds. Princeton Scientific, Princeton, New Jersey, pp. 249–255.

Black, W. D., and Claxton, M. J. (1979) A simple, reliable and inexpensive method for the collection of rat urine. *Lab. Anim. Sci.* 29, 253–254.

Blass, E. M. (1972) An improved rat metabolism cage. *Physiol. Behav.* 9, 681–683.

Bligh, J., and Johnson, K. G. (1973) Glossary of terms for thermal physiology. *J. of Appl. Physiol.* 35, 941–961.

Bock, K., Schirmer, G., Green, M., and Tehply, T. (1988) Properties of a 3-methylchoanthrene inducible phenol UDP-glucuronosyltransferase from rat liver. *Biochem. Pharmacol.* 37, 1439–1443.

Bodziony, J., and Schwille, P. O. (1985) Subcutaneous cannual in the jugular and femoral vein—a tool for frequent blood sampling and infusions in the rat. *Z. Versuchstierk.* 27, 29–32.

Boehm, N., Plas-Roser, S., Roos, M., and Aron, C. (1982) How different procedures of blood removal affect blood progesterone concentrations in the cyclic female rat. *J. Steroid Biochem.* 16, 339–342.

Bohensky, F. (1986) *Photo Manual and Dissection Guide of the Rat,* Avery Publishing Group, Wayne, New Jersey.

Bolton, W. K., Benton, F. R., Maclay, J. G., and Sturgill, B. C. (1976) Spontaneous glomerular sclerosis in aging Sprague-Dawley rats. *Am. J. Path.* 85, 277–302.

Bonkovsky, H., Hauri, H., Marti, U., Gasser, R., and Meyer, U. (1985) Cytochrome P-450 of small intestinal epithelial cells. Immunochemical characterization of the increase in cytochrome P-450 caused by phenobarbital. *Gastroenterology* 88, 458–467.

Boorman, G. A., and Hollander, C. F. (1973) Spontaneous lesions in the female WAG/Rij (Wistar) rat. *J. Gerontol.* 28, 152–159.

Boorman, G. A., Van Noord, M. J., and Hollander, C. F. (1972) Naturally occurring medullary thyroid carcinoma in the rat. *Arch. Pathol.* 94, 35–43.

Borbely, A. A., Tobler, I., and Steigrad, P. (1979) Chronic drug administration in behavioral studies by subcutaneous pellets. *Pharmacol. Ther.* 5, 451–453.

Borg, E., and Viberg, A. (1980) Role of heating in non-invasive blood pressure measurements in rats. *Acta Physiol. Scand.* 108, 73–75.

Borghoff, S., Stefanski, S., and Birnbaum, L. (1988) The effect of age on the glucuronidation and toxicity of 4,4'-thiobis(6- t-butyl-m-cresol). *Toxicol. Appl. Pharmacol.* 92, 453–466.

Born, C. T., and Moller, M. L. (1974) A simple procedure for long-term intravenous infusion in the rat. *Lab Anim. Sci.* 24, 355–358.

Boutin, J. (1987) Indirect evidences of UDP-glucuronosyl transferase heterogeneity: how can it help purification? *Drug Metab. Rev.* 18, 517–552.

Boutin, J., Antoine, B., Batt, A., and Siest, G. (1984) Heterogeneity of hepatic microsomal UDP-gllucuronososyl transferase activities: Comparison between human and mammalian species activities. *Chem. Biol. Interact.* 52, 173–184.

Boyd, M. (1980) Biochemical mechanisms in chemical-induced lung injury: Roles of metabolic activation. *CRC Crit. Rev. Toxicol.* 10, 103–176.

Boyer, T. (1989) The glutathione S-transferases: An update. *Hepatology* 9, 486–496.

Boyland, E., and Sydnor, K. L. (1962) The induction of mammary cancer in rats. *Br. J. Cancer* 16, 731–739.

Brandstaetter, J., and Terkel, J. (1977) Chronic double lumen intravenous cannulation of the unrestrained rat. *Lab. Anim. Sci.* 27, 999–1003.

Brick, J. O., Newell, R. F., and Doherty, D. G. (1969) A barrier system for a breeding and experimental rodent colony: Description and operation. *Lab. Anim. Care* 19, 92–97.

Broderson, J. R., Lindsey, J. R., and Crawford, J. E. (1976) The role of environmental ammonia in respiratory mycoplasmosis of rats. *Am. J. Pathol.* 85, 115–130.

Brouwer, K. L. R., Kostenbauder, H. B., McNamara, P. J., and Blouin, R. A. (1984) Phenobarbital in the genetically obese Zucker rat 2. In-vivo and in-vitro assessments of mirosomal enzyme induction. *J. Pharmacol. Exp. Ther.* 231, 654–659.

Brown, R. J., and Breckenridge, C. B. (1975) A technique for long-term blood sampling or intravenous infusion in the freely moving rat. *Biochem. Med.* 13, 280–286.

Brown, G. M., and Martin, J. B. (1974) Corticosterone, prolactine, and growth hormone responses to handling and new environment in the rat. *Psychosom. Med.* 36, 241–247.

Brown, Z. W., Amit, Z., and Weeks, J. R. (1976) Simple flow-thru swivel for infusions into unrestrained animals. *Pharmacol. Biochem. Behav.* 5, 363–365.

Budden, R., Buschmann, G., and Kuhl, U. G. (1981a) The rat ECG in acute pharmacology and toxicology, in *The Rat Electrocardiogram in Pharmacology and Toxicology,* Budden, R., Detweiler, D. K., and Zbinden, G., eds. Pergamon Press, Oxford, England, pp. 41–82.

Budden, R., Detweiler, D. K., and Zbinden G. (1981b) *The Rat Electrocardiogram in Pharmacology and Toxicology,* Pergamon Press, Oxford, England.

Bunag, R. D. (1973) Validation in awake rats of a tail-cuff method for measuring systolic pressure. *J. Appl. Physiol.* 34, 279–282.

Burhoe, S. O. (1940) Methods of securing blood from rats. *J. Hered.* 31, 445–448.

Burkhart, C. A., and Robinson, J. L. (1978) High rat pup mortality attributed to the use of cedar-wood shavings as bedding. *Lab. Anim.* 12, 221–222.

Burns, J., Horlington, M., Shaffer, M., and White, E. H. (1971) Miniature transmitters for heart rate measurements in groups of unrestrained rats. *Arch. Int. Pharmacodyn.* 193, 213–225.

Burschell, B., and Coughtrie, W. (1989) UDP-Glucuronosyltransferases. *Pharmacol. Ther.* 43, 261–289.

Bush, J. C., and Bush, C. M. (1971) A sacrifice apparatus for decapitation of laboratory animals. *Physiol. Behav.* 7, 647.

Bush, E., and Trager, W. (1985) Substrate probes for the mechanism of aromatic hydroxylation catalyzed by cytochrome P-450: Selectively deuterated analogues of warfarin. *J. Med. Chem.* 28, 992–996.

Butler, L. E., and Dauterman, W. C. (1988) The effect of dietary protein levels on xenobiotic biotransformations in F344 male rats. *Toxicol. Appl. Pharmacol.* 95, 301–310.

Buttner, D., and Wollnick, F. (1982) Spontaneous short-term fluctuations in the daily pattern of heart rate, body temperature, and locomotor activity in the laboratory rat. *Lab. Anim.* 16, 319–326.

Calabrese, E. J. (1984) Suitability of animal models for predictive toxicology: Theoretical and practical considerations. *Drug Metabol. Rev.* 15, 505–523.

Caldwell, J. (1981) The current status of attempts to predict species differences in drug metabolism. *Drug. Metab. Rev.* 13, 745–777.

Caldwell, J. (1982) Conjugation reactions in foreign-compound metabolism: Definition, consequences and species variations. *Drug Metab. Rev.* 13, 745–777

Cameron, T. P., Hickman, R. L., Korneich, M. R., and Tarone, R. E. (1985) History survival and growth patterns of B6C3F1 mice and F344 rats in the National Cancer Institute Carcinogenesis Testing Program. *Fund. Appl. Toxicol.* 5, 526–538.

Campbell, T. C., and Hayes, J. R. (1974) Role of nutrition in the drug-metabolizing enzyme system. *Pharmacol. Rev.* 26, 171–197.

Caprino, L., Borelli, F., Falchetti, R., Biader, U., and Franchina, V. (1978) A new computerized system to automatic ECG analysis: An application to hypoxic rat ECGs. *Comp. Biomed. Res.* 11, 195–207.

Carlton, W. W., and Gries, C. L. (1982) Adenoma and carcinoma, pars distalis, rat, in *Endocrine System,* Jares, T. C., Mohr, U., and Hunt, R. D., eds. Springer-Verlag, New York, pp. 134–145.

Carney, J. A., and Walker, B. L. (1973) Mode of killing and plasma corticosterone concentrations in the rat. *Lab. Anim. Sci.* 23, 675–676.

Carruba, M. O., Picotti, G. B., Miodini, P., Lotz, W., and DaPrada, M. (1981) Blood sampling by chronic cannulation technique for reliable measurements of catecholamines and other hormones in plasma of conscious rats. *J. Pharmacol. Meth.* 5, 293–303.

Cashman, J. (1989) Enantioselective N-oxidation of verapamil by the hepatic flavin-containing monooxygenase. *Mol. Pharmacol.* 36, 497–503.

Cassell, G. H., Lindsey, J. R., Baker, H. J., and Davis, J. K. (1979) Mycoplasmal and rickettsial diseases, in *The Laboratory Rat,* Vol. I, Baker, H. J., Lindsey, J. R., and Weisbroth, S. H., eds. Academic Press, New York, pp. 243–269.

Cate, C. C. (1969) A successful method for exsanguinating unanesthetized mice. *Lab. Anim. Care* 19, 256–258.

Cattley, R., and Popp, J. (1989) Differences between the promoting activities of the peroxisomal proliferator WY-14, 643 and phenobarbital in rat liver. *Canc. Res.* 49, 3246–3251.

Caulfield, M. P., Clover, K. F., Powers, D. A., and Savage, T. (1983) A rapid and convenient freehand method for the implication of cerebroventricular cannulae in rats. *J. Pharmacol. Meth.* 9, 231–236.

Celier, C., and Cresteil, T. (1989) Induction of drug metabolizing enzymes in Gunn rat liver: Effect of polycyclic aromatic hydrocarbons on cytochrome P-450 regulation. *Biochem. Pharmacol.* 38, 2825–2832.

Chadwick, R. W., Copeland, M. F., and Chadwick, C. J. (1978) Enhanced pesticide metabolism, a previously unreported effect of dietary fiber in mammals. *Food Cosmet. Toxicol.* 16, 217–225.

Chaiasson, R. B. (1988) *Laboratory Anatomy of the White Rat,* William C. Brown, Dubuque, Iowa.

Charles River (1988). Charles River 1989 Price List Charles River Laboratories, Inc., Massachusetts.

Charles River. *Spontaneous Neoplastic Lesions in the Crl:CD BR Rat.* Charles River Laboratories, Inc., Massachusetts.

Chasseaud, L. F., and Taylor T. (1974) Bioavailability of drugs from formulations after oral administration, in *Annual Review of Pharmacology,* Vol. 14, Elliott, H. W., ed. Illustrated Annual Reviews, pp. 35–46.

Chaube, S., Falahee, K. J., Rose, C. S., Siefried, H. E.. Taylor, T. J., and Winstead, J. A. (1982) *Dermatotoxicity.* EPA-560/11-82-002 United States Environmental Protection Agency, Office of Pesticides and Toxic Substances, Washington, DC.

Chengelis, C. (1988a) Paradoxical effects of cobaltous chloride on carbon disulfide hepatotoxicity in rats. *Res. Commun. Chem. Pathol. Pharmacol.* 61, 83–96.

Chengelis, C. (1988b) Changes in hepatic glutathione concentrations during carbon disulfide hepatotoxicity in the rat. *Res. Commun. Chem. Pathol. Pharmacol.* 61, 97–109.

Chengelis, C. (1988c) Age- and sex-related changes in the components of the hepatic microsomal mixed function oxidase system in Sprague-Dawley rats. *Xenobiotica* 11, 1221–1224.

Chengelis, C. (1988d) Age- and sex-related changes epoxide hydrolase, UDP-glucuronosyl transferase, glutathione S-transferase, PAPS sulfotransferase in Sprague-Dawley rats. *Xenobiotica* 11, 122–1237.

Chi, H. J., and Shin, S. H. (1978) The effect of exposure to ether on prolactin secretion and the half-life of endogenous prolactin in normal and castrated male rats. *Neuroendocrinology* 26, 193–201.

Chowdhury, J., Chowdhury, N., Falany, C., Tephly, T., and Arias, I. (1986) Isolation and characterization of multiple forms of rat liver UDP-glucuronosyltransferase. *Biochem. J.* 233, 827–837.

Christian, J. J., and Lemunyan, C. D. (1958) Adverse effects of crowding on lactation and reproduction of mice and two generations of their progeny. *Endocrinology* 1, 317–328.

Chu, K. (1977). *Percent Spontaneous Primary Tumors in Untreated Species Used at NCI for Carcinogen Bioassays.* NCI Clearing House.

Chu, K. C., Cueto, C., and Ward, J. M. (1981) Factors in the evaluation of 200 National Cancer Institute Carcinogen Bioassays. *J. Toxicol. Environ. Health* 8:251–280.

Chwalisz, K., Zou, J.-C., and Jungblut, P. W. (1983) A non-surgical technique for the transcervical administration of physiological and pharmacological agents into rat uteri. *Acta Endocrinol.* 103, 131–137.

Clark, P. A., and Harland, W. A. (1969) Device for intragastric fluid administration to the rat. *Lab. Anim.* 3, 61–63.

Clarke, H. E., Coates, M. E., Eva, J. K., Ford, D. J., Milner, C. K., O'Donoghue, P. N., Scott, P. P., and Ward, R. J. (1977) Dietary standards for laboratory animals: Report of the Laboratory Animals Centre Diets Advisory Committee. *Lab. Anim.* 11, 1–28.

Clough, G. (1976) The immediate environment of the laboratory animal, in *Control of the Animal House Environment. Laboratory Animal Handbook #7,* McSheeny, T., ed. Laboratory Animal Ltd., pp. 77–94.

Clough, G. (1982) Environmental effects on animals used in biomedical research. *Biol. Rev.* 57,487–523.

Cmarik, J., Inskeep, P., Meredith, M., Meyer, D., Ketterer, B., and Guengerich, F. (1990) Selectivity of rat and human glutathione S-transferases in activation of ethylene dibromide by glutathione conjugation and DNA binding and induction of unschedule DNA synthesis in human hepatocytes. *Cancer Res.* 50, 2747–2752.

Coates, M. E. (1984) Diets for germ-free animals. Part 1. Sterilization of diets, in *The Germ-free Animal in Biomedical Research,* Coates, M. E., and Gustafsson, B. E. eds. Laboratory Animals Ltd., pp. 85–90.

Coates, M. E. (1987). Feeding and watering, In *Laboratory Animals: An Introduction for New Experimenters,* Tuffery, A. A., ed. Wiley, pp. 203–223.

Cohen, B. J., Anver, M. R., and Ringler, D. H. (1978) Age-associated pathological changes in male rats. *Fed. Proc.* 37, 2848–2850.

Cojocel, C., Kramer, W., and Mayer, D. (1988) Depletion of cytochrome P-450 and alterations in activities of drug metabolizing enzymes induced by cephaloridine in the rat liver kidney cortex. *Biochem. Pharmacol.* 37, 3781–3785.

Coleman, G. L., Barthold, S. W., Osbaldiston, G. W., Foster, S. J., and Jonas, A. M. (1977) Pathological changes during aging in barrier-reared Fischer 344 male rats. *J. Gerontol.,* 32, 258–278.

Conahan, S. T., Narayan, S., and Vogel, W. H. (1985) Effect of decapitation and stress on some plasma electrolyte levels in rats. *Pharmacol. Biochem. Behav.* 23, 147–149.

Conner, M. W., and Newberne, P. M. (1984) Drug-nutrient interactions and their implications for safety evaluations. *Fund. Appl. Toxicol.* 4, S341–S356.

Conney, A., Davison, C., Gastel, R., and Burns, J. (1960) Adaptive increases in drug metabolizing enzymes induced by phenobarbital and other drugs. *J. Pharmacol. Exp. Therp.* 130, 1–8.

Conney, A. (1967) Pharmacological implications of microsomal enzyme induction. *Pharmacol. Rev.* 19, 317–366

Conney, A. (1986) Induction of microsomal cytochrome P-450 enzymes: The first Bernard B. Brodie lecture at Pennsylvania State University. *Life Sci.* 39, 2493–2528.

Conybeare, G. (1980) Effect of quality and quantity of diet on survival and tumor incidence of outbred swiss mice. *Food Cosmet. Toxicol.* 18, 65–75.

Conybeare, G., and Leslie, G. B. (1988) Improved oral dosing technique for rats. *J. Pharmacol. Meth.* 19, 109–116.

Cook, C., Karim, A., and Sollman, P. (1982) Stereoselectivity in the metabolism of disopyramide enantiomers in rat and dog. *Drug Metab. Dispos.* 10, 116–121.

Cotlove, E. (1961) Simple tail vein infusion method for renal clearance measurements in the rat. *J. Appl. Physiol.* 16, 764–766.

Cox, C. E., and Beazley, R. M. (1975) Chronic venous catheterization: A technique for implanting and maintaining venous catheters in rats. *J. Surg. Res.* 18, 607–610.

Cruickshanks, J., and Wood, L. C. (1970) Urine collection from individual rats. *J. Inst. Anim. Tech.* 21, 25–28.

Dairman, W., and Balazs, T. (1970) Comparison of liver microsome enzyme systems and barbiturate sleep times in rats caged individually or communally. *Biochem. Pharmacol.* 19, 951–955.

Dalton, R. G., Touraine, J. L., and Wilson, T. R. (1969) A simple technique for continuous intravenous infusion in rats. *J. Lab. Clin. Med.* 74, 813–815.

D'Amour, F. E., and Shaklee, A. B. (1955) Effect of audiogenic seizures on adrenal weight. *Am. J. Physiol.* 183, 269–271.

Dannan, G., and Guengerich, F. (1982) Immunochemical comparison and quantitation of microsomal flavin-containing monooxygenase in various hog, mouse, rat, rabbit, dog and human tissues. *Mol. Pharmacol.* 22, 787–794.

DeBoer, A. G., Breimer, D. D., Pronk, J., and Gubbens-Stibbe, J. M. (198) Rectal bioavailability of lidocaine in rats: Absence of significant first-pass elimination. *J. Pharm. Sci.* 69, 804–807.

Decker, C., Sugiyama, K., Underwood, M., and Correia, M. (1986) Inactivation of rat hepatic cytochrome P-450 by spironolactone. *Biochem. Biophys. Res. Commun.* 136, 1162–1169.

Decker, C., Rashed, M., Baille, T., Maltby, D., and Correia, M. (1989) Oxidative metabolism of spironolactone: Evidence for the involvement of electrophilic thiosteroid species in drug-mediated destruction of hepatic cytochrome P450. *Biochemistry* 28, 5128–5136.

Deftos, L. J., Boorman, G. A., and Roos, B. A. (1976) Immunoassay of calcitonin in rat medullary thyroid carcinoma. *Horm. Metab. Res.* 8, 83–84.

DeLeede, L. G. J., DeBoer, A. G., Roozen, C. P. J. M., and Breimer, D. D. (1983) Avoidance of "first-pass" elimination of rectally administered lidocaine in relation to the site of absorption in rats. *J. Pharmacol. Exp. Ther.* 225, 181–185.

DeLellis, R. A., Nunnemacher, G., and Bitman, W. R. (1979) C-Cell hyperplasia and medullary thyroid carcinoma in the rat. *Lab. Invest.* 40, 140–154.

DePass, L. R., Weil, C. S., Ballantyne, B., Lewis, S. C., Losco, P. E., Reid, J. B., and Simon, G. S. (1986) Influence of housing conditions for mice on the results of a dermal oncogencity bioassay. *Fund. Appl. Toxicol.* 7, 601–608.

Derelanko, M. J. (1987) Determination of erythrocyte life span in F-344, Wistar, and Sprague-Dawley rats using a modification of the [^{3}H]diisopropylfluorophosphate ([^{3}H]DFP) method. *Fund. Appl. Toxicol.* 9, 271–276.

Detweiler, D. K. (1967) Comparative pharmacology of cardiac glycosides. *Fed. Proc.* 26, 1119–1124.

Detweiler, D. K. (1981) The use of electrocardiography in Toxicological studies with rats, in *The Rat Electrocardiogram in Pharmacology and Toxicology,* Budden, R., Detweiler, D. K., and Zbinden, G., eds. Pergamon Press, New York, pp. 83–116.

Detweiler, D. K., Saatmon, R. A., and De Baecke, P. J. (1981) Cardiac arrhythmias accompanying sialodacryoadenitis in the rat in *The Rat Electrocardiogram in Pharmacology and Toxicology,* Budden, R., Detweiler, D. K., and Zbinden, G., eds. Pergamon Press, New York, pp. 129–134.

Devasagayam, T., Choliparambil, P., and Eapen, J. (1983) Changes in enzymes of hepatic rough and smooth microsomes during postnatal development and ageing of rats. *Mech. Age Dev.* 21, 365–375.

Dieke, S. H., and Richter, C. P. (1945) Acute toxicity of thiourea to rats in relation to age, diet, strain, and species variation. *J. Pharmacol. Exp. Ther.* 83, 195–202.

Dierickx, P. (1982) In vitro inhibition of the soluble glutathione S-transferase from rat liver by heavy metals. *Enzyme* 27, 25–32.

Doell, B. H., and Hegarty, P. V. J. (1970) The haemoglobin concentration of peripheral and central blood of the laboratory rat. *Br. J. Haematol.* 18, 503–509.

Dohler, K. D., Von Zur Muhlen, A., Gartner, K., and Dohler, Y. (1977) Effect of various blood sampling techniques on serum levels of pituitary and thyroid hormones in the rat. *J. Endocrinol* 74, 341–342.

Dohler, K. D., Wong, C. C., Gaudssuhn, D., Von Zur Muhlen, A., Gartner, K., and Dohler, U. (1978) Site of blood sampling in rats as a possible source of error in hormone determinations. *J. Endocrinol.* 79, 141–142.

Down, W., and Chasseaud, L. (1979) Effect of repeated oral administration of phenobarbitone or DDt on hepatic glutathione S-transferase activity in nonhuman primates: Comparison with the rat. *Biochem. Pharmacol.* 28, 3525–3528.

Driscoll, P. (1981) The normal rat electrocardiogram, in *The Rat Electrocardiogram in Pharmacology and Toxicology*, Budden, R., Detweiler, D. K., Zbinden, G., eds. Pergamon Press, New York, pp. 1–14.

Duignan, D., Sipes, G., Leonard, T., and Halpert, J. (1987) Purification and characterization of the dog hepatic cytochrome P-450 isozyme responsible for the metabolism of 2,2',4,4',5,5'-hexachlorobiphenyl. *Arch. Biochem. Biophys.* 255, 290–303.

Dutton, G. (1978) Developmental aspects of drug conjugation with special reference to glucuronidation. *Ann. Rev. Pharmacol. Toxicol.* 18, 17–35.

Dymsza, H. A., Miller, S. A., Maloney, J. F., and Foster, H. L. (1963) Equilibration of the laboratory rat following exposure to shipping stresses. *Lab. Anim. Care* 13, 60–65.

Early, J., and Schnell, R. (1972) Effects of glutathione depletion on selenium lethaolity and hepatic drug metabolism in male rats. *Toxicol. Lett.* 11, 253–257.

Edwards, G. S., Fox, J. S., Policastro, P., Goff, U., Wolf, M. H., and Fine, D. H. (1979) Volatile nitrosamine contamination in laboratory animal diets. *Cancer Res.* 39, 1857–1858.

Einheber, A., Wren, R. E., Carter, D., and Rose, L. R. (1967) A simple collar device for the protection of skin graphs in mice. *Lab. Anim. Care* 17, 345–348.

Eisenstein, E. M., and Woskow, M. H. (1958) Technique for measuring heart potentials continuously in a freely moving rat. *Arch. Neurol. Psych.* 80, 394–395.

Eisman, E. (1965) Technique for monitoring cardiac function without handling or restraining the animal. *Percept. Motor Skills* 20, 1093–1097.

Elovaara, E., Zitting, A., Nickels, J., and Aitio, A. (1987) m-Xylene inhalation destroys cytochrome P-450 in rat lung at low exposure. *Arch. Toxicol.* 61, 21–26.

Endou, H. (1983) Distribution and some characteristics of cytochrome P-450 in the kidney. *J. Toxicol. Sci.* 8, 165–176.

Ensor, C. R. (1946) The electrocardiogram of rats on vitamin E deficiency. *Am. J. Physiol.* 147, 477–480.

Enta, T., Lockey, S. D., Jr., and Reed, C. E. (1968) A rapid, safe technique for repeated blood collection from small laboratory animals. The farmer's wife method. *Proc. Soc. Exp. Biol. Med.* 127, 136–137.

Environmental Protection Agency (EPA) (1979) Proposed health effects test standards for toxic substances control act. Test rules. Good laboratory practice standards for health effects. *Fed. Reg.* Part 2, 27334–27375, Part 4, 44054–44093.

Environmental Protection Agency (EPA) (1985) Toxic Substances Control Act Testing Guidelines 40 CFR part 798 subpart G sections 798.6050 and 798.6200, *Fed. Reg.* 50

Epstein, A. N., and Teitelbaum, P. (1962a) Regulation of food intake in the absence of taste, smell, and other oropharyngeal sensations. *J. Comp. Physiol. Psychol.* 55, 753–759.

Epstein, A. N., and Teitelbaum, P. (1962b) A watertight swivel joint permitting chronic injection into moving animals. *J. Appl. Physiol.* 17, 171–172.

Evans, J. S. (1970) A technique for prolonged infusion of unanesthetized and relatively unrestrained rats. *J. Appl. Physiol.* 29, 275–277.

Eve, C., and Robinson, S. H. (1963) Apparatus for continuous long-term intravenous infusions in small animals. *J. Lab. Clin. Med.* 62, 169–174.

Everett, J. W., and Sawyer, C. H. (1956) The small saphenous vein as a route for intravenous injection in the white rat. *Nature* 178, 268–269.

Falabella, F. (1967) Bleeding mice: A successful technique for cardiac puncture. *J. Lab. Clin. Med.* 70, 981–982.

Fears, T. R., Tarone, R. E., and Chu, K. C. (1977) False-positive and false-negative rates for carcinogenicity screens. *Cancer Res.* 27, 1941–1945.

Feldman, D. B., and Seely, J. C. (1988) *Necropsy Guide: Rodents and the Rabbit.* CRC Press, Boca Raton, Florida, pp. 1–50.

Ferguson, H. C. (1962) Dilution of dose and acute oral toxicity. *Toxicol. Appl. Pharmacol.* 4, 759–762.

Ferguson, H. C. (1966) Effect of red cedar chip bedding on hexobarbital and pentobarbital sleep time. *J. Pharm. Sci.* 55, 1142–1143.

Ferrill, H. W. (1943) A simplified method for feeding rats. *J. Lab. Clin. Med.* 28, 1624–1625.

Flecknell, P. A. (1987) Non-surgical experimental procedures, in *Laboratory Animals: An In-*

troduction for New Experimentors, Tuffery, A. A., ed. Wiley, London, England, pp. 225–260.

Flynn, R. J. (1959) Studies on the etiology of ringtail of rats. *Proc. Animal Care Panel* 9, 155–160.

Food and Drug Administration (FDA) (1978) Nonclinical laboratory studies. Good laboratory practice regulations. *Fed. Reg.* Part 2 59986–60025.

Ford, D. (1976) The influence of sterilization processes on the protein quality of a laboratory rat diet. *Z. Versuchstierk.* 18, 160–161.

Ford, D. J. (1977) Influence of diet pellet hardness and particle size on food utilization by mice, rats, and hamsters. *Lab. Anim.* 11, 241–246.

Foster, C.H.L., Trexler, P. C., and Rumsey, G. (1967) A canned sterile shipping diet for small laboratory rodents. *Lab. Anim. Care* 17, 400–405.

Fowler, J.S.L., Brown, J. S., and Flower, E. W. (1980) Comparison between ether and carbon dioxide anaesthesia for removal of small blood samples from rats. *Lab. Anim.* 14, 275–278.

Fox, J. G., Aldrich, F. D., and Boylen, G. W., Jr. (1976) Lead in animal foods. *J. Toxicol. Environ. Health* 1, 461–467.

Fox, J. G., and Boylen, G. W., Jr. (1978) Analysis of lead in animal feed ingredients. *Am. J. Vet. Res.* 39, 167–169.

Fox, J. G., Thibert, P., Arnold, D. L., Krewski, D. R., and Grice, H. C. (1979) Toxicology studies. II. The laboratory animal. *Food Cosmet. Toxicol.* 17, 661–675.

Frape, D. L., Wilkinson, J., and Chubb, L. G. (1970) A simplified metabolism cage and tail cup for young rats. *Lab. Anim.* 4, 67–73.

Fraser, R. S., Harley, C., and Wiley, T. (1967) Electrocardiogram in the normal rat. *J. Appl. Physiol.* 23, 401–402.

Friedman, M., and Freed, S. C. (1949) Microphonic manometer for indirect determination of systolic blood pressure in the rat. *Proc. Soc. Exp. Biol. Med.* 70, 670–672.

Friedman, M., Byers, S. O., and Brown, A. E. (1967) Plasma lipid responses of rats and rabbits to an auditory stimulus. *Am. J. Physiol.* 212, 1174–1178.

Frolich, M., Walma, S. T., and Souverijn, J.H.M. (1981) Probable influence of cage design on muscle metabolism of rats. *Lab. Anim. Sci.* 31, 510–512.

Fuhrman, G. J., and Fuhrman, F. A. (1961) Effects of temperature on the action of drugs. *Ann. Rev. Pharmacol.* 1, 65–78.

Fukushima, M., Tsutsui, K., Kodama, J., Sakata, T., Goto, M., and Teranishi, T. (1979) New inexpensive device for estimating dry food intake in small animals. *Physiol. Behav.* 22, 1029–1032.

Fuller, G. C., Bousquet, W. F., and Miya, T. S. (1972) Effect of cold exposure on drug action and hepatic drug metabolism in the rat. *Toxicol. Appl. Pharmacol.* 23, 10–19.

Furner, R., Gram, T., and Stitzel, R. (1969) The influence of age, sex, and drug metabolism in four rat strains. *Biochemical Pharmacol.* 18, 1635–1641.

Furuhama, K., and Onodera, T. (1983) A simple technique for repeated blood collection from the tail vein of the rat. *J. Toxicol. Sci.* 8, 161–163.

Gad, S. C., and Chengelis, C. P. (1988) *Acute Toxicology Testing Perspectives and Horizons.* Telford Press, Caldwell, New Jersey, pp. 266–273, 503–509.

Gad, S. C., Smith, A. C., Cramp, A. L., Gavigan, F. A., and Derelanko, M. J. (1984) Innovative designs and practices for acute systemic toxicity studies. *Drug Chem. Toxicol.* 7, 5:423–434.

Galinsky, R. E., and Corcoran, G. B. (1986) Influence of advanced age on the formation and elimination of acetaminophen metabolites by male rats. *Pharmacology* 32, 313–320.

Galinsky, R. E., Kane, R. E., and Franklin, M. R. (1986) Effect of aging on drug-metabolizing enzymes important in acetaminophen elimination. *J. Pharm. Exp. Ther.* 237, 107–113.

Gallo-Torres, H. E., and Ludorf, J. (1974) Techniques for the *in vivo* catheterization of the portal vein in the rat. *Proc. Soc. Exp. Biol. Med.* 145, 249–254.

Gamble, M. R. (1982) Sound and its significance for laboratory animals. *Biol. Rev.* 57, 395–421.

Gamble, M. R., and Clough, G. (1976) Ammonia build-up in animal boxes and its effect on rat tracheal epithelium. *Lab. Anim.* 10, 93–104.

Garst, J., Wilson, W., Kristensen, N., Harrison, P., Corbin, J., Simon, J., Philpot, R., and Szabo, R. (1985) Species susceptibility to the pulmonary toxicity of 3-furyl isoamyl ketone (Perilla ketone): In vivo support for involvement of the lung monooxygenase system. *J. Anim. Sci.* 60, 248–257.

Gart, J. J., Chu, K. C., and Tarone, R. E. (1979) Statistical issues in interpretation of chronic bioassay tests for carcinogenicity. *J. Natl. Cancer Inst.* 62, 957–974.

Gartner, K., Buttner, D., Dohler, K., Friedel, R., Lindena, J., and Trautschold, I. (1980) Stress response of rats to handling and experimental procedures. *Lab. Anim.* 14, 267–274.

Geber, W. F. (1966) Developmental effects of chronic maternal audiovisual stress on the rat foetus. *J. Embryol. Exp. Morphol.* 16, 1–16.

Geber, W. F. (1973) Inhibition of fetal osteogenesis by maternal noise stress. *Fed. Proc.* 32, 2101–2104.

Geber, W. F., Anderson, T. A., and Van Dyne, B. (1966) Physiologic responses of the albino rat to chronic noise stress. *Arch. Environ. Health* 12, 751–754.

Germain, M. A., Webster, W. S., and Edwards, M. J. (1985) Hyperthermia as a teratogen: Parameters determining hyperthermia-induced head defects in the rat. *Teratology* 31, 265–272.

Gibson, J. E., and Becker, B. A. (1967) The administration of drugs to one day old animals. *Lab. Anim. Care* 17, 524–527.

Gibson, S. V., Besch-Williford, C., Raisbeck, M. F., Wagner, J. E., and McLaughlin, R. M. (1987) Organophosphate toxicity in rats associated with contaminated bedding. *Lab. Anim. Sci.* 37, 789–791.

Giner, M., Snyder, K., and Meguid, M. M. (1987) Chronic vascular access for repeated blood sampling in the unrestrained rat. *Am. J. Physiol.* 252, H992.

Glaister, J. (1986) *Principles of Toxicological Pathology*. Taylor & Francis, Philadelphia.

Golba, S., Golba, M., and Wilczok, T. (1974) The effect of trauma, in the form of intraperitoneal injections or puncture of the orbital venous plexus, on peripheral white blood cell counts in rats. *Acta Physiol. Pol.* 25, 339–345.

Gonzales, F. (1989) The molecular biology of cytohromes P450s. *Pharmacol. Rev.* 40, 243–288.

Goodman, D. G., Ward, J. M., Squire, R. A., Chu, K. C., and Linhart, M. S. (1979) Neoplastic and nonneoplastic lesions in aging F344 rats. *Toxicol. Appl. Pharmacol.* 48, 237–248.

Gorski, J. R., Arlotto, M. P., Klaassen, C. D., and Parkinson, A. (1985) Age-dependent and sex-dependent induction of liver microsomal benzo-a-pyrene hydroxylase activity in rats treated with pregnenolone 16-alpha-carbonitrile. *Carcinogenesis* (Lond.) 6, 617–624.

Gram, T., Guarino, A., Schroeder, D., Davis, D., Reagan, R., and Gillette, J. (1970) The effect of starvation on the kinetics of drug oxidation by hepatic microsomal enzymes from male and female rats. *J. Pharmacol. Exp. Ther.* 175, 12–21.

Grant, L., Hopkinson, P., Jennings, G., and Jenner, F. A. (1971) Period of adjustment of rats used for experimental studies. *Nature* 232, 135.

Gray, J. E. (1977) Chronic progressive nephrosis in the albino rat. *CRC Crit. Rev. Toxicol.* 5, 115–144.

Grazer, F. M. (1958) Technic for intravascular injection and bleeding of newborn rats and mice. *Proc. Soc. Exp. Biol. Med.* 99, 407–408.

Greaves, P., and Faccini, J. M. (1984) *Rat Histopathology: A Glossary for Use in Toxicity and Carcinogenicity Studies*, Elsevier, New York.

Green, R. S., and Turner, J. C. (1974) The manufacture of small quantities of rat food pellets in the laboratory. *Lab Anim.* 8, 131–132

Greenman, D. L., Oller, W. L., Littlefield, N. A., and Nelson, C. J. (1980) Commerical laboratory animal diets: Toxicant and nutrient variability. *J. Toxicol. Environ. Health* 6, 235–246.

Gregus, Z., Madhu, C., Goon, D., and Klaassen, C. (1988) Effect of glactosamine-induced hepatic UDP-glucuronic acid depletion on acetaminophen elimination in rats. Dispositional differences between hepatically and extrahepatically formed glucuronides of acetaminophen and other chemicals. *Drug Metab. Dispos.* 16, 527–533.

Gregus, Z., Varga, F., and Schmelas, A. (1985) Age-development and inducibility of hepatic glutathione S-transferase activities in mice, rats, rabbits and guinea-pigs. *Comp. Biochem. Physiol.* 80C (UK), 85–90.

Griffith, J. Q., Jr. (1934–1935) Indirect method for determining blood pressure in small animals. *Proc. Soc. Exp. Biol. Med.* 32, 394–396.

Guengerich, F. (1990). Purification and characterization of xenobiotic-metabolizing enzymes from lung tissue. *Pharmacol. Ther.* 45, 299–307.

Guengerich, F., Wang, P., Mitchell, M., and Mason, P. (1979) Rat and human liver microsomal epoxide hydratase. Purification and evidence for the existance of multiple forms. *J. Biol. Chem.* 254, 12248–12254.

Haggerty, G. C. (1989) Development of tier I neurobehavioral testing capabilities for incorporation into pivotal rodent safety assessment studies. *J. Amer. Coll. Toxicol.* 8, 53–69.

Hales, B., Jain, R., and Robaire, B. (1982) Differential regulation of male liver glutathione S-transferases. Effects of orchidectomy and hormone replacement. *Biochem. Pharmacol.* 31, 2389–2393.

Hall, R. I., Ross, L. H., Bozovic, M., and Grant, J. P. (1984) A simple method of obtaining repeated venous blood samples from the conscious rat. *J. Surg. Res.* 36, 92–95.

Halvorsen, O. (1983) Effects of hypolipidemic drugs on hepatic CoA. *Biochem. Pharmacol.* 32, 1126–1128.

Hamilton, C. L. (1967) Food and temperature, in *Alimental Canal*, Vol. 1, *Control of Food and Water Intake*, Code, C. F., and Heidel, W., eds. Williams & Wilkins, Baltimore, pp. 303–317.

Hansen, L., and Holm, H. (1971) Apparatus for collecting feces and urine from rats in metabolic experiments. *Lab. Anim.* 5, 221–224.

Harms, P. G., and Ojeda, S. R. (1974) A rapid and simple procedure for chronic cannulation of the rat jugular vein. *J. Appl. Physiol.* 36, 391–392.

Hart, R. W., and Fishbein, L. (1985) Interspecies extrapolation of drug and genetic toxicology data, in *Toxicological Risk Assessment*, Vol. I, Clayson, D. B., Krewski, D., and Munro, I., eds. CRS Press, Boca Raton, Florida, pp. 3–40.

Haseman, J. K., Huff, J. C., Rao, G. N., and Eustis, S. L. (1989) Sources of variability in rodent carcinogenicity studies. *Fund. Appl. Toxicol.* 12, 793–804.

Hasimoto, M., Davis, D. C., and Gillette, J. R. (1972) Effect of different routes of administration of cedrene on hepatic drug metabolism. *Biochem. Pharmacol.* 21, 1514–1517.

Hawkins, J., Jones, W., Bonner, F., and Gibson, G. (1987) The effects of peroxisomal proliferators on miccrosomal, peroxisomal, and mitochondrial enzyme activities in liver and kidney. *Drug Metab. Rev.* 18, 441–516.

Hayashi, S., and Sakaguchi, T. (1975) Capillary tube urinalysis for small animals. *Lab. Anim. Sci.* 25, 781–782.

Heimark, L., and Trager, W. (1985) Stereoselective metabolism of conformational analogues of warafarin by β-napththoflavone-inducible cytochrome P-450. *J. Med. Chem.* 28, 503–506.

Herd, J. A., and Barger, A. C. (1964) Simplified technique for chronic catheterization of blood vessels. *J. Appl. Physiol.* 19, 791–792.

Hermansen, K. (1970) A new method for determination of the systolic blood pressure in conscious rats. *Life Sci.* 9, 1233–1237.

Heston, W. E. (1975) Testing for possible effects of cedar wood shavings and diet on occurrence of mammary gland tumors and hepatomas in C3H-A and C3H-AfB Mice. *J. Natl. Cancer Inst.* 54, 1011–1014.

Hill, R., Howard, A. N., and Gresham, G. A. (1960) *Br. J. Exp. Pathol.* 41, 633–637.

Hjelle, J., Hazelton, G., and Klaassen, C. (1985) Acetaminphen decreases adenosine 3'-phosphate 5'phosphosulfate and uridine diphosphoglucuronic acid in rat liver. *Drug Metab. Dispos.* 13, 35–41.

Hock, F. J., and Beyhl, F. E. (1984) A novel method for the administration of the enzyme inducer phenobarbital to rats via an osmotic minipump. *IRCS Med. Sci.* 12, 661.

Hollander, C. F. (1968) Cartilaginous focus at the base of the non-coronary semilunar valve of the aorta in rats of different ages. *Exp. Gerontol.* 3, 303.

Howells, G. R., Wright, C. F., and Harrison, G. E. (1964) A new metabolic cage for rats. *J. Anim. Tech. Assoc.* 14, 137–140.

Hsu, C. K., New, A. E., and Mayo, J. G. (1980) Quality assurance of rodent models, 7th ICLAS Symp. Utrecht, 1979, in *Animal Quality and Models in Biomedical Research*, Gustav Fischer Verlag, pp. 17–28.

Huckle, K., Hutson, D., and Millburn. (1981) Species differences in the metabolism of 3-phenoxybenzoic acid. *Drug Metab. Dispos.* 9, 352–359.

Hulse, M., Feldman, S., and Bruckner, J. V. (1981) Effect of blood sampling schedules on protein drug binding in the rat. *J. Pharmacol. Exp. Ther.* 218, 416–420.

Hundley, J. M., Ashburn, L. L., and Sebrell, W. H. (1945) The electrocardiogram in chronic thiamine deficiency in rats. *Am J. Physiol.* 144, 404–414.

Hurwitz, A. (1971) A simple method for obtaining blood samples from rats. *J. Lab. Clin. Med.* 78, 172–174.

Hussain, A., Hirai, S., and Bawarshi, R. (1980) Nasal absorption of propranolol from different dosage forms by rats and dogs. *J. Pharm. Sci.* 69, 1411–1413.

Hysell, D. K., and Abrams, G. D. (1967) Complications in the use of indwelling vascular catheters in laboratory animals. *Lab. Anim. Care* 17, 273–280.

Igarashi, T., Satoh, T., Ueno, K., and Kitigawa, H. (1983) Sex-related differences in hepatic glutathione level and related enzyme activities in rat. *J. Biochem.* 93, 33–36.

ILAR Committee on Long-term Holding of Laboratory Rodents (1976) Long-term holding of laboratory rodents. *ILAR News* 19, L1–L25.

ILAR, NRC. (1985) Guide for the care and use of laboratory animals. NIH Publication No. 86–23, Washington, D.C., pp. 18–19.

Innes, J.R.M., and Stanton, M. (1961) Acute disease of the submaxillary and harderian glands (sialo-dacryoadenitis) of rats with cytomegaly and no inclusion bodies. *Am. J. Pathol.* 38, 455–468.

Ioannides, C., Parkinson, C., and Parke, D. (1981) Activation of benzo(a)pyrene to mutagens by microsomal preparations form different animal species: Role of cytochrome P-450 and P-448. *Xenobiotica* 11, 701–708.

Ito, N., Tatematsu, M., Hasegawa, R., and Tsuda, H. (1989) Medium-term bioassay system for detection of carcinogenicity and modifers of hepatocarcinogenesis utilizing the GST-P postive liver cell focus as an endpoint markker. *Toxicol. Pathol.* 17, 630–641.

Iversen, B. M., and Andersen, K. J. (1983) The effect of sampling conditions on rat plasma renin. *Comp. Biochem. Physiol.* 74A, 331–332.

Iwamoto, K., and Watanabe, J. (1985) Avoidance of first-pass metabolism of propranolol after rectal administration as a function of the absorption site. *Pharm. Res.* 2, 53–54.

Iwasaki, K., Lum, P., Ioannides, C., and Parke, D. (1986) Induction of cytochrome P-448 activity as exemplified by the O-deethylation of ethoxyresorufin. Effects of dose, sex, tissue and animal species. *Biochem. Pharmacol.* 35, 3879–3884.

Jacoby, R. O., and Barthold, S.W. (1981) Quality assurance for rodents used in toxicological research and testing, in *Scientific Considerations in Monitoring and Evaluation of Toxicologic Research*, Gralla, E. J., ed. Hemisphere, pp. 27–55.

Jacoby, R. O., Bhatt, P. N., and Jonas, A. M. (1979) Viral diseases, in *The Laboratory Rat*, Vol. I, Baker, H. J., Lindsey, J. R., and Weisbroth, S. H., eds. Academic Press, New York, pp. 271–306.

Jakobson, I., Warholm, M., and Mannervik, B. (1979) Multiple inhibition of glutathione S-transferase A from rat liver by glutathione derivatives: Kinetic analysis supporting a steady state random sequential mechanism. *Biochem. J.* 177, 861–868.

James, S., and Pheasant, A. (1978) Glutathione conjugation and mercapturic acid formation in the developing rat, in vivo and in vitro. *Xenobiotica* 8, 207–217.

Jansson, I., and Schenkman, J. (1973) Evicecne against participation of cytochrome b5 in the hepatic microsomal mixed function oxidase reaction. *Mol. Pharmacol.* 9, 840–845.

Jansson, I., Tamburini, P., Favreau, L., and Schenkman, J. (1985) The interaction of cytochrome b5 with four cytochrome P-450 enzymes from the untreated rat. *Drug Metab. Dispos.* 13, 453–458.

Johnson, H. D., and Voss, E. (1952) Toxicological studies of zinc phosphide. *J. Am. Pharm. Assoc.* 41, 468–472.

Jones, P. A., and Hynd, J. W. (1981) Continuous long-term intravenous infusion in the unrestrained rat—a novel technique. *Lab. Anim.* 15, 29–33.

Joy, R.J.T., Emma, C. P., and Mayer, J. (1967) New rat feeding jar: Use in study of relationships of food intake and body weight. *J. Appl. Physiol.* 23, 589–590.

Kahn, G. C., Rubenfield, M., Davies, D. S., Murray, S., and Boobis, A. R. (1985) Sex and strain differences in hepatic debrisoquine 4-hydroxylase activity of the rat. *Drug Metab. Dispos.* 13, 510–516.

Kahn, G. C., Rubenfield, M., Davies, D. S., and Boobis, A. R. (1987) Phenacetin O-deethylase activity of the rat: Strain differences and the effects of enzyme-inducing compounds. *Xenobiotica*, 17, 179–187.

Kai, K., Kobayashi, S., Uchida, E., Sakai, H., Tanaka, E., Kurata, N., and Yasuhara, H. (1988) The effects of molatilate on hepatic drug metabolizing systems in different strains of rats. *Comp. Biochem. Biophys* 90C, 13–19.

Kamataki, T., Maeda, K., Shimada, M., Kitani, K., Nagai, T., and Kato, R. (1985) Age-related alteration in the activities of drug-metabolizing enzymes and contents of sex-specific forms of cytochrome P-450 in liver microsomes from male and female rats. *J. Pharmacol. Exp. Ther.* 233, 222–228.

Kao, J., and Hudson, P. (1980) Induction of the hepatic cytochrome P-450-dependent monooxygenase system in young and geriatric rats. *Biochemical Pharmacol.* 29, 1191–1194.

Kapetanovic, I., Sweeney, D., and Rapoport, S. (1982) Age effects on haloperidol pharmacokinetics in male Fischer-344 rats. *J. Pharmacol. Exp. Ther.* 221, 434–438.

Kaplowitz, N., Aw, T., and Ookthens, M. (1985) The regulation of hepatic glutathione. *Ann. Rev. Pharmacol. Toxicol.* 25, 715–744.

Kato, R., and Takanaka, A. (1968) Metabolism of drugs in old rats (I). Activities of NADPH-linked electron transport and drug-metabolizing enzyme systems in liver microsomes of old rats. *Jpn. J. Pharmacol.* 18, 381–388.

Kato, R., Vassanelli, P., Frontino, G., and Chesara, E. (1964) Variation in the activity of liver microsomal drug-metabolizing enzymes in rats in relation to the age. *Biochem. Pharmacol.* 13, 1037–1051.

Kato, R., and Takanaka, A. (1968) Effect of phenobarbital on electron transport system, oxidation and reduction of drugs in liver microsomes of rats of different age. *J. Biochem.* 63, 406–408.

Kaufman, S. (1980) Chronic, nonocclusive, and maintenance-free central venous cannula in the rat. *Am. J. Physiol.* 239, R123–R125.

Keen, J., and Jakoby, W. (1978) Glutathine transferases. Catalysis of nucleophilic reactions of glutathione. *J. Biol. Chem.* 253, 5654–5657.

Keith, I. M., Olson, E. B. Jr., Wilson, N. M., and Jefcoate, C. R. (1987) Immunological identification and effects of 3-methylcholanthrene and phenobarbital on rat pulmonary cytochrome P-450. *Cancer Res.* 47, 1878–1882.

Kennedy, G. L. Jr. (1989) Inhalation toxicology, in *Principles and Methods of Toxicology*, Hayes, A. W., ed. Raven Press, New York, pp. 361–406.

Keplinger, M. L., Lanier, G. E., and Deichmann, W. B. (1959) Effects of environmental temperature on the acute toxicity of a number of compounds in rats. *Toxicol. Appl. Pharmacol.* 1, 156–161.

Kersten, H., Brosene, W. G., Jr., Ablondi, F., and SubbaRow, Y. (1947) A new method for the indirect measurement of blood pressure in the rat. *J. Lab. Clin. Med.* 32, 1090–1098.

Kesel, H. (1964) A simple aid in the intubation of small animals. *Lab. Anim. Care* 14, 499–500.

Khosho, F. K., Kaufmann, R. C., and Amankwah, K. S. (1985) A simple and efficient method for obtaining urine samples from rats. *Lab. Anim. Sci.* 35, 513–514.

Kizer, D. E., Clouse, J. A., Ringer, D. P., Hanson-Painton, O., Vaz, A. D., Palakodety, R. B., and Griffin, M. J. (1985) Assessment of rat liver microsomal epoxide hydrolase as a marker of hepatocarcinogenesis. *Biochem. Pharmacol.* 34, 1795–1800.

Klinger, W. (1982) Biotransformation of drugs and other xenobiotics during postnatal development. *Pharmacol. Ther.* 16, 377–429.

Knapp, S., Green, M., Tephly, T., and Baron, J. (1988) Immunohistochemical demonstration of isozyme- and strain-specific differences in the intralobular localizations and distributions of UDP-glucuronosyltransferases in livers of untreated rats. *Mol. Pharmacol.* 33, 14–21.

Koch, R., and Goldman, P. (1979) The anaerobic metabolism of metronidazole forms N-2-(hydroxyethyl)-oxamic acid. *J. Pharmacol. Exp. Therap.* 208, 406–10.

Koeslag, D., Humphreys, A. S., and Russell, J. C. (1984) A technique for long-term venous cannulation in rats. *J. Appl. Physiol.* 57, 1594–1596.

Kohn, D. F., and Barthold, S. W. (1984) Biology and diseases of rats, in *Laboratory Animal Medicine*, Fox, J. G., ed. Academic Press, New York, pp. 91–122.

Korol, B., and McShane, W. (1963) A new method for indirect recording of arterial pressure in unanesthetized rats. *J. Appl. Physiol.* 18, 437–439.

Koster, A. S., Nieuwenhuis, L., and Frankhuijzen-Sierevogel, A. C. (1989) Comparison of microsomal drug-metabolizing enzymes in 14 rat inbred strains. *Biochem. Pharmacol.* 38(5), 759–765.

Kraft, L. M. (1958) Observations on the control and natural history of epidemic diarrhea of infant mice (EDIM). *Yale J. Biol. Med.* 31, 121–137.

Kraus, A. L. (1979) Research Methodology, in *The Laboratory Rat*, Vol. II, Baker, H. J., Lindsey, J. R., and Weisbroth, S. H., eds. Academic Press, New York, pp. 2–42.

Kroll, D. J., Graichen, M. E., and Leonard, T. B. (1988) Strain difference in rat renal microsomal epoxide hydrolase elevation after mercuric chloride treatment. *Carcinogenesis* 9, 193–198.

Kudo, Y., Sokabe, H., and Zehr, J. E. (1981) A simple method to determine the ratio of cardiac to vascular β-receptor blockade in the rat in vivo. *J. Pharm. Dyn.* 4, 475–482.

Kupp, R. P., and Strolle, L. A. (1979) The effects of autolytic changes in animals on histologic interpretation. *Toxicol. Appl. Pharmacol.* 48, A145.

Kurata, N., Yoshida, T., and Kuroiwa, Y. (1989) Long term effects of phenobarbital on rat liver microsomal drug- metabolizing enzymes and heme-metabolizing enzyme. *Res. Commun. Chem. Pathol. Pharmacol.* 65, 161–179.

Laakso, M.-L., Johansson, G. Porkka-Heiskanen, T., and Peder, M. (1984) The effect of blood sampling on plasma levels of LH and FSH in male rats. *Acta Physiol. Scand.* 121, 233–239.

Lai, Y. L., Jacoby, R. O., and Bhatt, P. N. (1976) Keratoconjunctivitis associated with sialodacryoadenitis in rats. *Invest. Ophthalmol.* 15, 538–541.

Lai, Y. L., Jacoby, R. O., and Jonas, A. M. (1978) Age-related and light associated retinal changes in Fischer rats. *Invest. Ophthalmol. Vis. Sci.* 17, 634–638.

Laqueur, G. L. (1970) Contribution of intestinal macroflora and microflora to carcinogenesis, in *Carcinoma of the Colon and Antecedent Epithelium*, Burdette, W. J., ed. Thomas, Springfield, Illinois, pp. 305–313.

LaVail, M. W. (1976) Rod outer segment disk shedding in rat retina: Relationship to cyclic lighting. *Science* 194, 1071–1074.

Lax, E. R., Militzer, K., and Trauschel, A. (1983) A simple method for oral administration of drugs in solid form to fully conscious rats. *Lab. Anim.* 17, 50–54.

Lehr, D. (1945) Stomach-tube feeding of small laboratory animals. *J. Lab. Clin. Med.* 30, 977–980.

Leinweber, F. (1987) Possible physiological roles of carboxylic ester hydrolases. *Drug Metab. Rev.* 18, 379–440.

Leob, W. F., and Quimby, F. W. (1989) *The Clinical Chemistry of Laboratory Animals*, Pergamon Press, New York.

Leonard, R., and Ruben, Z. (1986) Hematology reference values for peripheral blood of laboratory rats, *Lab. Anim. Sci.* 36, 277–281.

Lesca, P., Fournier, A., Lecointe, P., and Cresteil, T. (1984) A dual assay for the specific screening of 3-methylchoanthrene- and phenobarbital-like chemical inducers of cytochrome P-450 monooxygenases. *Mutat. Res.* 129, 299–310.

Levine, W. (1983) Glutahione and hepatic mixed-function oxidase activity. *Drug Metab. Rev.* 14, 909–930.

Levine, G., Lewis, L. L., and Cember, H. (1973) A vacuum-assisted technic for repetitive blood sampling in the rat. *Lab. Anim. Sci.* 23, 556–558.

Lewis, R. E., Kunz, A. L., and Bell, R. E. (1966) Error of intraperitoneal injections in rats. *Lab. Anim. Care* 16, 505–509.

Ley, F. J., Bleby, J., Coates, M. E., and Patterson, J. S. (1969) Sterilization of laboratory animal diets using gamma radiation. *Lab. Anim.* 3, 221–254.

Lindeskog, P., Haaparanta, T., Norgard, M., Glaumann, H., Hansson, T., and Gustafsson, J. A. (1986) Isolation of rat intestinal microsomes: Partial characterization of mucosal cytochrome P-450. *Arch. Biochem. Biophys.* 244, 492–501.

Lindsey, J. R. (1979) Historical Foundations, in *The Laboratory Rat*, Vol. 1, Baker, H. J., Lindsey, J. R., and Weisbroth, S. H., Eds. Academic Press, New York, pp. 1–36.

Lipton, J. M. (1972) Superior saggital sinus as a chronic venous route in the rat. *J. Appl. Physiol.* 32, 701–702.

Lisella, F. S., Long, K. R., and Scott, H. G. (1971) Toxicology of rodenticides and their relation to human health. *J. Environ. Health* 33, 231–237, 361–365.

Litterst, C. C., Mimnaugh, E., Reagan, R., and Gram, T. (1975) Comparison of in vitro drug metabolism by lung, liver, and kidney of several common laboratory species. *Drug Metab. Dispos.* 3, 259–265.

Lombard, E. A. (1952) Electrocardiograms of small animals. *Am. J. Physiol.* 171, 189–193.

Longo, N., and Pellegrino, J. W. (1967) A simple telemetric method for monitoring cardiac function in small animals. *Percept. Motor Skills* 24, 512–514.

Loose, D. S., Kan, P. B., Hirst, M. A., Marcus, R. A., and Feldman, D. (1983) Ketoconazole blocks adrenal steroidogenesis by inhibiting cytochrome P450-dependent enzymes. *J. Clin. Invest.* 71, 1495–1499.

Losco, P. E., and Ward, J. M. (1984) The early stage of large granular lymphocyte leukemia of the F-344 rat. *Vet. Pathol.* 21, 286–291.

Lotlikar, P., Enomoto, M., Miller, J., and Miller, E. (1967) Species variations in the N- and ring -hydroxylation of 2-acetylaminofluorene and effects of 3-methylcholanthrene pretreatment. *Proc. Soc. Exp. Biol. Med.* 125, 341–346.

Loveless, B. W., Williams, P., and Heaton, F. W. (1972) A simple automatic feeding apparatus for rats. *Br. J. Nutr.* 28, 261–264.

Lower, G., and Bryan, G. (1973) Enzymatic N-acetylation of carcinogenic aromatic amines by liver cytosol of species displaying different organ susceptibilities. *Biochem. Pharmacol.* 22, 1581–1588.

Lu, A., and Miwa, G. (1980) Molecular properties and biological functions of microsomal epoxide hydrolase. *Ann. Rev. Pharmacol. Toxicol.* 20, 513–531.

Lu, A., and West, S. (1980) Multiplicity of mammalian microsomal cytochrome P-450. *Pharmacol. Rev.* 31, 227–295.

Lu, A., Somogyi, A., West, S., Kuntzman, R., and Conney, A. (1972) Pregnenolone-16α-carbonitrile: A new type of inducer of drug-metabolizing enzymes. *Arch. Biochem. Biophys.* 152, 457–462.

Lubet, R., Nims, R., Ward, J., Rice, J., and Diwan, B. (1989) Induction of cytochrome P-450b and its relationship to tumor promotion. *J. Am. Coll. Toxicol.* 8, 259–267.

Lumley, C. E., and Walker, S. R. (1985) The value of chronic animal toxicology studies of pharmaceutical compounds: A retrospective analysis. *Fund. Appl. Toxicol.* 5, 1007–1024.

Lumley, C. E., and Walker, S. R. (1986) A critical appraisal of the duration of chronic animal toxicity studies. *Reg. Toxicol. Pharmacol.* 6, 66–72.

Lushbough, C. H., and Moline, S. W. (1961) Improved terminal bleeding method. *Proc. Anim. Care Panel* 11, 305–308.

Lykke, A.W.J., and Cummings, R. (1969) Inflammation in healing. 1. Time-course and mediation of exudation in wound healing in the rat. *Br. J. Exp. Pathol.* 50, 309–318.

Maas, T., Pearson, R., Anderson, R., Woodson, L., Reiter, C., and Weinshilboum, R. (1982) Rat phenol sulfotransferase. Assay procedure, developmental changes and glucocroticoid regulation. *Biochem. Pharmacol.* 31, 849–856.

MacFarland, P. W., Kane, K. A., Podolski, M., and Winslow, E. (1981) Computer-assisted analysis of arrhythmias in the rat, in *The Rat Electrocardiogram in Pharmacology and Toxicology*, Budden, R., Detweiler, D. K., and Zbinden, G., eds. Pergammon Press, pp. 179–184.

MacPhail, R. C., Peele, D. B., and Crofton, K. M. (1989) Motor activity and screening for neurotoxicity. *J. Am. Coll. Toxicol.* 8, 117–125.

Makarananda, K., Fox, G., Price, S., and Hinton, R. (1987) Changes in plasma proteins in rats treated for short periods with hepatotoxins or with agents which induce cytochrome P450 isoenzymes. *Hum. Toxicol.* 6, 121–126.

Mannering, G. (1971) Microsomal Enyzme systems which catalyze drug metabolism, in *Fundamentals of Drug Metabolsim and Drug Disposition*, LaDu, B., Mandel, H., and Way, E., eds. Williams & Wilkins, Baltimore, pp. 206–252.

Mariani, L., and Bonanomi, L. (1978). Resistance of guinea pig to indomethacin ulcerogenesis. *Toxicol. Appl. Pharmacol.* 45, 637–639.

Maronpot, R. R., Montgomery, C. A., Boorman, G. A., and McConnell, E. E. (1986) National toxicology program nomenclature for hepatoproliferative lesions of rast. *Toxicol. Pathol.* 14, 263–273.

Matsui, M., and Watanabe, H. (1982) Developmental alteration of hepatic UDP-glucuronsyl transferase and sulfotransferase towards andosterone and 4-nitrophenol in Wistar rats. *Biochem. J.* 204, 441–447.

McAllister, F. F. (1938) The effect of ether anesthesia on the volume of plasma and extracellular fluid. *Am. J. Physiol.* 124, 391–397.

McClain, R. (1989) The significance of hepatic microsomal enzyme induction and latered thyroid function in rats: implications for thyroid gland neoplasia. *Toxicol. Pathol.* 17, 294–306.

McGarrity, G. J., and Coriell, L. L. (1973) Mass airflow cabinet for control of airborne infection of laboratory animals. *Appl. Microbiol.* 26, 167–172.

McGarrity, G. J., Coriell, L. L., Schaedler, R. W., Mandle, R. J., and Greene, A. E. (1969) Medical applications of dust free rooms. III. Use in an animal care laboratory. *Appl. Microbiol.* 18, 142–146.

McGee, M. A., and Maronpot, R. R. (1979) Harderian gland dacryoadenitis in rats resulting from orbital bleeding. *Lab. Anim. Sci.* 29, 639–641.

McKennis, H., Yard, A., Weatherby, J., and Hagy, J. (1959) Acetylation of hydrazine and the formation of 1,2-acetylhydrazine in vivo. *J. Pharmacol. Exp. Ther.* 126, 109–116.

McMartine, D., O'Connor, J., Fasco, M., and Kaminsky, L. (1980) Influence of aging and induction of rat liver and kidney microsomal mixed function oxidase systems. *Toxicol. Appl. Pharmacol.* 54, 411–419.

Mebus, C. A., and Piper, W. N. (1986) Decreased rat adrenal 21-hydroxylase activity associated with decreased addrenal microsomal cytochrome P-450 after exposure to 2, 3, 7,8-tetrachloro-dibenzo-p-dioxin. *Biochem. Pharmacol.* 35, 4359–4362.

Melnick, R. L., Jameson, C. W., Goehl, T. J., and Kuhn, G. O. (1987a) Application of microencapsulation to toxicology studies. I. Principles and stabilization of trichloroethylene in gelation-sorbital microcapsules. *Fund. Appl. Toxicol.* 8, 425–431.

Melnick, R. L., Jameson, C. W., Goehl, T. J., Maronpot, R. R., Collins, B. J., Greenwell, A., Harrington, F. W., Wilson, R. E., Tomoszewski, K. E., and Agarwal, D. K. (1987b) Application of microencapsulation for toxicology studies. II. Toxicity of microencapsulated trichloroethylene in Fischer 344 rats. *Fund. Appl. Toxicol.* 8, 432–442.

Meltzer, H. Y., Stanisic, D., Simonovic, M., and Fang, V. S. (1978) Ketamine as an anesthetic for obtaining plasma for rat prolactin assays. *Proc. Soc. Exp. Biol. Med.* 159, 12–15.

Menard, R., Guenthner, T., Kon, H., and Gillett, J. (1979) Studies on the destruction of adrenal and testicular cytochrome P-450 by spironolactone. Requirement for the 7-athio group and evidence for the loss of the heme and apoproteins of the cytochrome P-450. *J. Bio. Chem.* 253, 1726–33.

Meuleman, D. G., Vogel, G.M.T., and Van Delft, A.M.L. (1980) Effects of intra-arterial cannulation on blood platelet consumption in rats. *Thrombosis Res.* 20, 45–55.

Milakofsky, L., Hare, T. A., Miller, J. M., and Vogel, W. H. (1984) Comparison of amino acid levels in rat blood obtained by catheterization and decapitation. *Life Sci.* 34, 1333–1340.

Minasian, H. (1980) A simple tourniquet to aid mouse tail veinpuncture. *Lab. Anim.* 14, 205.

Mitchell, R., and Boyd, M. (1983) Localization of metabolic activation and deactivation systems in the lung: Significance to the pulmonary toxicity of xenobiotics. *Ann. Rev. Pharmacol. Toxicol.* 23, 217–238.

Mitruka, B. M., and Rawnsley, H. M. (1977) *Clinical Biochemical and Hematological Reference Values in Normal Experimental Animals.* Masson U.S.A., New York.

Miwa, G., West, S., and Lu, A. (1978) Studies on the rate-limiting enzyme component in the microsomal monooxygenase system: In corporation of purified NADPH-cytochrome c reductase and cytochrome P-450 into rat liver microsomes. *J. Biol. Chem.* 253, 1921–1929.

Moloney, W. C., Boschetti, A. E., and King, V. P. (1969) Observations on leukemia in Wistar Furth rats. *Cancer Res.* 29, 938–946.

Moloney, W. C., Boschetti, A. E., and King, V. P. (1970) Spontaneous leukemia in Fischer rats. *Cancer Res.* 30, 41–43.

Moron, M., DePierre, J., and Mannervik, B. (1979) Levels of glutathione, glutathione reductase and glutathione S-transferase activity in rat lung and liver. *Biochim. Biophys. Acta* 582, 67–68.

Moore, R. Y., Heller, A., Wurtman, R. J., and Axelrod, J. (1967) Visual pathway mediating pineal response to environmental light. *Science* 155, 220–223.

Moser, V. C. (1989) Screening approaches to Neurotoxicity: A functional observational battery. *J. Am. Coll. Toxicol.* 8, 85–93.

Moses, L. E. (1946) Heart rate of the albino rat. *Proc. Soc. Exp. Biol. Med.* 63, 58–62.

Mouzas, G., and Weiss, J. B. (1960) A survival technique for obtaining large volumes of blood from rodents. *J. Clin. Pathol.* 13, 264.

Mucha, R. F. (1980) Indwelling catheter for infusions into subcutaneous tissue of freely-moving rats. *Physiol. Behav.* 24, 425–428.

Mulder, G. (1970) The effect of phenobarbital on the submicrosomal distribution of uridine diphosphate glucuronyltransferase from rat liver. *Biochemical. J.* 117, 319–324.

Mulder, G. (1986) Sex related differences in drug conjugation and their consequences for drug toxicity; sulfation, glucronidation and glutathione conjugation. *Chem.-Biol. Interact.* 57, 1–15.

Muller, D., and Klinger, W. (1978) The influence of age on the inducer phenobarbital on the cytochrome P-450 dependent monoxygenation of drugs in rat liver. *Die Pharmazie* 33, 397–400.

Muller, P. J., and Vernikos-Danellis, J. (1970) Effect of environmental temperature on the toxicity of caffine and dextroamphetamine in mice. *J. Pharmacol. Exp. Ther.* 171, 153–158.

Muller, E., Forster, D., Dietze, H., Langenberg, R., and Klinger, W. (1973) The influence of age and barbital treatment on the content of cytochrome P-450 and b5 and the activity of glucose-6phosphatase in microsomes of the rat liver and kidney. *Biochem. Pharmacol.* 22, 905–910.

Mundy, L. A., and Porter, G. (1969) Some effects of physical environment on rats. *J. Inst. Anim. Tech.* 20, 78–81.

Murray, M. (1987) Mechanisms of inhibition of cytochrome P-450 mediated drug oxidation. *Drug Metab. Rev.* 18, 55–82.

Murrow, W. G. (1975) A method for intratracheal installation in the rat. *Lab. Anim. Sci.* 25, 337–340.

Nachtmann, R. G., Driscoll, T. B., Gibson, L. A., and Johnson, P. C., Jr. (1988) Commercial over-the-needle catheters for intravenous infusions and blood sampling in rats. *Lab Anim. Sci.* 38, 629–630.

Nair, V., and Casper, R. (1969) The influence of light on daily rhythm in hepatic drug metabolizing enzymes in rat. *Life Sci.* 8, 1291–1298.

Naslund, B. M., and Halpert, J. (1984) Selective inhibition by chloramphenicol of cytochrome P-450 isozymes in rat lung and liver involved in the hydroxylation of n-hexane. *J. Pharmacol. Exp. Ther.* 231, 16–22.

National Academy of Sciences (1977) *Drinking Water and Health.* National Academy of Sciences, Washington, D.C.

National Academy of Sciences (1978) Control of diets in laboratory animal experimentation. *ILAR News* 21, A1–A12.

National Research Council (1978) Nutrient requirements of the laboratory rat, in *Nutrient Requirements of Laboratory Animals* No. 10, National Academy Sciences/National Research Council, Washington, D.C., pp. 7–37.

Navia, J. M. (1977) Preparation of diets used in dental research, in *Animal Models in Dental Research.* University of Alabama Press, University, Alabama, pp. 151–167.

Nayfield, K. C., and Besch, E. L. (1981) Comparative responses of rabbits and rats to elevated noise. *Lab. Anim. Sci.* 31, 386–390.

NCI (1976) Guidelines for Carcinogen Bioassay in Small Rodents. *NCI Carcinogenesis Tech. Rep. Ser. No. 1.* Bethesda, Maryland, National Cancer Institute.

Nebert, D., Eisen, H., Negishi, M., Lang, M., Hjelmeland, L., and Okey, A. (1981) Genetic mechanisms controlling the induction of polysubstrate monooxygenase (P-450) activities. *Ann. Rev. Pharmacol. Toxicol.* 21, 431–462.

Neill, J. D. (1970) Effect of "stress" on serum prolactin and luteinizing hormone levels during the estrous cycle of the rat. *Endocrinology* 87, 1192–1197.

Nelson, N. S., and Hoar, R. M. (1969) A small animal balling gun for oral administration of experimental compounds. *Lab. Anim. Care* 19, 871–872.

Neptun, D. A., Smith, C. N., and Irons, R. D. (1985) Effect of sampling site and collection method on variations in baseline clinical pathology values in Fischer-344 rats. I. Clinical chemistry. *Fund. Appl. Toxicol.* 5, 1180–1185.

Nerenberg, S. T., and Zedler, P. (1975) Sequential blood samples from the tail vein of rats and mice obtained with modified Liebig condenser jackets and vacuum. *J. Lab. Clin. Med.* 85, 523–526.

Nevins, R. G. (1971) Design criteria for ventilation systems, in *Proceedings of the Symposium on Environmental Requirements for Laboratory Animals*, Besch, E. L., ed. Institute for Environmental Research Publication No. EIR-71-02. Kansas State University, pp. 28–43.

Newberne, P. M. (1975) Influence on pharmacological experiments of chemicals and other factors in diets of laboratory animals. *Fed. Proc.* 34, 209–218.

Newberne, P. M., and Rogers, A. E. (1973) Rat colon carinomas associated with aflatoxin and marginal vitamin A. *J. Natl. Cancer Inst.* 50, 439–448.

Newton, J. F., Yoshimoto, M. Bernstein, J., Rush, G. F., and Hook, J. B. (1983) Acetaminophen nephro toxicity in the rat. 1. Strain differences in nephrotoxicity and metabolism. *Toxicol. Appl. Pharmacol.* 69, 291–306.

Newton, J. F., Pasino, D. A., and Hook, J. B. (1985) Acetaminophen neurotoxicity in the rat: Quantitation of renal metabolic activation in vivo. *Toxicol. Appl. Pharmacol.* 78, 39–46.

Nielsen, E. B. (1981) Rapid decline of sterotyped behavior in rats during constant one week administration of amphetamine via implanted alzet osmotic minipumps. *Pharmacol. Biochem. Behav.* 15, 161–165.

Niems, A., Warner, M., and Loughnan, P. (1976) Developmental aspects of the hepatic cytochrome P450 monooxygenase system. *Ann. Rev. Pharmacol. Toxicol.* 16, 427–445.

Nightingale, C. H., and Mouravieff, M. (1973) Reliable and simple method of intravenous injection into the laboratory rat. *J. Pharm. Sci.* 62, 860–861.

NIH (1985) *Guide for the Care and Use of Laboratory Animals.* NIH Publication No. 86-23. National Institutes of Health, Bethesda, Maryland.

Nishihata, T., Takahagi, H., Yamamoto, M., Tomida, H., Rytting, J. H., and Higuchi, T. (1984) Enhanced rectal absorption of cefmetazole and cefoxitin in the presence of epinephrine metabolites in rats and a high-performance liquid chromatographic assay for cephamycin antibiotics. *J. Pharm. Sci.* 73, 109–112.

Nixon, G. A., and Reer, P. J. (1973) A method for preventing oral ingestion of topically applied materials. *Lab. Anim. Sci.* 23, 423–425.

Njaa, L. R., Utne, F., and Braekkan, O. R. (1957) Effect of relative humidity on rat breeding and ringtail. *Nature* 180, 290–291.

Nobunaga, T., Nakamura, K., and Imamichi, T. (1966) A method for intravenous injection and collection of blood from rats and mice without restraint and anesthesia. *Lab. Anim. Care* 16, 40–49.

Noell, W. K., Walker, V. S., Kang, B. S., and Berman, S. (1977) Retinal damage by light in rats. *Invest. Ophthal.* 5, 450–473.

Novin, D., Rezek, M., and Vanderweele, D. A. (1974) A cannula for infusion and withdrawal of fluids in unrestrained animals. *Physiol. Behav.* 12, 135–136.

Numazawa, S., Oguro, T., Yoshida, T., and Kuroiwa Y. (1989) Comparative studies on the inducing effects of cobalt chloride and co-protoporphyrin on hepatic ornithine decarboxylase and heme oxygenase in rats. *J. Pharmacobio-Dyn.* 12, 50–59.

Oesch, F. (1972) Mammalian Epoxide hydrases: Inducible enzymes catalysing the inactivation of carcinogenic and cytotoxic metabolites derived from aromatic and olefinic compounds. *Xenobiotica* 3, 305–340.

Oesch, F., Zimmer, A., and Glatt, H. R. (1983) Microsomal epoxide hydrolase in different rat strains. *Biochem. Pharmacol.* 32, 1783–1788.

Oesch, F., Hartmann, R., Timms, Ch., Strolin-Benedetti, M., Dostert, P., Worner, W., and Schladt, L. (1988) Time-dependence and differential induction of rat and guinea pig peroxisomal β-oxidation, palmitoyl-CoA hydrolase, cytosolic and microsomal epoxide hydrolase after treatment with hypolipidemic drugs. *J. Cancer Res. Clin. Oncol.* 114, 341–346.

Ogura, K., Sohotome, T., Sugiyama, A., Okuda, H., Hiratsuka, A., and Watabe, T. (1990) A rat liver cytosolic hydroxysteroid sulfotransferase catalyzing the formation of reactive sulfate esters from carcinogenic polycyclic hydroxymethyl-arenes. *Mol. Pharmacol.* 37, 848–854.

Okey, A. (1990) Enzyme induction in the cytochrome P-450 system. *Pharmacol. Ther.* 45, 241–298.

Oller, W. L., Gough, B., and Littlefield, N. A. (1980) Chemical surveillance and quality assurance for preparation of dosed (2-AAF) animal feed (ED01 study). *J. Environ. Pathol. Toxicol.* 3, 203–210.

Omaye, S. T., Skala, J. H., Gretz, M. D., Schaus, E. E., and Wade, C. E. (1987) Simple method for bleeding unanesthetized rat by tail venipuncture. *Lab. Anim.* 21, 261–264.

Ortiz de Montello, P. (ed.) (1986) *Cytochrome P-450: Structure, Mechanisms and Biochemistry.* Plenum Press, New York.

Osborne, B. E. (1973) A restraining device facilitating electrocardiogram recording in rats. *Lab. Anim.* 7, 158–188

Osborne, B. E. (1974) Uses and applications of electrocardiography in toxicology, in *Experimental Model Systems in Toxicology and Their Significance in Man*, Vol. XV. Excerta Medica, Amsterdam, pp. 85–97.

Oser, B. L. (1981) The rat as a model for human toxicological evaluations. *J. Toxicol. Environ. Health* 8, 521–542.

Oshinsky, R. J., and Strobel, H. W. (1987) Distributions and properties of cytochromes P-450 and cytochrome P-450 reductase from rat colon mucosal cells. *Int. J. Biochem.* 19, 575–588.

O'Steen, K. W. (1970) Retinal and optic nerve serotonin and retinal degeneration as influenced by photoperiod. *Exp. Neurol.* 27, 194–205.

Page, N. P. (1977) Concepts of a bioassay program in environmental carcinogenesis, in *Environmental Carcinogenesis*, Kraybill, H., and Mehlman, M., eds. Hemisphere, pp. 81–171.

Page, J. G., and Vesell, E. S. (1969) Hepatic drug metabolism in ten strains of Norway rat before and after pretreatment with phenobarbital. *Proc. Soc. Exp. Biol. Med.* 131, 256–261.

Pal, B. C., Ross, R. H., and Milman, H. A. (1984) *Nutritional Requirements and Contaminant Analysis of Laboratory Animal Feeds*, Report No. EPA 560/6-83-005. National Technical Information Service, Springfield, Virginia.

Parkinson, A., Thomas, P., Ryan, D., Reik, L., Safe, S., Robertson, L., and Levin, W. (1983a) Differential time course of rat liver microsomal cytochrome P-450 isozymes and epoxide hydrolase by aroclor 1254. *Arch. Biochem. Biophys.* 225, 203–215.

Parkinson, A., Thomas, P., Ryan, D., and Levin, W. (1983b) The in vivo turnover of rat liver microsomal epoxide hydrolase and both the apoprotein and heme moieties of specific cytochrome P-450 isozymes. *Arch. Biochem. Biophys.* 225, 216–236.

Pascóe, G., and Correia, M. (1985) Structure and functional assembly of rat intestinal cytochrome P-450 isozymes. Effects of dietary iron and selenium. *Biochem. Pharmacol.* 34, 599–608.

Pass, K. A., and Ondo, J. G. (1977) Dual cerebroventricular and vascular cannulation technique for use in conscious rats. *Physiol. Behav.* 18, 173–175.

Paulose, C. S., and Dakshinamurti, K. (1987) Chronic catheterization using vascular-access-port in rats: Blood sampling with minimal stress for plasma catecholamine determination. *J. Neurosci. Methods* 22, 141–146.

Pauly, J. E., and Scheving, L. E. (1969) in *Biorhythms in Clinical and Experimental Endocrinology*, Proceedings of the First International Symposium, Sayers, G., and Lunedei, A., eds. Rassegna di Neurologica Vegetativa, Florence

Pearce, K. A. (1957) A route of intravenous injection in the rat. *Nature* 180, 709.

Pekas, J. C. (1974) Gastrointestinal absorption and toxicology: Ingesta-exchange and simulated meal techniques. *Food Cosmet. Toxicol.* 12, 351–357.

Peplow, A. M., Peplow, P. V., and Hafez, E.S.E. (1974) Parameters of reproduction, in *Handbook of Laboratory Animal Science*, Vol. I, Melby, E. E., Jr., and Altmon, N. H., eds. CRC Press, Boca Raton, pp. 107–116.

Petty, C. (1982) *Research Techniques in the Rat.* Thomas, Springfield, Illinois, pp. 80–100, 108–116.

Pfeiffer, C. J. (1967) The physiologic effects of restricted activity in the rat: Stress effects of chronic restraint. *Exp. Med. Surg.* 25:201–217.

Philipeaux, J. M. (1856) Note sur l'extirpation des capsules survenales chez les rats albinos (*Mus rattus*). *C. R. Habd. Seances Acad. Sci. Paris,* 43, 904–906.

Phillips, W. A., Stafford, W. W., and Stuut, Jr., Jr. (1973) Jugular vein technique for serial blood sampling and intravenous injections in the rat. *Proc. Soc. Exp. Biol. Med.* 143, 733–735.

Picket, C., and Lu, A. (1989) Glutathione S-transferases: Gene structure, regulation, and biological function. *Ann. Rev. Biochem.* 58, 743–764.

Pleasants, J. R. (1984) Diets for germ-free animals. Part 2. The germ-free animal fed chemically defined ultra-filtered diets, in *The Germ-free Animal in Biomedical Research*, Coates, M. E., and Gustafsson, B. E., eds. Laboratory Animals, pp. 91–109.

Plummer, S., Boobis, A., and Davies, D. (1987) Strain related differences in the metabolic activation of aflatoxin B1 in the rat. *Xenobiotica* 17, 199–208.

Pompon, D., and Coon, M. (1984) On the mechanism of action of cytochrome P-450. Oxidation and reduction of the ferrous dioxygen complex of liver microsomal cytochrome P-450 by cytochrome b_5. *J. Biol. Chem.* 259, 15377–15385.

Pope, R. S. (1968) Small vessel cannulator. *J. Appl. Physiol.* 24, 276.

Popick, F. R. (1976) Application of a new intraventricular injection technique in rat brain norepinephrine studies. *Life Sci.* 18, 197–204.

Popovic, V., and Popovic, P. (1960) Permanent cannulation of aorta and vena cava in rats and ground squirrels. *J. Appl. Physiol.* 15, 727–728.

Powers, W. J., Jr., Peckham, J. C., Siino, K. M., and Gad, S. C. (1984) Effects of subchronic dietary caprolactam in renal function, in *An Industry Approach to Chemical Risk Assessment*. Industrial Health Foundation, pp. 77–96.

Proskauer, G. G., Neumann, C., and Graef, I. (1945) The measurement of the blood pressure in rats with special reference to the effect of changes in temperature. *Am. J. Physiol.* 143, 290–296.

Pucak, G. J., Lee, C. S., and Zaino, A. S. (1977) Effects of prolonged high temperature on testicular development and fertility in the male rat. *Lab. Anim. Sci.* 27, 76–77.

Pyykko, K. (1983) Age- and sex-related differences in rat liver microsomal enzymes and their inducibility by toluene. *Act. Pharmacol. Toxicol.* 53, 401–409.

Pyykko, K., Paavilainen, S., Metsa-Ketela, T., and Laustiola, K. (1987) The increasing and decreasing effects of aromatic hydrocarbon solvents on pulmonary and hepatic cytochrome P-450 in the rat. *Pharmacol. Toxicol.* 60, 288–293.

Quarterman, J., Williams, R. B., and Humphries, W. R. (1970) *Br. J. Nutr.* 24, 1049–1051.

Rabovsky, J., and Judy, D. (1989) The in vitro effects of alkanes, alcohols and ketones on rat lung cytochrome P-450 dependent alkoxyphenoxazone dealylase activities. *Toxicology* 63, 13–17.

Radzialowski, F. M., and Bousquet, W. F. (1968) Daily rhythmic variation in hepatic drug metabolism in the rat and mouse. *J. Pharmacol. Exp. Ther.* 163, 229–238.

Ralston Purina Co. *Certified rodent chow #5002, specifications*. Checkerboard Square, St. Louis, Missouri 63188.

Rampersaud, A., and Walz, F. (1986) Cytochrome P-450 polypeptides in pulmonary microsomes from rats. *Biochim. Biophys. Acta* 869, 293–303.

Rao, G. N. (1986) Significance of environmental factors on the test system, in *Managing Conduct and Data Quality of Toxicology Studies*, Hoover, B. K., Baldwin, J. K., Uelner, A. F., Whitmire, C. E., Davies, C. L., and Bristol, D. W., eds. Princeton Scientific, 173–186.

Rao, G. N., and Knapka, J. J. (1987) Contaminant and nutrient concentrations of natural ingredient rat and mouse diet used in chemical toxicology studies. *Fund Appl. Toxicol.* 9, 329–338.

Raynor, T. H., Steinhagen, W. H., and Hamm, T. E., Jr. (1983) Differences in the microenvironment of a polycarbonate caging system: Bedding vs raised wire floors. *Lab. Anim.* 17, 85–89.

Reddy, J., and Lalwani, N. (1983) Carcinogenesis by hepatic peroxisome proliferators: Evaluation of the risk of hypolipidemic drugs and industrial plasticizers to humans. *CRC Crit. Rev. Toxicol.* 12, 1–58.

Reed, D. (1990) Glutahione: toxicological implications. *Ann. Rev. Pharmacol. Toxicol.* 30, 603–31.

Reiter, L. W., and MacPhail, R. C. (1989) Motor activity: A survey of methods with potential use in toxicity testing. *Neurobehav. Toxicol.* 1, Suppl. 1, 53–66.

Renaud, S. (1969) Jugular vein technique for blood collection and intravenous injection in the rat. *Lab. Anim. Care* 19, 664–665.

Renton, K. (1980) Methyl red azo-reductase and its induction by 3-methylcholanthrene in the liver of different species. *Xenobiotica* 10, 243–246.

Reuber, M. D. (1977) Necropsy of animals for scientific research. *Clin. Toxicol.* 10, 111–127.

Rezek, M., and Havlicek, V. (1975) Chronic multipurpose cannulas and a technique for the cannulation of small veins and arteries. *Physiol. Behav.* 15, 623–626.

Rhodes, J., and Houston, J. (1983) Antipyrine metabolite kinetics in phenobarbital and β-naphthaflavone induced rats. *Drug. Metab. Dispos.* 11, 131–136.

Rhodes, M. L., and Patterson, C. E. (1979) Chronic intravenous infusion in the rat: A nonsurgical approach. *Lab. Anim. Sci.* 29, 82–84.

Rice, D. P., and Ketterer, D. J. (1977) Restrainer and cell for dermal dosing of small laboratory animals. *Lab. Anim. Sci.* 27, 72–75.

Richardson, B. P., Turkalj, I., and Fluckiger, E. (1984) Bromocriptine, in *Safety Testing of New Drugs*, Laurence, D. R., McLean, A.E.M., and Weatherall, M., eds. Academic Press, New York, pp. 19–63.

Richter, C. P. (1959) Rats, man, and the welfare state. *Am. Psychol.* 14, 18–28.

Rietjens, I., Dormans, J., Rombout, P., and van Bree, L. (1988) Qualitative and quantitive changes in cytochrome P-450 dependent xenobiotic metabolism in pulmonary microsomes and isolated Clara cel populations derived from ozone-exposed rats. *J. Toxicol. Environ. Health* 24, 515–31.

Rikans, L. (1984) Influence of aging on the susceptibility of rats to hepatotoxic injury. *Toxicol. Appl. Pharmacol.* 73, 243–249.

Rikans, L., and Notley, B. (1981) Substrate specificity of age-related changes in the inducibility of microsomal monooxygenases in middle-aged rats. *Mech. Age. Dev.* 16, 371–378.

Rikans, L., and Notley, B. (1982a) Age-related changes in hepatic microsomal drug metabolism are substrate specific. *J. Pharmacol. Exp. Ther.* 220, 574–578.

Rikans, L., and Notley, B. (1982b) Differential effects of aging on hepatic microsomal monooxygenase induction by phenobarbital and β-naphthaflavone. *Biochem. Pharmacol.* 31, 2339–2343.

Riley, V. (1960) Adaptation of orbital bleeding technic to rapid serial blood studies. *Proc. Soc. Exp. Biol. Med.* 104, 751–754.

Robineau, P. (1988) A simple method for recording electrocardiograms in conscious, unrestrained rats. *J. Pharmacol. Methods* 19, 127–133.

Robinsons, R., Cheng, C., Park, S., Gelboin, H. and Friedman, F. (1986) Structural comparison of monoclonal antibody immunopurified plumonary and hepatic cytochrome P-450 from 3-methylcholanthrene treated rats. *Biochem. Pharmacol.* 35, 3827–30.

Roe, F.J.C. (1987a) Opinions on animal selection for the assessment of carcinogenicity, in *Human Risk Assessment, the Role of Animal Selection and Extrapolation*, M. V. Roloff, ed. Taylor & Francis, pp. 31–44.

Roe, F.J.C. (1987b) The problem of pseudocarcinogenicity in rodent bioassays, in *Banbury Report 25: Nongenotoxic Mechanisms in Carcinogenesis*, Butterworth, B. E., and Slaga, T. J., eds. Cold Spring Harbor Laboratory, Cold Spring Harbor, New York, pp. 189–202.

Rogers, A. E. (1979) Nutrition, in *The Laboratory Rat*, Vol. I, Baker, H. J., Linsey, J. R., and Weisbroth, S. H., eds. Academic Press, New York, pp. 123–152.

Rogers, A. E., and Newberne, P. M. (1971) Diet and aflatoxin B_1 toxicity in rats. *Toxicol. Appl. Pharmacol.* 20, 113–121.

Rose, S., and Glow, P. H. (1965) Effects of intravitreous injection of drugs on the cholinesterase of the retina. *Aust. J. Exp. Biol. Med. Sci.* 43, 737–742.

Rose, S., and Nelson, J. F. (1955) A continuous long-term injector. *Austral. J. Exp. Biol.* 33, 415–420.

Rose, S., and Rabinov, D. (1967) Equipment and techniques for continuous infusion of drugs in humans and animals. *Cancer Chemother. Rep.* 51, 49–58.

Ross, A. R. (1977) Measurement of blood pressure in unrestrained rats. *Physiol. Behav.* 19, 327–329.

Rowberg, A., Franklin, D., and Van Citters, R. L. (1969) Nontraumatic method for measurement of blood pressure in animals with tails. *J. Appl. Physiol.* 27, 301–302.

Rowland, I. (1988) Factors affecting metabolic activity of the intestinal microflora. *Drug Metab. Reviews* 19, 243–262.

Runkle, R. S. (1964) Laboratory animal housing. Part II. *Am. Inst. Archit. J.* 41, 77–80.

Rusher, D. L., and Birch, R. W. (1975) A new method for rapid collection of blood from rats. *Physiol. Behav.* 14, 377–378.

Ryer, F. H., and Walker, D. W. (1971) An anal cup for rats in metabolic studies involving radioactive materials. *Lab. Anim. Sci.* 21, 942–943.

Sabaitis, C. P., Coombs, J. K., and Leong, B.K.J. (1989) Repeated oropharyngeal nebulization of drug to rats and dogs. *Toxicologist* 9, 184.

Sabine, J. R., Horton, B. J., and Wicks, M. B. (1973) Spontaneous tumors in C3H-A and C3H-AfB mice: High incidence in the United States and low incidence in Australia. *J. Natl. Cancer Inst.* 50, 1237–1242.

Sackler, A. M., Weltman, A. S., Bradshaw, M., and Jurtshuk, P., Jr. (1959) Endocrine changes due to auditory stress. *Acta Endocrinol.* 31, 405–418.

Sadjak, A., Klingenberg, H. G., Egger, G., and Supanz, S. (1983) Evaluation of the effects of blood smelling, handling, and anesthesia on plasma catecholamines in rats. *Z. Versuchstierk.* 25, 245–250.

Salen, H., Grossman, M. H., and Bilbey, D. L. (1963) Micro-method for intravenous injection and blood sampling. *J. Pharm. Sci.* 52, 794–795.

Salsburg, D. (1980) The effects of lifetime feeding studies on patterns of senile lesions in mice and rats. *Drug Chem. Toxicol.* 3, 1–33.

Sambhi, M. P., and White, F. N. (1960) The electrocardiogram of the normal and hypertensive rat. *Circ. Res.* 8, 129–134.

Sandiford, M. (1965) Some methods of collecting blood from small animals. *J. Anim. Tech. Assoc.* 16, 9–14.

Sansone, E. B., and Fox, G. (1977) Potential chemical contamination in animal feeding studies: Evaluation of wire and solid bottom caging systems and gelled feed. *Lab. Anim. Sci.* 27, 457–465.

Sansone, E. B., and Losikoff, A. M. (1978) Contamination from feeding volatile test chemicals. *Toxicol. Appl. Pharmacol.* 46, 703–708.

Sansone, E. B., Losikoff, A. M., and Pendleton, R. A. (1977) Potential hazards from feeding test chemicals in carcinogen bioassay research. *Toxicol. Appl. Pharmacol.* 39, 435–450.

Sass, B., Rabstein, L. S., Madison, R., Nims, R. M., Peters, R. L., and Kelloff, G. J. (1975) Incidence of spontaneous neoplasms in F344 rats throughout the natural life-span. *J. Natl. Cancer Inst.* 54, 1449–1456.

Schenkman, J., and Jansson, I. (1973) Evidence against the participation of cytochrome b5 in the hepatic microsomal mixed function oxidase reaction. *Mol. Pharmacol.* 9, 840–845.

Schmucker, D., and Wang, R. (1980a) Age-related changes in liver drug-metabolizing enzymes. *Exp. Gerontol.* 15, 423–431.

Schmucker, D., and Wang, R. (1980a) Effects of aging and phenobarbital of the rat liver drug-metabolizing system. *Mech. Ageing Dev.* 15, 189–202.

Schmucker, D., Vessey, D., Wang, R., James, J., and Maloney, A. (1984) Age-dependent alterations in the physiochemical properties of rat liver microsomes. *Mech. Ageing Dev.* 27, 207–217.

Schreiber, M., and Schmidt, F. H. (1979) Causes of artificially high blood glucose values in experiments with diabetic rats and mice. *Experientia* 35, 1552–1553.

Schreiber, H. P., Nettesheim, P., Lijinsky, W., Richter, C. B., and Walburg, H. E. (1972) Induction of lung cancer in germfree, specific-pathogen-free and infected rats by N-nitrosoheptamine: Enhancement by respiratory infection. *J. Natl. Cancer Inst.* 49, 1107–1111.

Schumacher, W., Budden, R., Buschmann, G., and Kuhl, U. G. (1981) A new method for the evaluation of ECG and blood pressure parameters in anesthetized rats by on-line biosignal processing, in *The Rat Electrocardiogram in Pharmacology and Toxicology*, Budden, R., Detweiler, D. K., and Zbinden, G., eds. Pergammon Press, New York, pp. 171–178.

Seidegard, J., and DePierre, J. (1983) Microsomal epoxide hydrolase. Properties, regulation and function. *Biochem. Biophys. Acta* 695, 251–270.

Sekura, R., and Jacoby, W. (1979) Phenol sulfotransferases. *J. Biol. Chem.* 254, 5658–5663.

Semler, D., Chengelis, C., Radzialowski, F. (1989) The effects of chronic ingestion of spironolactone on serum thyrotropin and thyroid hormones in the male rat. *Toxicol. Appl. Pharmacol.* 98, 263–268.

Serrano, L. J. (1971) Carbon dioxide and ammonia in mouse cages: Effect of cage covers, population, and activity. *Lab. Anim. Sci.* 21, 75–85.

Shani, J., Givant, Y., and Sulman, F. G. (1970) A capsule-feeder for small laboratory animals. *Lab. Anim. Care* 20:1154–1155.

Shay, H., and Gruenstein, M. (1946) A simple and safe method for the gastric instillation of fluids in the rat. *J. Lab. Clin. Med.* 31, 1384–1386.

Shefer, S., Hauser, S., and Mosbach, E. H. (1972) Stimulation of cholesterol 7 α-hydroxylase by phenobarbital in two strains of rat. *J. Lipid Res.* 13, 69–70.

Sherry, J. H., Johnson, P. B., and Colby, H. D. (1988) Species differences in adrenal spironolactone metabolism: Relationship to cytochrome P-450 destruction. *Biochem. Pharmacol.* 37, 355–357.

Shimamura, Y. O., and Shimamura, T. (1986) A convenient method for peroral administration of indocin to rats without the use of gastric gavage. *Kidney Int.* 29, 345.

Siegel, P. S. (1961) Food intake in the rat in relation to the dark-light cycle. *J. Comp. Physiol. Psychol.* 54, 294–301.

Simmons, M. L., and Brick, J. O. (1970) *The Laboratory Mouse, Selection and Management.* Prentice-Hall, Englewood Cliffs, New Jersey, pp. 153–156.

Simmons, M. L., Robie, D. M., Jones, J. B., and Serrano, L. J. (1968) Effect of a filter cover on temperature and humidity in a mouse cage. *Lab. Anim.* 2, 113–120.

Skett, P. (1988) Biochemical basis of sex differences in drug metabolism. *Pharmacol. Ther.* 28, 269–304.

Slack, C., and Jones, P. (1987) A technique for continuous long-term infusion in unrestrained rats. *Anim. Technol.* 38, 19–24.

Slanetz, C. A., Fratta, I., Crouse, C. W., and Jones, S. C. (1956) Stress and transportation of animals. *Proc. Anim. Care Panel* 7, 278–289.

Sloane-Stanley, G. H., and Chase, R. A. (1981) Intrathecal injections in rats by percutaneous lumbar puncture. *J. Pharm. Pharmacol.* 33, 480–482.

Smadja, C., Morin, J., Ferre, P., and Girard, J. (1988) Metabolic fate of a gastric glucose load in unrestrained rats bearing a portal vein catheter. *Am. J. Physiol.* 254, E407–E413.

Smith, S. G., and Davis, W. M. (1975) A method for chronic intravenous drug administration in the rat, in *Modern Pharmacology-Toxicology*, Vol. 5, *Methods in Narcotic Research*, Ehrenireis, S., and Neidle, A., ed. Marcel Decker, New York, pp. 3–32.

Smith, C. J., and Kelleher, P. C. (1973) A method for intragastric feeding of neonatal rats. *Lab Anim. Sci.* 23, 682–684.

Smith, C. N., Neptun, D. A., and Irons, R. D. (1986) Effect of sampling site and collection method of variations in baseline clinical pathology parameters in Fischer-344 rats. II. Clinical hematology. *Fund. Appl. Toxicol.* 7, 658–663.

Smith, P. C., Stanton, J. S., Buchanan, R. D., and Tanticharoenyos, P. (1968) Intestinal obstruction and death in suckling rats due to sawdust bedding. *Lab. Anim. Care* 18, 224–228.

Smith, D. M., Rogers, A. E., and Newberne, P. M. (1975) Vitamin A and benzo(a)pyrene carcinogenesis in the respiratory tract of hamsters fed a semisynthetic diet. *Cancer Res.* 35, 1485–1488.

Smith, P., McDonagh, A., and Benet, L. (1986) Irreversible binding of zomepirac to plasma proteins in vitro and in vivo. *J. Clin. Invest.* 77, 934–939.

Smyth, R. D., and Hottendorf, G. H. (1980) Application of pharmacokinetics and biopharmaceuticals in the design of toxicological studies. *Toxicol. Appl. Pharmacol.* 53, 179–195.

Smyth, R. D., Gaver, R. C., Dandekar, K. A., Van Harken, D. R., and Hottendorf, G. H. (1979) Evaluation of the availability of drugs incorporated in rat laboratory diet. *Toxicol. Appl. Pharmacol.* 50, 493–499.

Sobin, S. S. (1946) Accuracy of indirect determinations of blood pressure in the rat; relation to temperature of plethysmograph and width of cuff. *Am. J. Physiol.* 146, 179–186.

Solleveld, H. A., Hasemen, J. K., and McConnel, E. E. (1984) Natural history of body weight gain, survival, and neoplasia in the F344 rat. *Natl. Canc. Inst.* 72, 929–940.

Sontag, J. M., Page, N. P., and Saffiotti, U. (1976) Guidelines for carcinogen bioassay in small rodents. NIH Publication number 76-801, Bethesda, Maryland.

Sorg, D. A., and Buckner, B. (1964) A simple method of obtaining venous blood from small laboratory animals. *Proc. Soc. Exp. Biol. Med.* 115, 1131–1132.

Soulhaili–el Amri, Batt, A., and Siest, G. (1986) Comparison of cytochrome P-450 content and activities in liver microsomes of seven species, including man. *Xenobiotica* 16, 351–358.

Spaethe, S., and Jollow, D. (1989) Effects of cobalt protoporphyrin on hepatic drug-metabolizing enzymes. Specificity for cytochrome P-450. *Biochem. Pharmacol.* 38, 2027–2038.

Spear, J. F. (1982) Relationship between the scaler electrocardiogram and cellular electophysiology of the rat heart, in *The Rat Electrocardiogram in Pharmacology and Toxicology*, Budden, R., Detweiler, D. K., and Zbinden, G., eds. Pergammon Press, New York, pp. 29–40.

Squire, R. A., and Goodman, D. G. (1978) Tumors of laboratory animals, in *Pathology of Laboratory Animals,* Vol. 2, Jones, T. C., Garner, F. M., and Benirschke, K., eds. Springer-Verlag, New York.

Squire, R. A., and Levitt, M. H. (1975) Classification of specific hepatocellular lesions in rats: Report of a workshop. *Cancer Res.* 35, 3214–3223.

Steffens, A. B. (1969) A method for frequent sampling of blood and continuous infusion of fluids in the rat without disturbing the animal. *Physiol. Behav.* 4, 833–836.

Steiger, E., Vars, H. M., and Dudrick, S. J. (1972) A technique for long-term intravenous feeding in unrestrained rats. *Arch. Surg.* 104, 330–332.

Stern, J. A., Winokur, G., Eisenstein, A., Taylor, R., and Sly, M. (1960) The effect of group vs. individual housing on behavior and physiological responses to stress in the albino rat. *J. Psychosoma. Res.* 4, 185–190.

Stevens, K. R., and Gallo, M. A. (1989) Practical considerations in the conduct of chronic toxicity studies, in *Principles and Methods of Toxicology*, Hayes, A. W., ed. Raven Press, New York, pp. 237–250.

Stewart, R. D., and Sansilow, C. A. (1961) Silastic intravenous catheter. *New Engl. J. Med.* 265, 1283–1285.

Still, J. W., and Whitcomb, E. R. (1956) Technique for permanent long-term intubation of rat aorta. *J. Lab. Clin. Med.* 48, 152–154.

Strobel, H., Fang, W., and Oshinsky, R. (1980) Role of colonic cytochrome P-450 in large bowel carcinogenesis. *Cancer* 45, 1060–5.

Stuhlman, R. A., Packer, J. T., and Rose, S. D. (1972) Repeated blood sampling of *Mystromys albicaudatus* (white-tailed rat). *Lab. Anim. Sci.* 22, 268–270.

Suber, R. L., and Kodell, R. L. (1985) The effect of three phlebotomy techniques on hematological and clinical chemical evaluation in Sprague-Dawley rats. *Vet. Clin. Pathol.* 14, 23–30.

Sugita, O., Nagashima, K., Sassa, S., and Kappas, A. (1988) Immunochemical detection of cytochrome P450C-M/F and NADPH-cytochrome P450 reductase in rat liver and kidney. *Biochem. Biophys. Res. Commun.* 150, 925–930.

Sun, J., Lau, P., and Strobel, H. (1986) Aging modifies the expression of hepatic microsomal cytochromes P-450 after pretreatment of rats with β-naphthaflavone or phenobarbital. *Exp. Gerontol.* 21, 65–73.

Swan, A. G. (1975) Method for testing the effects of fluids on rat skin using acrylic chambers. *J. Invest. Dermatol.* 65, 231–234.

Swenberg, J. A. (1985) The interpretation and use of data from long-term carcinogenesis studies in animals. *CIIT Activ.* 5(6), 1–6.

Swenberg, J. A., Short, B., Borghoff, S., Strasser, J., and Charbonneau, M. (1989) The comparative pathobiology of α_2 μ-globulin nephropathy. *Toxicol. Appl. Pharmacol.* 101, 414–431.

Tamura, S., Kawata, S., Okamoto, M., and Tarui, S. (1988) Localization of cytochrome P-450 in the colonic mucosa of 3-methylcholanthrene pretreated and untreated rats. *Cell Tissue Res.* 252, 397–401.

Tarloff, J., Goldstein, R., Morgan, D., and Hook, J. (1988) Acetaminophen and p-aminophenol nephrotoxicity in aging male Sprague Dawley and Fischer 344 rats. *Fund. Appl. Tox.* 12, 78–91.

Tarloff, J., Goldstein, R., and Hook, J. (1989) Strain differences in acetaminophen nephrotoxicity in rats: Role of pharmacokinetics. *Toxicology* 56, 167–177.

Tarone, R. E., Chu, K. C., and Ward, N. J. (1981) Variability in the rates of some common naturally occurring tumors in Fischer 344 rats and (C57BL/6NXC3H/HEN)F[1] (B6C3F[1]) mice. *J. Natl. Canc. Inst.* 66, 1175–1181.

Teelmann, K., and Weihe, W. H. (1974) Microorganism counts and distribution patterns in air conditioned animal laboratories. *Lab. Anim.* 8, 109–118.

Teoh, T. B. (1961) The effects of methyl cellulose in rats with special reference to splenomegaly, anemia, and the problem of hypersplenism. *J. Pathol. Bacteriol.* 81, 33–44.

Tephly, T., Parks, R., and Mannering, G. (1964) Methanol metabolism in the rat. *J. Pharmacol. Exp. Ther.* 143, 292–300.

Tephly, T., Green, M., Puig, J., and Irshaid, Y. (1988) Endogenous substrates for UDP-glucuronsosyl transferases *Xenobiotica* 18, 1201–1210.

Thomas, P., Lu, A., West, S., Ryan, D., Miwa, G., and Levin, W. (1983) Accessibility of cytochrome P450 in microsomal membranes: Inhibition of metabolism by antibodies to cytochrome P450. *Mol. Pharmacol.* 13, 819–831.

Thomas, P., Reidy, J., Reik, L., Ryan, D., Koop, D., and Levin, W. (1984) Use of monoclonal antibody probes against hepatic cytochromes P-450c and P-450d to detect immunochemically related isozymes in liver microsomes from different species. *Arch. Biochem. Biophys.* 235, 239–253.

Thomsen, L. (1981) Bowl for feeding powdered diet to rats. *Lab. Anim.* 15, 177–178.

Timbrell, J., Mitchell, J., Sondgrass, W., and Nelson, S. (1980) Isoniazid hepatotoxicity: The relationship between covalent binding and metabolism in vivo. *J. Pharmacol. Exp. Ther.* 213, 364–369.

Tober-Meyer, B. K., Bieniek, H. J., and Kupke, I. R. (1981) Studies on the hygiene of drinking water for laboratory animals. 2. Clinical and biochemical studies in rats and rabbits during long-term provision of acidified drinking water. *Lab. Anim.* 15, 111–117.

Toftgard, R., Haaparanta, T., Eng, L., and Haplert (1986) Rat and liver microsomal cytochrome P-450 isozymes involved in hydroxylation of n-hexane. *Biochem Pharmacol.* 35, 3733–3738.

Tomkins, P. T., and O'Donovan, D. J. (1986) A fluorocarbon coated diuresis cage for rodents. *Lab. Anim.* 20, 16–21.

Tornquist, S., Sundin, M., Moller, M., Gustafsson, J., and Toftgard, R. (1988) Age dependent expression of cytochrome P-450b and metabolism of the potent carcinogen 2-nitroflourene in the rat lung. *Carcinogenesis* 9, 2209–2214.

Toth, B. (1979) 1-acetyl-2-phenylhydrazine carcinogenesis in mice. *Br. J. Cancer* 39, 584–587.

Traber, P., Chianale, J., Florence, R., Kim, K., Wojik, E., and Gumucio, J. (1988) Expression of cytochrome P-450b and P-450e genes in small intestinal mucosa of rats following treatment with phenobarbital, polyhalogenated biphenyls and organochlorine pesticides. *J. Biol. Chem.* 263, 9449–55.

Tsuda, H., Moore, M. A., Asamoto, M., Inoue, T., Fukushima, S., Ito, N., Satoh, K., Amelizad, Z., and Oesch, F. (1987) Immunohistochemically demonstrated altered expression of cytochrome P-450 molecular forms and epoxide hydrolase in N-ethyl-N-hydroxyethylnitrosamine-induced rat kidney and liver lesions. *Carcinogenesis* 8, 711–717.

Tsukamoto, H., Reidelberger, R. D., French, S. W., and Largman, C. (1984) Long-term cannulation model for blood sampling and intragastric infusion in the rat. *Am. J. Physiol.* 247, R595–R599.

Tucker, M. J. (1979) The effect of long-term food restriction on tumours in rodents. *Int. J. Cancer* 23, 803–807.

Tucker, S. P., Lovell, D. P., Seawright, A. A., and Cunningham, V. J. (1980) Variation in the hepatotoxic effects of carbon disulfide between different strains of rat. *Arch. Toxicol.* 45, 287–296.

Tynes, R., and Hodgson, E. (1983) Oxidation of thiobenzamide by the FAD-containing and cytochrome P-450-dependent monooxygenases of liver and lung microsomes. *Biochem. Pharmacol.* 32, 3419–3428.

Tynes, R., and Hodgson, E. (1985) Catalytic activity and substrate specificity of the flavin-containing monooxygenase in microsomal systems: Characterization of the hepatic pulmonary and renal enzymes of the mouse, rabbit, and rat. *Arch. Biochem. Biophys.* 240, 77–93.

Upton, R. A. (1975) Simple and reliable method for serial sampling of blood from rats. *J. Pharmacol. Sci.* 64, 112–114.

Upton, P. K., and Morgan, D. J. (1975) The effect of sampling technique on some blood parameters in the rat. *Lab. Anim.* 9, 85–91.

Utley, W., and Mehendale, H. (1989) Phenobarbital-induced cytosolic cytoprotective mechanisms that offset increases in NADPH cytochrome P450 reductase activity in menadione-mediated cytotoxicity. *Toxicol. Appl. Pharmacol.* 99, 323–333.

Van der Graff, M., Vermeulen, N., and Breimer, D. (1988) Disposition of hexobarbital: 15 years of an intriguing model substrate. *Drug Metab. Rev.* 19, 109–164.

Van Harken, D. R., and Hottendorf, G. H. (1978) Comparative absorption following the administration of a drug to rats by oral gavage and incorporation in the diet. *Toxicol. Appl. Pharmacol.* 43, 407–410.

Vainio, H., Aitio, A., and Hanninen, O. (1974) Action of transcription and translation inhibitors on the enhancement of drug hydroxylation and glucuronidation by 3-methylcholanthrene and phenobarbital. *Int. J. Biochem.* 5, 193–200.

Veltman, J. C., and Maines, M. D. (1986a) Alterations of heme, cytochrome P-450, and steroid metabolism by mercury in rat adrenal. *Arch. Biochem. Biophys.* 248, 467–478.

Veltman, J. C., and Maines, M. D. (1986b) Regulatory effect of copper on rat adrenal cytochrome P-450 and steroid metabolism. *Biochem. Pharmacol.* 35, 2903–2909.

Vetterlein, F., Sammler, J., Ri, H. D., and Schmidt, G. (1984) Method for measurement of heart rate in awake, noninstrumented small animals. *Am. J. Physiol.* 247, H1010–H1012.

Videm, S. (1980) A method for blood sampling and intravenous injection in rats. *Z. Versuchstierk.* 22, 101–104.

Vilageliu, J., Arano, A., and Bruseghini, L. (1981) Endothelial damage induced by polyethylene catheter in the rat. *Meth. Find. Exptl. Clin. Pharmacol.* 3, 279–281.

Wade, A. E., Holl, J. E., Hilliard, C. C., Molton, E., and Greene, F. E. (1968) Alteration of drug metabolism in rats and mice by an environment of cedarwood. *Pharmacology* 1, 317–328.

Wadsworth, R. M., and Ratnasooriya, W. D. (1981) Method for localized and sustained administration of drugs to the vas deferens of rats. *J. Pharmacol. Meth.* 5, 313–320.

Walz, F., Vlasuk, G., and Steggles, A. (1983) Species differences in cytochrome P-450 and epoxide hydrolase: Comparisons of xenobiotic-induced hepatic microsomal polypeptides in hamsters and rats. *Biochemistry* 22, 1547–1556.

Ward, J. M. (1975) Dose response to a single injection of azoxymethane in rats. Induction of tumors in the gastrointestinal tract, auditory sebaceous glands, kidney, liver and preputial gland. *Vet. Pathol.* 12, 165–177.

Watanabe, T., Horie, S., Yamada, J., Isaji, M., Nishigaki, T., Naito, J., and Suga, T. (1989) Species differences in the effects of bezafibrate, a hypolipidemic agent, on hepatic peroxisome-associated enzymes. *Biochem. Pharmacol.* 38, 367–371.

Watkins, P., Wrighton, S., Schuetz, E., Molowa, D., and Guzelian, P. (1987) Identification of glucocorticoid-inducible cytochromes P-450 in the intestinal mucosa of rats and man. *J. Clin. Invest.* 80, 1029–36.

Watkinson, W. P., Bruce, M. A., and Robinson, K. S. (1985) A computer-assisted electrocardiographic analysis system: Methodology and potential application to cardiovascular toxicology. *J. Toxicol. Environ. Health* 15, 713–727.

Waxman, D., Dannan, G., and Guengerich, F. (1985) Regulation of rat hepatic cytochrome P-450: Age-dependent expression, hormonal imprinting and xenobiotic inducibility of sex specific isozymes. *Biochemistry* 24, 4409–4417.

Waxman, D., Morrissey, J., and LeBlanc, G. (1989) Hypothesectomy differentially alters P-450 protein levels and enzyme activities in rat liver: Pituitary control of hepatic NADPH cytochrome P-450 reductases. *Mol. Pharmacol.* 35, 519–525.

Waynforth, H. B., and Parkin, R. (1969) Sublingual vein injection in rodents. *Lab. Anim.* 3, 35–37.

Waynforth, H. B., Holsman, J. W., and Parkin, R. (1977) A simple device to facilitate intragastric infusion per os in the conscious rat. *Lab. Anim.* 11, 129–131.

Weeks, J. R. (1972) Long-term intravenous infusion. *Meth. Psychobiol.* 2, 155–167.

Weeks, J. R., and Davis, J. D. (1964) Chronic intravenous cannulas for rats. *J. Appl. Physiol.* 19, 540–541.

Weeks, J. R., and Jones, J. A. (1960) Routine direct measurement of arterial pressure in unanesthetized rats. *Proc. Soc. Exp. Biol. Med.* 104, 646–648.

Weihe, W. H. (1973) The effect of temperature on the action of drugs. *Ann. Rev. Pharmacol.* 13, 409–425.

Weihe, W. H., Schidlow, J., and Strittmatter, J. (1969) The effect of light intensity on the breeding and development of rats and golden hamsters. *Int. J. Biometeorol.* 13, 69–79.

Weinshilboum, R. (1990) Sulfotransferase pharmacogenetics. *Pharmacol. Ther.* 45, 93–107.

Weisbroth, S. H. (1979) Bacterial and mycotic diseases, in *The Laboratory Rat*, Vol. I, Baker, H. J., Lindsey, J. R., and Weisbroth, S. H., eds. Academic Press, New York, pp. 193–241.

Weisbroth, S. H., Paganelli, R. G., and Salvia, M. (1977) Evaluation of a disposable water system during shipment of laboratory rats and mice. *Lab. Anim. Sci.* 27, 186–194.

Weisse, I., Stotzer, H., and Seitz, R. (1974) Age- and light-dependent changes in the rat eye. *Virchows Arch. A Pathol. Anat. Histol.* 362, 145–156.

Wen, S.-F., Tremblay, J. M., Qu, M., and Webster, J. G. (1988) An impedance method for blood pressure measurement in awake rats without preheating. *Hypertension* 11, 371–375.

Weyland, E., and Bevan, D. (1987) Species differences in disposition of benzo(a)pyrene. *Drug Metab. Dispos.* 15, 442–448.

White, W. W. (1971) A technic for urine collection from anesthetized male rats. *Lab. Anim. Sci.* 21, 401–402.

Wiberg, G. S., and Grice, H. C. (1965) Effect of prolonged individual caging on toxicity parameters in rats. *Food Cosmet. Toxicol.* 3, 597–603.

Williams, R. T. (1972) Toxicologic implications of biotransformation by intestinal microflora. *Toxicol. Appl. Pharmacol.* 23, 769–781.

Williams, J. R., Harrison, T. R. and Grollman, A. (1939) A simple method for determining the systolic blood pressure of the unanesthetized rat. *J. Clin. Invest.* 18, 373–376.

Winsett, O. E., Townsend, C. M., Jr., and Thompson, J. C. (1985) Rapid and repeated blood sampling in the conscious laboratory rat: A new technique. *Am. J. Physiol.* 249, G145–G146.

Winter, C. A., and Flataker, L. (1962) Cage design as a factor influencing acute toxicity of respiratory depressant drugs in rats. *Toxicol. Appl. Pharmacol.* 4, 650–655.

Wise, A. (1981) The standard stock diet—fact or fiction. *Nutr. Rep. Intern.* 23, 287–294.

Wise, A., and Gilburt, D. J. (1980) The variability of dietary fibre in laboratory animal diets and its relevance to the control of experimental conditions. *Food Cosmet. Toxicol.* 18, 643–648.

Wise, A., and Gilburt, D. J. (1981) Variation of minerals and trace elements in laboratory animal diets. *Lab. Anim.* 15, 299–303.

Wittgenstein, E., and Rowe, K. W., Jr. (1965) A technique for prolonged infusion of rats. *Lab. Anim. Care* 15, 375–378.

Wong, M. A., and Oace, S. M. (1981) Feeding pattern and gastrointestinal transit rate of rats under different room lighting schedules. *Lab. Anim. Sci.* 31, 362–365.

Wood, A., Ryan, D., Thomas, P., and Levin, W. (1983) Regio- and stereoselective metabolism of two C19 setoids by five highly purified and reconstituted rat hepatic cytochrome P-450 isozymes. *J. Biol. Chem.* 258, 8839–8847.

Woodnott, D. P. (1962) A simple technique for passing an oesophageal tube in the rat. *J. Anim. Tech. Assoc.* 12, 59.

Woods, J. E. (1978) Interactions between primary (cage) and secondary (room) enclosures, in *Laboratory Animal Housing*. Institute of Laboratory Animal Resources, National Academy of Science, Washington, D. C., pp. 65–83.

Worth, H. M., Kachmann, C., and Anderson, R. C. (1963) Intragastric injection for toxicity studies with newborn rats. *Toxicol. Appl. Pharmacol.* 5, 719–727.

Wostman, B. S. (1975) Nutrition and metabolism of the germfree animal. *World Rev. Nutr. Diet.* 22, 40–92.

Wright, B. A. (1970) A new device for collecting blood from rats. *Lab. Anim. Care* 20, 274–275.

Wurtman, R. J. (1975) The effects of light on man and other mammals. *Ann. Rev. Physiol.* 38, 467–483.

Wuttke, W., and Meites, J. (1970) Effects of ether and pentobarbital on serum prolactin and LH levels in proestrous rats. *Proc. Soc. Exp. Biol. Med.* 135, 648–652.

Yamada, J., Itoh, S., Horie, S., Watanabe, T., and Suga, T. (1986) Chain-shortening of xenobiotic acyl compound by the peroxisomal β-oxication system in rat liver. *Biochem. Pharmacol.* 35, 4363–4368.

Yamauchi, C., Fujita, S., Obara, T., and Ueda, T. (1981) Effects of room temperature on reproduction, body and organ weights, food and water intake, and hematology in rats. *Lab. Anim. Sci.* 31, 251–258.

Yeung, T., Sudlow, G., Koch, R., and Goldman (1983) Reduction of nitroheterocyclic compounds by mammalian tissues in vivo. *Biochem. Pharmacol.* 32, 2249–53.

Yoburn, B. C., Morales, R., and Inturrisi, C. E. (1984) Chronic vascular catheterization in the rat: Comparison of three techniques. *Physiol. Behav.* 33, 89–94.

Young, R. W. (1973) Renewal systems in rods and cones. *Ann. Ophthal.* 5, 843–854.

Zbaida, S., Stoddart, A., and Levine W. (1989) Studies on the mechanism of reduction of azo dye carcinogens by rat liver microsomal cytochrome P-450. *Chem.-Biol. Interact.* 69, 61–71.

Zbinden, F. (1981) Spontaneous and induced arrhythmias in rat toxicology studies, in *The Rat*

Electrocardiogram in Pharmacology and Toxicology, Budden, R., Detweiler, D. K., and Zbinden, G., eds. Pergamon Press, New York, pp. 117–128.

Zbinden, G., Kleinert, R., and Rageth, D. (1980) Assessment of emetine cardiotoxicity in a subacute toxicity experiment in rats. *J. Cardiovasc. Pharmacol.* 2, 155–164.

Ziegler, D. (1988) Flavin-containing monooxygenases: Catalytic activity and substrate specificities. *Drug Metab. Rev.* 19, 1–32.

Zucker, I. (1971) Light-dark rhythms in rat eating and drinking behavior. *Physiol. Behav.* 6, 115–126.

3

The Mouse

Toxicology: **James M. Andress**
G. D. Searle and Company
Skokie, Illinois

Pathology: **Charles H. Frith**
Toxicology Pathology Associates
Little Rock, Arkansas

Dawn G. Goodman
PATHCO, Inc.
Ijamsville, Maryland

Byron G. Boysen
Hazleton Wisconsin, Inc.
Madison, Wisconsin

Metabolism: **Chyung S. Cook**
G. D. Searle and Company
Skokie, Illinois

Toxicology   **James M. Andress**

HISTORY

The house mouse of North America and Europe *(Mus musculus)* is the most widely used animal in modern medical research. The mouse is a member of the order Rodentia, family Muridae, and subfamily Murinae.

The use of the mouse in biomedical research has been chronicled for several hundred years. William Harvey (1578–1657) published the results of his work on animal reproduction and blood circulation based in part on his work with mice (Harvey, 1616, cited in Morse, 1981). Joseph Priestly used mice in exploring the phlogiston theory (Priestly, 1775), and Antoine Lavoisier used mice in his studies of the physiology of respiration (Lavoisier, 1777) (both cited in Morse, 1981).

Mice were selectively bred for coat color for many centuries, but in the early 1900s efforts turned to breeding strains of mice that might mimic human disease states. Subsequently, inbred strains were derived that were particularly susceptible or resistant to various types of cancers and viruses. A strain is considered to be inbred when it has been derived by brother × sister matings for 20 or more consecutive generations (F_{20}), and can be traced to a single ancestral breeding pair in the 20th or subsequent generations. Certain other breeding systems (e.g., parent × offspring) may be substituted as long as the inbreeding coefficient achieved is at least equal to that at F_{20} (Lyon, 1981). The genetic groundwork was laid for most of the strains of inbred mice currently in use by researchers such as William E. Castle, Clarence C. Little, and Leonell C. Strong during the period of about 1900–1930 (Morse, 1981).

While highly inbred strains have proven invaluable in fields such as genetics and histocompatibility research, a school of thought developed that randombred or specifically outbred strains might more closely represent man in many areas of medical research. A random breeding program attempts to achieve a level of genetic variability similar to the initial (noninbred) population, and in so doing, preserve the "hybrid vigor" associated with heterozygosity.

Many of the inbred and outbred strains of mice currently in use are referred to as "Swiss" strains. All of these Swiss strains are traceable to a group of two male and seven female albino mice obtained from the noninbred stock of Dr. A. de Coulon of Lousanne, Switzerland, and imported into the United States by Dr. Clara Lynch of the Rockefeller Institute in 1926 for use in cancer research (Lynch, 1969, cited in Hill, 1983).

CHOICE OF THE MOUSE IN TOXICOLOGICAL RESEARCH

The choice of a species for toxicity testing is based on consideration of a large number of variables. Ideally, if toxicity testing is intended to provide information on the safety and/or safe use of a test article in or by humans, the species chosen for testing should be most similar to the human in the way it handles the test article pharmacodynamically. Substantial differences in absorption, distribution, metabolism, or elimination between test species and the target species, e.g., the human, will reduce the predictive value of the test results. From a practical standpoint, often the pharmacokinetics are not thoroughly understood in humans or the variety of available test species at the time of species selection. For this reason, testing is usually conducted in at least two species. At least one of those species is usually a rodent and one a nonrodent. The two most commonly used rodent species are mice and rats, and often toxicity testing is conducted in both of those species.

Mice have many advantages as test animals for toxicity testing. They are small, relatively economical to obtain, house, and care for, and they are generally easy to handle. Mice are generally more economical than rats in these respects. While mice may attempt to escape or bite handlers, with regular, gentle handling they are easily managed. Other advantages of the species include a short gestation period and a short natural life span. These characteristics allow studies that include evaluation of reproductive performance or exposure to a test article for periods approaching the expected life span (e.g., evaluation of carcinogenic potential) to be conducted in a practical time frame. High-quality, healthy mice are available from reliable commercial suppliers. Many genetically well-defined highly inbred, specifically or randomly outbred strains are available. Mice have been used in biomedical research for hundreds of years, and because of this, many technical procedures have been developed for use with the species, and a vast body of historical data is available for most strains. This historical database includes information on optimal nutritional and housing requirements in addition to data such as the expected background incidence of various diseases and types of tumors in untreated animals.

There are some disadvantages to using mice, and most are related to the small size of the animal. The smaller size and higher metabolic rate compared to the rat renders the species a bit less hearty than rats. Deviations in environmental conditions such as an air conditioning failure or failure in an automatic watering system typically have more severe effects on the smaller species such as mice than the same deviations have on rats. Owing to their high level of natural activity, most strains of mice will not become as docile or easy to handle as rats that have received equivalent handling. Small size also precludes or renders more difficult a number of procedures that are commonly conducted in toxicity testing, such as the collection of samples or repeated samples of blood and urine, electrocardiographic evaluation, and some necropsy evaluations.

This section will provide brief summaries of some of the normal physiological values and salient features of the species and some of the specific strains that may be useful in selecting an appropriate species and strain for toxicity testing.

Normal Physiological Values

Selected normal physiological values for mice are shown in Tables 1 and 2. Median survival of a number of groups of Charles River CD-1 outbred mice is shown in Table 3.

Table 1 Normal Physiological Values General and Reproductive

General	
life span	
average	1–3 years
maximum reported	4 years
adult weight	
male	20–40 g
female	18–40 g
surface area	0.03–0.06 cm^2
chromosome number (diploid)	40
food consumption	4–5 g/day
water consumption	5–8 ml/day ad libitum
body temperature	36.5°C
oxygen consumption	1.69 ml/g/hr
Reproductive	
age, sexual maturity	
male	50 days (20–35 g)
female	50–60 days, (20–30 g)
breeding season	continuous, cyclic
estrus cycle	4–5 days
gestation period	
average	19 days
range	17–21 days
litter size	
average	12
range	1–23
birth weight	1.5 g
age begin dry food	10 days
age at weaning	16–21 days (10–12 g)

Source: Data derived from Jacoby and Fox (1984), and from the *Animal Diet Reference Guide*, Purina Mills, Inc. (1987).

Table 2 Normal Physiological Values
Cardiovascular and Respiratory

Cardiovascular	
heart rate	
average	600/min
range	320–800/min
blood pressure	
systolic	133–160 mm Hg
diastolic	102–110 mm Hg
blood volume	
plasma	45 ml/kg
whole	78 ml/kg
hematocrit	41.5%
RBC life span	20–30 days
RBC diameter	6.6 microns
plasma pH	7.2–7.4
Respiratory	
rate	
average	163/min
range	84–230/min
tidal volume	
average	0.18 ml
range	0.09–0.38 ml
minute volume	
average	24 ml/min
range	11–36 ml/min

Source: Data derived from Jacoby and Fox
(1984), and from the Animal Diet Reference
Guide, Purina Mills, Inc. (1987).

These normal values will vary depending upon the strain of mouse, supplier, condition at arrival, type of feed, environmental and housing conditions, and in some cases, time of year. These data should be considered as a reference, but will not necessarily represent experience in any particular laboratory.

Species Differences

Mice are similar to other common laboratory animal species and to humans in many ways, yet the differences should not be underestimated. Mice have a high metabolic rate compared to other species. This fact alone may result in increased or decreased toxicity of a test article, depending on the specific mechanism of intoxication. In many cases, high metabolic rate may be associated with rapid absorption, distribution, metabolism, and elimination of a test article. Mice are obligate nose breathers, and have more convoluted nasal passages than humans. This may result in an excess of respirable test article deposited in the nasal passages, resulting in either increased or decreased relative toxicity, depending upon the most critical site of absorption. The small size of the mouse compared to other common laboratory species offers a significant advantage if the test article is expensive or in short supply. As an approximation, a mouse weighs about 10% as much as

Table 3 Median Survival of 16 Groups of Control Mice (%)

Sex	Period of time on study (months)			
	6	12	18	21
Male	98%	91%	63%	46%
Female	98%	95%	74%	68%

Data represent median survival of Charles River CD-1 outbred albino mice enrolled in 24-month chronic toxicity studies at pharmaceutical or contract toxicology laboratories.
Source: Adapted from Lang (1989).

a rat, about 5% as much as a guinea pig, about 1% as much as a rabbit, and less than 1% as much as a dog or primate. Material requirements to administer equivalent dose levels are usually proportional to body weight, so the test article savings associated with the mouse are evident. The small size of a mouse results in high surface area to body mass ratio, which in turn causes the mouse to be relatively intolerant of thermal and water balance stresses. The kidneys of a mouse have about twice the glomerular filtering surface per gram of body weight as a rat, and owing to the specific architecture of the murine kidney, they are capable of producing urine that is about 4 times as concentrated as the highest attainable human concentrations (Jacoby and Fox, 1984). These characteristics of renal architecture and function may be important to the toxicity of some test articles. Mice differ from most species by the formation of a persistent vaginal plug after mating. The presence of a vaginal plug is easily detected, is considered evidence of mating, and is a useful characteristic during the conduct of reproductive studies.

Strain Differences

In addition to differences between mice and other species, there are important differences among different strains of mice. The appropriate choice of a strain of mice for a particular toxicity study should consider the specific objectives of the study, and the specific characteristics of candidate strains that might assist or hinder in achieving those study objectives.

One difference among strains is in the normal body weights of various strains at different ages. These differences are summarized for selected strains available from the Charles River Breeding Laboratories in Table 4. Outbred strains tend to be larger at maturity than inbred strains, with the CD-1 strain reaching the highest mean weights at 56 days of age of those strains in Table 4. The CF1 strain has been reported to be highly resistant to mouse typhoid and to be relatively resistant to salmonellosis (Hill, 1981). Nude or athymic strains of mice are more sensitive to tumor development than heterozygous strains. These sensitive strains develop the same types of tumors as those seen in more conventional strains, but the incidences are higher and the latency periods shorter. There is a wide spectrum of susceptibility to spontaneous lung tumors in various strains of mice, and evidence suggests that there is a high correlation between spontaneous incidence and chemical inducibility in those various strains (Shimkin and Stoner, 1975).

Table 4   Normal Body Weights in Grams of Selected Strains of Mice

Age (days)	Outbred strains						Inbred strains						Hybrid	
	CD-1		CF-1		CFW		C3H		C57BL/6		BALB/c		B6C3F1	
	M	F	M	F	M	F	M	F	M	F	M	F	M	F
21	12	11	12	11	9	9	—	—	—	—	—	—	—	—
28	20	18	18	17	16	13	17	16	14	13	16	14	16	14
35	27	22	24	21	19	17	18	17	17	14	17	16	20	17
42	30	24	27	22	24	20	20	18	19	16	18	17	22	18
49	33	26	28	24	27	22	24	23	21	17	20	18	24	19
56	35	27	30	26	28	23	27	26	22	18	21	19	26	21

Source: Data derived from Charles River Growth Charts, Charles River Laboratories, ca. 1975.

The inbred strain A mouse appears to be the most susceptible to lung tumors, and forms the basis of a lung tumor bioassay, with tumors inducible within 8 weeks or less of treatment. Susceptibility of various strains to the initiation and/or promotion of skin tumors has also been shown to differ greatly (Chouroulinkov et al., 1988; Steinel and Baker, 1988). The incidences of selected spontaneously occurring neoplastic lesions in CD-1 (outbred) and B6C3F$_1$ (hybrid) strains are compared in Table 5.

The number of strain-related differences in susceptibility to various test articles and environmental conditions exceeds the scope of this chapter, but additional information is available (Nebert, 1981).

HUSBANDRY

Facilities

Facilities used to conduct toxicology studies in mice must have separate and adequate areas for the required laboratory procedures and for the housing and treatment of study mice. This discussion will be limited to facilities for the housing and treatment of mice. Several characteristics for an adequate facility for the conduct of toxicity studies intended to support regulatory approval of new drugs are listed in the Good Laboratory Practice regulations (CFR, 1988a). Such a facility should include enough animal rooms or areas to properly separate different species and projects. In addition, there should be facilities for the quarantine of incoming or sick animals, and for the isolation of any studies that involve use of hazardous materials. In practice, animal rooms used for toxicity studies in mice should not contain any other species of animals. Isolation of individual projects is generally interpreted to mean that an animal room should be dedicated to a single toxicity study. One exception to the requirement to conduct only one study per animal room is the case of acute or very short-term toxicity studies, each of which is limited to a small number of animals. Another exception is dermal carcinogenesis, or "skin painting" studies, which generally involve a relatively small number of animals treated for 30–40 weeks. A number of acute or dermal carcinogenesis studies may be run concurrently in a single room. For practical reasons, "adequate isolation" for acute or dermal carcinogenesis studies is typically interpreted to mean separate cage racks for each study and/or

Table 5 Incidence of Spontaneously Occurring Neoplastic Lesions

Lesions Occurring at Spontaneous Incidence of ≥1%
in Either Sex of Charles River CD-1 or B6C3F1 Mice

	Strain			
	CD-1		B6C3F1	
Location & lesion	M	F	M	F
Lymphoreticular tumors				
lymphosarcoma			6.0	12.0
lymphocytic leukemia			1.3	1.4
lymphoma	3.7	9.9		
histiocytic lymphoma			0.5	1.4
histiocytic sarcoma			0.1	1.4
lymphoblastic lymphoma	1.1	1.7	0.2	0.1
lymphocytic lymphoma	2.6	1.7	0.6	1.7
reticulum cell sarcoma	2.6	5.1	0.4	0.2
Skin/subcutis				
fibrosarcoma	0.2	0.5	1.0	0.5
Mammary gland				
adenocarcinoma		1.7		0.9
Lung				
bronchiolar/alveolar adenoma	4.0	2.9	8.3	3.3
bronchiolar/alveolar carcinoma	3.5	3.1	1.9	0.6
alveolar type II carcinoma	11.7	13.9	0.2	0.1
alveolar type II adenoma			2.5	1.2
adenoma			1.2	0.7
Liver				
nodular hepatocellular prolif.	5.4	1.7	0.5	0.1
hepatocellular adenoma	5.6	0.8	17.2	7.1
hepatocellular carcinoma	7.3	1.0	13.2	2.4
hemangioma	1.0	1.2	0.7	0.3
hemangiosarcoma	1.0	0.2	0.5	0.1
Reproductive system				
Ovary				
cystadenoma		1.1		0.3
Uterus				
endometrial stromal polyp		3.3		2.9
endometrial sarcoma		1.9		0.6
leiomyoma		1.0		0.4
leiomyosarcoma		1.0		0.3
hemangioma		1.0		0.9
Pituitary				
adenoma		3.4	0.3	7.9
Thyroid gland				
follicular cell adenoma	0.2		0.8	2.4
Adrenal				
cortical adenoma	8.6	1.0	0.4	0.3
Harderian gland				
cystadenoma			1.9	1.6
adenoma			1.5	0.6

Source: Data from Charles River Breeding Laboratories, compiled from control
animals on 24-month studies completed between 1978 and 1986.

isolation of multiple studies within the room by geographical location within the room. The intent of the requirements to isolate species and, in most cases, studies is to reduce the probability of cross-contamination between studies with the various test chemicals or disease entities, and to minimize the opportunity for accidental administration of the incorrect test substance to a group of animals. The concept of quarantining incoming animals can be met by having new animals delivered into a sanitized room that contains no other animals, then allowing the new mice an adequate period for acclimatization prior to initiation of the toxicity study. This procedure minimizes the risk of exposure of either new or existing animals to incoming or endemic diseases.

The physical conditions in an animal room are referred to as the macroenvironment. These conditions include such things as the temperature, relative humidity, lighting, ventilation, and concentrations of various gases (e.g. CO_2, ammonia). Many of the macroenvironmental parameters are routinely monitored in facilities that conduct toxicology studies. Abnormal fluctuations in some of these parameters can have a deleterious effect on the validity of toxicity data generated.

Temperature and Relative Humidity

Mice are quite sensitive to variations in temperature, and respond to those variations with important physiological changes. This sensitivity is caused by the large surface area to body weight ratio in mice, which causes them to radiate heat quickly in a cold environment. Mice respond to low temperature by nonshivering thermogenesis, and resting mice can generate heat at a rate about triple their basal metabolic rate. Group-housed mice can compensate for low temperatures by huddling in a group, a practice that is more effective in a solid-bottom cage containing bedding. Mice have a limited capacity to compensate for excessive heat, and do so primarily by vasodilation of the ears to increase heat loss, and by increasing body temperature by several degrees. In the wild, mice adapt to excessive temperatures by moving to cool burrows. Mortality is often observed if the ambient temperature reaches 37°C or higher. The range of environmental temperatures where an animal's oxygen consumption is minimal and virtually independent of changes in ambient temperature is called the thermoneutral zone. The thermoneutral zone for mice is one of the narrowest of species studied, and is about 30.0°C ± 0.5°C. Mice seem to be generally healthier at a temperature of about 21–25°C than they are within the thermoneutral zone (Jacoby and Fox, 1984). The recommended dry-bulb temperature for a mouse housing room is 18–26°C (ILAR, 1985).

Variations in environmental temperature can effect the results of toxicity studies in unpredictable ways. Muller and Vernikos-Danellis (1970) found that the acute toxicity of dextroamphetamine was reduced by 10-fold when the temperature was reduced to 15°C from a normal of 22°C, but was increased by two to threefold when the temperature was increased to 30°C. Conversely, the acute toxicity of caffeine was increased when the temperature was altered either up or down from 22°C. Food consumption is inversely related to ambient temperature, and the secondary effects of changes in food consumption can be complex.

The relative humidity in a mouse room is a significant factor in thermoregulation for the mice housed. At constant temperature, mice are more active at lower relative humidity than at higher humidity. This difference is believed to be a function of the mouse's ability to better dissipate heat under conditions of lower relative humidity (Stille et al., 1968). Low ambient relative humidity has been associated with increased transmission of a disease called ringtail in mice. High relative humidity leads to increased production of ammonia in the urine and feces. Increased ammonia concentrations have been associated with the development of respiratory diseases in rodents (Broderson et al., 1976). The recommended relative humidity for a room housing mice is 40–70% (ILAR, 1985).

Lighting

Any description of lighting in an animal facility must include a description of the intensity, wavelength or spectrum, and photoperiod of the light.

Light intensity is expressed in footcandles (ftc) (lumen/ft^2) or lux (lumen/m^2). Historically, lighting intensity was selected for convenience of the researchers, based on the assumption that what was good for people was good for mice. In fact, the *Guide for the Care and Use of Laboratory Animals* as recently as 1978 recommended light intensity of 100–125 ftc. Mice are nocturnal, however so it is not surprising that their eyes are better adapted to lower light levels. Continuous exposure to light at 100–125 ftc for 6 days has been found to cause loss of 90% of the photoreceptors in albino-beige mice (Robison and Kuwabara, 1978). Light levels of 25 ftc or lower have been recommended for mice (Robison et al., 1982). Amid this discussion of light levels, the specific design and location of individual cages within an animal room can have a substantial effect on the light level at the animal's level. Owing to the nocturnal nature of mice and the attenuation of light by the structure and location of individual cages, there is probably little or no actual injury to an animal housed in a room lighted to 100–150 ftc on a 12-hr light, 12 hr dark cycle.

The wavelength or spectrum of light found in a mouse room is generally a function of the type of fluorescent lighting in common use at the animal facility. While the lighting spectrum may not be of highest concern in designing toxicity studies, Spaulding et al. (1969) have shown that mice exhibited the highest level of voluntary wheel running activity under red light or in darkness, an intermediate level of activity under yellow, and the lowest under green, blue, or daylight. Recalling the nocturnal characteristics of mice, the proximity of red light to dusk/darkness and of blue light to ultraviolet and daylight on the visible spectrum is probably not a coincidence.

The photoperiod for mouse rooms used for toxicity studies is typically diurnal, with a cycle of about 12 hr light to 12 hr darkness. The photoperiod influences circadian rhythms, and is probably most often thought of in the context of influence on the estrus cycle. While the estrus cycle of the rat is synchronized by the photoperiod, the estrus cycle of the mouse is less easily influenced by photoperiod (Campbell et al., 1976).

Ventilation

Ventilation in an animal housing facility should be designed to provide sufficient fresh air to remove the thermal load generated by the animals, lights, and equipment, maintain acceptable levels of dust and odor, provide adequate oxygen, and contain any biohazards or intercurrent disease in the animal colony.

A common practice for animal facilities has been to design the heating, ventilation, and air conditioning system to provide 10–15 air changes per hour. In reality, this approach can be quite misleading because it depends upon the total volume of the animal room rather than the biological and thermal load. An animal room with 12-ft ceilings would require 50% more cubic feet of fresh air per minute to achieve 15 air changes per hour than would a room with 8-ft ceilings. Clearly the more important factor in this example is the number of cubic feet of fresh air per mouse (or kilogram of animals) housed rather than the number of air changes per hour. As a guide, an adequate ventilation rate for a mouse room is about 0.147 ft^3/min of fresh air per mouse, with a heat removal capacity of about 0.6 BTU per hour per mouse (Runkle, 1964).

If at all possible, supplied air should be 100% fresh outside air, introduced into the animal room at ceiling level, with exhaust air picked up at or near the floor to eliminate a maximum amount of heavier-than-air ammonia vapors. Supply air should minimally be drawn through a particle filter, and many facilities now include high-efficiency particle (HEPA) filters on supply air. Addition of HEPA filtration to an existing system will usually require a substantial increase in air conditioning blower power and/or capacity to overcome the added resistance of the filters. Supply of 100% fresh air at the ventilation rates discussed entails significant energy costs for heating and cooling. These costs can be reduced by the installation of a heat (cool) recovery system between the exhaust air and the incoming fresh air. The efficiencies of such a system are accrued during both the heating and the cooling seasons. If for some reason, 100% fresh air cannot be supplied, any recycled air must be passed through a complex filtration system to prevent reintroduction of (and cross-contamination by) biological or chemical contaminants and odors.

Relative air pressure between animal rooms and corridors should be considered as a prime mechanism for control of cross-contamination and communication of disease between animal rooms. In theory, if all animal rooms are either positive pressure relative to the corridor, or if all are negative relative to the corridor, there should be no communication of airborne contamination between rooms. If any hazardous substances or human pathogens will be used within the animal rooms, those rooms should be maintained negative to the corridor to prevent contamination of people.

Noise

There are no specific regulations or guidelines governing noise to which mice can or should be exposed. There are, however, numerous reports in the literature of adverse or abnormal effects of "stressful" noise on mice, including reduction in body weight (Fink and Iturrian, 1970); changes in immune response and tumor resistance (Jensen and Rasmussen, 1970); audiogenic seizures (Iturrian, 1973), which are seen in genetically susceptible mice and can also be induced in normal mice; unexpected responses to certain drugs (Iturrian and Johnson, 1975); actual hearing impairment; and others. In view of the variety of effects associated with noise, control of environmental noise in a facility used to conduct toxicity studies in mice should be addressed.

Noise should be described in terms of two dimensions: intensity and frequency. Sound intensity (sound pressure level or loudness) is measured in decibels (dB) and frequency (pitch) is measured in hertz (Hz). Hertz is the standard unit for cycles per second. While a "safe" intensity of sound has not been described, intensities of 90–100 dB have produced adverse effects, including inner ear damage, and it has been recommended that noise levels be maintained below 85 dB (Anthony, 1962). It is especially important to consider the frequency of environmental noise because the frequency spectrum for hearing in mice differs substantially from that in humans. High-frequency noise that is inaudible to humans can be disruptive or injurious to mice. The average human ear can hear sounds in the frequency range of about 20 Hz to 20 kHz, with maximum sensitivity at about 2 kHz. In contrast, mice can not hear sounds with frequencies as low as 1 kHz, clearly hear sounds at 50 kHz, and probably have an upper limit in the range of 60–70 kHz (Clough,

1982). Mice emit sound in these upper frequencies, apparently as a means of communication between mothers and young, and associated with mating and aggression. Environmental noise near these frequencies may disrupt normal behavior. Devices that emit sound in this spectrum include ultrasonic motion detectors (used for door openers and intrusion alarms), ultrasonic cleaning and mixing equipment, high-speed homogenizers, dropped or banged metallic devices (e.g., cages, pans, covers), and many others. Dogs and nonhuman primates create noise of an intensity and frequency as to be disruptive to mice.

Environmental noise should be controlled at two levels: at the design and selection of facilities and equipment and at establishment of procedures for animal husbandry and the conduct of laboratory activities that might produce noise at a disruptive intensity or frequency. As the noise of dogs and nonhuman primates is disruptive to rodents (ILAR, 1985), mice should not be housed in close proximity to these species. Loud noises (e.g, barking of dogs) can be transmitted from room-to-room, sometimes significant distances, through the ventilation system duct work. This transmission can be reduced by installing labyrinthine configurations and/or commercially available acoustic attenuators in the duct work that services noisy rooms. Mice should not be housed in close proximity to essentially noisy operations such as cage washing. Intense, high-frequency noise can be generated by the movement of cage racks, equipment carts, etc., in hallways adjacent to animal rooms. A variety of design considerations can improve this situation. A cage rack moving on rubber or synthetic cushioned wheels with well-lubricated bearings over a monolithic flooring will be much quieter than a similar rack on steel wheels with squeaky bearings moving over quarry tile or even concrete flooring. Procedures should be devised and personnel should be trained with an appreciation for the deleterious effects excessive noise may have on the well-being of mice, and consequently on the results of toxicity studies conducted with those animals.

Construction Parameters

Clearly a detailed discussion of the architectural and engineering aspects of a facility intended to house laboratory mice is beyond the scope of this text. Our experience has, however, suggested two areas that should receive top priority when new construction, renovation, or even routine maintenance is required.

Cleanability. Animal rooms are exposed to a wide variety of "soil" on a continuing basis. Sources include such things as feed dust, spilled water, animal waste, bedding, parasites (e.g., mouse pinworms), and various bacterial and viral strains that may infect the species housed. Consequently, animal rooms must be swept and mopped frequently, typically using a chemical detergent and disinfectant, and should be sanitized at least before each new study goes into a room, and on a regular basis if a long-term study is in progress. One of the most effective processes for sanitization uses a pressure sprayer to clean ceilings, walls, and floors with an effective disinfectant. This process requires that all surfaces (ceilings, walls, and floors) be coated with a durable, waterproof, chemical-resistant finish. That finish should withstand impacts, such as cage racks colliding with walls, and various objects being dropped on floors without damage to the flooring. In addition, all lighting fixtures, electrical outlets, switches, computer connections, thermostats, etc., should be either of waterproof construction, or should be equipped with waterproof covers which can be closed during sanitization.

Vermin Resistance. Animal rooms are notoriously attractive to insects such as cockroaches, flies, and other pests. The ready access to feed and water that is essential for the mice is an ideal environment for insect infestation as well. The use of toxicants to control pests in rooms housing animals on toxicity studies is discouraged for several reasons. Many common pesticides are known to induce the synthesis of hepatic microsomal enzymes, which in turn may alter the apparent toxicity of the substance being tested. As most toxicity studies are conducted on test substances with unknown or incompletely understood pharmacology, the possible interactions with a particular pesticide are unpredictable. Pests may consume a toxicant, then enter animal cages prior to dying, and be ingested by the study mice. This could lead to indirect intoxication of the study animals.

One environmental requirement for a successful insect population explosion is the availability of a concealed harborage for breeding. We have had remarkable success in controlling insect infestation in our facility by the simple process of sealing, caulking, closing, or eliminating every crack, crevice, hole, wall penetration, electrical outlet, and floor drain in our animal rooms. For this practice to be successful, contractors and maintenance people who work in these rooms must understand the purpose and importance of their task. Cracks in a wall behind a sink are just as useful as harborages as cracks in the middle of the wall, so each contractor and maintenance person must be watching for and eliminating these problems when they are found.

If elimination of harborage has not been implemented or is incomplete, it may be necessary to employ a toxicant on a carefully controlled basis. The study toxicologist should participate in the selection of a suitable toxicant, factoring in all that is known about the pharmacology of the substance being tested in the toxicity study and providing a best estimate of possible interactions with the toxicant. Accurate records should be kept of what toxicant was used, where and how much was applied, and how often it was applied. These factors should be reviewed and considered when the toxicity study is completed and the results are being interpreted.

Caging

The physical conditions in an animal cage (primary enclosure) are referred to as the microenvironment. These conditions (e.g., temperature, relative humidity, lighting, ventilation, concentrations of various gases [e.g., CO_2, ammonia]) may differ substantially from the conditions in the macroenvironment, depending upon the specific design and placement of the cage within the animal room. Microenvironmental parameters should be evaluated for various cage designs and locations within animal rooms, but are not routinely monitored in facilities that conduct toxicology studies.

Any caging used for mice in toxicology studies should be designed to provide adequate space for freedom of movement and a comfortable environment in terms of temperature, humidity, and ventilation that will minimize stress on the animals. The caging should be cleaned regularly to allow the mice to remain clean and dry. Caging should be as resistant to escape as possible to preserve the integrity of the study as well as the health and safety of the animals. Even if an escaped animal can be recovered and returned to its cage, the health of the animal and resultant impact on the integrity of the toxicity data generated remains in question, as the animal may have contacted toxic or interfering substances during its travels.

Cage Type

Two types of mouse caging most commonly used for toxicology studies are wire-bottom cages and solid-bottom cages.

Wire-Bottom Cages. Wire-bottom cages are typically suspended in rows on a movable rack with from 10 to 70 cages arranged on a side. Racks may be single sided or double sided, depending upon the configuration of the animal room and the number of animals that need to be housed. Most contemporary wire-bottom cages are fabricated of stainless sheet steel backs and sides, with stainless steel wire mesh fronts and floors. Sides and backs may have holes or slots stamped into them at manufacture to allow improved ventilation and access to an automatic watering system if one is available. Mesh fronts allow observation of the animals. Wire-bottom cages are also fabricated of polycarbonate or other rigid plastic product. Transparent plastic cages provide easier observation of animals, but typically offer reduced ventilation through the cage itself. Mesh floors allow urine, feces, and spilled food to drop through, typically to a waste pan or absorbent paper, which can be cleaned or replaced easily and regularly. Waste pans should be cleaned or papers replaced at least three times a week. A wire-bottom design has the advantage of keeping animals relatively free of contamination from urine and feces, whereas providing ease of cleaning. Wire-bottom cages should be rotated out of use and washed at least once every 2 weeks. This washing procedure should be monitored regularly, and should be adequate to produce negative results on microbiological swab testing. A procedure that achieves good microbiological test results in our facility for cages with average levels of soil employs removal (or emptying) of feeders, waste pans, and water bottles (if any). Then the racks with the suspended wire cages still in place are passed through a commercial rack washer which operates much like an automatic dishwasher. All cycle times are variable, but an effective combination for average soil is a wash cycle of about 10 min, followed by initial and final rinse cycles of about 3 min each. The wash cycle includes an effective disinfectant detergent (such as PRL-18, manufactured by Pharmacal Research Laboratories, Inc., Naugatuck, Connecticut). All water temperatures (wash, initial and final rinse) are maintained at or above 82°C (180°F), but this temperature is most important for the final rinse.

Solid-Bottom Cages. Solid-bottom cages, often referred to as shoe-box cages, may be suspended in a rack, like wire-bottom cages, or may be supplied with tops, and arranged on shelves, which are typically movable as a rack. Shoe-box cages are typically constructed of polycarbonate, which allows convenient observation of the animals, polypropylene, which is a translucent plastic, or sheet metal, such as stainless steel. Shoe-box cages provide a secure base for animals, and are essential if animals are to be allowed to deliver and suckle live litters. Solid-bottom cages can be provided with filter tops, which can significantly reduce airborne contamination of the environment within the cage. Filter tops do have a negative impact on ventilation within the cage, and levels of CO_2 and ammonia have been found to be substantially higher in cages with filter tops than in those with stainless steel rod tops (Serrano, 1971). There are a number of disadvantages associated with solid-bottom cages. These cages must be provided with some form of low-dust or dust-free absorptive bedding. This bedding must be changed regularly, which is labor intensive. If matings are conducted, vaginal plugs are often difficult or impossible to find in the bedding. As mice engage in coprophagy, a toxic substance or metabolite that is eliminated in the feces may be "recycled," thereby leading to an overestimate of the true toxicity of the substance. In addition, mice commonly ingest various types of bedding, such as wood chips, which renders impossible any serious estimate of food consumption. If an automatic watering system is in use, solid-bottom cages have the potential to fill with water if there is a malfunction, drowning the inhabitant(s).

In routine toxicology studies, solid-bottom cages, covers, feeders, etc., should be rotated out of use and washed once or twice a week, and their supporting racks should be washed at least once per month. This cage cleaning schedule should NOT be followed if reproductive procedures (mating, delivery and suckling of young) are being conducted, as constancy of home-cage odor is critical to reproductive efficiency and to reduce the likelihood of cannibalization of young. Cage washing may need to be suspended completely during the period of pregnancy and lactation. (See "Bedding" section of this section for special practices used with reproduction procedures.) The cage and accessory washing procedure should be monitored regularly, and should be adequate to produce negative results on microbiological swab testing. A procedure that achieves good microbiological test results in our facility for cages with average levels of soil employs passage through a tunnel washer on a steel mesh belt. The total transit or cycle time is typically about 3 min, with about 15 sec for prewash, and just under 1 min each for main wash, rinse, and drying cycles. The wash cycle includes an effective disinfectant detergent (such as Clout, manufactured by Pharmacal Research Laboratories, Inc., Naugatuck, Connecticut). The rinse water is heated to at least 82°C (180°F), and the drying cycle consists of exposure to high-temperature forced air. The belt speed in a machine such as this can be reduced (total transit time lengthened) for heavily soiled cages or increased (transit time shortened) for lightly soiled cages, but the single criteria which governs the minimum length of the transit time is the maintenance of negative results on the microbiological monitoring of the clean cages.

Cage Size

Mouse caging must be of adequate size to allow free movement and to avoid overcrowding. Minimum space requirements for mice are provided in the *Guide for the Care and Use of Laboratory Animals* (ILAR, 1985) on the basis of body weight. Those requirements are in Table 6. As a practical matter, to avoid the need for multiple-sized caging and frequent (e.g., perhaps weekly) changes in the size of caging occupied, the minimum specified for adults can be used for all ages.

Population

Mice may be housed singly (one to a cage) or in groups (several animals of the same treatment group caged together) for toxicity testing. It has long been recognized, however, that group housing can substantially alter the toxicity of some substances. Chance (1946) demonstrated that the acute toxicity of a group of sympathomimetic amines was increased by two- to 10-fold in mice that were group housed compared to mice housed singly. In addition, increased population in solid-bottom cages has been shown to lead to substantially higher levels of CO_2 and ammonia within the cage, even when open,

Table 6 Minimum Cage Space Requirements for Mice

Body weight	Floor area per mouse		Cage height	
(g)	in^2	cm^2	in	cm
<10	6.0	38.7	5	12.7
10–15	8.0	51.6	5	12.7
15–25	12.0	77.4	5	12.7
>25	15.0	96.8	5	12.7

stainless steel rod tops were used, but especially if filter tops were in place (Serrano, 1971). Increased levels of ammonia have been associated with hepatic microsomal enzyme induction, which can alter expected metabolism in a toxicity study.

Single Occupancy. Single housing of mice used in toxicity studies offers many advantages. Of paramount importance is the reduced likelihood of mistaking the identity of individuals when conducting various study procedures (weighing, dosing, collecting various observational, or other data). Singly housed mice are more quickly and easily identified and captured throughout the study. In addition, the risk of injury or cannibalism is eliminated in the event that one member of a group becomes debilitated. The biggest disadvantage to single housing is cost. Purchase price for individual caging for large numbers of mice is much higher than the cost for group housing. Individual caging requires much more floor space in the animal rooms than group caging for an equivalent number of animals, and the cost to provide animal care (food, water, cage cleaning, and sanitization) is much higher for single caging.

Group Housing. The biggest advantage to group housing is cost savings. Disadvantages include increased probability of mistaken identity, increased stress on animals as a result of establishment and testing of dominance hierarchy, and difficulty with individual animal identification systems. Group-housed mice tend to tear out each others ear tags, and tattooed markings may be obliterated as a result of repeated fighting for dominance. Measurement of food or water consumption is generally not useful for group-housed mice, as the distribution of food and water among animals of different hierarchical positions tends to be quite uneven. Group housing in solid-bottom cages effects microenvironmental parameters within the cage such as temperature, humidity, various gas concentrations (CO_2, ammonia), and others.

Bedding

Some form of bedding material is required in solid-bottom cages to allow mice to remain clean, dry, and free of urine and feces. The Good Laboratory Practice (GLP) regulations (CFR, 1988b) states that bedding should "not interfere with the purpose or conduct of the study" and should "be changed as often as necessary to keep the animals dry and clean." An appropriate bedding should absorb urine effectively, be as free of dust as possible to minimize pulmonary complications, be free of contaminating chemicals, and should have no unacceptable effect on the normal physiology or metabolism of the mice. Inhalation of aromatic hydrocarbons from cedar and pine bedding has been shown to cause induction of hepatic microsomal enzymes, which could seriously compromise the results of a toxicity study (Vesell, 1967; Wade et al., 1968). Opinions differ on whether the use of cedar wood shavings as bedding material contribute to the increased incidence of mammary gland tumors and hepatomas (Sabine et al., 1973, Heston, 1975). One of the most commonly used bedding materials for toxicity studies is hardwood chips derived from woods such as maple, birch, and beech (e.g., Absorb-Dri hardwood chips, Maywood, New Jersey). This selection is probably based on the properties of high absorption and low dust, coupled with an absence of proof that there are harmful interactions.

Bedding material should be changed at least once or twice weekly when cages are washed. More frequent bedding changes may be required if mice are group housed. An exception to this practice for bedding change occurs when reproductive procedures (mating, delivery and suckling of young) are involved in the study. A continuity of home-cage odor reduces maternal stress, is critical to reproductive efficiency, and reduces the likelihood of cannibalization of young. Therefore, during reproductive procedures, a portion (but not all) of the soiled bedding should be removed at regular intervals and replaced with clean bedding.

Animal Identification

Reliable identification of each animal used in a toxicity study is essential to the integrity of the study data and to the accurate interpretation of study results. The GLP regulations (CFR, 1988d) state that

> animals, excluding suckling rodents, used in laboratory procedures that require manipulations and observations over an extended period of time or in studies that require the animals to be removed from and returned to their home cages for any reason (e.g. cage cleaning, treatment, etc.), shall receive appropriate identification (e.g. tattoo, toe clip, color code, ear tag, ear punch, etc.).

And further, that "All information needed to specifically identify each animal within an animal-housing unit shall appear on the outside of that unit." The GLP regulation was amended (Federal Register, 1989) to eliminate toe clipping from the methods listed (above), and to discourage the use of toe clipping in nonclinical laboratory studies, as other, more humane methods are available. One new method, not listed in the GLP regulation, but which appears to offer some advantages is the implantable electronic microchip.

Cage Cards

In practice, the comprehensive information specified above for the outside of an animal-housing unit typically appears on a cage card. This information is relatively straightforward as long as animals are housed singly. The cage card should include complete identification of the study (study number is adequate if a unique coding system is used), identification of or references to the species, strain, sex, source, age, treatment group (e.g., substance tested and dose group), and individual animal number of the mouse (or mice) housed. The identification which appears on the mouse itself is limited to a few code letters and or numbers which can be cross-referenced to the cage card and raw data record for the study to obtain all of the information available about that individual mouse.

Ear Tags

Ear tags are durable, typically made of a noncorroding metal such as Monel, with letters and/or numbers stamped into the surface. The tags are quick and easy to apply, using a special plierslike applicator, and are easily read over a long period of time. One disadvantage to ear tags is that they can be torn out of the ear if they get caught on something in the cage, or especially, if mice are group housed. Group-housed mice seem to find each others' ear tags especially vulnerable to pulling and hierarchical conflict, and the incidence of tag loss in group-housed mice has proven unacceptably high in our facility. Conversely, the incidence of tag loss in singly housed mice (the norm for toxicity testing at our facility) is remarkably low, especially after the first few days of adaptation. When tags are lost from singly-housed mice, they are typically found in or under the cage, so the tag number can be confirmed and a replacement tag installed. A technique to increase tag retention is to avoid the edge of the ear, installing the piercing portion of the tag as near the center of the ear as possible. A useful tag for mice is a small ($\frac{5}{16}$ in long) self-piercing Monel tag ("V" shaped prior to application, crimped to a flattened "O" by installation) such as Style 4-1005, Size 1 from National Band and Tag, Newport, Kentucky. These tags can be ordered custom stamped with at least three numbers or letters on one surface, and four on the other surface (i.e., up to 10 million different numbers, more if letters are used as well).

Ear Notching or Punching

Ear notching or punching is a system of holes punched and/or notches cut into the edges of the ears based upon a predetermined numeric code. Figure 1 is an example of an ear-marking code (from Leard, 1984). Notching has the advantage of not offering a hard object that can be caught or pulled from the ear, such as an ear tag. Disadvantages include the requirement for substantially more time and care in initial identification of the animals. Clearly it takes longer and inflicts more pain on the mouse to punch and clip a precise pattern of from one to four or five holes and notches into the two ears of a mouse than to crimp on a single ear tag. Imprecisely positioned punches or notches may be difficult to read for the duration of the study. Group-housed mice may chew at each others ears, especially when the notches are fresh, rendering the code more difficult to read. Finally, most codes allow at most a few hundred nonrepeating numbers, meaning that patterns will have to be repeated within most facilities in a short time.

Tattoos

Mice can be tattooed on the tail or feet as a means of identification. Tattoos are permanent unless they become obliterated by chewing or injury. The process of applying alpha-numeric tattoos to the tails of mice is more time-consuming than ear tagging or notching, but more accessible than the feet. Another practical consideration is the size of a mouse tail. Very small letters are both more difficult and time consuming to apply to a mouse tail, and more difficult and time consuming to read at each subsequent identity check throughout the study. The size of the mouse tail and practical considerations of legibility limit the tattoo to four to five alpha-numeric characters on the dorsal (easily readable) surface of the tail. It is possible to tattoo an additional four to five alpha-numeric characters on the ventral surface of the tail if necessary. This surface is less easily read,

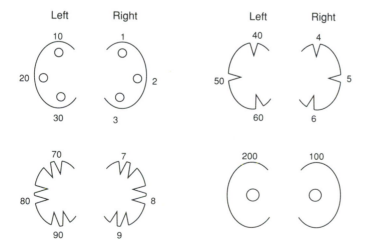

Figure 1 Example of an ear marking code which can be used for animal identification. (From Leard, 1984, used with permission.)

and can be used for study or facility code numbers that need not be read at each identity check.

While tattooing is a viable method of identification for longer toxicity studies because of its permanence, the amount of time required to both apply and read the tattoos makes this method impractical for shorter studies.

Color Coding of Skin or Hair

The skin or fur of a mouse can be quickly color coded using a variety of indelible felt-tip markers. A variety of combinations of colored markings on the tail or on the fur of the back are easily read without disturbing the animal. This procedure is particularly useful for toxicity studies of short duration. Owing to the fastidious grooming habits of mice, there is a tendency for colored marks to be groomed off quite quickly. This problem is exacerbated if the mice are group housed. A number of different brands and types of markers should be tested, as there is wide variability in their "durability" or resistance to grooming. This problem can be reduced somewhat by locating the color code in a place that is more difficult to groom, such as the top or back of the head. One substance that confers a durable stain on the fur is Bouin's fixative, but the color is limited to yellow, so the identity code must be based upon the location of the stain rather than the color. The number of possible easily distinguished colors and combinations of colors available for a color code and the maximum number of different sites that can be easily coded on a mouse limits the number of unique codes to a few hundred.

In general, color coding is a useful procedure for identifying mice in short studies. The toxicologist should evaluate each mouse and be prepared to "touch up" the color code on a daily basis.

Toe Clipping

Toe clipping for purposes of identifying mice involves amputation of various combinations of toes using a surgical scissor, nail clipper, or other suitable device to establish an identity code. Toe clipping has the advantage of permanence, but an individual may become "unreadable" through accident or injury that compromises unclipped toes. Toe clipping has many disadvantages, and no clear advantages over other methods such as ear tagging or notching. Most importantly, toe clipping is more traumatic than other methods, and has an increased likelihood of resulting in infection because it involves the feet. The method is time consuming to perform and the codes are difficult to read through the duration of the study because the mouse must be picked up and often the toes of each foot must be spread to facilitate accurate reading. As stipulated at the beginning of this section on animal identification, the Food and Drug Administration has amended the GLP regulations to eliminate toe clipping from the list of procedures recommended for identifying animals. Toe clipping may have some utility in neonatal (or very young) mice, in which the nervous system is not as well developed, and more conventional methods are impractical.

Implantable Electronic Microchips

A recent development in animal identification is the implantable electronic microchip (Bio Medic Data Systems, Maywood, New Jersey). The microchip is a transponder which has been sealed into a glass capsule about 1.0 cm in length and about 1.5 mm in diameter. This device is suitable for subcutaneous implantation in mice. The device is "energized" by one of a variety of portable or stationary readers, which emits a low-power radio-frequency signal. The transponder is stimulated to transmit its unique identification number back to the reader, where it can be both displayed and linked directly to a computer system. The microchips are easy to install, resistant to loss, and should perform well over the course of a longer-term study. The device has a capacity for up to 34 billion different numbers. Preliminary data from several laboratories suggest that the devices are well tolerated, and do not produce problematic histological changes at the implantation site. One disadvantage is that the devices must be read by the electronic reading equipment. The implication is that in the event of equipment failure, there is no means for manual decoding or reading of the chips. Possession of multiple readers should provide reasonable redundancy for most facilities.

Food

Nutritional Requirements

The explicit nutrient requirements for mice have not been extensively studied nor defined. What is known of these requirements has been estimated on the basis of a number of studies that have had other objectives. Some studies have focused on the effects of specific dietary deficiencies, and others have looked at "acceptable performance" in growth and reproductive parameters as evidence of nutrient adequacy. Mice have different nutrient requirements for growth, reproduction, and maintenance, and the many diverse genetic strains differ in their minimal requirements as well. Estimated minimum nutritional requirements for proper growth and reproduction of "conventional mice" have been compiled in Table 7 (NRC, 1978).

The estimated nutritional requirements for laboratory mice are published periodically by the National Research Council in a document titled *Nutrient Requirements of Laboratory Animals* (NRC, 1978). That document is revised when important new information becomes available, and is thus considered a current, authoritative source. The Third Revised Edition, published in 1978, is the most current source for this section. A subsequent edition is expected in 1992–1993.

Selection

The choice of a specific diet to be used in a mouse toxicity study should take into account all of the objectives and requirements of the study as well as the convenience, efficiency, cost, and availability of a particular diet. In general, diets obtained from well-known commercial suppliers with established procedures for quality control and documentation will be worth any added cost. One of the basic choices is whether to use pelleted diet or meal. Pelleted diet is generally easier and neater to handle, both for the people and the mice involved. The meal form of a diet is usually easier to use if the study design requires mixing of a test chemical with the diet, or if food consumption will be measured.

Mice can obtain adequate nutrition from a variety of types of diets. Diets are classified on the basis of the amount of refinement of the ingredients (NRC, 1978). Three types of diets will be described here. The types are natural ingredient diets, purified diets, and chemically defined diets.

Natural Ingredient Diets. These types of diets contain grains such as corn, wheat, oats, beet pulp, and other ingredients that have been subjected to minimal processing such as fish meal, soybean meal, wheat bran, and a variety of vitamin and mineral supplements. They also have been referred to as a cereal based, unrefined, nonpurified, or stock diets. Natural ingredient diets are the most widely used and are relatively economical. The principal objection to such diets is that they have had a tendency to vary widely in terms of

Table 7 Estimated Nutrient Requirements of Mice: National Research Council (1978)

Nutrient	Unit	Requirement
Linoleic acid	%	0.3
Protein (growth)	%	12.5
Protein (reproduction)	%	18.0
L-Amino acids		
Arginine	%	0.3
Histidine	%	0.2
Isoleucine	%	0.4
Leucine	%	0.7
Lysine	%	0.4
Methionine	%	0.5
Phenylalanine	%	0.4
Threonine	%	0.4
Tryptophan	%	0.1
Valine	%	0.5
Minerals		
Calcium	%	0.4
Chloride	(required, but not quantified)	
Magnesium	%	0.05
Phosphorus	%	0.4
Potassium	%	0.2
Sodium	(required, but not quantified)	
Chromium	mg/kg	2.0
Copper	mg/kg	4.5
Fluoride	(status uncertain for mice)	
Iodine	mg/kg	0.25
Iron	mg/kg	25.0
Manganese	mg/kg	45.0
Selenium	(required, but not quantified)	
Vanadium	(status uncertain for mice)	
Zinc	mg/kg	30.0
Vitamins		
A	IU/kg	500.0
D	IU/kg	150.0
E	IU/kg	20.0
K_1 equivalent	mg/kg	3.0
Biotin	mg/kg	0.2
Choline	mg/kg	600.0
Folacin	mg/kg	0.5
Inositol(myo-)	(bacterial synth. usually adequate)	
Niacin	mg/kg	10.0
Pantothenate (Ca)	mg/kg	10.0
Riboflavin	mg/kg	7.0
Thiamine	mg/kg	5.0
Vitamin B_6	mg/kg	1.0
Vitamin B_{12}	mg/kg	0.01

nutrient and contaminant content (Newberne, 1975; Wise and Gilburt, 1980; Wise, 1982; Rao and Knapka, 1987). Data have been compiled on key nutrient and contaminant concentrations for all of the lots of a commercially available natural ingredient rodent diet (Purina Certified Rodent Chow 5002, Purina Mills, Inc., St. Louis, Missouri) received at this facility over a period of 1 year. The variability of these concentrations from lot to lot is relatively low, as seen in Tables 8 and 9.

Purified Diets. These types of diets are formulated exclusively with refined ingredients. Dietary protein may be derived from sources such as casein or isolated soy protein, carbohydrate may be derived from sugar or starch, fat may be derived from vegetable oil or animal fat, and dietary fiber may be derived from some form of cellulose. Inorganic salts and pure vitamins are added to provide essential vitamins and minerals. Purified diets also have been referred to as semipurified, synthetic, or semisynthetic. They offer consistent nutrient concentrations and the ability to modify those concentrations to achieve specific nutritional deficiencies or excesses. Purified diets are less palatable for some animals, and food consumption should be monitored prior to study initiation and during the study to assure that adequate nutrition is being maintained.

Chemically Defined Diets. These types of diets are formulated entirely with chemically pure compounds. Amino acids, sugars, triglycerides, essential fatty acids, inorganic salts, and vitamins are blended to provide appropriate nutrition. These diets offer strict control of specific nutrient concentrations at the time of manufacturer, but the bioavailability of those nutrients may be altered by oxidation or interaction among nutrients. The availability of specific nutrients to the mice, then, may not be what the toxicologist believes is being providing. Chemically defined diets have the further disadvantages of being expensive and difficult to formulate, and have a very narrow appeal in toxicity testing.

In addition to the degree of refinement of ingredients, mouse diets are classified as closed formula or open formula on the basis of the availability of the quantitative as well as the qualitative aspects of the feed blend.

Closed Formula Diets. Manufacturers and vendors of closed formula diets typically provide a list of ingredients used to manufacture the diet, but not the actual proportions of each ingredient in the final blend. They also typically provide target or mean nutrient analyses from a number of batches. A reputable commercial vendor will analyze feed in production, and make minor adjustments to the quantitative aspects of the blend on a frequent basis to maintain nearly constant concentrations of key nutrients such as protein, fat, fiber, and minimal concentrations of potentially important contaminants (personal communication, D. Ettle, Purina Mills, Inc.).

Open Formula Diets. These types of diets are typically based on a published formulation for the quantity of each nutrient to be included, for example ground wheat: 230 g/kg, ground corn: 245 g/kg, and soybean meal: 120 g/kg. An example of an open formula, natural ingredient diet (Knapka et al., 1974) is in Table 10. It is often assumed that open formula diets provide more consistent nutrient and contaminant concentrations than equivalent closed formula diets because the relative proportions of ingredients stay fixed among lots, and across time. The opposite may be true. While it is true that the diet described in Table 10 will always contain 230 g/kg of ground wheat, it is also true that the actual protein and contaminant contents of that wheat (and of many other constituents) may vary widely during the year, depending upon climatic conditions during growth, geographical location of the source, and storage conditions since harvest (Greenman et al., 1980). These variables also affect lots from year to year.

Table 8 Content of Several Key Nutrients in Different Lots of a Closed Formula, Natural Ingredient Rodent Diet (Purina Certified Rodent Chow 5002)

	Protein (%)	Fat (%)	Fiber (%)	Calcium (%)	Phosphorus (%)
Pellets	20.8	5.75	4.46	0.781	0.680
	20.3	4.64	4.20	0.708	0.650
	20.3	5.08	4.14	0.684	0.633
	21.6	5.45	4.76	0.834	0.666
	20.3	5.40	4.28	0.893	0.661
	21.9	4.93	4.11	0.758	0.695
	20.8	5.00	4.60	0.774	0.588
	20.2	5.73	4.09	0.710	0.629
	20.1	5.82	3.77	0.760	0.607
	21.0	6.07	3.97	0.786	0.683
	20.2	5.94	4.36	0.768	0.599
	20.8	5.89	4.39	0.831	0.745
	20.6	5.80	3.95	0.841	0.592
	20.5	5.60	4.08	0.682	0.592
	20.3	5.74	3.75	0.763	0.606
	20.7	5.68	3.86	0.853	0.622
	20.3	5.90	3.87	0.726	0.536
	20.8	5.50	3.74	0.754	0.588
	20.8	6.17	3.81	0.860	0.600
means =	20.65	5.58	4.12	0.777	0.630
Meal	21.3	5.76	4.47	0.850	0.589
	21.9	5.45	4.45	0.924	0.716
	21.5	5.40	4.26	0.715	0.542
	21.7	4.82	3.84	0.877	0.696
	21.4	4.92	4.07	0.718	0.647
	20.3	5.74	4.00	0.632	0.561
	20.3	5.91	4.31	0.903	0.566
	20.7	6.43	3.68	0.741	0.676
	21.1	5.83	4.13	0.809	0.701
	21.1	6.02	4.03	0.681	0.587
	21.2	5.76	4.45	0.817	0.732
	21.2	6.15	3.99	0.880	0.576
	21.1	5.75	3.67	0.849	0.581
	21.5	6.33	3.93	0.832	0.605
	20.5	6.16	4.20	0.732	0.561
	20.4	5.81	3.97	0.790	0.602
means =	21.08	5.77	4.09	0.797	0.621
Combined means =	20.84	5.67	4.10	0.786	0.626
Range =	20.1–21.9	4.64–6.43	3.67–4.76	0.632–0.924	0.536–0.745

Table 9 Content of Several Key Contaminents in Different Lots of a Closed Formula, Natural Ingredient, Rodent Diet (Purina Certified Rodent Chow 5002) (in ppm)

	Arsenic	Cadmium	Lead	Mercury	Selenium
Pellets	0.334	0.0632	0.247	<0.05	0.119
	<0.200	0.0499	0.188	<0.05	0.190
	<0.200	0.0362	0.142	<0.05	0.221
	0.206	0.0711	0.139	<0.05	0.214
	<0.200	0.0647	0.136	<0.05	0.231
	<0.200	0.0620	0.138	<0.05	0.171
	<0.200	0.0779	0.181	<0.05	0.267
	<0.200	0.0551	0.132	<0.05	0.199
	<0.200	0.0838	0.146	<0.05	0.223
	0.210	0.0761	0.273	<0.05	0.267
	<0.200	0.0747	0.136	<0.05	0.243
	<0.200	0.0755	0.132	<0.05	0.176
	<0.200	0.0907	0.156	<0.05	0.243
	0.269	0.107	0.246	<0.05	0.178
	0.263	0.107	0.266	<0.05	0.214
	<0.200	0.111	0.147	<0.05	0.250
	<0.200	0.109	0.144	<0.05	0.161
	0.224	0.104	0.202	<0.05	0.205
	<0.200	0.105	0.147	<0.05	0.260
means =		0.0821	0.174	<0.05	0.212
Meal	0.255	0.0514	0.348	<0.05	0.258
	<0.200	0.0677	0.233	<0.05	0.280
	<0.200	0.0919	0.155	<0.05	0.283
	0.403	0.0498	0.145	<0.05	0.236
	<0.200	0.0427	0.214	<0.05	0.156
	<0.200	0.0520	0.147	<0.05	0.217
	<0.200	0.0804	0.117	<0.05	0.253
	0.321	0.0700	0.296	<0.05	0.208
	<0.200	0.0677	0.150	<0.05	0.212
	<0.200	0.0831	0.105	<0.05	0.224
	<0.200	0.0718	0.150	<0.05	0.228
	<0.200	0.0824	0.164	<0.05	0.216
	<0.200	0.122	0.131	<0.05	0.197
	<0.200	0.109	0.268	<0.05	0.214
	<0.200	0.120	0.153	<0.05	0.193
	<0.200	0.120	0.146	<0.05	0.199
means =		0.0801	0.183	<0.05	0.223
Combined means =		0.0802	0.178	<0.05	0.217
Range =	<0.200–0.403	0.0362–0.122	0.105–0.348	N/A	0.119–0.283

Table 10 Open Formula Natural Ingredient Mouse Diet

Ingredient	Amount per Ton
Major ingredients (lb)	
Dried skim milk	100
Fish meal (60% protein)	200
Soybean meal (49% protein)	240
Dehydrated alfalfa meal (17% protein)	80
Corn gluten meal (60% protein)	60
Ground #2 yellow shelled corn	490
Ground hard winter wheat	460
Wheat middlings	200
Brewer's dried yeast	40
Dry molasses	30
Soybean oil	50
Dicalcium phosphate	25
Salt	10
Ground limestone	10
Mineral and vitamin premixes	5
Mineral premix (g)	
Cobalt (cobalt carbonate)	0.4
Copper (copper sulfate)	4.0
Iron (iron sulfate)	120.0
Manganese (manganese oxide)	60.0
Zinc (zinc oxide)	16.0
Iodine (potassium iodate)	1.4
Vitamin premix	
Vitamin A (IU)	5500,000.
Vitamin D_3 (IU)	4600,000.
α-Tocopheryl acetate (IU)	20,000.
Vitamin K (menadione sodium bisulfite) (g)	2.8
Choline (choline chloride) (g)	560.0
Folic acid (g)	2.2
Niacin (g)	30.0
d-Pantothenic acid (calcium pantothenate) (g)	18.0
Riboflavin (g)	3.4
Thiamine (g)	10.0
Vitamin B_{12} (μg)	4000.0
Pyridoxine (g)	1.7

Source: Knapka et al. (1974).

Key nutrient and contaminant concentrations of an open formula natural ingredient diet (3–94 different lots of NIH-07) (Rao and Knapka, 1987) are compared to those of a commercially available closed formula diet (35 lots of Purina Certified Rodent Chow, 5002) in Table 11. Based upon the relative ranges of values for each of the constituents compared in this example, the closed formula diet was substantially less variable than the open formula diet in every constituent compared.

Table 11 Comparison of Nutrient and Contaminant Concentrations in an Open Formula Natural Ingredient Diet, NIH-07 (Rao and Knapka, 1987), and a Closed Formula Natural Ingredient Diet, (Purina Certified Rodent Chow, 5002)

Nutrient/contaminant		Open formula		Closed formula	
		mean	range	mean	range
Protein	(%)	23.86	21.6–26.3	20.84	20.1–21.9
Fat	(%)	4.89	3.3–6.0	5.67	4.64–6.43
Fiber	(%)	3.35	1.4–4.3	4.10	3.67–4.76
Ash	(%)	6.69	5.7–7.4	N/A	N/A
Calcium	(%)	1.30	0.81–1.69	0.786	0.632–0.924
Phosphorus	(%)	0.99	0.82–1.10	0.626	0.536–0.745
Arsenic	(ppm)	0.46	<0.05–1.06		<0.200–0.403
Cadmium	(ppm)	0.105	<0.05–0.40	0.0802	0.0362–0.122
Lead	(ppm)	0.85	0.33–3.37	0.178	0.105–0.348
Mercury	(ppm)	<0.05		<0.05	All <0.05
Selenium	(ppm)	0.28	0.10–0.52	0.217	0.119–0.283

Source: Open formula (Rao and Knapka, 1987); closed formula (Purina Certified Rodent Chow, 5002.

Provision of Feed and Feeders

Feed. Feed is typically provided on an ad libitum basis for toxicity studies. Healthy, adult mice will consume about 4–5 g of feed per day, and ordinarily they should be given a quantity adequate for at least 3–4 days. Typically, quantities sufficient to last more than a week are provided, with the balance discarded and replaced about weekly to maintain freshness. Two notable exceptions to ad libitum feeding are immediately prior to oral dosing in acute toxicity studies, and prior to blood collection for clinical laboratory analysis in studies of any duration.

The process of fasting mice presents a dilemma. Mice are nocturnal and, therefore, when food is available ad libitum, most of what they consume during a 24-hr period will be consumed during the dark phase of the light/dark cycle. Their stomachs are normally quite full in the morning, and empty slowly through the day. Any fasting procedure that begins in the morning and continues for up to about 12 hrs will result in a nutritional state (based on average stomach contents) that does not differ appreciably from fed mice. The next longer convenient interval is to fast animals overnight, from the end of one working day until the morning of the next (a period of about 15–16 hrs, which includes the normal feeding time). Overnight fasts are probably the norm for toxicity studies in mice. If food is available, young adult outbred albino mice (25–30 g) will gain about 7–10% of their "afternoon" body weight owing to feed consumption during that 16-hr period. If food has been removed, those same mice will lose about 8–10% of their "afternoon" body weight as a result of the fast (data from our laboratory). Fasting mice for a period of 24 hrs results in about a 30% reduction in absolute liver weight (liver/body weight ratios stay constant), a reduction of over 90% in hepatic glycogen content, and about a 50% reduction in reduced hepatic glutathione, but an increase of about 150% in total hepatic triglycerides (Strubelt, 1981). These changes were associated with increased hepatotoxicity from a variety of xenobiotics, and at least one author (Strubelt) believes that overnight fasting of mice should be avoided. The dilemma, then, is that if mice must be fasted, whether they should be fasted for a few hours during the day, which will be unlikely to achieve the needed effect, or overnight, which may have considerable effect on hepatic parameters.

Feeders. Feed is provided to mice in one of a very wide variety of feeders. One manufacturer alone (Lab Products, Inc.) lists over 25 different feeders suitable for mice. The mere existence of such a variety of designs testifies to the fact that no single design exists that satisfactorily solves all of the problems encountered in providing clean, dry feed to mice. Some of the basic problems include the fact that mice will, if given the opportunity, urinate, defecate, and sleep in their feeders as well as dig in it, play with it, and in almost any other conceivable way distribute feed outside of their feeders and even their cages. The challenge in feeder design, then, is to keep the mice out of (and off the top of) the feeder, minimize spillage (especially of meal), and still provide free access to the feed at all times. This challenge is more easily met for pelleted diet, especially when feed consumption is not being measured. In that situation, a feeder that is enclosed at the top and provides access to the feed through some form of slots of wire mesh at the bottom and sides is effective.

The more common situation in toxicity testing is that feed consumption will be measured. While this can be done with pelleted feed, and an inexpensive feeder has been reported (Dunn, 1978), meal is the more common dietary form when feed consumption will be measured. Feeders containing meal must be easy to install and remove from cages without spillage to facilitate weighing. They must be heavy enough and fit securely enough into the cage to prevent tipping or movement. A common form consists of a small glass jar or stainless steel bowl with a restrictive top plate to limit ease of entry. Various forms of feed followers (heavy washers with several holes, wire mesh, even marbles) can be placed on the surface of the feed to discourage digging or other means of expulsion of the feed.

Analysis

If toxicity studies are being conducted to support a safety claim to a regulatory agency (such as the U.S. Food and Drug Administration), the Good Laboratory Practice regulations should be considered. The GLP document (CFR$_b$, 1988c) stipulates that feed be analyzed periodically for levels of contaminants that might interfere with the toxicity study, and that documentation of such analyses be available. This consideration is particularly important for natural ingredient diets, which will almost certainly contain at least trace amounts of a variety of heavy metals, pesticides, and other environmental pollutants. The chemistry of the test article being studied should be evaluated for any special sensitivities to common contaminants, and if those sensitivities appear likely, special care should be taken to avoid those contaminants. In the absence of any suspected special sensitivities, diet should be screened on a regular basis for the well-known environmental contaminants such as heavy metals, aflatoxins, and various pesticides. One of the most practical (and common) solutions to the requirement for routine feed analysis is to purchase what is referred to as "certified" feed from one of the major commercial suppliers that offer such products. While more expensive than ordinary feed, certified feeds are analyzed for common contaminants by the supplier, and each lot is typically supplied with documentation of the results of those analyses which should meet regulatory requirements.

Water

Mice should be provided with ad libitum access to a source of clean, fresh water. For most toxicity studies, ordinary potable water available from a typical municipal water supply is appropriate. Some animal facilities are equipped to treat drinking water to alter pH, or to reduce chemical or microbiological contaminant levels. Treatment may include chlorination, reverse osmosis, distillation, or ion exchange.

Little is known about the mean quantitative water requirements for mice, but quantities of 6–7 ml/day are thought to be representative for adults (Jacoby and Fox, 1984). It is known that environmental temperature is the primary factor influencing water requirements (Knapka, 1983), with higher temperature and/or lower humidity leading to increased water consumption. The type of diet may also affect water consumption. The mouse has a biological half-time for turnover of water of 1.1 days, which is shorter than in larger animals (Jacoby and Fox, 1984). Owing to this short half-time, mice are particularly sensitive to water deprivation, and if they are maintained on a dry diet, may die within as little as 1 day of water deprivation. Any restriction in availability of water results in an immediate and dramatic reduction in food consumption and commensurate fecal output. This relationship is so reliable that a toxicology technician trained to be aware of reductions in fecal output on a regular basis will almost never miss a malfunction or deficiency in a watering system or feed source.

Water is typically distributed to individual caging by one of two methods: water bottles with sipper tubes attached to each cage, or an automatic watering system.

Water Bottles with Sipper Tubes. This type of watering device has the advantages of lower initial purchase cost and the ability to estimate water consumption on a per cage basis. Bottles have several disadvantages, including higher maintenance or use cost (bottles must be removed, disassembled, washed, refilled, and reinstalled at least once or twice per week to minimize bacterial contamination), some configurations make access to suspended caging more difficult, stoppers must be carefully installed to prevent leakage with resultant water deprivation, and some configurations require very careful installation of the bottle on the cage to assure that sipper tubes have an adequate downward slope to preclude air-lock and resultant water deprivation. Some cage designs allow mice to chew on water bottle stoppers, with the potential for ingestion of the debris.

Automatic Watering Systems. Such systems carry high initial purchase (and installation) costs, and generally lack the capacity to indicate water consumption per cage. Automatic watering systems for both the room and the cage rack distribution systems are usually constructed of stainless steel or PVC piping with stainless steel fittings. Stainless steel is more expensive, but also more durable. Automatic systems are supplied by some type of pressure-reduction station connected to the facility water supply, such that the water pressure at the cage is in the range of 1.5–4.0 lb/in^2 (psi). The pressure-reduction station can be fitted for automatic system monitoring (e.g., for leaks, overly high or low distribution pressure), and can provide connections for local water treatment such as chlorination. Racks are connected to the room distribution system by means of flexible hosing, and may include an air-gap isolator to prevent microbial contamination from traveling from a rack into the distribution system. Automatic watering systems require less labor while in use than water bottles, being limited to periodic checks that individual sipper fittings are functioning properly and that air has not been trapped in the rack distribution system. Whenever a rack is connected to the system, whether new to a room or reconnected after relocation, the rack should have all air bled from its distribution system and representative sippers should be checked to confirm the absence of air in the lines. Room distribution systems, particularly those in rooms with a small number of resident animals, have the potential to foster bacterial growth in the distribution system. This problem seems least severe in those rooms with the highest daily water flow rates. Automatic watering systems can be fitted with a central flushing system that provides a programmed flushing of the room distribution system at increased system pressure and flow rate. A program of daily flushing for about 5 min. has been found to produce an acceptable level of microbiological control.

Water Quality. This should be monitored by a regular system of chemical and micro-biological analyses. Samples should be collected from water bottles that have been in use for nearly the maximum allowable period, from clean bottles, and from the water source. Samples from automatic watering systems should be collected at sippers that have been in use in individual cages, at clean sippers, at one or more sources on the animal room distribution system, and at both the high- and low-pressure side of the pressure-reduction station. Water samples should be analyzed for the routine contaminants (e.g., heavy metals, pesticides) and for microbiological content (both type and plate count or concentration). Any special requirements of the toxicity study should be considered when selecting parameters for analysis. In general, water that is of acceptable quality for human consumption will be acceptable for mice.

Prevention of Infectious Diseases

The occurrence of an infectious disease during the conduct of a toxicity study will at best confer uncertainty about the interpretation of the study results, and at worst require the repetition of the entire study. The effect of even relatively benign infections on the health of mice that have been compromised by the administration of high doses of a potentially toxic test article can rarely be accurately predicted.

This section will discuss some of the fundamental considerations in the prevention of infectious disease in a mouse colony. A comprehensive discussion of infectious, neoplas-tic and noninfectious diseases in mice is beyond the scope of this chapter, but has been addressed elsewhere (Jacoby and Fox, 1984; Foster, et al, 1982).

Simplistically, infectious diseases can be prevented by obtaining high-quality, healthy mice from a reputable supplier, protecting those mice from exposure to infectious disease, and maintaining those animals in a clean, well-controlled environment with good-quality food and water.

It is fair to assume that the health status of mice will be no better than it is at the time they leave the breeding colony. Some commercial breeders are now offering mice that are free of antibodies to specific lists of mouse viruses as well as most important bacteria and parasites. These animals may be especially susceptible to infectious disease precisely because they lack antibodies to most common mouse diseases.

Periods when healthy mice are especially subject to exposure to infectious disease include the transit from the breeder to the user, and the introduction into the new home colony. Risk during transit is increased if the animals are transported by common carriers, such as commercial airlines and trucking companies. Often common carriers will be less cautious with animals than trained staff. The temptation exists to transport animals in "dirty" trucks because the animals are "dirty and smelly," or to leave them unattended at a warehouse or loading dock for several hours where the environmental conditions may be severe. These risks can be reduced if mice are shipped in filtered containers which exclude much of the biological contamination to which the container is exposed, and if they are shipped in a clean, environmentally controlled vehicle without intermediate transfer between shipper and receiver.

The largest risk upon receipt of mice at the new home colony is that the mice will be transported through or into an area that is inhabited by animals that are already infected with a contagious disease. This risk can be reduced by maintaining the integrity of the filtered shipping carton until the mice reach the room in which they will be housed. The room should have been previously sanitized to reduce the probability of infection from previous residents. It is generally a poor practice to introduce new mice into an animal room that already contains animals, especially if those animals have been in-house for any period of time or were received from another supplier. Different species should never be mixed in the same room. Environmental conditions, including temperature, humidity, and ventilation, and their contribution to animal health have been discussed earlier in this chapter.

Once clean, healthy animals have been introduced into a clean room stocked with clean caging, food, and water, their health status becomes a function of the quality and training of the animal care staff. A good understanding of the biology of mice, of infectious diseases, and of the kinds of things that can act as vectors for potential infection are invaluable assets for animal care staff. Handlers should be encouraged to wear gloves and laboratory coats or uniforms when working with mice, and to change those garments regularly. Proper hygiene is especially important when moving from one animal to another. In the event that an infectious disease is diagnosed in the colony, every reasonable effort should be made to isolate (or even eliminate) the infected animals to prevent spread. This might include maintenance by a handler or handlers who do not come into contact with important study animals.

STUDY DESIGN

Most toxicity and teratology studies conducted in mice are designed to provide information on potential human toxicity. Test substances are typically administered by the expected route of human exposure. A pharmaceutical product that is intended for oral administration (tablet, capsule, solution, or suspension), or a food additive would generally be administered by the oral route. Oral administration to mice is usually accomplished by administration of a solution or suspension by oral gavage, by mixture of the test substance with the diet, or less commonly added to the drinking water.

The specific design of toxicity studies should be tailored to the objective to be achieved and to any specific characteristics of the test substance. Many features of study design will be predicated on guidelines and practices of regulatory agencies such as the Food and Drug Administration (FDA) or Environmental Protection Agency (EPA) in the United States or their counterparts in other countries to which the results of the study will be submitted in support of a safety claim. Recommendations for study length (duration of dosing) fall in this category.

Toxicity studies are usually conducted in order of increasing duration of dosing, beginning with acute toxicity studies. When this regimen is followed, each study provides progressively more useful information for the selection of doses for the next, longer study.

Acute Toxicity Studies

Acute toxicity studies are conducted to evaluate the effects of single, high doses of the test substance. Usually each animal receives a single dose of the test substance in this study design. On rare occasion, repeated doses may be administered, but in any event, all doses are administered within 24 hrs or less. Historically, a primary objective of acute toxicity testing was to determine an LD_{50} dose, or that dose which would be lethal to 50% of the animals treated. To achieve this objective, groups of mice, often numbering 10 or more per sex, are treated with a single dose of the test substance. Depending upon the rate of survival in the initial group(s), additional groups are added to the study at higher and/or lower doses such that most animals die that receive the highest doses and most survive that receive the lowest doses. Survival is assessed at some predetermined interval after dosing, usually 7 or 14 days, but occasionally as early as 24 hr. The resultant dose-response data can be analyzed by a statistical method such as probit analysis (Finney, 1971) to provide an estimate of the median lethal dose (LD_{50}) and some measure of the precision of that estimate, such as the 95% fiducial limits. There are very few scientifically valid reasons to include determination of the LD_{50} as a significant objective of acute toxicity testing. Most regulatory agencies have dropped their requirements for a specific value for the LD_{50}, and animal welfare considerations preclude the use of the large numbers of animals previously required.

A more contemporary design for acute toxicity testing attempts to derive a maximum amount of information from a minimum number of animals. Study objectives include determination of the most important clinical signs attributable to high doses of the test substance, time of onset and remission of those signs, possible determination of a minimum lethal dosage, and in the event of lethality, the sequence and timing of effects leading to death or recovery. These objectives are achieved by means of a comprehensive schedule of animal observations following dosing. These objectives can usually be achieved by treating from one to three groups of three to five mice/sex/group at different doses.

Traditionally, acute toxicity testing of potential new pharmaceutical products is conducted in at least three species, with one being a nonrodent, and by at least two routes of administration, one of which is the intended clinical route. Mice are the most frequently selected rodent species for acute toxicity testing. The choice of routes of administration depends on the intended clinical route and on how much is already known about the oral bioavailability of the test substance. If the intended clinical route is oral, acute testing by oral gavage with a solution or suspension is of primary importance. If other clinical routes are anticipated (e.g., intravenous [iv] or dermal), they represent good secondary routes for acute testing. Ordinarily, at least one parenteral route is used for acute testing, and that route may be iv if the product is soluble in a fairly innocuous vehicle (e.g., water or saline) or intraperitoneal (ip) as a suspension if the product is insoluble in an aqueous (or other innocuous) vehicle. If the intended clinical route is not oral, the oral route is usually selected as a secondary route for acute toxicity testing to provide information relevant to accidental oral ingestion. A rough estimate of oral bioavailability can be based on a comparison of the acute toxicity associated with various doses administered by the oral and parenteral routes. Acute toxicity testing conducted for other purposes is usually more limited in scope. Most regulatory agencies no longer require a full complement of species and routes of administration to render decisions on acute toxicity.

There are a few characteristics of acute toxicity testing that are not common in other toxicity protocols. In a typical repeated dose toxicity study, several groups of animals are treated concurrently with predetermined doses of test substance and a control substance. To reduce animal use in acute toxicity testing, studies that include more than one dose group are usually dosed sequentially, with an interval of at least 24 hrs between dosing of subsequent groups. This allows the effects of the previous dose to be fully manifested, and allows selection of the subsequent dose to provide the highest probability of contributing more useful information. Another unusual aspect of acute toxicity studies is the nutritional status of the animals at dosing. Because some schools believe that the results of acute toxicity testing are more reliable if all animals are in a uniforn nutritional state, mice to be dosed orally are often fasted overnight prior to dosing. Fasting allows dose volumes to be higher than in repeated dose studies, and because dosing only occurs on 1 day, dietary stress is considered tolerable. The scientific merits of this practice are debatable, but fasting is "traditional" in oral acute toxicity studies. While the practice of conducting gross necropsies at the end of acute toxicity studies is growing in popularity, this practice rarely yields useful information. The toxicity resulting from acute exposure is usually associated with a biochemical or functional imbalance rather than with a change in the gross or microscopic architecture of an organ system. Changes observable at gross necropsy are more often associated with repeated dosing at sublethal levels. For similar reasons, microscopic examination of tissue is rarely conducted in acute toxicity studies unless there is some scientific reason to expect it would be useful.

The results of a well-designed acute toxicity study can help to predict likely target organ systems, possible outcome in the event of massive human overexposure, can help in establishing risk categories for EPA or Department of Transportation (DOT) classification, and can help in dose selection for the initial repeated dose toxicity tests to be conducted. An example of an acute toxicity study design is in Table 12.

Short-Term Toxicity Studies

The objective of short-term or subchronic toxicity studies is to describe and define the toxicity associated with repeated administration of high, but generally survivable doses of a test substance. This may include identification of target organs and systems, definition

Table 12 Typical Acute Toxicity Study Design for Mice

Number of mice/sex/dose group	3–5
Number of dose groups	1–3
Number of control groups	None
Dosing frequency	Single dose
Dosing days	1 day
Survival checks	Not done (part of Clin. Obs.)
Clinical observations	4 or more on day of treatment, then 1–2 daily
Physical examinations	Not done
Body weights	Prior to dosing
Feed consumption	Not done
Number of reversal mice	None
Duration of reversal period	Not applicable
Blood collection	Not done
Hematology parameters	Not done
Clinical chemistry parameters	Not done
Urine collection	Not done
Necropsy	Gross (increasingly, but rarely useful)
Tissue collection	Rarely (specific cause only)

of the maximum survivable repeated dose, and the highest "clean" or no effect dose. Short-term repeated dose studies also serve as dose range–finding studies for longer-term repeated dose studies.

Short-term toxicity studies range in duration of dosing from about 7–90 days. Mice typically receive a single, daily dose of the test substance, 7 days per week by the expected clinical route of administration. If the test substance is administered in the diet (or rarely, the drinking water), that admixture is available continuously. Short-term studies usually include three to four groups of mice exposed to different dose levels of the test substance, and an additional group exposed to the carrier to serve as a control for the effects of treatment. Group sizes for these studies are on the order of five to ten mice/sex/dose. Ideally, dose levels should be selected for these studies such that a few animals die at the highest dose prior to the completion of dosing (to assure exposure to the maximum survivable dose), and all survive at the lowest dose with minimal evidence of toxic effects. The middle dose or doses should be set at approximately equal log increments between the high and low doses. It is important to begin to identify the highest dose level that is free of serious toxic effects to determine whether the test substance is likely to be toxic to humans at the expected therapeutic dose or exposure level.

Parameters monitored in a typical short-term repeated dose study may include: daily observations for clinical signs of toxicity and mortality, weekly physical examinations, body weight and feed consumption, and terminal measurement of serum glucose and urea concentrations, serum aspartate aminotransferase, alanine aminotransferase, and alkaline phosphatase activity. Animals found dead or killed by design are typically submitted for gross necropsy, and selected tissues, such as adrenal gland, bone (sternum, including marrow), brain, heart, kidney, liver, lung, testis, and thymus are collected, weighed (except for bone and lung), and processed for routine microscopic examination by a qualified veterinary pathologist. An example of a short-term toxicity study design is in Table 13.

Table 13 Typical Short-term Toxicity Study Design for Mice

Number of mice/sex/dose group	5–10
Number of dose groups	3–4
Number of control groups	1
Dosing frequency	Once, daily
Dosing days	Daily for 7–90 days
Survival checks	1–2 daily
Clinical observations	Daily
Physical examinations	Weekly
Body weights	Weekly
Feed consumption	Weekly
Number of reversal mice	None
Duration of reversal period	None
Blood collection	Terminal, all animals
Hematology parameters	None
Clinical chemistry parameters	Limited
Urine collection	Not done
Necropsy	Gross, all animals
Tissue collection	Limited list, all animals

Chronic Toxicity Studies (26 weeks to 2 years)

The objective of chronic, or long-term, toxicity studies is to refine the description of the toxicity associated with long-term administration of high, survivable doses of a test substance. Chronic toxicity studies are more commonly conducted in rats than in mice, but such studies can be conducted in mice, and this discussion describes objectives and practices for conducting such studies in mice. Target organs and systems have usually been identified prior to the conduct of chronic studies, but it is the chronic studies that provide the best opportunities to understand the subtle changes associated with long-term administration of high doses, and to focus more closely on the highest "clean" or no effect dose. Chronic toxicity studies also serve to refine the doses to be administered in the carcinogenicity studies which typically follow them.

Chronic, or long-term, toxicity studies range in duration of dosing from about 26 weeks to as long as 2 years, but most do not exceed 1 year. Single, daily doses of the test substance are administered by the expected clinical route of administration. If the substance is intended for oral administration, the convenience and economy of administration in the diet (or rarely the water) becomes important. Diet admixtures are made available ad libitum unless they must be removed for a specific procedure during the study. Chronic studies usually include three groups of mice exposed to different dose levels of the test substance, and an additional group exposed to the carrier to serve as a control for the effects of treatment. Chronic toxicity studies often include "reversal groups," or subsets of each dose group which are not sacrificed immediately upon the completion of treatment. The purpose of the reversal groups is to determine whether any toxic effects associated with treatment are permanent or subject to recovery or reversal. Mice in the reversal groups may be allowed from 2 to 4 weeks of recovery time from the end of treatment until necropsy. Group sizes for chronic studies are on the order of 20–50 mice/sex/dose. Sizes of the reversal groups, if they are included, may be about 25–35% of the original dose groups. Dose levels should be selected for these studies such that there is substantial toxicity at the highest dose, but few if any treatment-related deaths. The low dose in chronic studies should confirm, or if necessary, refine previous estimates of the highest dose level that is free of serious toxic effects, and thereby reinforce previous estimates of the relative safety of the test substance at the expected human dose or exposure level. The middle dose should be the approximate geometric mean of the high and low doses.

Parameters monitored in a typical chronic toxicity study may include: daily observation for moribundity and mortality, weekly physical examinations, body weight and feed consumption, and terminal measurement of serum glucose and urea concentrations, serum aspartate aminotransferase, alanine aminotransferase, and alkaline phosphatase activity. Hematological parameters for mice are often limited to differential smear evaluations. While red blood cell counts, white blood cell counts, and hemoglobin concentrations can be determined, the values for mice are somewhat variable from many of the commonly used laboratory instruments, so these parameters are not always evaluated. Animals found dead or killed by design are typically submitted for gross necropsy, and a list of 30–50 selected tissues are collected, weighed (except for bone and lung), and processed for routine microscopic examination by a qualified veterinary pathologist. An example of a chronic toxicity study design is in Table 14.

Carcinogenicity Studies (18–24 months)

The objective of carcinogenicity studies is to determine whether the test substance is a carcinogen when administered at maximum tolerable doses for a period of time approach-

Table 14 Typical Chronic Toxicity Study Design for Mice

Number of mice/sex/dose group	20–50
Number of dose groups	3
Number of control groups	1
Dosing frequency	Once, daily
Dosing days	Daily 26–52 weeks
Survival checks	Daily
Clinical observations	Not done
Physical examinations	Weekly
Body weights	Weekly
Feed consumption	Weekly
Number of reversal mice	25–35% of main groups
Duration of reversal period	2–4 weeks
Blood collection	Terminal, all animals
Hematology parameters	Dif. smear, RBC, WBC
Clinical chemistry parameters	Limited list
Urine collection	Not done
Necropsy	Gross, all animals
Tissue collection	Comprehensive list, all animals

ing the life expectancy of the mouse. This objective is simpler in many respects than the objective of the longer toxicity studies. It is assumed that by the time carcinogenicity studies are undertaken, the chronic toxicity studies have been essentially completed, and the actual toxicity of the substance is about as well understood as it can be based on animal studies. Carcinogenicity studies are not usually encumbered by tests to further the understanding of toxicity, but rather are focused to maximize the ability to answer the single question of carcinogenicity.

Carcinogenicity studies in mice are generally designed to expose the animals for a period of 18 months to 2 years. Improvements in animal husbandry during the past decade have increased the life expectancy of most strains of mice, so there has been a tendency to extend carcinogenicity studies in mice to 2 years. The study design normally contains provisions to allow for termination of the study prior to the intended endpoint if excessive mortality is encountered. This provision is intended to ensure that an adequate number of survivors are sacrificed with successful collection of all necessary tissues for a meaningful, statistical analysis of tumor incidence. Carcinogenicity studies usually include three groups of mice exposed to different dose levels of the test substance, and an additional group exposed to the carrier to serve as a control for the effects of treatment. Group sizes for these studies are on the order of 50–70 mice/sex/dose.

The high dose in carcinogenicity studies should be the maximum tolerated dose. This dose should produce evident toxicity by the end of dosing. A commonly held minimum criteria for evident toxicity is a decrement in body weight or body weight gain of at least 10% from the control to the high-dose group. If the test substance is not very toxic, most regulatory agencies will accept a carcinogenicity study in which the high dose is the highest dose that can be practically administered, even though that dose does not produce evident toxicity. In this example, the animal has, in effect, "tolerated" the highest dose that could be administered.

The selection of lower doses is not as critical as in chronic studies because the concept of a "clean dose" of a known carcinogen is not widely accepted, and will be of little value in attempting to commercialize a product.

The middle dose may become important if the high dose has been inadvertently set too high, resulting in excessive toxicity and early mortality. In that case, a middle dose that elicits evident toxicity without excessive mortality may become an acceptable maximum tolerated dose and effectively "salvage" the study. As in chronic studies, the middle dose should be at the approximate geometric mean of the high and low doses.

The most important data generated in a carcinogenicity study are the histopathology data. Of particular importance are the data on the incidence of various types of malignancies in the different treatment groups. Control or even untreated mice normally will have some "background" incidence of various types of malignancies over the course of a carcinogenicity study. The key question then is whether the treated groups have a significantly higher incidence of "normally expected" tumor types than the control group, whether they have occurrences of "nonnormal" tumor types that are not seen (concurrently or historically) in control animals, and, most importantly, whether such incidence is attributable to the test substance.

Other parameters monitored in a typical carcinogenicity study may include: daily observation for survival and moribundity, periodic physical examinations, periodic examinations for palpable masses, body weight, and feed consumption (especially important in dietary admix studies), and for some studies periodic peripheral blood smears and terminal red and white blood cell counts. Animals found dead or killed by design are submitted for gross necropsy, and a comprehensive list of 40–50 prescribed tissues plus any tissue masses, suspected tumors, and identifiable regional lymph tissue are collected from each animal to be processed and examined histologically by a qualified veterinary pathologist for evidence of carcinogenicity. An example of a carcinogenicity study design is in Table 15.

Table 15 Typical Carcinogenicity Study Design for Mice

Number of mice/sex/dose group	50–70
Number of dose groups	3
Number of control groups	2
Dosing frequency	Once, daily
Dosing days	Daily for 18–24 months
Survival checks	Daily
Clinical observations	Not done
Physical examinations	Monthly during first year, 2×/month thereafter
Body weights	Weekly during first year, 2×/month thereafter
Feed consumption	Weekly during first 26 weeks, 2×/month second 26 weeks, then monthly
Number of reversal mice	None
Duration of reversal period	Not done
Blood collection	Optional periodic, terminal
Hematology parameters	Periodic peripheral smears, terminal smears, RBC, WBC
Clinical chemistry parameters	Not done
Urine collection	Not done
Necropsy	Gross, all animals (incl. palpable masses)
Tissue collection	Comprehensive list, all animals

Teratology Studies

Mice are used in teratology studies to assess the effects of test substances on congenital defects in the young when administered to pregnant females. Mice have a regular, short estrus cycle, a short gestation period, high fertility, and typically produce relatively large litters of young. Mice rank behind rats and rabbits as the species of choice for assessing teratology, but there may be good scientific reasons to use mice in some instances. The conduct of Segment II teratology studies in mice and rabbits with Segment I and III studies in rats provides an opportunity to evaluate teratogenicity in three species. While there is an advantage in conducting teratology studies in at least two species, preferably one of which is a nonrodent, some substances (e.g., certain antibiotics) are especially toxic to rabbits, making teratology testing impractical in that species. In that case, mice become the second best species available (behind rats) for teratology testing, and are usually the choice as the second species. A significant disadvantage in using mice for teratology studies is that they are much more cannibalistic than rats or rabbits. This characteristic renders the species unusable for Segment I and III studies, in which pregnant females are allowed to deliver their young, and limits them to use in Segment II studies, in which the young are delivered by cesarean section on gestation day 18, prior to delivery. Mating can be confirmed in mice by daily inspection of cohabitating females for the presence of a vaginal plug. The copulatory plug in mice is much more persistent than in rats, in which mating must be confirmed by vaginal lavage and microscopic examination.

Segment II Teratology Studies

A Segment II teratology study is conducted to assess the effects of a test substance on fetal survival and congenital malformations (teratology). Females are mated and monitored daily for the presence of copulatory plugs. The presence of a plug confirms that mating has occurred, and the day of discovery is defined as gestation day 1. Mated females are dosed with the test substance from gestation days 6 through 15, a period that begins soon after implantation (day 5), and continues through completion of organogenesis (day 13). This dose period exposes the young throughout the period of organogenesis, but tends to minimize preimplantation embryotoxicity and postorganogenesis maternal and fetal toxicity. Young are delivered by cesarean section on gestation day 18, prior to normal parturition on day 19, to avoid cannibalism. The maternal reproductive organs are examined for numbers of corpora lutea, implantations, resorptions, and live and dead fetuses. The fetuses are weighed, sexed, and examined for gross, visceral, and skeletal abnormalities. An example of a Segment II teratology study design is in Table 16.

Genetic Toxicity Studies

The objective of genetic toxicity testing is to identify and describe the effects of agents which specifically produce genetic alterations at subtoxic doses. Mice are used in a variety of genetic toxicity study designs in an effort to achieve this objective. Neither a comprehensive listing of genetic toxicity procedures using mice nor a comprehensive description of any number of those procedures is within the scope of this chapter. Rather, a few of the most commonly employed procedures will be summarized. The reader is referred to other sources such as Brusick (1980), Thorgeirsson (1982), and Dean (1983, 1984) for more detailed discussions of genetic toxicity, and more comprehensive descriptions of some of the specific tests used in that field.

TABLE 16 Typical Segment II Teratology Study Design for Mice

Number of female mice/dose group	20
Number of dose groups	3
Number of control groups	1
Dosing frequency	Once, daily
Dosing days	Days 6–15 of gestation
Survival checks	Daily
Clinical observations	Daily
Physical examinations	Not done
Body weights	1–3×/week
Feed consumption	Not done
Number of reversal mice	None
Duration of reversal period	Not done
Blood collection	Not done
Caesarean section	Day 18 of gestation
Necropsy	All dams gross, all fetuses external and ⅓ of fetuses visceral exam at caesarean section

Mouse Micronucleus Assay

The objective of the mouse micronucleus assay is to determine whether a test article causes disruption and separation or breakage of chromosomes. The mouse micronucleus assay is one of the most commonly conducted in vivo tests for genetic toxicity. Comparison of the incidence of micronuclei in proliferating cells from treated versus control mice provides an indirect measurement of chromosome damage in somatic cells. Micronuclei can only be formed as a result of disruption and separation or breakage of chromosomes, followed by cell division. The preferred cells for evaluation are newly formed erythrocytes in mouse bone marrow because the micronuclei formed in these cells are not expelled during the last division in which the nucleus is extruded from the normoblast.

One or more dose levels of test article and a control treatment are administered to separate groups of at least five mice per sex. The highest dose should be the maximum tolerated dose, or one that produces some evidence of cytotoxicity. It is important that high quality (e.g., specific pathogen–free) mice of known genetic stability and consistent species, strain, source, age, weight, and clinical condition be used to assure comparability with historical controls. Each animal typically receives a single dose of test or control article. Bone marrow samples are collected at a minimum of three different intervals after dosing, ranging from 12 to 72 hr. At least 1000 polychromatic erythryoctes are evaluated for the presence of micronuclei for each test and control mouse. An example of a mouse micronucleus assay study design is in Table 17.

Heritable Translocation Assay

The objective of the heritable translocation assay (HTA) is to assess the potential of a test article to induce reciprocal translocations between chromosomes in germ cells of treated male mice. This assay has the advantage of detecting transmissible genetic alterations, which are potentially more damaging to the gene pool than nontransmissible or lethal changes. Induced translocations can be detected by mating the F1 progeny of treated males with untreated, unrelated females. Translocations will be evidenced by a reduction in the number of viable fetuses sired by affected males. The presence of translocation

Table 17 Typical Mouse Micronucleus Assay Study Design

Number of mice/sex/dose group	5 or more
Number of dose groups	1 or more
Number of control groups	2, one positive, one negative
Dosing frequency	Single dose
Dosing days	One day
Survival checks	Daily
Clinical observations	Not done
Body weights	Prior to dosing
Feed consumption	Not done
Bone marrow collection	3 or more intervals, from 12–72 hr after dosing
Polychromatic erythrocytes evaluated/mouse:	1000 minimum

figures in meiotic metaphase serves as cytogenetic verification of the presence of reciprocal translocations.

The HTA typically consists of three groups of 30 male mice each, treated with different dose levels of the test article, and a negative control group treated with the dosing vehicle. A positive control group is optional. As the period of spermatogenesis in the mouse is about 7 weeks, all treated and control animals are dosed on a daily basis for 7 weeks. The dosing route is usually oral gavage, and the dose levels are selected on the basis of the oral LD_{50}. The high dose is typically one-eighth of the LD_{50}, the medium and low doses about one-third, and one-tenth of the high dose, respectively. Upon completion of dosing, each male is mated to two females. Two hundred healthy males are selected from the offspring of each of these groups of matings and allowed to reach sexual maturity, whereupon each male is mated to three virgin females. The females from this second mating are sacrificed about 3 weeks after cohabitation with the males was initiated, and the number of living fetuses and resorbing embryos present in the uteri are counted. Any male that produces 10 or more living fetuses in any one female is considered fertile, and no further matings are needed. Males falling below that criteria are mated to an additional set of three females, and the evaluation is repeated. Failing males may be remated up to three times. Males that never succeed in producing at least one litter of 10 or more living fetuses are considered sterile (or semisterile), are sacrificed, and their gonadal cells are examined for cytogenetic evidence of translocations. An example of a HTA study design is in Table 18.

Microbial Host-Mediated Assay

The objective of the microbial host-mediated assay is to determine the ability of a mammalian system (e.g., the mouse) to metabolically activate or detoxify a test article with respect to its mutagenic potential. The mutagenic potential is measured by means of one of a variety of microorganisms, depending on the specific types of mutations being investigated (e.g., base-pair substitution, frame shift). Some of the microorganisms used for this type of testing include various strains of *Salmonella typhimurium, Escherichia coli,* and *Neurospora crassa.* The results of the host-mediated assay can be compared with the direct effect of the test article on the same tester strain of microorganisms to determine whether the host (e.g., mouse) is metabolically activating, detoxifying, or having no effect on the mutagenic potential of the test article. The microbial host-mediated assay, then, is an attempt to combine the convenience of microorganisms for detecting hereditary changes with the metabolism of the test article gained by administration to a whole animal.

Table 18   Typical Mouse Heritable Translocation Assay Study Design

Number of male/mice/dose group	30
Number of dose groups	3
Number of control groups	1–2 (negative; pos. optional)
Dosing frequency	Once daily
Dosing days	Daily, 7 weeks
Survival checks	Daily
Clinical observations	Not done
Mating of dosed males	Upon completion of dosing
Number of F_1 males mated/group	200
Number of F_1s examined cytogenetically for translocations	All sterile and semisterile
Tissue collection	Testes

The microbial host-mediated assay consists of three groups of about 10 mice each, treated with different dose levels of the test article, a negative control group treated with the dosing vehicle, and a positive control group. Doses are administered daily for up to about 5 days. The high dose is usually about one-half of the LD_{50}, with the medium and low doses about one-third and one-tenth of the high dose, respectively. The preferred route of administration is oral, but intramuscular or intraperitoneal injection may be used if necessary. At the end of the period of test article administration, the tester strain of microorganism is administered, usually intravenously. Following appropriate incubation periods (e.g., 1, 2, and 4 hrs), mice are sacrificed and the microorganisms are collected, frequently from liver tissue. The collected microorganisms are grown on minimal agar plates to assess mutation rate. An example of a microbial host-mediated assay study design is in Table 19.

Special Studies

The diversity of toxicity study designs using the mouse as a test system to examine a specific hypothesis defies description. Many of these designs do not strictly fit within the major section headings chosen for this chapter, and might be referred to as "special studies." This chapter is intended to focus on the more commonly conducted types of toxicity studies conducted in mice, but it might be useful to describe two special study designs here as examples of some of the interesting endpoints that can be evaluated in this species.

Mouse Ear Swelling Test

The concept of a mouse ear swelling test (MEST) is that sensitization can be detected by measuring edema in the ear of a mouse that results from topical application of a test article to an animal that has been previously sensitized by means of dermal application to the abdomen.

The objective of the MEST is to provide an alternative test for dermal sensitization potential that makes more efficient use of animals, labor, and other resources than traditional study designs conducted in guinea pigs. A MEST test is often preceded by a dose-finding activity to identify the highest concentration of test article that is no more than minimally irritating to the abdominal skin, and the highest concentration that is nonirritating to the ear. These concentrations are then employed in the sensitization assay.

Table 19 Typical Mouse Microbial Host-Mediated Assay

Number of mice/dose group	10
Number of dose groups	3
Number of control groups	2 (one positive, one negative)
Dosing frequency	Once, daily
Dosing days	Daily for 5 days
Survival checks	Daily
Clinical observations	Not done
Body weights	Prior to dosing
Tester organism administered	After last dose
Tester organism recovered	e.g. 1, 2, and 4 hr after administration
Necropsy	Not done
Tissue collection	Liver or other appropriate tissue for organism recovery

The sensitization assay is carried out in three phases: an induction phase, a challenge phase and if necessary, a rechallenge phase. The sensitization assay requires 15 mice treated with the test article and 10 treated with a control substance, typically the vehicle used for the test article. During the induction phase (study day 1), the abdomen is shaved using a small animal clipper, and 20 μl of 1:1 emulsion of Freund's complete adjuvant in distilled water is injected intradermally at each of two abdominal sites on opposite sides of the ventral midline. Once daily on study days 1, 2, 3, and 4, the stratum corneum is stripped from the abdominal skin using adhesive tape, and the appropriate concentration of test article is applied to the abdomen at a volume of 100 μl.

On study day 11, the challenge phase is initiated. The appropriate concentration of test article is applied to the skin of the left ears of all treated and five of the ten control mice at a volume of 10 μl, and an equal volume of the control (vehicle) is applied to the right ears of those same animals. Thicknesses of both ears of all treated and the five selected control mice are measured on days 12 and 13. Any mouse with a left ear thickness $\geq$ 120% of its right ear thickness is considered to be a positive responder. If one or more mice are judged positive in the absence of primary irritation (any control mice with left ear thickness $\geq$ 110% of right ear thickness) on study day 12 or 13, the test article is considered to be a sensitizer. Evidence of primary irritation requires that the test be repeated using a lower concentration for the challenge dose.

If results are negative (all mice with a left ear thickness increases of < 10%) or equivocal (some mice with increases of 10–19%, but none $\geq$ 20%), a rechallenge is conducted on study days 17 through 20. Baseline ear thicknesses are measured on study day 17. The test article is applied to the right ears of all test mice and the control mice that were not used during the initial challenge on study day 18. Ear thicknesses of the right ears of all test mice and the new control mice are measured on study days 19 and 20, and are compared to the baseline thicknesses taken on day 17. The criteria for positive response are the same as for the initial challenge. An example of a MEST study design is in Table 20.

Dermal Carcinogenicity (Skin Painting) Study
The concept of the dermal carcinogenicity (or skin painting) study is that carcinogens, or of more recent interest, cocarcinogens and tumor promoters can be evaluated or their potencies compared in as little as a few months of testing.

Table 20 Typical Mouse Ear Swelling Test Study Design

Number of male/mice/dose group	15/treated group, 5/control group
Number of dose groups	1
Number of control groups	2
Dosing frequency	Once, daily
Dosing days	Days 1, 2, 3, and 4 (induction)
	Day 11 (challenge)
	Day 18 (optional rechallenge)
Survival checks	Daily
Clinical observations	Not done
Body weights	Not done
Ear thickness measured	Day 10, 12, and 13 (challenge)
	Day 17, 19, and 20 (rechallenge)
Necropsy	Not done
Tissue collection	None

The carcinogenicity of some chemicals (e.g., polycyclic aromatic hydrocarbons) can be detected easily by the production of papillomas or carcinomas. Mouse skin apparently functions in this system because it contains enzymes necessary to produce the active intermediates which lead to initiation. Tars from tobacco, coal, and various petroleum products show active carcinogenic potential in this system, although many of the same products are not carcinogenic when administered systemically. Hepatic detoxification of systemically administered doses probably accounts for this difference.

This study design has been especially useful in recent years in the study of cocarcinogens and tumor promoters. In a typical study design, groups of 25–50 mice might receive from one to a few systemic doses of a known tumor initiator. Following receipt of the initiator, the fur over the anterior portion of the back is shaved, and the suspected tumor initiators are applied to the skin of the back at a frequency of 2–3 times per week. Shaving will need to be repeated approximately weekly. Development of papillomas or carcinomas of the skin is readily visible in the shaved area. Active chemicals are often detected within a few months' treatment. This study is generally intended to continue treatment for a period of about 30–40 weeks, but may be continued for up to 2 years if necessary.

Obvious advantages of this study design include its relative efficiency in terms of animal numbers and labor, and its relative brevity compared to a conventional 18- to 24-month carcinogenicity bioassay. It is reasonable to conclude that positive findings of carcinogenicity in this test would make a conventional carcinogenicity bioassay unnecessary. Negative findings in a dermal carcinogenicity test, however, would not assure the absence of carcinogenic potential, and a conventional bioassay would still be necessary.

Disadvantages of this procedure include difficulty in accurate quantification of dose, as the topically applied dose can run off the animal, be scratched or licked off, or can accumulate as a crust, effectively reducing absorption. Another criticism centers around the fact that if treatment with a suspected promoter is interrupted after a period of 60 days or so, evident papillomas often regress, raising the question of whether they represented sites of true carcinogenicity.

DOSING TECHNIQUES

Techniques are available to administer test substances to mice by most routes of potential human exposure. The choice of a route of administration for a toxicity study should consider the expected route of human exposure and any other scientific objectives that need to be achieved to facilitate safe use of the test substance. Of the various routes available, most test articles will have the most rapid onset of effects and the greatest potency when administered by the intravenous route, followed in approximately descending order by the inhalation, intraperitoneal, subcutaneous, intramuscular, intradermal, oral, and topical routes (Klaassen and Doull, 1980). The expected route of human exposure is probably the most important single determinant of route for toxicity testing. In the discussion that follows, the most commonly employed routes for toxicity testing in mice will be discussed first, followed by the less commonly employed routes.

Oral Administration

Oral administration is probably the most frequently used route of exposure for toxicity testing in mice. Many products are intended for oral administration to humans, and many others are subject to accidental ingestion. Oral administration subjects the test substance to limitations of absorption and metabolism that are similar but not necessarily identical to those in humans. Mice, like rats, differ from many other species in that they do not have an emetic response. For this reason, large doses of substances that would cause emesis in dogs or primates will be retained in the stomachs of mice. While this characteristic facilitates testing at high doses and maximizes potential exposure to toxic effects, it may lead to an overestimate of potential human toxicity because the animal lacks the protective aspect of the emetic response. Another area in which mice differ from dogs and primates is that mice are nocturnal. This characteristic adds some pharmacokinetic variables to the equation for extrapolating toxicity findings from the mouse to the human. Doses that are administered during the day are administered to animals that are in the lower phase of their circadian metabolic cycles. This may mean slower absorption, slower metabolism to either more or less toxic metabolites, and/or slower elimination of the test substance. Conversely, test substances administered in the diet or drinking water will be largely consumed at night, as that is when mice consume most of their daily intake of food and water. While this regimen more closely approximates human consumption during the active part of the day, it makes observation of the animals during the period of peak exposure and metabolism difficult. Three means of oral administration are oral gavage, dietary admix, and mixture with the drinking water.

Gavage

Oral gavage offers the advantages of precisely measured doses which can be administered at precise times. Doses can be administered during the day so animals can be conveniently observed for toxic effects during the first few hours after dosing. Volatile substances and those that lack stability over longer periods in the presence of diet, air, or water can be effectively administered by this method. Gavage allows administration of unpalatable substances that might not be accepted in the diet or water. There are disadvantages associated with gavage administration. The test substance must either be a liquid or must be soluble or suspendable in a liquid vehicle system. The method is relatively labor-intensive compared to diet admix. The processes of daily handling and intubation of all animals engenders the risk of injury during the intubation process, including esophageal puncture and aspiration of test article. In addition, the process of frequent handling causes stress to the animals. While it is convenient to administer doses during the day, daytime is the period of lowest metabolic activity for nocturnal species such as mice. This circadian effect may not be most representative of diurnal species such as humans.

Description of Technique. Gavage administration entails intubation of the mouse with an intubation needle attached to a graduated hypodermic syringe. The dose is administered into the esophagus. Intubation needles for mice are typically constructed of stainless steel tubing with a stainless steel ball tip to reduce the probability of esophageal perforation and reflux and aspiration of the dose. Acceptable tubing sizes range from 22 to 18 gauge, with the larger bore reserved for older mice (e.g., ≥25 g). Tubing length is not critical, but may range from 1 to 3 in. The ball tip is typically 1.25–2.25 mm in diameter. Intubation needles are available commercially (e.g., Popper & Sons, Inc., New Hyde Park, New York) in straight and curved configurations. The choice of shape is a question of personal preference on the part of the dosing technician. Examples of curved and straight intubation needles suitable for use in mice are pictured in Figure 2. Prior to dosing, the test substance must be prepared in a liquid form at an appropriate concentration. Liquid test substances may require dilution. Solid substances will require either dissolution or suspension in an innocuous vehicle. The preferred vehicle is water. If the substance is insoluble in water, various agents may be added to improve wetting (e.g., 0.1% v/v polysorbate 80) and to reduce settling (e.g., 0.5% w/v methylcellulose). Suspensions should be analyzed prior to administration to assure proper concentration, homogeneity, and stability of the substance in the suspending vehicle. Appropriate dose volumes for gavage administration are in the range of 5–10 ml/kg of body weight, but volumes as high as 20 ml/kg can be administered carefully, particularly in acute studies in which the mice have been fasted prior to dosing.

For the actual process of dose administration, the mouse should be weighed, and the individual dose calculated. The appropriate dose volume should be drawn into the dosing syringe and any air bubbles should be expelled. The mouse is then picked up by the skin of the back and neck, and the head tipped back to form a straight line from the nose through the back of the throat and to the stomach, as illustrated in Figure 3. The in-

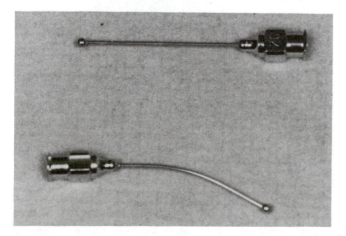

Figure 2 Examples of curved and straight intubation needles suitable for administration of oral gavage doses to mice. Both needles shown are 20 gauge × 1.50 in., and have a 2.25 mm diameter ball tip.

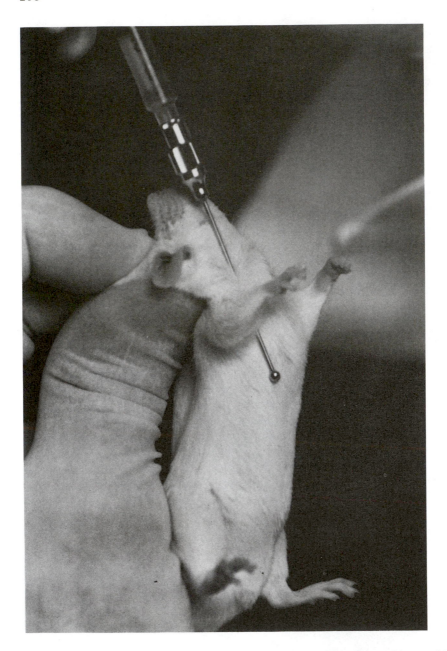

Figure 3   An appropriate means of holding a mouse for oral intubation with a straight intubation needle. Note the relatively straight line from the animals nose through the back of the throat to the stomach.

tubation needle is inserted to the back of the mouth, then gently tipped back, if necessary, to enter the esophagus. The mouse will generally facilitate entry into the esophagus by swallowing the ball of the needle. One successful approach is to envision the tip of the sternum as a "target" for the tip of the intubation needle. When properly positioned, the tube can easily be inserted to a reasonable depth, but it need not reach the stomach. When in position, the dose should be administered slowly to avoid reflux, but promptly to reduce the likelihood that the mouse will struggle and injure itself. A properly intubated mouse is illustrated in Figure 4.

Dietary Admix

Oral administration by dietary admix offers several advantages, including ease of administration, minimal handling of animals for dosing, and elimination of the risk of injury

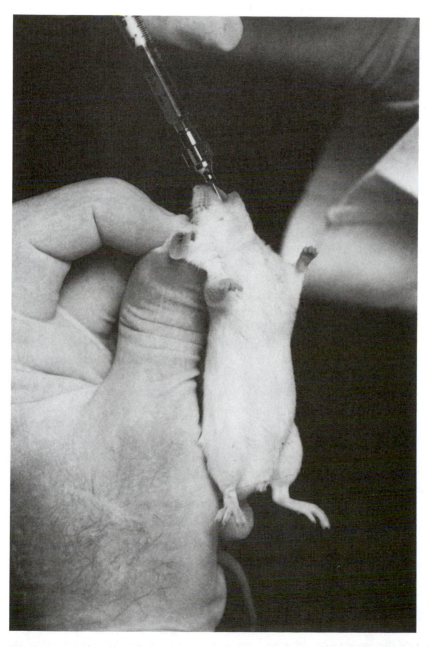

Figure 4   A mouse is shown with a straight oral intubation needle properly inserted. The syringe is being loosely held in this illustration to show the natural angle of the intubation needle.

associated with intubation. The method offers relatively precise dose administration for the group (better than water mix; not as good as gavage), as both mean food consumption and mean body weight for periods of a week or longer are easily measured. Dry, insoluble substances can be administered easily, and administration of test substances to mice during the "awake" phase of their circadian cycle is an advantage. There are disadvantages associated with dietary admix. Accuracy of individual doses is lower than with gavage, and there is not a single identifiable time of dosing. Volatile substances and those that lack stability over periods of at least 4–7 days in the presence of diet, air, or water are precluded from this method. Diet admixtures must be sampled and the samples analyzed periodically to assure proper concentration and homogeneity of the mixture during the course of the study. Unpalatable test substances typically result in reduced dietary intake, which leads to an increase in the concentration of test substance in diet during subsequent weeks in an attempt to reachieve the desired doses. The increased concentrations may be even less palatable, leading to further reduction in dietary intake, and in some cases, eventually to malnutrition. In any dietary study, results should be evaluated carefully to discriminate between changes associated with altered nutritional status and true test substance toxicity.

Description of Technique.   Oral administration by dietary admix entails presentation of a mixture of the test substance in diet in place of the normal diet received by the animals. The concentration of test article in diet is adjusted, based upon the most recently collected data on mean body weight and food consumption for each sex and dose group, to provide the desired doses of test article during the period in question. Early in a study, when body weight and food consumption are changing due to rapid growth of the animals, projections of the mean body weight and food consumption for the coming period should be based upon both the most recent measurements and the rate of change (slope of the plot) of those parameters over several recent periods. If test article stability permits, a convenient period for measurement of body weight and food consumption is about 1 week.

Test substances are usually mixed with the meal form of rodent diet in one or more of a variety of mechanical blenders. Common types of blenders include the Turbula, paddle style, and twin shell or "V" blenders. Turbula and paddle blenders are illustrated in Figures 5 and 6. When large quantities of diet admix are required, it may be advantageous to blend the test substance with the diet in two steps, preparing a premix of 1–2 kg in a blender such as a Turbula, then adding the premix to a larger-scale blender, such as a paddle blender. This procedure often produces a more homogeneous mix in a shorter blending period.

Following mixing, the appropriate concentration of blend is dispensed into animal feeders for presentation to the mice. Feeders are weighed when they are placed in the cages and when they are removed to determine the average amount of feed consumed per day. Mice are weighed at the same times, both to determine body weight gain over the period and to calculate the food consumption in grams per kilogram of body weight per day. Based upon this calculation, the concentration of test substance in diet may be varied up or down to more closely approach the intended doses of test substance in milligrams per kilograms per day.

Among potential problems that may be encountered in conducting dietary admix studies, two may lead to inappropriate calculations of feed consumption, leading to incorrect calculation of concentrations for future periods. These problems are excessive feed spillage, which may result from mice digging or playing in their feeders, and contamination of the feeder with urine and feces, which may result from mice living in

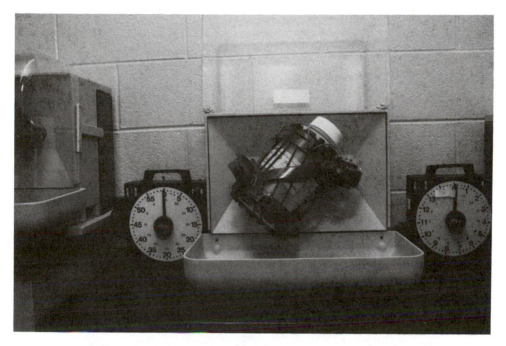

Figure 5 Example of a Turbula blender commonly used to prepare premixes of diet and test article in quantities of about 1 kg. The mixing container effectively rolls and tumbles.

their feeders. Feeders should be checked daily for excessive spillage at the time survival checks and/or observations are conducted, and excessive spillage should be documented. Contamination with urine and feces will lead to an incorrectly high feeder weight at the end of the feed consumption period, and an underestimate of true feed consumption. Excessive contamination should be documented. Animals with excessive spillage and those with excessive contamination of feeders should be excluded from the calculations of mean body weight and food consumption used to prepare future concentrations of diet admix.

Drinking Water

Administration of a water-soluble test substance in the drinking water has many of the same advantages as administration of a dietary admix. This method is rarely used for toxicity studies, however, because of the difficulty in accurately measuring the quantity of water actually consumed. While graduated water bottles can be used, spillage due to mice rubbing against sipper tubes, inefficient drinking, evaporation, vibration, and leaking bottles makes these measurements imprecise. If that practical problem could be solved, administration in the drinking water would bear little conceptual difference from dietary admix. Stability of environmental temperature and humidity is essential to the conduct of a study in which the test article is mixed in the drinking water, as increased temperature and/or lowered humidity lead to increased water consumption. Water consumption must remain relatively stable to allow calculation of appropriate concentrations of test article in water to achieve study objectives.

Description of Technique. From a practical standpoint, administration of test article in

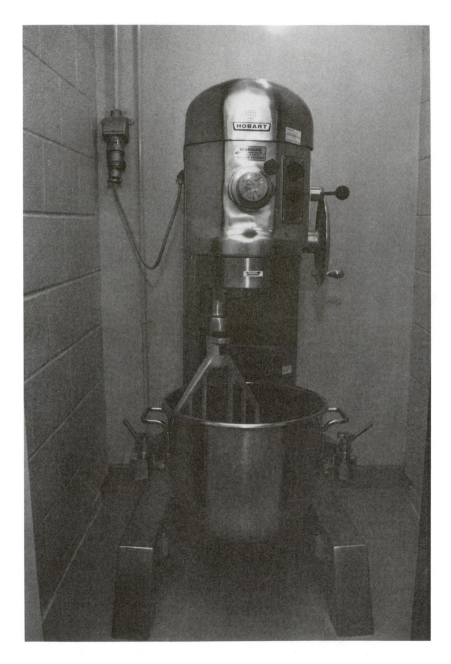

Figure 6   Example of a paddle blender used in preparing final mixes of diet and test article. This blender works on the principle of a low speed, rotating paddle.

the drinking water has many similarities to administration by dietary admix. It is essential that the test article be both soluble and chemically stable in water for the period of presentation. That period should be in the range of about 2 days to a maximum of about 1 week. Water remaining in a water bottle for periods in excess of a week may become heavily contaminated with bacteria. Analogous to the situation with diet admix, the precision of dose administration is directly related to the accuracy with which average daily water consumption and body weight can be measured. Concentrations of test article in water should be adjusted, if necessary, after each measurement of average daily water consumption and body weight to assure precise dose administration.

As solubility in water is a prerequisite for this method, mixing procedures are usually simpler than for diet admixes. Homogeneity analysis should not be required for a true solution, but samples should be analyzed regularly to confirm that concentrations are what they were intended to be.

Water can be provided in graduated bottles. The contents of the bottles should be recorded at the beginning of the consumption period (but after the bottles are placed on the cages to accommodate spillage during that operation), and again at the end of the consumption period to determine average daily water consumption. Evidence of spillage or leakage should be documented. Difficulty in accurately measuring the amount of water actually consumed by the mice is the largest disadvantage to this method of administration.

Intravenous Injection

Intravenous (iv) injection offers the advantages of immediate, complete systemic availability of a precise dose at a known point in time. The process of absorption is eliminated, as is the possibility that some or all of the test article may be metabolized by the liver prior to distribution to the systemic circulation and target organs. Most substances exhibit the highest potency and rapidity of onset of activity of all routes of administration when administered intravenously. Intravenous administration provides a useful benchmark against which absorption and bioavailability from administration by other routes can be compared.

It is essential that test articles administered intravenously be in solution at the time of administration, and remain in solution after injection. Solutions that are subject to precipitation by changes in pH, temperature, or osmolarity should be confirmed at physiological conditions to assure that they will not precipitate after injection. Introduction of insoluble particles, such as those in a suspension, introduces a high probability of embolism, particularly in the pulmonary capillary bed, which will produce severe moribundity or death. The toxicologist is left with the problem of differentiating such moribundity or mortality from the true toxicity of the test article.

Other characteristics of an iv solution that should be evaluated prior to undertaking an iv toxicity study involving repeated dosing include the potential for the solution to cause hemolysis or vascular or subcutaneous irritation. Hemolysis may be a result of the administration of solutions of inappropriate osmolarity (hypotonic solutions are particularly damaging); in which case the problem can be resolved by adjusting the osmolarity of the solution.

Ideally, solutions for iv administration should be isotonic to blood, and have a pH of about 7. Usually a pH in the range of about 5–9 will be acceptable. Solutions that cause appreciable vascular or subcutaneous irritation may result in sufficient injury to the veins and surrounding tissue to preclude repeated administration.

The rate of iv injection is an important variable which must be controlled fairly precisely to achieve reproducible results within a study. If the iv toxicity of two or more test articles is to be compared, it is essential that each be administered at the same rate. Intravenous injections can be administered as a bolus over a period as short as a few seconds, as a continuous, 24-h/day infusion, or over just about any interval in between.

There is nothing particularly magical about any specific dosing period, but it is critical that it remain constant. As a practical matter, an injection period of about 2 min is a reasonable upper limit for hand-held injections into caudal veins of reasonable numbers of mice. Longer periods lead to very slow injections, increase the risk of extravasation, are time consuming, and are difficult and tiring for the toxicologist. Injection periods much shorter than 1 min increase the likelihood that an inordinately high peak plasma concentration that may precede mixing with the total blood volume may compromise the survival of the animal. A corollary to the artificially high peak plasma concentration associated with a short injection period can occur if the injection is administered at an uneven rate. It is particularly critical that the rate of injection not be increased during the last half of the injection period, as this is a time when the animal has already received an initial "loading", and the deleterious effect of increasing the rate of administration will be amplified. In our laboratory, we have found that administration of volumes of 5–10 ml/kg body weight (0.15–0.30 ml for a 30-g mouse) administered evenly over a period of 2 min represents a good compromise. One of the biggest disadvantages of iv administration is that it is a very labor-intensive procedure, requiring more time per animal than any other route. In addition, repeated, daily administration to caudal veins of mice for periods longer than 2–4 weeks becomes technically difficult owing to the accumulation of scar tissue and occasional trauma.

Long duration or continuous, 24-hr per day infusions, while possible, are technically difficult, and will not be discussed in detail here. As a practical matter, long-duration injections or continuous infusions are typically administered through a surgically im-planted catheter using an infusion pump. The catheter is usually placed in a large, superficial vein such as the jugular or femoral vein, then exteriorized at a site such as between the scapulae, which is difficult for the animal to chew or scratch. The surgical procedure is relatively simple. The difficulty lies in keeping the cannula patent and secure in the vein during recovery after surgery, then through the period of dosing. The maximum volume of infusion, even over a continuous 24-hr period should not exceed about 20–30 ml/kg/day, which will typically be less than 1 ml administered over a 24-hr period. This infusion rate is so slow as to be difficult to administer, even with a high-quality infusion pump. The catheter must be attached to the mouse in a way that prevents mutilation of the catheter by the animal without undue limitation of mobility. Long duration or continuous infusions are rarely used for toxicity testing in mice.

Description of Technique.   Intravenous administration entails injection of the desired dose into an appropriate vein. In a typical study, mice will receive a single injection daily over a period of about 2 min or less. Such injections are usually administered into a lateral caudal (tail) vein, using a hypodermic needle attached to a graduated syringe. Hypoder-mic needles used for caudal vein injections in mice are usually no more than 1 in long, and are in the range of about 23–25 gauge. The smallest hypodermic syringe that will contain the full dose volume will provide the greatest precision in dose measurement, but 1-cc disposable syringes are often used.

The needle should be installed on the syringe such that the bevel of the needle faces the graduations on the syringe that will be used to measure the dose. This will allow the syringe graduations to be read easily when the needle has been inserted into the vein in a "bevel up" configuration. Typical needles and syringes are shown in Figure 7. A stopwatch that is easy to read is useful for timing dose administration, and an electronic timer that is activated by a foot pedal is most convenient. A convenient restrainer should hold the mouse securely, but without undue risk of suffocation or injury, while allowing

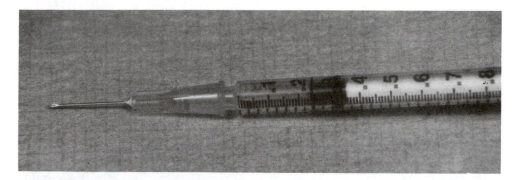

Figure 7   Typical needle and syringe used for intravenous administration into a mouse caudal vein. Shown is a 1-cc disposable hypodermic syringe with a 23 gauge × 0.75 in disposable needle. Note that the needle is installed with the bevel facing the graduations on the syringe. This facilitates reading the graduations during the injection process with the needle inserted in the "bevel up" configuration.

free access to the tail. Examples of a useful restrainer, timer, and foot-activated switch are shown in Figure 8. A source of warm water and/or a tourniquet device are useful, as is a supply of small gauze sponges. A tourniquet which can be easily operated with one hand is pictured in Figure 9. This tourniquet can be constructed from a disposable plastic syringe and a piece of suture. The larger the syringe size, the more pressure it is able to exert on the suture loop. Relatively large (e.g., size 0) braided silk suture should be used for the loop to minimize the risk of cutting the skin of the tail. The suture loop is attached to the plunger inside the barrel of the syringe, then threaded out through the tip of the syringe.

Prior to dosing, the dosing solutions should be prepared. Solutions should be analyzed periodically to assure that proper concentrations are being attained. Each mouse should be weighed, and its dose calculated. As previously noted, doses in the range of 5–10 ml/kg are acceptable for injection over periods of about 30 sec to 2 min. The mouse is placed into the restrainer, and the appropriate dose is drawn into the syringe. Any air bubbles should be expelled from the syringe. This is most important for iv injections. A tourniquet device can be applied at this point, but should not be applied too tightly. The objective is to block venous return, but not arterial supply, thus dilating the veins. As an alternative to a tourniquet, some toxicologists prefer to warm the tail with a gauze sponge wetted in warm (not hot) water to enhance vasodilation. The tail is now held in one hand while the needle is inserted with the other. The needle should be inserted with the bevel up to minimize the chance of puncturing through both sides of the vein. Successful venipuncture will result in the reflux of a small amount of blood into the hub of the needle. Owing to the small volume of blood that usually refluxes, this phenomenon will be most easily visualized if needles are used that have transparent "flashback" hubs. The initial attempt at venipuncture should be made toward the tip of the tail, such that if the vein is missed, a subsequent attempt can be made closer to the base of the tail without risk that the dose will leak out of the initial hole. When the needle is securely in the vein, it can be held with the "tail-holding hand" while the plunger of the tourniquet is depressed to open the vein with the "dosing hand."

Now that the needle is in the vein and the vein is open, the timer can be started, and the

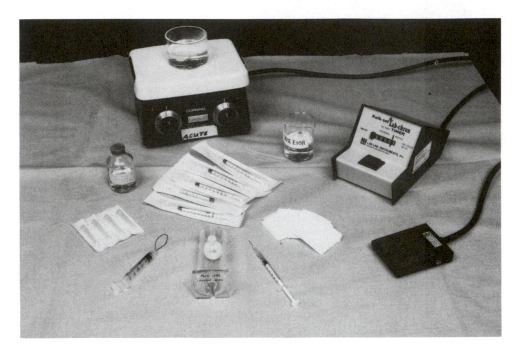

Figure 8   Some of the equipment used in intravenous dosing of mice includes a useful restrainer, a timer, and a foot-activated switch for the timer.

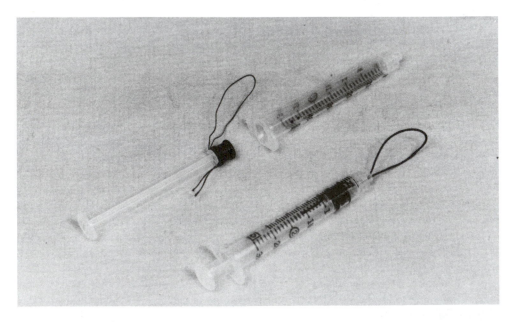

Figure 9   Illustration of a tourniquet for the tail of a mouse which can be easily operated with one hand. The tourniquet can be made by attaching a loop of relatively heavy suture material to the plastic plunger of a disposable syringe.

dose can be administered. A photograph of a mouse receiving an iv dose is shown in Figure 10. One convenient method to assure even dose administration is to divide the dosing period and the dose volume into a convenient number of parts. A 2-min dosing period might be divided into eight 15-sec intervals, and the dose volume divided by eight. The doser can then administer one-eighth of the total dose volume over each 15-sec interval for 2 min to assure a relatively even rate of injection. When the full dose has been administered, a clean, dry gauze sponge should be pinched over the injection site, and the needle should be withdrawn. Maintaining pressure on the site of the injection for 10–30 sec after withdrawal of the needle is usually adequate to prevent bleeding. The mouse can now be removed from the restrainer. As iv injections typically result in a rapid onset of activity, it is often appropriate to observe a mouse for the first few minutes after dosing for clinical signs of toxicity.

Intraperitoneal Injection

The intraperitoneal (ip) route of administration generally offers the second most rapid absorption of a test article among the parenteral routes, with systemic availability second only to intravenous injection. Rapid absorption is conferred by the large surface area of the lining of the peritoneal cavity, and by the rich blood supply to that area. Intraperitoneal administration leads to absorption primarily through the portal circulation. As a result, test articles that are metabolized by the liver are subjected to extensive (or even complete) metabolism prior to reaching systemic circulation and target organs, unless, of course, the target organ is the liver, in which case toxicity may even be amplified. Test articles that are excreted in the bile are similarly subject to elimination prior to reaching the systemic circulation and target organs. Water-insoluble mixtures,

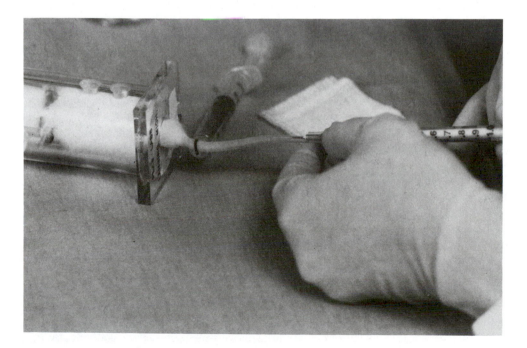

Figure 10 Photograph of a mouse receiving an intravenous dose into a caudal vein.

aqueous suspensions, for example, can be administered by the ip route. This may provide the opportunity for rapid systemic absorption of lipid-soluble or certain other test articles. Solutions or suspensions for ip injection should be adjusted to a pH in the range of about 5–9 to reduce the potential for irritation. Osmolarity of the dosing formulation is not critical, as it is for iv injection. Dose volumes for ip administration are in the range of 5–10 ml/kg/day, but volumes as high as 20 ml/kg/day are acceptable, particularly if the study is of limited duration, or if it is known that the test article will be absorbed by the ip route.

One of the most significant disadvantages of ip administration is the risk of peritonitis. Peritonitis can result from any of three primary causes: physical irritation caused by accumulation of a truly insoluble or irritating test article in the peritoneal cavity, introduction of exogenous microbiological contamination, or microbiological contamination resulting from injury to the gastrointestinal tract or urinary bladder. The potential for a test article to produce physical irritation or chemical peritonitis can be assessed in studies of 1 to a few days in duration. While physical or chemical peritonitis is the most frequently seen form of peritonitis in toxicity studies, it is still found with only a small percentage of test articles. Mice are relatively resistant to microbiological infection, so microbiological peritonitis is even less common than physical or chemical peritonitis. Peritonitis resulting from injury during the injection process is extremely rare when injections are administered by qualified toxicologists. There is a slight risk to the animals of physical injury to a major organ or vessel during the injection process, but again this is extremely rare in the hands of qualified dosers.

Description of Technique.   Intraperitoneal injections are administered into the peritoneal cavity using a hypodermic needle attached to a graduated syringe. Each mouse receives a single daily dose, administered as a bolus, for the duration of the toxicity study. The injection should be administered into the animal's lower, right abdominal quadrant to minimize the risk of injury to the liver, spleen, and bladder. For initial training purposes in dosing by the ip route, it is useful to sacrifice a mouse, then open the abdominal cavity to expose the internal organs that may be susceptible to injury during the injection procedure. This will allow a novice to hold the animal in a dosing position and clearly visualize where the lobes of the liver, the spleen, and the urinary bladder will be, and the area of less vulnerability between these organs. Hypodermic needles used for ip injections to mice need be no longer than about 5/8 in, and should be the smallest diameter that will allow easy injection of the dose volume to minimize the trauma to the abdominal wall with commensurate potential for leakage. Needles in the range of 23–25 gauge are appropriate for use with solutions and suspensions of low viscosity. Suspensions of high viscosity may require the use of needles with a larger bore. Needles as large as 19–20 gauge can be used, but require great care to avoid injury and leakage of the test article from the injection site.

Prior to initiation of a toxicity study, dosing formulations should be prepared, and samples analyzed for concentration and homogeneity of suspensions, if appropriate. Each mouse should be weighed and its dose calculated. The appropriate dose is then drawn into a syringe, and air bubbles are expelled. The mouse is picked up with one hand, and held with the ventral surface toward the doser, as shown in the photograph in Figure 11. Movement of the animals right hind leg should be restricted to limit interference with the syringe and needle during dosing. The needle should be inserted at an angle of about 30–45 degrees into the abdominal cavity to facilitate penetration of the abdominal wall.

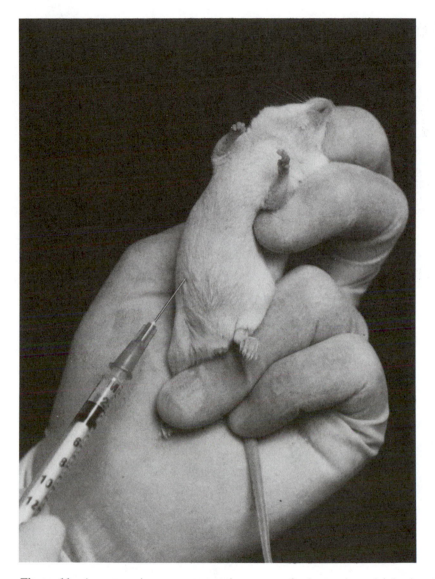

Figure 11 An appropriate way to restrain a mouse for intraperitoneal injection. Note that the movement of the right hind leg has been restricted to limit interference with the syringe and needle during dosing.

The location should be to the right of the midline (to avoid the spleen) at a position about midway between the lower edge of the liver and the urinary bladder to a depth of about 1 cm (3/8 in). A properly inserted needle is shown in the photograph in Figure 12. Following insertion, the needle is withdrawn slightly, moved about, and the angle of insertion is reduced to assure that the tip has not penetrated or snagged any internal organs. The dose is now administered as a bolus and the needle withdrawn. If a large-bore needle has been used, it may be necessary to apply gentle finger pressure over the injection site for a few seconds to prevent leakage of the dose.

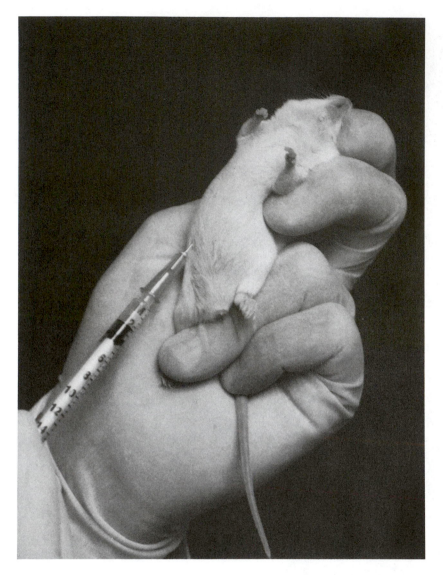

Figure 12 A mouse receiving an intraperitoneal injection. Note that following insertion of the needle at an angle of about 30 to 45 degrees through the abdominal wall, the angle has been reduced to minimize probability of penetrating an internal organ. The injection site is to the right of the midline (to avoid the spleen) at a position about midway between the lower edge of the liver and the urinary bladder to a depth of about 1 cm (0.625 in).

Intramuscular Injection

The intramuscular (im) route of administration is less commonly used in toxicity testing, but it may be appropriate if the test article is intended for intramuscular administration to humans. The im route generally results in slower absorption of a test article, with lower peak plasma levels, but more sustained effects than intravenous or intraperitoneal injection. The rate of absorption can be influenced by the amount of vascular perfusion of the tissue surrounding the injection, the vehicle, and the injected volume, which indirectly may alter the surface area of tissue available for absorption. Coadministration of a vasodilator generally increases the rate of absorption, whereas coadministration of a vasoconstrictor generally decreases that rate. Administration of the test article as a solution or suspension in a viscous, poorly absorbed vehicle generally retards absorption. The ability to control the rate of absorption can be a significant advantage in some cases, as it allows the toxicologist to administer a dose of a test article that may be absorbed over a period of many hours or even days. This can be especially useful in the case of test articles that have short half-lives after absorption, as a result of rapid metabolism and/or elimination. Limitations to im dosing include the limited number of muscle groups in the mouse that are large enough to accept dosing; e.g., the muscles of the posterior aspect of the femoral region, and the small dose volume that can be administered. If possible, the same injection sites should not be treated every day to allow time for absorption and recovery from the trauma of dosing. This means that while a single acute dose might be divided into both hind limbs, repeated daily doses should be administered into alternate limbs. The dose volume should not exceed 1.0 ml/kg per injection site, or about 0.03 ml for a 30-g mouse, and smaller volumes are preferable. An acute study, in which each animal is dosed once, would allow 1 ml/kg to be administered into each hind limb, for a total dose volume of 2 ml/kg. This dose volume coupled with the limit of solubility or suspendability of the test article in the vehicle selected may restrict the maximum dose of test article below toxic levels. A further limitation on toxicity testing by the im route is that the formulation to be injected must not cause significant local irritation, particularly if repeated doses will be administered. This limitation may require that a separate study be conducted to assess im irritation potential prior to initiation of a repeated dose study by this route. Intramuscular injection is more labor intensive than most other routes with the exception of iv injection.

Description of Technique. Intramuscular injections are administered into the large muscle groups of the posterior aspect of the femoral region using a hypodermic needle attached to a graduated syringe. Each mouse receives a single daily dose, administered as a bolus into alternate hind limbs for the duration of the study. Hypodermic needles used for im injection should be the smallest diameter that will allow injection, but in the range of 27 gauge up to a maximum of about 23 gauge. Prior to dosing, the same procedures for formulation, analysis, weighing of mice, and calculation of doses should be followed as those recommended for ip dosing. The dose is drawn into a syringe, and air bubbles are expelled. The mouse may be held by an assistant, and the needle inserted to the approximate center of the muscle mass, as shown in the photograph in Figure 13. The dose is injected as a bolus, and the needle is withdrawn. The muscle may be massaged gently to distribute the dose prior to returning the mouse to its cage.

Subcutaneous Injection

The subcutaneous (sc) route of administration is not commonly used in toxicity testing, but may be appropriate if the test article is intended for sc administration to humans, or as a more practical substitute for im testing in mice. The sc route is similar in many characteristics of absorption to the im route, and generally results in slower absorption of a test article, with lower peak plasma levels, but more sustained effects than ip administration. The rate of sc absorption can also be influenced by the amount of vascular perfusion of the tissue surrounding the injection, the vehicle, and the injected volume, which indirectly may alter the surface area of tissue available for absorption. Coadministration of

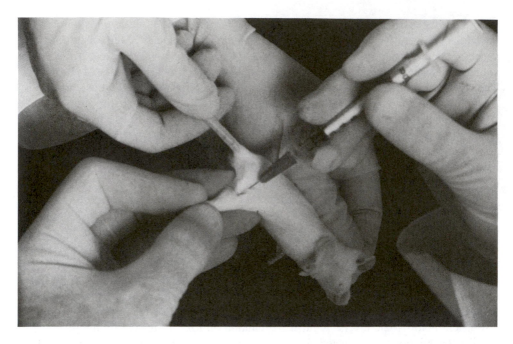

Figure 13 Example of a mouse receiving an intramuscular injection. The mouse may be held by an assistant, and the needle inserted to the approximate center of the muscle mass.

a vasodilator generally increases the rate of absorption, whereas coadministration of a vasoconstrictor generally decreases that rate. Administration of the test article as a solution or suspension in a viscous, poorly absorbed vehicle generally retards absorption. The ability to control the rate of absorption is similar to that seen with im injection, and can offer the same advantages, as it may allow the toxicologist to administer a dose of a test article that may be absorbed over a period of many hours or even days. Some limitations to im dosing do not apply to sc dosing. Subcutaneous doses can be injected at a wide variety of sites, if necessary. In addition, dose volumes of up to 10–20 ml/kg/day may be administered repeatedly if they are well absorbed and do not cause excessive local irritation. These large dose volumes allow administration of much higher total doses than can be administered im. It may still be necessary to conduct a separate study to assess sc irritation potential prior to initiation of a repeated dose toxicity study. Subcutaneous injections can easily be administered to mice without assistance.

Description of Technique.   Subcutaneous injections are administered into the region beneath the skin using a hypodermic needle attached to a graduated syringe. Each mouse receives a single daily dose, administered as a bolus. Daily doses may be administered at the same site if absorption is complete and irritation is minimal, but subcutaneous trauma may be reduced if the injection site can be changed from day-to-day. Hypodermic needles used for sc injection should be the smallest diameter that will allow injection, but in the range of about 26 gauge up to a maximum of about 20 gauge. While larger volumes can be administered, dose volumes of about 10 ml/kg/day are preferable.

Prior to dosing, the same procedures for formulation, analysis, weighing of mice, and calculation of doses should be followed as those recommended for ip dosing. The dose is drawn into a syringe, and air bubbles are expelled. The mouse is grasped by a fold of skin, as shown in the photograph in Figure 14. One of the most convenient injection sites is the skin in the mid-scapular region, which allows the restraint and dosing of the mouse with minimal risk of being bitten. The needle is inserted through the skin into the subcutaneous region, as shown in the photograph in Figure 15. The dose is injected as a bolus, and the needle is withdrawn. The injection site may be pinched for a few seconds to prevent leakage, and the area around the injection site may be massaged gently to distribute the dose prior to returning the mouse to its cage.

Intradermal Injection

Intradermal (id) injection is not a route that is commonly used for toxicity studies. It may be appropriate to test products intended for id administration to humans by that same route in mice, and studies of limited duration are technically feasible. The id route offers the advantage of slow absorption owing to the poor vascular perfusion of the skin relative to tissues in other areas of potential administration. This slow absorption is typically associated with longer time to onset of effects and lower peak plasma levels, but more sustained effects than routes that result in faster absorption. To the extent that the test article may be metabolized by the skin, the id route would be expected to offer greater opportunity for such metabolism than subcutaneous injection, but less than topical administration. Injected volume for id dosing should be limited to about 1 ml/kg per injection site or less, with smaller volumes preferred if repeated doses will be adminis-

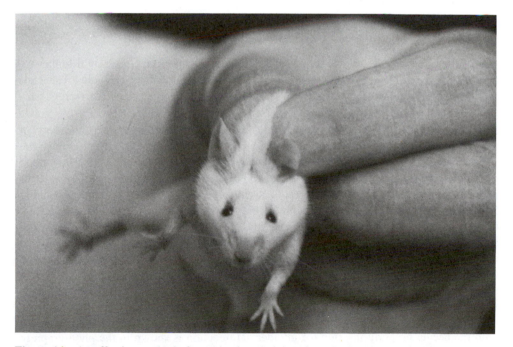

Figure 14   An effective method of restraint for administration of subcutaneous doses. As the skin is grasped, a roughly triangular surface is created between the thumb and forefinger of the holding hand which can be easily penetrated with the hypodermic needle. One of the most convenient injection sites is the skin in the mid-scapular region, which allows the restraint and dosing of the mouse with minimal risk of being bitten.

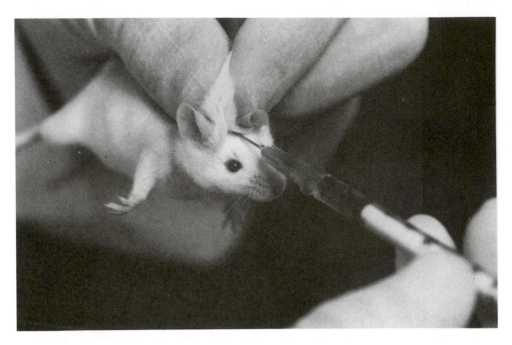

Figure 15 A mouse receiving a subcutaneous injection. The needle is inserted through the skin into the subcutaneous region.

tered. It is acceptable to administer id doses at multiple sites simultaneously if higher total doses are required. Irritating formulations of the test article must be avoided, especially if multiple doses will be administered, as ulceration and necrosis of the skin can result.

Description of Technique.   Intradermal injections can be administered at a variety of accessible sites, but the skin of the abdomen or back is often used. The area in which the injections will be administered should be shaved with a small animal clipper to allow good visualization during and after dosing. Doses can be administered using a small hypodermic needle attached to a graduated tuberculin syringe. Needle diameter should be limited to 27 gauge or smaller, and 30 gauge is preferable. The use of a needle with an intradermal bevel is not necessary. Prior to dosing, the same procedures for test article preparation and analysis of formulations, weighing of mice, and calculation of doses should be followed as recommended for ip dosing. The dose is drawn into the syringe and air bubbles are expelled. The mouse is held in one hand, and the needle is inserted into the skin at a shallow angle with the bevel of the needle up to avoid penetration into the subcutaneous space. With practice, the toxicologist can feel the needle penetrate into the subcutaneous space, if that happens by accident, and can relocate the needle prior to injection. A mouse with the needle properly inserted for intradermal injection is shown in the photograph in Figure 16. A properly administered intradermal dose will appear as a small bleb on the surface of the skin. An example of such a bleb is shown in the photograph in Figure 17. A dose administered into the subcutaneous space will not appear as a bleb, as the dose will be distributed over a larger area.

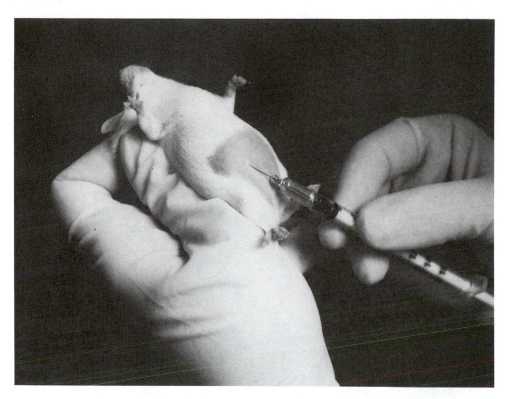

Figure 16 A mouse with the needle properly inserted for intradermal injection. Note the angle of the needle to the skin. The bevel of the needle is up to reduce the likelihood of penetration into the subcutaneous space.

Topical Administration

The topical route of administration is occasionally used for toxicity testing. This choice of route may be appropriate for testing the systemic and local toxic effects of substances intended for human topical administration or which are likely to come into accidental contact with human skin. Data suggest that the mouse is one of the less appropriate species for extrapolation of percutaneous toxicity to the human, as the permeability of mouse skin (as well as rat and rabbit skin) is substantially higher than the permeability of human skin (Maibach and Wester, 1989). Nevertheless, topical application to mice may be appropriate in special cases, such as the conduct of the mouse ear swelling test (MEST) for dermal sensitization potential (Gad *et al.*, 1986).

Historically, the skin was perceived as a barrier to absorption. It is now clear that lipophilic compounds are readily absorbed into and across the skin, and further that the skin may be a source of significant metabolism of some chemicals (Maibach and Wester, 1989). Variables in addition to lipophilicity that are likely to effect dermal absorption include the integrity of the skin at the treatment site, the vehicle employed for dosing, occlusion, and/or restraint of the mouse after treatment, and whether the test article is washed off after some prescribed period. Variations on the integrity of the skin include totally intact skin, skin from which the outer epidermal layers have been tape

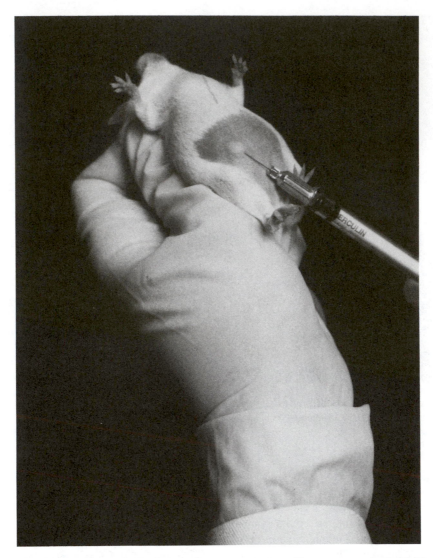

Figure 17   A properly administered intradermal dose will appear as a small "bleb" on the surface of the skin immediately upon completion of the injection. Absence of such a "bleb" probably indicates that the intended dose went into the subcutaneous space.

stripped using a surgical adhesive tape (e.g., Dermiclear), and skin that has been abraded. The presumption is that nonlipophilic test articles will penetrate stripped (thinned) or abraded (interrupted) skin more extensively than they would intact skin. The proper choice of a vehicle may enhance the permeability of the skin to a nonlipophilic chemical. Occlusion of the treatment site and/or restraint of the mouse after application of a topical dose improves retention of the dose in contact with the skin and reduces the probability that the animal will orally ingest the topical dose. Washing excess test article from the treatment site after a prescribed time will limit the exposure period to a known interval. The appropriate choices for the above (and other variables) in topical toxicity study design are a function of the specific objectives of the study, and the physical and chemical characteristics of the test article.

Description of Technique. As the number of procedural variables for topical dosing is so great, the procedures described for topical dosing in the mouse ear swelling test (Gad et al., 1986) will be described as a representative technique. In that procedure, the hair is clipped from the treatment site (e.g., abdomen or back) on the first day of treatment, and the epidermal layer is tape stripped until the site has a slightly shiny appearance, typically 10–20 applications and removals of a surgical adhesive tape such as Dermiclear (Johnson & Johnson Co., New Brunswick, NJ). The tape-stripping procedure is shown in Figure 18. Next, a fixed volume, e.g., 100 μl, of the test article in a volatile solvent such as ethanol is applied to the treatment site. The solvent is allowed to dry using a warm air blower if necessary, and the animal is returned to its cage. On subsequent treatment days the tape-stripping operation can be reduced to about 5–10 applications of adhesive tape to achieve the shiny appearance.

Inhalation

The inhalation route of administration offers the most rapid absorption of most test articles, with systemic availability second only to intravenous injection. Efficiency of absorption by the inhalation route is conferred by the large surface area of the respiratory system, the close proximity of the inner alveolar surface to the blood circulating through the lungs, and the fact that the entire cardiac output passes through the lungs with each circuit of the blood through the body. Absorption of inhaled agents proceeds via one or more of the following mechanisms depending upon specific characteristics of the agent: direct absorption into the blood stream, absorption from the gastrointestinal tract following deposit in the nasopharynx or transport by mucociliary escalation and swallowing, and/or lymphatic uptake following deposit in the alveoli.

Inhalation studies are particularly useful in estimating the risk of accidental or occupational exposure to a gas, vapor, dust, fume, or mist as well as in evaluating the toxicity of agents that are intended to be administered by inhalation. Administration by inhalation is the most technologically complex means of routine exposure, and a comprehensive description of the procedures is beyond the scope of this chapter. The reader is referred to other works (e.g., McClellan and Henderson, 1989; Menzel and McClellan, 1980; Kennedy and Trochiomowicz, 1982) for further description. Rather this discussion will be limited to some of the advantages, disadvantages, and variables to be considered in inhalation testing. The primary advantage of inhalation is rapid, effective absorption. The primary disadvantage is the technological complexity of the method, with the associated risk of technical error and disregard of an important variable.

For a mouse to inhale a test article, the mouse must be placed in an environment which contains the test article in the form of a gas, vapor, dust, fume, or mist. The test article must exist in a particle size that is inspirable, generally having an aerodynamic diameter from 1 to about 10 μ. Particle size dictates where in the respiratory tract the test article will be deposited and absorbed. Larger particles are deposited in the nasopharyngeal region, with successively smaller particles deposited in the trachea, bronchial, bronchiolar, and finally the alveolar region for particles of about 1 μ or less. The technology of particle generation and uniform distribution through the exposure apparatus is complex in itself. In addition to generating and uniformly distributing the test atmosphere, care must

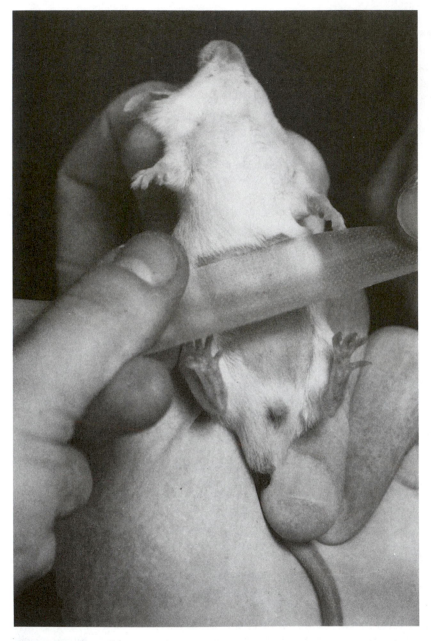

Figure 18   Illustration of the procedure for removal of the stratum corneum by tape stripping prior to administration of a topical dose to the abdomen of a mouse.

be exercised to capture the exhaust from the exposure apparatus, such that the test article can be contained without contamination of the laboratory or environment. Exposure periods can range from a few minutes, appropriate for test articles that may pose only an acute exposure risk to continuous exposure over a prolonged period, appropriate for test articles that may pose a risk of long-term environmental or occupational exposure.

Exposure apparatus generally takes the form of a chamber which contains the whole animal or groups of animals, or a device which exposes only the head or nose of the animal(s) to the experimental atmosphere.

Chamber (Whole Body)

Inhalation chambers allow relatively large numbers of mice to be exposed simultaneously without restraint. The aerodynamic considerations are complex, but simpler than for a head-only or nose-only exposure system. Flow rate through a chamber must be adequate to provide temperature and humidity control. Disadvantages of whole body chambers include the tendency for test article to accumulate in the fur, from which it can be ingested; on the skin and eyes, which may interfere with the intended route of exposure; and the difficulty in monitoring respiratory volume and rate of individual animals.

Head/Nose Exposure (Head Only/Nose Only)

Head- or nose-only exposure apparatus limits exposure of the mouse to the test article by routes other than inhalation, as only a small amount of skin and fur are exposed to the test environment. In addition, it is possible to monitor respiratory volume and rate of individual animals with some of the head- or nose-only equipment. Disadvantages to this equipment include the fact that a relatively small number of animals can be simultaneously exposed, and those animals must be restrained in a position which keeps their heads or noses in close contact with the exposure apparatus. This restraint imposes stress on the animals, and virtually precludes continuous exposure, as the processes of eating and drinking are not possible with most of this equipment. The restrainer may limit the animals ability to dissipate excess body heat.

DATA COLLECTION TECHNIQUES

Types of data that are routinely collected during the conduct of toxicity studies in mice fall into three broad categories: clinical observations and physical examinations, clinical laboratory evaluations, and postmortem procedures. Cardiovascular parameters are not measured in routine toxicology studies. Heart rates in awake mice have been measured in the range of 300 to more than 800 beats/min (Kaplan *et al.*, 1983). Reliable blood pressure measurements are best made by cannulation of a major artery, such as the carotid. Such procedures require anesthesia and surgery, neither of which is especially desirable during the course of a study that may be of long duration and involve many animals.

Clinical Observations and Physical Examinations

Clinical observations entail the recording of effects that can be detected by direct observation, such as abnormal gait and body weight. For the sake of this discussion, a variety of parameters that can be observed or measured directly will be discussed in this section. Clinical observations often provide the first indication of which physiological systems are being affected by the test article.

Mice should be observed regularly throughout the in-life portion of a toxicity study. The type and frequency of these observations should be tailored to meet the scientific objectives of the specific study. Most effects observed following administration of acute (single) doses occur within a relatively short time after dosing. As acute intravenous doses are often associated with almost immediate effects, it might be appropriate to observe treated mice within 5 min, at about 15, 30, and 60 min, and again at 2 and 4 hr after dosing. Observations should be repeated at least once daily on all subsequent study days throughout the post-dosing observation period. This schedule should provide information on the times of onset, peak activity, and remission from toxic effects as well as information on the sequence and severity of effects observed. The high intensity of data collection on the day of dosing in acute studies requires that the system for conducting and recording observations be simple and time efficient. Typically, a system of "exception reporting" is used, in which observations of exceptions from the norm are recorded, and the absence of comment on a system (e.g., respiration) implies that parameter is normal. Clinical observations in repeated dose studies should be conducted at approximately the same time each day to assure that changes in findings over the course of the study can be attributed to the accumulation of or adaptation to toxic effects rather than incidental changes attributable to circadian rhythm or time after dosing. Minimally, all animals should be observed early in the day, prior to daily dosing, and it is highly desirable to conduct at least one additional daily observation at 2–4 hr after dosing (or late in the day) to be aware of effects that may be associated with higher blood levels of test article usually found from a few minutes to a few hours after dosing.

The simplest form of clinical observation is an observation for survival and moribundity. This or a higher level of observation must be conducted at least once daily in all toxicity studies. The next level of observation is an observation for clinical signs of toxicity, such as abnormal level of spontaneous motor activity, abnormal gait, abnormal respiration, and abnormal quantity or quality of fecal output.

The next level of observation is more structured, and is typically conducted about once weekly during studies of a few weeks' duration to as infrequently as about once monthly during the later phases of 26-week to 2-year studies. During the conduct of a physical examination, specific parameters are evaluated, such as quality of coat, body orifices (for excessive or unusual discharges), eyes, respiratory sounds, and in studies longer than about 26 weeks, animals are examined carefully for evidence of visible or palpable masses. Body weight and feed consumption are typically monitored in studies longer than a few days. An appropriate interval for measuring body weight and feed consumption is about a week. These two parameters should be measured concurrently, such that changes in one can be compared directly to changes in the other. In longer studies, in which the mice have reached maturity and body weight gain has approached zero, the frequency at which body weight and feed consumption are measured can be reduced to as infrequently as once per month. The interval over which they are measured would remain at about a week, however.

Clinical Laboratory Evaluations

Clinical laboratory evaluations of mice refer to evaluations of blood and urine. Blood is routinely collected at sacrifice in repeated dose studies, and small quantities (e.g., about 0.10 ml) of blood can be collected at interim periods during the course of the study for the purpose of evaluating differential smears or other limited objectives. Interim (nonterminal) blood samples can be collected by retro-orbital venous plexus puncture, cardiac puncture, and tail snip, among other techniques. Each of these techniques has certain disadvantages. Retro-orbital puncture is technically difficult, and may require anesthesia or immobilization of the animal. Cardiac puncture typically requires anesthesia, and cardiac injury may compromise the histological evaluation of cardiac tissue. Tail snip often yields samples that are contaminated with extravascular, extracellular fluids. Any administration of anesthetic agents during the study of a test article that is not thoroughly understood engenders some risk to the interpretation of the study, as potential interactions of the anesthetic with the metabolism or direct effect of the test article are nearly impossible to predict. Blood collected at the time of sacrifice is typically drawn from the inferior vena cava or the abdominal aorta while the mouse is under anesthesia. In the case of terminal blood collection, potential interaction of the anesthetic agent with the test article, induction of liver enzymes, etc., is not an issue.

Parameters evaluated in blood samples drawn from mice include evaluation of differential smears for morphological abnormalities and differential white counts, measurement of serum glucose and urea concentrations, serum aspartate aminotransferase, alanine aminotransferase, and alkaline phosphatase activity. Red blood cell counts, white blood cell counts, and hemoglobin concentrations can be measured, but these parameters are quite variable for mice on many of the commonly used laboratory instruments, so they are often omitted. In addition, bone marrow smears may be prepared, but are usually only prepared at sacrifice in mice. Bone marrow smears may help in understanding hematological changes. Caution should be exercised in comparing experimental data with results obtained from the literature or with results obtained on different instrumentation or by different procedures. For greatest utility, a set of normal values should be compiled for the laboratory procedures and equipment used to produce the data in the toxicity study.

As a practical matter, urine is not usually collected in routine toxicity studies. The primary difficulty in conducting urinalysis is that the mouse produces a very small volume of urine during a reasonable collection period (e.g., 16–24 hr), and of that volume, considerable and variable quantities are lost to evaporation and on the surfaces of the collection apparatus. As a result, attempts to evaluate urinary concentrations of practically anything can be very misleading.

Postmortem Procedures

Postmortem procedures, literally those procedures performed after the death of the animal, include confirmation of the identification number and sex of the animal, an external examination, examination of the significant internal organs in place prior to removal, then removal, weighing of appropriate organs, and collection of tissue specimens for histological processing and microscopic examination. The microscopic examination of tissue specimens by a qualified veterinary pathologist may be the single most important source of information in understanding the toxicity of a test article. The pathologist's findings should be carefully integrated with the other study data (e.g., clinical observations, body weights, feed consumption, and clinical laboratory findings) to fully comprehend the effects of the test article on the mouse under the conditions of study.

Ordinarily the list of tissues to be routinely weighed, collected, and processed for histological examination will be specified in the study protocol. In addition to the tissues specified in the protocol, specimens are usually collected of all lesions or target organs that have been identified during the course of the study or at gross necropsy. It is important to provide the necropsy staff with a current list of abnormal clinical observations, especially any evidence of visible or palpable masses, as this is the time when the visible and palpable lesions can be linked to the histopathological evaluation of those lesions. Every effort should be made to locate all lesions described, and collect representative tissue from those sites.

A detailed description of necropsy procedures is beyond the scope of this discussion. It should be emphasized that the necropsy process, particularly when conducted on a large number of animals at the scheduled termination of a study, is a process in which a large number of tissue samples may be collected, and a similarly large quantity of data may be gathered during a short period of time. As such, this process presents many opportunities for loss or misidentification of samples and data. A rigorous system of accounting for which tissues have been collected from each animal, and for tracking the samples and data collected is critical to the accurate interpretation of the toxicity study.

SUMMARY

In summary, the mouse is one of the most useful species for toxicity testing. Mice have been used in biomedical research for hundreds of years. As a result of long usage, many techniques have been developed to dose and evaluate mice, and a wealth of historical data has been accumulated in the literature. A wide variety of genetic strains have been developed for specific purposes. It is often possible to select a strain for testing that is particularly vulnerable or resistant to either the test article or a particular type of lesion that might be expected to be associated with that test article. The small size of the mouse confers economy in acquisition, husbandry, handling, and test article consumption. The relatively short gestation period and life span of the mouse are useful in conducting reproductive studies, or studies in which the test article will be administered for a high percentage of the lifetime of the animal.

The small size of the mouse is responsible for most of the disadvantages of the species as well. The species is relatively susceptible to environmental stress. Small size and blood volume makes it difficult or impossible to collect multiple samples of blood and urine over short periods of time. Assays that might require large volumes of blood or urine are precluded. Certain physiological evaluations, such as electrocardiograms, are difficult owing to the small size and high activity level of the species.

Pathology   **Charles H. Frith, Dawn G. Goodman, and
                         Byron G. Boysen**

As they age, animals of all species, including humans, develop a variety of lesions, both neoplastic and nonneoplastic. Such lesions are usually referred to as spontaneous or age-associated lesions. These lesions are most frequently proliferative, degenerative, or inflammatory in nature. Each species and strain of animal has certain characteristic lesions which are commonly observed with aging. The purpose of this chapter is to discuss those age-associated lesions which are frequently observed in various strains and stocks of mice and those lesions which might interfere with interpretation of toxicology studies. The B6C3F1 hybrid mouse strain and the CD-1 mouse stock are the two strains/stocks of mice most commonly used in toxicology studies in the United States. The National Toxicology Program (NTP) utilizes the B6C3F1 mouse, whereas private industry utilizes primarily the CD-1 strain for toxicology studies. Both strains have their advantages and their disadvantages. Data are available regarding the time of onset and incidences of age-associated lesions found in these strains/stocks. This chapter will primarily discuss lesions found in B6C3F1 and CD-1 mice.

The B6C3F1 mouse is the F_1 hybrid of two inbred strains, C57BL/6 females and C3H/HeN males and is designated (C57BL/6 x C3H/HeN)F_1. The C57BL/6 strain was originated by Little in 1921. The C3H strain was originated by Strong in 1920 (Anonymous, 1981). When the C3H strain was obtained by Heston in 1941, it was designated as the C3H/HeN. Subsequently, the strain was established behind the specific pathogen–free (SPF) barrier. The mouse mammary tumor virus (MTV), which is transmitted through the milk, was not transmitted to the offspring, which were caesarean-derived and maintained behind the barrier. The strain was then designated as C3H/HeN-MTV-. This strain is used to provide the male parent for the B6C3F1 mouse used by the National Toxicology Program (NTP) and, therefore, does not carry the MTV (Goodman et al., 1985). The B6C3F1 mouse from the Charles River Laboratories is likewise MTV- (Anonymous, 1982). However, it is possible that B6C3F1 mice from other sources may be derived from C3H mice carrying the MTV.

The CD-1 mouse is an outbred stock maintained at the Charles River Laboratories. The full designation for this stock is Crl:CD-1(ICR)BR. The CD-1 mouse was derived from Swiss stock (Anonymous, 1982). The so-called Swiss mouse was imported to the United States in 1926 by C. J. Lynch of the Rockefeller Institute for Medical Research, and was derived from a noninbred stock maintained in Europe. Subsequently, the stock was given to other researchers and commercial laboratories (Lynch, 1969). The Swiss stock used by the Charles River Laboratories to establish the CD-1 mouse was obtained from Hauschka and Mirand of Roswell Park Memorial Institute (HaM/ICR) in 1959. The CD-1 mouse was caesarean derived at that time and, subsequently, maintained behind an SPF barrier (Anonymous, 1982).

In evaluating toxicology studies, it is important to be aware of the types of age-associated lesions observed in untreated animals of the strain/stock of mouse used in the study, at what age such lesions are generally observed, the incidences observed, and the degree of severity. Generally, few if any lesions are encountered in CD-1 and B6C3F1 mice less than 6 months of age. Those that are encountered are usually sporadic in occurrence and minimal to mild in severity. Neoplasms of any type are rarely seen in animals of this age, although they can occur. Most acute and subchronic toxicity studies in mice are conducted in animals less than 6 months of age. Thus, spontaneous lesions rarely complicate interpretation of data from these types of studies. After a year of age, spontaneous lesions start to appear, increasing in frequency and severity with advancing age. Most long-term toxicology studies are terminated at 18 months or 2 years with CD-1 or B6C3F1 mice, respectively. B6C3F1 mice have good longevity with 75–80% surviving to the end of 2-year studies (Goodman et al., 1985). At 2 years only 50% of CD-1 mice are still alive (Anonymous, 1982).

For the B6C3F1 mouse, extensive data have been published on the incidences of spontaneous neoplasms (Ward et al., 1979; Goodman, et al., 1985; Haseman et al., 1984, 1985; Anonymous, 1989). Although the CD-1 mouse is used in many laboratories which have developed their own databases for disease incidences, relatively little data have been published in a concise form (Lang, 1987; Percy and Jonas, 1971; Homburger, et al., 1975). For both the CD-1 and the B6C3F1 mice, there is little published data on the incidences of nonneoplastic diseases.

It is well known that factors such as nutrition, husbandry, and genetic background can affect the development of many spontaneous lesions. Necropsy protocols, tissue sampling procedures, and diagnostic criteria can also have an impact on the reported incidences of lesions; thus, it is important that each laboratory develop its own historical incidence data. Nomenclature and diagnostic criteria have been published for neoplastic lesions, providing some degree of standardization. For nonneoplastic lesions, nomenclature and diagnostic criteria are not well established. In addition, some pathologists may use a single diagnosis for a specific disease entity, i.e., nephropathy, whereas others may diagnose each of the components of the disease process. Some pathologists do not diagnose common spontaneous lesions, particularly if the lesions are minimal to mild in severity. All of these factors make it difficult to compare incidences of spontaneous nonneoplastic lesions between laboratories and even between studies evaluated by different pathologists.

Since there is some standardization of neoplastic lesions, incidence data derived from other laboratories for specific neoplasms for untreated animals of the same strain and sex can be relevant. Data from different laboratories can be used to determine whether the in-house laboratory controls really do reflect the incidences of specific neoplasms in the overall population. Such controls are also useful when little in-house laboratory data are available. With this in mind, historical control data for neoplasms with an incidence of greater than 0.5% are presented for B6C3F1 mice (Table 21) and for CD-1 mice (Table 22).

The historical control data presented in Table 21 for B6C3F1 mice are based on data from the NTP (Haseman et al., 1984, 1985). These data are derived from studies conducted at several contract laboratories. Although the data are collected from multiple laboratories, some variables have been minimized. The derivation and source of the animals as well as the diet used are controlled by the NTP. The data include only untreated controls. The data are based on all animals placed on study regardless of date of death. The NTP conducts an extensive review of the pathology portion of their studies for neoplastic lesions. Thus, the terminology for neoplastic lesions is generally comparable between studies and laboratories (Goodman et al., 1985).

The historical control data presented in Table 22 for CD-1 mice have been obtained from Hazleton Washington, Vienna, Virginia (courtesy of S. Jones and S. Weymouth). All studies were conducted between 1984 and 1989 and were dietary studies lasting approximately 78 weeks. The data are based only on animals killed at terminal sacrifice and does not include animals dying on study.

Table 21 Incidences of Primary Tumors in Untreated Control B6C3F1 Mice[a] 2-Year Studies[b]

	Male		Female	
	number of tumors (%)	Range (%)	number of tumors (%)	Range (%)
Circulatory system[c]	(1791)[d]		(1791)[d]	
Hemangioma	23(1.3)	0–14	28(1.6)	0–6
Hemangiosarcoma	56(3.1)	1–10	38(2.1)	0–8
Digestive system				
Liver[c]	(1784)[d]		(1781)[d]	
hepatoclr adenoma	179(10.0)	0–44	68(3.8)	0–18
hepatoclr carcinoma	377(21.1)	8–32	82(4.6)	0–15
Total	540(30.3)	14–58	147(8.3)	0–20
Forestomach[e]	(2252)[d]		(2336)[d]	
Squamous cell papilloma	6(0.3)	—f	12(0.5)	—f
Small intestine[e]	(2148)[d]		(2234)[d]	
adenocarcinoma	14(0.7)	—f	2(0.1)	—f
Endocrine system				
Adrenal[c]	(1716)[d]		(1722)[d]	
cortical adenoma	33(1.9)	0–8	5(0.3)	0–4
cortical carcinoma	2(0.1)	0–4	1(0.1)	0–2
pheochromocytoma	19(1.1)	0–6	13(0.8)	0–4
Pituitary[c]	(1464)[d]		(1542)[d]	
adenoma	10(0.7)	0–6	133(8.6)	0–30
carcinoma	1(0.1)	0–2	7(0.5)	0–5
Thyroid[c]	(1680)[d]		(1661)[d]	
follicular cell adenoma	26(1.5)	0–7	36(2.2)	0–8
follicular cell carcinoma	2(0.1)	0–2	7(0.4)	0–6
Hematopoietic System[c]	(1791)[d]		(1791)[d]	
Lymphoma/leukemia	224(12.5)	2–32	506(28.3)	12–62
Integumentary System[c]	(1791)[d]		(1791)[d]	
Fibroma/neurofibroma	29(1.6)	0–12	0	—
Fibrosarcoma/neurofibrosarcoma	59(3.3)	0–24	16	0–8
Sarcoma	40(2.2)	0–12	15	0–10
Musculoskeletal system[e]	(2343)[d]		(2486)[d]	
Osteosarcoma	3(0.1)	—f	14(0.6)	—f
Rhabdomyosarcoma	12(0.5)	—f	2(0.1)	—f
Reproductive system				
Ovary[e]			(2167)[d]	
Tubular adenoma			19(0.9)	—f
Uterus[c]			(1756)[d]	
endometrial stromal polyp			22(1.3)	0–6
endometrial stromal sarcoma			9(0.5)	0–4
Mammary gland[c]	(1791)[d]		(1791)[d]	
fibroadenoma	0(0.0)	—	6(0.3)	0–6
adenocarcinoma	0(0.0)	—	31(1.7)	0–12
Respiratory system[c]	(1780)[d]		(1777)[d]	
Alveolar/bronchiolar adenoma	215(12.1)	2–28	87(4.9)	0–14
Alveolar/bronchiolar carcinoma	87(4.9)	0–17	36(2.0)	0–6

Table 21   *(continued)*

	Male		Female	
	number of tumors (%)	Range (%)	number of tumors (%)	Range (%)
Special sense organs				
Harderian gland[c]	(1791)[d]		(1791)[d]	
adenoma	49(2.7)	0–12	25(1.4)	0–6
carcinoma	3(0.2)	0–2	2(0.1)	0–2

[a]Tumors with an incidence of 0.5% or greater in one or both sexes.
[b]Includes moribund sacrifice, spontaneous death, and terminal sacrifice animals.
[c]Data taken from Haseman et al., 1985.
[d]Number of animals examined.
[e]Data taken from Haseman et al., 1984.
[f]Data not available.

As mentioned above, there is little published data on the incidences of spontaneous nonneoplastic lesions in mice. Some of the more common lesions observed in CD-1 and B6C3F1 mice as well as some of the more common lesions in other strains of mice are described in the text, although incidences are generally not given. With current husbandry practices, infectious diseases are uncommon in laboratory mice and are generally not considered further in this chapter.

At necropsy, organ weights are usually taken for a number of organs. Historical control data on this information are sadly lacking in the literature. These data are included for B6C3F1 and CD-1 mice in this chapter. There can be problems in interpreting such data, and these are discussed in the section on organ weights.

CARDIOVASCULAR SYSTEM

Vessels

Nonneoplastic Lesions

Vascular Ectasia (Angiectasis).   Vascular ectasia can occur in a variety of organs and consists of dilatation of the capillaries in a focal area of the organ affected. Microscopically, angiectasis consists of dilated vascular spaces or sinusoids lined by flattened or slightly plump endothelial cells. This lesion is often seen in the ovary of aged mice. Vascular ectasia is also often seen in the mesenteric lymph node. The affected lymph nodes are often enlarged and dark red. Microscopically, there are dilated vascular channels filled with red blood cells and lined by well-differentiated endothelium. The lining of the vascular channels is sometimes incomplete. The lesion is more prominent in the medulla but can affect the cortex and, occasionally, the perimesenteric fat as well. This lesion has been referred to as mesenteric disease (Dunn, 1954). Vascular ectasia in any organ must be distinguished from vascular tumors (i.e., hemangioma or hemangiosarcoma).

Polyarteritis.   Polyarteritis in the mouse has been compared to periarteritis nodosa in man. The etiology of both is unknown, but an immune origin is suspected. In mice, the lesion involves small muscular arteries and is usually evident in multiple sites. Organs

Table 22 Incidences of Primary Tumors in Untreated Control CD-1 Mice[a] 18-Month Studies[b,c]

	Male		Female	
	Number of tumors (%)	Range (%)	Number of tumors (%)	Range (%)
Circulatory system	(363)[d]		(391)[d]	
hemangioma	5(1.4)	0–8	5(1.3)	0–3
hemangiosarcoma	9(2.5)	0–6	10(2.6)	0–12
Digestive system				
liver	(362)[d]		(391)[d]	
hepatocellular				
adenoma	35(9.7)	0–16	5(1.3)	0–5
carcinoma	19(5.2)	0–16	2(0.5)	0–3
Endocrine system				
adrenal	(362)[d]		(391)[d]	
cortical adenoma	3(0.8)	0–5	0(0.0)	—
Pituitary	(362)[d]		(391)[d]	
adenoma	0(0.0)	—	3(0.8)	0–3
Thyroid	(362)[d]		(391)[d]	
follicular cell				
adenoma	2(0.6)	0–4	0(0.0)	—
Hematopoietic system	(362)[d]	(391)[d]		
mixed cell lymphoma	2(0.6)	0–5	6(1.5)	0–6
histiocytic sarcoma (lymphoma)	0(0.0)	—	4(1.0)	0–2
lymphocytic lymphoma	8(2.2)	0–11	15(3.8)	0–17
Reproductive system				
testis	(362)[d]			
interstitial cell tumor	3(0.8)	0–5		
ovary			(391)[d]	
cystadenoma			3(0.8)	0–5
luteoma			4(1.0)	0–3
uterus			(391)[d]	
endometrial stromal polyp			14(3.6)	0–10
endometrial stromal sarcoma			2(0.5)	0–3
leiomyoma			7(1.8)	0–4
leiomyosarcoma			5(1.5)	0–5
mammary gland	(362)[d]		(391)[d]	
fibroadenoma	0(0.0)	—	1(0.3)	0–4
adenocarcinoma	0(0.0)	—	4(1.0)	0–3
Respiratory system	(362)[d]		(391)[d]	
alveolar/bronchiolar adenoma	47(13.0)	0–30	33(8.4)	0–19
alveolar/bronchiolar carcinoma	10(2.8)	0–8	8(2.0)	0–8
Special sense organs				
harderian gland	(335)[d]		(359)[d]	
adenoma	7(2.1)	0–6	3(0.8)	0–5
carcinoma	0(0.0)	—	1(0.3)	0–2

[a]Tumors with an incidence of 0.5% or greater in one or both sexes.
[b]Includes only terminal sacrifice animals.
[c]Data supplied by Ms. S. Weymouth and Dr. S. Jones of Hazelton Washington, Vienna, Virginia, 1990.
[d]Number of animals examined.

commonly involved include the heart, tongue, uterus, testis, kidney, and urinary bladder. The media of the affected vessels is homogeneous and intensely eosinophilic with hematoxylin and eosin (H&E) stain. Both fibrosis and an infiltration of mononuclear cells occur around the affected vessels. This disease is uncommon in the B6C3F1 and CD-1 strains, but it has been reported in BALB/c mice (Frith and Ward, 1988).

Neoplastic Lesions

General. Tumors of endothelial cells (hemangioma, hemangiosarcoma) can be found at any site in the body. The most common sites are the spleen and liver. The subcutis, skeletal muscle, and female reproductive tract are also other common sites (Strandberg and Goodman, 1982). Lymphangiomas and lymphangiosarcomas, tumors of lymphatics, are rare.

Hemangioma. Hemangiomas are benign tumors arising from endothelial cells lining blood vascular channels. Microscopically, they consist of dilated vascular spaces or thin-walled capillaries lined by a single layer of endothelial cells. The endothelial cells are well-differentiated and usually slightly plump. No mitotic figures are present. The connective tissue stroma is often delicate but may consist of dense collagenous tissue, particularly around the dilated spaces.

Hemangiosarcoma. Hemangiosarcomas are malignant neoplasms arising from endothelial cells lining blood vascular channels. These neoplasms may be pleomorphic. They consist of dilated vascular spaces of varying sizes which may or may not be filled with red blood cells. The cells lining the vascular spaces are plump with oval basophilic nuclei and with indistinct cell borders. There is often piling up of the lining cells. In areas of the tumor, there may be solid sheets of cells. Particularly in the spleen, the tumors may be predominantly solid. Necrosis, hemorrhage, and thrombosis are frequent. Hemangiosarcomas may metastasize, although it is usually difficult to determine the primary site. Often, there may be multiple primary sites. This is one of the reasons that the incidence of vascular tumors is calculated using the number of animals with vascular tumors regardless of site.

Heart

Nonneoplastic

General. Spontaneous nonneoplastic lesions of the heart are uncommon in CD-1 and B6C3F1 mice.

Epicardial and Myocardial Mineralization. Mineralization of the myocardium and epicardium occurs in some strains of mice as early as 1 month of age, and is more common in males than in females; it occurs most often on the right ventricle. Microscopically, the mineralized foci are characterized by distinctly basophilic areas after H&E staining, by black areas when stained with von Kossa, and red areas when stained with Alizarin Red. The mineralization may be minimal or quite extensive, covering most of the epicardial surface of the right ventricle. The mineralized areas may be surrounded by fibrosis, but an inflammatory component is minimal. The exact etiology is unknown, but the lesion appears to have a genetic predisposition (DiPaola et al., 1964; Brownstein, 1983).

Mineralization of the myocardium is also a common lesion in a number of strains of mice (Rings and Wagner, 1972). The mineralized areas are focal and may involve the myocardium of both ventricles and the interventricular septum. The atria are usually spared. The lesion appears to be a distinct entity and different from the epicardial mineralization. Microscopically, the mineralized areas stain distinctly basophilic with H&E. The focal areas of mineralization are often surrounded by fibrous connective tissue and a minimal infiltrate of mononuclear inflammatory cells is present.

Atrial Thrombosis. Atrial thrombosis is not a common lesion, but occurs as both a spontaneous and an induced lesion in mice (Schieferstein et al., 1985). The thrombus more commonly involves the left atrium. Grossly, the involved atrium is enlarged and red. Microscopically, the distended atrium contains an organizing mural thrombus. The degree of organization depends upon the age of the thrombus. Some of the thrombi may contain focal areas of cartilaginous metaplasia. If the thrombi are large, they may lead to a secondary chronic passive congestion of the lungs.

Neoplastic

Primary tumors of the heart are extremely rare in mice (Strandberg and Goodman, 1982).

DIGESTIVE SYSTEM

Salivary Glands

General

The mouse as well as many other species has three paired salivary glands—submaxillary (submandibular), parotid, and sublingual (Frith and Townsend, 1985). All three major salivary glands are closely associated and located in the subcutaneous tissue of the ventral neck area.

Sexual Dimorphism

The submandibular, or submaxillary, salivary gland is distinctly different morphologically in adult male and female mice. Immature mice of both sexes present a pattern similar to that in adult female mice, suggesting that the difference in adult males is due to the production of testosterone. In the female mouse, the acini are small and epithelial cells have centrally located nuclei and only a few cytoplasmic granules. In the adult male, the acini are much larger and the tall columnar lining epithelial cells have basally located nuclei and abundant eosinophilic cytoplasmic granules. This sexual dimorphism is not present in the rat.

Nonneoplastic Lesions

Lobular Hyperplasia and Atrophy. Lobular hyperplasia and atrophy are seen in both the submaxillary and parotid salivary glands, but are rare in the sublingual. The lesion commonly involves a single lobule in which some acini are atrophied and replaced by hyperplastic ducts.

Basophilic Foci. Chiu and Chen (1986) described the occurrence of basophilic hypertrophic foci in the parotid glands in both rats and mice. They were characterized by focal hypertrophy and hyperchromasia of acinar cells in Sprague-Dawley rats and Swiss mice. The incidence in the Swiss mice was 4.8%. The lesions were considered to be spontaneous, and their morphology and growth pattern suggested that they were neither degenerative, necrotic, hyperplastic, preneoplastic, nor neoplastic. The investigators considered them to be a distinct pathological entity of an unknown nature.

Neoplastic Lesions

Spontaneous neoplasms of the major salivary glands of mice occur relatively infrequently (Frith and Heath, 1985). Because mammary tumors often arise in the neck area immediately adjacent to the salivary glands, they have sometimes been mistakenly identified as salivary gland tumors. Careful dissection of a tumor and the contiguous normal tissues in the neck and head region, followed by histological demonstration of actual involvement of a salivary gland by the tumor is, therefore, essential if one is to have reasonably sound evidence of salivary gland origin. Any spontaneous tumor in the neck region of a female mouse of strain BALB/c, A, C58, CF-1, or any hybrid of the C and A strains is most likely to be a salivary gland tumor of myoepithelial type.

Spontaneous neoplasms of the salivary gland are extremely rare in all strains of mice (Frith and Heath, 1985). The National Toxicology Program (NTP) Carcinogenesis Bioassay Data System reported only 30 epithelial tumors from 40 chronic studies using the B6C3F1 mouse, representing approximately 8000 animals. All of these neoplasms were not personally confirmed by the authors, and some of them could have been mammary tumors. One of the authors (C.H.F.) can only recall two or three epithelial salivary gland tumors in over 20,000 BALB/c female mice from the National Center for Toxicological Research (NCTR).

Myoepithelioma. Myoepithelioma of the salivary glands is rare in mice except in certain strains (Peters et al., 1972; Delaney, 1977). It is extremely rare in the B6C3F1 and the CD-1 strains. The neoplasm may occur at a low incidence in the BALB/c mouse and is more common in the female. It develops most frequently in the submaxillary or parotid salivary glands and is rare in the sublingual gland. Myoepitheliomas have also been reported in the human parotid gland (Leifer et al., 1974). The myoepithelioma is believed to be derived from the myoepithelial cells in the salivary glands. The tumors become quite large and grossly are often cystic. Microscopically, they are composed of large pleomorphic cells, suggesting both an epithelial and a mesenchymal origin. The larger tumors commonly metastasize to the lung.

Other Tumors. Spontaneous tumors of the mouse salivary glands other than myoepitheliomas are extremely rare. Mouse polyoma virus causes salivary gland tumors, including a mesenchymal, an epithelial and a mixed epithelial/mesenchymal type (Dawe, 1979). Polyoma virus infection does not occur as a spontaneous disease.

Pancreas

Nonneoplastic Lesions

Acinar Atrophy and Fatty Replacement. Atrophy of the acinar pancreas with fatty replacement occurs at a low incidence in mice and may be lobular or diffuse. The existing islets appear normal and are embedded in a stroma of adipose tissue. Occasionally, the adipose tissue contains a chronic inflammatory cell infiltrate. The occurrence of the lesion only in aged mice suggests that it is a true atrophy and not hypoplasia.

Neoplastic Lesions

Acinar Cell Tumors. Acinar cell tumors have been described in the rat (Boorman and Eustis, 1985), but they are extremely rare in the mouse (Prejean et al., 1973; Cavaliere et al., 1981).

Esophagus

Nonneoplastic

Esophageal Rupture. Rupture of the esophagus is seen in mice as a result of oral intubation and gavage. If the animal survives, an associated inflammatory reaction is present. The lesion is usually fatal.

Neoplastic Lesions

Papilloma and Squamous Cell Carcinoma.   Papillomas and squamous cell carcinomas have been reported in the rat (Cardesa and Ovelar, 1985; Ovelar and Cardesa, 1985), but appear to be rare in the mouse. The experimental production of papillomas has been reported in the mouse (Horie et al., 1965).

Stomach

Normal Anatomy

The stomach of both the mouse and the rat is divided into a glandular (forestomach) and a nonglandular stomach. The two regions are separated by a ridge around the entrance of the esophagus. The ridge is formed by the thickened lamina propria of the nonglandular stomach. The nonglandular stomach is lined by stratified squamous epithelium, and the glandular stomach is lined by glandular epithelium. The glandular region contains three types of glands: cardiac, pyloric, and fundic.

Nonneoplastic Lesions

Glandular Hyperplasia.   Hyperplasia of the glandular gastric mucosa may occasionally be seen in mice (Rehm et al., 1987). The lesion may be either focal of diffuse in nature.

Squamous Cell Hyperplasia of the Forestomach.   The forestomach (nonglandular stomach) of the mouse is lined by stratified squamous epithelium which may occasionally become hyperplastic. This lesion may result from the oral administration of toxic irritants.

Neoplastic Lesions

Adenoma and Adenocarcinoma of the Glandular Stomach.   Adenoma and adenocarcinoma of the gastric mucosa are rare in mice. Adenomas are usually well circumscribed and delineated from the normal mucosa. The cells within the adenomas are well differentiated. Gastric adenocarcinomas are invasive and infiltrate into the lamina propria and muscularis.

Squamous Cell Papilloma and Carcinoma of the Forestomach.   Squamous cell papilloma and carcinoma occur in the nonglandular stomach. Papillomas are composed of a stalk with a vascular connective tissue core covered by neoplastic squamous epithelium. Squamous cell carcinomas are usually relatively well differentiated and produce keratin. They are locally invasive and may occasionally metastasize to the lungs.

Intestine

Noneoplastic Lesions

Intussusception and Rectal Prolapse.   Intussusception may occur in both the large and small intestines and may lead to intestinal obstruction, inflammation, necrosis and death. Prolapse of the rectum may be associated with a pinworm infestion or *Citrobacter* infection (Barthold, 1978); it is characterized by an eversion of the mucosal surface of the rectum exposed through the anus.

Pinworms.   Pinworms in mice commonly involve two species, *Syphacia obvelata* and *Apicularis tetraptera*. They are usually found in the colon and sections of the parasite may be seen microscopically in the colonic lumen of infected mice. Pinworms are not usually associated with any pathological changes in the large intestine, but occasionally intussusception or rectal prolapse may occur.

Neoplastic Lesions

Adenoma and Adenocarcinoma.   Adenomas of the small intestine are frequently small and may not be detected if the intestine is unopened during gross examination. They are especially common in the duodenum. Microscopically, the adenoma appears as a poly-poid epithelial growth projecting into the lumen of the intestine. The epithelium is relatively well differentiated, but usually appears more basophilic than adjacent normal epithelium. Adenocarcinomas are composed of more anaplastic or pleomorphic cells, which may project into the lumen as well as infiltrate into and beyond the submucosa and tunica muscularis. Adenocarcinomas frequently are cystic or papillary and microscopically show many mitotic figures.

Leiomyoma and Leiomyosarcoma. Smooth muscle tumors of the small intestine are relatively uncommon. Leiomyomas are usually well-circumscribed lesions composed of well-differentiated smooth muscle cells. Leiomyosarcomas are not well circumscribed and neoplastic smooth muscle cells may infiltrate the submucosa and serosa.

ENDOCRINE SYSTEM

Adrenal Gland

Nonneoplastic Lesions

Subcapsular Cell Hyperplasia. Many strains of mice develop proliferations of spindle cells in the subcapsular region of the adrenal cortex (Dunn, 1970; Goodman, 1983). The proliferating cells may extend downward into and through the zona glomerulosa and zona fasciculata. The cells are fusiform or oval with spindle-shaped nuclei and scant basophilic cytoplasm. The spindle cells have been referred to as type A cells (Dunn, 1970) and are the most common type seen. Type B cells are occasionally found. These are large polygonal cells with abundant eosinophilic cytoplasm and round vesicular nuclei.

This lesion is rare in young mice but increases in incidence and severity with age. It is more common in females than in males. The actual incidence is not well documented as many pathologists do not report this lesion unless severe. Gonadectomy or gonadal atrophy often enhances development of this lesion.

Cortical Hyperplasia and Hypertrophy. Small focal lesions are occasionally found involving primarily the zona fasciculata of the adrenal cortex. There may be increased numbers of cells per unit area within the focus compared to the adjacent cortex (hyperplasia). These cells are smaller than normal cortical cells. In other foci, the cells may be enlarged with abundant eosinophilic cytoplasm (hypertrophy). Some foci contain both types of cells. Compression is minimal or nonexistent. These lesions must be distinguished from cortical adenomas.

Medullary Hyperplasia. Foci of small- to normal-size pheochromocytes with basophilic cytoplasm are occasionally found in the adrenal medulla. There is little if any compression of surrounding tissue and the edges of the focus blend in with adjacent medullary parenchyma.

Lipofuscin. Pigmented macrophages are commonly observed at the corticomedullary junction in aged mice of many strains. This lesion has also been referred to as ceroid deposition, or "brown degeneration" (Dunn, 1970; Frith, 1983c). At first, the pigment appears as yellow-brown faintly granular material in the cortical cells adjacent to the medulla. As the lesion increases in severity, the cells become enlarged with abundant foamy brown to yellow cytoplasm and small pyknotic nuclei. Occasional multinucleate giant cells are found. The pigment is PAS positive and acid fast. This lesion is often not diagnosed unless severe, so accurate incidence figures are unavailable.

Other Nonneoplastic Lesions. Amyloidosis of the adrenal cortex may be seen in the adrenal cortex, usually in the zona fasciculata (Sass, 1983). Amyloidosis is discussed under the section on Multisystem Diseases. Accessory adrenal cortical tissue, often in close approximation to the adrenal gland, is observed sporadically (Sass, 1983).

Neoplastic Lesions

Subcapsular Cell Adenoma (A-Cell Adenoma). These tumors are nodular masses composed of spindle-shaped (type A) cells comparable to those seen in subcapsular cell hyperplasia and causing compression of the adjacent adrenal cortex. Large polygonal type B cells are often found interspersed among the spindle cells, either singly or in nests.

Cortical Adenoma (B-Cell Adenoma). Cortical B-cell adenomas consist of nodules of well-differentiated cortical cells which are demarcated from and compress the adjacent parenchyma (Frith, 1983a). There is distortion and loss of the normal cord arrangement. The cells are polygonal with abundant eosinophilic cytoplasm and round vesicular nuclei. The presence of mitoses is variable.

Pheochromocytoma. Pheochromocytomas are tumors of the adrenal medulla (Frith, 1983d), and are composed of polyhedral cells with amphophilic or basophilic cytoplasm and basally located nuclei. The cells are arranged in trabeculae or nests separated by dilated vascular spaces. There is compression of the adjacent tissue. It is difficult to distinguish benign from malignant pheochromocytomas on the basis of cytology. By convention, tumors which have invaded the adrenal capsule or have spread beyond the adrenal gland are diagnosed as malignant. Those still within the adrenal gland, even if replacing most of the adrenal cortex, are considered benign.

Other Neoplasms. Malignant tumors of the adrenal gland, subcapsular cell carcinoma, cortical carcinoma, or malignant pheochromocytomas are uncommon. They resemble their benign counterpart morphologically, but they may exhibit more atypia, loss of architecture, and evidence of invasion or metastasis. Ganglioneuromas have been reported infrequently.

Pituitary Gland

Nonneoplastic Lesions

Pituitary Cysts and Cystoid Degeneration. True pituitary cysts, lined by epithelium, have been described in mice, primarily in the anterior lobe (Carlton and Gries, 1983). These cysts are usually microscopic and lined by ciliated cuboidal to columnar epithelium. Variable-sized foci, where there is a loss of parenchymal cells, are frequently seen in the anterior pituitary of mice. These spaces are frequently referred to as cysts, although cystoid degeneration (Cameron and Sheldon, 1983) might be more appropriate. The spaces are lined by the cells normally found in the anterior pituitary and are usually filled with faintly granular eosinophilic material. This lesion is often seen in association with hyperplasia or adenomas of the pituitary.

Hyperplasia of the Anterior Pituitary. Hyperplasia of the anterior pituitary may be either focal or diffuse. Focal hyperplasia is more common and more easily recognized. The cells comprising the focus are of a single cell type and may be any of the cell types found in the anterior pituitary. Most frequently, they resemble chromophobes; i.e., large, pale cells with round nuclei. The borders of the foci blend into the adjacent parenchyma with little if any compression.

Neoplastic Lesions

Adenoma of the Anterior Pituitary. Adenomas of the anterior pituitary are common in female B6C3F1 and CD-1 mice and are infrequent in males. Adenomas of the anterior pituitary, like the hyperplasias, are composed of a single cell type, usually one which appears to be a chromophobe. The cells are arranged in solid sheets or in cords, often separated by dilated blood-filled sinusoids. There is compression of the adjacent parenchyma. Cellular atypia may be present. It is difficult to distinguish between adenomas and carcinomas on cytology alone. By convention, if the tumor has invaded the brain or adjacent bone, it is considered malignant. If confined to the pituitary even if causing compression of the brain, it is regarded as benign, even if atypia is present.

Other Neoplasms. Occasional neoplasms of the pars intermedia have been reported (Goodman et al., 1981).

Thyroid Gland

Nonneoplastic Lesions

Cystic Follicles. Individual follicles may become enlarged and distended with colloid. The cystic follicles are lined by a single layer of cuboidal or flattened follicular epithelium. Large follicles are normally found at the periphery of the thyroid.

Follicular cell Hyperplasia. The lesion may be focal, multifocal, or diffuse. The affected follicles are of variable sizes. The epithelium is cuboidal to tall columnar, hyperchromatic, and at times multilayered, although this is not a prominent feature. The hyperplastic epithelium may form papillary projections into the lumen or form multiple small follicles within an enlarged follicle (cystic hyperlasia).

Neoplastic Lesions

Follicular cell Adenoma. Adenomas are discrete, well-circumscribed, but nonencapsulated lesions which often cause compression of the adjacent parenchyma. The tumors may have papillary, follicular, or solid patterns (Heath and Frith, 1983). The cells are hyperchromatic, variable in size, and often have a high nuclear to cytoplasmic ratio. The cells are often multilayered, and nuclear crowding is common. The mitotic rate is usually low.

Follicular cell Carcinoma. Carcinomas may have a papillary, solid, or follicular pattern or combinations thereof (Heath and Frith, 1983). The lesion is often at least partially encapsulated with a dense scirrhous reaction and neoplastic cells or follicles within the capsule. The cells are pleomorphic with a high nuclear to cytoplasmic ratio. The mitotic rates are variable but often high. Invasion of adjacent structures is common.

Other Neoplasms. C-Cell adenomas and carcinomas are extremely uncommon in mice (Squire et al., 1978; Russfield, 1982; Frith and Heath, 1983; van Zwieten et al., 1983).

Parathyroid

Spontaneous lesions, both neoplastic and nonneoplastic, are uncommon in mice (Squire et al., 1978; Russfield, 1982).

Pancreatic Islets

Nonneoplastic Lesions

Islet Cell Hyperplasia. Hyperplasia of the pancreatic islets usually involves more than one islet (multifocal), and may involve all islets visible in a histologic section. Certain mouse strains have high incidences of this lesion (Sass et al., 1978). The islets are much enlarged owing to an increased number of cells, which morphologically are similar to those in smaller normal islets. The specific cell type is difficult to identify at the light microscopic level, and the histochemistry and electron microscopy are often needed. Immunoperoxidase staining of the hyperplastic islets has revealed that most of the cells contain insulin and some contain somatostatin.

Neoplastic Lesions

Islet Cell Adenoma.   Islet cell adenomas in mice commonly involve a single islet within a histological section (Frith and Sheldon, 1983), are larger than hyperplastic islets, and compress adjacent normal pancreas. The cells form ribbons along sinusoidal, thin-walled vessels, and the adenomas often appear more vascular than hyperplastic islets. The cells stain lightly eosinophilic with hematoxylin and eosin; the nuclei demonstrate a delicate chromatin pattern. The cells are well differentiated, and mitotic figures are few in number.

Islet Cell Carcinoma.   Islet cell carcinomas are invariably larger than adenomas and are commonly visible grossly. The cells vary from well-differentiated cells to extremely pleomorphic and anaplastic cells (Frith and Sheldon, 1983). Well-differentiated islet cell carcinomas usually invade locally and occasionally metastasize. Most tumors are probably insulinomas. The cytoplasm of the neoplastic cells is eosinophilic and the nuclei are vesicular. Nucleoli are prominent and may be multiple. Mitotic figures are evident and pleomorphism may be prominent. Some anaplastic carcinomas may be difficult to classify with certainty as islet cell in origin.

FEMALE GENITAL SYSTEM

Ovary

Nonneoplastic Lesions

Ovarian Cysts.   Cysts of the ovary and paraovarian tissues are extremely common in aged females of most strains of mice (Goodman, et al., 1981; Burek, et al., 1982; Frith and Ward, 1988). They may be focal or multifocal and may become quite large, compressing and replacing most of the ovary in some instances. Because of this, it is often difficult to interpret possible toxic lesions of the ovary in aged animals. The cysts are lined by flattened to low cuboidal epithelium which occasionally may become hyperplastic, forming small papillary fronds. There are often foci of chronic inflammatory cells in the capsule. Pigment-laden macrophages are also common. The cysts may be filled with clear fluid or may be hemorrhagic.

Lipofuscin.   Lipofuscin or aging pigment is common in the ovarian stroma of aged female mice. Lipofuscinosis is characterized by large round cells with abundant foamy pale yellow pigmented cytoplasm present in the ovarian stroma. The pigment is acid fast and PAS positive.

Tubular Hyperplasia.   Tubular hyperplasia consists of a proliferation of the germinal epithelium into the ovarian stroma forming foci of tubules and cleftlike spaces lined by cuboidal to low columnar epithelium. The cells have small round nuclei and scant cytoplasm.

Interstitial Cell (Stromal/Luteal) Hyperplasia.   The lesion consists of enlargement and increased number of interstitial cells. The cells contain abundant foamy cytoplasm and are arranged in nests and packets by delicate stromal fibers.

Neoplastic Lesions

Tubular Adenoma. These neoplasms arise by downgrowth of the germinal epithelium into the ovarian stroma. The tubules are similar to those seen in tubular hyperplasia. The tubular structures replace the entire ovary and occasionally invade paraovarian fat (Carter, 1968; Frith et al., 1981; Goodman, et al., 1981; Goodman and Strandberg, 1982; Morgan and Alison, 1987b; Frith and Ward, 1988). These tumors are the most common ovarian tumor seen in the B6C3F1 mouse. They are also the most common type of tumor induced, either alone or in combination with granulosa cell tumors.

Cystadenoma. Ovarian cystadenomas are sporadically seen in many strains of mice (Carter, 1968; Frith et al., 1981a; Goodman et al., 1981; Goodman and Strandberg, 1982; Morgan and Alison, 1987a; Frith and Ward, 1988). Microscopically, they are cystic tumors lined by cuboidal to columnar epithelium with basal nuclei. There are usually simple to complex papillary structures projecting into the lumen and lined by similar epithelium.

Luteoma. Luteomas are composed of large polygonal cells with abundant pale cyto-plasm and round central nuclei. The cells are arranged in nests and cords. The tumors are generally well circumscribed, although not encapsulated, and often involve the greater portion of the ovary (Carter, 1968; Frith et al., 1981a; Goodman, et al., 1981; Goodman and Strandberg, 1982; Frith and Ward, 1988). These tumors are the most common type of ovarian tumor seen in the CD-1 mouse.

Other Neoplasms. Granulosa cell tumors and teratomas are occasionally seen in mice. Dysgerminomas and Sertoli cell tumors are extremely rare (Carter, 1968; Frith et al., 1981a; Alison and Morgan, 1987a,b; Frith and Ward, 1988).

Uterus

Nonneoplastic Lesions

Cystic Endometrial Hyperplasia. This lesion is extremely common in aged female mice (Goodman, et al., 1981; Burek et al., 1982; Frith and Ward, 1988). There is both proliferation and dilatation of the endometrial glands. The glands are lined by columnar epithelium and the lumens are often filled with eosinophilic material. In severe lesions, large cysts may develop. These are lined with low cuboidal or flattened epithelium.

Hydrometra. Marked dilatation of the lumen of the uterus with fluid or mucoid material is termed hydrometra. The wall of the uterus is thinned and there is loss of the endometrial glands. The lumen is filled with faint fibrillar eosinophilic fluid or mucoid material. The cause of the hydrometra often cannot be determined microscopically.

Neoplastic Lesions

Endometrial Stromal Polyp. These neoplasms occur frequently in many strains of mice (Goodman and Strandberg, 1982). They are small morbid excrescences that project into the uterine cavity. Microscopically, the mass consists of an edematous stroma composed of spindle-shaped or stellate cells and varying numbers of endometrial glands, which may be cystic. The stroma is often highly vascular. The surface is covered by a single layer of simple columnar epithelium.

Endometrial Stromal Sarcoma. These neoplasms arise in the endometrium and are composed of sheets of spindle cells with scant pale eosinophilic cytoplasm and elongated, hyperchromatic, fusiform nuclei. Cell borders are usually indistinct. The cells may be organized in fasciculi which run at angles or perpendicular to one another and in which the nuclei, cut in cross-section, may appear round or oval. Occasional areas may be present in which the fusiform nuclei may appear plump and contain vacuoles. Areas of necrosis are common. Cellular atypia and mitotic figures may be present but are variable. Spread is by infiltration into the myometrium, cervix, and serosa. Metastasis is infrequent. It is necessary to distinguish endometrial stromal sarcoma from mesenchymal tumors such as leiomyosarcoma or fibrosarcoma (Goodman and Strandberg, 1982) as well as histiocytic sarcoma (Frith et al., 1981b).

Leiomyoma. Leiomyomas are benign tumors of smooth muscle which are well circumscribed. They are composed of interlacing, compact bundles of fusiform smooth muscle fibers which frequently run perpendicular to each other. The nuclei are elongate with round to blunt ends and are centrally located. These tumors are seen more frequently in CD-1 mice than in B6C3F1 mice.

Leiomyosarcoma. These neoplasms are malignant tumors of smooth muscle. They infiltrate the uterine wall and invade through the serosa. The cells are less well-differentiated smooth muscle cells than those seen in leiomyomas and are arranged in interlacing or whirling patterns. Mitotic activity is variable.

Vagina

Spontaneous lesions of the vagina are rare in mice of all strains. (Goodman and Strandberg, 1982; Frith and Ward, 1988).

Mammary Gland

Nonneoplastic Lesions

Spontaneous nonneoplastic lesions of the mammary gland are uncommon in B6C3F1 and CD-1 mice. Ectasia of mammary ducts or focal hyperplasia of the acinar tissue are occasionally observed.

Neoplastic Lesions

Adenocarcinoma. Adenocarcinomas in mice have been traditionally classified as adenocarcinoma types A, B, or C, adenoacanthoma, or carcinosarcoma (Dunn, 1959), although other types have been reported (Sass and Dunn, 1979; Medina, 1982). In many toxicology studies, the type of carcinoma is not specified. In the B6C3F1 mouse, the type seen most frequently is the adenocarcinoma type C. This neoplasm is characterized by variable-sized cystic structures surrounded by abundant, delicate connective tissue. The glands are lined by a single layer of low cuboidal epithelium with oval nuclei arranged at various angles to the basement membrane. The glands are surrounded by one to several layers of spindle cells, presumably myoepithelial cells. Metastases are rare. In the CD-1 mouse, the most common mammary adenocarcinoma is adenocarcinoma type B. These tumors are pleomorphic in appearance, with a variety of morphological patterns. They may be composed of nests and acini, solid sheets of cells, or they may form papillary or cystic structures. The cells are cuboidal with oval or round nuclei and scant cytoplasm. The amount of stroma is variable. These neoplasms may metastaze to the lungs.

Clitoral Gland

Nonneoplastic Lesions

Cystic Ducts (Ectasia). Dilatation of the ducts of the clitoral glands occurs frequently and may be associated with inflammatory changes, either acute or chronic.

Neoplastic Lesions

Neoplasms of the clitoral gland are very uncommon. They must be distinguished from sebaceous gland tumors.

HEMATOPOIETIC SYSTEM

Nonneoplastic Lesions

Thymic Cysts

Thymic cysts have been seen in a number of strains of mice and they generally increase in incidence with age (Frith and Wiley, 1981). The cysts are lined by a simple cuboidal epithelium and the lumen is usually empty. They are more commonly located in the medulla.

Thymic Atrophy

Atrophy of the thymus increases with age and in response to certain toxicants, viruses, or irradiation. In the severely atrophic thymus, the distinction between cortex and medulla cannot be made, and all cell types are decreased in number. Historical data from carcinogenicity studies usually do not reflect the true incidence of atrophy because the lesion is expected and many pathologists do not identify the change as a lesion.

Ectopic Thymus

Ectopic thymus has been reported by investigators adjacent to or in association with the parathyroid gland. The ectopic tissue is predominantly cortical thymic tissue.

Accessory Spleen

A small accessory spleen is occasionally noted in mice. The accessory spleen is usually near the normal spleen and may be embedded in the pancreas. Normal red and white pulp may be present.

Splenic Pigmentation

Both hemosiderin and melanin pigment may occur in the spleens of mice. Hemosiderin is golden brown and usually present in the cytoplasm of macrophages or reticular cells. It stains positively with iron stains such as Prussian blue. Hemosiderin is found to some extent in mice of all ages and increases in amount with age. Its presence is usually not diagnosed unless severe, although this may vary with the pathologist. When diagnosed inconsistently in a study, false-positive or false-negative trends may develop. Melanin pigment may occur in the spleen of mice with pigmented skin. It is slightly darker than hemosiderin and has a characteristic elongated or stringy appearance. It is not associated with macrophages and is iron negative.

Extramedullary Hematopoiesis

Extramedullary hematopoiesis is normally found in the spleen of mice. The degree of hematopoiesis may vary from strain-to-strain. The erythropoietic activity is characterized by foci of immature erythrocytic precursors with small darkly staining nuclei in the red pulp. Certain neoplastic conditions may markedly stimulate erythropoietic activity.

The erythropoietic activity in the spleen may or may not be associated by an increase in the granulopoietic activity. A generalized increase in granulopoiesis may be accompanied by granulopoietic elements in a variety of other organs, including the liver, adrenals, and lymph nodes. This is also referred to as a leukemoid reaction. A marked increase in granulopoietic activity must be distinguished from granulocytic leukemia. In granulopoiesis, the complete series of developing cells, including the mature neutrophils, are usually present. In granulocytic leukemia, the developing stage of the neoplastic granulo-cytes may vary from animal-to-animal, but typically a single stage predominates (Dunn, 1954). In addition, marked hyperplasia of granulocytic elements is usually accompanied by lesions responsible for the hyperplasia including abscesses, ulcerative tumors, or other inflammatory lesions.

Sinus Histiocytosis

Accumulations of histiocytes may occur in the subcapsular and medullary sinuses of lymph nodes. The histiocytes have dark basophilic nuclei and abundant distinctly eosinophilic cytoplasm. They may contain hemosiderin and other pigments, erythrocytes, and other phagocytized material.

Plasmacytosis

Plasmacytosis is an increased number of normal-appearing plasma cells in lymph nodes. The plasmacytosis may be a reaction to an adjacent chronic inflammatory lesion or to tumor antigens. The most common lymph node involved is the submandibular lymph node.

Lymphoid Hyperplasia

Hyperplasia of a variety of cell types may occur in hematopoietic tissue of mice. Lymphoid hyperplasia of the lymph nodes is one of the more common lesions, but it is rare in mice under 12 months of age. The incidence increases slightly with age and is slightly greater in females than in males in most strains. Hyperplasia may be seen in the B-cell areas (follicles, germinal centers), T-cell thymic-dependent areas (paracortex), and medullary cords or sinuses. In the common hyperplastic lymph node, the normal corti-comedullary division is usually not apparent (paracortical hyperplasia) and the marginal sinus is often filled with lymphocytes. The lymphocytes are usually small and normal in appearance. The lesion is difficult to distinguish from the lymphoblastic type of malignant lymphoma if only a single node is involved; but the lymphocytes are mature, few mitotic figures are observed, and the "starry sky" effect found in lymphoblastic lymphomas is not seen. Thickening of the medullary cords often is noted and is characterized by the presence of many plasma cells (plasmacytosis), occasionally resembling plasmacytoma. The plasmacytosis is a reaction to chronic inflammatory lesions or tumor antigens.

Mastocytosis

An increase in mast cells (mastocytosis) may occur in either the spleen or in lymph nodes. Occasionally, focal accumulations of mast cells may occur in other organs such as the ovary or uterus. Investigators have also noted mast cells associated with certain tumors (Cramer and Simpson, 1944). The number of mast cells normally found in a specific organ may vary from strain-to-strain (Dunn, 1969).

Miscellaneous Lesions

Megakaryocytosis, bone marrow atrophy, necrosis, and atrophy and mineralization of lymph nodes may occur in mice, but all are rare in both trhe CD-1 and B6C3F1 strains.

Neoplastic Lesions

Dunn (1954) described neoplasms of the reticular system in the mouse as arising from stem cells, granulocytes, lymphocytes, reticular cells, and plasmacytes. She recom-mended that the term *leukemic* be used to denote these lesions irrespective of whether or not malignant cells were found in the peripheral blood. The authors of this chapter would prefer to classify individual neoplasms as either leukemic or nonleukemic, but this designation assumes less importance with the immunological classification illustrated in Table 23 adapted from Pattengale and Frith (1983).

Lymphoblastic Lymphoma

Using immunocytochemical techniques and the newer classification of murine malignant lymphomas (Pattengale and Frith, 1983, 1986; Pattengale and Taylor, 1983; Frederickson et al., 1985; Frith et al., 1985) the lymphoblastic type is comparable to Dunn's lymphocytic leukemia. This disease is one of the more common hematopoietic neoplasms in many strains of mice and may occur as early as 1 month of age (T lymphoblastic). It may develop from either T or B lymphocytes, it may be spontaneous, or it may be induced by retroviruses, chemicals, or irradiation. The incidence of lymphoblastic lymphoma usually increases slightly in all strains with age and at 3–6 months may have a slight peak (T lymphoblastic) in some strains such as the BALB/c and a major peak in AKR mice. The incidence is generally higher in female than in male mice. Lymphoblastic lymphoma often involves a number of organs, most commonly the liver, spleen, thymus, lymph nodes, bone marrow, and lungs, but it often arises in the thymus (T lymphoblastic). The disease results in an enlargement of most involved organs owing to the proliferation of neoplastic lymphoid cells. Neoplastic lymphocytes are often present in the blood, and in such cases the neoplasm should be classified as leukemic. The neoplastic lymphocytes have large or small nucleoli, round vesicular nuclei, and a small amount of cytoplasm. This is the most common hematopoietic tumor in the CD-1 mouse, and it is often referred to as lymphocytic lymphoma.

Follicular Center Cell Lymphoma

Dunn's (1954) reticulum cell sarcoma type B has been referred to as malignant lymphoma, mixed cell type (Frith and Wiley, 1981), or pleomorphic cell type, and more recently has been identified as a follicular center cell lymphoma (FCC) of B-cell origin (Pattengale and Frith, 1983; Pattengale and Taylor, 1983; Frederickson et al., 1985). The spleen, mesenteric lymph nodes, and Peyer's patches of the ileum are the most commonly involved sites. The disease is rare before 12 months of age and may increase dramatically

Table 23 Immunomorphological Classification of Murine Lymphomas, Related Leukemias or Tumors

Morphological type	Immunological type			
	B cell	T cell	Non-B, Non-T	Histiocyte
Follicle center cell				
small cell type	+	–	–	–
large cell type	+	–	–	–
large and small (mixed) cell type	+	–	–	–
Plasma cell	+	–	–	–
Immunoblast	+	(+)[a]	(+)	–
Small lymphocyte	+	(+)	(+)	–
Lymphoblast	+	+	+	–
Histiocyte	–	–	–	+

[a]Parentheses indicate that the disease has been seen in humans, but to date has not been reported in the mouse.
Source: Adapted from Pattengale and Frith (1983).

in some strains after 18 months. This neoplasm is slightly more common in female than in male mice. This is the most common hematopoietic neoplasm in B6C3F1 mice. Many references still use the term *mixed cell lymphoma* for this neoplasm.

Microscopically, FCC lymphomas present a background of large, pale transformed B lymphocytes. In the spleen, the lesion originates in the germinal centers of the follicles in the B-cell areas of the white pulp and often results in a grossly nodular appearance. These lymphomas may be composed of small follicular center cells, large follicular center cells, or a mixture of small and large follicular center cells. The small and large cell mixture appears to be the most common type. In lymphomas of small FCCs, the cells are cohesive and nuclei are markedly irregular in size and shape with scant cytoplasm. In lymphomas composed of large FCCs, the cells are large and cohesive with irregularly shaped folded and notched nuclei (cleaved) and moderate amounts of cytoplasm. The B-cell nature of these cells has been confirmed using immunoperoxidase techniques with Bouin's or B-5 fixed tumors demonstrating the presence of cytoplasmic or cell surface immunoglobulin (CIg) of the various isotypes. The FCC lymphoma also commonly involves the mesenteric lymph nodes.

Histiocytic Sarcoma

Dunn's (1954) reticulum cell neoplasm type A, or malignant lymphoma (Frith et al., 1981b), histiocytic type, or histiocytic lymphoma, has been recently classified as histiocytic sarcoma (Pattengale and Frith, 1983). Other investigators have described the lesion as endometrial sarcoma (Chouroulinkov et al., 1969; Dawson et al., 1974) or malignant schwannoma (Stewart et al., 1974). Research findings have suggested that the neoplastic cells are derived from histiocytic cells of uncertain origin (tissue histiocytes, Kupffer's cells, macrophages) (Frith et al., 1981). Histiocytic sarcomas are rare until 12 months of age and, again, slightly more common in females than in males. The liver is the most commonly involved organ in male mice; in females, the uterus and vagina as well as the liver are often involved, suggesting these tissues as sites of origin. Other organs less frequently involved include the spleetn, lymph node, bone marrow, lung, kidney, and ovaries. Metastatic lesions to the lungs occur in a high percentage of cases with liver involvement. This neoplasm is common in both CD-1 and B6C3F1 mice.

Other Neoplasms

Plasma cell lymphomas occur infrequently in control mice. The lymph nodes, spleen, and liver may be involved. The cells are large with amphophilic cytoplasm, some are binucleated, the mitotic index is high, and the cells retain a characteristic plasma cell appearance. Spontaneous plasma cell myelomas are rare, but intraperitoneal plasma cell tumors can be induced with intraperitoneal injections of mineral oil.

Immunoblastic lymphoma of B-cell origin is rare in the mouse (Pattengale and Frith, 1983). It is characterized by noncohesive, large lymphoid cells with round to oval vesicular nuclei with prominent and distinct nucleoli. In addition, the nuclei are sometimes eccentric and have clumped, peripherally marginated clock face–like chromatin, and the cytoplasm is moderately dense and amphophilic (plasmacytoid features).

The term thymoma is usually used in the mouse to classify a lesion characterized by the presence of a neoplastic epithelial component with or without neoplastic lymphocytes. The epithelial component appears to be derived from the epithelial cells in Hassall's corpuscles or thymic reticular tissue. This type of tumor is rare in all strains of mice.

Other rare nonlymphoid hematopoietic neoplasms in the mouse include, mast cell tumor (Deringer and Dunn, 1947; Dunn, 1969; Frith et al., 1976), granulocytic leukemia (Dunn, 1954; Frith and Wiley, 1981), and erythroleukemia (Frith et al., 1990).

INTEGUMENT

Nonneoplastic Lesions

Alopecia

Alopecia or hair loss on the face and back is common in mice and appears to be associated with friction contact with feeding jars. Alopecia also occurs on the thorax and abdomen of B6C3F1 mice, the cause of which is unknown (Burek et al., 1982).

Neoplastic Lesions

General

Subcutaneous mesenchymal tumors are much more common in mice than are epithelial neoplasms (Goodman, et al., 1981; Holland and Fry, 1982). Malignant mesenchymal tumors are usually characterized by the predominant or most malignant pattern observed. However, in mice, these neoplasms appear to represent a spectrum. Because of this, some pathologists do not separate the different types and may group these tumors under a single term such as fibrosarcoma or sarcoma NOS (sarcoma not otherwise specified). These tumors are common in male B6C3F1 mice, and there is some evidence that they may be associated with fighting and chronic trauma in group-housed male mice (Squire, 1990).

Fibroma

These tumors are composed of fusiform or stellate cells with pale, ovoid, or rounded nuclei. The cells produce interlacing bundles of collagen fibers, which may be densely packed or loosely arranged as if separated by edema or a mucinous ground substance. The tumors are relatively well circumscribed and noninvasive.

Fibrosarcoma

These tumors are the malignant counterpart of the fibromas. Fibrosarcomas are more cellular than fibromas and produce less collagen. They are locally invasive and may metastasize.

Neurofibrosarcoma

These neoplasms are similar to fibrosarcomas and are characterized by bundles of cells and fibers that are arranged in whorls which when cut longitudinally produce a herring bone pattern. They are believed to arise from nerve sheaths. Many pathologists do not differentiate these tumors from fibrosarcomas.

Sarcomas (not otherwise specified, NOS)

Sarcomas NOS are extremely cellular tumors which may contain large bizarre nuclei, mitotic figures, and multinucleated giant cells. A pattern of interwoven bundles of fusiform cells may be apparent but collagen fibers are difficult to demonstrate in any quantity even with polarized light. They may be locally invasive and metastasize.

LIVER AND BILIARY SYSTEM

Liver

Nonneoplastic Lesions

Extramedullary Hematopoiesis. Extramedullary hematopoiesis is normally present in both the fetal and neonatal mouse liver. The lesion may also occur in the adult mouse liver secondary to either an infectious disease or neoplasia. When the predominant cell type is the granulocyte, granulopoietic hyperplasia may be specified, and if nucleated erythrocytes are the prominent cells, erythropoietic hyperplasia is an appropriate term. In the mouse liver, the granulocytic activity seems maximal in the sinusoids adjoining the portal vein (Dunn, 1954). Megakaryocytes may be associated with the areas of hematopoiesis.

Fatty Metamorphosis. Fatty metamorphosis may occur in mice as a response to a toxicant. It is also seen in old obese controls and is more common in male than in female mice. The degree of fatty metamorphosis may vary and usually starts with a centrilobular distribution. The empty clear vacuoles with the peripherally located compressed nuclei represent lipid which has been removed during tissue processing. The lipid can be confirmed by staining frozen sections with Oil Red O or Sudan Black B.

Hemosiderosis. Hemosiderin pigment may be found in Kupffer's cells within the liver. The pigment is a distinctive granular, golden color within the cytoplasm of Kupffer's cells. Occasionally special stains such as Prussian Blue may be used to confirm the presence of iron to differentiate it from other pigments such as bile or ceroid.

Ceroid Pigment (Lipofuscin). Ceroid is a lipofuscin pigment which is acid fast and periodic acid Schiff (PAS) positive. An increase of ceroid pigmentation has been associated with aging mice in certain organs, including the ovaries and adrenals. Ceroid pigment in the liver may also occur as a result of hepatic toxicants. The pigment is slightly darker brown than hemosiderin, and is usually present in the cytoplasm of Kupffer's cells adjacent to portal areas.

Necrosis. Focal hepatic necrosis is a nonspecific entity quite often encountered as an incidental finding in the liver of mice. It can be the result of viruses (mouse hepatitis), bacteria (*Bacillus piliformis*), toxicants, and ischemia; however, the etiology is often unknown. It may involve single cells, single or multiple lobules, and it may vary in distribution. Coagulation necrosis with distinct eosinophilic cytoplasm and pyknotic or absent nuclei is the typical morphological feature. Cell outlines are usually distinct and an associated inflammatory reaction depends upon the duration of the lesion.

Microgranulomas. Microgranulomas are commonly seen in small numbers in the livers of many strains of mice. They consist of small collections of macrophages and lymphocytes within the sinusoids or surrounding a single necrotic hepatocyte. The cause of these lesions is unknown. Periodic showering of bacteria from the intestine through the blood stream has been suggested as a possible cause.

Karyomegaly and Cytomegaly. A striking histological feature of the livers of aged mice is the presence of hepatic cells with enlarged nuclei of variable size. The enlarged nuclei may be rounded or elongated and generally are two or more times normal in size. The polyploid cells appear with increasing frequency as aging occurs (Jones, 1967). This increase in nuclear size (karyomegaly) may or may not be associated with an increase in cell size (cytomegaly), and cytomegaly may occur either with or without an increase in the size of the nucleus. These changes have also been seen in mice treated with DDT, phenobarbital (Ward et al., 1983), Aroclor 1254 (Kimbrough and Linder, 1974), and other chemicals; and in mouse hepatitis virus–infected cells (Ward et al., 1977). Toxins also often induce binucleate and multinucleated hepatocytes as well.

Inclusion. Both intranuclear and intracytoplasmic inclusions are frequently observed within normal and neoplastic mouse hepatocytes. Intranuclear inclusions are round, often filling most of the nucleus, and are distinctly eosinophilic in appearance. These inclusions have been reported to increase in incidence with age and are usually considered to be invaginations of the cytoplasm into the nucleus (Andrew, 1962; Herbst, 1976).

Cytoplasmic inclusions are somewhat less common, and are most frequently seen in hepatocytes in or adjacent to hepatocellular neoplasms. Intracytoplasmic inclusions are round, vary markedly in size, and are usually eosinophilic. Some investigators have reported these intracytoplasmic inclusions to be aggregates of smooth endoplasmic reticulum (Hruban et al., 1966), or Mallory bodies. These types of intracytoplasmic inclusions have been reported in mice (Frith and Ward, 1980).

Bile Duct and Ductular Hyperplasia.   Proliferation of hepatic bile ducts may occur in response to toxicants and is sometimes associated with an inflammatory reaction. The lesion is usually diffuse and many bile ducts are usually present in portal triads). Bile ductules (cholangioles, oval cells) may become hyperplastic in response to toxicants as well. Normal and hyperplastic bile ducts and ductules stain for keratin.

Cholangiofibrosis (Adenofibrosis).   Cholangiofibrosis is characterized by focal areas of basophilic, atypical ducts in a fibrous stroma. It is rarely seen in control mice. The lesion is controversial and much less commonly induced in the mouse than in the rat. Adenofibrosis has been described in the mouse induced by Aroclor 1254 (Kimbrough and Linder, 1974).

Cirrhosis.   Hepatic cirrhosis, whether postnecrotic, biliary, pericellular, or of some other type, is uncommon spontaneously in mice. It may be seen after a variety of toxicants, including carbon tetrachloride and chronic mouse hepatitis infection in nude mice (Ward et al., 1977). It often takes the form of a focal or diffuse increase of fine reticular fibers rather than distinct fibrous collagenous bands (Ward et al., 1979a).

Cholangitis.   Cholangitis is inflammation of the bile ducts and is characterized by the presence of inflammatory cells (polymorphonuclear leukocytes and/or mononuclear cells) within the ducts and periductular tissue.

Hepatocellular Foci of Cellular Alteration.   Foci of cellular alteration in mice are somewhat similar to those described in the rat (Squire and Levitt, 1975) and may be seen in mice exposed to some carcinogens, including benzidine (Frith and Dooley, 1976), Aldrin and Dieldrin (Reuber, 1976), N-nitrosodimethylamine, N-nitrosodiethylamine (Ward et al., 1983, Ward, 1984) and other chemicals (Frith and Ward, 1980). They are occasionally seen in control mice. The primary alteration involves tinctorial qualities and textural appearances of the cytoplasm and size of hepatocytes. There is no obvious disruption of the liver architecture, and the affected hepatocytes merge with adjacent hepatocytes without compressing adjacent normal parenchyma. Foci of cellular alteration may be classified as eosinophilic, basophilic, vacuolated, clear cell, or mixed. They may progress to adenomas and occasionally to carcinomas (Ward, 1984; Frith et al., 1980a).

Clear cell foci consist of cells with a clear, ground-glass, or sometimes a lacy cytoplasm containing much glycogen. The clear areas stain with PAS stain prior to but not after diastase digestion, suggesting the presence of glycogen. The nuclei of the affected cells are not flattened against the cell membrane as in the vacuolated cells, but often are located in the center of the involved cells and surrounded by clear cytoplasm. Often, clear cell foci contain many hepatocytes with basophilic or clear cytoplasm.

Mixed cell foci contain, in varying proportions, two or more of any of the cell types described in the preceding paragraphs.

Focal Fatty Change.   Focal fatty change consists of focal areas of hepatocytes which contain lipid-laden, distinct cytoplasmic vacuoles of variable size. The nuclei of these vacuolated cells in microscopic sections are either absent or are flattened against the cytoplasmic membrane. Some pathologists use the term *vacuolated cell foci of cellular alteration* for this lesion.

Neoplastic Lesions

General. Hepatocellular neoplasms—induced or spontaneous—are among the most common tumors in the mouse. The incidence of liver tumors in mice is very high in some strains, and the incidence can be affected by various factors. Consequently, the mouse liver tumor has been criticized as an inappropriate endpoint in carcinogenesis bioassays. There is probably no other tumor that has created more difficulty and confusion in the interpretation of its morphology, biology, and significance (Tomatis et al., 1973; Frith et al., 1979; Turusov and Takayama, 1979; Ward et al., 1979c; Popp, 1984). The terminology used to describe liver tumors in the mouse has been quite varied and inconsistent. Up to now, some pathologists have considered a hepatocellular neoplasm to be a "true" tumor only if it metastasizes, whereas others diagnose all mouse liver neoplasms as hepatocellular carcinoma irregardless of their morphology and biological behavior.

A variety of terms, including hyperplastic nodule, nodular hyperplasia, neoplastic nodule, hepatoma, liver cell tumor, liver cell adenoma, hepatocellular adenoma, liver cell carcinoma, and hepatocellular carcinoma have been used to describe neoplastic hepatocellular lesions of mice. *Hepatocellular neoplasm* is a collective term used to describe the progressive stages of tumor development from the benign hepatocellular adenoma to the morphologically and biologically malignant hepatocellular carcinoma. Inasmuch as experimental pathologists, particularly those involved in carcinogenicity testing, need to distinguish between nontumors and tumors as well as between benign and malignant tumors, and since special biological and histochemical methods are either not helpful or simply cannot be used in large-scale studies, an attempt has been made to classify hepatocellular neoplasms on a purely morphological basis. The preferred term is *hepatocellular adenoma* for benign tumors and *hepatocellular carcinomas* for malignant tumors (Frith and Ward, 1980).

Hepatocellular Adenoma. The term *hepatocellular adenoma* is the preferred term for the morphologically and biologically benign liver cell neoplasm (Reuber, 1971; Butler and Newberne, 1975; Gellatly, 1975; Ward and Vlahakis, 1978; Vesselinovitch and Mihailovich, 1983; Ward, 1984). Adenomas are progressively growing focal lesions and may represent early stages in the formation of carcinomas (Ward and Vlahakis, 1978; Frith et al., 1980a). Synonyms for this lesion include benign hepatoma, hyperplastic nodule, nodular hyperplasia (Butler and Newberne, 1975), type A nodule (Walker et al., 1972), type 1 or 2 nodule (Gellatly, 1975), liver tumor (Tomatis et al., 1972), neoplastic nodule (Squire and Levitt, 1975), and hepatocellular carcinoma (Stewart, 1974; Stewart et al., 1980). Hepatocellular adenomas are usually 1–10 mm in diameter, consist of cells resembling relatively normal hepatocytes, and usually contain cells similar to those in the foci of cellular alteration. Adenomas exist as distinct nodules which compress adjacent parenchyma and may bulge from the liver surface. Histologically, they are composed of a uniform population of well-differentiated cells which form a solid nodule and which may be composed of larger or smaller than normal hepatocytes that have cytoplasm which is basophilic, eosinophilic, or vacuolated. Adenomas may form regular plates one cell thick. They do not invade adjacent parenchyma or vessels, the lesions do not metastasize, and the small nodules have a lower degree of transplantability than do carcinomas (Reuber, 1967; Gellatly, 1975; Williams, 1979). Transplantability is evidence of their neoplastic nature. More recently, they have been shown to be of clonal origin (Rabes et al., 1982), and some tumor cells contain α-fetoprotein, which is also evidence of neoplasia (Koen et al., 1983a). Some chemicals induce either eosinophilic (Ward et al., 1979a; Hoover et al., 1980; Ward, 1984) or basophilic adenomas (Vesselinovitch et al., 1978; Ward et al., 1979). Naturally occurring hepatocellular carcinomas can arise within adenomas (Frith and Dooley, 1976; Ward and Vlahakis, 1978; Ward, 1984). These foci of carcinoma within adenomas appear identical to carcinomas described below.

Hepatocellular Carcinoma.   The diagnosis of hepatocellular carcinoma is often made on a distinct trabecular or adenoid pattern as well as on cytological features characteristic of malignancy. Synonyms for this lesion include type B nodule (Walker et al., 1972), type 3 nodule (Gellatly, 1975), trabecular carcinoma, and malignant hepatoma. The liver cell plates are more than one cell layer thick, irregular, and composed of well to poorly differentiated hepatocytes. The well-differentiated tumors are composed of uniform cells with a fair amount of cytoplasm. The moderately well-differentiated hepatocellular carcinomas are composed of larger hepatocytes which vary more in size and shape and form plates or a solid pattern. The poorly differentiated tumors are composed of cells with less cytoplasm and more immature nuclei forming prominent plates or a solid pattern; some have extremely large anaplastic cells.

The incidence of metastases has generally been considered very low for mouse hepatocellular tumors, but more recent studies indicate that a thorough examination of step or serial sections of the lung reveals a much higher incidence than previously expected, especially for tumors induced by dimethylnitrosamine (Kyriazis et al., 1974). Metastases are frequently uncommon (0–5%) in mice with spontaneous hepatocellular carcinomas (Butler and Newberne, 1975), but they may be seen in up to 40% of male B6C3F1 or C3H mice with hepatocellular carcinoma that are allowed to live out their life span. Metastases usually occur only when tumors are large (over 10 mm) and increased in weight (Frith et al., 1980a). Some chemicals cause highly metastatic tumors, whereas other cause carcinomas with a low metastatic rate (Ward, 1984). Pulmonary metastases may share the trabecular pattern often seen in the primary hepatocellular carcinomas, or they may be more solid in appearance.

Hepatoblastoma.   Hepatoblastomas have been described in mice as occurring spontaneously and are rarely experimentally induced. Turusov et al. (1973) described liver tumors in mice which resembled human hepatoblastomas. These tumors are almost invariably found within or adjacent to hepatocellular carcinomas and are readily distinguished by their basophilia with H&E stain. The tumors frequently consist of organoid structures lined by vascular channels. The channels are surrounded by several layers of tumor cells arranged either radially or concentrically. In some areas, the cells are arranged in rows, rosettes, sheets, or ribbons. Foci of osseous metaplasia are occasionally seen. The cell of origin for this particular mouse neoplasm is uncertain, although it has been suggested that this type is of fetal origin (Turusov et al., 1973). While similar neoplasms occur in children, however, hepatoblastomas only occur in aged mice. Other pathologists have referred to similar lesions as poorly differentiated cholangiocarcinomas (Reuber, 1967) and cholangiomas (Vlahakis and Heston, 1971; Jones and Butler, 1975). Recently, the presence of keratin in hepatoblastomas has been demonstrated in aged mice but not α-fetoprotein, suggesting their duct or ductular origin rather than their hepatocellular origin.

Cholangioma and Cholangiocarcinoma.   Cholangiomas and cholangiocarcinomas are relatively rare in mice compared to the common occurrence of hepatocellular neoplasms (Reuber, 1967; Vlahakis and Heston, 1971). Some hepatocellular carcinomas assume a distinctly adenoid or glandular pattern suggestive of an adenocarcinoma, yet in some cases, when the transition is not evident, it is sometimes difficult to differentiate a hepatocellular adenocarcinoma from a cholangiocarcinoma. Mixed carcinomas, or carcinomas containing distinct areas of both trabecular hepatocellular carcinoma and cholangiocarcinoma, have also been described.

Metastatic Tumors. Metastatic tumors of the livers are rare compared to metastatic tumors of the lung. The most common are the hematopoietic neoplasms, including lymphoblastic lymphoma and follicular center cell lymphoma. Histiocytic sarcoma may occur as either a metastatic or a primary neoplasm of the liver. Metastatic tumors which have been seen in the liver include the alveolar/bronchiolar adenocarcinoma, urinary bladder transitional cell carcinoma, osteosarcoma, and pancreatic islet cell carcinoma (Frith, 1983).

Gallbladder

Nonneoplastic Lesions

Gall Stones. Gall stones are rare in mice. The stones have not been seen frequently enough to be chemically characterized. Stones are present in the lumen and consist of concentric laminations or lamellae.

Crystals. Distinct eosinophilic crystals of obscure etiology are occasionally seen in the cytoplasm of the epithelial cells and in the lumen of the gallbladder of mice. They may be similar in etiology to those described in the lungs, and may be products of the epithelium, since the acidophilic cytoplasm of the epithelial cells stains and reacts the same as the extracellular crystals (Yang and Campbell, 1964).

Neoplastic Lesions

Papilloma and Carcinoma. Gallbladder papillomas are rare tumors in the mouse. They consist of papillary projections covering a connective tissue core. A single gallbladder carcinoma has been seen in a control mouse at NCTR, and a small number have been seen in the B6C3F1 mouse (Yoshitomi et al., 1986).

MALE GENITAL SYSTEM

Testes

Nonneoplastic Lesions

Hypospermia. Hypospermia (immaturity of the seminiferous tubules) is a normal condition in very young mice (<4 weeks of age), but it may be induced in older mice with toxicants. The testicles appear morphologically normal, but maturing and mature spermatozoa are absent from both the testes and the epididymis.

Testicular Atrophy. Testicular atrophy occurs as an aging lesion in mice and may also be due to other factors such as exposure to specific toxic compounds, irradiation, and hypoxia. The lesion may be focal or diffuse. The seminiferous tubules and germinal epithelial cells are reduced in number and the testis may also be reduced grossly in size. A relative increase of Sertoli cells, interstitial cells, or multinucleated cells may be seen. The lipofuscin pigment ceroid may be associated with the atrophy. Ceroid is acid fast and PAS positive.

Testicular Mineralization. Focal dystrophic mineralization of the seminiferous tubules may occur occasionally. It may represent previous areas of injury. The mineralization is composed of basophilic concentric masses which may be amorphous or concentrically laminated.

Hyperplasia of Interstitial Cells. An increase in the relative number of interstitial cells may be associated with testicular atrophy. Focal hyperplasia of interstitial cells may also occur and possibly represent a preneoplastic condition.

Neoplastic Lesions

Interstitial Cell Tumors.   Both benign and malignant spontaneous tumors of the interstitial cells of Leydig are rare in most strains of mice, but can be seen in the CD-1 mouse. The neoplasms can be induced with synthetic or natural estrogens in certain strains, particularly BALB/c mice. The cytoplasm of the neoplastic cells is distinctly eosinophilic. Small, well-circumscribed tumors are adenomas and large tumors which are invasive or metastasize are referred to as carcinomas. The larger carcinomas occasionally metastasize to the lungs.

Accessory Sex Glands

Nonneoplastic Lesions

Spermatocele of Epididymis.   Spermatocele of the epididymis is a dilatation of a duct of the epididymis with the lumen filled with spermatozoa. If the duct ruptures, the release of spermatozoa in surrounding tissues may result in the formation of spermatic granuloma.

Preputial and Clitoral Gland Ectasia.   The preputial and clitoral glands are each one of the accessory sex glands of the male and female mouse, respectively. The gland is smaller in the female mouse. It is composed of modified sebaceous acini and squamous ducts. The glands may become markedly dilated (ectasia) and acute suppurative and chronic inflammation is common.

Preputial Gland Abscess.   Abscesses of the preputial gland are frequently seen in male mice as a consequence of fighting. The abscess is characterized by the presence of numerous neutrophils and liquefactive necrosis. Grossly, the exudates are frequently green in color.

Neoplastic Lesions

Neoplasms of Accesory Sex Glands.   Neoplasms of all of the male accessory sex glands (prostate, seminal vesicles, preputial and coagulating glands) are extremely rare. Adenocarcinomas of the prostate may be composed of relatively well-differentiated neoplastic cells. Squamous metaplasia may occasionally be seen. Adenomas and carcinomas of the seminal vesicle and coagulating gland have been reported very infrequently. Squamous cell carcinomas are very occasionally seen in the preputial gland.

Nervous System

Nonneoplastic Lesions

Cerebral Mineralization.   Mineralized deposits detected in the cerebrum generally occur in the region of the medial, ventral, and posterior thalamic nuclei (Morgan et al., 1983). These deposits are very common. However, the incidence is quite variable and can depend upon the level of the brain from which the sections were taken. They vary from single, rounded bodies up to 100 μM in diameter to very extensive, irregular, but usually rounded masses, which in most cases are found to be associated with blood vessels. The deposits exhibit faint to intense basophilia, and distinct concentric laminations are often evident. The most intense basophilia is associated with the larger deposits. The deposits stain negative for amyloid and iron, and are weakly positive with Alcian blue, the reaction being confined primarily to the periphery of the deposits. They stain densely dark brown black with very distinct lamination by Verhoeff's method. Alizarin red stains them black at the periphery and faint red in the core. X-Ray microanalysis spectra have been obtained from selected representative regions, including the dense peripheral zone of a large mineralized deposit, the shredded core of a large mineralized deposit, and a small mineralized deposit (Morgan et al., 1983). Significant peaks for calcium and phosphorus were obtained from the dense peripheral zone of a large mineralized deposit.

Inclusion Cyst. The inclusion cyst may occur rarely as a spontaneous lesion in the brain and spinal cord. Cysts range in size from very small to quite large, but the morphological appearance is similar. The cyst is lined by flattened squamous epithelium and is filled with eosinophilic desquamated keratin.

Hydrocephalus. Hydrocephalus usually involves the lateral ventricles, is bilateral, and is characterized by increased fluid in the ventricular system. The ventricles may be so enlarged as to cause a dome shape to the cranium. The sulci and gyri may be flattened and almost indiscernible in advanced cases. Microscopically, the ventricles are enlarged at the expense of the flattened cerebral cortex. Hydrocephalus is sometimes associated with large pituitary tumors.

Vacuolization of the White Matter–Central Nervous System. Vacuoles are a common entity in the white matter of the brains of mice, particularly in the cerebellum. It has been suggested that this may be an artifact associated with the collection and processing of the brain. It has also been suggested that this may be a degenerative lesion and may increase with age.

Infarct. Infarcts are rare in the central nervous system, but occasionally occur in the cerebrum. They more commonly occur at the surface or less frequently deeper within the parenchyma.

Neoplastic Lesions

Oligodendroglioma. Tumors of the central nervous system of the mouse are extremely rare lesions (Morgan et al., 1984). The most common tumor is the oligodendroglioma which occurs in the cerebrum and/or diencephalon. It is usually ventrolateral in location and involves much of the thalamus, hypothalamus, and amygdaloid. The oligodendroglioma comprises a poorly demarcated mass of proliferating oligodendrocytes with variable degrees of neuronal satellitosis, nuclear palisading, and mitoses. These cells have scanty cytoplasm, with a distinct perinuclear halo in some cases; the single round to oval nuclei are often hyperchromatic.

Astrocytoma. Astrocytomas occur much less frequently than oligodendrogliomas in mice. The neoplasms comprise cells with indistinct cytoplasmic boundaries and large, oval or slightly folded nuclei. The margins of the tumor mass are indistinct and there may be areas of edema, hemorrhage, and microcystic damage. Hemorrhage and necrosis are seen more frequently in astrocytomas than in oligodendrogliomas.

Lipoma. Lipomas have been seen associated both with the meninges and choroid plexus (Morgan et al., 1984). These consist principally of discrete, well-demarcated, small to large clusters or masses of mature adipocytes. They may be present in the interstitium of the choroid plexus of the lateral ventricles and are extremely small (10–12 cells per section). Occasionally, a small mass of cartilagelike material is present among the fat cells. The cell or tissue of origin of these lesions is unknown.

Meningioma. Meningiomas also occur rarely in the mouse and can assume a variety of patterns as in other species. These neoplasms comprise a regular pattern of loosely interwoven bundles of delicate spindle cells, with single small hyperchromatic oval nuclei. The nuclei in some areas palisade in an irregular fashion. These cells lay in a faintly basophilic finely granular ground substance. In some cases, the neoplasms infiltrate the ventral brain along the adventitia of small blood vessels.

Metastatic Tumors. Leukemias and lymphomas commonly metastasize to the brain. Mesenchymal tumors (sarcomas) may also occasionally spread to the brain.

RESPIRATORY SYSTEM

Upper Respiratory Tract (Nasal Cavity, Larynx, Trachea)

Spontaneous nonneoplastic and neoplastic lesions of the nasal cavity, larynx, and trachea are uncommon in mice.

Lung

Nonneoplastic Lesions

Alveolar Epithelial Hyperplasia. Alveolar epithelial hyperplasia is characterized by a single layer of nonciliated cuboidal cells lining all or part of the alveolar wall. The cells are found on the scaffold of existing stroma and the normal architecture remains intact. There are no papillary projections into the lumens nor are there solid masses of cells filling alveolar spaces. The proliferating cells are type II pneumocytes (Goodman et al., 1981). These lesions can be precursor lesions for the alveolar/bronchiolar neoplasms.

Lymphocytic Infiltrates. Lymphocytic infiltrates are very common around blood vessels and bronchioles or in the pleura as focal lesions. These lesions are usually minimal to mild in severity and are not diagnosed by some pathologists. Lymphoid tissue is normally present in association with the bronchi.

Neoplastic Lesions

General. The most common lung tumors observed in B6C3F1 and CD-1 mice are alveolar/bronchiolar adenomas and carcinomas. Many of these arise from type II pneumocytes. Tumors arising from Clara cell have also been described (Kaufman, et al., 1979; Theiss and Shimkin, 1982 Kaufman and Sato, 1985a,b). On H&E sections, these two tumor types can be difficult to differentiate morphologically. Consequently, in most toxicology studies, the terms alveolar/bronchiolar (A/B) adenoma and carcinoma are used routinely. Squamous cell carcinomas of the lung can be induced by various agents, but they are extremely uncommon spontaneously.

Alveolar/bronchiolar Adenoma. Alveolar/bronchiolar adenomas microscopically may be circumscribed and compress adjacent tissue or the edges may be irregular where the neoplastic cells extend into adjacent airways. The lesion is composed of cells with a normal nuclear/cytoplasmic ratio that are cuboidal or columnar and resemble normal lining cells of the lower airway. Proliferating cells may form papillary projections into alveoli or completely fill them. The central portions of these tumors tend to be more solid than the periphery.

Alveolar/bronchiolar Carcinoma. Alveolar/bronchiolar carcinomas tend to be larger than adenomas. There is cellular and nuclear pleomorphism, increased nuclear/cytoplasmic ratio, hyperchromatic nuclei, and an increase in mitotic figures. There may be multiple solid areas within the tumor; invasion of airways, blood vessels, lymphatics, and pleural surfaces; extension throughout the mediastinum; coelomic and distant metastases. Necrosis is common. When these tumors metastasize, they may have a sarcomatous pattern.

SPECIAL SENSES

Eye

Nonneoplastic Lesions

Nonneoplastic lesions of the eye are occasionally observed in aged CD-1 and B6C3F1 mice. Most commonly observed, although infrequent and sporadic in incidence, are cataracts and retinal atrophy.

Retinal Atrophy. Age-related retinal atrophy in the mouse consists of atrophy or loss of the rods, since the mouse does not possess cone cells. The incidence varies from less than 2% in the BALB/c strain to 100% in the C3H strain. The lesion may occasionally be unilateral or partial and is characterized by atrophy of the layer of rods as well as the outer plexiform and outer nuclear layers.

Cataract. Cataract is an occasional lesion seen in the lens of the eyes of mice. Morphologically, cataracts appear as multiple globoid circumscribed bodies within the substance of the lens, especially at the periphery or capsular surface.

Neoplastic Lesions

Primary tumors of the eye are extremely rare in all mouse strains (Squire et al., 1978).

Harderian Gland

Nonneoplastic Lesions

Small focal lymphocytic infiltrates and ectasia of the ducts are occasionally observed.

Neoplastic Lesions

Harderian Gland Adenoma. These tumors are frequently well-demarcated lesions that cause compression of the adjacent parenchyma, but usually do not have a well-defined capsule. The architecture consists of pseudoglandular structures from which arborizing and folded fingerlike fronds project into the lumen. The fronds are composed of a delicate fibrovascular core covered by cells which are usually tall columnar with foamy amphophilic cytoplasm. The cells usually form a single layer, but areas are frequently present that give the appearance of having a basal layer of normal-appearing cells "capped" by smaller cells adjacent to the lumen.

Harderian Gland Adenocarcinoma. These tumors may be well differentiated, differing from adenomas by greater cellular atypia, invasion, and metastases. Undifferentiated adenocarcinomas contain areas of varying size which are solid and composed of pleomorphic cells, many of which contain a single large vacuole. Mitotic figures are uncommon.

URINARY SYSTEM

Kidney

Sexual Dimorphism of the Kidney. The glomerular tuft of the adult male mouse kidney of certain strains has a unique morphological characteristic that is not a pathological lesion. In most animals, the parietal layer of Bowman's capsule is composed of a single layer of flattened epithelium. In the male mouse, the parietal layer of most of the glomeruli is composed of simple cuboidal epithelium. This characteristic is seen only in adult male mice and is not present in each glomerulus. The proportion of glomeruli showing this characteristic varies in different strains.

Nonneoplastic Lesions

Double Renal Pelvis. The kidney of the mouse contains a single large renal papilla surrounded by the renal pelvis. Very rarely, a congenital anomaly consisting of a double renal pelvis may occur.

Renal Infarct. Renal infarcts in the mouse are morphologically comparable to renal infarcts in other species. They quite commonly appear as triangular-shaped areas of coagulation necrosis which extend from the capsular surface through the cortex to or into the medulla. The tubules may be intensely eosinophilic, and fibrosis may be present in older lesions. The surface of the infarct is depressed below the normal renal surface. In recent lesions, polymorphonuclear leukocytes may infiltrate the border and some tubules may contain hemoglobin casts.

Renal Papillary Necrosis.   Necrosis of the renal papilla may occur in the mouse kidney and is usually associated with renal amyloidosis or toxins.

Hydronephrosis.   Hydronephrosis may follow obstruction of one or both ureters or the urethra of the urinary bladder. Causes of hydronephrosis include calculi, tumors or inflammation (Bendele and Carlton, 1986). It may be minimal and result in only a slight dilatation of the renal pelvis, or it may be severe enough to cause marked compression atrophy of the kidney. Hydroureter may be present proximal to the blockage.

Chronic Nephritis.   Chronic nephritis is a common entity in some strains of mice, particularly in the CD-1 strain. The lesion is characterized by the presence of numerous proteinaceous casts within the tubules and areas of tubular atrophy, regeneration and dilatation; interstitial fibrosis; and chronic inflammation. The degree of nephropathy may be graded as minimal, mild, moderate, or severe. The cause is unknown.

Membranous Proliferative Glomerulonephritis.   This lesion is characterized by proliferation of the mesangial cells of the glomeruli and thickening of glomerular basement membranes. The severity may vary from mild to marked. An eosinophilic homogeneous material is present within the glomeruli. The etiology of the disease is unknown, but it may be autoimmune or viral in origin. It occurs sporadically in most mouse strains.

Renal Calculi.   Mineral concretions may occur in the renal pelvis of mice. The lesion is uncommon, and the stones have not been characterized chemically. Calculi consist of concentric laminations of basophilic material.

Tubluar Hyperplasia.   Tubular changes which might be interpreted as precursors of renal epithelial tumors in mice have been described on several occasions (Terracini et al., 1966; Terracini and Testa; 1970; Lombard et al., 1974; Resnik et al., 1979; Shinohara and Frith, 1980). They were not recognizable macroscopically and histologically appeared as dilated tubules lined by large epithelial cells with nuclei showing no or minor irregularities, occasionally piled up in two to three layers or forming a few short papillae. The borderline between hyperplastic tubules, papillary cysts, and papillary adenomas can be established only on an arbitrary basis. In addition, hyperplastic tubules with very moderate formation of papillae have been occasionally seen in untreated Swiss mice in which adenomas are extremely rare (Terracini et al., 1966).

Neoplastic Lesions

General.   Renal neoplasms are reported to be "rare" in the mouse (Dunn, 1967; Cohen and Friedell, 1982). This may simply be a consequence of the fact that animals developing tumors at other sites have been considered more suitable for the study of fundamental aspects of neoplasia. More recent reports in the mouse have been published suggesting that both spontaneous and induced renal tumors in mice may not be as rare as previously reported (Lombard et al., 1974; Shinohara and Frith, 1980; Turusov et al., 1985; and Li et al., 1987).

Tubular Cell Adenoma.   Most renal tubular cell adenomas are singular and can be morphologically classified as cystic, papillary, or solid (Shinohara and Frith, 1980). The papillary type is the most common and exhibits a pronounced papillary pattern. If the pattern appears predominantly cystic without a prominent proliferative papillary pattern, the adenoma may be classified as cystic. The cells forming the adenomas are uniformly cuboidal with eosinophilic cytoplasm and relatively small nuclei. Mitotic figures are rare. The cystic and papillary adenomas are usually encapsulated. Some adenomas form a solid pattern and are classified as solid type. They are usually well demarcated from adjacent renal parenchyma, but are not encapsulated. Cells primarily form a solid pattern interspersed with a small amount of fibrous connective tissue containing blood capillaries. The cytoplasm of the cells forming the solid adenomas is usually acidophilic, and the nuclei are small. Adenomas may grow in size and progress to carcinomas (Shinohara and Frith, 1980). They may originate from focal tubular hyperplasia. In the cystic-papillary adenomas, the number of papillae and the extent of cellular proliferation vary markedly and may be difficult to distinguish on purely morphological grounds from early hyperplastic lesions. Cystic, papillary, and solid aspects may coexist in the same tumor. Cellular proliferation may also be diffuse with no formation of tubules or traebeculae. The tumors are usually sharply defined, often with some compression of the surrounding parenchyma. Cells can be either acidophilic, occasionally foamy, or basophilic and granular. Nuclei are vesicular, and more or less regular. In some tumors, the papillary pattern can be so marked as to raise the question of an origin from the transitional epithelium. Cytological features may be of help in this case, since tubular cells contain more cytoplasm and are not arranged in a transitional pattern.

Renal Tubular Cell Carcinoma.   Renal cell tumors may occur as spontaneous lesions (Shinohara and Frith, 1980) or as induced lesions (Lombard et al., 1974). They may be solid, tubular, or anaplastic in morphological pattern. Renal tubular cell carcinomas are composed of epithelial cells with either granular eosinophilic or basophilic-staining cytoplasm. The cells vary from small and uniform to large and pleomorphic. The nuclei are usually small and round or oval in the uniform cells, but show various sizes and shapes and prominent nucleoli in the pleomorphic cells. The mitotic index in the tubular cell carcinomas varies from tumor-to-tumor. The arrangement of tumor cells in these carcinomas shows a basic tubular pattern. Sometimes these tumors form irregular tubular structures composed of tumor cells with various sizes and shapes. Mitoses are frequent, and sometimes single or multiple cystlike structures with pale eosinophilic material are seen.

Tubular cell carcinomas may be anaplastic and consist of pleomorphic cells that form irregular tubular structures. Some of these tumors contain areas of sarcomatous change. The nuclei tend to be hyperchromatic and multinucleated giant cells are common. The mitotic index is high, and areas of necrosis and/or hemorrhage are common. Carcinomas occasionally metastasize to the lungs.

Ureter

Nonneoplastic

Ureteral Diverticulum.   Diverticula are not common spontaneous lesions in the mouse but have been associated with inflammation and the administration of 4-ethylsulfonyl naphthelene-1-sulfonamide (ENS), acetazolasmide, and oxamide (Jackson et al., 1979; Frith et al., 1984). The lesion exists as a downgrowth into the ureteral wall which may be confused with a carcinoma. Downgrowths of the surface epithelium may extend through the muscularis to the adventitia. The lesion appears to be associated with the crystalluria.

Urinary Bladder

Nonneoplastic

Bladder Calculi.   Urinary calculi may occur spontaneously or may be associated with the administration of such compounds as ENS (Jackson et al., 1979; Frith et al., 1984). The calculi are usually accompanied by chronic cystitis, and may also result in papillary and nodular urothelial hyperplasia.

Lymphoid Aggregates.   Focal lymphoid aggregates may occur in the lamina propria of the urinary bladder. Their incidence and severity increase with age.

Urothelial Hyperplasia.   The microscopic evaluation of hyperplasia of the urinary bladder can be best performed in urinary bladders that have been inflated with fixative. The fixative can be instilled through the urethra with a 22- to 23-gauge needle. It may be necessary to ligate the neck of the bladder after inflation to prevent loss of the fixative. The bladder can be bisected after fixation, examined grossly with a dissecting microscope, and then processed for microscopic evaluation.

Hyperplasia of the transitional epithelium of the mouse urinary bladder is a rare spontaneous lesion, but a common finding in animals treated with bladder carcinogens and may be either focal, multifocal, diffuse, simple, papillary, or nodular (Frith, 1979). Hyperplasia may also be associated with chronic cystitis, calculi formation, and in response to such toxic compounds as cyclophosphamide or methyl or ethyl methanesulfonate. Simple hyperplasia may be either focal or diffuse and mild, moderate, or marked. Lesions may be classified as mild hyperplasia when the urothelium averages four transitional cell layers in thickness, as moderate hyperplasia when it averages five to six cell layers, and marked hyperplasia when it averages seven or more cell layers.

Focal nodular hyperplasia (epithelial downgrowths) may occur in conjunction with either simple or papillary hyperplasia and consists of nodular downgrowths which extend into the lamina propria of the bladder. It may be focal or multifocal. Nodular hyperplasia is comparable morphologically to von Brunn's nests or cystitis cystica in humans (Frith, 1979). Although the areas of nodular hyperplasia often appear to have no connection with the surface epithelium, serial sections usually reveal such a connection. The lesion may regress if the etiological stimulus is removed (Frith and Rule, 1978).

Neoplastic Lesions

Urinary Bladder Papilloma.   Naturally occurring benign epithelial lesions of the urinary bladder are rare in mice and occur as papillary formations projecting into the lumen. The epithelium shows no plemorphism, atypia, or anaplasia and is well differentiated. Papillomas induced with 2-acetylaminofluorene (2-AAF) may have a slender narrow stalk or a broad base (Frith, 1979).

Urinary Bladder Carcinoma.   Naturally occurring bladder carcinomas are extremely rare in mice (Frith et al., 1980c). Experimentally induced malignant neoplasms of the urothelium may be classified according to histological pattern, cell type, and depth of invasion (Frith et al., 1980c). Malignant epithelial lesions classified by histological pattern may be divided into papillary and nonpapillary (solid, polypoid) carcinomas. Papillary carcinomas project into the lumen and may or may not show invasion (Frith et al., 1980c). Nonpapillary or solid carcinomas grow down into (invade) the bladder wall.

Bladder carcinomas classified according to histological cell type are divided into transitional cell, transitional cell with squamous metaplasia), squamous, undifferentiated, and adenocarcinoma types. The most common type induced is the transitional cell carcinoma, but this may depend on the type and the dose level of the carcinogen (Frith et al., 1980c).

Transitional cell carcinoma with squamous metaplasia and squamous cell carcinomas tend to be more aggressive and infiltrative than transitional cell carcinomas (Frith et al., 1980c). Urinary bladder carcinomas commonly invade locally, but only very occasionally metastasize to the lungs.

Urinary Bladder Mesenchymal Tumors.   Spontaneous mesenchymal tumors of the urinary bladder are rare. Experimentally induced primary mesenchymal tumors of the mouse urinary bladder occur much less frequently than epithelial tumors. The most comon are the vascular tumors such as hemangioma and hemangiosarcoma. Hemangiosarcomas may occasionally occur in conjunction with transitional cell carcinomas. Mesenchymal tumors of muscle origin are extremely rare. Occasionally tumors resembling sarcomas are seen, but these may be undifferentiated carcinomas. Chandra and Frith (1991) described leiomyosarcomas occurring as a spontaneous lesion in CD-1 mice.

MUSCULOSKETAL SYSTEM

Bone

Nonneoplastic Lesions

Fibro-osseous Lesion, Bone.   This lesion has been called by a variety of terms: fibro-osseous lesion, myelofibrosis, fibrous osteodystrophy, senile osteodystrophy, or osteoporosis (Sass and Montali, 1980; Goodman, et al., 1981; Burek, et al., 1982; Frith and Ward, 1988). This lesion is seen in the sternum and other bones in aging mice, particularly in females. There is replacement of all or part of the marrow cavity with an eosinophilic fibrillar matrix containing abundant collagen fibers. Fibroblastlike cells and osteoclasts are present throughout the matrix. Small foci of normal marrow may be present. Although the lesion resembles fibrous osteodystrophy associated with renal disease, the pathogenesis appears to be different as both kidneys and parathyroids are normal. Similar lesions have been induced with estrogen administration.

Ankylosis.   Ankylosis of the hock joints have been reported in group-caged male B6C3F1 mice (Rao and Lindsey, 1988). The incidence of ankylosis increases rapidly after 6 months of age. The cause is unknown but the incidence decreased when mice were individually caged. The joints are enlarged. Microscopically, there are bony proliferations (exostoses) on the tarsal bones. There is bridging of the joint and in severe cases obliteration of the joint with new bone.

Other Nonneoplastic Lesions.   Osteoarthrosis and bone necrosis with associated fractures have also been reported sporadically (Burek et al., 1982).

Neoplastic Lesions

Osteomas and osteosarcomas, tumors of bone, are occasionally observed in mice. Cartilaginous tumors, chondromas, and chondrosarcomas are extremely rare in mice (Lombard, 1982).

Muscle

Both neoplastic and nonneoplastic spontaneous lesions of skeletal muscle are uncommon in laboratory mice (Squire, et al., 1978; Burek et al., 1982; Lombard, 1982).

MULTIPLE SYSTEM

Nonneoplastic Lesions

Amyloidosis

The CD-1 mouse is widely used for chronic toxicology studies. The major cause of death of aged CD-1 mice is amyloidosis. Amyloidosis occurs much less frequently in other strains of mice. It is uncommon in B6C3F1 mice. The disease appears to begin as a deposition of amyloid in the submucosa of the duodenum, jejunum, and ileum. In severe cases, many other organs are also involved. Involvement of the glomeruli of the kidneys is usually the cause of death in animals that die with amyloidosis.

Incidence and Distribution.   The incidence of the disease in a 2-year chronic study in mice that died on study (DOS) and animals that were sacrificed (SAC) is presented in Table 24. In the 0- to 8-month-old animals, amyloidosis was only present in the duodenum, jejunum, ileum mesenteric lymph node, and ovaries. As the animals aged, amyloidosis was also present in the adrenal gland, gallbladder, heart, kidney. liver, mammary region, pancreas, thyroid, parathyroid, spleen, glandular stomach, and testes. Amyloidosis was more common in the animals that died on study than in the animals that were sacrificed at 24 months. In the animals that died on study from 12–24 months, the highest incidence of amyloidosis occurred in the ileum, kidney, and adrenal gland. The incidence of the various organs increased with age. The incidence was slightly higher in female than the male mice.

Morphology.   With the light microscope and H&E stain, amyloid apears as an amorphous, eosinophilic, hyaline, extracellular substance, with progressive accumulations encroaches on and produces pressure atrophy of adjacent cells. Special stains sometimes used to confirm the presence of amyloid include thioflavin T (secondary fluorescence with ultraviolet light) and metachromasia with crystal or methyl violet. The most common stain used to confirm amyloid is Congo Red, which imparts a pink or red color to amyloid. Congo Red stain also results in a green birefringence with polarized light.

Amyloid deposition in the small intestine (duodenum, jejunum, and ileum) and glandular stomach generally occurs in the lamina propria and submucosa. In the adrenal glands, amyloid deposits are common in the inner cortex surrounding the medulla. Lymph node involvement is primarily in the mesenteric lymph node and the amyloid deposits occur at the periphery of the node in the subcapsular sinuses. Amyloid deposits in the thyroid and parathyroid involve the interstitium in a diffuse fashion. Amyloid deposits in the kidney primarily involve the glomeruli. Renal amyloidosis appears to be the primary cause of death in many animals that die on study.

ORGAN WEIGHTS

Experimental Design

General

Organ weight data continue to be an essential component of classic and regulated toxicology studies in laboratory animals such as the mouse and the rat. Although a voluminous amount of organ weight data has been collected in studies prepared for regulatory agencies, very little of that data has been published in the literature. This has resulted in a sparsity of historical data for supporting interpretations pertaining to organ

Table 24 Incidence of Amyloidosis in CD-1 Mice (12–24 Months)

Dose groups	Males								Females							
	1		2		3		4		1		2		3		4	
Interim	DOS (22)[a]	SAC (25)	DOS (23)	SAC (23)	DOS (19)	SAC (24)	DOS (30)	SAC (16)	DOS (29)	SAC (20)	DOS (23)	SAC (25)	DOS (30)	SAC (18)	DOS (37)	SAC (12)
Incidence																
Adrenal Gland	(7)	(0)	(15)	(1)	(7)	(0)	(7)	(2)	(13)	(1)	(11)	(0)	(13)	(1)	(14)	(2)
Duodenum	(6)	(0)	(11)	(1)	(7)	(1)	(9)	(1)	(10)	(1)	(10)	(0)	(12)	(3)	(11)	(3)
Gall Bladder	(0)	(0)	(2)	(0)	(0)	(0)	(0)	(0)	(2)	(0)	(3)	(0)	(3)	(0)	(0)	(0)
Heart	(8)	(0)	(13)	(0)	(7)	(0)	(6)	(1)	(7)	(1)	(10)	(0)	(13)	(1)	(12)	(2)
Ileum	(8)	(3)	(15)	(2)	(8)	(6)	(9)	(3)	(14)	(2)	(10)	(3)	(13)	(6)	(14)	(3)
Jejunum	(5)	(0)	(9)	(1)	(5)	(1)	(7)	(2)	(10)	(1)	(8)	(1)	(12)	(3)	(10)	(3)
Kidney	(7)	(0)	(15)	(1)	(6)	(0)	(7)	(2)	(15)	(1)	(14)	(0)	(15)	(3)	(14)	(2)
Liver	(8)	(0)	(12)	(0)	(3)	(0)	(7)	(2)	(11)	(0)	(7)	(0)	(11)	(1)	(9)	(1)
Lymph Node	(3)	(0)	(12)	(1)	(4)	(1)	(4)	(3)	(9)	(1)	(7)	(1)	(12)	(1)	(10)	(3)
Mammary Region	(0)	(0)	(0)	(0)	(0)	(0)	(0)	(0)	(1)	(0)	(0)	(0)	(6)	(0)	(2)	(0)
Ovary	—		—		—		—		(11)	(1)	(8)	(0)	(11)	(1)	(12)	(2)
Pancreas	(0)	(0)	(0)	(0)	(0)	(0)	(0)	(0)	(0)	(2)	(0)	(2)	(0)	(1)	(0)	(2)
Parathyroid	(0)	(0)	(6)	(0)	(3)	(0)	(4)	(1)	(6)	(1)	(5)	(0)	(9)	(0)	(5)	(1)
Spleen	(5)	(0)	(10)	(0)	(4)	(0)	(4)	(0)	(10)	(1)	(8)	(1)	(13)	(0)	(6)	(0)
Stomach	(0)	(0)	(3)	(0)	(1)	(0)	(1)	(0)	(0)	(0)	(3)	(0)	(8)	(0)	(6)	(0)
Testis	(4)	(0)	(5)	(0)	(2)	(0)	(2)	(0)	—		—		—		—	
Thyroid	(8)	(0)	(15)	(0)	(6)	(0)	(6)	(0)	(11)	(1)	(11)	(0)	(12)	(1)	(11)	(2)

Abbreviations: DOS, died on study; SAC, sacrifice. Number of tissues examined.
Source: Frith and Chandra, 1991.

weight data. To help fulfill a need, relative organ weight data (organ weight-to-body weight percentage) for CD-1(ICR)BR mice and B6C3F1 mice (Table 25) is included in this chapter. (Data provided by S. Weymouth and S. Jones from Hazleton Washington, Vienna, Virginia).

Controllable Variables in Design

As with any well-designed experiment, the protocol should be carefully planned to avoid bias, decrease the number of variables, decrease the amount of biological variation, and ensure that sample size will provide adequate power for the statistical analysis.

Because body and organ weights are absolute numbers, bias can be controlled more easily than with many other types of biological data. Scales should be calibrated and validated to ensure that results are precise and accurate. Whenever possible, animals should be fasted overnight to minimize body and organ weight variation at the time of necropsy. For scientific and humane reasons, the animals should be given free access to water. Body weights should be taken immediately before necropsy. Animals should be necropsied randomly to ensure that the necropsy times are evenly distributed throughout the day. In rats, percent liver weight loss is greater than percent body weight loss during a routine work day for rats that have been fasted (Rothacker et al., 1988). Percent renal weight loss occurs in proportion to body weight loss during the same period of time. This may also apply to mice. It reinforces the fact that all variables should be controlled insofar as possible.

As soon as the animals are anesthetized, they should be rapidly and uniformly exsanguinated. The absolute hepatic and renal weights of exsanguinated rats are 23 and 15% lower, respectively, than those of rats that were not exsanguinated (Kanerva et al., 1982). In addition, the standard deviation of organ weights from exsanguinated rats is much lower than that of nonexsanguinated rats, which increases the sensitivity of the statistical analyses. The lower blood content of exsanguinated organs probably results in faster fixation of tissue and decreases the difficulty of microscopic evaluation. Although these data came from studies in rats, the same is likely to hold true for mice.

Organs should be collected and weighed quickly to avoid excessive or nonuniform dehydration and autolysis. To minimize the standard deviation in liver weights, bile should be drained from the gallbladder. In mice, the heart should be incised at the junction of the major vessels with the organ. Attempts to remove or retain blood in the chambers of the heart should be uniform to ensure that variation in absolute weights is minimized. Many pathologists prefer that the heart not be opened and that no attempt be made to remove blood from the chambers before weighing.

Immediately before weighing, excessive fat and fascia should be trimmed from organs and the organ should be gently blotted with filter paper to remove excess blood or other body fluid. Organ collection and weighing procedures should be uniform from animal-to-animal, organ-to-organ and study-to-study.

Excessive handling of small tissues during necropsy may result in autolysis, dehydration, or crushing of tissue, which increases the difficulty of microscopic examination. To avoid these problems, some investigators prefer to fix organs before weighing them. In one rat study, comparisons between fresh organ weights and those of organs fixed in 10% neutral buffered formalin indicated that fixation had a statistically significant effect on the weights of liver, kidneys, brain, lungs, spleen, and testes (Kanerva et al., 1983). The direction and magnitude of the differences varied among organs and sexes. However, the changes were consistent throughout sampling of each specific organ, indicating that in

Table 25 Organ-to-Body Weight Percentages for Mice

Organ	Strain	CD-1(ICR)BR				B₆C₃F₁	
	Age (wks)	>26		>78		>104	
	Sex	M	F	M	F	M	F
Adrenals	no.	10.00000	9.000000	173.0000	173.0000	40.00000	37.00000
	mean	0.022131	0.051612	0.015188	0.038021	0.015694	0.028338
	SD	0.005880	0.012019	0.005756	0.016269	0.005048	0.008327
	min	0.015260	0.034188	0.004918	0.015528	0.008333	0.016691
	max	0.031402	0.066791	0.036246	0.181185	0.035959	0.052360
Adrenal left	no.	0.000000	0.000000	85.00000	88.00000	0.000000	0.000000
	mean	0.000000	0.000000	0.007609	0.019007	0.000000	0.000000
	SD	0.000000	0.000000	0.003101	0.009582	0.000000	0.000000
	min	0.000000	0.000000	0.002357	0.008125	0.000000	0.000000
	max	0.000000	0.000000	0.018149	0.097909	0.000000	0.000000
Adrenal right	no.	0.000000	0.000000	84.00000	88.00000	0.000000	0.000000
	mean	0.000000	0.000000	0.008199	0.019365	0.000000	0.000000
	SD	0.000000	0.000000	0.003310	0.008681	0.000000	0.000000
	min	0.000000	0.000000	0.002809	0.004348	0.000000	0.000000
	max	0.000000	0.000000	0.020809	0.084669	0.000000	0.000000
Brain with stem	no.	10.00000	9.000000	234.0000	230.0000	40.00000	38.00000
	mean	1.511034	1.967633	1.497889	1.762074	1.490836	1.751111
	SD	0.134687	0.112187	0.172740	0.219994	0.136324	0.165646
	min	1.259053	1.722420	0.750435	1.085106	1.205426	1.172165
	max	1.710801	2.064639	1.965157	3.304563	1.737681	2.093913
Heart	no.	10.00000	9.000000	156.0000	148.0000	40.00000	38.00000
	mean	0.516713	0.543047	0.570298	0.559882	0.623888	0.617364
	SD	0.089502	0.052309	0.173607	0.082109	0.097599	0.084789
	min	0.395543	0.444030	0.300267	0.269504	0.462500	0.405412
	max	0.658621	0.596958	2.407547	0.850000	0.890657	0.811913
Kidney	no.	10.00000	9.000000	266.0000	261.0000	40.00000	38.00000
	mean	1.856140	1.461251	1.989803	1.705876	2.153085	1.700563
	SD	0.211315	0.323940	0.272915	0.223887	0.179888	0.178426
	min	1.584958	0.660448	0.985507	0.945137	1.648937	1.056701
	max	2.293729	1.821168	2.775919	2.545324	2.525598	2.246377
Kidney, left	no.	0.000000	0.000000	82.00000	79.00000	40.00000	38.00000
	mean	0.000000	0.000000	1.010117	0.843651	1.049165	0.818899
	SD	0.000000	0.000000	0.164602	0.136978	0.104168	0.090006
	min	0.000000	0.000000	0.439420	0.496454	0.804255	0.479897
	max	0.000000	0.000000	1.301754	1.245791	1.273189	1.086232
Kidney, right	no.	0.000000	0.000000	82.00000	79.00000	40.00000	38.00000
	mean	0.000000	0.000000	1.016143	0.882472	1.105696	0.882914
	SD	0.000000	0.000000	0.159915	0.126808	0.101921	0.091439
	min	0.000000	0.000000	0.536232	0.632911	0.844415	0.564691
	max	0.000000	0.000000	1.497659	1.277305	1.298635	1.147101
Liver	no.	10.00000	9.000000	78.00000	72.00000	0.000000	0.000000
	mean	4.273273	4.607630	4.867694	4.174702	0.000000	0.000000
	SD	0.307200	0.253697	1.173389	0.659241	0.000000	0.000000
	min	3.910863	4.216418	3.644231	3.486486	0.000000	0.000000
	max	4.732674	4.985765	12.69625	7.314815	0.000000	0.000000

Table 25 *(continued)*

| Organ | Sex | CD-1(ICR)BR | | | | B₆C₃F₁ | |
| | | >26 | | >78 | | >104 | |
		M	F	M	F	M	F
Liver/gallbladder	no.	0.000000	0.000000	187.0000	189.0000	31.00000	35.00000
	mean	0.000000	0.000000	4.764636	5.074481	4.281195	5.187510
	SD	0.000000	0.000000	0.987223	0.838878	0.559082	0.845616
	min	0.000000	0.000000	3.116845	2.552837	3.607254	3.075773
	max	0.000000	0.000000	10.28333	8.433775	6.299268	8.249035
Lung	no.	0.000000	0.000000	96.00000	98.00000	0.000000	0.000000
	mean	0.000000	0.000000	0.739844	0.828337	0.000000	0.000000
	SD	0.000000	0.000000	0.163484	0.136278	0.000000	0.000000
	min	0.000000	0.000000	0.539683	0.613415	0.000000	0.000000
	max	0.000000	0.000000	1.973898	1.406688	0.000000	0.000000
Ovary	no.	0.000000	9.000000	0.000000	114.0000	0.000000	37.00000
	mean	0.000000	0.105872	0.000000	0.295774	0.000000	0.124293
	SD	0.000000	0.022158	0.000000	0.452975	0.000000	0.177313
	min	0.000000	0.062044	0.000000	0.028485	0.000000	0.013918
	max	0.000000	0.137457	0.000000	3.181046	0.000000	0.903860
Pituitary	no.	0.000000	0.000000	20.00000	20.00000	40.00000	38.00000
	mean	0.000000	0.000000	0.006986	0.009237	0.005464	0.018458
	SD	0.000000	0.000000	0.003352	0.004006	0.002612	0.040184
	min	0.000000	0.000000	0.001786	0.003896	0.001194	0.003093
	max	0.000000	0.000000	0.014887	0.021683	0.016955	0.251111
Spleen	no.	10.00000	9.000000	71.00000	65.00000	0.000000	0.000000
	mean	0.249674	0.400824	0.353948	0.399419	0.000000	0.000000
	SD	0.062327	0.102932	0.419416	0.196157	0.000000	0.000000
	min	0.185897	0.231939	0.107843	0.162162	0.000000	0.000000
	max	0.365517	0.582090	3.172840	1.209965	0.000000	0.000000
Testes with epididymis	no.	10.00000	0.000000	198.0000	0.000000	40.00000	0.000000
	mean	1.110965	0.000000	1.103165	0.000000	1.210666	0.000000
	SD	0.109933	0.000000	0.235581	0.000000	0.233962	0.000000
	min	0.932927	0.000000	0.602564	0.000000	0.662271	0.000000
	max	1.241379	0.000000	3.140186	0.000000	1.736709	0.000000
Testes/epididymis, left	no.	0.000000	0.000000	28.00000	0.000000	0.000000	0.000000
	mean	0.000000	0.000000	0.517644	0.000000	0.000000	0.000000
	SD	0.000000	0.000000	0.092702	0.000000	0.000000	0.000000
	min	0.000000	0.000000	0.370270	0.000000	0.000000	0.000000
	max	0.000000	0.000000	0.799427	0.000000	0.000000	0.000000
Testes/epididymis, right	no.	0.000000	0.000000	28.00000	0.000000	0.000000	0.000000
	mean	0.000000	0.000000	0.536953	0.000000	0.000000	0.000000
	SD	0.000000	0.000000	0.098499	0.000000	0.000000	0.000000
	min	0.000000	0.000000	0.336364	0.000000	0.000000	0.000000
	max	0.000000	0.000000	0.747851	0.000000	31.000000	35.000000
Testis	no.	0.000000	0.000000	68.00000	0.000000	4.000000	5.000000
	mean	0.000000	0.000000	1.072484	0.000000	0.000000	0.000000
	SD	0.000000	0.000000	0.251187	0.000000	0.000000	0.000000
	min	0.000000	0.000000	0.398147	0.000000	0.000000	0.000000
	max	0.000000	0.000000	1.550802	0.000000	0.000000	0.000000

Testis, left	no.	0.000000	0.000000	58.00000	0.000000	0.000000	0.000000
	mean	0.000000	0.000000	0.551385	0.000000	0.000000	0.000000
	SD	0.000000	0.000000	0.083158	0.000000	0.000000	0.000000
	min	0.000000	0.000000	0.297361	0.000000	0.000000	0.000000
	max	0.000000	0.000000	0.724713	0.000000	0.000000	0.000000
Testis, right	no.	0.000000	0.000000	58.00000	0.000000	0.000000	0.000000
	mean	0.000000	0.000000	0.598274	0.000000	0.000000	0.000000
	SD	0.000000	0.000000	0.112681	0.000000	0.000000	0.000000
	min	0.000000	0.000000	0.313197	0.000000	0.000000	0.000000
	max	0.000000	0.000000	0.966845	0.000000	0.000000	0.000000
Thyroid/parathyroid	no.	0.000000	0.000000	20.00000	20.00000	40.00000	38.00000
	mean	0.000000	0.000000	0.019254	0.020708	0.018504	0.027063
	SD	0.000000	0.000000	0.007277	0.007090	0.005399	0.007526
	min	0.000000	0.000000	0.006757	0.011862	0.006460	0.017690
	max	0.000000	0.000000	0.037879	0.033721	0.032722	0.051136
Uterus	no.	0.000000	0.000000	0.000000	32.00000	0.000000	0.000000
	mean	0.000000	0.000000	0.000000	2.930984	0.000000	0.000000
	SD	0.000000	0.000000	0.000000	1.642410	0.000000	0.000000
	min	0.000000	0.000000	0.000000	0.706625	0.000000	0.000000
	max	0.000000	0.000000	0.000000	6.771605	0.000000	0.000000

toxicology studies with rats, valid statistical analyses can be applied to fixed organ weight data to compare differences among groups.

Statistical Procedures.

As expected with any well-designed scientific experiment, the protocol design or standard operating procedures should define statistical methods and procedures. Although protocols may be designed to compare data at different times in an experiment, it is probably more common in toxicology studies to comapre organ weight data from groups of rats necropsied at the same time. Although one may be tempted to do so, organ weight values should not be excluded from statistical analyses unless criteria are defined in the protocol or standard operating procedures are applied uniformly to all organ weight values. This is especially critical in carcinogenicity studies where tumors or chronic inflammatory processes may have a significant effect on organ weights. It would be erroneous to exclude from statistical analyses the weights of organs having tumors that may have been caused by the test material. Likewise, it may also be advisable to exclude those weights if the tumors were not caused by treatment. To avoid bias and the awkward situations listed above, it may be preferable to include all organ weight values in the initial statistical analyses except those values that are not scientifically believable or are associated with a mechanical or technical error that can be specifically identified. After completing and evaluating those analyses and other data generated in the study, new criteria can then be defined and uniformly applied to the organ weight data to exclude appropriate values before repeating the analyses.

Interpretation of Organ Weight Data

General

As with any biological variable, it is dangerous to interpret organ weight data without considering other data in the study. Likewise, it is dangerous to consider the potential effects of treatment on groups of animals until data from each animal have first been evaluated as a single unit. Food consumption, body weight gain, and absolute body weight data often provide useful information when interpreting organ weight data. Although one tends to rely on the results of light microscopic data, it is not unusual to have test material–related organ weight differences without evidence of a light microscopic effect. If the effect on individual cells causes uniform enlargement or shrinkage of cells, the pathologist may not observe differences between groups until those differences are dramatic. Likewise, pathological processes tend to change with time and organ weights may increase or decrease depending on the stage of the process.

Results of Statistical Analyses

In toxicological studies, the error rate (number of false positives or negatives) for statistical results or organ weights is probably much higher than is desirable. Often these changes in weight cannot be confirmed microscopically. This observation is based primarily on the results of analyses on individual organ weights for paired organs. Too often, group differences for one paired organ are statistically significant without there being a similar statistical difference for the opposite organ. One cause for the problem is probably the relatively low number of animals in each group. Although the causes for this problem may not be fully understood, one must not overinterpret the statistical results for the data. One should evaluate all of the other data as well as the statistical results before making a final judgment regarding a test material–related effect.

Metabolism   **Chyung S. Cook**

The mouse is the most extensively used experimental animal in biomedical research. In contrast to its popularity as an animal model, information on xenobiotic metabolism in the mouse is much less available compared with information in the rat and dog. This makes proper assessment of the suitability of this species for predicting xenobiotic metabolism in humans difficult. Although the metabolic patterns of some xenobiotics in the mouse are similar to those in the rat, there are many examples where xenobiotic metabolism is quantitatively and qualitatively different between these species, resulting in a difference in toxicity. The mouse is, in general, a more active oxidizer compared to the rat. Sex differences in xenobiotic metabolism are much less frequently observed in the mouse than in the rat.

Kato (1966) studied species differences in cytochrome P-450 content in relation to the activity of hepatic microsomal mixed function oxidase. Among the species studied (male and female mice, male and female rats, male rabbits, and male cats), the mouse has the highest content of cytochrome P-450 with the highest activity of NADPH oxidase, aminopyrine N-demethylase, and aniline hydroxylase (Kato, 1979). The mouse has the highest liver/body weight ratio (66.2 ± 2.8 g/kg body weight) among the commonly used laboratory animals (e.g., rat, 40.4 g/kg; guinea pig, 40.2 g/kg; rabbit, 34.5 g/kg; dog, 23.2 g/kg) but the microsomal protein concentration in the mouse liver (22.3 mg/g liver) was similar to that of the other species (Gregus et al., 1983). Consequently, the amount of cytochrome P-450 (0.5–1.1 nmol/mg) in the mouse (Table 26) was similar to that in the rat and guinea pig when calculated on the basis of milligrams of protein (Chhabra et al.,

Table 26 Summary of Hepatic Xenobiotic Drug Metabolizing Enzymes in Mice

Enzyme	Concentration or activity	Comments and References
Cytochrome P-450 (nmol/mg protein)	1.1[a], 0.48[b] 1.08 ± 0.05 for M & 1.04 ± 0.07 for F[c], 0.6 ± 0.02[d]	[a]Chhabra et al. (1974) [b]Souhaili-el Amri et al. (1986) [c]Kato (1979) [d]Flyn et al. (1972)—determined at 27°C for 1 hr
Cytochrome b (nmol/mg protein)	0.3 ± 0.01[d], 0.543 ± 0.069[e]	[d]Flyn et al. (1972)—determined at 27°C for 1 hr [e]Gregus et al. (1983)
NADPH:Cytochrome c reductase (nmol/min/mg protein)	113.0[a], 127.5[b], 109[f], 28.0 ± 1.4[d]	[a]Chhabra et al. (1974), [b]Souhaili-el Amri et al. (1986), [f]Litterst et al. (1975) [d]Flyn et al. (1972)—determined at 27°C for 1 hr
NADPH:Cytochrome P-450 reductase (nmol/min/mg protein)	1.43 ± 0.18[d]	[d]Flyn et al. (1972)—determined at 27°C for 1 hr
Hydroxylase (nmol/min/mg)		
aniline hydroxylase	16.1 ± 0.1[a], 1.5[f], 1.21 ± 0.06 for M & 1.18 ± 0.06 for F[c], 0.53 + 0.02[d]	[a]Chhabra et al. (1974), [f]Litterst et al. (1975), [c]Kato, (1979) [d]Flyn et al. (1972)—determined at 27°C for 1 hr
benzo[a]pyrene hydroxylase	114 ± 11 unit/mg/min[a]	[a]Chhabra et al. (1974)
biphenyl-4-hydroxylase	6.35 ± 0.67[a] 2.8[f]	[a]Chhabra et al. (1974) [f]Litterst et al. (1975)
hexobarbital hydroxylation	1.51 ± 0.10 for M & 1.53 ± 0.07 for F[c]	[c]Kato (1979)
Sotyrene 7,8-oxide hydrolase		
Ethoxycoumarin O-demethyl N-Demethylase (nmol/min/mg)	1.4[g]	[g]Oesch and Wolf (1989)
Aminopyrene N-demethylation	11.0 ± 1.9[f], 2.33 ± 0.14[d]	[f]Litterst et al. (1975) [d]Flyn et al, 1972—determined at 27°C for 1 hr
Ethylmorphine N-demethylation	6.75 ± 0.64[a]	[a]Chhabra et al. 1974
N-hydroxylase		
dibenzylamine	0.627 ± 0.0.13[h]	[h]Beckett and Gibson (1975)
UDP-Glucuronosyl Transferase (nmol/min/mg)		
1-naphthol	2.6[e]	[e]Gregus et. al. (1983)
4-nitrophenol	6.1[e]	[e]Gregus et. al. (1983)

Table 26 *(continued)*

Enzyme	Concentration or activity	Comments and References
Glutathion S-transferase (nmol/min/mg)		
1-chloro-2, 4-dinitrobenzene	617[g] (cytosol), 147–15[g,i] (microsomes)	[g]Oesch and Wolf (1989), [i]Morgenstern et al. (1984)
Herachloro-1,3-butadiene	0.109[g] (cytosol),	[g]Oesch and Wolf (1989)
Protein estimates		
microsomal	34.3 ± 9.4[f]	[f]Litterst et al. 1975
(mg/g)	22.3 ± 1.3[e]	[e]Gregus et al. (1983)
cytosolic	79.0 ± 3.2[e]	[e]Gregus et al. (1983)
(mg/g)		

1974; Litterst et al., 1975, 1976; Gregus et al., 1983). However, the value in mouse liver was slightly higher than that in the dog (0.347 nmol/mg). The level of NADPH-cytochrome c reductase activity (109 ± 33 nmol/mg/min) was much lower in the mouse compared with the rat (187 ± 51 nmol/mg/min). The activities in mixed function oxidase measured by hydroxylase activity for aniline and biphenyl were about twofold higher in the mouse than in the rat. Aminopyrine N-demethylase activity was similar in these species. In contrast, the activities of benzo(a)pyrene hydroxylase and ethylmorphine N-demethylase in the mouse were about half the activities in the rat (Chhabra et al., 1974).

Souhaili-el Amri et al. (1986) compared the contents and activities of cytochrome P-450 in liver microsomes in six laboratory animal species and humans, and confirmed the results reported by Litterst et al. (1975, 1976). They also reported that the contents of cytochrome P-450 and NADPH-cytochrome c reductase in the male mouse (0.48 ± 0.04 and 127.5 ± 6.5 nmol/mg/min, respectively) were slightly higher than those in human males (0.31 ± 0.09 and 99.8 ± 14.4 nmol/mg/min). In contrast, the content of cytochrome b_5 in the male mouse (0.20 ± 0.02 nmol/mg/min) was slightly lower than that in human (0.29 ± 0.11 nmol/mg/min).

The distribution pattern of mixed function oxidases for xenobiotics between the smooth and rough microsomal membranes of the liver is known to be species dependent. In the mouse liver microsomes, concentrations of all components of a mixed function oxidase system were approximately the same between smooth and rough membranes (Gram et al., 1971), whereas in some animals (e.g., monkey, guinea pig), the concentrations were approximately twofold higher in the smooth membrane.

It has been shown that the levels of mixed function oxidase are generally highest in the mammalian liver compared with the levels in other organs. In the mouse, the content of cytochrome P-450 was approximately four- and twofold higher in the liver than in the lung and kidney, respectively. Activity of NADPH-cytochrome c reductase was similar in these organs. Hydroxylase activity for aniline and biphenyl and aminopyrine N-demethylase activity were much higher in the liver than in the lung and kidney. However, beta-glucuronidase activity for phenolphthalein in the mouse spleen was 3- to 10-fold higher than that in the liver depending on the strains.

Sex difference in the activity of microsomal mixed function oxidase is a peculiar phenomenon which is observed clearly in the rat with higher activity in the male than in the female. However, sex differences in mice are not consistently observed (Westfall et al., 1964, Davies et al., 1969; Kato, 1974) and appear to be strain dependent. There was no sex difference in the contents of cytochrome P-450, NADPH-cytochrome c reductase or NADPH oxidase in the mouse. Sex differences were not evident in aminopyrine N-demethylase and aniline hydroxylase activities (Souhaili-El Amri et al., 1987), whereas clear sex differences were demonstrated in the hexobarbital hydroxylase (Castro and Gillette, 1967; MacLeod et al., 1986) and N-demethylation activity of ethylmorphine (Kato and Onoda, 1966; Catz and Yaffe, 1967; MacLeod et al., 1987) with significantly higher maximal velocities (V_{max}) in female than in male mice of some strains. UDP-Glucuronyltransferase activity in the male mouse was similar to or significantly greater than that in the female depending on the strain of the mouse (Boutin, 1984).

Strain differences in the metabolism of xenobiotics are frequently observed in the mouse as also observed in the rat and rabbit. For example, a marked strain difference in the oxidative metabolism of hexobarbital was observed in mice. The duration of sleeping time after a single dose of the drug, which is determined by the rate of its oxidation, ranged from 20 min in the CS7BL mouse strain to 60 min in the 129J strain. Interestingly, there appears to be an inverse relationship between toxicity and sleeping time in the strains of mice studied. This relationship in time correlates with the strain-dependent rates of hepatic metabolism, perhaps suggesting an intermediate toxic product.

The mouse is known to have a high activity of oxidative enzymes compared with other laboratory animals and humans. The biological half-life of oxidative metabolism of hexobarbital in the mouse is 20–60 min whereas the half-lives in the rabbit, rat, dog, and human are 60, 140, 260 and 360 min, respectively.

As discussed in another chapter (see Xenobiotic section in Chap. 8), N-dealklyation is most frequently used by the dog and human and least frequently used by the rat. The mouse uses this pathway for many compounds and appears to have high N-dealkylase activity in general. For example, the mouse has been shown to excrete major amounts of the N-dealkylated metabolite of tiaramide (Schwarz, 1973), whereas the other species (rat, dog, and monkey) favor N-oxide formation and/or side chain oxidation. Oxamniquine has been shown to be metabolized by N-dealkylation in the mouse but not in the rat. When N-demethylation activity for aminopyrine was examined in the mouse, rat, rabbit, and cat, the enzyme activity in the mouse was highest and at least threefold higher than that in the male rat (Kato, 1966). In addition, there was no sex difference in the N-demethylase activity in the mouse, whereas the enzyme activity in the male rat was approximately fourfold higher than that in the female rat. Castro and Gillette (1967) studied species difference in N-demethylation of ethylmorphine using hepatic microsomes of the mouse, rat, guinea pig, and monkey. Ethylmorphine N-demethylase activity in the male and female mouse was higher than that in the other species except for the male rat. N-Demethylase activity in the male mouse (V_{max} of 139 mmol/mg/10 min) was approximately half the activity in females. Later Van Den Berg et al. (1977) found that ethylmorphine N-demethylase activity differed between the sexes in one strain of mouse (CPB-SE) but not in another strain (CPB-V). In the rat, the ethylmorphine N-demethylase activity in males (V_{max} of 203 mmol/mg/10 min) was approximately fivefold higher than that in females.

Diazepam is metabolized oxidatively by two metabolic pathways; one is ring hydroxylation, which is the main pathway in the rat, and the other is oxidative N-demethylation, which is the main pathway in the mouse and man. Although concentrations of diazepam in blood and brain are similar in the mouse and rat, antimetrazol activity is longer lasting in the mouse than in the rat owing to the accumulation of active N-demethylated metabolite in the mouse brain (Marcucci et al., 1968). In humans, the N-demethylated metabolite was the major metabolite detected in plasma.

Amphetamine is metabolized oxidatively by two metabolic pathways: one is ring hydroxylation and the other oxidative deamination (Dring et al., 1976). N-Deamination of amphetamine occurs in the mouse as in humans (Caldwell, 1976). In the rat, amphetamine was shown to be extensively metabolized by aromatic hydroxylation and poorly metabolized by oxidative deamination. Based on the available metabolism data, the mouse appears to be a relatively good animal model, in general, for N-dealkylation and N-deamination. However, the extents of N-dealkylation and N-deamination are highly compound dependent and caution must be exercised for this generalization.

There are several microsomal aromatic hydrocarbon hydroxylases (AHHs) whose occurrence depends not only upon species, but also on the nature of the aromatic compound. Generally, the activities of these enzymes are much greater in the mouse than in humans as observed with amphetamine and benzo(a)pyrene (Souhaili-el Amri et al., 1986). Aromatic hydroxylation of amphetamine occurred to the extent of 10–19% in the mouse and about 3% in humans. In the rat, it was about 60% (Parke, 1968). In contrast to amphetamine hydroxylase activity, the activity of benzo(a)pyrene hydroxylase in the mouse was approximately threefold higher than that of the male inbred SD rat (Oesch et al., 1973). The AHH activity in human liver was approximately 30–60% of the hepatic activity of the male rat (Pelkonen et al., 1975). Although the bezo(a)pyrene hydroxylase activity was similar in male and female mice, a sex difference has been shown in the rat, with the female displaying about 20–40% of the hepatic activity of the male.

Biphenyl was metabolized in the mouse to 2-hydroxybiphenyl as well as 4-hydroxybiphenyl, which is the metabolite of all species examined (Creaven, et al, 1965). However, in rats the 2-hydroxy metabolite was formed only in young animals but not in the adults, although rats are known to be a good animal model for aromatic hydroxylation. Therefore, the distribution and activity of the microsomal hydroxylases among species can not be predicted for all compounds. If a difference is found among species with a given compound, then it is likely, but not always certain, that a similar species difference may consistently occur with its derivatives (Williams, 1974).

Many unreactive compounds may be metabolized to chemically highly reactive intermediates and act as mutagenic/carcinogenic agents. Unreactive aromatic hydrocarbons and olefinic compounds are converted to highly active arene oxides and alkene oxides which are formed from the epoxidation of double bonds in aromatic rings and olefinic double bonds, respectively. The mouse is reported to have high epoxygenase activity (Gregus et al., 1983). In a comparative in vitro metabolism study of naphthalene using microsomal preparations from lung, liver, and kidney of mice, rats, and hamsters, it has been shown that metabolism of naphthalene to an epoxide was most extensive with microsomal preparations from the mouse lung (Buckpitt et al., 1987). Furthermore, metabolism of naphthalene was stereoselective to form (1R,2S)-naphthalene 1,2-oxide with the mouse lung, which is the target tissue for acute toxicity in this species. In contrast, with microsomal preparations from the mouse liver and kidney, and with all microsomal preparations from the rat and hamster, metabolism was not stereoselective.

The epoxides are metabolized to much less reactive vicinal diols by epoxide hydrolases and to glutathione conjugates by glutathione S-transferase. Therefore, the level and activity of epoxide hydrolases among species may be of great importance for the mutagenic/carcinogenic risks. With styrene oxide as the substrate the epoxide hydrolase activity in the mouse (1.4 nmol/mg protein/min) was less than one-fortieth of that in humans (59.3 nmol/mg protein/min) and less than one-fourth the activity in the rat (5.5 nmol/mg protein/min) (Oesch and Wolf, 1989). However, in the diabetic mouse (male and female db/db strain) the styrene oxide hydrolase activity was increased approximately threefold (Watkins and Klueber, 1988). In addition, genetic polymorphism of microsomal epoxide hydrolase activity in the mouse has been reported (Lyman et al., 1980).

A species, such as mice, having high epoxygenase activity (Gregus et al., 1983) but low epoxide hydrolase activity (Oesch and Wolf, 1989) may be much more susceptible than the human to toxicity related to epoxide formation. However, epoxides are also detoxified via glutathione conjugation. The mouse liver has a high level of glutathione transferase activity (149 ± 13 nmol/mg/min) compared to that of rats (87 ± 10 nmol/mg/min) and humans (25 ± 4 nmol/mg/min) (Pacifici et al., 1981). For example, following acrylonitrile administration, concentrations of an oxide metabolite (2-cyanoethylene oxide) in rat blood were 6–11 times higher than those in the mouse, although mouse liver oxidized acrylonitrile to the oxide at a much greater rate (approximately 3 times) than rat liver (Kedderis, 1989). Acrylonitrile was metabolized to thiodiglycolic acid, a metabolite of the glutathione conjugate, 7 times faster in the mouse than in the rat. Therefore, to what extent these interspecies difference in the epoxide toxicity will occur for other substrates remains to be further evaluated.

It has been reported that N-hydroxylase activity is predominately mediated via the polycyclic hydrocarbon-inducible P1-450 (Felton et al., 1976) and is of great importance for toxicity evaluation. The mouse is the most susceptible to acetaminophen-induced hepatic injury and the rat had the lowest susceptibility. This difference in toxicity was found to be related to the rates of N-hydroxylation of the drug by the hepatic microsomes (Davis et al., 1974). An increase in N-hydroxylation enhances the need for reduced glutathione and glutathione depletion in the liver precedes marked increases in covalently bound acetaminophen. Formation of metabolites covalently bound to microsomal protein and depletion of hepatic glutathione were highest in the mouse but only minor extents of covalent binding and depletion of glutathione were observed in the rat. As a result, in the mouse acetaminophen induced hepatotoxicity. Increases in covalently bound metabolites of the drug were found to be highly correlated with the Ah[b] allele (Thorgeirsson et al., 1977).

Lotlikar et al. (1967) studied species differences in the relative N- and ring hydroxylation of 2-acetylaminofluorene by liver microsomes of the mouse and other species. The N-hydroxylase activity in the mouse was lower than that in hamster and rabbit but higher than that in the rat and guinea pig. The N-hydroxy metabolite was practically undetectable in the guinea pig, which explains resistance of the guinea pig to hepatoma induction by 2-acetylaminofluorene. Later Razzouk and Roberfroid (1982) reported that V_{max} values for N-hydroxylase of aminofluorene and acetylaminofluorene in the mouse (510 and 225 pmol/mg/min, respectively) were higher than those in the hamster (260 and 140 pmol/mg/min, respectively) and at least 10-fold higher than those in the rat (41 and 14 pmol/min/min, respectively). N-Hydroxylase activities were also studied in several species with dibenzylamine (Beckett and Gibson, 1975) and 4-aminobiphenyl (McMahon, et al., 1980). In contrast to acetylaminofluorene N-hydroxylase activity, N-hydroxylase activity of dibenzylamine (18.8 nmol/mg/30 min) and 4-aminobiphenyl (13.2 μmol/80 min) in the mouse were approximately twofold lower compared with guinea pig liver. The activity of dibenzylamine N-hydroxylase in the mouse was slightly higher than that in the rat (12.5 nmol/mg/30 min), whereas 4-aminobiphenyl N-hydroxylase activity in the mouse was fivefold higher than that in the rat (2.4 μmol/80 min). Thus, based on the limited information available, N-hydroxylase activity in the mouse is moderate and similar to or higher than that of the rat.

The mouse is not reported to display any defects in conjugation reactions such as those observed in the cat (glucuronidation), pig (sulfation), and dog (acetylation). In acetylation of certain aromatic amines, both fast and slow acetylators have been identified with some mouse strains such as C57BL/6J and A/J as with the human population (Elves et al., 1985). Lower and Bryan (1973) studied acetylation of the carcinogens 2-aminofluorene, 4-aminobiphenyl, and 2-aminonaphthalene by the mouse liver cytosol enzymes. The most readily acetylated carcinogen was 2-aminofluorene (332 $\pm$ 25 nmol/50 mg liver/5 min), followed by 4-aminobiphenyl (215 $\pm$ 15 nmol/50 mg liver/5 min) and 2-aminonaphthalene (209 $\pm$ 9 nmol/50 mg liver/5 min). These enzyme activities in the mouse liver were about half the activities in the hamster liver but 6–10 times higher than those in the rat liver. Recently, Calabrese (1988) reported that the mouse was about 4.6-fold more efficient acetylator than the human fast acetylator for 2-aminofluorene. The rat displayed about half the activity of the human fast acetylator and sevenfold greater activity to acetylate 2-aminofluorene than the human slow acetylator, which is consistent with previous findings (Lower and Bryan, 1973).

Lower and Bryan (1976) also studied deacetylase activites of the acetylated derivatives of each of the above same three compounds in the mouse, hamster, rat, guinea pig, and dog. Deacetylase activity of 4-acetylaminobiphenyl was highest in the mouse and more than 20 times that observed in the rat. However, deacetylase activities for 2-acetylaminofluorene (54.7 $\pm$ 6.3 nmol/mg/hr) and 2-acetylaminonaphthalene (21.1 $\pm$ 6.3 nmol/mg/hr) in the mouse were approximately three- and sixfold lower compared with those of hamster liver. The guinea pig and rat were generally the least efficient in deacetylation of these compounds. The relative capacity of the animal model to acetylate and deacetylate is an important variable with respect to arylamine-induced cancer. In the mouse, as in the rat, the ratio of N-acetyltransferase to deacetylase activity is very high relative to the dog. This may provide rodents with some protection against bladder cancer, but not hepatocarcinogenesis.

Surprisingly there is little information available for glucuronidation activity of drugs in the mouse. Based on limited information, UDP-glucuronosyltransferase activities in rodents and primates are generally high compared with that in the cats (Caldwell, 1978). Gregus et al. (1983) studied hepatic UDP-glucuronosyltransferase activity toward 11 acceptors in the mouse, rat, guinea pig, rabbit, cat, quail, and trout. The transferase activity in the mouse, when compared to the activity in other species, was high toward phenolphthalein, diethylstilbestrol, morphine, valproic acid, and bilirubin, whereas the activity was medium or low toward 1-naphthol, p-nitrophenol, testosterone, estrone, chloramphenicol, and digitoxigenin. Therefore, the UDP-glucuronyltransferase activity appears to be highly substrate specific and no general pattern in its activity could be established among the species studied. Considerable evidence has accumulated which suggests that multiple forms of UDP-glucuronyl transferase exist, and this may explain why glucuronidation activity is high for some substrates but not for others.

A strain difference in UDP-glucuronosyltransferase activity in the mouse has been reported (Tsyrlov and Lyakhovich, 1978). After pretreatment with 3-methylcholanthrene, the microsomal UDP-glucuronosyltransferase activity increased threefold in C57BL mice but not in AKR mice, although the transferase activity in the control animals was similar between these two strains.

Hydrolysis of glucuronide conjugates is carried out by the lysosomal enzyme beta-glucuronidase, which is present in most tissues, particularly liver, kidney, spleen, intestine tract, endocrine, and reproductive organs. The level of beta-glucuronidase in multiple tissues has been studied in a variety of animal species as well as in humans. Genetic polymorphism of beta-glucuronidase activity was observed in the various tissues of the mouse in which the activity in the high-activity strain is 4–10 times greater than that of the low activity strain. The enzyme levels in the liver, kidney, and spleen of the high-activity strain of the mouse were similar to the activity in the respective human tissues, whereas the activities in the rat were approximately 10-fold higher than those in humans. The beta-glucuronidase of the cecal contents and feces were also similar in mice and humans (Rowland et al., 1986). However, beta-glucuronidase activity in the mouse intestine was much higher than that in humans and rats. The activities of beta-glucuronidase in the spleen were similar to or higher than those in the liver regardless of species and strain of mouse.

As discussed earlier, GSH transferase activity in the mouse liver was reported to be higher than that in the rat with 1-chloro-2,4-dinitrobezene as a substrate (Igarashi et al., 1983, 1986) and also higher than human liver with styrene oxide as a substrate (Pacifici et al., 1981). Recently, Oesch and Wolf (1989) determined glutathione transferase activities in liver microsomes and cytosol from various species, including mice and humans with hexachloro-1,3-butadiene and 1-chloro-2,4-dinitrobenzene. Contrary to the earlier findings, the glutathione transferase activities in the mouse were lower than those in the rat with the same substrate and also lower than those in humans. This difference may be, in part, due to strain difference of the mouse and substrate difference in humans among the studies. The transferase activity in the microsomes (0.16 nmol/min/mg) and cytosol (0.109 nmol/min/mg) were similar in the mouse, whereas in humans the enzyme activity was much greater in microsomes (1.17 nmol/min/mg) than in cytosol (0.031 nmol/min/mg) with hexachloro-1,3-butadiene as a substrate (Oesch and Wolf, 1989). However, with 1-chloro-2,4-dinitrobenzene, GSH transferase activity in the cytosol fraction in mice (617 nmol/min/mg) and humans (1666 nmol/min/mg) was about 11- and 30-fold higher than the activities in the microsomal fraction, respectively. Therefore, the GSH transferase activity appears to be highly compound specific and it is difficult to make any broad generalization.

Thiol methylation is an important pathway in the metabolism of many sulfhydryl drugs. At least two enzymes, thiol methyltransferase (TMT) and thiopurine methyltransferase (TPMT) can catalyze the thiol methylation. Thiol methyltransferase is membrane associated and catalyzes the S-methylation of aliphatic sulfhydryl compounds such as 2-mercaptoethanol, captopril, and D-penicillamine. It is inhibited by SKF 525A but not by the benzoic acid derivatives that are potent inhibitors of TPMT. Otterness et al. (1986) studied TMT activity in hepatic microsomes from 10 different strains of mice using 2-mercaptoethanol as the methyl acceptor substrate and compared the activity with that in human red blood cell membranes and kidney microsomes. Since the properties of TMT in the mouse liver were similar to those of the enzyme in the human tissues, the authors concluded that the inbred mouse is a useful experimental animal model to study the regulation and function of TMT.

Very little work has been reported on the conjugation reactions of xenobiotics with sulfate, taurine, and aminoacids in the mouse. Based on the limited information, the mouse appears to have moderate sulfate conjugation capability as illustrated with acetaminophen and 4-hydroxy-3-methoxyphenyl ethanol. The concentration of adenosine 3'-phosphate-5'-phosphosulfate (PAPS), which is required for sulfation reactions as the sulfate donor, in the male mouse liver (29.4 ± 1.6 mmol/g of tissue) was lower than that of rats (67.9–76.8 mmol/g), similar to hamsters and rabbits, but much higher than that in the dog (16.1–17.3 mmol/g). The concentrations of PAPS in the mouse kidney, lung, and intestine were approximately half that of liver.

Emudianughe et al., (1978, 1987) studied amino acid conjugation of the isomeric naphthylacetic acids in seven subprimate animal species, including the mouse. With 2-naphthylacetic acid, the taurine conjugate was the major urinary conjugated metabolite (57%), whereas the glucuronide conjugate was 40% of the urinary conjugated metabolites. However, with 1-naphthylacetic acid, the majority of the urinary conjugate metabolites in the mouse was the glucuronide (68%) and the glycine conjugate was minor (16%). In general the dog appears to be the most extensive taurine conjugator, man and rhesus monkey are weak species for this conjugation pathway, and the mouse is intermediate. An exception to this is the conjugation metabolism of an arylacetic acid, oxepinac. Oxepinac was metabolized to the taurine conjugate in the mouse as well as in the rat (Hakusui, 1978). However, in the dog and man it was conjugated with glucuronic acid, although the dog is known to be an extensive taurine conjugator with some other compounds. Glutamine conjugates of naphthylacetic acids were not detected in the mouse urine, although other rodents such as the rat and hamster formed substantial amount of this conjugate.

The drug-metabolizing enzymes in the mouse are generally induced or inhibited with compounds known to be enzyme inducers or inhibitors, respectively, in the other species. An exception to this is that DDT, an enzyme inducer for the rat, pig, and sheep did not produce any enhancement of the oxidative metabolism of drugs in the mouse (Hart & Fouts, 1965; Gabliks & Maltby-askari, 1970). Furthermore, with some inducers marked strain differences were observed in the induction of xenobiotic metabolism in the mouse (Glass and van Lier, 1988). A typical example includes AHH induction by polycyclic hydrocarbons. The AHH assay is a reliable, simple, and very sensitive assessment of aromatic hydrocarbon responsiveness following treatment of animals with polycyclic hydrocarbon inducers. Using AHH induction as an indicator of phenotype at the Ah locus, several laboratories have found that about half or slightly more than half of all inbred mouse strains examined were responsive and the remaining mouse strains were nonresponsive (Nebert et al., 1979).

SKF-525A inhibited aminopyrine N-demethylase and hexobarbital hydroxylase in mouse hepatic preparations as in rat hepatic preparations. However, the inhibition was quasicompetitive in the mouse, whereas in the rat it was competitive, thus indicating differences in the nature of the monooxygenases between these two species.

Not many in-depth works have been published about stereoselectivity in metabolism and toxicity of xenobiotics in the mouse. One interesting example, however, is stereoselective toxicity of thalidomide. Both S-(–)thalidomide and the R-(+)-enantiomer are transformed into 1-N-phthaloylglutamine and 1-N-phthaloylglutaminic acid in various species. Although conflicting reports have been published on potential racemization of thalidomide enantiomers and the sensitivity of different mice and rat strains as to thalidomide toxicity, in SWS mice only the glutaminic acid metabolite derived from the S-(–)-enantiomer and not the one derived from the R-(+)-isomer was shown to be embryotoxic and teratogenic (Ockzenfelz et al., 1976).

Species differences in toxicity of a compound may be due to factors other than metabolism differences. Some of these factors include protein binding and biliary excretion in addition to absorption and elimination. When protein binding of some drugs (clofibric acid, etodolac, tolrestat, perrinone, benoxaprofen) was examined in the rat, mouse, dog, rabbit, rhesus monkey, and human, the binding was, in general, highest in human serum, weakest in the mouse, and somewhat variable with other species.

Differences in biliary excretion may have pronounced toxicological implications, especially when followed by reabsorption; i.e., enterohepatic circulation takes places. For example, the intestinal toxicity of indomethacin in five species of laboratory animals (rat, dog, monkey, guinea pig, and rabbit) is inversely proportional to the exposure of the intestinal mucosa to the drug as a consequence of enterohepatic circulation. In general, the mouse, rat, and dog are very efficient in biliary excretion, and guinea pigs, monkeys, and human are relatively inefficient. For example, the biliary excretion rate of methyl mercury was substantially higher in the mouse, rat, and hamster (approximately 0.8 nmol/min/kg) compared with that in the guinea pig and rabbit (0.15 and 0.03 nmol/min/kg, respectively) (Stein et al., 1988). The biliary excretion rate of GSH-related thiols and disulfides was also highest in the mouse.

As reported for other species, the drug-metabolizing enzymes in newborn mice are not fully developed. When phenobarbital was injected in mice of various ages, the newborn animals failed to metabolize any of the drug over a 3-hr period. One-week-old mice metabolized about 18% and 3-week-old mice about 22%. A hexobarbital sleeping time study also revealed striking differences with age (Jondorf et al., 1958). The sleeping time of 1-week-old mice was about 107 mins, whereas the sleeping time of adult was less than 5 mins.

REFERENCES

Alison, R. H., and Morgan, K. T. (1987a) Granulosa cell tumor, ovary, mouse, in *Genital System*, Jones, T. C., Mohr, U., and Hunt, R. D., eds. Springer-Verlag, New York, pp. 22–30.

Alison, R. H., and Morgan, K. T. (1987b) Teratoma, ovary, mouse, in *Genital System*, Jones, T. C., Mohr, U., and Hunt, R. D., eds. Springer-Verlag, New York, pp. 46–52.

Andrew, W. (1962) An electron microscopic study of the age changes in the liver of the mouse. *Am. J. Anat.* 110, 1–18.

Andrews, B. S., Eisenberg, R. A., Theofilopoulos, A. N., Izui, S., Wilson, C. B., McConahey, P. J., Murphy, E. D., Roths, J. B., and Dixon, F. J. (1978) Spontaneous murine lupus-like syndromes. *J. Exp. Med.* 148, 1198–1215.

Anonymous (1981) *NIH Rodents 1980 Catalog, Strains and Stocks of Laboratory Rodents.* Provided by the NIH Genetic Resources, NIH Publication No. 81-606.

Anonymous (1982) *Charles River Technical Bulletin.* Charles River Laboratories, Wilmington, Massachusetts.

Anonymous (1989) *Spontaneous Neoplastic Lesions in the B6C3F1/Cr1BR Mouse.* Charles River Laboratories, Wilmington, Massachusetts.

Anthony, A. (1962) Criteria for acoustics in animal housing. *Lab. Anim. Care* 13, 340–347.

Barthold, S. (1978) Transmissible murine colonic hyperplasia. *Vet. Pathol.* 15, 223–236.

Beckett, A. H. and Gibson, G. G. (1975) Microsomal N-hydroxylation of dibenzylamine, *Xenobiotica* 5, 677–686.

Bendele, A. M., and Carlton, W. W. (1986) Incidence of obstructive uropathy in male B6C3F1 mice on a 26-month carcinogenicity study and its apparent prevention by ochratoxin A. *Lab. Anim. Sci.* 36, 282–285.

Benson, A. M., Hunkeler, M. J., and York, J. L. (1989) Mouse hepatic glutathione transferase isozymes and their differential induction by anticarcinogens. *Biochem. J.* 261, 1023–1029.

Boorman, G. A., and Eustis, S. L. (1985) Acinar-cell carcinoma, pancreas, rat, in *Monographs on Pathology of Laboratory Animals: Digestive System.* Jones, T. C., Mohr, U., and Hunt, R. D., eds. Springer-Verlag, Berlin, pp. 219–224.

Boutin, J. A., Antoine, B., Batt, A. M., and Siest (1984) Heterogeneity of hepatic microsomal

UDP-glucuronyltransferase(s) activities: Comparison between human and mammalian species activities. *Chem. Biol. Interact.* 52, 173–184.

Broderson, J. R., Lindsey, J. R., and Crawford, J. E. (1976) The role of environmental ammonia in respiratory mycoplasmosis of rats. *Am. J. Pathol.* 85, 115–130.

Brownstein, D. G. (1983) Genetics of dystrophic epicardial mineralization in DBA/2 mice. *Lab. Anim. Sci.* 33, 247–248.

Brusick, D. (ed.) (1980) *Principles of Genetic Toxicology.* Plenum Press, New York.

Buckpitt, A. R., Castagoli, N., Jr., Nelson, S. D., Jones, A. D., and Bahnson, L. S. (1987) Stereoselectivity of naphthalene epoxidation by mouse, rat, and hamster pulmonary, hepatic, and renal microsomal enzymes. *Drug Metab. Dispos.* 15, 491–498.

Burek, J. D., Molello, J. A., and Warner, S. D. (1982) Selected nonneoplastic diseases, in *The Mouse in Biomedical Research*, Vol. II, Foster, H. L., Small, J. D., and Fox, J. G., eds. Academic Press, New York. pp. 425–439.

Butler, W. H., and Newberne, P. M. (eds.) (1975) *Mouse Hepatic Neoplasia.* Amsterdam, Elsevier, pp. 195.

Byzeznicka, E. A., Hazelton, G. A. and Klaassen, C. D. (1987) Comparison of adenosine 3'-phosphate 5'-phosphosulfate concentrations in tissues from different laboratory animals. *Drug Metab. Dispos.* 15, 133–135.

Calabrese, E. J. (1988) Comparative biology of test species. *Environ. Health Perspect.* 77, 55–62.

Caldwell, J. (1976) The metabolism of amphetamines in mammals. *Drug Met. Rev.* 5, 219–280.

Caldwell, J. (1978) Structure-metabolism relationships in the amino acid conjugations, in *Conjugation Reactions in Drug Biotransformation*, Aitio, A., ed. Elsevier/North-Holland Biomedical Press, Amsterdam.

Cameron, A. M., and Sheldon, W. (1983) Cystoid degeneration, anterior pituitary, mouse, in *Endocrine System*, Jones, T. C., Mohr, U., and Hunt, R. D., eds. Springer-Verlag, New York, pp. 165–168.

Campbell, C. S., Ryan, K. D., and Schwartz, N. B. (1976) Estrus cycles in the mouse: Relative influence of continuous light and the presence of a male. *Biol. Reprod.* 14, 292–299.

Cardesa, A., and Ovelar, M. Y. (1985) Squamous cell carcinoma, esophagus, rat, in *Monographs on Pathology of Laboratory Animals: Digestive System*. Jones, T. C., Mohr, U., and Hunt, R. D., eds. Springer-Verlag, Berlin, pp. 268–272.

Carlton, W. W., and Gries, C. L. (1983) Cysts, pituitary; rat, mouse, and hamster, in *Endocrine System*, Jones, T. C., Mohr, U., and Hunt, R. D., eds. Springer-Verlag, New York, pp. 161–163.

Carter, R. L. (1968) Pathology of ovarian neoplasms in rats and mice. *Eur. J. Cancer* 3, 537–543.

Castro, J. A., and Gillette, J. R. (1967) Species and sex differences in the kinetic constants for the N-demethylation of ethylmorphine by liver microsomes. *Biochem. Biophys. Res. Commun.* 28, 426–430.

Catz, C. S., and Yaffe, S. Y. (1967) Strain and age variations in hexobarbital response. *J. Pharmacol. Exp. Ther.* 155, 152–156.

Cavaliere, A., Bacci, M., and Fratini, D. (1981) Spontaneous pancreatic adenocarcinoma in a mouse *(Mus musculus)*. *Lab. Anim. Sci.* 31, 502–503.

Cayan, M. N. (1987) Retrospective evaluation of appropriate animal models based on metabolism studies in man, in *Human Risk Assessment—The Role of Animal Selection and Extrapolation*, Roloff, N. W., ed. Taylor & Francis, London.

CFR (21 CFR Part 58) (1988a) Good Laboratory Practice for Nonclinical Laboratory Studies, Subpart E, paragraph 58.43 Animal Care Facilities. April 1988.

CFR (21 CFR Part 58) (1988b) Good Laboratory Practice for Nonclinical Laboratory Studies, Subpart E, paragraph 58.90 Animal Care, item (h). April 1988.

CFRb (21 CFR Part 58) (1988c) Good Laboratory Practice for Nonclinical Laboratory Studies, Subpart E, paragraph 58.90 Animal Care, item (g). April 1988.

CFR (21 CFR Part 58) (1988d) Good Laboratory Practice for Nonclinical Laboratory Studies, Subpart E, paragraph 58.90 Animal Care, item (d), April 1988.

Chance, M.R.A. (1946) Aggregation as a factor influencing the toxicity of sympathomimetic amines in mice. *J. Pharmacol. Exp. Therapeut.* 87, 214–219.

Chandra, M., and Frith, C. H. (1991) Spontaneously occurring leiomyosarcomas in the mouse urinary bladder. *Toxicol. Pathol.* 19:164–167.

Chhabra, R. S., Pohl, R. J., and Fouts, J. R. (1974) A comparative study of xenobiotic-metabolizing enzymes in liver and intestine of various animal species, *Drug Metab. Dispo.*, 2, 443–447.

Chiu, T., and Chen, H. C. (1986) Spontaneous basophilic hypertrophic foci of the parotid glands in rats and mice. *Vet. Pathol.* 23, 606–609.

Chouroulinkov, I., Lasne, C., Phillips, D., and Grover, P. (1988). Sensitivity of the skin of different mouse strains to the promoting effect of 12-O-tetradecanoyl-phorbol-13-acetate. *Bull. Cancer*, 75, 557–565.

Clough, C. (1982) Environmental effects on animals used in biomedical research. *Biol. Rev.* 57, 487–523.

Cohen, S. M., and Friedell, G. H. (1982) Neoplasms of the urinary system, in *The Mouse in Biomedical Research* Foster, H. L., Small, J. D., and Fox, J. G., eds. Academic Press, New York, pp. 439–463.

Creaven, P. J., Parke, D. V., and Williams, R. T. (1965) A fluorimetric study of the hydroxylation of biphenyl in vitro by liver preparations of various species. *Biochem. J.*, 96, 879–885.

Davis, D. S., Gigon, P. L., and Gillett, J. R. (1969) Species and sex differences in electron transport system in liver microsomes and the relationship to ethylmorphine demethylation. *Life Sci.*, 8, 85–91.

Davis, C. D., Potter, W. Z., Jollow, D. J., and Mitchell, J. R. (1974) Species differences in hepatic glutathione depletion, covalent binding and hepatic necrosis after acetaminophen. *Life Sci.* 14, 2099–2109.

Dawe, C. J. (1979) Tumors of the salivary and lachrymal glands, nasal fossa and maxillary sinuses, in *Pathology of Tumors in Laboratory Animals*, Vol. 11—*Tumors of the Mouse*, Turusov, V. S., ed. International Agency for Research on Cancer, Lyon, p. 91.

Debackere, M., and Uehleke, H. (1964) C- and N-hydroxylation of aromatic amines by isolated liver microsomes of different species, in *Some Factors Affecting Drug Toxicity*, pp. 40–44, Spanjaard, K., ed. *Proceedings of the European Socity for the Study of Drug Toxicity*, Vol. 4, Excerpta Medica Foundation, Amsterdam.

Dean, B. J. (ed.). (1983) *Report of the UKEMS Sub-committee on Guidelines for Mutagenicity Testing*, Part I, *Basic Test Battery*, etc., United Kingdom Environmental Mutagen Society.

Dean, B. J. (ed) (1984) *Report of the UKEMS Sub-Committee on Guidelines for Mutagenicity Testing*, Part II, *Supplemental Tests*, etc., United Kingdom Environmental Mutagen Society.

Delaney, W. E. (1977) Transplantable murine salivary gland carcinomas (myoepithelioma). Biologic behavior and ultrastructural features. *J. Natl. Cancer Inst.* 58, 61–65.

Deringer, M. K., and Dunn, T. B. (1947) Mast cell neoplasia in mice. *J. Natl. Cancer Inst.* 7, 289–298.

DiPaola, J. A., Strong, L. C., and Moore, G. E. (1964) Calcareous pericarditis in mice of several genetically related strains. *Proc. Soc. Exp. Biol. Med.* 115, 496–497.

Dring, L. G., Smith, R. L., and Williams, R. T. (1966) The fate of amphetamine in man and other animals. *J. Pharm. Pharmacol.* 18, 402–404.

Dunn, T. B. (1954) Normal and pathologic anatomy of the reticular tissue in laboratory mice. *J. Natl. Cancer Inst.* 14, 1281–1433.

Dunn, T. B. (1959) Morphology of mammary tumors in mice, in *The Pathophysiology of Cancer*, Homburger, F., and Fishman, W. H., eds. Hoeber-Harper, New York, pp. 38–84.

Dunn, T. B. (1967) Renal disease of the mouse, in *Pathology of Laboratory Rats and Mice* Cotchin, E., and Roe, F.J.C., eds. Oxford and Edinburgh, Blackwell Scientific, pp. 149–176.

Dunn, T. B. (1969) Mast cell neoplasia in mice. *Natl. Cancer Inst. Monogr.* 32, 285–287.

Dunn, T. B. (1970 Normal and pathologic anatomy of the adrenal gland of the mouse, including neoplasms. *J. Natl. Cancer Inst.* 44, 1323–1389.

Dunn, J. R., and Stern, J. S. (1978) Feeder for measuring food intake in the mouse. *Lab. Anim. Sci.* 28, 97–98.

Eddy, B. E. (1969) Polyoma virus. *Virol. Monogr.* 7, 1–114.

Edsbacker, S., Andersson, P., Lindberg, C., Paulson, J., Ryrfeldt, A., and Thalen, A. (1987) Liver metabolism of Budesonide in rat, mouse, and man: Comparative aspects. *Drug Metab. Dispos.* 15, 403–411.

Elves, R. G., Ueng, T., and Alvares, A. P. (1985) Regulation of hepatic monooxygenases by phenobarbital, 3-methylcholathrene, and polychlorinated biphenyls in rapid and slow acetylator mice. *Drug Metab. Dispos.* 13, 354–358.

Emudianughe, T. S., Caldwell, J., Dixon, P.A.F., and Smith, R. L. (1978) *Xenobiotica* 8, 525.

Emudianughe, T. S., Caldwell, J., and Smith, R. L. (1987) Studies on the metabolism of arylacetic acids, 6., Comparative metabolic conjugation of 1- and 2-naphthylacetic acid in the guinea pig, mouse, hamster and gerbil, *Xenobiotica* 17, 815–821.

Federal Register, Vol. 54 (75), April 20, 1989. Rules and Regulations: p. 15923.

Felton, J. S., Nebert, D. W., and Thorgeirsson, S. S. (1976) Genetic difference in 2-acetylamino-fluorene mutagenicity in vitro associated with mouse hepatic aryl hydrocarbon hydroxylase activity induced by polycyclic aromatic compounds. *Mol. Pharmacol.* 12, 225.

Fink, G. B., and Iturrian, W. B. (1970) Influence of age, auditory conditioning and environmental noise on sound induced seizures and seizure threshold in mice, in *Physiological Effects of Noise*, Welch, B. L., and Welch, A. S., eds. Plenum Press, New York, pp. 211–226.

Finney, D. J. (1971) *Probit Analysis*, 3rd ed. Cambridge University Press, pp. 50–80, 100–124.

Flyn, E. L., Lynch, M. and Zannon, V. G. (1972) Species difference in drug metabolism, *Biochem. Pharmac.* 21, 2577–2590.

Foster, H. L., Small, J. D., and Fox, J. G. (eds.) (1982) *The Mouse in Biomedical Research*, Vol. II, *Diseases*. Academic Press, New York.

Frederickson, T. N., Morse III, H. C., Yetter, R. A., Rowe, W. A., Hartley, J. W., and Pattengale, P. K. (1985) Multiparameter analysis of spontaneous nonthymic lymphomas occurring in NFS/N mice congenic for ecotropic murine leukemia viruses. *Am. J. Pathol.* 121, 349–360.

Frith, C. H. (1979) Morphologic classification of inflammatory, degenerative and proliferative lesions of the urinary bladder of mice. *Invest. Urol.* 16, 435–444.

Frith, C. H. (1983a) Adenoma and carcinoma, adrenal cortex, mouse, in *Endocrine System*, Jones, T. C., Mohr, U., and Hunt, R. D., eds. Springer-Verlag, New York, pp. 49–56.

Frith, C. H. (1983b) Incidence of hepatic metastases for various neoplasms in several strains of mice. *Toxicol. Pathol.* 11, 120–128.

Frith, C. H. (1983c) Lipogenic pigmentation, adrenal cortex, mouse, in *Endocrine System*, Jones, T. C., Mohr, U., and Hunt, R. D., eds. Springer-Verlag, New York, pp. 60–63.

Frith, C. H. (1983d) Pheochromocytoma, adrenal medulla, mouse, in *Endocrine System*, Jones, T. C., Mohr, U., and Hunt, R. D., eds. Springer-Verlag, New York, pp. 27–29.

Frith, C. H., and Chandra, M. (1991) Incidence, distribution and morphology of amyloidosis in Charles River CD-1 mice. *Toxicol. Pathol.* 19, 123–127.

Frith, C. H., and Dooley, K. (1976) Hepatic cytologic and neoplastic changes in mice given benzidine dihydrochloride. *J. Natl. Cancer Inst.* 56, 679–682, March.

Frith, C. H., and Heath, J. E. (1983a) Adenoma of the thyroid of the mouse, in *Monographs on Pathology of Laboratory Animals: Endocrine System*, Jones, T. C., Mohr, U., and Hunt, R. D., eds. Springer-Verlag, New York, pp. 184–187.

Frith, C. H., and Heath, J. E. (1983b) Adenoma, thyroid, mouse, in *Endocrine System*, Jones, T. C., Mohr, U., and Hunt, R. D., eds. Springer-Verlag, New York, pp. 188–191.

Frith, C. H., and Rule, J. E. (1978) The effects of discontinuing administration of high levels of

2-acetylaminofluorene on the transitional epithelium of the mouse urinary bladder. *J. Environ. Pathol. Toxicol.* 1, 581–585.

Frith, C. H., Pattengale, P. K., and Ward, J. M. (1985) *A Color Atlas of Hematopoietic Pathology of Mice.* Toxicology Pathology Associates, Little Rock, AR, pp. 7–13.

Frith, C. H., and Sheldon, W. D. (1983) Hyperplasia, adenoma and carcinoma of pancreatic islets of the mouse, in *Monographs on Pathology of Laboratory Animals: Endocrine System,* Jones, T. C., Mohr, U., and Hunt, R. D., eds. Springer-Verlag, Berlin, pp. 297–303.

Frith, C. H., and Townsend, J. W. (1985) Histology and ultrastructure, salivary gland, mouse, in *Monographs on Pathology of Laboratory Animals: Digestive System,* Jones, T. C., Mohr, U., and Hunt, R. D., eds. Springer-Verlag, Berlin, pp. 177–184.

Frith, C. H., and Ward, J. M. (1980) A morphologic classification of proliferative and neoplastic hepatic lesions in mice. *J. Environ. Pathol. Toxicol.* 3, 329–351.

Frith, C. H., and Ward, J. M. (1988) *Color Atlas of Neoplastic and Non-neoplastic Lesions in Aging Mice.* Elsevier, New York.

Frith, C. H., and Wiley, L. D. (1981) Classification and incidence of hyperplastic and neoplastic hematopoietic lesions in mice. *J. Gerontol.* 36, 534–545.

Frith, C. H., Sprowls, R. W., and Breeden, C. R. (1976) Mast cell neoplasia in mice. *Lab. Anim. Sci.* 26, 478–481.

Frith, C. H., Baetcke, K. P., Nelson, C. J., and Schieferstein, G. (1979) Importance of the mouse liver tumor in carcinogenesis bioassay studies using benzidine dihydrochloride as a model. *Toxicol. Lett.* 4, 507–518.

Frith, C. H., Baetcke, K. P., Nelson, C. J., and Schieferstein, G. (1980a) Sequential morphogenesis of liver tumors in mice given benzidine dihydrochloride. *Eur. J. Cancer* 16, 1205–1216.

Frith, C. H., Boothe, A. D., Greenman, D. L., and Farmer, J. H. (1980b) Correlations between gross and microscopic lesions in carcinogenic studies in mice. *J. Environ. Pathol. Toxicol.* 3, 139–153.

Frith, C. H., Farmer, J. H., Greenman, D. L., and Shaw, G. W. (1980c) Biologic and morphologic characteristics of urinary bladder neoplasms induced in BALB/c female mice with 2-acetylaminofluorene. *J. Environ. Pathol. Toxicol.* 3, 103–119.

Frith, C. H., Zuna, R. E., and Morgan, K. (1981a) A morphologic classification and incidence of spontaneous ovarian neoplasms in three strains of mice. *J. Natl. Cancer Inst.* 67, 693–702.

Frith, C. H., Davis, T. M., Zolotor, L. A., and Townsend, J. W. (1981b) Histiocytic lymphoma in the mouse. *Leukemia Res.* 4, 651–662.

Frith, C. H., Highman, B., Burger, G., and Sheldon, W. D. (1983a) Spontaneous lesions in virgin and retired breeder BALB/c and C57BL/c and C57BL/6 mice. *Lab. Anim. Sci.* 33, 273–286.

Frith, C. H., Wiley, L. D., and Shinohara, Y. (1983b) Sequential morphogenesis of bladder tumors in BALB/c female mice fed 2-acetylaminofluorene. *Invest. Urol.* 28, 1071–1076.

Frith, C. H., West, R. W., Stanley, J. W. and Jackson, C. D. (1984) Urothelial lesions in mice given 4-ethylsulfonyl-naphthalene-1-sulfonamide, acetazolamide, and oxamide. *J. Exp. Pathol. Toxicol. Oncol.* 5, 25–38.

Frith, C. H., McConnell, and Johnson, A. N. (1990) Erythroleukemia in a mouse: A case report. *Lab. Anim. Sci.* 40, 418–419.

Gabliks, J. and Maltby-Askari, E. (1970) The effect of chlorinated hydrocarbons on drug metabolism in mice. *IMS Ind Med. Surg.*, 39, 347–50.

Gad, S. C., Dunn, B. J., Dobbs, D. W., Reilly, C., and Walsh, R. D. (1986) Development and validation of an alternative dermal sensitization test: The mouse ear swelling test (MEST). *Toxicol. Appl. Pharmacol.* 84, 93–114.

Gellatly, J.B.M. (1975) The natural history of hepatic parenchymal nodule formation in a colony of C57BL mice with reference to the effect of diet, in *Mouse Hepatic Neoplasia,* Butler, W. H., and Newberne, P. W., eds. Amsterdam, Elsevier, pp. 77–108.

Glass, S. J., and van Lier, R.B.L. (1988) Metabolism of 7-ethoxyresorufin by phenobarbital or Aroclor 1254 pretreated mice. *Drug Metab. Dispos.* 16, 333–4.

Goodman, D. G. (1983) Subcapsular-cell hyperplasia, adrenal, mouse, in *Endocrine System*, Jones, T. C., Mohr, U., and Hunt, R. D., eds. Springer-Verlag, New York, pp. 66–68.

Goodman, D. G., and Strandberg, J. D. (1982) Neoplasms of the female reproductive system, in *The Mouse in Biomedical Research*, Vol. IV, Foster, H. L., Small, J. D., and Fox, J. G., eds. Academic Press, New York, pp. 397–411.

Goodman, D. G., Bates, R. R., Ward, J. M., Frith, C. H., Sauer, R. M., Jonse, S. R., Strandbert, J. D., Squire, R. A., Montali, R. J., and Parker, G. A. (1981) Common lesions in aged B6C3F1 (C57BL/6N xC3H/HeN)F1 and BALB/cStCrlf-C3H/Nctr mice. *Reg. Vet. Pathol.* AFIP, Washington, D.C.

Goodman, D. G., Boorman, G. A., and Strandberg, J. D. (1985) Selection and use of the B6C3F1 mouse and F344 rat in long-term bioassays for carcinogenicity, in *Handbook of Carcinogen Testing*, Milman, H. A., and Weisburger, E. K., eds. Noyes, Park Ridge, NJ, pp. 282–325.

Gram, T. E., Schroeder, D. H., Davis, D. C., Regan, R. L., and Guarino, A. M. (1971) Enzymic and biochemical composition of smooth and rough microsomal membranes from monkey, guinea pig and mouse liver. *Biochem. Pharmacol.* 20, 1371–1381.

Greenman, D. L., Oller, W. L., Littlefield, N. A., and Nelson, C. J. (1980) Commercial laboratory animal diets: Toxicant and nutrient variability. *J. Toxicol. Environ. Health* 6, 235–246.

Gregus, Z., Watkins, J. B., Thompson, T. N., Harvey, M. J., Rozman, K., and Klaassen, C. D. (1983) Hepatic phase I and II biotransformations in quail and trout comparison to other species commonly used in toxicity testing. *Toxicol. Appl. Pharmacol.* 67, 430–441.

Hakusui, H., Susuki, W., Takegoshi, T., Saito, T., and Sano, M. (1978) Studies on pharmacokinetics and biotransformation of oxepinac in mouse, rat, dog, and man.

Hart, L. G., and Fouts, J. R. (1965) Further studies on the stimulation of hepatic microsomal drug-metabolizing enzymes by DDT and its analogues. *Arch. Exp. Pathol. Pharmacol.*, 249, 486–500.

Harvey, W. E. (1616) *Prelectiones Anatomie Universalis.*

Haseman, J. K., Huff, J. E., and Boorman, G. A. (1984) Use of historical control data in carcinogenicity studies in rodents. *Toxicol. Pathol.* 12, 126–135.

Haseman, J. K., Huff, J. E., Rao, G. N., Arnold, J. E., Boorman, G. A., and McConnell, E. E. (1985) Neoplasms observed in untreated and corn oil gavage control groups of F344/N rats and (C57BL/6N X C3H/HeN)F1 (B6C3F1) mice. *J. Natl. Cancer Inst.* 75, 975–984.

Heath, J. E., and Frith, C. H. (1983) Carcinoma, thyroid, mouse, in *Endocrine System*, Jones, T. C., and Hunt, R. D., eds. Springer-Verlag, New York, pp. 188–191.

Herbst, M. (1976) Glycogenous hepatonuclear inclusions in the aged mouse: An electron microscopical study of the histogenesis of nuclear inclusions. *Pathol. Eur.* 11, 69–79.

Heston, W. E. (1975) Testing for possible effects of cedar wood shavings and diet on occurrence of mammary gland tumors and hepatomas in C3H-A^{vy} and C3H-A^{vy}fB mice. *J. Natl. Cancer Inst.* 54, 1011–1014.

Hietanen, E., and Vainio, H. (1973) Interspecies variations in small intestinal and hepatic drug hydroxylation and glucuronidation. *Acta Pharmacol. Toxicol.* 33, 57–64.

Hill, B. F. (ed.) (1981) The CF1 mouse, history and utilization, in *Charles River Digest*, 20(2), Charles River Breeding Laboratories, Wilmington, Massachusetts.

Hill, B. F. (ed.) (1983) The CD-1 mouse, history and utilization, in *Charles River Digest*, 22(1), Charles River Breeding Laboratories, Wilmington, Massachusetts.

Hjelle, J. J., Hazelton, G. A., and Klaassen, C. D. (1985) Increased UDP-glucuronosyltransferase Activity and UDP-glucuronic Acid Concentration in the small intestine of butylated hydroxyanisole treated mice. *Drug Metab. Dispos.* 13, 68–70.

Holland, J. M., and Fry, R.J.M. (1982) Neoplasms of the integumentary system and harderian glands, in *The Mouse in Biomedical Research*, Vol. IV, Foster, H. L., Small, J. D., and Fox, J. G., eds. Academic Press, New York, pp. 3-528.

Homburger, F., Russfield, A. B., Weisburger, J. H., Lim, S., Chak, S. P., and Weisburger, E. K.

(1975) Aging changes in CD-1 HaM/ICR mice reared under standard laboratory conditions. *J. Natl. Cancer Inst.* 55, 37–45.

Hoover, K. L., Ward, J. M., and Stinson, S. F. (1980) Histopathologic differences between liver tumors in untreated (C57BL/6 x C3H)F1(B6C3F1) mice and nitrofen treated mice. *J. Natl. Cancer Inst.* 65, 937–948.

Horie, A., Hohchi, S., and Kuratsune, M. (1965) Carcinogenesis in the esophagus. II. Experimental production of esophageal cancer by administration of ethanolic solution of carcinogens. *Gann* 56, 429–441.

Hruban, Z., Kirsten, W. H., and Slesers, A. (1966) Fine structure of spontaneous hepatic tumors of male C3HfGs mice. *Lab. Invest.* 15, 577–588.

Hukusui, H., Suzuki, W., Takegoshi, T., Saito, T., and Sano, M. (1978) *Arzneim. Forsch.* 28, 456.

Igarashi, T., Satoh, T., Ueno, K., and Kitagawa, H. (1983) Species difference in glutathione level and glutathione related enzyme activities in rats, mice, guinea pigs and hamsters, *J. Pharm. Dyn.* 6, 941–949.

Igarashi, T., Tomihari, N., Ohmori, S., Ueno, Koichi, Kitagawa, H., and Satoh, T. (1986) Comparison of glutathione S-transferases in mouse, guinea pig, rabbit, and hamster liver cytosol to those in rat liver. *Biochem. Int.* 13, 641–648.

ILAR (Institute of Laboratory Animal Resources) Committee on the Care and Use of Laboratory Animals (1985) *Guide for the Care and Use of Laboratory Animals.* NIH Publication No. 86-23. Washington, D.C., U.S. Department of Health and Human Services.

Ioannou, Y. M., Sanders, J. M., and Mathews, H. B. (1988) Species-dependent variations in metabolism and clearance in rats and mouse. *Drug Metab. Dispos.* 16, 435–440.

Iturrian, W. B. (1973) *The Effect of Noise on Immature Rodents.* Carworth Letter, no. 92, Carworth, Division of Becton, Dickinson and Company, New York.

Iturrian, W. B., and Johnson, H. D. (1975) Infantile auditory exposure and unusual response to antipsychotic drugs. *Proc. Soc. Exp. Biol. Med.* 148, 219–223.

Jackson, C. D., Frith, C. H., West, R. W., and Stanley, J. W. (1979) Effects of 4-ethylsufonylnaphthelene-1-sulfonamide, acetazolamide, and oxamide on the mouse urinary tract, in *Toxicology and Occupational Medicine*, Elsevier, North-Holland, New York, pp. 233–242.

Jacoby, R. O., and Fox, J. G. (1984) Biology and diseases of mice, in *Laboratory Animal Medicine*, Fox, J. G., Cohen, B. J., and Loew, F. M., eds. Academic Press, New York, pp. 31–89.

Jensen, M. M., and Rasmussen, A. F., Jr. (1970) Audiogenic stress and susceptibility to infection, in *Physiological Effects of Noise*, Welch, B. L., and Welch, A. S., eds. Plenum, New York, pp. 7–19.

Jondorf, W. R., Maickel, R. P., and Brodie, B. B. (1958) Inability of newborn mice and guinea pigs to metabolize drugs. *Biochem. Pharmacol.*, 1, 352–354.

Jones, J. C. (1967) Pathology of the liver of rats and mice, in *Pathology of Laboratory Rats and Mice*, Cotchin, E., and Roe, F.J.C., eds. Blackwell, London, pp. 1–23.

Kanerva, R. L., Alden, C. L., and Wyder, W. E. (1982) The effect of uniform exsanguination on absolute and relative organ weights, and organ weight variation. *Toxicol. Pathol.* 10, 43–45.

Kanerva, R. L., Lefever, F. R., and Alden, C. L. (1983) Comparison of fresh and fixed organ weights of rats, *Toxicol. Pathol.* 11, 129–131.

Kaplan, H. M., Brewer, N. R., and Blair, W. H. (1983) Physiology, in *The Mouse in Biomedical Research*, Vol. III, Foster, H. L., Small, J. D., and Fox, J. G., eds. Academic Press, New York, pp. 247–292.

Kato, R. (1966) Possible role of P-450 in the oxidation of drugs in liver microsomes. *J. Biochem.* Tokyo 59, 574–583.

Kato, R. (1974) Sex-related differences in drug metabolism. *Drug Metab. Rev.* 3, 1–32.

Kato, R. (1979) Characteristics and differences in the hepatic mixed function oxidases of different species. *Pharmacol. Ther.* 6, 4–98.

Kato, R., and Onoda, K. (1966) Effect of morphine administration on the activities of microsomal drug-metabolizing enzyme systems in liver of different species. *Jpn. J. Pharmacol.* 16, 217–219.

Kauffman, S. L., Alexander, L., and Sas, L. (1979) Histologic and ultrastructural features of the Clara cell adenoma of the mouse lung. *Lab. Invest.* 40, 708–716.

Kauffman, S. L., and Sato, T. (1985a) Alveolar type II Cell adenoma, lung, mouse, in *Respiratory System*, Jones, T. C., Mohr, U., and Hunt, R. D., eds. Springer-Verlag, New York, pp. 102–107.

Kauffman, S. L., and Sato, T. (1985b) Bronchiolar adenoma, lung, mouse, in *Respiratory System*, Jones, T. C., Mohr, U., and Hunt, R. D., Springer-Verlag, New York, pp. 107–111.

Kedderis, G. L. (1989) The biotransformation of acrylonitrile: Implications of metabolic studies for risk assessment. *CIIT Activ.* 9, 1–5.

Kennedy, G. L. Jr., and Trochimowicz, H. J. (1982) Inhalation toxicology, in *Principles and Methods of Toxicology*, Hayes, A. W., (ed). Raven Press, New York, pp. 185–207.

Kimbrough, R. D., and Linder, R. E. (1974) Induction of adenofibrosis and hepatomas of the liver in BALB/c mice by polychlorinated biphenyls (Aroclor 1254). *J. Natl. Cancer Inst.* 53, 547–552.

Klaassen, C. D., and Doull, J. (1980) Evaluation of safety: Toxicologic evaluation, in *Casarett and Doull's Toxicology: The Basic Science of Poisons*, 2nd Ed., J. Doull, C. D. Klaassen, and M. O. Amdur, eds. Macmillan, New York, pp. 13–14.

Knapka, J. J. (1983) Nutrition, in *The Mouse in Biomedical Research*, Vol. III, Foster, H. L., Small, J. D., and Fox, J. G., eds. Academic Press, New York, pp. 51–67.

Knapka, J. J., Smith, K. P., and Judge, F. J. (1974) Effect of open and closed formula rations on the performance of three strains of laboratory mice. *Lab. Anim. Sci.* 24, 480–487.

Koen, H., Pugh, T. D., Nychka, D., and Goldfarb, S. (1983a) Presence of alphafetoprotein positive cells in hepatocellular foci and microcarcinomas induced by single injections of diethylnitrosamine in infant mice. *Cancer Res.* 43, 702–708.

Kulkarni, A. P., and Hodgson, E. (1980) Comparative toxicology, in *Introduction to Biochemical Toxicology*, Hodgson, E., and Guthrie, F. E., eds. Elsevier, New York, pp. 106–132.

Kulkarni, A. P., Smith, E., and Hodgson, E. (1976) Occurrence and characterization of microsomal cytochrome P-450 in several vertebrate and insect species. *Comp. Biochem. Physiol.* 54B, 509–513.

Kyriazis, A. P., Koka, M., and Vesselinovitch, S. D. (1974) Metastatic rate of liver tumors induced by dimethylnitrosamine in mice. *Cancer Res.* 34, 2881–2886.

Lang, P. L. (1987) Spontaneous neoplastic lesions in the Crl:CD-1(ICR)BR mouse. *Charles River Monograph*, Charles River Laboratories, Wilmington, Massachusetts, February.

Lang, P. L. (1989a) Spontaneous Neoplastic Lesions in the B6C3F$_1$/CrlBR mouse. *Charles River Monograph*, Charles River Laboratories, Wilmington, Massachusetts, February.

Lang, P. L. (1989b) Survival of Crl:CD-1 BR Mice During Chronic Toxicology Studies, *Charles River Laboratories Reference Paper*, Wilmington, Massachusetts, *Fall*.

Lavoisier, A. (1777) *Experiments on the Respiration of Animals*.

Leard, B. L. (1984) The mouse, in *Manual for Assistant Laboratory Animal Technicians*, Sapanski, W. B. Jr., and Harkness, J. E., eds. American Association for Laboratory Animal Science, Cordova, TN, p. 143.

Leifer, C. L., Miller, A. S., Putong, P. B., Harwick, R. (1974) Myoepithelioma of the parotid gland. *Arch. Pathol.* 98, 312–319.

Li, J., Okada, S., Hamazaki, S., Ebina, Y., and Midorikawa, O. (1987) Subacute nephrotoxicity and induction of renal cell carcinoma in mice treated with ferric nitrilotriacetate. *Cancer Res.* 47, 1867–1869.

Litterst, C. L., Mimnaugh, E. G., Regan, R. L., and Gram, T. E. (1975) Comparison of in vitro drug metabolism by lung, liver and kidney of several common laboratory species. *Drug Metab. Dispos.* 3, 259–265.

Litterst, C. L., Gram, T. E., Mimnaugh, E. G., Leber, P., Emmerling, D., and Freudenthal, R. I. (1976) A comprehensive study of in vitro drug metabolism in several laboratory species. *Drug Metab. Dispos.* 4, 203–207.

Lombard, L. S. (1982) Neoplasms of musculoskeletal system, in *The Mouse in Biomedical Research*, Vol. IV, Foster, H. L., Small, J. D., and Fox, J. G., eds. Academic Press, New York, pp. 501–511.

Lotlikar, P. D., Enomoto, M., Miller, J. A., and Miller, E. C. (1967) Species variations in the N- and ring-hydroxylation of 2-acetylaminofluorene and effects of 3-methylcholanthrene pretreatment. *Proc. Soc. Exp. Biol. Med.* 125, 341–346.

Lower, G. M., and Bryan, G. T. (1973) Enzymatic N-acetylation of carcinogenic aromatic amines in liver cytosol of species displaying different organ susceptibilities. *Biochem. Pharmacol.* 22, 1581–1588.

Lower, G. M., and Bryan, G. T. (1976) Enzymatic deacetylation of carcinogenic arylacetamides by tissue microsomes of the dog and other species. *J. Toxicol. Environ. Health* 1, 421.

Lyman, S. D., Poland, A., and Taylor, B. A. (1980) Genetic polymorphism of microsomal epoxide activity in the mouse. *J. Biol. Chem.* 255, 8650–8654.

Lynch, C. J. (1969) The so-called Swiss mouse, *Lab. Anim. Care* 19, 214–220.

Lyon, M. F. (1981) Nomenclature, in *The Mouse in Biomedical Research*, Vol. I, Foster, H. L., Small, J. D., and Fox, J. G., eds. Academic Press, New York, pp. 27–38.

Maceleod, J. N., Sorensen, M. P., and Shapiro, B. H. (1987) Strain independent evaluation of hepatic monooxygenase enzymes in female mice. *Xenobiotica* 17, 1095–1102.

Maibach, H. I., and Wester, R. C. (1989) Percutaneous absorption: In vivo methods in humans and animals. *J. Am. Coll. Toxicol.* 8, 803–813.

Marcucci, F., Guaitani, A., Kvetina, J., Mussini, E., and Garattini, S. (1968) Species difference in diazepam metabolism and anticonvulsant effect. *Eur. J. Pharmacol.* 4, 467–470.

McClellan, R. O., and Henderson, R. F. (eds.) (1989) *Concepts in Inhalation Toxicology*, Hemisphere, New York.

McMahon, R. E., Turner, J. C., and Whitaker, G. W. (1980) The N-hydroxylation and ring-hydroxylation of 4-aminobiphenyl in vitro by hepatic mono-oxygenases from rat, mouse, hamster, rabbit and guinea pig. *Xenobiotica* 10, 469–481.

Medina, D. (1982) Mammary tumors, in *The Mouse in Biomedical Research*, Vol. IV, Foster, H. L., Small, J. D., and Fox, J. G., eds. Academic Press, New York, pp. 373–396.

Menzel, D. B., and McClellan, R. O. (1980) Toxic responses of the respiratory system, in *Casarett and Doull's Toxicology: The Basic Science of Poisons*, 2nd ed., Doull, J., Klaassen, C. D., and Amdur, M. O. eds. Macmillan, New York, pp. 246–274.

Moldeus, P. (1978) Paracetamol metabolism and toxicity studied in isolated hepatocytes from mouse, in *Conjugation Reactions in Drug Biotransformation*, Aitio, A., ed. Elsevier/North-Holand Biomedical Press, Amsterdam.

Morgan, K. T., and Alison, R. H. (1987a) Cystadenoma, ovary, mouse, in *Genital System*, Jones, T. C., Mohr, U., and Hunt, R. D., eds. Springer-Verlag, New York, pp. 42–46.

Morgan, K. T., and Alison, R. H. (1987b) Tubular adenoma, ovary, mouse, in *Genital System*, Jones, T. C., Mohr, U., and Hunt, R. D., eds. Springer-Verlag, New York, pp. 36–41.

Morgan, K. T., Johnson, B. P., Frith, C. H. and Townsend, J. (1983) An ultrastructural study of spontaneous mineralization in the brains of aging mice. *Acta Neuropathol.* 58, 10–124.

Morgan, K. T., Frith, C. H., Crowder, D., and Swenberg, J. (1984) Incidence of primary neoplasms of the nervous system in control mice. *J. Natl. Cancer Inst.* 72, 151–160.

Morgenstern, R., Lundvist, G., Andersoon, G., Balk, L., and Desierre, J. W. (1984) The distribution of microsomal glutathione transferase among different organelles, different organs, and different organisms. *Biochemical Pharmacol.* 33, 3609–3614.

Morse, H. C., III (1981) The laboratory mouse—a historical perspective, in *The Mouse in Biomedical Research*, Vol. I, Foster, H. L., Small, J. D., and Fox, J. G., eds. Academic Press, pp. 1–16.

National Research Council (NRC) (1978) *Nutrient Requirements of Laboratory Animals*, *10*, 3rd revised ed. National Academy of Sciences, Washington, D.C.

Nebert, D. W. (1981) Selected aspects of pharmacogenetics, in *The Mouse in Biomedical Research*, Vol. I, Foster, H. L., Small, J. D., and Fox, J. G., eds. Academic Press, pp. 285–298.

Nebert, D. W., and Jensen, N. M. (1979) The Ah locus: Genetic regulation of the metabolism of carcinogens, drugs and other environmental chemicals by cytochrome P-450–mediated monooxygenases. *CRC Crit. Rev. Biochem.* Vol. 6, pp. 401–437.

Newberne, P. M. (1975) Influence on pharmacological experiments of chemicals and other factors in diets of laboratory animals. *Fed. Proc. Fed. Am. Soc. Exp. Biol.* 34, 209–218.

Ockenfels, H., Kohler, F., and Meise, W. (1976) Teratogenic effect and stereospecificity of a thalidomide metabolite, *Pharmazie*, 31, 492–493.

Oesch, F., and Wolf, C. R. (1989) Properties of the microsomal and cytosolic glutathione transferases involved in hexachloro-1:3-butadiene conjugation. *Biochem. Pharmacol.* 38, 353–359.

Otterness, D. M., Keith, R. A., Kerremans, A. L., and Weinshilboum, R. M. (1986) Mouse liver thiol methyltransferase: Assay conditions, biochemical properties, and strain variation. *Drug Metab. Dispos.* 14, 680–688.

Ovelar, M. Y., and Cardesa, A. (1985) Squamous cell papilloma, esophagus, rat, in *Monographs on Pathology of Laboratory Animals*: *Digestive System*, Jones, T. C., Mohr, U., and Hunt, R. D., eds. Springer-Verlag, Berlin, pp. 263–265.

Pacifici, G. M., Boobis, A. R., Brodie, M. J., McManus, M. E., and Davies, D. S. (1981) Tissue and species differences in enzymes of epoxide metabolism. *Xenobiotica* 11, 73–79.

Parke, D. V. (1960) The metabolism of [^{14}C]aniline in the rabbit and other animals. *J. Biochem.* 77, 493–503.

Parke, D. V. (1968) *The Biochemistry of Foreign Compounds*. Pergamon, New York.

Pattengale, P. K., and Frith, C. H. (1983) Immunomorphologic classification of spontaneous lymphoid cell neoplasms occurring in female BALB/c mice. *J. Natl. Cancer Inst.* 70, 169–179.

Pattengale, P. K., and Frith, C. H. (1986) Contributions of recent research to the classification of spontaneous lymphoid cell neoplasms in mice. *CRC Crit. Rev. Toxicol.* 16, 185–212.

Pelkonen, O., Kaltiala, E. H., Karki, N. T., Jaalonen, K., and Pyorala, K. (1975) Properties of benzpyrene hydroxylase from human liver and comparison with the rat, rabbit and guinea pig enzymes. *Xenobiotica* 5, 501–509.

Percy, D. H., and Jonas, A. M. (1971) Incidence of spontaneous tumors in CD-1 HaM/ICR Mice. *J. Natl. Cancer Inst.* 46: 1045–1065.

Peters, R. L., Rabstein, L. S., Spahn, G. J., Mdison, R. M., and Huebner, R. J. (1972) Incidence of spontaneous neoplasms in breeding and retired breeder BALB/c Cr mice throughout the natural life span. *Int. J. Cancer* 10, 273–282.

Popp, J. A. (1984) *Mouse Liver Neoplasia, Current Perspectives*. Hemisphere, Washington, pp. 1–184.

Prejean, J. D., Peckham, J. C., Casey, A. E., Griswald, D. P., Weisberger, E. K. and Weisberger, J. H. (1973) Spontaneous tumors in Sprague-Dawley rats and Swiss mice. *Cancer Res.* 33, 2768–2773.

Priestly, J. (1775). *Experiments and Observations*. Vol. I, J. Johnson, London, p. 87.

Quinn, G. P., Axelrod, J. and Brodie, B. B. (1958) Species, strain and sex differences in metabolism of hexobarbitone, amodopyrine, antipyrine and aniline. *Biochem. Pharmacol.* 1, 152–159.

Rabes, H. M., Bucher, T., Hartmann, A., Linke, I., and Dunnwald, M. (1982) Clonal growth of carcinogen-induced enzyme-deficient preneoplastic cell populations in mouse liver. *Cancer Res.* 42, 3220–3227.

Rao, G. N., and Knapka, J. J. (1987) Contaminant and nutrient concentrations of natural ingredient rat and mouse diet used in chemical toxicology studies. *Fund. Appl. Toxicol.* 9, 329–338.

Rao, G. N., and Lindsey, J. R. (1988) Ankylosis of hock joints in group caged mice B6C3F1 mice. *Lab. Anim. Sci.* 38, 417–421.

Razzouk, C. and Roberfroid, M. B. (1982) Species differences in the biochemical properties of liver microsomal arylamine and arylamide N-hydroxylases. *Chem. Biol. Interact.*, 41, 251–264.

Remmer, H. (1970) Induction of drug metabolizing enzymes in different animal species. *Proc. Eur. Soc. Drug Toxicity* 11, 14–18.

Reuber, M. D. (1967) Poorly differentiated cholangiocarcinomas occurring spontaneously in C3H and C3H x y hybrid mice. *J. Natl. Cancer Inst.* 38, 901–907.

Reuber, M. D. (1971) Morphologic and biologic correlation of hyperplastic and neoplastic lesions occurring "spontaneously" in C3H x hybrid mice. *Br. J. Cancer* 25, 538–543.

Reuber, M. D. (1976) Histopathology of carcinomas of the liver in mice ingesting Dieldrin or Aldrin. *Tumori* 62, 463–472.

Rings, R. W., and Wagner, J. E. (1972) Incidence of cardiac and other soft tissue mineralized lesions in DBA/2 Mice. *Lab. Anim. Sci.* 22, 344–352.

Robison, W. G. Jr., and Kuwabara, T. (1978) A new albinobeige mouse: Giant granules in retinal pigment epithelium. *Invest. Ophthalmol. Vis. Sci.* 17, 365–370.

Robison, W. G. Jr., Kuwabara, T., and Zwaan, J. (1982) Eye research, in *The Mouse in Biomedical Research*, Vol. IV, Foster, H. L., Small, J. D., and Fox, J. G., eds. Academic Press, New York, p. 76.

Roebuck, B. D., and Wogan, G. N. (1977) Species comparison of in vitro metabolism of aflatoxin B_1. *Cancer Res.* 37, 1649–1656.

Rothacker, D. L., Kanerva, R. L., Wyder, W. E., Alden, C. L., and Maurer, J. K. (1988) Effects of variation of necropsy time annd fasting on liver weights and liver components in rats. *Toxicol. Pathol.* 16, 22–26.

Rowland, I. R., Mallett, A. K., Bearne, C. A., and Farthing, M.J.G. (1986) Enzyme activities of the hindgut microflora of laboratory animals and man. *Xenobiotica* 16, 519–523.

Runkle, R. S. (1964) Laboratory animal housing. Part II. *Am. Inst. Archit. J.* 41, 77–80.

Russfield, A. (1982) Neoplasms of the endocrine system, in *The Mouse in Biomedical Research*, Vol. IV, Foster, H. L., Small, J. D., and Fox, J. G., eds. Academic Press, New York. pp. 465–475.

Sabine, J. R., Horton, B. J., and Wicks, M. B. (1973) Spontaneous tumors in C3H-A[vy] and C3H-A[vy]fB mice: High incidence in the United States and low incidence in Australia. *J. Natl. Cancer Inst.* 50, 1237–1242.

Sass, B. (1983a) Accessory adrenocortical tissue, mouse, in *Endocrine System*, Jones, T. C., Mohr, U., and Hunt, R. D., eds. Springer-Verlag, New York, pp. 12–15.

Sass, B. (1983b). Amyloidosis, adrenal, mouse, in *Endocrine System*, Jones, T. C., Mohr, U., and Hunt, R. D., eds. Springer-Verlag, New York, pp. 57–59.

Sass, B., and Dunn, T. B. (1979) Classification of mouse mammary tumors in Dunn's miscellaneous group, including recently reported types. *J. Natl. Cancer Inst.* 62, 1287–1293.

Sass, B., and Montali, R. J. (1980) Spontaneous fibro-osseous lesions in aging female mice. *Lab. Anim. Sci.* 30, 907–908.

Sass, B., Vernon, M. L., Petesr, R. L., and Kelloff, G. J. (1978) Mammary tumors, hepatocellular carcinomas and pancreatic islet cell changs in C3H mice. *J. Natl. Cancer Inst.* 60, 611–621.

Schieferstein, G., Littlefield, N., Sheldon, W. W., Gaylor, D., and Burger, G. (1985) Carcinogenesis of 4-aminobiphenyl in BALB/cStCrlfC3H/Nctr mice. *Eur. J. Clin. Oncol.* 21, 865–873.

Schwarz, M. A., Postma, E., Kolins, S. J., and Leon, A. S. (1973) Metabolites of bromazepam, a benzodiazepine, in the human, dog, rat and mouse. *J. Pharm. Sci.*, 62, 1776–1779.

Serrano, L. J. (1971) Carbon dioxide and ammonia in mouse cages: Effect of cage covers, population, and activity. *Lab. Anim. Sci.* 21(1), 75–85.

Shimkin, M. B. and Stoner, G. D. (1975) Lung tumors in mice: Application to carcinogenesis bioassay. *Adv. Cancer Res.* 21, 1–58.

Shinohara, Y., Frith, C. H. (1980) A morphologic classification of benign and malignant renal cell tumors in aged BALB/c mice. *Am. J. Pathol.* 100, 455–457.

Souhaili–el Amri, H., Batt, A. M., and Siest, G. (1986) Comparison of cytochrome P-450 content and activities in liver microsomes of seven animal species, including man. *Xenobiotica* 16, 351–358.

Spalding, J. F., Archuleta, R. F. and Holland, L. M. (1969) Influence of the visible color spectrum on activity in mice. *Lab. Anim. Care* 19, 50–54.

Squire, R. A. (1990) Personal communication.

Squire, R. A., and Levitt, M. H. (1975) Report of a workshop of classification of specific hepatocellular lesions in rats. *Cancer Res.* 35, 3214–3223.

Squire, R. A., Goodman, D. G., Valerio, M. G., Fredrickson, T., Stranberg, J. D., Levitt, M. H., Lingeman, C. H., Harshburger, J. C., and Dawe, C. J. (1978) Tumors, in *Pathology of Laboratory Animals*, Vol. II, Benirschke, K., Garner, F. M., and Jones, T. C., eds. Springer-Verlag, New York, pp. 1051–1284.

Stein, A. F., Gregus, Z., and Klaassen, C. D. (1988) Species variations in biliary excretion of glutathione-related thiols and methyl mercury. *Toxicol. Appl. Pharmacol.* 94, 351–359.

Steinel, H. H., and Baker, R.S.U. (1988) Sensitivity of HRA/Skh hairless mice to initiation/promotion of skin tumors by chemical treatment. *Cancer Lett.* 41, 63–68.

Stewart, H. L., Deringer, M. K., Dunn, T. B., and Snall, K. C. (1974) Malignant schwannomas of nerve root, uterus, and epididymis in mice. *J. Natl. Cancer Inst.* 53, 1749–1758.

Stille, G., Brezowsky, H., and Weihe, W. H. (1968) The influence of the weather on the locomotor activity of mice. *Arzneimittelforschung* 18, 892–893.

Strandberg, J. D., and Goodman, D. G. (1982) Neoplasms of the cardiovascular system, in *The Mouse in Biomedical Research*, Vol. IV, Foster, H. L., Small, J. D., and Fox, J. G., eds. Academic Press, New York, pp. 539–545.

Strubelt, O., Dost-Kempf, E., Siegers, C.-P. Younes, M., Volpel, M., Preuss, U., and Dreckmann, J. G. (1981) The influence of fasting on the susceptibility of mice to hepatic injury. *Toxicol. Appl. Pharmacol.* 60, 66–77.

Terracini, B., and Testa, M. C. (1970) Carcinogenicity of a single administration of N-nitrosomethylurea: Comparison between newborn and 5-week-old mice and rats. *Br. J. Cancer* 24, 588–598.

Terracini, B., Palestro, G., Ramella Gigliardi, M., and Montesano, R. (1966) Carcinogenicity of dimethylnitrosamine in Swiss mice. *Br. J. Cancer* 20, 871–876.

Theiss, J. C., and Shimkin, M. B. (1982) Neoplasms of the respiratory system, in *The Mouse in Biomedical Research*, Vol. IV, Foster, H. L., Small, J. D., and Fox, J. G., eds. Academic Press, New York, pp. 477–484.

Thorgeirsson, S. S. (1982) Chemical mutagenesis, in *The Mouse in Biomedical Research*, Vol. IV, Foster, H. L., Small, J. D., and Fox, J. G., eds. Academic Press, New York, pp. 329–339.

Thorgeirsson, S. S., Wirth, P. J., Nelson, W. L., and Lamber, G. H. (1977) Genetic regulation of metabolism and mutagenicity of 2-acetylaminofluorene and related compounds in mice, in *Origins of Human Cancer*, Hiatt, H. H., Watson, J. D., and Winsten, J. A., eds. Cold Spring Harbor Laboratory, Cold Spring Harbor, New York, pp. 869.

Tomatis, L., Turusov, V., Charles, R. T., Biocchi, M., and Gati, E. (1972) Liver tumors in CF-1 mice exposed for limited period to technical DDT. *Z. Krebsforsch.* 32, 25–35.

Tomatis, L., Partensky, C., and Montesano, R. (1973) The predictive value of mouse liver tumor induction in carcinogenicity testing—a literature survey. *Int. J. Cancer* 12, 1–20.

Tsyrlov, I. B., and Lyakhovich, V. V. (1978) Genetic variation of cytochrome P-450 (P-448) catalytic ceters activities in relation to subsequent conjugation reactions, in *Conjugation Reactions in Drug Biotransformation*, Aitio, A., ed. Elsevier/North Holland, Amsterdam.

Turusov, V. S., and Takayama, S. (1979) Tumours of the liver, in *Pathology and Tumours in*

Laboratory Animals, Vol. II—*Tumours of the Mouse*. International Agency for Research on Cancer, Lyon, pp. 1–669.

Turusov, V. S., Chemeris, G. Y., and Parfenov, Y. D. (1985) Perirenal angiosarcoma induced in male mice by 1,2-dimethylhydrazine—a model for studying androgens in chemical carcinogenesis. *Carcinogenesis* 6, 325–331.

Van Den Berg, A. P., Noordhoek, J., Savenije-Chapel, E. M., and Koopman-Kool, E. (1977) Sex- and strain-dependent hepatic microsomal ethylmorphine N-demethylation in mice: the roles of type 1 binding and NADPH-cytochrome P-450 reductase. *Chem. Biol. Interact.*, 19, 185–195.

Vesell, E. S. (1967) Induction of drug-metabolizing enzymes in liver microsomes of mice and rats by softwood bedding. *Science* 157, 1057–1058.

Vesselinovitch, S. D., and Mihailovich, N. (1983) Kinetics of diethylnitrosamine hepatocarcinogenesis in the infant mouse. *Cancer Res.* 43, 4253–4259.

Vesselinovitch, S. D., Mihailovich, N., and Rao, K. V. (1978) Morphology and metastatic nature of induced hepatic nodular lesions in C57BL x C3H F1 mice. *Cancer Res.* 38, 2003–2010.

Vlahakis, G., and Heston, W. E. (1971) Spontaneous cholangiomas in strain C3H-AXy-fB Mice and their hybrids. *J. Natl. Cancer Inst.* 46, 677–683.

Wade, A. E., Holl, J. E., Hilliard, C. C., Molton, E., and Greene, F. E. (1968) Alteration of drug metabolism in rats and mice by an environment of cedarwood. *Pharmacology* 1, 317–328.

Walker, A.I.T., Thorpe, E., and Stevenson, D. E. (1972) The toxicology of Dieldrin (HEOD). Long-term oral toxicity studies in mice. *Food Cosmet. Toxicol.* 11, 415–432.

Ward, J. M. (1984) Morphology of potential preneoplastic hepatocyte lesions and liver tumors in mice and a comparison with other species, in *Current Perspectives in Mouse Liver Neoplasia*, Popp, J. A., ed Hemisphere, Washington, D.C., pp. 1–26.

Ward, J. M., and Vlahakis, G. (1978) Evaluation of hepatocellular neoplasms in mice. *J. Natl. Cancer Inst.* 61, 807–811.

Ward, J. M., Collins, M. J. Jr., and Parker, J. C. (1977) Naturally occurring mouse hepatitis virus infection in the nude mouse. *Lab. Anim. Sci.* 27, 372–376.

Ward, J. M., Bernal, E., Buratto, B., Goodman, D. G., Strandberg, J. D., and Schueler, R. (1979a) Histopathology of neoplastic and nonneoplastic hepatic lesions in mice fed diets containing tetrachlorvinphos. *J. Natl. Cancer Inst.* 63, 111–118.

Ward, J. M., Goodman, D. G., Squire, R. A., Chu, K. C., and Linhart, M. S. (1979b) Neoplastic and nonneoplastic lesions in aging (C56BL/6N x C3H/HeN) F1 (B6C3F1) mice. *J. Natl. Cancer Inst.* 63, 849–854.

Ward, J. M., Griesemer, R. A., and Weisburger, E. K. (1979c) The mouse liver tumor as an endpoint in carcinogenesis tests. *Toxicol. Appl. Pharmacol.* 51, 389–397.

Ward, J. M., Rice, J. M., Cresia, D., Lynch, P., and Riggs, C. (1983) Dissimilar patterns of promotion by di-(2-ethylhexyl)phthalate and phenobarbital of hepatocellular neoplasia initiated by diethylnitrosamine in B6C3F1 mice. *Carcinogenesis* 4, 1021–1029.

Ward, J. M., Diwan, B. A., Oshima, M., Hu, H., Schuller, H. M., and Rice, J. M. (1985a) Tumor-initiating and promoting activities of di(2-ethylhexyl)phthalate in vivo and in vitro. *Environ. Health Perspect.* 65, 279–291.

Ward, J. M., Singh, A., Katyal, S. L., Anderson, L. M., and Kovatch, R. M. (1985b) Immunocytochemical localization of the surfactant apoprotein and Clara cell antigen in chemically induced and naturally occurring pulmonary neoplasms of mice. *Am. J. Pathol.* 118, 493–499.

Watkins III, J. B., and Klueber, K. M. (1988) Hepatic phase II biotransformation in C57B1/KsJ db/db mice: Comparison to that in Swiss Webster and 129 REJ mice. *Comp. Biochem. Physiol.* 90C, 417–421.

Westfall, B. A., Boulos, B. M., Shields, J. L., and Carb, S. (1964) *Proc. Soc. Exp. Biol. Med.*, 115, 509.

Williams, R. T. (1974) Inter-specied variations in the metabolism of xenobiotica. *Biochem. Soc. Trans.* 2, 359–377.

Williams, G. M., Hirota, N., and Rice, J. M. (1979) The resistance of spontaneous mouse hepatocellular neoplasms to iron accumulation during rapid iron loading by parenteral administration and their transplanatability. *Am. J. Pathol.* 94, 65–74.

Wise, A. (1982) Interaction of diet and toxicology—the future role of purified diet in toxicological research. *Arch. Toxicol.* 50, 287–299.

Wise, A., and Gilburt, D. J. (1980) The variability of dietary fiber in laboratory animal diets and its relevance to the control of experimental conditions. *Food Cosmet. Toxicol.* 18, 643–648.

van Zwieten, M. J., Frith, C. H., Nooteboom, A. L., Wolfe, H. J., and DeLellis, R. A. (1983) Medullary thyroid carcinoma in female BALB/c mice. A report of 3 cases with ultrastructural, immunohistochemical and transplantation data. *Am. J. Pathol.* 110, 219–229.

Yoshitomi, K., Alison, R. H., and Boorman, G. A. (1986) Adenoma and adenocarcinoma of the gallbladder in aged laboratory mice. *Vet. Pathol.* 23, 523–527.

4

The Hamster

Toxicology: **Anne C. Costello**
                   S. C. Johnson & Son, Inc.
                   Racine, Wisconsin

Pathology: **Frederick G. Hess**
                   American Cyanamid Company
                   Princeton, New Jersey

Metabolism: **Christopher P. Chengelis**
                   WIL Research Laboratories, Inc.
                   Ashland, Ohio

Toxicology   **Anne C. Costello**

Presently, the hamster is the third most popular laboratory animal behind the rat and mouse (Renshaw, 1975). The hamster is an excellent laboratory animal because of its reproduction ease, unique anatomical and physical features, rapid physiological development, short life span, low incidence of spontaneous diseases, and a high susceptibility to induced pathological agents. Hamsters have been used in various research fields, especially in carcinogenesis because of its low incidence of spontaneous tumors. Hamsters have also played an important role in blood vessel physiology because their cheek pouches with thin vascularized walls are very accessible. Research with hamsters has provided much information concerning several disease states in humans.

TAXONOMY AND HISTORY

Hamsters belong in the subfamily Cricetinae of the family Cricetidae in the order Rodentia. There are 50 species of hamsters in the Cricetinae, of which eight species are maintained for medical research. Members of Cricetidae (also including the lemming, deer mice, and gerbils) are characterized by thick bodies, short legs, and large cheek pouches that are used to transport and store food. They have incisors that grow continuously and cuspidate molars which do not.

The Syrian hamster was first described as a new species (*Cricetus auratus*) in 1839. For almost 100 years, no hamsters were caught in the wild. The only proof that the species existed was the preservation in alcohol of two hamsters, one in London and the other in Beirut. Specimens were finally obtained from the wild starting in the 1900s.

SPECIES

The following is a discussion of the eight hamster species maintained in the laboratory. Table 1 lists these hamsters' common and scientific names and their chromosome numbers.

Syrian Hamster

The Syrian hamster is the most common laboratory hamster. Ninety percent of all hamsters used in research are Syrian. The remaining 10% are Chinese, European, Armenian, Rumanian, Turkish, South African, and Dzungarian hamsters. The Syrian was originally native to the arid, temperate regions of Southeast Europe and Asia Minor. It lives in deep tunnels which ensure cool temperatures and increased humidity. It is a nocturnal animal. The Syrian is virtually tailless and has smooth short hair. Normal coloration is reddish gold with a grayish white ventral portion. The dorsal side may have a black stripe. The ears are pointed with dark coloration; and the eyes are small, dark and bright. The average life span is 2 years, but these animals can live up to 3 years. The animal is 14–19 cm in length and weighs 114–140 g at adulthood. The female is usually heavier and longer than the male.

The Syrian hamster was introduced into the laboratory in 1930 to study the Mediterranean disease kala-azar. Israel Aharoni (Hebrew University, Jerusalem, Israel) collected 11 young golden hamsters from Syria in 1930 while on a zoological expedition. The litter with their mother had been found in their burrow 2.5 meters under a wheat field. Aharoni and his wife kept the hamsters in their house until one night when they all escaped. Nine hamsters were recovered and given to the animal facilities supervisor of the Weizmann &

Table 1 Common and Species Names and Chromosome Number

Common name	Species name	Chromosome number
Syrian (Golden)	*Mesocricetus auratus*	44
European (Common, Black, Field)	*Cricetus cricetus*	22
Chinese (Striped back)	*Cricetus griseus* or *barabensis*	22
South African	*Mystromys albicaudatus*	32
Rumanian (Newtoni's)	*Mesocricetus newtoni*	38
Turkish (Kurdanti)	*Mesocricetus auratus*	42/44
Armenian (Gray, Migratory	*Cricetulus migratorius*	22
Dzungarian (Hairy-footed)	*Phodopus sungorus*	28

Seiff Institute, Jerusalem, Israel. Of the nine, five escaped the first night in the new facility, leaving only one female. The female was mated and gave birth to a litter of healthy pups. In a year's time, these hamsters produced more than 300 offspring and were the forbearers of today's laboratory-bred Syrian hamster. Interestingly, as of 1972 there is no record of any further captures of Syrian hamsters from the wild.

The Syrian has been involved in oncology, virology, endocrinology, physiology, parasitology, genetics, and pharmacology research. The cheek pouch of the Syrian hamster has provided the technology for studying microcirculation and the growth of human tumors.

Chinese Hamster

The Chinese hamster is native to China. It is 39–46 g in weight and 9 cm long at adulthood. Its life span is 2.5–3.0 years under laboratory conditions. Though the Chinese hamster is smaller than the Syrian, its testicles, spleen, and brain are larger.

The Chinese hamster was originally used for the first time in 1919. Mice were extremely scarce at the time so hamsters were used to determine the best therapy for the patients with pneumonia. The Chinese hamster was also used to study TB, influenza, diphtheria, and rabies. Robert B. Watson, in December 1948 (right before the Communist takeover of China), was given 10 female and 10 male hamsters from C. H. Hu of the Peking Union Medical College. Watson placed the hamsters on what he believes was one of the last Pan Am flights out of China to San Francisco. From San Francisco, the hamsters were sent to New York. V. Schwenter of the Harvard Medical School obtained the hamsters and eventually successfuly bred them in the laboratory. Of the original 20 hamsters, four of the females and three of the males produced offspring which gave rise to the present Chinese hamster population. The Harvard colony has since become extinct; however, colonies were established at the Upjohn Company, Kalamazoo, Michigan, and the C. H. Best Institute in Toronto, Ontario, in the 1960s.

The Chinese hamster has been used primarily in research for cytogenetics because of its low chromosome number (Fenner, 1986), and in diabetes mellitus because some strains have very high incidences of the disease and because the course of the disease in this species is similar to that seen in humans.

European Hamster

The European hamster was first found in a West Germany industrial area. Its natural habitat is the lowlands of Central and Eastern Europe. The European hamster is a very aggressive animal, and in the wild each adult lives in its own burrow. It has a white face and feet, bodies are dorsally reddish brown and ventrally black with white patches laterally. They are about the size of a guinea pig, averaging 27–32 and 22–25 cm in length and weighing 450 and 350 g for males and females, respectively. Males reach sexual maturity at 60 days of age, whereas females at 80–90 days of age. This hamster is mainly a seed eater. In the wild, it hibernates in the winter months. In their natural habitat, European hamsters can live up to 8 years, whereas under laboratory conditions, the average life span is 5 years. This reduction is believed to be due to the lack of hibernation afforded a laboratory-raised European hamster (Mohr et al., 1987).

The European hamster has been used only in hibernation studies and in inhalation studies because its tidal volumes are the largest of any laboratory rodent species.

Armenian Hamster

The Armenian hamster is native to the Union of the Soviet Socialist Republic (U.S.S.R.). Its body size, weight, care, and maintenance are similar to that of the Chinese hamster.

The Armenian hamster was first introduced as a laboratory animal in 1963. It was brought to the United States as a part of the U.S.A.-U.S.S.R. Cultural Exchange Program. Scientists in the United States wanted to find more species of the dwarf hamster (like the Chinese), and the Armenian species was the only species found.

Although the Armenian hamster has been used on a limited basis, its research use has been in cytogenetics and oncology.

Turkish Hamster

The Turkish hamster is native to Iran and Turkey. It was originally trapped in 1962. As an adult, its average body weight is 150 g and its average life span is a little less than 2 years, though they have lived as long as 4 years.

Some populations of the Turkish hamster have a diploid number of 42 and others number of 44. These hamsters interbred readily and produce offspring with a diploid number of 44. Hamsters with diploid number of 42 hibernate less than those with 44. Besides hibernation research, Turkish hamsters have been used in immunology, genetics, and reproductive behavior research (Yerganian, 1972; Cantrell et al., 1987).

Rumanian Hamster

The Rumanian hamster was initially trapped and described in 1965. It is native to the Bucharest area and is used in the laboratories surrounding that area. Its care, size, and management are similar to that of the Syrian hamster, though it does not reproduce as well as the Syrian. The Rumanian hamster adult averages 100 g in weight. Its face is more pointed and ratlike than the Syrian hamster, but it is similar in appearance to the Turkish hamster.

Dzungarian Hamster

The Dzungarian hamster is very timid. The males are 11 cm long and 40–50 g in weight; the females are 9 cm long and weigh 30 g at maturity. The Dzungarian hamster has a short tail about 1 cm in length, which is usually hidden by the body fur. The fur on the dorsal side is gray with a dark-brown or black stripe from the nape of the neck to the base of the tail. The ventral fur is white. The average life span has been reported to 1 year by Herberg et al. (1980) and 2 years by Heldmaier and Steinlechner (1981).

The Dzungarian hamster, native to the U.S.S.R., was originally trapped in Siberia and provided to the United States by the U.S.S.R. The present Dzungarian hamster population is the result of the mating of one female to two males who were domesticated in 1965.

The Dzungarian has been used in research involving photoperiodism, the pineal gland and thermoregulation.

South African Hamster

The South African is the only member of its genus and the only hamster native to Africa. The first colony was established in South Africa in 1941. In its natural habitat, South African hamsters are nocturnal, solitary burrowing rodents. Unlike other hamsters, it does not have cheek pouches. The hamster has gray to brown fur on its dorsal aspect with white on the ventral surface, feet, and tail. The tail is 5–8 cm long. Its ears are erect and the eyes are dark and bright. Adult males and females weigh 145 and 95 g, respectively (Hall et al., 1967). The average life span is 2.4 years, with a maximum life span of 6.2 years (Davis, 1963).

The U.S. received its first S. African hamster in 1962. These hamsters have not had much of an impact in biomedical research except in diabetes mellitus and infectious disease research.

HUSBANDRY

Housing, Caging, and Bedding

Hamsters should be housed singularly unless they have been housed together since weanlings. If raised together, hamsters will occasionally fight, though they tend not to cause each other too much physical harm. European hamsters should be housed one animal per cage and only brought together for breeding purposes.

Caging requirements are described in Table 2. Caging material is usually rigid plastic (polycarbonate, polystyrene, polypropylene), galvanized metal, stainless steel, glass, and hard alloys of aluminum, but never wood (it will only take a hamster a short time to be free of a wooden cage, as they are great chewers). Cages may have solid or open wire

Table 2 Space Recommendations and Regulations for Hamsters

Recommendations of the Laboratory Animal Resources National Research Council Guide for the Care and Use of Laboratory Animals (1985)

Weight of animal (g)	Type of housing	Floor area/ animal (cm^2)	Height (cm^2)
<60	Cage	64.5 (10 in^2)	15.24 (6.0 in^2)
60–80	Cage	83.9 (13.0 in^2)	15.24 (6.0 in^2)
81–100	Cage	103.2 (16.0 in^2)	15.24 (6.0 in^2)
>100	Cage	122.6 (19.0 in^2)	15.24 (6.0 in^2)

Regulations of Animal Welfare Act (PL89-544 as amended PL91-579) and the Animal Welfare Act, Code of Federal Regulations (1985).

Age	Minimum space per hamster (in^2)		Maximum population/ enclosure
	dwarf	other	
Weanling to 5 weeks	5.0	10.3	20
5–10 weeks	7.5	12.5	16
≥ 10 weeks	9.0	15.0	13

The interior height of the cage should be 5.5 in for hamsters other than the dwarfs and 5 in for the dwarfs.

mesh bottoms; however, hamsters tend to have fewer stress-related deaths and more rapid growth in solid-bottom cages with direct bedding.

If solid-bottom cages are used, materials such as straw, beet pulp, peat moss, hard wood chips, or wood (treated) shavings should be provided in the cage so that the hamster is able to build a nest to sleep in during the day. Straw may also be provided in cages with open wire-mesh bottoms so that the hamsters may nest.

Pregnant females should not be housed in suspended cages with open wire mesh bottoms. They should be housed separately in solid-bottom cages with a caging material as described above. A nursing female and her young should have at least 121 in^2 of floor space. With dwarf hamsters, there should be at least 25 in^2 of floor space for the mother and her young.

Temperature, Humidity, and Lighting Requirements

Hamsters are generally more adversely affected by higher temperatures than lower ones. Temperature ranges for the nonbreeding hamster are 69–75°F (20–24°C) (Fox, 1980) and for breeding 72–74°F. If temperatures fall below 4°C, the hamster will start to hibernate (Schermer, 1967).

Humidity requirements are 40–60% with a lighting cycle of 12 hr light and 12 hr dark. This lighting also fulfills the requirement necessary for breeding. In uncontrolled light and temperature environments, failures in hamster reproduction have been observed in winter owing to decreased light and in the summer to increased temperatures.

WATER AND DIET

Water

Water should be available ad libitum. Water can be provided by a automatic watering system with a lixit accessible to the smallest hamster or by a water bottle with a sipper tube. Fluid requirements are 30 ml/day for the Syrian hamster, 11–13 ml/100 g/day for the Chinese hamster, and 5 ml/100 g/day for the European hamster.

Diet

The best diet for a hamster is one which is 16–24% protein, 60–65% carbohydrates, and 5–7% fat. Most animal facilities use standard rodent chow for hamsters, though hamsters do have a higher requirement for zinc (0.6%), copper (10 ppm), and potassium (20 ppm) than rats (Newberne et al., 1979). Copper may need to be increased during studies when the hamster may be extremely stressed. This should be determined by the principal investigator. Some studies have shown that a soybean meal may offer better nutritional efficiency for hamsters. During lactation, nutritional requirements for female hamsters may increase, such as is seen in the rat. The female will show signs of extreme weight loss and maternal cannibalism during lactation if not enough nutrition is being provided.

Hamsters start eating solid food at days 7–10 of age. Syrian hamsters consume 5.5–7.0 g of food during their growth and development. Adult and pregnant hamsters usually consume 10–15 g/day. Unlike rats, males and females consume nearly the same amounts of food. Hamsters, like other rodents, are coprophagic.

Feed is usually provided ad libitum. Hamsters do most of their eating at night, usually every 2 hours. Hamsters are hoarding animals and, therefore, will remove the food pellets from the feeder and pile them in a corner of the cage. The corner is usually opposite of the corner used for urination and defecation. Because of this trait, exact feed consumption for hamsters is difficult to determine. Feeders should have slots large enough to allow the hamster with its broad muzzle access to the food.

If hamster are fasted for several hours or up to 4 days, they do not increase their food intake to compensate for the loss. If food is only available a certain time each day, a hamster will eat exactly as much as they would ordinarily eat if the food were ad libitum; however, hoarding activity is increased. This is in sharp contrast to the rat, which will compensate for periods of fasting.

DISEASES AND SPONTANEOUS TUMORS

Amyloidosis

Amyloidosis is a noninfectious disease which occurs in aging hamsters. It is the principal cause of death of hamsters on long-term studies (Renshaw, 1975). In one report, a colony had an 88% incidence of the disease after 18 months of age. The onset of the disease may be due to a defect in the immune system because the first histopathological sign is deposition of immune globulins in blood vessels. Edema, proteinuria, hypercholesteremia, and ascites have also been associated with the disease.

The incidence of amyloidosis varies from colony-to-colony. The amyloidosis is found in the liver, kidney, stomach, adrenal, thyroid, and spleen. The clinical signs and histopathological findings are similar to that seen in humans with the nephrotic syndrome.

Amyloidosis can be induced in adult Syrian hamsters by 1-ml sc injections (5 times a week, once a day) of 50% casein Hammerstein in 0.3 M $NaHCO_3$, pH 7.5 (Gruys et al., 1979). Amyloidosis was induced in 8 weeks, first seen in the liver, spleen, and then the kidney. Amyloidosis can also be induced in animals treated with diethylstilbestrol.

Antibiotic-Associated Enterocolitis

After treatment with gram-positive selective antibiotics, moribundity and mortality have been reported in hamsters. The cause of the disease may be due to the change of the intestinal microflora.

Calcinosis

Calcinosis is characterized by mineralization of connective tissue in almost every organ of the hamster and is seen especially in the arteries. The early stage of the disease is characterized by the precipitation of mineralized material in the elastic fibers in the arteries. In the later stage, the lesions spread to larger areas of the vessel.

Multifocal Retinal Dysplasia

Multifocal retinal dysplasia is found to have a 2% incidence in LAK:LVG Syrian hamsters. The disease can be detected from ophthalmoscopic examination in hamsters as young as 6 weeks of age and as old as 9 months. Ophthalmoscopically, the dysplasia foci are seen as either retinal streaks or small, circular areas of cream-colored depigmentations. Histologically, the focal dysplasias are manifested as invaginations and rosettelike structures composed of elements of the photoreceptor layer, outer-limiting membrane, and outer nuclear layer (Schiavo, 1980).

Polycystic Disease

Hamsters have a cyst incidence of 76% at ages over 1 year (Gleiser et al., 1970). The liver is the most common site of the cysts (Renshaw, 1975). The lesions appear to be due to development defects of normal ductal structures such as the bile duct (Van Hoosier et al., 1984). No clinical signs have been reported.

Hamster Enteritis

Hamster enteritis, or wet tail or wet tail disease, has also been called terminal ileitis, proliferative ileitis, and enzootic adenocaracinoma, among other terms. It is the most common and important disease of hamsters, especially the Syrian species. Hamster enteritis is a disease state in which the animals are excoriated, lethargic, irritable, anorexic, emaciated, and the caudal area is wet due to the diarrhea associated with the disease. After the onset of symptoms, death is usually 48 hr to a week later. The lesions seen are ulcerations of the cecal mucosa, inflammatory lesions of the ileum, cecum, jejunum, and colon, and the rectum contains yellow semifluid material. The specific cause is not known, but *Escherichia coli* has been associated with the etiology. It occurs at all ages, but it is seen especially just after weaning. The epizootiology and transmission is through direct contact and formites. The best prevention and control of the disease is to obtain hamsters from suppliers with a minimal history of the disease. Orally administered antibiotics are the most commonly recommended treatment for this disease (Frisk, 1987).

Pneumonia

Next to wet tail, pneumonia is the most common disease affecting hamsters. The common causes are *Pasteurella pneumotropica, Streptococcus pneumoniae,* and *Streptococcus agalactiae*. The role of *Mycoplasm* sp. in pneumonia in hamsters, though defined in mice and rats, has not been defined in hamsters. The clinical signs include anorexia, nasal and ocular discharge, and respiratory distress. Stress and significant variations in environmental conditions may be contributing and predisposing factors in the disease. Stressful situations should be avoided and affected animals should be isolated. The diagnosis is made through assessment of clinical signs, lesions, and microbiology laboratory results. If treatment is necessary, antibiotics to which the etiological agent is sensitive should be used.

Lymphadenitis

Lymphadenitis in the hamster is consider to be analogous to the condition seen in guinea pigs. In the hamster, the agent of etiology is either *Staphylococcus aureus,* β-hemolytic *Streptococcus* Lancefield group C, or *Streptobacillus moniliformis*. Cervical lymphadenitis is a chronic disease in which clinical signs appear several weeks after infection. Anorexia and death follow the observation of neck swelling owing to cervical lymph node abscesses.

Tyzzer's Disease

Tyzzer's disease is seen more frequently in the mouse than in the hamster. The etiological agent is *Bacillus piliformis*. The clinical signs are diarrhea, dehydration, and lethargy. Lesions seen are enterocolitis, multiple white myocardial nodules, dilated cecum, colon containing semifluid stools, lymphadenitis, and multifocal necrotizing hepatitis (Zook et al., 1977). The diagnosis of the disease is by demonstration of *B. piliformis* in affected tissues following Giemsa or silver staining. Death is within 48 hr.

Salmonellosis

Salmonellosis is very rare in the hamster. The etiological organism is *Salmonella enteritidis*. The disease has a quick onset with death in a few days. Lesions seen are multifocal necrosis of the liver and septic thrombi involving the veins and venules. Affected animals, food, and bedding should be isolated to prevent further colony infections.

Lymphocytic Choriomenigitis

Lymphocytic choriomenigitis (LCM), which is transmittable to humans, is caused by a ribonucleic acid (RNA) virus of the arenavirus group. The clinical signs vary with the strain of the virus and of the hamster, the hamster's age, and the time of infection. Transmission is through direct contact, aerosol exposure, or formites. Fifty percent of those infected as newborns or congenitally develop a chronic progressive fatal disease characterized by inactivity or weight loss (wasting disease). Findings at necropsy of those who develop the disease are chronic glomeruonephropathy and widespread vasculitis (Genovesi et al., 1987). To control for the disease, hamster colonies should be tested for antibodies and infected animals eliminated. Hamsters implanted with tumors developed LCM and were shown to be antibody positive to the virus. The causative agent was the tumors. Students and staff working with the infected hamsters developed LCM, as did naive hamsters located near them. The spread of infection was halted by elimination of the infected hamsters and tumor cell lines (Biggar et al., 1977).

Sendai Virus Infection

Sendai virus infection is caused by parainfluenza 1 (Sendai). This virus is an RNA agent of the paramyxoivirus group, which is related to the human virus hemadsorption type-2 (HA-2). Mice are believed to be the natural host, though rats, hamsters, and guinea pigs are susceptible to natural infections. Clinical signs are apparently asymptomatic. Others infected in vitro or as newborns or young adults develop subchronic infections. Consolidation of the lungs seen at necropsy have been reported in the hamster. In the absence of more reports, it is anticipated that gross and microscopic lesions would be similar to those seen in the mouse; i.e., an acute, interstitial pneumonia. The control and treatment of this virus in the hamster is the same as for the mouse.

Type C Virus Infection

Type C virus seems to be similar to the retrovirus type C oncovirus. The agent was first observed in human adenovirus-induced hamster tumors. One report indicates that lymphomas in hamsters may be associated with this agent. Transmission of type C virus is unclear, and it is believed that the agent may not be expressed until activation by chemical or physical agents or by infections caused by other oncoviral agents. In a study by Yabe et al. (1972), an untreated adult male hamster had an osteocarcinoma which contained particles resembling type C virus. Yabes attempted to transmit the tumor with tissue extracts, but was not successful.

Parasitic Infections

Protozoa

Fecal smears of hamsters show the presence of a vast number and variety of protozoa. Protozoa may have a role in enteric diseases, though this is unclear because similar numbers and kinds of protozoa are found in both healthy and sick animals. Table 3 lists the protozoa found most often in hamsters and the location and prevalence of these protozoa in a hamster colony (Wantland, 1955).

Nematodes

The major nematode infections in hamsters are caused by *Syphacia obvelata* (mouse pinworm) and *Syphacia muris* (ratoxyurid). The occurrence of *Syphacia obvelata* is less than 1%; however, infection rates can be very high in individual colonies. The pinworm is found in the intestine and the gross lesion is inflammation of the large intestine. Treatment is with 10 mg/ml piperazine citrate (in drinking water) twice in a 7-day period (Unay et al., 1980). *Syphacia muris* is the consequence of direct contact with infected rats.

Mites

Acariasis in hamsters is caused by infestation by one of two species, *Demodex cricetic* or *D. aurato*. Infection rates are high, though clinical signs of skin disease are very rare. Clinical signs seen included alpoecia on the rump and back with dry, scaly skin.

Ear mites in the hamster are caused by the *Notoedres* sp., tropical rat mite (*Srnithonysaus baacote*), and the nasal mite (*Spleorodens clethrionomys*).

Cestodes

Hymenolepis nana, the dwarf tape worm, and *H. diminuta* are found in the small intestine and are usually benign infections; however, when in large numbers they may cause impactions and obstructions. Infection may also produce a mucoid or catarrhal inflammation of the bowel (enteritis). Diagnosis of the infection is by the observation of eggs in the feces or mature worms in the intestine. Newly acquired animals should be quarantined, and infected animals are isolated and treated with niclosamide.

SPONTANEOUS TUMORS

Table 4 lists the most common spontaneous tumors in hamsters by incidence and their incidence. The most frequent tumors are seen in the adrenal cortex and intestinal tract, followed by the lymphoreticular system, the endometrium, endocrine system, and

Table 3 Location and Prevalence of Protozoa in the Hamster

Organism	Location	Prevalence (%)
Trichomonas sp.	Cecum, colon	99
Endamoeba muris	Cecum	33
Giardia sp.	Small intestine	9
Chilomastix bettencoutri	Cecum	9
Hymenolepis nana	Small intestine	>1
Syphacia obvelata	Intestine	>1

Table 4   Incidence of Spontaneous Tumors in Syrian Hamsters

Neoplasm	Males	Females	Total
Adrenal adenoma	12.7	9.4	11.0
Lymphoreticular neoplasm	3.7	2.3	3.0
Uterus endometrial polyp		3.0	
Uterus endometrial carcinoma		3.0	
Adrenal carcinoma	3.0	2.0	2.5
Pancreas islet cell adenoma	3.7	1.3	2.5
Vagina papilloma		2.0	
Stomach papilloma	1.7	1.7	1.7
Thyroid carcinoma	1.0	2.0	1.5
Uterus leiomyoma		1.0	
Small intestine adenocarcinoma	0.3	1.3	0.8
Pituitary adenoma	0.0	1.3	0.7
Pancreas islet cell carcinoma	0.7	0.7	0.7
Ovary fibroma		0.7	
Ovary theca cell tumor		0.7	

ovaries of aging females (Sher, 1982). The benign tumors found are usually adenomas of the adrenal cortex and polyps of the intestinal tract. In a study by Dontenwill et al. (1973), adenocarcinomas were age related with a rate of greater than 50% in hamsters over 100 weeks of age. The rate of small intestinal adenocarcinomas (0.8%) seen by Fabry (1985) was higher in hamsters than in rats or mice. Lymphosacromas are the most common malignant tumors of the Syrian hamster. Tumors of the liver, pituitary, lung, urinary bladder, and mammary gland are practically unknown in the hamster, but these do occur spontaneously in older rats and mice (Homburger et al., 1979). Genetic drifts seen in many colonies of hamsters may influence the rate of spontaneous tumors as in the rat and mouse.

ANIMAL IDENTIFICATION

Hamsters are usually identified by tagging, punching, or coding of the ear or ear tattooing, which is done aseptically.

DOSING AND RESTRAINING

Oral Administration

To dose a hamster orally (po), the animal is grasped by the skin of the neck and back. The gavage tube (metal 18- or 20-gauge) or a polyethylene cather (2–3 cm in length) is passed into the mouth via the interdental space. The tube is passed gently into the esophagus and the fluid administered. The method is similar to the procedure done in the mouse and rat.

Subcutaneous Administration

The hamster is restrained for subcutaneous (sc) dosing as described for oral dosing. The needle is placed into the skin that is tented by the holding method. The injection is made into the skin parallel to the back. The hamster's loose skin enables large volumes to be injected sc in comparison to other rodent species of the same size (Collins, 1979).

Intradermal Administration

To administer an agent intradermally (id), the skin over the injection is shaved. The needle (30-gauge) is advanced just a few millimeters into the skin. If there is suddenly no resistance, then the needle has been pushed through the skin. Withdraw and advance the needle again. Following administration of the material, a small welt will be visible.

Intramuscular Administration

To administer an intramuscular (im) dose, the muscles of the posterior and anterior thighs of the hamster are the most frequently used sites. The animal is restrained as described for oral dosing by an assistant and one leg is held by the doser. The quadriceps are held between the forefinger and the thumb of the doser. The material is injected into the muscle mass.

Intraperitoneal Administration

To dose a hamster intraperitoneally (ip), the animal is grasped as described for oral dosing. The needle is pushed parallel to the line of the leg through the abdominal wall into the peritoneal cavity. Following the leg line avoids administration into the urinary bladder and the liver. Administration may occur when there is no resistance to the needle passage.

Intravenous Administration

It is best that the hamster is anesthetized to administer materials intravenously (iv). The three veins which can be used are the femoral, jugular, and cephalic. The areas must be shaved, a skin incision made to expose the vein, and then a needle may be placed into the vein and the material administered.

BLOOD COLLECTION TECHNIQUES

Retro-orbital Method

The retro-orbital is the method of choice for collecting blood from the hamster. The method used is that as described for the rat. A 23-gauge needle or a microhematocrit tube may be used to obtain the blood. Three milliliters of blood may be collected retro-orbitally; however, for repeated sampling a volume of 0.5 ml is best for the animal. The use of anesthesia is preferable in the hamster.

Cardiac Puncture

Cardiac puncture in hamsters requires practice because the heart can be difficult to locate or can rotate away from the needle. A 25-gauge ⅜-in needle is the suggested equipment. A safe volume to draw from the heart with minimal damage is 1–2 ml. Repeated sampling from the heart is not advised because the mortality rate due to the blood withdrawn can be high (Wechster, 1983). The use of anesthesia is suggested in the hamster. Upon exsanguination, 5 ml can be withdrawn from a 95-g hamster (Schermer, 1967).

Tail Clipping Method

Tail clipping is a method only good for a maximum of six samples because the tail is so short. To facilitate blood flow, place a suction bell (which is connected to a water pump) on the base of the tail. Anesthesia is not necessary if the hamster is placed in a narrow tube with the hind legs protruding so they can be held.

Femoral Vein Method

To collect blood from the femoral vein, a tourniquet is placed above the stifle and the fur over the area clipped. A skin incision is made to expose the vein and a 25-gauge ⅝-in needle is placed into the vein. The blood is collected from the needle hub with a capillary microcontainer or a microhematocrit tube.

Jugular Vein Method

To collect blood from the jugular vein, the hamster should be anesthetized, the area shaved over the jugular, a skin incision made, and a 25-gauge ⅝-in needle placed into the vein and the blood withdrawn.

URINE COLLECTION

The best method is to collect the urine over 17–24 hr as the animal voids. A preservative such as thymol can be added to the collection vessel before starting. Catherization of the ureter can be done; however, there is always the chance of blood or tissue contamination. A hamster's urine is normally a thick, milky fluid.

ANALGESIA AND ANETHESIA

Analgesia

Buprenorphine (0.5 mg/kg/sc) given every 8 hr provides good analgesia for the hamster.

Hamsters are easily restrained if held by an experienced handler and usually preanesthesia is not necessary; however, preanesthesia will be discussed.

Preanesthesia

Hypnorm (1ml/kg/ip) provides sufficient analgesic for superficial procedures, and diazepam (5ml/kg/ip) provides sedation, but no analgesia.

Anesthesia

Table 5 lists the concentrations of suggested anesthesias, site of administrations, and length of sedation (Flecknell, 1987).

Inhalation Anesthesia

To use inhalation anesthesia, the method is the same as described for the rat. The first choice for the hamster is methoxyflurane, followed by ether, halothane, and enflurane.

Table 5 Anesthesia Data for Hamsters[a]

Compounds	Concentration	Time of sedation (min)
Fentanyl-fluanisone[b] + diazepam	1 ml/kg	60
Fentanyl-fluanisone-midazolan[b]	4 ml/kg	30–40
Ketamine-xylazine[b]	200:10 mg/kg	70
Pentobarbital sodium	35 mg/kg	30–60
Thiopental sodium	40 mg/kg	
Alphaxolone-alphadolone[c]	15 mg/kg	20–60
Pentobarbitone[c]	36 mg/kg	20–50

[a]Administered intraperitoneally.
[b]Provides surgical anesthesia.
[c]Provides sedation/light anesthesia.

EUTHANASIA

The hamster may be euthansized by inhalation and by physical and parenteral methods. The best method is asphyxiation with carbon dioxide from dry ice or a gas cylinder followed by ether, halothane (respiratory arrest in 30 sec), or methoxyflurane. The physical methods are cervical dislocation and decapitation with a guillotine (this method should only be done by a experienced researcher to prevent unnecessary pain and distress to the animal). Sodium pentobarbital (150 mg/kg) may be given iv, ip, intracardically (which may be painful), or into the thoracic cavity.

PHYSICAL PARAMETERS

Neonatal Body Weights

At birth, Syrian hamsters weigh 2–3 g and Chinese hamsters weigh 1.5–2.5 g. Neonate hamsters are hairless with the ears and eyes closed. Table 6 lists information about the early development of the eight laboratory hamsters.

Body Weights and Weight Gains

Figure 1 charts the average weight of male and female Syrian hamsters over an average life span.

The average adult body weight for each of the species is discussed in the species section of this chapter.

In a study by Borer et al. (1977), Syrian hamsters gained 2 g/day from birth to 5 weeks of age. From days 30 (weight = 65 g) to 70 the hamsters gained 1 g/day. From day 70–88 the hamsters gained 0.3 g/day. Syrian hamsters at maturity weighed from 100 to 135 g.

Dentition

The dentition of a Syrian hamster is monophyodont, bunodont, and brachyodont. The incisors of the Syrian species grow irregularly depending on age and sex of the hamster.

Table 6 Neonatal Data for Hamsters

Species	Birth weight (g)	Day eyes open	Day ears open	Day pups solid food	Day weaned	Teeth at birth
Syrian	2–3	15	5	7–10	21	Yes
Chinese	1.5–2.5	10–14	10–14		21–25	
Dzungarian	1.8	10	3–4	10	16–18	Yes
European						No[a]
Armenian		14	14	14	18	
Rumanian						
Turkish		12–13		12–13	20	
South African	6.5	16–25	3–5	21	25	No[a]

[a]Incisors erupt at 3–5 days.

The adult European hamster has one set of permanent teeth which consists of four continuously growing incisors and 12 molars.

Life Spans

The average life spans for each of the laboratory species are discussed in the species section of this chapter.

Sexual Maturity

Sexual maturity for female hamsters begins at 4–6 weeks of age. At this time, there are 10 mature and 25 reserve follicles in each ovary. A female's first spontaneous estrus and ovulation are at 4–5 weeks and 30 days, respectively. In young immature females (4 weeks of age), ovulation may be artificially induced with 30 IU pregnant horse serum

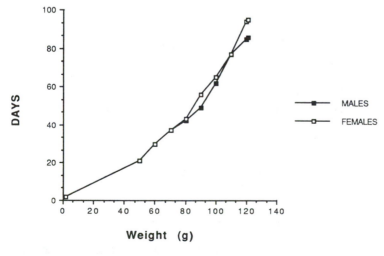

Figure 1 Weight vs age in syrian hamsters.

(Magalhaes, 1970). The estrus cycle is 94 hr or > 4 days in length with four distinct stages: proestrus, estrus, metestrus, and diestrus. Identification of the stage can be determined from differentiation of a vaginal smear through examination of cell types. During estrus (which occurs before and after ovulation) the female will show lordosis and will mate. The end of estrus is the appearance of a copious postovulatory discharge. The discharge is creamy, white, opaque, and very viscous with a pungent cheesy odor. Ovulation occurs regularly every 4 days, 9–10 hr after the peak concentrations of luteinizing hormone (LH). The breeding life of a hamster is usually about 10–12 months, or after the production of six litters.

Syrian hamster males reach sexual maturity at 6–7 weeks of age and have a breeding life of about 1 year. The testicles of male Syrian and Chinese hamsters descend at day 26 and 30, respectively.

The secondary sex characteristic of the Syrian hamster is a scent organ (flank organ) which is located on the flank. The male touches the female's organ with his paws during copulation. The intensity of the pigmentation is an indication of androgen activity. The males have a darker pigmentation than females. The pigmentation is first seen at 25 days of age and is more marked at 35 days of age.

BREEDING

Environmental Effects

With most laboratory hamster colonies maintained in controlled environments, seasonal changes in reproduction are rarely observed. In uncontrolled light and temperature environments, failures in hamster reproduction such as small litter sizes and lack of pregnancies have been seen in winter due to decreased light and in the summer due to increased temperatures.

Copulation

When a female in heat is placed with a male, there is a short period of investigation before mating. A female will demonstrate her willingness to mate by assuming lordosis, a posture where the back is held flat and firm with the legs braced and the tail is held erect and vertical. The male will groom the female and himself before mating. A male and female will repeatedly mate for 20–60 min with mounting and copulation taking place several times a minute. Rarely does a male attack a female during mating. An unreceptive female will attack a male and bite him on the face or scrotum. Females may also become aggressive after mating and will attack the male as described above.

Sperm penetration is usually 2–4 hr after ovulation. Fifty-six to 343 million sperm can be recovered from the female reproduction tract after copulation. This is approximately 40–45% of the number of spermatozoa present in the vas deferens and epidymis of a mature male (Magalhaes, 1970). The observation of a copulation plug is an indication of successful mating. Examination for postovulatory discharge on days 5 and 9 of pregnancy will also confirm pregnancy. If a discharge is present, the female is having a normal estrus and therefore is not pregnant. If a discharge is present on day 10, the female is having a pseudopregnancy. In pseudopregnancy, the corpora lutea persist and function, but for a shorter time than a normal pregnancy. It is the result of copulation with a sterile male. Pseudopregnant females are excellent models to study decidual cell response and the formation of diciduas.

Table 7 Reproductive Data for Hamsters

Species	Litter size (pups)	Gestation period (days)	Sexual maturity	
			males	females
Syrian	11	16	6–7 wks	4–6 wks
Chinese	5	21	8–12 wks	12 wks
Dzungarian	4	18	35–40	90–139
European	7–9	15–17	60 dys	80–90 dys
Armenian	6–7	18–19		
Rumanian		16		
Turkish	6	14–15	7–8 wks[a]	7–8 wks
South African	3	38	4–7 mths	4–7 mths

[a]Occasionally do not reach maturity until 5–6 months of age, and then they may undergo spontaneous testicular regression.

Pregnancy

If copulation is successful (breeding day is day 0), on day 10 the female hamster shows an increase in body weight and a characteristic abdominal distension. Pregnancy length is 15 days and 7–17 hr. Gestation periods for Syrian hamster over 6 months of age and 1 year are over 16 and 17 days, respectively.

Parturition

Hours before delivery, the pregnant female becomes restless, alternates between eating, grooming, and nest building and shows an increased respiratory rate. Hamsters that build small or tiny nests frequently have smaller litters or none at all. Active licking of the perineal region indicates the onset of birth. Young are born either breech or head first. They are licked clean and separated from the membranes and umbilical cord by their mother. Placentas are eaten immediately or stored as food. Litter sizes vary with the age of the female, genetic factors, types of diet, light, temperature, nesting material, and caging material. Litter sizes usually decrease in breeders older than 14 months. The male-to-female ratio at birth is almost equal.

During lactation the mother shows excessive weight loss, which can be reduced if humidity is kept over 40% and animals have adequate water and food. Maternal cannibalism is common, particularly during the neonates' first week of life. The young appear to be biting the mother and the mother retaliates by killing and eating the young. Other reasons for cannibalism include stress to the mother, especially if there are strange, loud noises, or if the litter is too large and the female reduces it to a manageable size. With Dzungarian hamsters, the mother and the young can be housed with the father. Both parents participate in the care of the offspring. The infants of a South African hamster remain attached to the mother's nipples and travel with her until they are 15–20 days of age. Since the female only has four nipples, the maximum litter size is four.

Respiratory Rate and Oxygen Consumption

The minimum respiratory rate (breaths/min) is 33, the maximum is 127. The average respiratory rate is 74 and the mean resting respiratory rate is 30–33 breaths/min (Robinson, 1968). Hamsters are nose breathers and have a resting oxygen consumption of 2.3 ml/g/hr.

BODY TEMPERATURE

Rectal temperature for Syrian hamsters is 99.5°F (37.5°C) and 36–37°Celsius for the Dzungarian hamster.

BLOOD PRESSURE

The blood pressure measured by cannulation of the carotid artery of the hamster is 111 mmHg (Sroia et al., 1954). The blood pressure measured on the cheek pouch by Berman et al. was 90 ± 11.3 mmHg. Another measurement of blood pressure by photoelectric tensiometry was 108 mmHg. Though there can not be a direct comparison of these measurements because of the techniques used, the values obtained are similar and can be used as reference values for each method described.

HEART RATE

The mean heart rate (beats/min) of the Syrian hamster is 450 with a range of 300–600.

ECG PATTERNS

The rate of contraction in the Syrian hamster is 350–500 beats/min. The P-Q interval is 48 msec with a range of 40–60, the QRS interval is 15 msec with a range of 13 to 20, the T- and P-wave amplitude are 0.33 ± 0.07 mV and 0.19 ± 0.03 mV, respectively. For measurement of ECGs, the hamster needs to be anesthetized because of its aggressive behavior. The ECG tracings of hamsters resemble human ECG tracings (Lossnitzer et al., 1977).

CLINICAL LABORATORY

Clinical chemistry values for Syrian hamsters are listed in Table 8. The following will be a discussion of several interesting aspects of the hamster and its clinical chemistry values.

In comparison to humans, the hamster has lower bilirubin, cholesterol, alkaline phosphatase, creatine phosphokinase, lactic dehydrogenase, and A/G ratio values and higher blood urea nitrogen, bicarbonate, phosphorus, amylase, acid phosphatase, aspartate aminotransferase, and α_2-globulin values.

Since hamsters are such deep day sleepers, blood collection times should be noted because during light photoperiods clinical chemistry values can be variable. The anesthesia used may also affect clinical chemistry values. These must be taken into account when analyzing clinical chemistry data.

Glucose

Thiobarbiturate anesthesia may produce glucose levels as high as 300 mg/dl in adult male Syrian hamsters. The hyperglycemia can exist for up to 5 hr after anesthesia exposure and

Table 8 Clinical Chemistry Values for Syrian Hamsters

Test	Units	Male mean values	Female mean values	Range both sexes
Bilirubin	(mg/dl)	0.42	0.36	0.20–0.74
Cholesterol	(mg/dl)	54.8	51.5	10.0–80.0
Creatinine	(mg/dl)	1.05	0.98	0.35–1.65
Glucose	(mg/dl)	73.4	65.0	32.6–118.0
Urea Nitrogen	(mg/dl)	23.4	20.8	12.5–26.0
Uric Acid	(mg/dl)	4.58	4.36	1.80–5.30
Sodium	(mEq/L)	128	134	106–146
Potassium	(mEq/L)	4.66	5.30	4.0–5.9
Chloride	(mEq/L)	96.7	93.8	85.7–112.0
Bicarbonate	(mEq/L)	37.3	39.1	32.7–44.1
Phosphorus	(mg/dl)	5.29	6.04	3.4–8.24
Calcium	(mg/dl)	9.52	10.4	7.4–12.0
Magnesium	(mg/dl)	2.54	2.20	1.9–3.5
Amylase	(Somogyi units/dl)	175	196	120–250
Enzymes				
alkaline phosphatase	(IU/L)	17.5	15.4	3.2–30.5
acid phosphatase	(IU/L)	7.45	6.90	3.9–10.4
alanine transaminase	(IU/L)	26.9	20.6	11.6–35.9
aspartate transaminase	(IU/L)	124	77.6	37.6–168
creatine phosphokinase	(IU/L)	101	85.0	50–190
creatine kinase	(IU/L)	23.1		
lactic dehydrogenase	(IU/L)	115	110	56.0–170.0
Serum proteins				
total protein	(g/dl)	6.94	7.25	4.3–7.7
albumin	(g/dl)	3.23	3.50	2.63–4.10
α_1-globulin	(g/dl)	0.64	0.55	0.30–0.95
α_2-globulin	(g/dl)	1.85	1.70	0.9–2.70
β-globulin	(g/dl)	0.56	0.83	0.1–1.35
γ-globulin	(g/dl)	0.71	0.67	0.15–1.28
A/G ratio		0.87	0.93	0.58–1.24

Source: Mitruka, B. M., and Rawnsley, H. M. (1981) *Clinical Biochemical and Hematological Reference Values in Normal Experimental Animals and Humans*. 2nd ed. Masson, New York.

there is no relationship to the length of hyperglycemia compared to the duration of the anesthesia. Hyperglycemia has also been reported in hibernating hamsters (Newcomer et al., 1987).

Lipids

The lipids found in the hamster are cholesterol, phospholipids, triglycerides, and fatty acids. Cholesterol concentrations in hamsters are the highest when compared to other laboratory animals, but lower than human levels. Short photoperiods (10 hr or less) can cause a decrease in cholesterol, but other lipids such as plasma triglycerides are not affected. Serum lipids do increase in the hamster during hibernation. A strain of spontaneous hypercholesterolemic Syrian hamsters show increases in cholesterol when exposed to low temperatures.

Urea Nitrogen

Hamsters who develop kidney disease during the aging process have increased urea nitrogen levels as seen in other laboratory animals.

ENZYMES

Serum obtained by cardiac puncture may be contaminated by aspartate aminotransferase (AST), lactic dehydrogenase (LDH), alanine aminotransferase (ALT), and creatine phosphokinase owing to the high concentrations of these enzymes already present in the heart.

Alkaline Phosphatase

The alkaline phosphatase in the hamster is composed of isoenzymes from bone, liver, and intestine. Alkaline phosphatase is a more sensitive indicator of liver damage than bilirubin or alanine aminotransferase. Dramatic increases are usually indicative of bile duct obstruction. Immature hamsters have elevation of values two- to threefold compared to adults.

Alanine Aminotransferase

Alanine Aminotransferase is specific for liver damage in dogs, cats and rats. In the hamster, ALT levels are increased in both acetaminophen-induced and viral-induced hepatic necrosis.

Aspartate Aminotransferase

The activity of AST is low but increases following muscle injury. Increased AST levels have been seen in hamsters with liver neoplasms.

Creatine Kinase and Lactic Dehydrogenase

Cardiomyopathic Syrian hamsters show elevated creatine kinase and lactic dehydrogenase activities. Normal creatine kinase levels are 23.1 IU/L whereas in cardiomyopathic hamsters the levels are 730 IU/L.

Thyroid Hormones

Thyroid hormones are of interest because of the hamster's hibernation. Basal T_3 and T_4 decrease with age. T_4 levels in 3-month-old hamsters are 6.75 ± 0.75 μg/dl and 3.59 ± 0.16 μg/dl in 20-month-old hamsters. T_3 levels in 3-month-old hamsters are 62 ± 2 ng/dl and 42 ± 3 ng/dl in 20 month-old-hamsters. These changes are also seen in humans and in other rodent species. Older hamsters show less of an increase in T_3 and T_4 levels after thyroid-stimulating hormone (TSH) administration. During short photoperiods there is a decrease in TSH, T_3, and T_4. Lower temperatures also cause decreases in T_3 and T_4 levels, whereas in cold conditions there is an increase T_3 and a decrease in T_4. Pregnant hamsters may metabolize thyroid hormones differently because there is a decrease in protein-bound iodine during pregnancy.

Reproductive Hormones

During estrus there is one luteinizing hormone (LH) surge and the follicle-stimulating hormone (FSH) is biphasic. The first burst of FSH occurs concurrently with LH. The second burst is thought to be responsible for the initiation and/or maintenance of follicular growth for the next estrus cycle. Maintenance of functional corpora lutea is believed to be performed a combination of prolactin, FSH, and a small amount of LH.

Progesterone is the dominant hormone during the first 2 days of estrus, decreasing on day 3 but rising again on day 4. The levels of progesterone on days 1–2 are dependent on LH. Estradiol levels are low for the first 2 days and increase and decrease on day 4.

Adrenal Hormones

In the hamster, corticosterone and cortisol are secreted by the adrenal cortex. Corticosterone levels are 3 to 4 times higher than cortisol during the day. Adrenocorticotropic hormone (ACTH) stimulation increases both hormones; however, cortisol levels are stimulated at a higher rate. Basal cortisol levels are 0.45 ± 0.04 μg/dl and 0.38 ± 0.09 μg/dl in males and females, respectively, and corticosteriod levels are 7.4 ± 1.9 mg/dl (Tomson et al., 1987). Pregnant hamsters can produce large quantities of cortisol (30 μg/dl), whereas nonpregnant females have relatively low levels (0.3 μg/dl) in comparison to other species. Increased plasma cortisol levels are seen after exposure to chronic stress.

Glucocorticord levels follow the circadian pattern seen in other rodents.

PROTEINS

Chinese hamsters with spontaneous diabetes have 10–30% of their total proteins being α_2, whereas control hamster have only 3–8%. Asymptomatic hamsters with significantly elevated α_2 proteins do develop chemical or clinical diabetes later on.

HEMATOLOGY VALUES

Hematological values for Syrian hamsters are listed in Table 9. Hematological values for European and Chinese hamsters are listed in Table 10. The blood volume of a hamster is 6–9% of body weight. The maximum safe volume for one bleeding is 5.5 ml/kg. The practical volume from adult hamsters for diagnostic use is 1 ml. Hematological values for a hamster vary considerably because they are deep day sleepers, though values between males and females are similar. The variations seen are changes in blood volume and quantity of blood components.

Erythrocytes

Erythrocytes in the hamster have a diameter of 5 to 7 μm. South African hamsters have larger erythrocytes than other hamsters and laboratory rodents. A small portion of erythrocytes show polychromasia (Schermer, 1967). Erythrocytes have a life span of 50–78 days. Desai (1968) saw an increase in erythrocyte longevity during hibernation. Nucleated or basophilic cells are rare, but reticulocytes are found from 3–4.9%.

Leukocytes

Hamster leukograms are similar to those of other laboratory rodents. During photoperiods the total leukocyte counts range from 5000 to 10,000/μl, whereas during hibernation counts drop to 2500/μl. During sleep, the lymphocyte:neutrophil ratio is 45%:45%, whereas in awake animals the neutrophil percentage varies between 17 and 35%.

Table 9 Hematological Values for Syrian Hamsters

Test	Units	Male mean	Male range	Female mean	Female range
RBC	x10E6/mm^3	7.5	4.7–10.3	6.96	3.96–9.96
HgB	g/dl	16.8	14.4–19.2	16.0	13.1–18.9
MCV	μ^3	70.0	64.8–77.6	70.0	64.0–76.0
MCH	$\mu\mu$g	22.4	19.9–24.9	23.0	20.2–25.8
MCHC	%	32.0	27.5–36.5	32.6	27.8–37.4
Hct	%	52.5	47.9–57.1	49.0	39.2–58.8
Sedimentation Rate	mm/hr	0.64	0.32–0.96	0.50	0.30–0.70
Platelets	x10E3/mm^3	410	367–573	360	300–490
WBC	x10E3/mm^3	7.62	5.02–10.2	8.56	6.48–10.6
Neutrophils	x10E3/mm^3	1.68	1.11–2.25	2.48	1.88–3.08
Eosinophils	x10E3/mm^3	0.07	0.04–0.12	0.06	0.04–0.08
Basophils	x10E3/mm^3	0.08	0.05–0.10	0.04	0.03–0.05
Lymphocytes	x10E3/mm^3	5.6	3.69–7.51	5.81	4.41–7.20
Monocytes	x10E3/mm^3	0.19	0.12–0.26	0.20	0.16–0.25

Source: Mitruka, B. M., and Rawnsley, H. M. (1981) *Clinical Biochemical and Hematological Reference Values in Normal Experimental Animals and Humans.* 2nd ed. Masson, New York.

Coagulation

Hamster blood starts to coagulate at 15–20 sec (Schermer, 1967) with a mean coagulation time of 142 sec (Desai, 1968).

Trypanosomes

Hamster frequently have trypanosomes in the blood. These microorganisms are parasitic but not pathogenic. They have been observed in other laboratory animals, including sheep and monkeys, but not in the large numbers as seen in the hamster. The counts of trypanosomes can be very large, sometimes equaling the leukocyte counts. Prof. Enigk of the Bernhardt-Nocht Institute, Germany (personal communication) found that 50% of his hamster colony had typanosomes. Transmission is not known; however, trypanosomes are not considered harmful and will not interfere with the outcome of a hamster study (Schermer, 1967).

BLOOD GASES AND pH

The values for blood gases are PaO_2 71.8 ± 4.9 mmHg, $PaCO_2$ 41.1 ± 2.4 mmHg, HCO_3^- 29.9 ± 2.9 mEq/L, and the blood pH is 7.48 ± 0.03. Measurements of exercising hamsters show a increase of 12.9 ± 7.9 in PaO_2, a decrease of 6.6 ± 2.6 $PaCO_2$, and a decrease of 3.5 ± 2.3 in HCO_3^- concentrations.

URINE VALUES

The range of urine volume is 5.1–8.5 ml/24 hr in normal hamsters. In diabetic Chinese hamsters, the urine volume can be as high as 25 ml/day. Sodium and potassium con-

Table 10 Hematological Values for European and Chinese Hamsters

Parameter	Units	European range	Chinese range
RBC	x10E6/mm^3	6.04–9.10	4.4–9.1
HgB	g/dl	13.4–15.5	10.7–14.1
MCV	μ^3	58.7–71.4	53.6–65.2
MCH	$\mu\mu$g	18.6–22.5	15.5–19.1
MCHC	%	26.4–32.5	27.0–32.0
Hct	%	44.0–49.0	36.5–47.7
WBC	x10E3/mm^3	3.4–7.6	2.7–9.6
Neutrophils	x10E3/mm^3	3.5–41.6	14.8–23.6
Eosinophils	x10E3/mm^3	0–2.1	0.3–3.1
Basophils	x10E3/mm^3	0–0.2	0.0–0.5
Lymphocytes	x10E3/mm^3	50.0–95.0	68.1–84.8
Monocytes	x10E3/mm^3	0–1.0	0–2.4

Source: Mitruka, B. M., and Rawnsley, H. M. (1981) *Clinical Biochemical and Hematological Reference Values in Normal Experimental Animals and Humans.* 2nd ed. Masson, New York.

centrations are 70 and 120 mmol/L, respectively. The pH is basic, proteins are excreted about 10 times the rate of humans, and cholesterol is the main lipid excreted.

SPECIES PECULIARITIES

The hamster cheek pouch is unique because it accepts heterologously neoplastic tissue but rejects normal human tissue. This led to the discovery that a biological difference existed between malignant and nonmalignant tissues. The cheek pouch has been used for the transplanting of neoplastic tissue for evaluation of growth. When this method was standardized, it became a screening tool for chemotherapeutic agents (Newcomer et al., 1987).

The cheek pouch is transparent and very accessible. It is ideally suited for in vivo studies of microcirculation and the behavior of formed blood elements.

STRAIN-RELATED CONSIDERATIONS

In a study by Althoff and Mohr (1973) comparing the chronic respiratory response of the Chinese, Syrian, and European hamsters to diethylnitrosamine (DEN) and dibutylnitrosamine (DBN), strain-related differences were found. In the Chinese hamster, DEN did not produce neoplasms in the respiratory tract. In the Syrian species, DEN caused tumors in the trachea and lungs followed by the nasal cavity. In European hamsters, DEN produced benign and malignant tumors in the respiratory tract and caused death after 15 weeks of daily treatment.

In the Chinese hamster, DBN caused papillary tumors and malignant neoplasms in the nasal and paranasal cavities. In the Syrian species, DBN caused tumors, primarily in the trachea, then the nasal cavities and lungs. At the high dosages in European hamsters, DBN caused carcinogenic effects in the trachea, lungs, and nasal cavities, whereas low dosage groups had lung carcinomas.

As indicated by this study, hamsters are good models to study respiratory carcinogenesis; however, different species can have different responses to a chemical. The spontaneous rate of respiratory tumors, metabolism, and nature of chemical need to be known before cross-species extrapolation can be done.

TYPICAL STUDY PROTOCOLS

Carcinogenicity Toxicity Testing

Hamsters are excellent animals for carcinogenicity testing because they have a low incidence of spontaneous tumor development, but they are highly susceptible to experimentally induced carcinogenesis. The incidence of spontaneous tumors in Syrian hamsters is reported to be lower than the incidence seen in mice or rats (Homburger et al., 1979a; Mohr, 1979). Though the hamster does have a short lifespan, substance-related effects and neoplasms develop rapidly, during which spontaneous diseases and tumors may not occur.

The carcinogenicity protocols used for rats are satisfactory for hamster studies. Changes that need to be incorporated are that blood collections should be kept to a minimum and the length of the study may need to be shortened owing to the hamster's shorter life span.

Hamsters are specifically recommended for long-term testing with aromatic amines, polycyclic hydrocarbons, and other agents suspected of being pulmonary carcinogens. Urinary bladder carcinomas induced by aromatic amines can take up to 7 years to induce in dogs, but can cause neoplasms in less than 1 year in hamsters.

Nitrosamines caused tumors in the hamster forestomach, liver, pancreas, nasal cavity, lung, trachea, and occasionally the esophagus. The common site for nitrosamine tumor induction in the rat is the esophagus, demonstrating species specificity for a target organ site. Hamsters are not more susceptible to nitrosamines because some nitrosamines are more toxic in the rat than the hamster and vice versa (Newcomer et al., 1987). The hamster does show a nitosamine-induced pancreatic tumor that is similar to pancreatic tumors in humans.

The use of hamsters in diet admix studies has been very limited and, therefore, there is not a large database to study.

Inhalation and Intratracheal Studies

Inhalation studies constitute the majority of the toxicological research using the hamster as the test species. The hamster is deemed useful because it has a lower incidence of spontaneous respiratory tumors and of respiratory diseases (Werner, 1979), and its respiratory epithelium is more similar to that of the human than other laboratory rodents. In studies with cigarette smoke, certain in-bred species of the hamster are the only laboratory rodents where carcinogenesis can be induced. A laryngeal cancer in the hamster is caused by tar fractions or cigarette smoke. This cancer has been found to be histologically identical to the cancer seen in humans (Homburger et al., 1979a).

Acute and subacute inhalation toxicity studies using the hamster have studied nickle monoxide (NiO), cobaltous oxide (CoO), and chrysotile asbestos. Hamsters exposed to asbestos for 11 months developed asbestoses and those exposed to NiO developed pneumoconiosis, disease states seen in humans.

For inhalation study designs, the exposure chamber has to be large enough to allow an adequate number of animals to be exposed simultaneously. It should be equipped with the means to regulate temperature and humidity and have identical chambers for all treatment groups. The hamsters should be housed separately; however, if there are space limitations, animals may be housed in groups. The position of the cages should be rotated from exposure-to-exposure. The animals should be housed in an area other than the inhalation chamber when not being treated. This will reduce the contamination of the exposure chamber by bodily fluids.

Animals are randomly distributed to test groups based on body weights as performed in other types of animal studies. The animals should have free access to water at all times. Feed should be available when animals are not being exposed unless exposure times are very lengthy. If feed is provided during exposure, then the feed is also being exposed to the test materials and may be an important aspect of the study. The number of exposures whether once or several times a day and the length of exposure time can be decided by the investigator; however, once decided, exposure time should remain consistent throughout the study. The concentration and particle size of the aerosol should be determined periodically and the aerosols should be evenly distributed in the chamber (Raabe et al., 1973) Data may be collected concerning clinical signs, body weights, pharmacokinetics, mortality, hematological and clinical chemistry functions, organ weights, and gross and microscopic observations.

For intratracheal instillation studies, the same procedures as described for inhalation studies are used except animals are exposed to the control and test articles via intratracheal administration. The common dose volume is 0.2 ml per animal and the animal is usually anesthetized during dose administration. The number of treatments per day and the length of the study may be decided by the principal investigator.

Teratology Studies

The hamster is an excellent tool for teratology studies because of its predictable estrus, short pregnancy period, rapid embryonic development, and a low incidence of spontaneous malformations.

Retinoic acid (vitamin A) has been shown to be a teratogen in hamsters. Thaliomide was found to be a teratogen in certain in-bred strains of the Syrian hamster. Other hamster teratogens are hydrocortisone, colchicine, vincristine, vinblastine, heavy metals such as cadmium compounds, organic and inorganic mercury, 2,4,5-T (2,4,5-trichlorophenoxyacetic acid), and 2,4-D (2,4-dichlorophenoxyacetic acid) alone or contaminated with dioxin (Newcomer et al., 1987).

The study design for teratology studies should take into account the embryonic development of the hamster, the strain-specific fertility seen in hamsters, and the age of the mother.

Toxicology Studies

The protocols used for rats in acute and long-term toxicity studies are satisfactory for the hamster; however, blood collection should be kept to a minimum and the length of the test may need to be shorten owing to the shorter life span of the hamster.

The majority of toxicology work involving hamsters has been inhalation and respiratory studies. The hamster has been found to be a useful model in the study of toxicity; however, it has some biochemical and physiological characteristics not seen in other rodent species. The hamster has a strong resistance to certain pharmacological agents such as barbiturates, morphine, and colchine. The hamster oral LD_{50} of colchicine is 600 times the lethal dose known to humans, whereas morphine when given to hamsters at the LD_{50} does not produce a narcotic reaction. These characteristics should not be considered a barrier to the use of hamsters in toxicology studies.

Of 304 compounds evaluated by the IARC, 130 were carcinogenic in at least one rodent species. Of the 130, only 38 compounds were tested in both hamsters and rats, 35 were tested in hamsters and mice, and 78 tested in both rats and mice. Of those tested in hamsters and rats, 84% of the compounds had similar results in both species, 86% in both mice and hamsters, and in mice and rats 90% had similar results. Based on this information, hamsters are not more or less sensitive to toxicity than other rodent species used in long-term testing (Arnold et al., 1979).

CHINESE HAMSTER OVARY (CHO) CELL CHROMOSOME ABERRATIONS

The purpose of this assay is to evaluate the ability of a compound to induce chromosome aberrations in the Chinese hamster ovary (CHO) cells.

The CHO cells used in this assay may be obtained from the American Tissue Culture Collection, Rockville, Maryland (Brusick, 1982). The original cells were obtained from a Chinese hamster.

The assay is divided into two parts, nonactivation and activation, with S9 rat liver as the activating agent. EMS (0.5 $\mu l/ml$) is the positive agent for the nonactivation, whereas for the activating studies it is dimethylnitrosamine (DMN) at 0.5 $\mu l/ml$. The solvent used to dissolve the test article is used as the solvent vehicle for the control and positive control articles. The dosages selected for the test article are one toxic (loss of growth potential) and four lower (usually in a half-log series) concentrations. These dosages are determined in a range-finder with the cells exposed to the test article for 4 hr and incubated for 24 hr.

The CHO cells are grown in 10% fetal calf serum (FCS)/Ham's F12 media. The cell density should be kept at 1.5×10^6 per 75 cm^2 plastic flask. For the assay, approximately 0.25×106 cells per well per test article concentration are tested. The cells are exposed to the test article for 2 hr at 37° C. Cells used in the activation section receive the S9 rat liver along with the test article before the 2-hr activation. The cells are then washed with sterile saline and given fresh media. For each of the test article dosages, half of the plates per treatment group will receive 5-bromo-2'-deoxyuridine (BrdU) at a concentration of 10 μM. The cells are then incubated for 24 hr with colcemid (2×10^{-7} M) added at hour 17. After incubation, the metaphase cells are collected by mitotic shake-off. These cells are swollen with 0.0075M KCl solution, washed with a methanol: acetic acid (3:1) fixative, dropped onto glass slides, and air dried.

The slides are stained with 10% Giemsa (pH 6.8) and the slides are scored for chromosomal aberrations such as chromatid and chromosome gaps, breaks, and chromatid deletions.

MODELS OF DISEASES

Cardiomyopathy

Cardiomyopathy in hamsters originates from a genetically (recessive autosomal gene) determined metabolic defect that induces degenerative lesions in all striated muscles with particular intensity and consistency in the heart (Bajusz, 1969; Gertz, 1973). The clinical and pathological aspects of the disease resemble nonvascular myocardial disease in man. Animals appear normal, though there is cardiac muscle degeneration. The lesions appear histologically in both sexes at 35–40 days of age for males and 25–30 days for females. The first lesion is an acute myolysis with primary dissolution of the myofilaments. This lesion is healed and replaced by connective tissue by day 100 (Gertz, 1973). The disease becomes clinically apparent with a whole body subcutaneous edema; however, there are no ECG changes to foretell edema formation or to tell degree of lesion formation. The ECG changes are observed after lesion formation and consist of alterations in pathways of cardiac excitation and high-frequency alterations in the QRS interval. In the late stages of the disease, ascites, hydrothorax, and hydopericardium appear. In the terminal stage, animals are hyperneic and cyanotic. At necropsy, the liver, spleen, kidney, heart, and other visceral organs show congestive changes such as enlargement and increases in volumes. Cardiomyopathic hamsters show an edema respond to therapy with digitalis, diuretics, and salt restrictions. The average life span of hamsters with this disease is 146 days.

Since this model responds to therapy in a manner similar to humans and the disease state has similar manifestations, it is considered well suited to study heart failure in humans due to cardiac muscle impairment.

Dental Caries

Caries is a disease of poorly developed and poorly calcified teeth in the hamster. It is considered transmissible and infectious. It can be induced in normal hamsters by inoculation with cariogenic microflora. Animals are infected by adding microflora to drinking water or exposing the animals to infected feces. The carious lesions are in the molars. The lesions start with changes in enamel translucency, surface depressions, and fissures. The disintegration goes into the dentine with eventual exposure of the pulp. Bacterial (putrefactive) infections, inflammation, and complete necrosis of the molar occurs.

With the testing of this model, fluoride was found to beneficial to hamsters and this prompted clinical trials in humans (Keyes et al., 1966).

Diabetes Mellitus

Diabetes mellitus was first described in 1959 and in 1969 in the Chinese hamster and South African hamsters, respectively (Stuhlman, 1979). Only certain strains of the Chinese species are affected, and the disease is probably transmitted by a recessive gene. The disease in the Chinese hamster has a rapid onset between 1 and 3 months of age. The indications of the disease are polyuria, polydipsia, glycosuria, and ketonuria. A normal Chinese hamster has glucose levels of 110 ± 6 mg/100 ml, whereas a diabetic hamster has levels of 200 to 800 mg/ml. The diabetes mellitus seen in the Chinese hamster is very similar to the disease state in humans. There is a variation in the syndromes (chronic, insulin dependent), the occurrence of secondary manifestations (cataracts), discrepancies in established parameters of native insulin values, and what the role of heredity plays in the disease.

In the South African hamster, which has a 22% incidence of diabetes mellitus, the disease is inherited as a non–sex linked polygenic trait. With the South African hamster, the hyperglycemia varies in incidence, age of onset, degree of severity, and rate of progression, as in humans, but it is not influenced by age, sex, or state of obesity. Obesity is not a feature seen in the diabetic South African hamster, though it is seen in the Chinese hamster.

Either one of these models will provide insight into diabetes mellitus. These models can be used to study the disease pathogenesis, development of secondary complications, exact genetic mechanisms, and possible therapeutic regimens.

Leprosy

The hamster was first injected with leprosy bacilli in 1937. It was the first time a laboratory animal was found to be susceptible to the agent. In recent years, leprosy bacilli has been grown in cell culture systems and in the tail and foot pads of the mouse, so the role of the hamster in leprosy research has declined (Frenkel, 1987).

Muscular Dystrophy

The muscular dystrophy (MD) syndrome can be induced in hamsters by feeding them a diet deficient in vitamin E from weaning until death. The gross appearance of the disease state does not occur before the eleventh or twelfth month. Strains of cardiomyopathic Syrian hamsters (BIO 14.6 and BIO 53.38) do have genetic dispositions for this disease. The clinical signs appear 60–200 days after birth, and all skeletal muscles, including the heart, are affected. The lesions are pleomorphic, characterized by focal degeneration of myofibrils, coagulation necrosis, the formation of contraction clots, and alignment of muscle nuclei in chainlike rows within the fiber (Homburger, 1970). In the final stage of the syndrome, the myofibrils convert to granular mass in which the nuclei have disintegrated. Earliest changes occur at 33 days of age with death usually by 220 days due to cardiac failure. These hamsters have morphological manifestations of muscular dystrophy.

This model is excellent to study the mechanism of MD from an in vivo system to intact animals.

Osetoarthritis and Degenerative Joint Disease

Osteoarthritis and degenerative joint disease are diseases that a hamster may develop in old age. These diseases are rare in hamsters under 2 years of age. The diseases are characterized by separation of the zone of calcification of the cartilage with sclerosis and dislocation of the bone, fibrillation of ligaments, and fibrosis of the synovial membrane. Organisms such as *Mycoplasma, Streptobacillus moniliformis, Corynebacterium kutscheri,* hormonal imbalances, and chemical and physical agents are associated with the disease.

The disease in hamsters is similar to that seen in humans (Handler, 1965), which makes this an excellent model to study.

Pancreatic Cancer

Pancreatic cancer is a very difficult neoplasm to induce in laboratory animals. It can be induced in Syrian hamsters with nitrosamines. The neoplasms, histogenesis, and enzymatic patterns seen in human pathogenesis are similar to those in the hamster. Occasionally, hamsters develop diabetes during the pancreatic carcinogenesis, as is also seen in the pathogenesis in humans.

Pulmonary Emphysema

Pulmonary emphysema was induced in Syrian hamsters by pulmonary instillation of an aerosol of papain. The lesions and extent of formation correlate with dosage and time of exposure. The lesions found in the hamster correspond to those found in humans (Martorana, 1976).

Syphilis

The hamster expresses both primary and secondary infections of syphilis after inoculation with the etiological agent, *Treponema pallidumbosnia* A. The rabbit is the only other laboratory animal which shows infections, though neither the hamster nor rabbit express the tertiary lesions seen in humans. Rabbits are a problem in the study of syphilis because they can have a spontaneous incidence of *Treponema* infections which may interfere with the study. The hamster was useful in determing the importance of cellular immune mechanisms with syphilis infections (Frenkel, 1987).

Thrombosis

Arterial thrombosis in the hamster is the only spontaneous animal model of thrombosis. There are similarities between human thrombosis and the hamster model, such as an increasing incidence with age and the thrombi in the hamster occurs in the right atrium, whereas in humans the atrial thrombosis is a complication of right heart failure.

Hamster strains with a high incidence of spontaneous thrombosis are a good model to study the possible mechanism of human thrombosis.

SUMMARY

The hamster has not become the animal of choice in toxicity testing because it has a reputation as a difficult animal to handle, a poor breeder, and a species very susceptible to disease. The hamster is not aggressive when handled properly by a trained individual, the average litter size is 10–11 pups, and actually the hamster has probably the lower incidence of spontaneous tumors and diseases than other common laboratory rodents.

Hamsters are very desirable for carcinogenesis testing because of their relatively short life span with physiological growth occurring early in life, and they have no significant difference in carcinogenesis susceptibility than the rat or mouse. Actually, the spontaneous neoplasms (pituitary, mammary, hepatic, and pulmonary tumors) found to interfere with the interpretation of data obtained from carcinogenesis testing with common strains of mice and rats are rarely seen in the hamster (Homburger et al., 1979a).

The hamster may be the test species of choice for toxicity testing of special compounds whose metabolism and target organ sites are similar in both the hamster and the human.

Pathology   **Frederick G. Hess**

BACKGROUND—MILESTONES IN THE HAMSTER LIFE CYCLE

A newborn Syrian hamster *Mesocricetus auratus* weighs approximately 2–3 g; an adult of 6 months weighs approximately 150 g. For males, spermatogenesis commences at approximately day 25 of age; sexual maturity is reached at day 40. For females, earliest ovulation occurs from weeks 4–8. The average estrus cycle is 4 days, whereas gestation occurs in 16 days.

Litters vary in size from four to 12 pups. Females of some strains are able to produce six litters or more (Van Hoosier and Ladiges, 1984). Normal weaning time is 21–28 days. Breeding capability for males and females is approximately 12 months.

The average life span for these naturally nocturnal animals is approximately 2 years, with a 3-year maximum life expectation (Van Hoosier and Ladiges, 1984). However, specific closed colonies have had mean survival times of 63–79 weeks for males and 50–63 weeks for females (Slauson et al., 1978; Pour et al., 1979; Redman et al., 1979).

SPECIAL ANATOMICAL FEATURES

Anatomically, a unique morphological feature of the Syrian hamster is its well-developed cheek pouches, which are highly distendible evaginations of the lateral buccal walls. The hamster utilizes them to transport and store food. For experimental purposes, these readily accessible structures are eversible and may be utilized as sites for normal/abnormal tissue transplants (including tumor implantations). Immunological rejection does not occur owing to the absence of an intact lymphatic drainage pathway (Van Hoosier and Ladiges, 1984).

The upper gastrointestinal tract is unusual in that the esophagus enters between the forestomach and glandular stomach. Also at this junction, the limiting ridge of the hamster stomach represents a distinct constriction, forming the two separate compartments.

NONNEOPLASTIC LESIONS

The published incidence rates of the most frequent nonneoplastic lesions of untreated outbred Syrian hamsters are listed in Table 11. Since most of these lesions were tabulated using only one or two references and proper historical control data have not been published, the actual incidences are probably lower than those given in Table 11. Various factors, which are known to increase frequency rates, include age, sex, diet, breeding methods, genetic drift, hormonal imbalance, the presence of transmissible bacterial, viral, or parasitic agents, and the extent of gross necropsy and histopathological evaluations.

Amyloidosis

Systemic amyloidosis is a principal cause of death in aging hamsters (Van Hoosier and Ladiges, 1984). In one colony, a high frequency of 88% occurred in hamsters over 18 months of age and a lower frequency of 42% in hamsters 13–18 months of age (Gleiser et al., 1971). In another colony, systemic amyloidosis was noted as the cause of death of approximately 25% of males that were sacrificed at week 53 and 33% of females that were sacrificed at week 40 (Slauson et al., 1978).

Table 11 Incidence of Various Nonneoplastic Lesions in Untreated Outbred Syrian (Golden) Hamsters

Organ	Lesion	Incidence (%)		Reference
		male	female	
Adrenal glands	Cortical cyst	2	8	Pour *et al.* (1976c)
	Cortical hyperplasia	15	5	Pour *et al.* (1976c)
Arteries	Vascular calcinosis	5–13	10	Pour *et al.* (1976a)
Colon/cecum/ileum	Enteritis (colitis/typhlitis/ proliferative ileitis)	38–90	36–90	Pour *et al.* (1976a, b) Frisk and Wagner (1977)
Heart	Thrombosis	13–73	20–73	Pour *et al.* (1976a) McMartin (1977) McMartin and Dodds (1982) Doi *et al.* (1987)
Kidneys	Arteriolar nephrosclerosis	72	80	Slauson *et al.* (1978)
	Nephrocalcinosis	25–31	16–20	Pour *et al.* (1976a)
	Pyelonephritis, acute/ chronic	6–13	8–13	Pour *et al.* (1976a)
Liver	Cholangiectasis	12–31	12–35	Pour *et al.* (1976b)
	Cholangitis	30–49	29–31	Pour *et al.* (1976a, b)
Pancreas	Islet cell hyperplasia	37–64	30–81	Pour *et al.* (1976c)
Parathyroid glands	Hyperplasia (principal cells)	83	22	Pour *et al.* (1976c)
Ovaries	Cyst	—	6	Pour *et al.* (1976c)
Stomach/(forestomach/ glandular-pylorus region)	Erosions/ulcerations	4–8	5–20	Pour *et al.* (1976a, b)
Vertebra	Chondrosis	30–83	10–81	Pour *et al.* (1976a)
Multiple organs	Amyloidosis	16–88	16–88	Gleiser *et al.* (1971) Pour *et al.* (1976a)

By analysis of serum electrophoretic patterns, there was a decrease in albumin and a concomitant increase in total globulin, primarily a sharp transient rise in α_2 serum globulin, as detected in 12-month-old hamsters (Van Hoosier and Ladiges, 1984). By transmission electron microscopy, amyloid deposits were identified as finely granular, amorphous material that was located in the mesangial matrix and between endothelial cells and the basement membranes of glomeruli.

By light microscopy, the initial lesion appears to be located in the walls of glomerular capillaries, forming so-called "wire-loop" lesions. In addition, amyloid accumulation in epithelium/connective tissue has been seen primarily in hepatic periportal areas, adrenal cortex, pancreas, and adjacent to splenic lymphoid follicles. Less frequent sites are the lungs, ovaries, testes, and epididymides.

For positive diagnosis by light microscopy, Congo Red stain and the birefringence of these areas in polarized light are utilized (Gleiser et al., 1971). Biochemically, AA and AP proteins have been identified in isolated amyloid fibrils from aged hamsters (Brandwein et al., 1981). Since amyloidosis in mice is strain related, genetic factors are suspected to play an important role in the pathogenesis of the disease in the hamster.

Arteriolar Nephrosclerosis

Arteriolar nephrosclerosis was observed at approximately 75% incidence of control animals (Slauson et al., 1978). Progressive renal arteriolar sclerosis with subsequent glomerulosclerosis (fibrinoid necrosis) and tubular degeneration/atrophy with fibrosis were described. Degenerative vascular changes (fibrinoid necrosis) were seen in the testes, ovaries, and uterus. Although limited serological analyses for anti-LCM antibody were negative, chronic viral infection was considered as the potential cause of the disease.

Atrial Thombosis

Certain colonies of Syrian hamsters have been maintained and utilized as prospective animal models. For instances, a high incidence (73%) of aging, male and female acromelanic Syrian hamsters had atrial thrombosis, accompanied by a consumption coagulopathy (McMartin, 1977; McMartin and Dodds, 1982).

The thrombi were located primarily in the left atrium, resulting from localized hemostasis secondary to cardiac failure. Atrioventricular valvular thickening and bilateral ventricular hypertrophy were often present. Pulmonary edema and pleural effusion were commonly seen at gross necropsy, which correlated clinically to hyperpnea, tachycardia, and cyanosis. Microscopically, myocardial degeneration/necrosis was associated with calcification and fibrosis.

Similar cardiac lesions were noted at a frequency of 40% per sex in a closed colony of APA strain, random-bred hamsters (Doi et al., 1987). Glomerulonephrosis was also noted with no apparent correlation to the cardiac thrombosis as well as chronic renal disease characterized by tubular dilatation/atrophy and proteinaceous casts.

A cardiomyopathic hamster model with progression to myocardial failure has been described (Bajusz et al., 1969; Gertz, 1973). Within 65 days of age, hamsters of both sexes of the inbred strain BIO 14.6 developed myocardial degeneration/necrosis with calcification as well as generalized myodystrophy. At 9–12 months of age, marked ventricular hypertrophy, thrombosis of the left atrium, and hepatic chronic passive congestion were seen, indicative of an animal model for congestive heart failure.

Generalized Vascular Calcinosis

Generalized vascular calcinosis was noted in the aorta and coronary and renal arteries (Pour et al., 1976a). Later, this abnormality was ameliorated by modifications in the diet (Pour and Birt, 1979; Birt and Pour, 1983).

Hemorrhagic Necrosis

In the late 1970s, spontaneous hemorrhagic necrosis (SHN) was described in late-term fetal hamsters at days 14–15 of gestation (Keeler and Young, 1978; Young and Keeler, 1978). It was characterized by multifocal but coalescent zones of parenchymal hemorrhage, edema, and necrosis affecting the subependymal capillary vasculature of the forebrain, thalamus, medulla, and spinal cord. Litter viability was decreased.

Fetal brain development and differentiation were influenced by intrauterine environmental factors, especially diet deficient in vitamin E. Supplementation of diet with vitamin E throughout gestation and lactation completely prevented SHN and fully restored litter viability to normal levels (Keeler and Young, 1979). Cross-breeding of susceptible/ nonsusceptible strains eliminated the disease (Keeler and Young, 1978).

BACTERIAL INFECTIONS

Hamster Enteritis

Several important bacterial infectious agents have been known to affect the health status of the Syrian hamster as well as to produce complications in histopathological evaluations. Foremost, hamster enteritis (HE) remains a disease entity of great concern. It is usually manifested early as an epizootic disease with a high mortality of approximately 90% of weanling hamsters from 3 to 8 weeks of age (Frisk and Wagner, 1977a).

In this chapter, hamster enteritis will be the term used to describe wet tail, or wet tail disease, which also has been referred to as proliferative ileitis, regional enteritis, terminal ileitis, atypical (transmissible) ileal hyperplasia, and enzootic intestinal adenocarcinoma (with localized invasion to adjacent muscularis). Hamster enteritis appears to include a spectrum of various stages of these lesions.

Clinical symptoms/signs include diarrhea, dehydration, lethargy, anorexia, and irritability. The disease progresses to staining of the perineum, tail, and ventral abdomen. Death occurs from 48 hr to 1 week after the onset of symptoms.

Gross necropsy lesions range from mild acute changes such as ileal hyperemia/ hemorrhage to marked distension of segments of the ileum. Mucosal areas may become ulcerative and necrotic, eventually penetrating into the muscular layers, resulting in multiple abscesses of the subserosa. Enlargement of the mesenteric lymph nodes and peritonitis with adhesions also develop. Intussusception of the colon and prolapse of the rectum have been described for hamsters that recovered from HE (Jacoby et al., 1975).

Microscopic lesions range from mild acute enteritis with epithelial hyperplasia of the columnar cells to marked epithelial hyperplasia associated with chronic inflammation and fibrosis. Other regions of the mucosa have epithelial degeneration/necrosis and hemorrhages, ulcerations, and/or abscesses (Frisk and Wagner, 1977a). Associated lesions include lymphadenitis of the mesenteric lymph nodes (Amend et al., 1976).

Etiologically, intracytoplasmic bacteria have been demonstrated by transmission electron microscopy (Wagner et al., 1973; Frisk and Wagner, 1977b; Johnson and Jacoby, 1978; Frisk et al., 1981). Intracytoplasmic particles resembling rod-shaped bacteria have been detected with indirect fluorescent-antibody technique using serum from hamsters with HE (Jacoby et al., 1975; Jacoby, 1978; Frisk et al., 1981).

Specifically, the bacterium *Escherichia coli* has been isolated from the intestinal tract of hamsters with HE (Amend et al., 1976; Frisk et al., 1978, 1981; McNeil et al., 1986). In one facility, *E. coli* was isolated early in the disease process, whereas *Campylobacter* sp. was observed in later stages within hyperplastic epithelial cells (Frisk and Wagner, 1977a). In addition, Jacoby (1978) demonstrated by immunofluorescence an intracellular antigen morphologically compatible with gram-negative rods like *Campylobacter fetus*. Thus, two or more organisms may act synergistically to produce the disease, since neither *E. coli* nor *C. fetus* cultured alone could reproduce the natural disease (Van Hoosier and Ladiges, 1984).

Similar gross and microscopic changes as described above for HE were noted predominantly in the ceca of Syrian hamsters (Barthold et al., 1978; Rehg and Lu, 1982).

The most effective treatment for HE has been oxytetracycline in the drinking water, as compared to neomycin, dimetridazole, and tetracycline hydrochloride (McNeil et al., 1986). Other antimicrobials, i.e., clindamycin, lincomycin, ampicillin, vancomycin, erythromycin, cephalosporins, and gentamycin, caused fatal gastrointestinal toxicity to hamsters with clinical symptoms, including diarrhea, dehydration, anorexia, and hypothermia (Bartlett et al., 1977, 1978; Lusk et al., 1978; Hawkins et al., 1984). The anaerobe *Clostridium difficile* was found to be the direct cause of the enterocolitis, producing overgrowth of the ileal/colonic/cecal flora. Gross pathology consisted of distension, hyperemia, and hemorrhage of the ileum, cecum, and ascending colon. Histological sections revealed mucosal acute and chronic inflammation and congestion/hemorrhages as well as luminal collections of inflammatory cells, mucin, and sloughed epithelial cells.

Tyzzer's Disease

As compared to HE, Tyzzer's disease has been noted much less frequently. The only outbreak of Tyzzer's disease in a colony bred in the United States was reported in 1977 (Zook et al.). Two other epizootics were reported in Japan (Takasaki et al., 1974; Nakayama et al., 1975).

Clinical symptoms include the sudden onset of diarrhea, dehydration, and lethargy; deaths occur within 48 hr. At gross necropsy, the most common lesion is yellow-white foci (1–2 mm diameter) in the liver, corresponding microscopically to areas of necrosis with inflammatory infiltrates. Secondary changes are thickened and discolored portions of the terminal ileum, cecum, and colon. These regions correspond microscopically to coagulative necrosis associated with epithelial cell sloughing, submucosal edema, polymorphonuclear and mononuclear cellular infiltrates, multinucleated giant cells, and fibrosis.

The causative agent is a gram-negative, pleomorphic bacterium, *Bacillus piliformis*. Positive diagnosis has been demonstrated with PAS and Giemsa stain within the cytoplasm of intestinal epithelial cells as well as hepatocytes and myocardial fibers.

Other Bacterial Infections

The possible roles of bacteria (e.g., *Pasteurella pneumotropica* and *Streptococcus pneumoniae*) as well as *Mycoplasma pulmonis* in the etiology of pneumonia in Syrian hamsters have not been clearly defined (Van Hoosier and Ladiges, 1984).

VIRAL INFECTIONS

Lymphocytic Choriomeningitis

Syrian hamsters and contaminated tumor cell lines were likely sources of the infectious ribonucleic acid (RNA) lymphocytic choriomeningitis (LCM) virus, which infected various laboratory personnel between 1965 and 1974, as well as other naive hamsters (Biggar et al., 1977; Skinner and Knight, 1979). Commercial distribution of the cell lines ceased in 1974.

Clinical signs/symptoms of LCM occur rarely in hamsters, even in those with chronic infections for months. However, ataxia, conjunctivitis, dehydration, and tremors have been noted in a few hamsters. Death occurs following chronic progressive infection characterized by viremia, viruria, and high titers of virus in tissues (Parker et al., 1976).

Experimentally, complement-fixing antibodies have been detected in young adult hamsters by 10 days after inoculation.

Microscopic lesions include conjunctivitis, chronic glomerulonephritis, generalized vasculitis, and lymphocytic cellular infiltrates in the liver and kidneys.

Sendai Virus

Parainfluenza 1 (Sendai) is an RNA agent of the paramyxovirus group which has been implicated as a cause of hamster pneumonia. An enzootic form of the disease was reported at a research facility (Profeta et al., 1969). At gross necropsy complete consolidation of the lungs has been observed. Occasional deaths have been reported in suckling hamsters (Van Hoosier and Ladiges, 1984).

FUNGAL INFECTIONS

Hamsters are susceptible to various fungal infections. Histoplasmosis, for example, has been studied extensively; hamsters are highly sensitive and, therefore, useful for diagnostic purposes. Most fungi grow in the spleen, lymph nodes, and liver (Van Hoosier and Ladiges, 1984).

PARASITIC INFECTIONS

Cestodes

Hymenolepis nana, the dwarf tapeworm, is the most prevalent internal parasite found in hamsters (Van Hoosier and Ladiges, 1984). Their size varies from 25–40 mm in length, and they are usually found in the small intestine.

Although the consequences of infection are usually benign, impactions followed by deaths have been observed, dependent on the number of parasites and degree of intestinal occlusion.

Preventative measures rely on routine sanitation of cages and effective insect and vermin control. Yomesan (niclosamide) has been reported as effective and safe for treatment of cestode infections in hamsters (Ronald and Wagner, 1975). Laboratory personnel should be aware of the possible transmissible potential and receive proper hygienic procedures.

Mites

Two species of mites (*Demodex aurati* and *D. criceti*) have been identified in hamster epidermis (Flatt and Kerber, 1968; Owen and Young, 1973). *D. aurati* resides in hair follicles, whereas *D. criceti* inhabits folds in the epidermis.

Both species appear to be asymptomatic, low-grade pathogens. However, clinical skin disease in which *D. aurati* was identified, resulted in demodectic mange consisting of marked alopecia and scab formation in 50% incidence of male hamsters (Estes et al., 1971). Predisposing factors included sex, age, and stress.

NEOPLASTIC LESIONS

The incidence rates of naturally occurring tumors in untreated outbred Syrian hamsters are generally low. The most frequent tumor types are listed in Table 12, as reported in

Table 12 Incidence of Various Neoplasms in Untreated Outbred Syrian (Golden) Hamsters

Organ	Tumor type	Incidence (%)		Reference
		male	female	
Adrenal glands	Cortical adenoma	10–12	2–7	Pour *et al.* (1976c)
	Pheochromocytoma	3	2	Pour *et al.* (1976c)
Colon/cecum	Adenocarcinoma[a]	7	20	Fabry (1985)
Harderian gland	Adenoma	3	—	Pour *et al.* (1976b)
Liver	Cholangioma	4	7	Pour *et al.* (1976b)
	Hepatocellular adenoma	4	0	Pour *et al.* (1976b)
Lymphoreticular system	Malignant lymphoma (lymphosarcoma)	2–53	2–53	Ambrose and Coggin (1975)
				Pour *et al.* (1976c)
				Coggin *et al.* (1983)
Ovaries	Granular cell tumor/thecoma	—	3	Pour *et al.* (1976c)
Pancreas	Islet cell adenoma	4–14	2–3	Pour *et al.* (1976c)
Parathyroid glands	Adenoma	2–5	4–7	Pour *et al.* (1976c)
Skin	Melanoma	2	2	Turusov (1982)
Spleen	Hemangioendothelioma	1–3	—	Pour *et al.* (1976d)
Stomach (forestomach)	Papilloma	5–8	3–5	Pour *et al.* (1976d)
Uterus	Endometrial carcinoma	—	5	Pour *et al.* (1976c)
	Endometrial polyp	—	12	Pour *et al.* (1976c)
	Leiomyoma	—	3	Pour *et al.* (1976c)
Vagina	Papilloma	—	4	Pour *et al.* (1976c)

[a]Associated with background incidence of inflammatory changes/infectious diseases.

references from 1970 to 1989. Significant low spontaneous tumor rates ($<2\%$) are noted for the respiratory tract, pituitary gland, and mammary gland of both sexes and the genital tract of male hamsters. Such low incidences establish the Syrian hamster as a good candidate for chemical carcinogenicity studies, including morphological studies utilizing electron microscopy, cytology, and histochemistry (Schreiber et al., 1974; Becci et al., 1978; Hess et al., 1981a, b).

Since most of the tumor types in Table 12 are listed with only one or two references and factual historical data have not been published, the actual incidence rates are probably lower than those given. Various factors that cause these differences include diet, water quality, survival age, sex, breeding methods, genetic drift, hormonal imbalances, extent of gross necropsy and microscopic examinations, and the presence of transmissible agents.

One or more of these predisposing factors may become relatively predominant and complicate the frequency of historical tumor data. For example, in one report the majority (75%) of lymphosarcomas was horizontally transmitted, suggestive that infectious agent(s) were involved (Van Hoosier and Trentin, 1979). Similarly, five epizootics of poorly differentiated lymphocytic lymphomas (53% incidence) were horizontally transmitted in two facilities by a viroidlike agent (Coggin et al., 1983). The predominant sites were the large and small intestines with involvement of mesenteric and cervical lymph nodes.

Metabolism   **Christopher P. Chengelis**

HEPATIC MICROSOMAL MIXED FUNCTION OXIDASE

There are two or three strains of hamsters used in biomedical research. Much of the work pertaining to xenobiotic metabolism, however, has concentrated on the Syrian or Syrian golden strain. Therefore, the reader should assume that most of the following discussion is based on this particular strain. As in all other species studied, the liver is the major site and the microsomal mixed function oxidase (MMFO) system is the major system involved in xenobiotic metabolism in the hamster. Some of the salient enzyme activities are summarized on Table 13. The liver-to-body weight ratio on the nonfasted hamster is slightly higher than that of the rat, and may range from 3.5 to 5.4% depending on sex, age, and protein content of the diet (Birt et al., 1983). Cytochrome P-450 concentrations are higher than that of rats, ranging between 0.95 and 1.35 nmol/mg microsomal protein in most published reports. A concentration of 1.85 nmol/mg (for naive hamsters) has been reported (Chaing and Steggles, 1983). As in all species, cytochrome P-450 in hamsters exists as a family of isozymes, but the number of different isozymes has not been as well characterized in the hamster as in other rodent species. Chaing and Steggles (1983) studied the effect of different inducing agents and identified at least three different cytochrome P-450 isozymes. Using different inducing agents, Ardies et al. (1987) demonstrated the existence of at least five different isozymes of cytochrome P-450 in the hamster. Concentrations of cytochrome b_5 also tend to be somewhat higher than those of the rat, ranging from 0.43 to 0.58 nmol/mg. The activity of NADPH:cytochrome C reductase is in the same range as that of the rat; i.e., 200–320 nmol/min/mg. It has not been established if this enzyme in the hamster plays the rate-limiting role in MMFO activity that it does in the rat.

The saturating activities of the hamster MMFO with various common model substrates are also summarized on Table 13. In general, activity tends to be higher than that of the rat. Few differences in qualitative species MMFO substrate selectivity have been identi-fied between the rat and hamster. There are interesting and important quantitative differences. For example, the fact that carbon tetrachloride has been reported to be a hepatocarcinogen in hamsters but not in rats is apparently due to differences in the rates of metabolism. Castro et al. (1989) have demonstrated that hamsters have a much higher rates (both in vivo and in vitro) of production of reactive metabolites of CCl_4 that bind to nuclear protein than rats. Weyand and Bevan (1987) examined the in vivo disposition of benzo(a)pyrene in different rodent species. The major difference between the hamster and the other species was that increased amounts of radioactivity were retained in the lungs of hamsters at lower doses with a proportional decrease in the amount of radioactivity excreted into the bile. Bergman et al. (1984) studied species differences in α-naphthafla-vone microsomal metabolism. Total metabolism was essentially the same in rats and hamsters, and the same three chemicals made up the majority of the metabolites in both species (ANF-5,6-oxide, ANF-6-phenol, and ANF-7,8-dihydrodiol). The oxide, howev-er, was the major metabolite in rats and the dihydrodiol was the major metabolite in hamsters, indicating a site-selective species difference.

Birt et al. (1983) studied the effects of age, gender, and dietary protein on the hepatic MMFO in hamsters. In general, a high protein diet (10% vs 40% lactalbumin) tended to

Table 13 Summary of Hepatic Xenobiotic Metabolizing Enzymes in Hamsters

Enzyme	Concentration or activity	Comments and references
Cytochrome P-450	0.95–1.35 nmol/mg	Burke and Prough (1976), Smith et al. (1986), Ardies et al. (1987), Mc-Cody and Koop (1988, Blaich et al. (1988)
Cytochrome b$_5$	0.43–0.58 nmol/mg	Blaich et al. (1988), DeMarco and McCoy (1985), Smith et al. (1986)
NADPH: cytochrome P-450 reductase	200–320 nmol/min/mg	Blaich et al. (1988), Burke and Prough (1976), Smith et al. (1986)
MMFO acitvites		
aniline	0.50–1.2 nmol/min/mg	Burke and Prough (1976), Fuji et al.
benzphetamine	6.0–12.5 "	(1985), Smith et al. (1986), Ardies et al.
7-ethoxycoumarin	5.0–14 "	(1987), McCoy and Koop (1988), Blaich
benzo(a)pyrene	0.3–2.5 "	et al. (1988)
Epoxide hydrolase (with styrene oxide) microsomal	12.6–25.9 nmol/min/mg	Pacifici et al. (1981), Oesch and Woolf (1989)
UDP-glucuronosyl transferase (with 4-nitrophenol)	40–50 nmol/min/mg	Hietanen and Vainio (1976) (untreated microsomes; no trypsin or detergents)
Glutathione S-transferase (with chlorodinitrobenzene)		Igarashi et al. (1986), Lam (1988), Morgenstern et al. (1989)
cytosolic	7–8 μmol/min/mg	
microsomal	0.9–1.0 μmol/min/mg	
Protein estimates		Birt et al. (1983), Lechner et al. (1975)
microsomal	25–35 mg/gram liver	
cytosolic	?	

mg = mg protein

cause slight increases in the levels of microsomal protein and tended to cause the most pronounced sex- and age-related differences. When the results only of the low protein diet (which would be most representative of standard hamster chow) were evaluated, some interesting observations become apparent. In general, microsomal protein tended to increase as a function of age, while MMFO activity either increased or remained about the same in comparing activity in young versus old hamsters. While a few isolated differences were identified, consistent and convincing differences between sexes were not demonstrated. Cytochrome P-450 also tended to increase as a function of both dietary protein content and age. Changes in cytochrome P-450, however, were not reflected in equivalent increases in MMFO activity. For example, in 18-week-old female rats (10% lactoglobulin) the cytochrome P-450 concentration was 0.58 nmol/mg protein and AHH activity was 132 ng/min/mg, whereas in 60-week-old rats (40% lactoglobulin) cytochrome P-450 content was 1.62 nmol/mg and AHH activity was 126 ng/mg/min. This suggests the possibility that there are age- and/or dietary-related variations in the iso-zymic character of cytochrome P-450 in hamsters.

MICROSOMAL INDUCTION

As amply reviewed elsewhere (see Chap. 1), in vivo treatment of mammals with a wide variety of organic chemicals can result in increases in MMFO activity by a process called enzyme induction. The prototypical inducing agent is phenobarbital, and its effects in hamsters have been well documented. Lechener and Gomez (1975) reported treatment of hamsters with phenobarbital (80 mg/kg/day for 2 days, po) induced about a 20% increase in microsomal protein, a 75% increase in cytochrome P-450, and significant increase in MMFO activity with both aminopyrene and aniline. McCoy et al. (1981) compared the effect of both phenobarbital and 3-methylcholanthrene (3-MC) in both rats and hamsters. Both treatments caused increases in cytochrome P-450 in both species, although there were slight quantitative differences in amount induced. When benzo(a)pyrene metabolism was examined, however, there was a marked difference in species response: Phenobarbital increased metabolism in hamsters, but 3-MC did not, whereas phenobarbital did not increase this activity in rats, but 3-MC caused a two orders of magnitude increase. Steggles and Chaing (1983) used an inducing regimen of a single intraperitoneal dose of phenobarbital (50 mg/kg) followed by 4 days of treatment with 0.1% phenobarbital in the drinking water. This resulted in a 40% increase in cytochrome P-450. The MMFO activity on a milligram protein basis was significantly increased with all substrates; with benzphet-amine and 7-ethoxycoumarin, activity on a nanomole P-450 basis was significantly increased as well. Smith et al. (1986) treated hamsters with phenobarbital (70 mg/kg ip for 4 days) and observed a 65% increase in cytochrome P-450 as well as a significant increase in cytochrome b_5 that were accompanied by increases in MMFO activity toward both benzphetamine and ethoxycoumarin. This increase in cytochrome b_5, however, has not been confirmed by other investigators (Blaich et al. 1988). Blaich et al. (1988) directly compared the inducing effects of phenobarbital on MMFO activity of both rats and hamsters. As expected, significant induction of activity toward ethoxycoumarin (the prototypical substrate for the isozyme of cytochrome P-450x induced in the rat by phenobarbital) was obtained in both species. In contrast, phenobarbital induced slight increases in rats toward both benzo(a)pyrene and ethoxyresorufin (substrates of P-448 induced by 3-MC in rats), whereas in hamsters phenobarbital increased activity only toward benzo(a)pyrene. Hence, phenobarbital is an effective inducing agent in hamsters, but the response of hamsters is somewhat different than in rats. In general, phenobarbital effectively induces the activity in both species toward substrates, such as benzphetamine and ethoxycoumarin, of rat cytochrome isozyme P-450e. In contrast, phenobarbital and 3-MC are equally efficacious in hamsters in inducing increases in the metabolism of substrates, such as benzo(a)pyrene, of rat cytochrome isozyme P-450d (P-448). As will be detailed below, hamsters and rats differ considerably in their induction with 3-MC–type agents.

The effect of traditional cytochrome P_1-450– or P-448–inducing agents has been studied in the hamster and the response of the hamster to some of these agents has been shown to be different from that of the rat. Russel and Prough (1976) noted that treatment of hamsters with 20 mg/kg ip once daily for 3 days of 3-methylcholanthrene (a classic or prototype inducing agent of cytochrome P_1-450 in rats) did not increase MMFO activity toward benzo(a)pyrene, ethylmorphine, or benzphetamine, but did increase activity toward biphenyl 2.4- to 3.4-fold. The activity of NADPH:cytochrome P-450 reductase was not induced, and this is an observation that has been generally confirmed by most subsequent investigations on MMFO induction in the hamster.

Hietanen and Vainio (1976) examined the inducing effect of DDT (1,1,1-trichloro-2,2-bis([p-chlorophenyl])ethane) on in vitro benzo(a)pyrene metabolism in four different species, including the hamster. In terms of baseline activity, the animals had the following rank: guinea pig>hamster>mouse>rat. Treatment with DDT (single dose, 160 mg/kg po), however, increased the activity twofold in hamsters, whereas actually causing slight decreases in the other species. These early papers suggest that hamsters are relatively resistant to 3-MC induction, while still responding to halogenated aromatics. This was confirmed by Chaing and Steggles (1983), who noted that 3-MC induced increases in microsomal cytochrome P-450 (and thereby did induce some increases in MMFO activity on a milligram protein basis), but did not increase MMFO activity per nanomole of cytochrome P-450 toward benzphetamine, 7-ethoxycoumarin, benzo(a)pyrene, or p-nitrophenetole.

Blaich et al. (1988) also reported data which suggest that while 3-MC induces increases in microsomal benzo(a)pyrene metabolism, these increases seem to be due mostly to increases in total microsomal protein rather than a specific isozyme. Comparable treatment of rats with 3-MC induces much larger increases in microsomal benz(a)pyrene metabolism.

On the other hand, Chaing and Steggles (1983) reported that polychlorinated-biphenyls (single dose, 300 mg/kg ip) induced large increases in cytochrome P-450 and had about the same effect on benzo(a)pyrene metabolism as 3-MC, but (unlike 3-MC) increased MMFO activity per nanomole cytochrome P-450 toward benzphetamine and p-nitrophenetole. Interestingly, β-naphthalflavone (BNF), which in the rat is considered to be a 3-MC–type inducer, induced a different pattern in hamsters than 3-MC did, in that it induced increases in microsomal 7-ethoxycoumarin metabolism, both on a milligram microsomal protein and nanomole cytochrome P-450 basis, but actually decreases benzphetamine metabolism (Chaing and Steggles, 1983; Smith et al., 1986; Ardies et al., 1987). Across the board, 7-ethoxyresorufin deethylation is induced by 3-MC, BNF, and polyhalogenated hydrocarbons in hamsters as it is in rats (Chaing and Steggles, 1983; Smith et al., 1986; Blaich et al., 1988). The response is much greater in rats; 3-MC induces a 30-fold increase in rats as opposed to a threefold increase in hamsters (Iwasaki et al., 1985). Thus, with regard to cytochrome P_1-450 or P-448 induction in the hamster, three points should be kept in mind. First, 3-MC–type agents are less effective in inducing aromatic hydrocarbon hydroxylase (AHH)–type activity in hamsters than in rats. Second, different agents of this class have more selective effects on MMFO activity than in rats (e.g., BNF induces activity different than 3-MC). Third, halogenated hydrocarbons are the most effective members of this class in inducing generalized increases in MMFO activities and, hamsters may, in fact, be the most sensitive rodent to these agents (e.g., DDT).

The prototypical type 3, or steroidal inducing agent, pregnenolone-16(α)-carbonitrile has no effect on MMFO activity in hamsters (Chaing and Steggles, 1983).

SEX-RELATED DIFFERENCES

Unlike the situation in the rat, there is no consistently reported marked sex-related differences in cytochrome P-450 concentrations or in MMFO activity. There are some suggestive hints in the literature, however. Blaich et al. (1988) examined MMFO induction in male and female hamsters, and found that 3-MC increased the cytochrome P-450 content in both sexes: 1.34–2.27 nmol/mg for males and 1.24–2.58 nmol/mg for females. Cytochrome b_5, in contrast, was increased only in females: from 0.43 to 0.48 in nmol/mg males and from 0.53 to 0.71 nmol/mg in females. As in the rat, MMFO induction was accompanied by large increases in ethoxyresorufin deethylation: from 0.14 to 1.16 nmol/min/mg for males and from 0.08 to 1.39 nmol/min/mg for females. With regard to ethoxycoumarin deethylation, however, activity was significantly increased in males (5.37–7.47 nmol/min/mg) but decreased in females (5.27–3.23 nmol/min/mg). Phenobarbital had the same inducing effect regardless of the sex in hamsters.

What are the toxicological consequences of MMFO induction in hamsters? There are a few examples in the literature that can be discussed here. Blaich and Metzler (1988) studied the effects of microsomal enzyme induction on diethylstilbestrol metabolism and toxicity in hamsters. They observed that pretreatment of male hamsters with 7,8-benzoflavone decreases the incidence of kidney tumors but increases the incidence of liver tumors.

Ioannides et al. (1981) compared baseline and induced (with phenobarbital and 3-MC) mutagen (benzo(a)pyrene and 2-acetylaminofluorene) activation of the hamster, guinea pig, mouse, and rat in the Ames assay, which uses the S9 liver fraction (a combination of cytosol and microsomes). In all three species, 3-MC induction increased the mutagenicity of benzo(a)pyrene, whereas phenobarbital decreases it. Given the previous discussion that phenobarbital and 3-MC have approximately the same effect on microsomal benzo(a)pyrene metabolism (Chaing and Steggles, 1983), these results would suggest that there are other factors involved in mutagenicity microsomal metabolism.

Santhanam and Lotlikar (1989) reported that pretreatment of hamsters with BNF increased the extent of aflatoxin B_1 binding to hepatic deoxyribonucleic acid (DNA) in vivo. They further reported that this response differentiates the hamster from the rat (in which BNF decreases aflatoxin "activation") and may make the hamster an attractive model to study aflatoxin-induced carcinogenesis.

ETHANOL INDUCTION AND METABOLISM

The role of the MMFO in ethanol metabolism is the subject of some debate. There is ample evidence to demonstrate, however, that ethanol induces a specific isozyme of cytochrome P-450. As it has been reported that the hamster more avidly drinks ethanol than the rat (Ardies et al., 1987), the hamster may be a more attractive model for the study of ethanol metabolism and toxicity. Thus, the inducing effect of ethanol in the hamster has been studied by several investigators.

DeMarco and McCoy (1985) compared the effect of two different 28-day ethanol treatment regimens (drinking water vs liquid diet) in hamsters. They observed that only the liquid diet regimen was effective in increasing cytochrome P-450 content, but this increase was accompanied by a decrease in cytochrome b_5 content and benzo(a)pyrene hydroxylase activity.

Fuji et al. (1985) used the drinking water regimen (10% ethanol v/v for 3 weeks) and also noted that ethanol causes modest increases in cytochrome P-450 in hamsters which was accompanied by decreases in MMFO activity on (a nanomole cytochrome P-450 basis) with benzphetamine, 7-ethoxycoumarin, and benzo(a)pyrene. In contrast, there were increases in aniline hydroxylation, dimethylnitrosamine demethylation, and ethanol oxidation activity. As discussed by Fuji et al. (1985), these data are sufficient to conclude that ethanol induction in the hamster is different from that observed in the rat, in which a large specific increase in 7-ethoxycoumarin deethylation occurs. These data also suggest that ethanol induces a specific isozyme of cytochrome P-450 at the expense of other isozymes in the hamster.

Ardies et al. (1987) compared the effect of ethanol with other inducing agents (phenobarbital, BNF, and isoniazid) in hamsters. The resultant MMFO of each inducing agent was distinctive with regard to the composite picture produced by the ethyl isocyanide binding spectrum, induction of cytochrome b_5 effects on activity with specific substrates and pattern produced by SDS-PAGE on microsomal protein. Consistent with previous publications, the MMFO of ethanol-treated (10% v/v ethanol in drinking water) hamsters had increased activity with ethanol and aniline but not with benzphetamine or 7-ethoxycoumarin (Ardies et al., 1987).

Using both SDS-PAGE and immunoprotein methods, McCoy and Koop (1988) further confirmed the existence of a distinctive cytochrome P-450 induced by ethanol in hamsters. Hence, ethanol does induce a specific cytochrome P-450 in hamsters which, depending on treatment regimen may or may not be reflected by an increased total cytochrome P-450, that has a rather narrow substrate specificity.

TCDD METABOLISM AND INDUCTION

Rat and hamsters display a 100-fold difference in sensitivity to 2,3,7,8-tetrachlorodibenzodioxin (TCDD). Hamsters are, in fact, among the least sensitive species studied, having an LD_{50} between 1 and 5 mg/kg to this chemical. This observation has stimulated work comparing and contrasting the metabolism and the inducing effect of TCDD in hamsters and rats. Wroblewski and Olson (1988) studied the metabolism and inducing effects of TCDD in isolated rat and hamster hepatocytes. Interestingly, hepatocytes isolated from uninduced animals of both species had approximately the same rates of TCDD metabolism, and pretreatment with both 3-MC (50 mg/kg ip for 3 days) or TDCC (single doses; 5 μg/kg in rats and 500 μg/kg in hamsters) caused approximately the same five- to sixfold increase in TCDD metabolism in both species. TCDD pretreatment, however, induced increases in benzo(a)pyrene metabolism in rats and not hamsters. The cytochrome P-450–specific inhibitors metyrapone and α-naphthaflavone (ANF) both had inhibitory effects on TCDD metabolism in rats, with ANF being far more effective. In hamsters, metyrapone had no effect and ANF had only a slight and transitory effect on TCDD metabolism. In an earlier work, Wroblewski et al. (1987) noted that neither 3-MC or TCDD induced increases in benzo(a)pyrene metabolism (when expressed on nanomole cytochrome P-450 basis), but both cause large increases in ethoxyresorufin metabolism in the hamster. These data suggest that TCDD has different inductive effect in rats and hamsters, but do not readily support the hypothesis that the species differences in TCDD toxicity are due to differences in metabolism.

PEROXISOMAL PROLIFERATION

Hepatomegaly is a commonly used indicator of enzyme induction. However, hepatomegaly can also accompany induced increases in hepatic peroxisomes. The basic biology of these agents has been reviewed elsewhere. While rats and mice are very sensitive to these agents, Lake et al. (1984) reported that hamsters were far less sensitive to such agents. For example, equivalent doses of clofibrate (500 mg/kg) induced an 18-fold increase in carnitine acetyl transferase activity (a standard peroxisomal marker) in rats, but only a 2.5-fold increase in hamsters. Other data presented in this paper were consistent with this observation. This group (Lake et al., 1989a,b) expanded upon these observations with studies on nafenopin. They observed, for example, that when rats, hamsters, and guinea pigs were treated under the same dosage regimen (50 mg/kg/day by gavage for 3 weeks), the resulting increases in palmitoyl-CoA transferase were 10-fold in rats, 1.5 in hamsters, and none in the guinea pig. Watanabe et al. (1989) obtained similar results in their studies on the species differences in peroxisomal proliferation associated with bezafibrate. Thus, the hamster is far less sensitive to peroxisomal proliferating agents than the rat and, therefore, may be a more appropriate model than the rat in assessing the toxicity of peroxisomal proliferating agents.

EPOXIDE HYDROLASE

Aromatic groups frequently are oxidized to arene-oxides or epoxides by the MMFO, which are in turn inactivated by hydrolysis to dihydrodiols by epoxide hydrolase. This is an important enzyme that has been intensely studied in a wide variety of species, except for hamsters. Initial work by Pacifici et al. (1981) suggests that the hamster may have relatively high epoxide hydrolase activity (12.6 nmol/min/mg microsomal protein) in comparison to other rodent species (hamster = guinea pig > rat > mouse). In comparison to nonrodent species, the rankings were baboon > hamster = human > dog. Interestingly, the hamster had the highest activities of renal and pulmonary epoxide hydrolase. Oesch and Wolf (1989), in their studies on hexachloro-1:3-butadiene metabolism, confirmed that hamsters had higher epoxide hydrolase activity than other rodent species but obtained a higher saturating activity than Pacifici et al. (1981); i.e., 25.9 nmol/min/mg. Rigorous exploration of the substrate specificities, inhibitors, and other enzymological aspects of this enzyme in hamsters remains to be done.

AROMATIC AMINE OXIDATION

Hamsters have proven to be convenient species for studying the oxidation of aromatic (primary or secondary) amines and amides. Lotlikar et al. (1967) noted that of the five most studied rodents (rat, hamster, mouse, rabbit, and guinea pig), hamsters had the highest baseline activity in the in vitro N-hydroxylation of 2-acetylaminofluorene, and that such activity was highly inducible by pretreatment with 3-MC. Razzouk and Roberfroid (1982) confirmed that the hamster had higher activity than the rat with 2-AAF (and 2-aminofluorene), but observed that the mouse had higher activity than the hamster. The difference between the two papers may be due to the difference in mouse strains examined. The Razzouk paper did not specifically examine the relative contributions of the MMFO versus the flavine mixed function oxidase (FMFO) system N-hydroxylation in the hamster, but did present data from experiments using inhibitors that the FMFO was at least partially involved.

Becket and Gibson (1975) examined the species-related differences in N-hydroxylation of dibenyzlamine and noted (consistent with Lotlikar et al., 1967, and Razzouk and Roberfroid, 1982) that the hamster had higher activity than either the rat or the mouse (but not as high as the rabbit or the guinea pig).

McMahon et al. (1980) examined N-hydroxylation of 4-aminobiphenyl in various species. N-Hydroxybiphenyl is the major metabolite of this chemical in the rat, guinea pig, C3H mouse, and hamster. The highest initial rates (in vitro) were seen in the hamster, whereas the lowest were seen in the rat. In contrast to the previous discussion on induction, these authors also reported that PCB treatment induced large increases in N-hydroxylation in the rat but had no effect in the hamster.

Gorrod and co-workers (1983, 1987) studied the metabolism of N-benzyl-4-substituted anilines, and observed that hamsters had the highest N-hydroxylation activity, although it should be mentioned that the hamster also had the highest N-debenzylation activity. As discussed by Gemborys and Mudge (1981), the hamster has a high rate of N-hydrooxylation with acetaminophen, which contributes to the sensitivity of this species to acetaminophen hepatotoxicity. Little work has been reported on the FMFO in hamsters, but the data reported by Gorrod and Patterson is consistent with the hypothesis that the FMFO is largely responsible for N-hydroxylation in the hamster.

Ioannides et al. (1981), in their studies on the effects of different inducing agents on the activation of 2-acetylaminofluorene, concluded that a system other than the MMFO is involved in this process in hamsters as well as in other species. McKoy et al. (1986) studied the microsomal metabolism of nicotine in hamsters. Nicotine N'-oxide was one of the major metabolites in their studies, and using a combination of inhibitor and protease treatments, they were able to conclude that this reaction was mediated via the FMFO. In contrast, Nwosu and Crooks (1988) were unable to detect any nicotine N'-oxide as a urinary metabolite when nicotine was administered in vivo to hamsters. The reasons for the differences between these two papers is not evident, but the N-oxide could either be further metabolized and/or simply not excreted via the urine. In general, when the combined literature is considered, the hamster has a relatively high capacity, especially compared to the rat, for the oxidation of aromatic amines and amides, and this activity is mediated, at least in part, by the FMFO.

N-ACETYLATION

The acetylation of aromatic amines to aromatic amides is generally considered to be the first step in the activation of aromatic amines to hepatocarcinogens (e.g., the conversion of 2-aminofluorene to 2-acetylaminofluorene). Lower et al. (1973) reported that the hamster has higher in vitro rates of aromatic amine acetylation than the guinea pig, mouse, and rat. For example, with 4-aminobiphenyl, the activity in hamster cytosolic preparations was 2.4-fold higher than that of the rat. Ioannides et al. (1981) compared the metabolic activation of 2-acetylaminofluorene to mutagens by the microsomes from different species. Hamster microsomes were extremely active in this regard, whereas rat microsomes displayed very weak activity. Given that the hamster has greater activity in the acetylation of aromatic amines and the subsequent oxidative activation of these to mutagenic intermediates, the hamster would probably be a better model than the rat in the study of the metabolism and toxicity of aromatic amines.

Interestingly, homozygous "rapid" and "slow" acetylator inbred strains of hamster has been identified and characterized (Hien et al., 1986; Trinidad et al. 1989). The slow acetylator strain has only 3% of the N-acetyl transferase activity with aminofluorene as the rapid strain, whereas the activities of other enzymes involved in aromatic amine "activation" are similar (Hien et al., 1986). Additional work (Trinidad et al., 1989) further established that the difference was consistent for a variety of aromatic amines (e.g., p-aminobenzoic acid) but not for nonaromatic amines (e.g., isoniazid).

GLUTATHIONE S-TRANSFERASE

Glutathione and the glutathione S-transferase (GST) enzymes comprise one of the most important systems in the phase II metabolism or deactivation of active metabolites. The capacity of this system is controlled by the amounts of glutathione available and the activity of the GSTs. As reported by James and Harbison (1982), there is little difference between rats, guinea pigs, and hamsters with regard to the concentration of reduced glutathione, ranging from 6.5 to 9.3 μmol/g liver. They also reported that SKF 525-A as well as other chemicals that form metabolic intermediate complexes with cytochrome P-450 cause decreases in glutathione in the hamster. Stein et al. (1988) reported a broader range; 4.4 (rat) to 10.6 μmole/g (mouse), with a mean for the hamster of 5.4 μmole/g. Igarashi et al. (1983) reported a similar range; 3.5 (guinea pig) to 7.8 μmol/g (mouse), with the mean for hamsters of 5.4 μmol/g. Fasting had no effect on glutathione concentrations in hamsters, but provoked decreases of 47–65% in the other species examined. Igarashi and co-workers (1986) have also examined GST for species-specific differences. When glutathione S-transferase activity was examined using crude cytosol as the enzyme source and 1-chloro-2,4-dinitrobenzene (CDNB) as a substrate, hamsters had the highest activity compared to the rat, mouse, guinea pig, and rabbit. The GST of the hamster is made up of three different subunits ranging in weight from 27 to 28.5 Da, as identified by SDS-PAGE (Igarashi et al., 1986). On S-sepharose column chromatography, hamster GST activity eluted as four apparent isozymes (presumably different combinations of subunits). Rigorous exploration of the substrate specificities of the different hamster isozymes has not been reported. Lam (1988) reported a value for GST activity (7.73 $\pm$ 0.46, measured under saturating conditions that was in good agreement with that reported by Igarashi et al. (1986). They also reported that the hamster differs from other species in that subchronic treatment with BHT does not cause an increase in GST. In summary, the hamster possesses an active multizymic cytosolic GST system and adequate amounts of glutathione for this system to a play role in xenobiotic metabolism and toxicity, but it has not been thoroughly explored.

Glutathione S-Transferase is generally considered to be a cytosolic enzyme. As reviewed by Morgenstern et al. (1984), however, the existence of a distinct microsomal GST has been known since the early 1980s. There is sufficient evidence that this is a distinct enzyme and not a contaminant of microsomal preparations by cytosolic remnants. For example, in in vitro assay systems it is allosterically activated by N-ethylmaleimide, and only with such activation does the specific activity approach that of the cytosolic enzymes with the more traditional substrates, such as CDNB. As reported by Morgenstern et al. (1984), the hamster has the highest specific activity for microsomal GST of any of the common laboratory species. For example, male hamsters have an activity of 957 $\pm$ 58 nmol/min/mg (with CDNB in N-ethylmaleimide–stimulated hepatic microsomes), whereas male rats have an activity of 540 $\pm$ 25 nmol/min/mg under the same conditions. While on the basis of specific activity and total amounts, the microsomal GST comprises only a small portion of the total hepatic GST, it can still play an important role in the metabolism and toxicity of specific chemicals. For example, in hamsters hexachloro-1,3-butadiene is preferential metabolized by the microsomal GST by a ratio of 22.7 to 1.0 over the cytosolic enzyme (Oesch and Wolff, 1989). Similar ratios were 37.7 and 3.3., for human and rat preparations, respectively. The hamster may, therefore, be a better species than the rat in the study of this enzyme.

CONJUGATION REACTIONS: GLUCURONIDE, SULFATE, AND AMINO ACIDS

Enzyme systems other than GST are involved in Phase II reactions. As a loose rule of thumb, these other systems tend to act on more stable chemicals, such as aromatic acetates, phenols or primary amines, than GST. These other systems catalyze the formation of glucuronic acid, sulfate, and amino acid conjugates. This would also include acetylation, which has been previously discussed. The activity of these systems have been at least partially examined in the hamster. Huckle et al. (1981a) studied the species differences in the in vivo metabolism of 3-phenoxybenzoic acid. Glucuronide conjugates predominated in the hamster, whereas the sulfates predominated in rat. They noted that the hamster, like other rodents and unlike the cat or ferret, form a very low percentage of amino acid (glycine and taurine) conjugates. In fact, the hamster has the lowest activity of any rodent of glycine N-acyl transferase activity measured in vitro under optimum conditions (Huckle et al., 1981b). Emudianughe et al. (1987a) examined the in vivo metabolism of 1-naphthylacetic acid, and observed that the predominant urinary metabolite in hamsters was the glucuronide (64%), whereas the glycine conjugate comprised a smaller percentage (10%). One could generalize that if a functional group could be conjugated with either glucuronic acid or an amino acid, the former will always predominate in the hamster. This, however, is not the case. Emudianughe et al. (1987a,b) compared the metabolism of 1- versus 2-naphthylacetate, and found that this chemical was such a poor substrate for uridine-diphospho-glucoronosyl (UDP-glucuronosyl) transferase that even in the hamster amino acid conjugates (glycine and glutamine) were the major metabolites. Hence, depending on the substrate or metabolite available, the hamster will tend to form glucuronide metabolites at the expense of amino acid conjugates, but there are exceptions.

In the last few years, relatively little work has been done on the UDP-glucuronosyl transferase (a microsomal enzyme) in hamsters. Hietanen and Vainio (1976) compared the in vitro activity of UDP-glucuronosyl transferase in the rat and hamster using p-nitrophenol as the substrate. They observed that on a microsomal protein basis, the hamster had higher activity, but when corrected for the microsomal protein and expressed on a gram liver basis, the activity of the two species was about the same (8–12 nmol/min/g). Rats have somewhat higher UDP-glucuronosyl activity with thyroid hormone (T_4), a natural substrate, than hamster (Henry and Gasiewicz, 1987), and TCDD treatment induced increases in both species. Interestingly, TCDD provokes completely different changes in circulating thyroid hormone concentrations in rats (decreases) and hamsters (increases); a difference than can not be accommodated by the difference in UDP-glucuronosyl transferase. Based on the available data, there appears to be quantitative differences in the activity of this enzyme between the rat and the hamster that will require additional work to delineate.

ACETAMINOPHEN METABOLISM AND TOXICITY

UDP-Glucuronosyl transferase and 3' phosphoadenosine-5' phosphosulfate (PAPS) sulfotransferase (a cytosolic enzyme) frequently act on the same substrates, and the differences in substrate specificity and the availability of cosubstrate (PAPS availability is often limiting) determine which conjugate is preferentially formed. This has been studied in the hamster in the metabolism of acetaminophen. As mentioned, the hamster is among the most sensitive of species to the hepatotoxic effect of acetaminophen, a phenomenon believed to be due, at least partly, to the higher rates of N-hydroxylation by hamsters. This was convincingly demonstrated by Green et al. (1984), who examined the metabolism and toxicity of acetaminophen in hepatocytes isolated from various species. As expected, the hamster produced a higher ratio of toxic to nontoxic (i.e., sulfates and glucuronides) metabolites than other species. This was confirmed by Tee et al. (1987), who demonstrated (1) that hepatocytes isolated from several different species, including the hamster, were equally sensitive to cell injury when exposed to the putative toxic metabolite of acetaminophen, N-acetyl-p-benzoquinoneimine, and (2) hamsters have higher rates of production of this metabolite than other species. Even in hamsters, however, the majority of acetaminophen is disposed of via conjugation to nontoxic metabolites.

As demonstrated by Roberts et al. (1985), sulfate formation is the preferred conjugative pathway of acetaminophen metabolism in isolated hamster hepatocytes. Miller and Jollow (1987) also demonstrated that the sulfate was the preferred conjugate in hamster hepatocytes, especially in incubations fortified with inorganic sulfate. Further, pretreatment of intact hamsters with an inhibitor of PAPS sulfotransferase (2,6-dichlorodinitrophenol; 10 mg/kg ip given 30 min before acetaminophen) greatly enhanced acetaminophen induced liver injury. In vivo, however, the glucuronide is the preferred conjugate. Miller and Jollow (1987) concluded that this was due to the capacity (as evidenced by the K_m) of the sulfotransferase, and not the availability of PAPS. Brezenicka et al. (1987) measured the concentrations of PAPS and observed that the concentration in hamster was about half that in rats (approximately 68 vs 33 nmol/g liver). These observations are not mutually exclusive, and it is likely that both the capacity of sulfotransferase and the availability of PAPS are the reasons that the sulfotransferase does not play a greater role in the metabolism (and, therefore, protection against hepatotoxicity) of acetaminophen in hamsters.

DIETHYLSTILBESTROL METABOLISM AND TOXICITY

The sensitivity of hamsters to the heptotoxicity of acetaminophen is an example of a quantitative species difference in toxicity that has a metabolic explanation. The response of hamsters to diethylstilbestrol (DES) meanwhile is an example of a qualitative species difference; that is, DES causes kidney tumors in male hamsters, but not in any other species studied. Gottschlich and Metzler (1980) extensively studied the metabolism of DES in hamsters and could not identify any species or sex-related differences in the metabolism of DES to explain the difference in toxicity. This work was continued (Blaich and Metzler, 1988a,b) and has produced some interesting findings. For example, cotreatment of hamsters with 7,8-benzoflavone and DES lead to a reduction in the kidney tumor incidence and a rise in liver tumor incidence. There is still, however, no evidence that the metabolism of DES plays a role in the induction of renal tumors by this chemical in hamsters. The more rapid hepatic metabolism of DES induced by 7,8-benzoflavone probably plays a role in the protection to the kidney afforded by this treatment regimen.

EXTRAHEPATIC METABOLISM

Up to this point, this section has focused on hepatic xenobiotic metabolism as the liver is quantitatively the most important organ in xenobiotic transformations. Other organs can also possess metabolic capacity that can play a role in xenobiotic metabolism and toxicity. Those of the hamster will be briefly mentioned here. Burke and Prough (1976) examined the MMFO activity of hamster liver and lung with a variety of different substrates. In general, the lung had much lower activity (e.g., 0.05% for AHH), but for a few substrates activity in the lung can approach that of the liver (e.g., 77% with biphenyl), and MMFO activity in the hamster lung is essentially unresponsive to induction by 3-methylcholanthrene. Smith et al. (1986) demonstrated that the kidney contains cytochrome P-450 (and the other components of the MMFO) at about 10% (on a microsomal protein basis), and that increases in the activity of the renal MMFO was not induced by common hepatic MMFO inducing agents. Li et al. (1983) demonstrated that AHH activity of the male hamster kidney is about 20% of that of the kidney, and that various antiandrogenic and/or estrogenic treatments will depress the activity of the kidney but not the liver. Wiebkin et al. (1984) reported that isolated hamster pancreatic acinar cells have low (16- to 210-fold less than the rat) but measurable rates of MMFO activity with a variety of different substrates. Pretreatment of hamsters with common inducers had no effect on acinar MMFO activity. Hietanen and Vainio (1976) reported that unlike other species examined, the hamster has no measurable intestinal (duodenum) AHH activity, but does have UDP-glucuronosyl transferase activity (about 25% on a microsomal basis when compared to hepatic activity). Hein et al. (1986) demonstrated that the hamster kidney has higher levels of sulfotransferase than the liver. Kawakubo et al. (1988) reported that hamster skin has a surprisingly high N-acetyl transferase activity that could play a role in carcinogen activation in this species. Hadley and Dahl (1983) reported that the MMFO activity of hamster nasal tissue to be higher than any other species examined.

GUT FLORA METABOLISM

As reviewed by Rowland et al. (1986), the gut flora can also play a role in xenobiotic metabolism and toxicity. The gut flora metabolic activity in rodents tends to be lytic (β-glucosidase and β-glucuronidase) or reductive (azo, nitro, and nitrite reductases) in nature. The rat and hamster have essentially equivalent activities of β-glucosidase (30–35 μmol/hr/g feces), azo reductase (2–3 μmol/hr/g feces), and nitroreductase (3.8–4.2 μmol/hr/g feces). The rat has much higher activities with β-glucuronidase (156 vs 60.8 μmol/hr/g feces) and nitrate reductase (3.9 vs 1.7 μmol/hr/g feces).

REFERENCES

Adler, S. (1948) Origin of the golden hamster *Cricetus auratus* as a laboratory animal. *Nature* 162, 256–257.

Althoff, J., and Mohr, U. (1973) Comparative studies in three hamster species related to respiratory carcinogenesis, in *The Laboratory Animal in Drug Testing*, Spiegel, A., ed. Gustav Fischer Verlag, Stuttgart, pp. 229–232.

Ambrose, K. R., and Coggin, J. H. (1975) An epizootic in hamsters of lymphomas of undetermined origin and mode of transmission. *J. Natl. Cancer Inst.* 54, 877–879.

Amend, N. K., Loeffler, D. G., Ward, B. C., and Van Hoosier, G. L. (1976) Transmission of enteritis in the Syrian hamster. *Lab. Anim. Sci.* 26, 566–572.

Ardies, C., Lasker, J., and Lieber, C. (1987) Characterization of the cytochrome monoxygenase system of hamster liver microsomes, effects of prior treatment with ethanol and other xenobiotics. *Biochemical Pharmacol.* 21, 3613–3619.

Arnold, D. L., and Grice, H. C. (1979) The use of the Syrian hamster in toxicology studies, with emphasis on carcinogenesis bioassay. *Prog. Exp. Tumor Res.* 24, 222–234.

Bajusz, E. (1969) Hereditary cardiomyopathy: A new disease model. *Am. Heart J.* 77(5), 686–696.

Bajusz, E., Homburger, F., Baker, J. R., and Bogdonoff, P. (1969) Dissociation of factors influencing myocardial degeneration and generalized cardiocirculatory failure. *Ann. N.Y. Acad. Sci.* 156, 396–420.

Barthold, S. W., Jacoby, R. O., and Pucak, G. J. (1978) An outbreak of cecal mucosal hyperplasia in hamsters. *Lab. Anim. Sci.* 28, 723–727.

Bartlett, J. G., Onderdonk, A. B., Cisneros, R. L., and Kasper, D. L. (1977) Clindamycin-associated colitis due to a toxin-producing species of *Clostridium* in hamsters. *J. Infect. Dis.* 136, 701–705.

Bartlett, J. G., Chang, T. W., Moon, N., and Onderdonk, A. B. (1978) Antibiotic-induced lethal enterocolitis in hamsters: Studies with eleven agents and evidence to support the pathogenic role of toxin-producing clostridia. *Am. J. Vet. Res.* 39, 1525–1530.

Becci, P. J., McDowell, E. M., and Trump, B. F. (1978) The respiratory epithelium. VI. Histogenesis of lung tumors induced by benxo(a)pyrene-ferric oxide in the hamster. *J. Natl. Cancer Inst.* 61, 607–618.

Beckett, A., and Gibson, G. (1975) Microsomal N-hydroxylation of dibenzylamine. *Xenobiotica* 5, 677–686.

Bergman, H., Bryant, B., and Nesnow, S. (1984) Metabolism of A-naphthaflavone by rat, mouse, rabbit, and hamster microsomes. *Toxicol. Appl. Pharmacol.* 72, 469–475.

Berman, H. J., Lutz, B. R., and Fulton, G. P. (1955) Blood pressure of golden hamsters as affected by Nembutal Sodium and X-irradiation (abstract). *Am. J. Physiol.* 183, 597.

Biggar, R. J., Schmidt, T. J., and Woodall, J. P. (1977) Lymphocyte choriomeningitis in laboratory personnel exposed to hamsters inadvertently infected with LCM virus. *J. Am. Vet. Med. Assoc.*, 171(9), 829–832.

Birt, D. F., and Pour, P. M. (1983) Influence of dietary fat on spontaneous lesions of Syrian golden hamster. *J. Natl. Cancer Inst.* 71, 401–406.

Birt, D., Hruza, D., and Baker, P. (1983) Effects of dietary protein level on hepatic microsomal mixed-function oxidase systems during aging in two generations of Syrian hamsters. *Toxicol. Appl. Pharmacol.* 68, 77–86.

Blaich, G., and Metzler, M. (1988a) Effect of pretreatment with 7,8-benzoflavone and diethystilbestrol in the male Syrian golden hamster *in vivo*. *Biochem. Pharmacol.* 37, 3565–3570.

Blaich, G., and Metzler, M. (1988b) The effect of pretreatment with 7,8-benzoflavone on drug-metabolizing enzymes and diethylstilbestrol metabolism in male hamster liver microsomal preparations. *Xenobiotica* 18, 199–206.

Blaich, G., Gottlicher, M., Cikrty, P., and Metzler, M. (1988) Induction of P-450 isoenzyme factivities in Syrian golden hamster liver compared to rat liver as probed by the rat of 7-alkoxyresorufin-O-dealkylation. *Chem. Biol. Int.* 67, 129–138.

Brandwein, S. R., Skinner, M., and Cohen, A. S. (1981) Isolation and characterization of spontaneously occurring amyloid fibrils in aged Syrian (golden) hamsters. *Fed. Proc., Fed. Am. Soc. Exp. Biol.* 40, 789 (Abstr. No. 3182).

Brusick, D. (1982) Genetic toxicology, in *Principles and Methods of Toxicology*, Hayes, A. W., ed. Raven Press, New York, pp. 223–272.

Brzenznicka, E., Hazleton, G., and Klaassen, C. (1987) Comparison of adenosine 3'-phosphate 5'-phosphosulfate concentrations in tissues from different laboratory animals. *Drug Metab. Dispos.* 15, 133–135.

Burke, M., and Prough, R. (1976) Some characteristics of hamster liver and microsomal aryl hydrocarbon (biphenyl and benzo(a)pyrene) hydroxylation reactions. *Biochem. Pharmacol.* 25, 2187–2195.

Cantrell, C. A., and Padovan, D. (1987) Other hamsters: Biology, care and use in research, in *Laboratory Hamsters*, Van Hoosier, G. L., and McPherson, C. W., eds. Academic Press, Orlando, Florida, pp. 369–386.

Castro, G., Gomez, M., and Castro, A. (1989) Species differences in the interaction between CC14 reactive metabolites and liver DNA or nuclear protein fractions. *Carcinogenesis* 10, 289–294.

Chiang, J., and Steggles, A. (1983) Identification and partial purification of hamster microsomal cytochrome P-450 isoenzymes. *Biochem. Pharmacol.* 32, 1389–1397.

Coggin, J. H., Bellomy, B. B., Thonas, K. V., and Pollock, W. J. (1983) B-cell and T-cell lymphomas and other associated diseases induced by an infectious DNA viroid-like agent in hamsters *(Mesocricetus auratus)*. *Am. J. Pathol.* 110, 254–266.

Collins, G. R. (1979) Hamster, in *The Manual for Laboratory Animal Technicians*. American Association Laboratory Animal Science, Publication 67-3, Joliet, Illinois, pp. 121–130.

Davis, D.H.S. (1963) Wild rodents as laboratory animals and their contributions to medical research in South Africa. *S. Afr. J. Med. Sci.* 28, 53–69.

DeMarco, G., and McCoy, G. (1985) Involvement of cytochrome b_5 in hepatic microsomal metabolism of benzo(a)pyrene. *Biochem. Biophys. Res. Comm.* 128, 621–627.

Desai, R. G. (1986) Hematology and microcirculation, in *The Golden Hamster Its Biology and Use in Medical Research*, Hoffman, R., Robinson, P. E., and Magalhaes, H., eds. Iowa State University Press, Ames, pp. 185–191.

Doi, K., Yamamoto, T., Isegawa, N., Doi, C., and Mitsuoka, T. (1987) Age-related non-neoplastic lesions in the heart and kidneys of Syrian hamsters of the APA strain. *Lab. Anim.* 21, 241–248.

Dontenwill, W., Chevallier, H. T., Harke, H. R., Lafrenzl, U., Rechzeh, C., and Schneider, B. (1973) Investigations of the effect of chronic cigarette-smoke inhalation in the Syrian golden hamster. *JNCI* 51, 1781–1832.

Emudianughe, T., Caldwell, J., and Smith, R. (1987a) Studies on the metabolism of arylacetic acids. 6. Comparative metabolic conjugation of 1- and 2-naphthylacetic acid in the guinea pig, mouse, hamster, and gerbil. *Xenobiotica* 17, 815–821.

Emudianughe, T., Caldwell, J., and Smith, R. (1987b) Studies on the metabolism of arylacetic acids. 7. The influence of varying dose size upon the conjugation pattern of 2-naphthylacetic acid in the guinea pig, mouse and hamster. Xenobiotica 17, 823–828.

Estes, P. C., Richter, C. B., and Frankling, J. A. (1971) Demodectic mange in the golden hamster. *Lab. Anim. Sci.* 21, 825–828.

Fabry, A. (1985) The incidence of neoplasms in Syrian hamsters with particular emphasis on intestina neoplasia. *Arch. Toxicol. Suppl.* 8, 124–127.

Fenner, F. (1986) *Viral and Mycoplasm Infections of Laboratory Rodents: Effects on Biomedical Research*, Bhatt, P. N., Jacoby, R. O., Morse, M. C., and New, A. E., eds. Academic Press, San Diego, pp. 24–25.

Flatt, R. E., and Kerber, W. T. (1968) Demodectic mite infestation in golden hamsters. *Lab. Anim. Dig.* 4, 6–7.

Flecknell, P. A. (1987) *Laboratory Animal Anaesthesia: An Introduction for Research Workers and Technicians*. Academic Press, San Diego, pp. 94, 174, 225–26, 261–301, 283.

Fox, J. G. (1979) Selected aspects of animal husbandry and good laboratory practices. *Clin. Toxicol.* 15(5), 539–553.

Frenkel, P. A. (1987) Experimental biology: Use in infectious disease research, in *Laboratory Hamsters*, Van Hoosier, G. L., and McPherson, C. W., eds. Academic Press, Orlando, Florida, pp. 227–249.

Frisk, C. S., and Wagner, J. E. (1977a) Hamster enteritis: A review. *Lab. Anim.* 11, 79–85.

Frisk, C. S., and Wagner, J. E. (1977b) Experimental hamster enteritis: An electron microscopic study. *Am. J. Vet. Res.* 38, 1861–1868.

Frisk, C. S., Wagner, J. E., and Owens, D. R. (1978) Enteropathogenicity of *Escherichia coli* isolated from hamsters *(Mesocricetus auratus)* with hamster enteritis. *Infect. Immunol.* 20, 319–320.

Frisk, C. S., Wagner, J. E., and Owens, D. R. (1981) Hamster *(Mesocricetus auratus)* enteritis caused by epithelial cell-invasive *Escherichia coli*. *Infect. Immunol.* 31, 1232–1238.

Frisk, C. S. (1987) Bacterial and mycotic diseases, in *Laboratory Hamsters,* Van Hoosier, G. L., and McPherson, C. W., eds. Academic Press, Orlando, FL, pp. 111–133.

Fuji, H., Ohmaachi, T., Sagami, I., and Watanabe, M. (1985) Liver microsomal drug metabolism in ethanol-treated hamsters. *Biochem. Pharmacol.* 34, 3881–3884.

Gemborys, M., and Mudge, G. (1981) Formation and disposition of the minor metabolites of acetaminophen in the hamster. *Drug Metab. Dispos.* 9, 340–351.

Genovesi, E. V., and Peters, C. J. (1987) Susceptibility of inbred Syrian hamsters to lethal disease by lymphocytic choriomeningitis virus. *Proc. Soc. Exp. Biol. Med.* 185(3), 250–261.

Gertz, E. W. (1973) Animal model of human disease. Animal model: cardiomyopathic Syrian hamster. *Am. Jour. Pathol.* 70, 151–154.

Gleiser, C. A., Van Hoosier, G. L., and Sheldon, W. G. (1970) A polycystic disease of hamsters in a closed colony. *Lab. Anim. Care* 20(50), 923–929.

Gleiser, C. A., Van Hoosier, G. L., Sheldon, W. G., and Read, W. K. (1971) Amyloidosis and renal paramyloid in a closed hamster colony. *Lab. Anim. Sci.* 21, 197–202.

Gorrod, J., and Gooderham, N. (1987) The metabolism of N-benzyl-4-substituted anilines: Factors influencing *in vitro* C- and N-oxidation. *Xenobiotica* 17, 165–177.

Gorrod, J., and Patterson, L. (1983) The metabolism of 4-substituted N-ethyl- N-methylanilines. III. The effect of various potential inhibitors, activators and inducers on a-C- and N-oxidation. *Xenobiotica* 13, 521–529.

Gottschlich, R., and Metzler, M. (1980) Metabolic fate of diethylstilbestrol in the Syrian hamster, a susceptible species for diethylstilbestrol carcinogenicity. *Xenobiotica* 10, 317–327.

Green, C., Dabbs, J., and Tyson, C. (1984) Metabolism and cytotoxicity of acetaminophen in hepatocytes isolated from resistant and susceptible species. *Toxicol. Appl. Pharmacol.* 76, 139–149.

Gruys, E., Timmermans, H.J.F., and Van Ederen, A. M. (1979) Desposition of amyloidin the liver of hamsters: An enzyme-histochemical and electron microscopic study. *Lab. Anim.* 13, 1–9.

Guide for the Care and Use of Laboratory Animals (Revised 1985) Animal Resources Program, Division of Research Resources, NIH, Bethesda, Maryland.

Hadley, W., and Dahl, A. (1983) Cytochrome P-450-dependent monooxygenase activity in nasal membranes of six species. *Drug Metab. Dispos.* 11, 275–276.

Hall, A., Persing, R. L., White, D. C., and Ricketts, R. T. (1967) Mystromys albicaudatus as a laboratory species. *Lab. Anim. Care* 17(2), 180–188.

Hallett, A. F., and Politzer, W. M. (1972) Diabetes mellitus in Mystromys albicaudatus. *Arch. Pathol.* 93(2), 178.

Handler, A. H. (1965) Spontaneous lesions of the hamster, in *The Pathology of Laboratory Animals*, Ribelin, W. E., and McCoy, J. R., eds. Thomas, Springfield, Illinois, pp. 210–240.

Hawkins, C. C., Buggy, B. P., Fekety, R., and Schaberg, D. R. (1984) Epidemiology of colitis induced by *Clostridium difficile* in hamsters: Application of a bacteriophage and bacteriocin typing system. *J. Infect. Dis.* 149, 775–780.

Hein, D., Kirlin, W., Ogolla, F., Trinidad, A., Thompson, L., and Ferguson, (1986) The Role of acetylator genotype-on hepatic and extrahepatic acetylation, deacetylation, and sulfation of 2-aminofluorene, 2-acetylaminofluorene, and N-hydroxy-2-acetylaminofluorene in the inbred hamster. *Drug Metab. Dispos.* 14, 566–572.

Heldmaier, G., and Steleinlechner, S. (1981) Seasonal pattern and energetics of short daily torpor in the Dzungarian hamster, Phosupua aunfoeua. *Oceologia* 48, 265–270.

Henry, E., and Gasiewicz, T. (1987) Changes in thyroid hormones and thyroxine glucuronidation in hamsters compared with rats following treatment with 2,3,7,8-tetrachloro-diobenzo-p-dioxin. *Toxicol. Appl. Pharmacol.* 89, 165–174.

Herberg, L., Buchanan, K. D., Herbetz, L. M., Kern, H. F., and Klex, H. K. (1980) The Dzungarian hamster, a laboratory animal with inappropriate hyperglycemia. *Comp. Biochem. Physiol.* A65A, 35–60.

Hess, F. G., McDowell, E. M., and Trump, B. F. (1981a) The respiratory epithelium. VIII. Interpretation of cytologic criteria for human and hamster respiratory tract tumors. *Acta Cytol.* 25, 111–134.

Hess, F. G., McDowell, E. M., Resau, J. H., and Trump, B. F. (1981b) The respiratory epithelium. IX. Validity and reproducibility of revised cytologic criteria for human and hamster respiratory tract tumors. *Acta Cytol.*

Hietanen, E., and Vainio, H. (1976) Effect of administration route on acute toxicity and on drug biotransformation in various rodents. *Arch. Environ. Contam.* 4, 201–216.

Homburger, F., and Bajusz, E. (1970) New models of human disease in Syrian hamsters. *J.A.M.A.* 212(4), 604–610.

Homburger, F., and Bernfeld, P. (1979) Cigarette smoke-induced laryngeal cancer: A model for bronochogenic carcinoma in humans. *New Engl. J. Med.* 862.

Homburger, F., Adams, R. A., and Soto, E. (1979a) The special suitability of inbred hamsters for carcinogenesis testing. *Arch. Toxicol. Suppl.* 2, 445–450.

Homburger, F., Adams, R. A., Soto, E., and Van Dongen, C. Gg. (1979b) Susceptibility and resistance to chemical carcinogenesis in inbred Syrian hamsters. *Prog. Exp. Tumor Res. 2*, 215–221.

Huckle, K., Hutson, D., and Millburn, P. (1981a) Species differences in the metabolism of 3-phenoxybenzoic acid. *Drug Metab. Dispos.* 9, 352–359.

Huckle, K., Tait, G., and Millburn, P. (1981b) Species variation in the renal and hepatic conjugation of 3-phenoxybenzoic acid with glycine. *Xenobiotica* 11, 635–644.

Igarashi, T., Tomihari, N., Ohmori, S., Ueno, K., Kitagawa, H., and Satoh, T. (1983) Comparison of glutathione S-transferase and related enzyme activities in mouse, guinea pig, rabbit, and hamster liver cytosol to those in rat liver. *Biochem. Int.* 13, 641–648.

Ioannides, C., Parkinson, C., and Parke, D. (1981) Activation of benzo(a)pyrene and 2-acetamidofluorene to mutagens by microsomal preparations from different animal species: Role of cytochrome P-450 and P-448. *Xenobiotica* 11, 701–708.

Iwasaki, K., Lum, P., Ioannides, C., and Parke, D. (1986) Induction of cytochrome P-448 as exemplified by the O-deethylation of ethoxyresorufin. *Biochem. Pharmacol.* 35, 3879–3884.

Jacoby, R. O. (1978) Transmissible ileal hyperplasia of hamsters. I. Histogenesis and immunocytochemistry. *Am. J. Pathol.* 91, 433–450.

Jacoby, R. O., Osbaldiston, G. W., and Jonas, A. M. (1975) Experimental transmission of a typical ileal hyperplasia of hamsters. *Lab. Anim. Sci.* 25, 465–473.

James, R., and Harbison, R. (1982) Hepatic glutathione and hepatotoxicity. Effects of cytochrome P-450 complexing compounds SKF 525–A, L-a-acetyl-methadol (LAAM), nor-LAM, and piperonyl butoxide. *Biochem. Pharmacol.* 31, 1829–1835.

Johnson, E. A., and Jacoby, R. O. (1978) Transmissible ileal hyperplasia of hamster. II. Ultrastructure. *Am. J. Pathol.* 91, 451–468.

Kaufmann, D. G., and Madison, R. H. (1974) Synergistic effects of benzo(a)pyrene and M-methyl-N-nitrosurea on respiratory carcinogenesis in Syrian golden hamsters, in *Experimental Lung Cancer: Carcinogenesis and Bioasays*, Karbe, E., and Park, J. F., eds. Springer-Verlag, New York.

Kawakubo, Y., Manabe, S., Yamazoe, Y., Nishikawa, T., and Kato, R. (1987) Properties of cutaneous acetyltransferase catalyzing N-N-hydroxyarylamines. *Biochem. Pharmacol.* 37, 265–270.

Keeler, R. F., and Young, S. (1978) Multifactorial contributions to the etiology of spontaneous hemorrhagic necrosis of the central nervous system of fetal hamsters. *Teratology* 17, 285–292.

Keeler, R. F., and Young, S. (1979) Role of vitamin E in the etiology of spontaneous hemorrhagic necrosis of the central nervous system of fetal hamsters. *Teratology* 20, 127–132.

Keyes, P. H. (1960) The infectious and transmissible nature of experimental dental caries. *Arch. Oral Biol.* 1, 304–320.

Lake, B., Gray, T., Foster, J., Stubberfield, C., and Gangolli, S. (1984) Comparative studies on di-(2-ethylexyl)phthalate-induced hepatic petoxisome proliferation in the rat and hamster. *Toxicol. Appl. Pharmacol.* 72, 46–60.

Lake, B., Evans, T., Foster, J., Stubberfield, C., and Gangolli, S. (1989a) Comparative studies on di-(2-ethylexyl)phthalate-induced hepatic peroxisome proliferation in the rat and hamster. *Toxicol. Appl. Pharmacol.* 99, 148–160.

Lake, B., Evans, J., Gray, T., Korosi, S., and North, C. (1989b) Comparative studies on nafenopin-induced hepatic peroxisome proliferation in the rat, syrian hamster, guinea pig, marmoset. *Toxicol. Appl. Pharmacol.* 99, 148–160.

Lam, L. (1988) Effects of butylated hydroxyanisole on glutathione S-transferase and catechol O-methyltransferase activities in Syrian golden hamster. *Biochem. Pharmacol.* 37, 3011–3016.

Lechner, M., and Gomes, F. (1975) Enzyme induction by phenobarbital and liver RNAse activities in mice, hamsters, and guinea pigs. *Gen. Pharmacol.* 6, 127–132.

Li, S., Lam, L., and Li, J. (1983) Effect of steroid hormone treatment on aryl hydrocarbon hydroxylase activity in the Syrian hamster kidney. *Biochem. Pharmacol.* 32, 2847–2850.

Lossnitzer, K., Grewe, N., Konrad, A., and Adler, J. (1977) Electographic changes in cardiomyopathic Syrian hamsters (strain BIO 8262). *Basic Res. Cardiol.* 72, 421–435.

Lotlikar, P., Enomoto, M., Miller, J., and Miller, E. (1967) Species variations in the N- and ring-hydroxylation of 2-acetylaminofluorene and effects of 3-methylcholanthrene pretreatment. *Proc. Soc. Exp. Bio. Med.* 125, 341–346.

Lower, G., and Bryan, G. (1973) Enzymatic N-acetylation of carcinogenic aromatic amines by liver cytosol of species displaying different organ susceptibilities. *Biochem. Pharmacol.* 22, 1581–1588.

Lusk, R. H., Fekety, R., Silva, J., Browne, R. A., Ringler, D. H., and Abrams, G. D. (1978) Clindamycin-induced enterocolitis in hamsters. *J. Infect. Dis.* 137, 464–475.

Magalhaes, H. (1970) Hamsters, in *Reproduction and Breeding Techniques for Laboratory Animals*, Hafez, E.S.E., ed. Lea & Febiger, Philadelphia, pp. 258–272.

Martorana, P. A. (1976) The hamsters as a model for experimental pulmonary emphysema. *Lab. Anim. Sci.* 26, 352–354.

McCoy, G., and Koop, D. (1988) Biochemical and immunochemical evidence for the induction of an ethanol-inducible cytochrome P-450 in male Syrian golden hamster. *Biochem. Pharmacol.* 37, 1563–1568.

McCoy, G., Chen, C., and Hecht, S. (1981) Influence of mixed-function oxidase inducers on the *in vitro* metabolism of N'nitrosonornicotine by rat and hamster liver microsomes. *Drug Metab. Dispos.* 9, 168–169.

McCoy, G., Howard, P., and DeMarco, G. (1988) Characterization of hamster liver nicotine metabolism. I. Relative rates of microsomal C and N oxidation. *Biochem. Pharmacol.* 35, 2767–2773.

McMahon, R., Turner, J., and Whitaker, G. (1980) The N-hydroxylation and ring-hydroxylation of 4-aminobiphenyl *in vitro* by hepatic mono-oxygenases from rat, mouse, hamster, rabbit and guinea pig. *Xenobiotica* 10, 469–481.

McMartin, D.N. (1977) Spontaneous atrial thrombosis in aged syrian hamsters. I. Incidence and pathology. *Thromb. Haemostasis* 38, 447–456.

McMartin, D. N., and Dodds, W. J. (1982) Atrial thrombosis in aged Syrian hamsters. *Am. J. Pathol.* 107, 277–279.

McNeil, P. E., Al-Mashat, R. R., Bradley, R. A., and Payne, A. P. (1986) Control of an outbreak of wet-tail in a closed colony of hamsters *(Mesocricetus auratus)*. *Vet. Rec.* 119272–119273.

Miller, M., and Jallow, D. (1987) Relationship between sulfotransferase activity and susceptibility to acetaminophen-induced liver necrosis in the hamster. *Drug Metab. Dispos.* 15, 143–150.

Mitruka, B. M., and Rawnsley, H. M. (1981) *Clinical Biochemical and Hematological Reference Values in Normal Experimental Animals and Humans.* 2nd ed. Masson, Publishing, New York.

Mohr, U. (1979) The Syrian golden hamster as a model in cancer research. *Prog. Exp. Tumor. Res.* 24, 245–252.

Mohr, U., and Ernst, H. (1987) The European Hamster: Biology, care and use in research, in

Laboratory Hamsters, Van Hoosier, G. L, and McPherson, C. W., eds. Academic Press, Orlando, Florida, pp. 351–366.

Morgenstern, R., Lundquvist, G., Anderson, G., Balk, L., and DePierre, J. (1984) The distribution of microsomal glutathione transferase among different organelles, different organs, and different organisms. *Biochem. Pharmacol.* 33, 3609–3614.

Nakayama, M., Saegusa, J., Itoh, K., Kiuchi, Y., Tamura, T., Ueda, K., and Fujiwara, K. (1974) Transmissible enterocolitis in hamsters caused by Tyzzer's organism. *Jpn. J. Exp. Med.* 45, 33–41.

Newberne, P. M., and McConnell, R. G. (1979) Nutrition of the Syrian golden hamster. *Prog. Exp. Tumor. Res.* 24, 127–138.

Newcomer, C. E., Fitts, D. A., Goldman, B. D., Murphy, M. R., Rao, G. N. Shklar, G., and Schwartz, J. L. (1987) Experimental biology: Other research uses of Syrian hamsters, in *Laboratory Hamsters*, Van Hoosier, G. L., and McPherson, C. W., eds. Academic Press, Orlando, Florida.

Nwosu, C., and Crooks, P. (1988) Species variation and stereoselectivity in the metabolism of nicotine enantiomers. *Xenobiotica* 18, 1361–1372.

Oesch, F., and Wolff, C. (1989) Properties of the microsomal and cytosolic glutathione S-transferases involved in hexachloro-1,3-butadiene conjugation. *Biochem. Pharmacol.* 38, 353–359.

Owens, D., and Young, C. (1973) The occurrence of Demodex aurati and Demodex criceti in the Syrian hamster *(Mesocricetus auratus)* in the United Kingdom. *Vet. Rec.* 92, 282–284.

Pacifici, G., Boobis, A., Brodie, M., McManus, M., and Davies, D. (1981) Tissue and species differences in enzymes of epoxide metabolism. *Xenobiotica* 11, 73–79.

Parker, J. C., Igel, H. J., Reynolds, R. K., Lewis, A. M., and Rowe, W. P. (1976) Lymphocytic choriomeningitis virus infection in fetal, newborn, and young adult Syrian hamsters *(Mesocricetus auratus)*. *Infect. Immunol.* 13, 967–981.

Pour, P., and Birt, D. (1979) Spontaneous diseases of Syrian hamsters—Their implications in toxicological research: Facts, thoughts and suggestions. *Prog. Exp. Tumor Res.* 24, 145–156.

Pour, P., Mohr, U., Althoff, J., Cardesa, A., and Kmoch, N. (1976c) Spontaneous tumors and common diseases in two colonies of Syrian hamsters. III. Urogenital system and endocrine glands. *J. Natl. Cancer Inst.* 56, 949–961.

Pour, P., Mohr, U., Althoff, J., Cardesa, A., and Kmoch, N. (1976d) Spontaneous tumors and common diseases in two colonies of Syrian hamsters. IV. Vascular and lymphatic systems and lesions of other sites. *J. Natl. Cancer Inst.* 56, 963–974.

Pour, P., Kmoch, N., Greiser, E., Mohr, U., Althoff, J., and Cardesa, A. (1976a) Spontaneous tumors and common diseases in two colonies of Syrian hamsters. I. Incidence and sites. *J. Natl. Cancer Inst.* 56, 931–935.

Pour, P., Mohr, U., Cardesa, A., Althoff, J., and Kmoch, N. (1976b) Spontaneous tumors and common diseases in two colonies of Syrian hamsters. II. Respiratory tract and digestive system. *J. Natl. Cancer Inst.* 56, 937–948.

Pour, P., Ii, Y., and Althoff, J. (1979) Comparative studies on spontaneous tumor incidence based on systematic histologic examination of rat and hamster strains of the same colony. *Prog. Exp. Tumor Res.* 24, 199–206.

Profeta, M. L., Lief, F. S., and Plotkin, S. A. (1969) Enzootic Sendai infection in laboratory hamsters. *Am. J. Epidemiol.* 89, 316–324.

Raabe, O. G., Bennick, J. E., Light, M. E., Hobbs, C. H., Thomas, R. L., and Tillery, M. I. (1973) An important apparatus for acute inhalation exposure of rodents to radioactive aerosols. *Toxicol. Appl. Pharmacol.* 26, 264–273.

Razzouk, C., and Roberfroid, M. (1982) Species differences in the biochemical properties of liver microsomal arylamine and arylamide N-hydroxylases. *Chem.-Biol. Interact.* 41, 251–264.

Redman, H. C., Hobbs, C. H., and Revar, A. H. (1979) Survival distribution of Syrian hamsters *(Mesocricetus auratus,* Sch:SYR) used during 1972–1977. *Prog. Exp. Tumor Res.* 24, 108–117.

Regulations of Animal Welfare Act (PL89-544 as amended PL91-579) and the Animal Welfare Act, Code of Federal Regulations (1985).

Rehg, J. E., and Lu, Y. S. (1982) Clostridium difficile typhlitis in hamsters not associated with antibiotic therapy. *J. Am. Vet. Med. Assoc.* 181, 1422–1423.

Renshaw, H. W., Van Hoosier, G. L., and Amend, N. K. (1975) Survey of naturally occurring diseases of the Syrian hamster. *Lab. Anim.* 9, 179–191.

Roberts, S., Price, V., and Jollow, D. (1986) The mechanisms of cobalt chloride induced protection against acetaminophen hepatotoxicity. *Drug Metab. Dispos.* 14, 25–33.

Robinson, P. F. (1968) General aspects of physiology, in *The Golden Hamster Its Biology and Use in Medical Research*, Hoffman, R., Robinson, P. E., and Magalhaes, H., eds. Iowa State University Press, Ames, pp. 111–118.

Ronald, N. C., and Wagner, J. E. (1975) Treatment of Hymenolepsis nana in hamsters with Yomesan® (niclosamide). *Lab. Anim. Sci.* 25, 219–220.

Rowland, I., Mallett, A., Bearne, C., and Farthing, M. (1986) Enzyme activities of the hindgut microflora of laboratory animals and man. *Xenobiotica* 16, 519–523.

Santhanam, K., and Lotlikar, P. (1989) Effect of β-naphthalflavone on the metabolism of aflatoxin B1 in hamsters. *Cancer Lett.* 45, 129–134.

Schermer, S. (1967) The golden hamster, in *The Blood Morphology of Laboratory Animals*, F. A. Davis, Philadelphia, pp. 75–84.

Schiavo, D. M. (1980) Multifocal retinal dysplasia in the Syrian hamster LAK:LVG (SYR). *J. Environ. Pathol. Toxicol.* 3(5–6), 569–576.

Schreiber, H., Sacomanno, G., Martin, D. H., and Brennan, L. (1974) Sequential cytological changes during development of respiratory tract tumors induced in hamsters by benzo(a)pyrene-ferric oxide. *Cancer Res.* 34, 689–698.

Sher, S. P. (1982) Tumors in control hamsters, rats and mice: literature tabulation. *CRC Crit. Rev. Toxicol.* 10(1), 51–59.

Skinner, H. H., and Knight, E. H. (1979) The potential role of Syrian hamsters and other small animals as reservoirs of lymphocytic choriomeningitis virus. *J. Small Anim. Pract.* 20, 145–161.

Slauson, D. O., Hobbs, C. H., and Crain, C. (1978) Arteriolar nephrosclerosis in the Syrian hamster. *Vet. Pathol.* 15, 1–11.

Smith, J., Rush, G., and Hook, J. (1986) Induction of renal and hepatic mixed function oxidases in the hamster and guinea pig. *Toxicology* 38, 209–218.

Stein, A., Gregus, Z., and Klaassen, C. (1988) Species variations in biliary excretion of glutathione-related thiols and methylmercury. *Toxicol. Appl. Pharmacol.* 93, 351–359.

Stuhlman, R. A. (1979) Animal model: Spontaneous diabetes mellitus in Mystromys albicaudatus. *Am. J. Pathol.* 94, 685–688.

Stroia, L. N., Bohr, D. F., and Vocke, L. (1954) Experimental hypertension in the hamster. *Am. J. Physiol.* 179, 154–158.

Takasaki, Y., Oghiso, Y., Sato, K., and Fujiwara, K. (1974) Tyzzer's disease in hamsters. *Jpn. J. Exp. Med.* 44, 267–270.

Tee, L., Davies, D., Seddon, C., and Boobis, A. (1987) Species differences in the hepatotoxicity of paraacetamol are due to differences in the rate of conversion to its cytotoxic metabolite. *Biochem. Pharmacol.* 36, 1041–1052.

Tomson, F. N., and Wardrop, K. J. (1987) Clinical chemistry and hematology, in *Laboratory Hamsters*. Van Hoosier, G. L. and McPherson, C. W. eds Academic Press, Orlando, Florida, pp. 43–59.

Trinidad, A., Kirlin, W., Ogolla, F., Andrews, A., Yerokun, T., Ferguson, R., Brady, P., and Hein, D. (1989) Kinetics characterization of the acetylator genoatype-dependent and -independent N-acetyltransferase in homozygous rapid and slow acetylator inbred hamster liver cytosol. *Drug Metab. Dispos.* 17, 238–247.

Turusov, V. S. (ed.) (1982) Vol. III. Tumors of the Hamster, in *Pathology of Tumours in Laboratory Animals*. WHO, IARC Scientific Publications No. 34, Lyon, France, pp. 1–450.

Unay, E. S., and Davis, B. J. (1980) Treatment of Syphacia Obvelata in the Syrian hamster (Mesocricetus auratus). *Am. J. Vet. Res.* 41(11), 1899–1900.

Van Hoosier, H. L., and Ladiges, W. C. (1984) Biology and diseases of hamsters, in *Laboratory Animal Medicine*, Academic Press, Orlando, Florida, Fox, J. G., Cohen, B. J., and Loew, F. M., eds. pp. 123–147.

Van Hoosier, G. L., and Trentin, J. J. (1979) Naturally occurring tumors of the Syrian hamster. *Prog. Exp. Tumor Res.* 23, 1–12.

Wagner, J. E., Owens, D. R., and Troutt, H. F. (1973) Proliferative ileitis of hamsters: Electron microscopy of bacteria in cells. *Am. J. Vet. Res.* 34, 249–252.

Wantland, W. W. (1955) Parasitic fauna of the golder hamster. *J. Dent. Res.* 34, 631–648.

Wardrop, K. J., and Van Hoosier, G. L. (1989) The hamster, in *The Clinical Chemistry of Laboratory Animals*, Loeb, W. F., and Quimby, F. W. eds. Pergamon Press, New York, pp. 31–39.

Watanabe, T., Horie, S., Yamada, J., Isaji, M., Nishigaki, T., Naito, J., and Suga, I. (1989) Species differences in the effects of bezafibrate, a hypolipidemic agent on hepatic peroxisome-associated enzymes. *Biochem. Pharmacol.* 38, 367–371.

Wechsler, R. A. (1983) Blood collection techniques and normal values for ferrets, rabbits, and rodents: A review. *Vet. Med. Small Anim. Clin.* 78(5), 713–717.

Werner, A. P., Stuart, B. O., and Sanders, C. L. (1979) Inhalation studies with Syrian golden hamsters. *Prog. Exp. Tumor Res.* 24, 177–198.

Weyland, E., and Bevan, D. (1987) Species differences in disposition of benzo(a)pyrene. *Drug Metab. Dispos.* 15, 442–448.

Wroblewski, V., and Olson, J. (1988) Effect of monooxygenase inducers and inhibitors on the hepatic metabolism of 2,3,7,8-tetrachlorodiobenzo-p-dioxin in the rat and hamster. *Drug Metab. Dispos.* 16, 43–51.

Wroblewski, V., Gessner, T., and Olson, J. (1988) Qualitative and quantitative differences in the induction and inhibition of hepatic benzo(a)pyrene metabolism in the rat and hamster. *Biochem. Pharmacol.* 37, 1509–1517.

Yabe, Y., Katoaka, N., and Koyama, H. (1972) Spontaneous tumors in hamsters: Incidence, morphology, transplantation and virus studies. *GANN* 63, 329–336.

Yerganian, G. (1972) History and cytogenetics of hamsters. *Prog. Exp. Tumor Res.* 16, 2–41.

Young, S., and Keeler, R. F. (1978) Hemmorrhagic necrosis of the central nervous system of fetal hamsters: Litter incidence and age-related pathological changes. *Teratology* 17, 293–302.

Zook, G. C., Huang, K., and Rhorer, R. G. (1977) Tyzzer's disease in Syrian hamsters. *J. Am. Vet. Med. Assoc.* 171(9), 833–837.

5

The Guinea Pig

Toxicology: **Shayne Cox Gad**
                   Becton Dickinson and Company
                   Research Triangle Park, North Carolina

Pathology: **John C. Peckham**
                   Experimental Pathology Laboratories, Inc.
                   Research Triangle Park, North Carolina

Metabolism: **Christopher P. Chengelis**
                   WIL Research Laboratories, Inc.
                   Ashland, Ohio

Toxicology   **Shayne Cox Gad**

Journalists often refer to human research subjects as "human guinea pigs," and the public mind has long regarded the guinea pig as the classic laboratory animal for all biomedical research and safety assessment. Actually, their use is now proportionately constant at 2% of the annual total of laboratory animals. This makes them only the third or fourth most popular species in toxicology/safety assessment.

Though not used in the numbers perceived by the general public, guinea are important research animals that are used primarily in studies of immunology, audiology, and infectious diseases. They are relatively expensive, usually costing 3–5 times as much as rats and often more than rabbits; however, perhaps their greatest disadvantage for research use is the lack of readily accessible peripheral veins for intravenous injections and collection of blood and serum samples. As will be seen, however, they are more widely used in safety assessment than most believe.

SPECIES AND CHARACTERISTICS

The scientific name of the guinea pig is *Cavia porcellus*. Guinea pigs are hystricomorph rodents (suborder Hystricomorpha, order Rodentia) originating from South America. They are more closely related to porcupines and chinchillas than to mice or rats.

Guinea pigs have long been used as experimental animals in biomedical research because they are small, tame, and easy to handle. Of the three natural varieties (English, Abyssinian, and Peruvian), the albino form of the short-haired English variety is the most commonly utilized in the laboratory. The Harley strain of this variety is by far the most commonly used in toxicology. Recently, the Charles River Laboratories has also developed a fertile, euthymic hairless strain which offers advantages for use in dermal studies.

The popularity of the guinea pig as a pet and research animal owes much to their docile nature. They seldom bite or scratch and will respond to attention with frequent and gentle handling. At the same time, they tend to be messy in their habits, and the development of human allergies to guinea pigs is not uncommon (in the toxicology laboratory, probably only allergies to the rabbit and rat are more common).

In many ways, this roly-poly rodent is the most attractive laboratory animal. Exceptionally curious, the guinea pig investigates any activities outside of its cage by attempting to watch, and expressing itself by a wide range of sounds from a deep chortle to a shrilling whistle. They are unable to climb, but they can jump short distances.

Guinea pigs are alert, full bodied, and have smooth, shiny skin. Their coat is dense, with the hair being clean and not marked by discharge from the nose, eyes, or ears. If allowed to feed freely, guinea pigs can become quite large over time. Males will commonly reach 1 kg at 1 year, and can weigh several kilograms at a later age.

HISTORY

The guinea pig was first scientifically described by Gesner (1516–1605) and Aldrovandus (1522–1607) in about 1580 (Wagner, 1979). The use of the guinea pig as a test animal for biomedical research goes at least back to Lavoisier in 1780 (Lane-Petter, 1963), who used it to measure heat production by animals.

In 1979, Collins reported that (for 1965) about 2.5 million guinea pigs were used annually for research in the United States. Over the more than 20 years since, this figure has undoubtedly decreased. By 1983, total use of guinea pigs in research was 521,237 (of which 28,753 were used in toxicology).

UTILIZATION AS A TEST ANIMAL

In the broad range of biomedical research, the guinea pig has been employed as the test animal in a wide range of investigations: nutrition, pharmacology, allergy, radiology, and immunology. Complement, a substance originally isolated from the blood of guinea pigs, is a key component in serological work.

The guinea pig can be easily infected by human tuberculosis germs, and is indeed the animal of choice for diagnosis of tuberculosis in humans. Another disease that the guinea pig shares with its fellow mammal, the human, is scurvy. This diesase is noninfectious, being caused by a deficiency of vitamin C in the diet. An idle but interesting fact is that the only other animal subject to scurvy, the monkey, is also very susceptible to human-type tuberculosis.

In safety assessment/toxicology studies, however, the use of the guinea pig is a bit narrower. Table 1 summarized these uses. Specific protocols for some of these tests will be discussed later in this chapter.

BASIC BIOLOGICAL CHARACTERISTICS

During the course of all the different kinds of toxicology studies that need to be designed and conducted, a complete knowledge of the fundamental biological characteristics is

Table 1 Toxicological Endpoints Evaluated Using The Guinea Pig as a Model

Endpoint	References
Delayed contact dermal sensitization (Coombs type IV) Buehler, Draize, Landsteiner, Guinea pig maximization (GPMT), etc., test designs	Landsteiner and Chase (1937, 1940, 1941, 1942) Draize et al. (1944) Buehler (1964) Magnusson and Kligman (1969)
Immediate hypersensitization	Ayala et al. (1988)
Photosensitization Armstrong and Harber and Shalita tests	Ichikawa et al. (1981) Harber and Shalita (1975)
Ototoxicity (because of early findings with antibiotics and nonsteroidal anti-inflammatory drugs)	Brummett (1983) Cayals and Guilhaume (1985) Parravicini et al. (1983)
Cataractogenesis (induction of cataracts by dermal and/or oral application of test substances)	Melnikova and Radionov (1979)
Pulmonary irritation and sensitization	Emerson and Cole (1983) Karol et al. (1980)
Systemic toxicity (in place of traditional species such as rat, mouse, and dog). Usually due to efficacy data being developed in carrageenan colitis model in this species	Adrian et al. (1976) Lee and Thomsen (1982)
Host resistance assay (for generalized screen of effect on immune competence, in place of traditional mouse model in same assay)	
Teratology	Hoar (1979)
Inhalation	Firpo et al. (1988)

essential. Also, most studies are conducted with the measurement of various parameters to determine if a test material has had any (particularly any adverse) effect on the animals. Such measurements must start from a position of knowledge of what normal values are, and of what kind of variability is commonly seen.

Tables 2–9 summarize a range of basic biological characteristics of the guinea pig. Most of these were gained from the review of general sources (e.g., Collins, 1979), though a number of special references are cited in the tables. The tables summarize physiological (Table 2), reproductive (Table 3), hematology (Table 4), clinical chemistry (Table 5), serum enzyme (Table 6), serum protein component (Table 7), organ weight (Table 8), and deoxyribonucleic acid (DNA) repair (Table 9) characteristics. Figure 1 shows growth curves for male and female animals.

Table 2 Physiological Parameters

Life span	2–6 years
Rectal temperature	38.6–40.0°C
Respiration rate	69–160/min
Heart rate	240–277 (Fara and Catlett, 1971) or 130–190 (Collins, 1971)/min
Daily food consumption	8 g/100 g body weight
Daily water consumption	10 ml/100 g body weight
Percent of total life span	Embryonic 1.8% Gestational 4.4% Puberty 4.2%
Oxygen consumption	0.76 ml O_2/g/hr
Tidal volume	1.8 ml
Minute volume	0.16 L
Mean blood pressure (mm Hg)	Systolic 76.7 Diastolic 46.8
Metabolic rates (resting)	3–5 weeks of age 34.0 cal/m²/hr 7–9 weeks of age 33.25 11–13 weeks of age 32.95 5–6 months 30.8 11–12 months 29.54

HUSBANDRY

Guinea pigs represent an intermediate species in terms of ease and expense of care. While they are considerably easier to house and maintain than primates, dogs, or rabbits, they also are clearly more expensive and difficult than rats or mice.

    The objective of all that is done for the husbandry of laboratory animals can be distilled

Table 3 Reproductive Parameters

Puberty	45–70 days
Breeding age	12–14 weeks
Gestation	59–70 days; 63 average
Weaning age	21–28 days
Diploid chromosome number	64
Litter size	1–8; 3–4 average
Estrus cycle	16–18 days

Table 4   Hematology Parameters

Plasma volume	30.6–38.2 ml/kg body weight
Whole blood volume	75 ml/kg body weight
RBC diameter	7.1 μ
RBC sedimentation rate	0.5–1.5 mm/hr
Blood pH	7.35
RBC	4.5–7.0 × 10^6/mm^3
Hematocrit	42.0–55.2 ml/100 ml
Platelets	3.4–10.0 × 10^5/mm^3
Hemoglobin	11.7–14.5/100 ml
WBC	9.9–10 × 10^3/mm^3

Differential:		
	Neutrophils	4.2 × 10^3/mm^3
	Eosinophils	0.4
	Basophils	0.07
	Lymphocytes	4.9
	Monophils	0.43

PVC (%)	43
MCV (cuμ)	81
MCH ($\mu\mu$g)	25
MCHC (%)	30
Reticulocytes (%)	0.9–1.0
Red blood cell: Diameter	7.1 μ (Scarborough, 1931; Ponder, 1948)
Life span	
	60–80 days (Edmendson and Wyburn, 1963)

Table 5   Clinical Chemistry Parameters

Plasma	Calcium	5.3 mEq/L
	Sodium	145–152 mEg/L
	Chloride	105 mEq/L
	Phosphorus	5.3 mg/100 ml
	Potassium	6.8–8.9 mEq/L
	Magnesium	2.3 mg/100 ml
	Cholesterol	21–43 mg/100 ml
	Serum protein	5.4 g/100 ml
	Albumin	2.8–3.9 g/100 ml
	Globulin	1.7–2.6 g/100 ml
	Protein-bound iodine	1.8–2.2 mμg/100 ml
Whole blood	Glucose	82–107 mg/100 ml
	Bilirubin	22–39 mg/100 ml
	Non–protein-bound nitrogen	30–51 mg/100 ml
	Creatinine	0.99–1.77 mg/100 ml
	Blood urea nitrogen	8–28 mg/100 ml
	Glucose	79–107 mg/100 ml
	Uric acid	1.3–5.6 mg/100 ml
	Total lipids	94–245 mg/100 ml
	Phospholipids	25–77 mg/100 ml
	Triglycerides	0–145 mg/100 ml
	Progesterone	0–2.75 ng/100 ml
	Estrogen	0–54 pg/100 ml

Table 6 Serum Enzyme Activities

	Values			
	male		female	
Enzyme	mean	SD	mean	SD
Amylase (Somogyi units/dl)	295.	31.0	269.	28.0
Alkaline phosphatase (IU/L)	74.2	6.92	65.8	5.46
Acid phosphatase IU/L)	32.2	2.59	28.7	3.20
Alanine transaminase (SGPT) (IU/L)	44.6	6.75	38.8	7.15
Aspartate transaminase (SGOT) (IU/L)	48.2	9.50	45.5	7.00
Creatine phosphokinase (CPK) (IU/L)	0.95	0.15	1.10	0.20
Lactic dehydrogenase (LDH) (IU/L)	46.9	9.50	52.1	11.2

Source: Data from Albritton (1952); Altman and Dittmer (1964, 1971); Nomura et al. (1975).

Table 7 Serum Protein Components of the Normal Guinea Pig

	Values			
	male		female	
Fractions	mean	SD	mean	SD
Total protein (g/d)	5.60	0.28	4.80	0.34
Albumin (g/dl)	2.73	0.30	2.42	0.27
(%)	48.8	5.50	50.5	5.40
α_1-Globulin (g/dl)	0.11	0.04	0.10	0.02
(%)	1.90	0.38	2.20	0.19
α_2-Globulin (g/dl)	0.33	0.08	0.23	0.06
(%)	5.90	1.25	4.80	1.42
β-Globulin (g/dl)	1.14	0.20	0.82	0.17
(%)	20.4	4.10	17.1	3.60
γ-Globulin	1.29	0.26	1.22	0.15
(%)	23.1	4.60	25.4	3.25
Albumin/globulin	0.95	0.16	1.02	0.18

Source: Data from Spector (1961); Burns and Lannoy (1966); Altman and Dittmer (1974); Dimopoullos (1972); Moreland (1974).

Table 8 Organ Weights in Two Strains of Guinea Pigs[a]

Organ	Weight (g) ± SD			
	strain 2 male	strain 2 female	strain 13 male	strain 13 female
Body	802 ± 65	780 ± 69	1044 ± 69	940 ± 99
Liver	25.37 ± 2.9	29.21 ± 4.83	33.7 ± 3.89	35.5 ± 8.50
Lungs[b]	5.21 ± 0.97	5.18 ± 1.22	7.23 ± 0.94	7.44 ± 0.88
Heart	2.12 ± 0.28	2.07 ± 0.27	2.42 ± 0.33	2.26 ± 0.23
Thyroid[c]	0.061 ± 0.013	0.058 ± 0.007	0.078 ± 0.017	0.074 ± 0.924
Kidney[c]	2.94 ± 0.56	2.79 ± 0.38	2.57 ± 0.24	2.33 ± 0.15
Adrenal[c]	0.402 ± 0.13	0.394 ± 0.110	0.310 ± 0.050	0.284 ± 0.041
Spleen	0.78 ± 0.12	1.03 ± 0.27	0.73 ± 0.07	0.93 ± 0.16

[a]N = 20 in all cases.
[b]Weight of both lungs.
[c]Weight of left organ only.
Source: From Breazile and Brown (1976).

to maintaining healthy animals in as stable an environment as possible, and as humanely as possible.

One set of broad principles which should be taken into account when assessing whether animals are being humanely maintained and utilized are the so called "five freedoms" (Webster, 1986). These are:

1. Freedom from thirst, hunger, and malnutrition—achieved by readily accessible fresh water and diet to maintain full health and vigor
2. Appropriate comfort and shelter
3. Freedom from injury and disease—achieved by prevention or rapid diagnosis and treatment
4. Freedom of movement and the opportunity to express most normal patterns of behavior
5. Freedom from fear

Table 9 DNA Repair Activity (erg/mm^2 UV light equiv.)

IQ	9.4
MCIQ	1.7
2 - AF	14.2
IQ/2-AF	5.5
MeIQ/2-AF	0.7

Source: Loury and Byard, 1985.

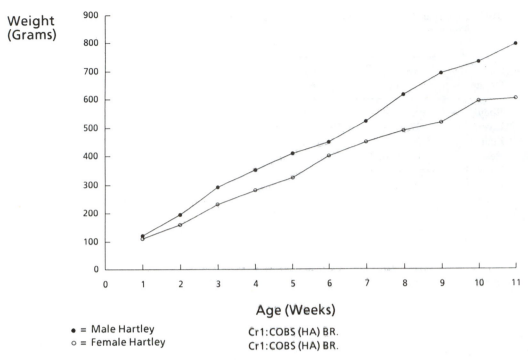

Figure 1 Guinea pig weight curves.

Though in toxicological research some of these five principles are not strictly possible, to the extent possible they should guide the researcher's actions.

Housing and Caging

Eveleigh (1988) has recently reviewed the history of the development of caging for several laboratory species, including the guinea pig, and the interested reader is directed to that source.

Since guinea pigs do not climb, they can be kept in open-sided boxes or pens, provided that the sides are at least 10 in high.

Guinea pigs may be housed indoors in pens on the floor, in fixed or portable tiered compartments, or in cages. Floor pens, despite their disadvantages (such as waste of space and spread of infection), are commonly used because of the simplicity and ease of cleaning and inspection. The general size of a pen is 40 × 96 in, and it can be placed on each side of the room, leaving a passage of about 24 in wide. Another arrangement uses only one-half of the available space each day.

Tiered compartments may also be used. These are permanent compartments made of concrete or wooden shelves or portable metal units. The permanent type are not much more economical in space than the floor pens, and they are generally more expensive and difficult to clean and disinfect. The portable type, up to four tiers, are space saving and easy to clean.

The initial cost of a caging system is greater than boxes, pens, or tiered compartments, but it is space saving. Generally, 30 × 30 × 14 in cages made out of a single aluminum alloy sheet are ideal. These cages can be divided by panels if needed. Each cage can hold a harem of four sows and one boar. The cages will hold 12 young animals up to 350 g in weight, and the number may be reduced to 10, eight, and six as the weight increases. The cages for experimental animals are 10 × 10 × 10 in and are made up of 3/4 in wire mesh to hold individual animals, and a 24 × 16 in floor area may be enough for 10 guinea pigs. The most common bedding material is seasoned softwood shavings. Peat moss, though more expensive, is highly recommended. Treated flax and corncobs are also good, as they have highly absorbent and deodorant properties. Cereal straw should not be used because it may be irritating to the animals and may act as a source of contamination.

The ILAR (Institute of Laboratory Animal Resources) guidelines as to floor space to be provided per animal did not change with the 1985 revision of the *Guide for the Care and Use of Laboratory Animals*. Caging or housing of whatever form should provide (as a minimum) the following space for each animal (NIH, 1985).

Weight (g)	Floor Area per animal (cm²)	Height (cm)
Up to 250	277 (43 in.)	17.8 (7 in.)
250–350	374 (58 in.)	17.8 (7 in.)
Over 350	652 (101 in.)	17.8 (7 in.)

Attention to the details of thorough cleaning is an essential component of the husbandry of guinea pigs. Obnoxious odors, the accumulation of mineral scale from the high concentration of mineral salts in guinea pig urine, and the spread of infectious diseases between animals and cages are minimized with proper sanitation of cages and racks.

Cages in which bedding is used should be cleaned and sanitized often enough to prevent an accumulation of excreta or debris. This generally means that cages should be sanitized at least once each week, and all new bedding should be added each time the cage is sanitized. Although wire floor cages do not have to be cleaned as frequently, they should be sanitized at least once every 2 weeks. The pan under the cage, however, must be cleaned frequently to prevent the accumulation of excreta. If large numbers of animals are maintained in each cage, daily cleaning of the pans may be necessary to maintain a high level of sanitation. Soiled bedding should be disposed of promptly either by incineration or in a way that will not contaminate other animal areas or areas of human habitation.

Temperature, Ventilation, and Humidity Control

Strict attention should be given to air-handling systems to control temperature, humidity, air velocity, and air pressure within the animal room. Guinea pigs are extremely susceptible to respiratory disease, and well-designed, efficiently operating system provides the essential environmental stability for respiratory disease control.

There should be 10–15 changes of air per hour and no air should be recirculated unless it has been filtered to remove airborne contaminants. Care must be taken to control the velocity and direction of airflow to produce a draftless and even distribution of air to all areas of a room. An ideal state of mass air displacement is, in some instances, difficult to achieve in a room filled with animals and cages, and in these circumstances cages can be designed or arranged to minimize drafts.

Ideally, room temperatures should be maintained between 65 and 75°F (20–25°C) and relative humidity at approximately 45–55%.

Breeding

It is general practice now to purchase guinea pigs for toxicological research from specialized venders, and generally it is not cost effective to try to raise stocks for use in tests. However, there are specialized cases (teratology and reproductive toxicity studies, for example) where successful breeding is an essential component of the test. In such cases, guinea pigs are best mated when they are approximately 3 months old or weight from 450 to 600 gs. Specific considerations of experimental design will generally dictate the details of arrangements for mating, but it should be kept in mind that the reproductive potential of the guinea pig is high and that most simple pair cohabitations result in pregnancy.

Mating in the guinea pig is normally detected by either the presence of sperm in the vagina or by the presence of a vaginal plug. The plug consists of a central core formed by a mixture of secretions from the male's vesicular and coagulating glands and is enclosed by a mass of flat epithelial cells apparently derived from the vaginal wall (Stockard and Papanicolaou, 1919). The plug usually fills the vagina from cervix to vulva. A few hours after its formation, the plug falls out of the vagina and can often be observed as a waxy mass on the cage floor. The efficiency of utilizing plugs to predict pregnancy is usually high. Live sperm, on the other hand, can be found routinely in vaginal smears for only a few hours after copulation.

Watering

Most facilities supply water to guinea pigs either from suspended water bottles or from an automatic system through sipper tubes. If bottles are used, it is frequently the practice to supply ascorbic acid in the water. Whichever of these supply methods is utilized, however, the use of either distilled or deionized water rather than chlorinated tap water is recommended as it will reduce the endogenous rate of vitamin C deactivation. Guinea pigs do have a tendency to play with water tubes, which can result in the flooding of cages.

Nutrition

Among the commonly used laboratory species, only guinea pigs and primates require a dietary source of vitamin C (ascorbic acid). Collins and Elvehjem (1958) reported the ascorbic acid requirement for growth of immature guinea pigs is 0.5 mg/100 g body weight per day. Nungester and Ames (1948) indicated that a 300-g guinea pig requires a daily intake of approximately 6 mg of vitamin C to provide adequate protection against infection. Under intensive breeding conditions, the requirement of the adult female that is pregnant or lactating during most of her breeding life is as least 20 mg/day (Bruce and Parker, 1947).

Commercial pelleted diets are manufactured to meet the requirements of the guinea pig for ascorbic acid. Additionally, they are usually fortified to compensate for ascorbic acid losses in storage, but careful attention must be paid to manufacturing dates on such food. Laboratory animal feeds must not be maintained too long in storage and must be fresh when used. Ideally, guinea pig feeds should be stored in rooms where the temperature is 50°F or less, and should not be stored in the animal room. The date of manufacture is commonly given or coded on each feed bag, and a strong effort should be made to store feed for no longer than 4–6 weeks from the date of manufacture. This is especially important where no green vegetable supplement is offered. Feeders should be designed to prevent guinea pigs from climbing into them. For this purpose the standard J-type feeder works very well.

Feeding guinea pigs green vegetables in addition to the pelleted diet has been a subject of continuing controversy. A "green" supplement on a regular basis may provide insurance against vitamin C deficiency; however, such supplements offer benefits beyond this one advantage. These benefits are most apparent in a production colony under an intensive breeding system where there is heavy stress on the pregnant or lactating female. Such supplements enhance the ability of breeding animals to maintain body weight. Based on the results of feeding experiments in which four different commercially prepared diets were compared using large numbers of animals held for breeding periods of 18–24 months. It has been observed that the feeding of a green supplement resulted in an average increase of 10–44% in weaned offspring over the same pelleted feeds without a green supplement.

Guinea pigs do have some rather specific requirements for amino acids and vitamins in their diets (Navia and Hunt, 1976). Besides vitamin C, they are also very susceptible to vitamin E deficiencies and diets with 30–33% protein are recommended.

Diseases

Scurvy

Signs of scurvy usually appear with 2 weeks after guinea pigs are deprived of vitamin C. The guinea pig diet should provide 15–20 mg vitamin C/kg body weight for maintenance (Clark and Baker, 1975a); vitamin C deficiencies frequently occur when guinea pigs are fed rabbit chow. Although rabbit pellets resemble guinea pig pellets in appearance, rabbit pellets lack vitamin C, are lower in protein, and therefore do not meet the dietary requirements of guinea pigs.

Clinical signs of a vitamin C deficiency are reluctance to move, an unkempt appearance, swellings around the joints, diarrhea, and cutaneous sores. Animals often succumb to secondary bacterial infections before the classic signs of scurvy are evident. The most prominent gross lesions seen at necropsy are hemorrhages in the muscle and periosteum, particularly around the stifle joint and rib cage, and epiphyseal enlargement, best noted at the costochondral junction.

Vitamin E Deficiency

Guinea pigs are very susceptible to vitamin E deficiencies, usually resulting in the development of skeletal muscle necrosis, but a deficiency is unlikely in animals fed commercially produced diets (Wagner, 1979)

Alopecia

A diffuse loss of hair over the flanks and back develops to a degree in all sows in late pregnancy. It is more marked with an intensive breeding program. Around the time of weaning, a thinning of the hair occurs during the transition from baby fur to more mature hair (Wagner, 1976). Alopecia also seems to be associated with other stress conditions, although the exact cause is not known. Nutritional and genetic factors are probably involved to some degree.

Loss of hair with a distinctive pattern or patchy distribution can result from a hair-chewing vice termed barbering. Animals may chew their own hair or that of a cage mate. The location of hair loss can usually provide a clue as to whether it is self-inflicted or has resulted from barbering by a cage mate.

Circumanal Sebaceous Accumulations

Excessive accumulations of sebaceous secretions occur in the folds of the circumanal and genital region in adult male guinea pigs. These folds must be cleansed periodically to preclude infection and unpleasant odors. At times, the sebaceous secretions form a plug that accumulates in the folds between the two halves of the scrotum. It can be removed after softening with soap and water (Williams, 1976).

Preputial Infection and Vaginitis

Male guinea pigs occasionally develop preputial infections caused by lodging of foreign material in the preputial folds. Breeding males on bedding may be affected when pieces of bedding adhere to the moist prepuce following copulation and are drawn into the preputial fornix. Treatment primarily involves removing the particle and cleansing the area.

Vaginitis in female guinea pigs is usually caused by entrapment of wood chips or their bedding in the vagina, causing a foreign body reaction. The problem is corrected by washing the area carefully and wiping away the chips. It may be desirable to place the animal on a different type of bedding until the area has healed.

Water Deprivation

Sometimes animals die of water deprivation even when ample water seems to be available. This may occur when (1) water is provided by a device with which the animal is not familiar or does not know how to operate, (2) water devices are placed too high or are otherwise inaccessible, particularly for small weanlings, (3) water is unpotable because of impurities or odors in the container or the water itself, or (4) automatic watering systems become plugged or jammed.

Table 10 provides an overview of the major infective and parasitic diseases seen in laboratory guinea pigs. Guinea pigs are highly susceptible to factors in the environment that lower their resistance to infection. Among these are poor sanitation, overcrowding, mixing of species, improper temperature and humidity control, inadequate diet (especially insufficient vitamin C), transportation, and experimental procedures.

DOSING TECHNIQUES

Before any dose may be administered, an animal must first be picked up and manipulated. Guinea pigs should be lifted by grasping the trunk with one hand while supporting the rear quarters with the other. Support is particularly important with adults and pregnant animals. Injured lungs may result if an animal is grasped too firmly over its back.

Oral Dosing (Gavage)

Guinea pigs can be stomach tubed using a technique similar to that for the rat. An assistant restrains the animal by grasping it around the shoulders and supporting the hindquarters to prevent undue struggling. A blunted 15-16-gauge hypodermic needle, polyethylene catheter (3–4 figure) or commerically manufactured dosing needle ("Popper tube") as used for rats, is introduced into the mouth through the interdental space and advanced gently into the esophagus. A small gag made from a solid plastic rod with a hole drilled centrally may be used to prevent the animal from biting a plastic catheter.

Subcutaneous Injection

The animal should be restrained by an assistant as described above, and a small area of skin on the flank tented by the operator. The needle is introduced into the raised skin,

Table 10   Some Common Infectious and Parasitic Diseases of the Guinea Pig

Name	Pathogenic agents	Symptoms—appearing singly or in various combinations	Gross lesions
Virus pneumonia	Virus	Acute—unthrifty, emaciated Latent—no change	Lungs
Pseudo tuberculosis	Bacterial—*Yersinia* or *Pasteurella pseudotuberculosis*	Acute—rapid breathing, rales, diarrhea, enlarged lymph nodes, emaciation, unthrifty Latent—no change (organisms may be recovered from throat)	Lungs, liver spleen show whitish, caseous abcesses
Bacterial pneumonia	*Bordetella bronchiseptica and Streptococcus pneumonia*	Acute—rales, discharge from nose, enlarged lymph nodes Latent—no change (organisms may be recovered from throat)	Lungs
Lymphadenitis	Bacterial—*Streptococcus pyogenes* Group C	Acute—gross swelling of lymph nodes in neck region; unthrifty, emaciation Latent—no change (organisms may be recovered from throat)	Lymph nodes, pericardium
Salmonellosis	Bacterial—*Salmonella typhimurium, Salmonella enteritidis*	Acute—slight diarrhea, unthrifty, emaciation Latent—no change (organisms may be recovered from feces)	Enlargement of gallbladder and liver
Wasting disease	Unknown (probably a virus)	Acute—inappetence, rapid loss of weight, unthrifty Latent—no change	None
Salivary gland virus	Cytomegalovirus	Acute—large eosinophillic intranuclear inclusion of the salivary gland ductal epithelium, loss of appetite Latent—none	Swollen glands

Scientific name	Common name	No. of legs (may be rudimentary)	Food	Remarks
Gyropus ovalis	Louse	6	Blood	Adults visible to naked eye
Gliricola porcelli	Louse	6	Blood	Adults visible to naked eye

Scientific name	Common name	Shape	Host tissue invaded	Remarks
Paraspidodera unicata	Round worms	long, narrow smooth body	Intestines	Eggs may be seen (microscopically) in feces. Adults may be seen by naked eye in feces
Two species: 1. *Emieria caviae* 2. *Balantidium caviae*	Coccidia	Spherical	Intestines	Eggs (oocysts) may be seen (microscopically) in feces

parallel to the body wall. The skin of the guinea pig is thicker than in smaller rodents and provides more resistance to needle passage, hence injection is easier if a short (0.5–1.0 in) 21- to 23-gauge needle is used.

Intradermal Injection

Intradermal injection carried out as described for rats. The thicker skin of the guinea pig makes the technique relatively easy in this species. As described previously, the presence of a small bleb of material indicates successful intradermal rather than subcutaneous injection.

Foot Pad Injection

The footpads are occasionally used as injection sites, particularly of material intended to act as an antigen for antisera preparation. The animal should be restrained by an assistant as described above and injection made into the large central pad of the foot. In view of the considerable swelling that often ensues, only one pad should be inoculated, so that the animal can avoid placing full weight on that limb. Since there is little evidence to suggest that foot pad inoculation of antigen results in any better antibody production than does inoculation at other sites, it is preferable to avoid using this technique.

Intraperitoneal Injection

A similar technique to that described in the rat and the mouse is used for intraperitoneal injection of guinea pigs. The animal should be restrained by a second individual. The operator extends one of the animal's legs and introduces the needle along the line of the thigh, into the center of the posterior quadrant of the abdomen.

Intramuscular Injection

As with other rodents, the anterior and posterior thigh are the sites most frequently used for intramuscular injection, although it is also possible to inject into the triceps muscles on the anterior aspect of the shoulder. To inject into the thigh, the animal should be restrained by an assistant as for intraperitoneal injection, and one leg held firmly by the operator. If the quadriceps muscles are to be used, they should be held between the thumb and forefinger and the needle introduced at right angles to the skin into the center of the muscle mass.

Intravenous Injection

Guinea pigs have few superficial veins; those which are reasonably accessible are the ear veins and the penile vein (in males). These veins are small and fragile, and hence intravenous injection is difficult in this species. In large (>500 g) guinea pigs, the ear veins should be used. The ear should first be swabbed with a small quantity of xylene to dilate the vessels, and the animal restrained by an assistant on a firm surface.

The ear should be held firmly at one edge, and a suitable vein selected. A very fine needle (29–30 gauge) should be used, and once positioned in the vein, the syringe can be steadied using the remaining fingers of the hand restraining the ear. Any movement of the animal during this procedure is likely to result in damage to the vein, and to avoid this it may be preferable to anesthetize the animal. Following successful venipuncture, the xylene should be removed from the ear using a wet swab.

Penile vein injections should always be carried out in anesthetized animals, since the procedure may cause considerable discomfort. The penis is extruded from beneath the inguinal skin by pressure at either side of the genital opening. The tip should then be grasped between the thumb and forefinger and the organ extended and rotated so that the dorsal penile vein lies uppermost. When introducing the needle, care should be taken to avoid damaging the fragile vein.

A second approach is to use the saphenous vein or the dorsolateral vein of the penis. A cut-down may be required for exposure of the saphenous vein. Guinea pig skin is tough, especially over the back, and subcutaneous injections require a degree of force.

COMMON TECHNIQUES

Blood Collection and Measuring Blood Flow and Blood Pressure

Obtaining blood samples from guinea pigs is almost as difficult as intravenous injections. Methods commonly employed include cutting the nail bed; puncture of the dorsal metatarsal vein of the marginal ear vein; puncture of the orbital sinus; vacuum-assisted bleeding of either the lateral marginal vein of the hind limb, or the lateral metatarsal vein, cardiac puncture; or via an indwelling cannula technique. Carbon dioxide anesthesia increase the yields of blood and serum particularly when exsanguinating the animal. A method of obtaining 3–6 ml of blood from the femoral artery has been described by Simpson et al. (1967) and Burnett et al. (1968).

Blood flow throught he spleen has been determined with xenon-133, based on the measurement of the rate of the disappearance of xenon-133 from the spleen. Similarly, uterine blood flow was measured near term and a technique for recording the blood pressure of fetal guinea pigs was described briefly by Davitaya and Nadirashvili (1971).

Guinea pigs lack readily accessible peripheral veins, having deeply placed vessels often covered by layers of fat. A small amount of blood can be collected from the orbital sinus or by clipping a toenail. Larger amounts of blood can be obtained from the femoral artery or vein or directly from the heart. Cardiac puncture is best carried out with the animal lightly anesthetized. The guinea pig can either be placed on its right side and the needle inserted at the site of the apex beat around the fourth intercostal space, or on its back and the needle inserted in the zyphoid area, aiming for the left ventricle. Cardiac punctures in the guinea pig, however, involve a significant element of risk.

Shaving and Tape Stripping

Two main techniques are common to most dermal toxicity studies performed in the guinea pig. These are shaving (for the removal of hair from an area that it is desired to apply test material to) and tape stripping (for the removal of the stratum corneum, or barrier layer, of the skin).

Shaving

The Oster Model A5 electric clippers with detachable blades are most commonly used to shave guinea pigs, rabbits, and rodents.

1. The guinea pig is restrained manually with sufficient downward pressure on the anterior (neck and shoulder) area and posterior (haunches and rump) area of the animal.
2. Initially, the Oster Model A5 electric clipper with blade size 10 is used. Size 10 cuts the hair to a length of approximately 1/16 in.

3. The clipper blade is held parallel to the animal's skin. Proceeding slowly, the hair is shaved against the grain of hair growth, giving the blade a chance to feed and cut. The skin of the animal is stretched to remove wrinkling, which both facilitates shaving and reduces the risk of cutting or tearing the skin.
4. An assistant, helping to restrain the animal with one hand, uses the other hand to guide the nozzle of a vacuum cleaner in front of the electric clipper to remove hair clippings during the shaving process. The hair which is collected in the vacuum is emptied into a plastic bag and disposed of as waste.
5. After the hair of the back and both flanks of the guinea pig have been clipped to a length of 1/16 in, the size 10 blade is removed and a size 40 blade is attached to cut the remaining hair to a length of approximately 1/130 inch following steps 3 and 4, above.
6. The blades should be changed periodically to reduce overheating and resultant skin irritation.

Each guinea pig is examined for any signs of abrasion/irritation which may have occurred during shaving. If abrasion is present, this should be recorded.

Blade Maintenance

Proper maintenance of cutting blades is essential. Cutting blades used in one toxicity study should never be used in another toxicity study unless they are first cleaned thoroughly with an appropriate solvent, such as acetone or ethanol. Once the blades are cleaned with the solvent and oiled with clipper oil, they may be used in a different toxicity study. If several toxicity studies are performed simultaneously, it is important to use a different blade set for each individual study in order to prevent cross-contamination. One blade set may be identified for shaving all control animal groups of different studies.

Cleaning Blades. Should cutting blades fail to cut, examine the cutting surfaces of the upper and lower cutting blade units. If hair or foreign matter is present, remove it; blades will not cut when hair or foreign matter is present. Brush the blades with the small brush supplied with the clippers to remove the hair and/or foreign matter build-up.

If more extensive cleaning is needed, the cutting blades should be detached from the clipper. Without separating, slide the upper blade approximately half way to either side. (Do not remove tension spring fastened to lower blade by two screws; doing so will disturb the cutting tension.) New blades or very dirty blades should be cleaned prior to use. This material will remove congealed preservatives from new blades and hard-to-remove foreign matter from used blades. Repeat the cleaning procedure by sliding the upper blade in the opposite direction. Wipe blades completely dry. If blades should separate, lift the spring with the fingertip just enough to slide the upper blade into position. Run the motor when reattaching the blade assembly. Apply a thin film of Oster oil and wipe excess oil from blade surfaces prior to use.

Oiling Blades. Apply oil several times during use to maintain a light film on the mating faces of the blades and the tension spring guide. Always wipe excess oil from blade surfaces prior to use.

Sharpening Blades. Dull blades, improper sharpening, and excessive tensioning (to force dull blades to cut) reduce cutting efficiency and can cause the clipper to heat, slow down, and reduce the motor and blade life. When cutting blades no longer cut smoothly and cleanly, sharpening is necessary.

Tape Stripping

Tape stripping (or denuding of the skin) is performed using a tacky transparent tape product such as 1-in wide Dermiclear (Johnson & Johnson Products, Inc.). After shaving, an assistant holds the animal while successive 10-in lengths of tape are employed. Successive portions of the length of tape are pressed firmly over the region of skin from which it is desired to remove the outer layer of the epidermis. This is repeated until the skin is observed to become glossy in appearance.

The permeability of guinea pig skin is generally closer to that of the human than either the rabbit or rat (Tregear, 1966).

Anesthesia

Guinea pigs are among the most difficult rodents in which to achieve safe and effective anesthesia, and they are generally considered poor risks for it. Their response to many injectable anesthetics is very variable and postanesthetic complications such as respiratory infections, digestive disturbances and generalized depression and inappetance are frequently seen. Many of these problems can be avoided by careful selection of anesthetic agents and a high standard of intra- and postoperative nursing care. At times, guinea pigs may exhibit a peculiar squirming movement during administration of volatile anesthetics. This movement does not signify return to consciousness, and caution should be exercised in administering additional anesthetic (Flecknell, 1987).

Preanesthetic Medication

Guinea pigs are nonaggressive animals that are generally easy to handle and restrain. When frightened they run around their cage at high speed, making safe handling difficult. It is important to approach guinea pigs quietly and handle them gently but firmly. They should be picked up around the shoulders and thorax and the hindquarters supported as they are lifted clear of their cage. Intramuscular or intraperitoneal injection of anesthetic agents can then be carried out. Preanesthetic medication is therefore not usually required, but if an anesthetic is to be administered by intravenous injection into an ear vein, initial sedation is advantageous.

The following drugs can be used to produce sedation and restraint:

1. Fentanyl/fluanisone (1 ml/kg im) will produce restraint, sedation, and sufficient analgesia for minor procedures such as skin biopsy.
2. Diazepam (5 mg/kg ip) produces heavy sedation and immobility, but no analgesia. The animal is easily roused by painful stimuli or other disturbances such as noise. This agent can be useful in providing sufficient sedation to allow local anesthetic techniques to be used humanely.
3. Ketamine (100 mg/kg im) immobilizes guinea pigs but does not produce good analgesia.
4. Alphaxalone/alphadolone (40 mg/kg im) produces deep sedation but requires a large volume of drug to be injected (2–3 ml for an adult guinea pig).
5. Atropine (0.05 mg/kg sc) should be administered prior to any general anesthetic to minimize the volume of bronchial and salivary secretions. It is particularly useful in guinea pigs because of their relatively narrow airways, which are prone to obstruction.

General Anesthesia

Intravenous administration of anesthetics is difficult to achieve in guinea pigs and drugs are usually administered by the intraperitoneal, subcutaneous, or intramuscular routes. The animals should be carefully weighed and dose rates calculated accurately.

The anesthetic combination of choice is fentanyl/fluanisone together with diazepam or midazolam. This combination provides surgical anesthesia with good muscle relaxation lasting about 45 min. If a longer period of anesthesia is required, further doses can be given (approximately 0.5 ml/kg im every 20–30 min). Following the completion of surgery, the anesthesia can be reversed using naloxone (0.1 mg/kg iv) or buprenorphine (0.1 mg/kg iv).

An effective alternative is to administer ketamine (40 mg/kg ip) and xylazine (5 mg/kg ip). This combination provides about 30 min of surgical anesthesia, although the level of analgesia may be insufficient for major surgery in some animals.

Alphaxalone/alphadolone produces only light surgical anesthesia even when administered by the iv route. If additional anesthetic is administered, severe respiratory depression frequently ensues.

If sodium pentabarbitol is to be used, this is best administered at a dose of 25 mg/kg ip to sedate and immobilize the animal and anesthesia should then be deepened using a volatile agent such as methoxyflurane. Use of the higher dose rates of pentobarbitone (37 mg/kg ip) which are needed to produce surgical anesthesia are frequently associated with an unacceptably high mortality.

Induction of anesthesia by an inhalational agent can be either by use of an anesthetic chamber or administration via a small face mask. Following induction, it is usually most convenient to maintain anesthesia using a face mask, since endotracheal intubation is an extremely difficult technique to carry out in guinea pigs.

Methoxyflurane is the volatile anesthetic of choice in guinea pigs as it has a wide margin of safety and is nonirritant. Holothane can be used successfully, but it can produce profound hypotension even at normal maintenance concentrations. Ether is unsuitable for use in guinea pigs, since it is highly irritant to their respiratory tract, producing increased bronchial secretions that tend to occlude the narrow airways. In addition, bronchospasm may be produced during induction of anesthesia with ether.

Anesthetic Management

Care must be taken to prevent the development of hypothermia. Postoperative recovery is aided by administering 10–15 ml of warmed dextrose-saline (0–18% saline, 4% dextrose) sc to correct any fluid deficiency. A warm (25–30°C) recovery area should be provided and the animal given additional subcutaneous fluid for the next few days if its appetite is depressed.

Breeding

Generally, guinea pigs should be bred in the laboratory only if such breeding represents an integral part of the study. This usually means only for reproduction and developmental toxicology studies, for which the guinea pig is an infrequent subject.

Any breeding stock should be obtained from reliable sources. Soon after weaning, any offspring for follow-on generations should be quarantined and placed in the breeding quarters early in order to avoid any breeding setback due to environmental changes.

Puberty in the females may occur in 4–5 weeks; they weigh about 250–400 g at puberty. The males mature at about 8–10 weeks, weighing about 400–600 g. The first mating, however, should be done around 12 weeks of age, when the female and male weigh about 450 and 500 g, respectively. The guinea pig experiences postpartum estrus, and mating at this time will considerably reduce the interval between litters. The gestation period varies between 59 and 72 days, with an average ot 63 days. The weight of the guinea pig at birth depends on the nutritional status of the sow and the number of pups in the litter. For single births, the weight may be 150 g; however, for three to four youngsters, the weight is generally between 85 and 90 g. If the live birth weight is below average, the chances of survival are generally very poor. There are usually three to four litters per gestation. Development of young guinea pigs is rapid; they gain 3–5 g of weight per day for the first 2 months. Mature adults may weight 700–750 g at 5 months of age.

Nonintensive Method

In this procedure, the individual sows (five to 10 per boar) may be isolated throughout their breeding span (2 years). The method is wasteful of space, and generally the annual number of offspring is lower (12 per sow per year). However, it has the advantage of allowing the keeping of correct breeding records, and it is excellent for inbreeding and disease control.

Communal Farrowing

In this system of breeding, the heavily pregnant sows are removed from mating pens and allowed to litter and to rear the young communally. When the youngsters are 180 g in weight, the mothers are removed and returned to mating pens. The preferred system is to have one boar and up to 20 sows; the boar can be rotated every week if desired. Such a system yields an average of seven litters per 2-year life span.

Intensive System

Monogamous or polygamous systems can be followed. Monogamous systems are expensive, since a large number of boars have to be maintained, and the yields are lower. In the polygamous system, the yields may be as high as 14–16 young per sow per year.

DEVELOPMENTAL TOXICITY

Guinea pigs have characteristics which make them unlike any of the other species commonly used for developmental toxicity studies (rabbits, rats, and mice). Their endocrine control of reproduction is similar to that of the human even to its trimester characteristics, and yet pregnancy is preceded by estrus. The placenta is capable of the full range of endocrine activity, but it is labyrinthine and its functions are supplemented by a yolk sac exposed to uterine secretions. Estrus, ovulation, and fertilization can be accurately timed, as with most rodents, and data are available defining or describing most of the aspects of gestation and embryonic development. For example, normal resorption activity involves the loss of approximately 5.8–6.3% of implanted embryos as determined by differences between the number of implantation sites and functioning corpora lutea (Hoar and King, 1967; Hoar, 1969). Normal embryonic development of the guinea pig through the twenty-sixth day of gestation has been described by Scott (1937). The process of ossification of the entire skeleton of the guinea pig has been detailed by Petri (1935).

Structural malformations have been induced in guinea pigs in a variety of ways. Thalidomide given ip as a saline suspension, by gavage, or in dry feed for three consecutive generations produced a "conspicuous number of cleft palates and deformities of the outer ear and shortened limbs" as well as reducing the litter size, increasing prenatal deaths, and producing smaller individual offspring, particularly from those mothers fed thalidomide in the diet (Arbab-Zadeh, 1965).

Trypan blue (an azo dye) produces deleterious effects in the fetus. Pregnant guinea pigs received a single subcutaneous injection of 2 ml of 1% trypan on a single day during the period of days 6–13 of gestation and their offspring were recovered on day 30 of gestation or allowed to deliver. The response seen at 30 days included an increased resorption rate, growth retardation, and gross abnormalities with the maximum incidence of abnormalities (57%) resulting from injection on day 11. Every embryo from treated females was affected by the dye, with the response varying from shorter crown-rump length to gross abnormalities. The malformations found included: cyst of the anterior thoracic wall (49.3%), spina bifida (33.8%), microphthalmia (5.6%), hydrocephaly (4.2%), edema (2.8%), meningocele (1.4%), and assorted other defects (2.8%). Fifty percent of the retarded and/or malformed embryos displayed a posterior cleft palate. Treated females going to term had a reduced litter size, their offspring displaying only those abnormalities (5.3%) which were compatible with life (Hoar and Salem, 1961).

Hypervitaminosis A produces malformations in the guinea pig. Giroud and Martinet (1959a,b) gave pregnant guinea pigs 50,000 IU of vitamin A on days 12–14 of gestation and reported an increased number of spontaneous abortions, resorptions, and a case of mandibular fissure combined with a bifid tongue. Robens (1970) gave guinea pigs 200,000 USP units/kg of vitamin A palmitate as a single dose on selected days (14–20) during organogenesis. Most of the females were allowed to deliver, although some were terminated at 50 days of gestation. Multiple structural defects, involving primarily the head region, were seen in 60.8% of offspring born following maternal treatment on days 14–16. Missing coccygeal vertebrae and agnathia (38.5% of offspring) were seen following treatment on day 17 of gestation. Limb defects (37.2%) were the most frequent abnormalities resulting from treatment on days 18–20, whereas only one of 226 control offspring was abnormal.

Edwards (1967, 1969a,b) examined effects of hyperthermia applied early during gestation on reproduction and fetal development in guinea pigs. He noted that resorptions appeared to be most common following hyperthermia on about days 11–15, whereas abortions, occurring at a mean of 32.4 4.85 days of gestation, appeared most frequently (83%) following hypothermia on days 11–18. Of 251 offspring recovered at delivery, the following malformations were noted: microencephaly (41%), hypoplastic digits (13%), exomphalos (7%), talipes (4%), hypoplastic incisors (4%), cataract (3%), renal agenesis (2%), and amyoplasia (2%). A detailed evaluation of prenatal retardation of brain growth at various times during gestation was also conducted by Edwards (1969c). The incidence of reduced brain weight and microencephaly increased most markedly following hyperthermia for 4 or 8 days during days 15–32 of gestation. Following 2 successive days of hyperthermia, the effects were most marked on days 20–23 of gestation.

COMMON PROTOCOLS

As presented in Table 11 the guinea pig is used in a wide variety of studies in toxicology. The most common are the various sensitization and photosensitization studies. The rationale for the use of guinea pigs in these designs has previously been reviewed (Gad and Chengelis, 1988). Typical or prototype protocols for these more common designs are as follows.

Table 11 Dosage Tables for Pharmaceuticals Commonly Used in Guinea Pigs

Antibiotics	
penicillin—do not administer.	
cephaloridine—25 mg/kg IM daily.	
sulfamethazine—333 mg/liter drinking water for 300 gram animal.	
tetracycline—255 mg/liter drinking water for 300 gram animal.	
Antihistamines	
diphenhydramine (Benadryl)	5.0 mg/kg sc
tripelennamine	5.0 mg/kg po or im
Tranquilizers	
chlorpromazine	0.5 mg/kg im
promazine HCl	0.5–1.0 mg/kg im
meprobamate	100 mg/kg im
Anesthetics	
pentobarbitol sodium	30 mg/kg iv; 40 mg/kg ip
thiopental sodium	20 mg/kg iv; 55 mg/kg ip
ketamine	22–44 mg/kg im
droperidol-fentanyl	0.66–0.88 mg/kg im
urethane	1,500 mg/kg ip
Analgesics	
aspirin	269 mg/kg ip
meperidine	2 mg/kg im
Miscellaneous	
atropine	0.05 mg/kg sc, im
heparin	5 mg/kg iv

Modified Buehler Procedure

The modified Buehler procedure is a closed patch procedure for evaluating test substances for potential delayed contact dermal sensitization in guinea pigs. The procedure, based on that described by Buehler (1965), is practical for test substances that cannot be evaluated by the traditional intradermal injection procedure of Landsteiner and Jacobs or by the guinea pig maximization test (GMPT) for skin sensitization testing. The closed patch procedure is performed when a test substance either is highly irritating to the skin by the intradermal injection route of exposure or it cannot be dissolved or suspended in a form allowing injection. It is also the method of choice for some companies. This procedure, which is one version of the Buehler test, complies with the test standards set forth in the Toxic Substances Control Act (TSCA) and other regulatory test rules. There are other versions which also comply.

Animals

1. Young albino female Hartley strain guinea pigs, weighing between 300 and 400 g, are currently the standard animals used. Studies sponsored by the Charles River Laboratories have shown that their hairless guinea pigs are just as responsive, however.

2. Although several proposed test rules suggest the use of male guinea pigs, the female sex is preferred because the aggressive social behavior of males may result in considerable skin damage that might interfere with the interpretation of challenge reactions. This concern occurs because animals are commonly group housed (Marzulli and Maibach, 1983).

3. Animals that show poor growth or are ill in any way are not usd, since illness can markedly decrease the response. Animals with skin marked or scarred from fighting are avoided. The guinea pigs are observed for at least 2 weeks prior to test to detect any illness before starting a study.

4. The guinea pigs are identified by a cage card and marking pen or any other suitable method. There is no regulatory requirement, however, for the identification of individual animals.

5. The guinea pigs are randomly assigned to test and negative control groups consisting of at least 15 and six animals each, respectively. If a pretest group is necessary, as many animals as needed for that group are randomized also.

Pretest Screen

1. If practical, the dermal irritation threshold concentration should be established for the test substance prior to the first induction application. A concentration of the test substance that produces minimal or no irritation (erythema and/or edema formation) is determined. The highest concentration that produces no irritation is preferred for the dermal sensitization study challenge dose.

2. Those animals randomly assigned to the pretest group are used.

3. Each animal is prepared by clipping a 1-in square area of hair from the left upper flank using a small animal clipper with a size 40 blade.

4. The test substance is diluted, emulsified, or suspended in a suitable vehicle. Vehicles are selected on the basis of their solubilizing capacity for the test substance and on their ability to penetrate the skin.

5. Different concentrations of the test substance are tested on the pretest group of guinea pigs; a few animals are used for each concentration tested.

6. A volume of 0.5 ml is applied to a patch consisting of a cotton pad (1 in × 1 in) occluded with impermeable surgical tape, or placed in a Hilltop-style occlusive "chamber."

7. The patch is applied to the shaved left flank of a guinea pig. The patch is held firmly in place for 24 hr by wrapping the trunk of the animal with a 3-in wide elastic bandage. A 2-in wide strip of tape is used to line the center adhesive side of the bandage in order to prevent skin damage from the adhesive.

8. After 24 hrs of exposure, the wrappings and patches are removed.

9. Observations of skin reactions (erythema and/or edema formation) are recorded 48 hrs after application.

10. A judgment is made as to which concentration will be used for the dermal sensitization study based on the dermal irritation data which have been collected. The highest concentration that produces minimal or no dermal irritation is selected.

Induction Phase

1. Test group and control group guinea pigs are weighed at the beginning of the study and weekly thereafter.

2. Test control group guinea pigs are shaved as described earlier.

3. If the test substance is a liquid (solution, suspension, or emulsion), a volume of 0.5

Table 12 Evaluation of Skin Reactions

Skin reaction	value
Erythema and eschar formation:	
no erythema	0
very slight erythema (barely perceptible)	1
well-defined erythema	2
moderate to severe erythema	3
severe erythema (beet redness) to slight eschar formation (injuries in-depth)	4
necrosis (death of tissue)	+N
eschar (sloughing)	+E
Edema formation:	
no edema	0
very slight edema (barely perceptible)	1
slight edema (edges of area well-defined by definite raising)	2
moderate edema (raised approximately 1 millimeter)	3
severe edema (raised more than 1 millimeter and extending beyond the area of exposure)	4

Source: Draize (1959).

ml of the highest concentration found to be nonirritating in a suitable vehicle (as determined in the pretest portion of this procedure) is applied to a patch consisting of a cotton pad (1 in × 1 in) occluded with impermeable surgical tape. If the test substance is a solid or semisolid, 0.5 g* is applied. If the test substance is a fabric, a 1-in square is moistened with 0.5 ml of physiological saline before application.

4. The first induction patch is applied to the clipped left flank of each test group guinea pig. The patch is held firmly in place for 24 hr by wrapping the trunk of each animal with a 3-in wide elastic bandage. A 2-in wide strip of tape is used to line the center adhesive side of the bandage in order to prevent skin damage from the adhesive. A 2-in length of athletic adhesive tape is placed over the bandage wrap as a precautionary measure to prevent unraveling.

5. After 24 hr of exposure, the wrappings and patches are removed and disposed of in a plastic bag.

6. Each dermal reaction, if any, is scored on the basis of previously designated values for erythema and edema formation such as the Draize scale (Draize et al., 1959; see Table 12). Observations are made 48 hrs after initiation of the first induction application. Resulting dermal irritation scores are recorded.

7. After the initial induction application, subsequent induction applications (two to nine) are made on alternate days (3 times weekly) until a total of 10 treatments has been administered. Each of these patches is removed after 6 hrs of exposure. It should be noted that some investigators use a modification which calls for one application per week for 3 weeks.

---

*When the test substance is in flake, granule, powder, or other particulate form, the weight of the test substance that has a volume of 0.5 ml (after compacting as much as possible without crushing or altering the individual particles, such as by tapping the measuring container) is used whenever this volume weighs less than 0.5 g.

8. Observations are made 24 and 48 hrs after initiation of each subsequent induction application. Dermal scores of the remaining nine induction applications are recorded.

9. Clipping the hair from the left flank induction sites of test group animals and corresponding sites on negative control group animals is performed just prior to each subsequent induction application. Only the test group guinea pigs receive the induction applications.

Challenge Phase

1. Fourteen days after the tenth induction application, all 10 test group and three of six control group guinea pigs are prepared for challenge application by clipping a 1-in square of hair from the right side (the side opposite that which was clipped during the induction phase).

2. A challenge dose, using freshly prepared test substance (solution, suspension, emulsion, semisolid, solid, or fabric), is applied topically to the right side (which had remained untreated during the induction application) of test group animals. The left side, which had previously received induction applications, is not challenge dosed.

3. The concentration of the challenge dose is the same as that used for the first induction application. (It must be a concentration that does not produce dermal irritation after one 24-hr application.)

4. Each of three negative control group guinea pigs is challenge dosed on the right flank at approximately the same time that the test group guinea pigs are challenge dosed. This is, in effect, a check for unexpected primary irritation.

5. All patches are held in contact with the skin for 24 hrs before removal.

6. The skin sites are evaluated using the previously selected scoring system for erythema and edema formation, such as that presented in Table 12. Observations are made 48, 72, and 96 hr after initiation of the challenge application and the skin reactions are recorded.

Rechallenge Phase

1. If the test substance is judged a nonsensitizing agent after the first challenge application, or causes dermal sensitization in only a few animals, or causes dermal reactions that are weak or questionable, then a second and final challenge application will be performed on each test animal 7 days after the initiation of the first challenge dose.

2. Controls from the first challenge application are not rechallenged because they have been exposed to the test substance and are no longer true negative controls. The three remaining naive control group animals (not used for the first challenge) are challenged for comparison to the test group animals.

3. The procedure used for the first challenge applications will be used for the second challenge application (including reclipping, patching method, and duration of exposure). Either the same concentration or a new concentration (higher or lower) of test substance may be used, depending on the results of the first challenge. Observations are made 48, 72, and 96 hr after initiation of the rechallenge application and skin reactions are recorded.

4. When a rechallenge application is performed, the data from both challenges are compared. If neither challenge produces a positive dermal reaction, the classification of the test substance is based on both challenge applications. If one challenge application (whether it is the first or second) produces a greater number of positive dermal reactions than the other, the classification of the test substance is based on the challenge with the most positive responses.

5. Two or more unequivocally positive responses in a group of 15 animals should be considered significant. A negative, equivocal, or single response probably assures that a substance is not a strong sensitizer, although this is best confirmed by further testing with human subjects (NAS, 1977).

Interpretation of Results

1. Judgment concerning the presence of absence of sensitization is made for each animal. The judgment is made by comparing the test animal's challenge responses to its first induction treatment response as well as to those challenge responses of negative control animals.

2. Challenge reactions to the test substance that are stronger than challenge reactions to negative controls, or to those seen after the initial induction application should be suspected as results of sensitization (NAS, 1977). A reaction that occurs at 48 hr, but resolves by 72 hr or 96 hr, should be considered a positive response as long as it is stronger than that which is displayed by controls at the same time interval.

Strengths and Weaknesses

There are a number of both advantages and disadvantages to the Buehler methodology, which has been in use for over 20 years. The relative importance and merits of each depend on the intended use of the material. The four advantages are:

1. Virtually no false positives (in fact, in the experience of the author, when the pretest is properly conducted, there are no false positives), compared to human experience, are generated by test.
2. The techniques involved are easy to learn and very reproducible.
3. The Buehler-style test does not overpredict the potency of sensitizers. That is, materials which are identified as sensitizers are truly classified as very strong, weak, or in between—not all (or nearly all) as very strong.
4. There is a large database in existence for the Buehler-style test. Unfortunately, the vast majority is not in the published literature.

Likewise, there are three disadvantages associated with the Buehler-style test.

1. The test gives a high rate of false negatives for weak sensitizers and a detectable rate of false negatives for moderate sensitizers. That is, the method is somewhat in-sensitive—particularly if techniques for occlusive wrapping are inadequate.
2. The test takes a long time to complete. If animals are on-hand when started, the test is 5–6 weeks long. As few laboratories keep a "pool" of guinea pigs on-hand (especially as they are the most expensive of the common lab species), the usual case is that 8–10 weeks is the minimum time required to get an answer from this test.
3. The test uses a relatively large amount of test material. In the normal acute "battery," the guinea pig test systems use more material than any other test systems unless an acute inhalation study is included. With 10 induction applications, this is particularly true for the Buehler-style test.

Guinea Pig Maximization Test

The guinea pig maximization test (GPMT) was developed by Magnusson and Kligman (1969, 1970, 1975) and is considered a highly sensitive procedure for evaluating test substances for potential dermal sensitization.

Animals

1. Young adult female guinea pigs weighing between 250–350 g at the initiation of the study are used.

2. Animals that show poor growth or are ill in any way are not used, since illness may markedly decrease the response. Animals with skin marked or scarred from fighting are avoided. The guinea pigs are observed for at least 2 weeks to detect any illness before starting a study.

3. The guinea pigs are randomly assigned to two groups: (1) a test group consisting of 15 animals, and (2) a control group consisting of six animals. If a pretest group is necessary, as many animals as needed for that group also are randomized.

4. Test and control group guinea pigs are weighed 1 week prior to dosing (day 7), on the day of dosing (day 0), and weekly thereafter.

Pretest

1. Several animals are used to pretest the test substance and vehicles to determine the topical dermal irritation threshold concentration.

2. These animals are shaved on the left flank, to which is applied a 2 × 2 cm filter paper patch which contains 0.1 ml of the test concentration.

3. The trunks of the animals are wrapped for 24 hr with a 3-in wide elastic bandage to hold the patch in contact with the skin.

4. Wrappings are removed after the 24 hr exposure and, based on skin reactions at 48 hr, a concentration of the test substance to be used on the test is determined. Dermal irritation values are recorded for future reference.

5. In addition, several guinea pigs are utilized to determine a concentration (generally between 1 and 5%) of test substance in vehicle and in Freund's Complete Adjuvant (FCA) emulsion that can be injected id (intradermally) without eliciting a strong local or systemic toxic reaction.

6. The hair is clipped in an area of approximately 4 × 6 cm from the upper shoulder region of these animals.

7. Several concentrations of the test substance (ranging between 1 and 5%) can be injected in the same animal to compare local dermal reactions produced by the different concentrations.

8. However, if sytemic toxicity is suspected, then each concentration should be tested in separate animals to determine local and systemic effects.

9. The dermal reactions (erythema, edema and diameter) are recorded 24 hr after the id injections.

Induction Stage 1 (Day 0)

1. The hair in an area of 4 × 6 cm is clipped from the shoulder region of each test and control group guinea pig on day 0.

2. Three pairs of intradermal (id) injections are made with a glass 1-ml tuberculin syringe with a 26-gauge needle, each pair flanking the dorsal midline.

3. The three pairs of id injections for test group animals are as follows:

    a. 0.1 ml test substance in appropriate vehicle
    b. 0.1 ml FCA emulsion alone
    c. 0.1 ml test substance in FCA emulsion

4. The three pairs of id injections for control group animals are as follows:

    a. 0.1 ml vehicle alone
    b. 0.1 FCA emulsion alone
    c. 0.1 ml vehicle in FCA emulsion

5. Injections (a) and (b) in the above two steps are given close to each other and nearest the head; injection (c) is given most posteriorly.

6. The date, time, and initials of those individuals performing the id injections are recorded.

7. Immediately before injection, an emulsion is prepared by blending commercial FCA with an equal volume of house distilled water or other solvent as appropriate.

    a. Water-soluble test materials are dissolved in the water phase prior to emulsification.
    b. Oil-soluble or water-insoluble materials are dissolved or suspended in FCA prior to adding water.
    c. Paraffin oil, peanut oil, or propylene glycol can be used for dissolving or suspending water-insoluble materials.
    d. A homogenizer is used to emulsify the FCA alone and the test substance in either FCA or vehicle prior to the id injections.
    e. The concentration of the test substance for id injections is adjusted to the highest level that can be well tolerated locally and generally.

8. The adjuvant injection infiltration sometimes causes ulceration, especially when the injection is superficial. This ulceration lasts several weeks. These lesions are undesirable but do not invalidate the test results except for lowering the threshold level for skin irritation.

Induction Stage 2 (Day 7)

1. Test substance preparation:

    a. The concentration of the test substance is adjusted to the highest level that can be well tolerated.
    b. If the test substance is an irritant, a concentration is chosen that causes a weak to moderate inflammation (as determined by the pretest).
    c. Solids are micronized or reduced to a fine powder and then suspended in a vehicle, such as petrolatum or propylene glycol.
    d. Water- and oil-soluble test substances are dissolved in an appropriate vehicle.
    e. Liquid materials are applied as such, or diluted if necessary.

2. The same area over the shoulder region that received id injections on day 0 is again shaved on both test and control guinea pigs.

3. A volume of 0.3 ml of a mildly irritating concentration (if possible) of the test substance (determined by the pretest) is spread over a 1 × 2 in filter paper patch in a thick, even layer.

4. The patch is occluded with surgical tape and then is secured to test group animals with an elastic bandage, which is wrapped around the torso of each test group animal.

5. The control group animals are exposed to 0.3 ml of 100% vehicle using the same procedure.

6. The date, time, and initials of those individuals performing the second induction should be recorded.

7. The dressings of both groups are left in place for 48 hr before removal.

Challenge Stage (Day 21)

1. An area of hair (1.5 × 1.5 in) on both flanks of the guinea pigs (15 test and three controls) is shaved.

2. A 1 × 1 in patch with a nonirritating concentration of test substance in vehicle (as determined by the pretest) is applied to the left flank and a 1 × 1 in patch with 100% vehicle is applied to the right flank.

3. The torso of each guinea pig is wrapped in an elastic bandage to secure the patches for 24 hr.

4. The date, time, and initials of those individuals performing the challenge dose are recorded.

5. The patches are removed 24 hr after application.

Rechallenge (Day 28)

1. If the first challenge application of test substance does not cause dermal sensitization, or causes dermal sensitization in only a few animals, or causes dermal reactions that are weak or questionable, then a second challenge application of test substance to the 15 test group guinea pigs should be conducted on day 28 (week after the first challenge). The three remaining naive control group animals (not used for the first challenge) are challenged for comparison to the test group animals.

2. The three negative control group animals used on day 21 will not be rechallenged. These animals will be discontinued from the study because they were exposed to the test substance during the first challenge and are no longer negative controls.

3. A 1 × 1 in patch with a nonirritating concentration of test substance in vehicle is applied to the right flank of test and control group animals. The left flanks are not dosed.

4. The date, time, and initials of those individuals performing the rechallenge dose should be recorded.

5. Steps 3 and 5 are followed as for challenge stage (day 21).

Observations—Challenge and/or Rechallenge Readings

1. Twenty-one hours after removing the patch, the challenge area on each flank is cleaned and shaved, if necessary.

2. Twenty-four hours after removing the patch, the first reading of dermal reactions is taken.

3. The dermal reactions are scored on a 4-point scale:

    0—No reaction
    1—Scattered and mild redness
    2—Moderate and diffuse redness
    3—Intense redness and swelling

4. Forty-eight hours after removing the patch, the second reading is taken and the scores are recorded.

Interpretation of Results

1. Both the intensity and duration of the test responses to the test substance and the vehicle are evaluated.

2. The important statistic in the GPMT is the frequency of sensitization and not the intensity of challenge responses. A value of 1 is considered just as positive as a value of 3 (as long as the values for controls are zero).

3. The test agent is a sensitizer if the challenge reactions in the test group clearly outweigh those in the control group. A reaction that occurs at 24 hr but resolves by 48 hr after removal of patches, should be considered a positive response, as long as it is stronger than that which is displayed by controls. The sensitization rate (% of positive responders) is based on the greatest number of animals showing a positive response, whether it is from the 24-hr data or the 48-hr data after removal of patches.

4. When a second challenge application is performed, the data from both challenges are compared. If neither challenge produces a positive dermal reaction, the classification of the test substance is based on both challenge applications. If one challenge application (whether it is the first or second) produced a greater number of positive dermal reactions than the other, the classification of the test substance is based on the challenge with the most positive responses.

5. Under the classification scheme of Kligman (1966) (see Table 13) the test substance is assigned to 1 of 5 classes, according to the percentage of animals sensitized, ranging from a weak grade I to an extreme grade V.

The advantages and disadvantages of the GPMT can be summarized as follows. First, the advantages:

1. The test system is sensitive and effectively detects weak sensitizers. It has a low false-negative rate.
2. If properly conducted, there are no false positives—that is, materials which are identified as potential sensitizers will act as such at some incidence level in humans.
3. There is a large database available on the evaluation of compounds in this test system, and many people are familiar with the test system.

The disadvantages, meanwhile are:

1. The test system is sensitive; it overpredicts potency for many sensitizers. There is no real differentiation between weak, moderate, and strong sensitizers; virtually all positive test results identify a material as strong.
2. The techniques involved (particularly the intradermal injections) are not easy. Some regulatory officials have estimated that as many as 35% of the laboratories which try cannot master the system to get it to work reproducibly.

Table 13 Sensitization Severity Grading Based on Incidence of Positive Responses

Sensitization rate (%)	Grade	Classification
0– 8	I	Weak
9– 28	II	Mild
29– 64	III	Moderate
65– 80	IV	Strong
81–100	V	Extreme

Source: Kligman (1966).

3. The test, though not as long as the Buehler-style test, still takes a minimum of 4 weeks to produce an answer.
4. The test uses a significant amount of test material.
5. One cannot evaluate fibers or other materials which cannot be injected (such as either solids which cannot be finely ground and/or suspended, or which are highly irritating or toxic by the iv route).
6. The irritation pretest is critical. Failure to detect irritation in this small group of animals does not guarantee against irritation in test animals at challenge.

Split Adjuvant Test

The guinea pig split adjuvant dermal sensitization procedure for detecting contact allergenicity is based on that developed by Maguire (1967, 1972, 1973a, b, 1975), and is sensitive and effective for the detection of substance and products with weak allergic potential and will serve as a useful alternative for testing materials that cannot be injected intradermally (e.g., fabrics, nonsoluble solids, and extremely irritating or toxic materials). A concise outline of the split adjuvant technique has been published (Klecak, 1983).

Animals

1. Young adult female guinea pigs weighing between 250 and 350 g at the initiation of the study are used.
2. Animals that show poor growth or are ill in any way are not used, since illness markedly decreases the response. Animals with skin marked or scarred from fighting are avoided. The guinea pigs are observed for at least 2 weeks to detect any illness before starting a study.
3. The guinea pigs are randomly assigned to two groups: (1) a test group consisting of 10 animals; and (2) a control group consisting of six animals. If a pretest group is necessary, as many animals as needed for that group also are randomized.
4. Test and control group guinea pigs are weighed and the weights are recorded 1 week prior to dosing (day 7), on the day of dosing (day 0), and weekly thereafter.

Pretest

1. Several animals are used to pretest the test substance and vehicles to determine the dermal irritation threshold concentration.
2. These animals are shaved on the left flank (2 × 2 cm).
3. Then 0.2 ml of ointment (semisolid) or 0.1 ml of liquid is spread onto a 1.5 × 1.5 cm Whatman No. 3 filter paper patch, which is occluded on the opposite side with surgical tape.

    a. Solid test substances are micronized or reduced to a fine powder and then suspended in a vehicle, such as petrolatum or propylene glycol.
    b. Water- and oil-soluble test substances are dissolved in an appropriate vehicle.
    c. Liquid test substances are applied as such (100%), or diluted if necessary.

4. The pretest patch is then applied to the left flank. The trunk of each animal is wrapped for 24 hr with a 3-in-wide elastic bandage to hold the patch in contact with the skin.
5. Wrappings are removed after 24 hr of exposure. Based on skin reactions at 48 hr, a concentration of the test substance to be used on test is determined. Dermal irritation values are recorded for later reference.

Induction Stage

The date, time, and initials of those individuals performing the induction applications should be recorded.

Day 0

1. The hair in an area 1 × 1 in is clipped behind the shoulder girdle of each test and control group guinea pig.

2. Dry ice is applied for 5 sec to the skin site of each test and control animal. Dry ice is used only for the day 0 induction application.

3. Then 0.2 ml of ointment (semisolid) or 0.1 ml of liquid is spread onto a 0.5 × 0.5 in Whatman No. 3 filter paper patch, which is occluded on the opposite side with surgical tape.

   a. The test substance is tested at a concentration that is minimally irritating (if possible), as determined by the pretest.
   b. If the substance is mixed in petrolatum or ointment, 0.2 ml is dispensed onto the patch.
   c. In the case of liquids, 0.1 ml is used.
   d. If a fabric is to be tested, a 1.5 × 1.5 cm sample is cut, moistened with 0.2 ml of physiological saline, and then is applied under a filter paper patch.

4. Control group animals are dosed with vehicle only, not test substance.

5. The trunk of each animal is wrapped for 48 hr with a 3-inch-wide elastic bandage to hold the patch in contact with the skin.

Day 2

1. The wrapping and patch is removed from each test and control group animal 48 hr after the initial induction application.

2. A fresh patch is applied to the same site using the same procedure as described for induction day 0 (without dry ice). Test group animals receive test substance in vehicle, and control group animals receive vehicle alone for a 48-hr period.

Day 4

1. The wrapping and patch is removed from each test and control group animal 48 hr after the application of the day 2 induction patch.

2. An emulsion of FCA emulsion is prepared by blending commercial FCA with an equal volume of house distilled water.

3. Two volumes of 0.1 ml of FCA emulsion are injected id into the induction site of each test and each control group animal with a glass 1-ml tuberculin syringe and a 26-gauge needle. These two injections flank the dorsal midline.

4. A fresh patch is applied to the same site using the same procedure as described on induction day 2. Test group animals receive test substance in vehicle, and control group animals receive vehicle alone for a 48-hr period.

Day 6

The wrapping and patch are removed from each test and control group animal 48 hr after the application of the day 4 induction patch.

Day 7

A fresh patch is applied to the induction site using the same procedure as described on induction day 2. Test group animals receive test substance in vehicle, and control group animals receive vehicle alone for a 48-hr period.

Day 9
The wrapping and patch are removed from each test and control group animal 48 hr after the application of the day 7 induction patch.

Challenge Stage

Day 21
1. An area of hair (1 × 1 in) on both flanks of the guinea pigs (10 test and three controls) is shaved.
2. A 0.5 × 0.5 in filter paper patch with the highest nonirritating concentration of test substance in vehicle (as determined by the pretest) is applied to the left flank and 1.5 × 1.5 cm patch with 100% vehicle is applied to the right flank.

   a. If the test substance is liquid, 0.1 ml is applied to the patch.
   b. If the test substance is mixed in petroleum or ointment, 0.2 ml is dispensed onto the patch.
   c. If the test substance is a fabric, a 0.5 × 0.5 in sample is cut, moistened with physiological saline, and then is applied under a patch.

3. The torso of each guinea pig is wrapped with an elastic bandage to secure the patches for 24 hr.
4. The date, time, and initials of those individuals performing the challenge dose should be recorded.
5. The patches are removed on day 22 and the challenge area on each flank is cleaned and clipped atraumatically.

Challenge Readings

1. On day 23, 24 hr after removing the patch, the first reading of dermal reactions is taken, and results are recorded.
2. Readings of the challenge site are taken again 48 hr after removing the patch, and results are recorded.
3. The intensity of the skin reaction is classified according to the following rating scale used by Maguire (1973b).

$$0 = \text{Normal skin}$$
$$+ = \text{Very faint, nonconfluent pink}$$
$$+ = \text{Faint pink}$$
$$++ = \text{Pale pink to pink, slight edema}$$
$$+++ = \text{Pink, moderate edema}$$
$$++++ = \text{Pink and thickened}$$
$$+++++ = \text{Bright pink, markedly thickened}$$

Interpretation of Results

1. The frequency, intensity and duration of the test responses to the test substance and the vehicle are evaluated.
2. The test substance is a sensitizer if the challange reactions in the test group clearly outweigh those in the control group.
3. Two or more unequivocally positive responses (at least a + on the rating scale) in a group of 10 animals should be considered significant. A negative, equivocal, or single response probably assures that a substance is not a strong sensitizer, although this is best confirmed by further testing with human subjects (NAS, 1977).

Rechallenge (Day 28)

1. If the first challenge application does not cause dermal sensitization, then a second application of the 10 test group guinea pigs will be conducted on day 28 (1 week after the first challenge). The remaining naive control group animals (not used for the first challenge) are challenged for comparison to the test group animals.

2. The three negative control group animals used on day 21 will not be rechallenged. These animals will be discontinued from the study because they were exposed to the test article during the first challenge and are no longer negative controls.

3. A 0.5 × 0.5 in patch with the highest nonirritating concentration of test substance in vehicle is applied to the right flank of test and control group animals. The left flanks are not dosed.

4. The date, time, and initials of those individuals performing the rechallenge dose are recorded.

5. Steps 3 and 5 of the challenge procedure are repeated here.

Strengths and Weaknesses

The advantages and disadvantages of the split adjuvant test can be summarized as below. The advantages are:

1. The test system has a lower false-negative rate for moderate and weak sensitizers than does the Buehler design.

2. If properly conducted, there are no false positives.

3. Fibers and other materials which cannot be injected intradermally can be evaluated here.

As elsewhere, there is also a list of disadvantages. These include:

1. The techniques involved (particularly the intradermal injection) are not easy ones.

2. The sensitivity of the test system is "bought" at the expense of making relative hazard predictions not necessarily accurate. The test system tends to overpredict potency.

3. The test still both takes a relatively long time to complete and uses a significant amount of test material.

4. There is a limited published database on test system performance, and relatively few people have experience with it.

Photosensitization Tests

There are at least five in vivo photosensitization test methods. Only two of these (Harber and Shalita method and the Armstrong assay) will be presented here. The other three (the Vinson and Borselli method, the Guillot et al. method, and a method using mice) are beyond the scope of this text.

Though the pattern of evolution of predictive animal tests is not as clear as that of dermal sensitization tests, the two methods presented here each represent a distinct phase of that development.

Harber and Shalita Method

This is the older of the two methods and uses dermal exposure without any adjuvant to increase the response. This method was originally published by Harber and Shalita in 1972.

Animals

1. Young adult female Hartley strain guinea pigs weighing between 300 and 400 g at the start of the study are used.

2. Animals that show poor growth or are ill in any way are not used, since illness markedly decreases the response. Animals with skin marked or scarred from fighting are avoided. The guinea pigs are quarantined and observed for at least 2 weeks to detect any illness before starting a study.

3. The guinea pigs are randomly assigned to a test group of 10 animals and negative control group of six animals. If a pretest group is necessary, as many animals as needed for that group also are randomized.

4. Test and control group guinea pigs are weighed 1 week prior to dosing (day 7), on the day of dosing (day 0), and weekly thereafter.

Pretest (If Necessary)

1. Several animals are used to pretest different concentrations of test substance in vehicle (usually acetone) to determine the topical dermal irritation threshold concentration on skin that is exposed to ultraviolet B (UVB) and ultraviolet A (UVA) irradiation sequentially and on skin tht is exposed to UVA irradiation alone.

2. The hair of these animals is shaved over the whole dorsal region.

3. A volume of 0.2 ml of each test concentration is applied twice to each guinea pig: (1) to the nuchal region; and (2) to the dorsal lumbar region.

4. Thirty minutes after application, the treated nuchal sites are irradiated with sunlamp emissions (UVB) for 30 min while the lumbar sites are shielded with elastoplast tape.

5. After the UVB exposure, the tape is removed from the lumbar region, and both the treated nuchal sites and lumbar sites are irradiated with black light emissions (UVA) for 30 min.

6. The animals are returned to their respective cages after the UVA exposure.

7. Twenty-four hours after the initial exposure to the test substance, the nuchal and lumbar skin sites are scored for erythema formation.

8. A concentration is chosen for induction applications that causes a mild or weak erythema response at the nuchal sites. If the test substance does not cause an erythema response, then the highest concentration level that is practical should be used for induction.

9. The highest concentration of the test substance that is nonirritating to the lumbar sites is used for challenge application. Two lower concentrations of the test substance, prepared by serial dilution from the highest concentration, are also used for the challenge application.

Induction Stage (Days 0, 2, 4, 7, 9, 11)

1. The hair in an area of approximately 1×1 in is clipped from the nuchal region of each test and control group guinea pig.

2. A volume of 0.2 ml of a relatively high concentration of the test substance in either acetone or ethanol is applied to the shaved nuchal region of each test group guinea pig. The concentration will be the highest level that can be well tolerated locally, and generally by the guinea pig, as determined by a pretest for dermal irritation.

3. A volume of 0.2 ml of solvent (acetone or ethanol) is applied to the shaved nuchal region of each control group guinea pig.

4. Thirty minutes after application, the treated nuchal sites of test and control guinea pigs are irradiated with sunlamp emissions for 30 min and black light emissions for 30 min, successively. The lumbar region of the back is shielded from the light sources during the irradiation procedures with an elastic bandage which is wrapped around the torso of each animal.

5. The clipping, topical exposure to test substance, and irradiation procedures are repeated 6 times during a 12-day period (typical study days are 0, 2, 4, 7, 9, and 11).

Challenge Stage (Day 32)

1. Elicitation of contact photosensitivity is performed 21 days from the last sensitizing (induction) exposure.

2. The hair of the dorsal lumbar region of each of 10 test group and three of six control group guinea pigs is clipped for the first time.

3. Three different concentrations of test substance using the solvent used for induction, as determined from the pretest, are applied topically to this region; test and control animals are treated alike. Each concentration is applied to the right and left side of the dorsal mid-line.

4. The torso of each test and control guinea pig is wrapped in Saran Wrap (1-layer thick) after the test chemical is applied. The Saran Wrap is held in place at the ends with athletic adhesive tape. The same tape is used to shield the left side of each animal from the UVA light source.

5. Thirty minutes after application, the right side of each animal is exposed to nonerythrogenic (> 320 nm) UVA emissions for 30 min. The radiation is passed through a pane of window glass 3 mm thick in order to eliminate passage of radiation lower than 320 nm.

6. After the black light exposure, all animals are unwrapped, returned to their respective cages, and placed in a darkened room for 24 hr.

Challenge Readings

1. If the test substance leaves a colored residue, the excess test material is removed by washing with a suitable solvent at 24 hr so that the area of challenge skin can be evaluated accurately.

2. All test sites, both irradiated and nonirradiated, are scored and interpreted 24 and 48 hr after the initial test substance application and subsequent exposure to black light irradiation.

3. Erythema is scored as follows:

   0—No erythema
   1—Minimal, but definite erythema
   2—Moderate erythema
   3—Considerable erythema
   4—Maximal erythema

4. Erythema scores are recorded.

Rechallenge

1. If the test substance is judged a nonphotosensitizing agent after the first challenge application, a second and final challenge application will be performed on each test group animal 7 days after the initiation of the first challenge dose.

2. Controls from the first challenge application are not rechallenged because they have been exposed to the test substance and are no longer true negative (naive) controls. The three remaining naive control group animals (not used for the first challenge) are challenged for comparison to the rechallenge of test group animals.

3. The procedure used for the first challenge application will be used for the second application, either the same or a new concentration of test substance, including reshaving, the same patching method, and the same duration of exposure. Observations are again made 24 and 48 hr after the second challenge application and skin reactions are recorded.

Interpretation of Results

1. The negative control group of animals, having received no previous photosensitive (induction) exposures, serves to identify any phototoxic or primary irritant (nonphototoxic) substances.

2. An erythema score of 1 or more is considered a positive response.

3. Interpretation of data is based on the dermal score for erythema (see Gad and Chengelis, 1988, for details).

Armstrong Assay

This method, originally published by Ichikawa, Armstrong, and Harber (1981), introduced the use of adjuvents in a photosensitization test system.

This assay has been recommended by the Cosmetic, Toiletries and Fragrances Association. It is of interest that the Environmental Protection Agency (EPA) has not made public a concern about photoallergens, since several pesticides have similar chemical structures to fragrances and numerous pesticides are known to form reactive species in the presence of UV light.

Lights. The Armstrong assay uses UVA light (320–400 nm) in the induction and challenge phase. The UVA lights are commonly known as "black lights" and can be purchased as "BLB" fluorescence-type bulbs from major lighting manufacturers. However, the selection of the light source is critical, since the range of wavelengths emitted by the bulb is controlled by the phosphor coating and different manufacturers use different phosphors to produce BLB lights. There may even be different phosphors used by the same manufacturer, and there is no code on the bulbs to indicate which phosphor is being used. The General Electric BLB emits effective energy only at wavelengths longer than 350 nm, whereas the entire spectrum between 315 and 400 nm is covered by the Sylvania BLB bulb. Less than 2% of the total energy emitted by the General Electric BLB light is between 250 and 350 nm, whereas 42% of the energy from the Sylvania BLB light falls in this range. There are known photoallergens which require the energy contained in the spectrum below 345 nm for activation and thus give a false negative if the incorrect light source is used. The best precaution is to determine the emission spectrum of the lights which are to be used in the assay.

It is necessary to determine the total energy being emitted by the lights in order to calculate the proper jaules per square centimeter (J/cm^2) exposure. An International Light Model 700 provides a relatively inexpensive means of measuring the light energy when fitted with a cosine-corrected UVA detector (W150s quartz diffuser, UVA pass filter SEE015 detector). The device has a peak sensitivity of 360 nm and a width of 50 nm. A bank of eight bulbs is readily prepared by bolting together two industrial 4-bulb (48 in long) reflectors. Two sets of these will allow 40 animals to be treated at one time. The lights are allowed to warm 30 min before use. They are turned off just before the animals are placed under them and then turned back on. The light intensity is measured at several locations at the level of the top of the backs of the animals and the correct exposure time then calculated. The lights are adjusted to be between 4 and 6 in above the back and 10 J/cm^2 is the proper exposure.

Patching. The Hill Top Chamber (see the earlier description of the Buehler assay) provides a good patching system in this assay. A volume of 0.3 ml is used. The animal restrainers described in the description of the Buehler assay work well for holding the animals during the patching and the exposure to the light as well as in providing excellent occlusion.

Induction Site Preparation. The majority of hair is removed from the intended patching site with a small animal clipper fitted with a #40 blade. The assay has a frequent requirement for the complete removal of hair using a depilatory which (such as that available from Whitehall Laboratories, New York, New York) is applied and left in contact with the skin for no more than 15 min. It must be washed away completely with a stream of warm running water. The animals are dried with a towel and the inside of the cages wiped clean of any depilatory before returning the guinea pigs.

When required, the epidermis is partially removed by tape stripping. The skin must be completely dry or the stripping will be ineffective. A length of tape approximately 8 in long is used. Starting at one end of the tape, it is placed against the skin and rubbed with the finger a few times to cause good adhesion. It is then pealed away, taking with it some dry epidermal cells. A new section of the tape is then applied to the skin and the procedure repeated 4 or 5 times. The skin will have a shiny appearance owing to the leakage of moisture from the dermis. The tape should not be jerked away from the skin as this can cause the rupture of dermal capillaries.

The potential of the animal to respond to a sensitizer is enhanced by the injection of Freund's complete adjuvant (Calbio-chem, San Diego, California, or Difco, Detroit, Michigan). The adjuvant is diluted 1:1 with sterile water before using. The injections must be intradermal. In the Armstrong assay, a pattern of four 0.1-ml injections are given just prior to the first induction patching in the nuchal area. All four injections should fit under the edge of the area to be covered by the Hill Top Chamber. It is advisable to perform the skin-stripping operation before the injections, since adjuvant can leak onto the skin and prevent effective removal of the epidermis.

The occlusion of the patches is done in the same manner as described for the Buehler assay. The test site(s) is exposed to the UVA light after 2 hr of occlusion. The animal is left in the restrainer and the dental dam above the test site to be exposed is cut and the patch removed. Sites not to be exposed are left patched. Excess material is wiped from the site to be exposed and the remaining parts of the animal are covered with aluminum foil. All patches are removed after the light-exposure step, and patched areas wiped free of excess material, and the animal returned to its cage.

Grading. The grading is the same as used in the Buehler assay.

Vehicles. With the exception of water, it is desirable to use a vehicle for the inductions which is different from the one used at the challenge (see Buehler assay). Since the control animals in the Armstrong assay are sham treated (including any vehicle), one can patch the test and control animals with vehicle at the time of challenge if the same vehicle must be used for both the induction and the challenge. It is advantageous to use a vehicle which dissolves the test material, though suspensions may not be avoidable in all cases.

Irritation Screens. The irritation screen is used to determine acceptable concentrations for the induction phase (i.e., one which does not produce eschar with repeated exposure or systemic toxicity) and the challenge phase (no more than slightly irritating). Each concentration must be tested with and without exposure to UVA light, as both conditions are used in the challenge. Thus, to evaluate four concentrations requires that eight animals be used. Each animal receives a pair of patches, with each pair being a different concentration (i.e., each concentration is patched on four animals). One of each pair of patches is placed on the left side and the corresponding concentration on the remaining patch is placed on the right side. The hair is removed by depilation the day of patching. The patches on the right side are removed after 2 hr of occlusion, the remaining parts of the animal covered with foil, and the right side exposed to 10 J/cm^2 of UVA light. Animals are returned to their cages after the exposure. If different solvents are being used in the induction and challenge phase, then two separate screens need to be run.

Conducting the Armstrong Assay.   Combining the discussed techniques in a specific regimen yields the assay as follows:

1. Irritation/toxicity pretest (eight animals)
    Day 0: Remove the hair from the lumbar region by clipping and depilitation. Apply to concentration on each animal on adjacent left side/right side locations for a total of four dose concentrations. Occlude the patches for 2 hr (± 15 min). Expose the right side to 10 J/cm^2 of UVA light after removing the patches on the right side. Remove the remaining patches and excess material after the exposure to light.
    Day 1: Grade all test sites 24 hr ($\pm$ 1 hr) after removal of all patches (24-hr grade).
    Day 2: Repeat the grading 48 hrs (+2 hr) after removing the patches (48-hr grade).
2. Induction (20 test + 10 sham controls + any rechallenge controls)
    Day 0: Weigh all test and control animals. Remove the hair from the nuchal area with clippers and depilatory. Remove the epidermis by stripping 4–5 times with tape. Make four 0.01-ml id injections of a 1:1 dilution of FCA in an area to be covered by the patch. Cover this area on the test animals with a Hill Top Chamber which has 0.3 ml of test material preparation in it. Patch the sham controls with water or solvent on the patch. Occlude with dental dam and restrain in a holder for 2 hr (± 15 min). Remove the patches, cover the nonpatched areas with foil, and exposure to 10 J/cm^2 of UVA light for 30 min.
    Days 2, 4, 7, 9, 11: Repeat the activity of day 0 with the following exceptions: Do not weigh animals and do not inject adjuvant. Move the patch back when the original induction site becomes too damaged but remain in the nuchal area. Dipilation may not be needed at each induction.
3. Challenge (20 test + 10 sham control animals 9–13 days after last induction exposure)
    Day 0: Weigh all animals, clip the lumber region free of hair and dipilate. Do not strip the skin. Patch each animal with a pair of adjacent patches (one on the left side and one on the right side) containing 0.3 ml of a nonirritating concentration of test material in a Hill Top Chamber. Occlude the patches and restrain the animal for 2 hr (± 15 min). Remove the patches from the right side and cover the rest of the animal's body with foil. Expose the right side to 10 J/cm^2 of UVA light. Remove the remaining patch and any excess material.
    Day 1: Grade all challenge sites, keeping separate the grades of the site exposed to light and those not exposed to light 24 hr (± 1 hr) after removal of the patches (24-hr grade).
    Day 2: Repeat the grading 48 hr (± 2 hr) after removal of the patches (48-hr grade).
4. Rechallenge
    All or selected animals may be rechallenged with the same or a different test material 7–12 days after the challenge. Use 10 new sham-treated controls and naive test sites on all animals following the same procedure as used in the challenge.
5. Interpretation of results
    Determine the number of positive responders (number of animals with a score >1 at either the 24- or 48-hr grading or with a score 1 unit higher than the highest score in the control). Determine the average score at 24 hr and at 48 hr for the test and control

groups using face values. Keep the data for the sites exposed to light separate from the data from sites not exposed to light.

Strengths and Weaknesses. The Armstrong Assay was found to give responses in the guinea pig which were consistent with what has been observed in humans: positive responses for 6-methyl coumarin and musk ambrette. One major disadvantage is that the procedure is time consuming with six induction exposures; additional work might demonstrate that fewer exposures will yield the same results.

The procedure is very stressful on the animals because of the injection of adjuvant and the multiple skin strippings and depilation.

As with any assay involving the intradermal injection of adjuvant, there is often a problem with using the results of the irritation screen in naive animals to accurately predict the results that will be seen in the sham controls at the challenge. If the material being tested is a nonirritant, or if one selects a concentration of an irritant which is far below the irritating concentration, then the screen does an adequate job of predicting the background irritation level in the challenge controls. However, if a slightly irritant concentration of an irritant is used, then the screen often underpredicts the irritation response and a high background level of irritation is observed at the challenge in the sham controls. The interpretation of the results of the challenge becomes difficult. The use of animals in the irritation screen which have had a prior injection of adjuvant might provide a viable alternative and reduce the number of times that rechallenges must be run because of high background levels of irritation.

The Armstrong assay was designed to evaluate materials for their photoactivated sensitization potential and not their potential to be nonphotoactivated dermal sensitizers. At this time, there is no background data which will allow for properly positioning results of the Armstrong assay with regard to human risk if the assay indicates that a test material is a sensitizer or that a material is both a sensitizer and a photoallergen. Thus, it is highly recommended that a "standard" sensitization assay which can be related to humans be run before or in conjunction with the photosensitization assay. The use of a subjective grading system can be a source of significant verification.

Host Resistance Test

The guinea pig can also be used for the host resistance assay, a primary immunotoxicity screen. A protocol for such an assay is as follows.

Test System

1. Male Hartley guinea pigs (Charles River Breeding Laboratories; Portage, Michigan) are used. The guinea pigs should be 7–8 weeks old at the time of dosing. Animals will be acclimatized for at least 14 days prior to dosing.

2. Animals that appear abnormal should be rejected prior to dosing or assignment to a test group.

3. Animals are randomly selected from the pool of available animals and assigned to each dosage group.

4. Each animal is identified by a cage card.

Challenge Organism

1. *Pseudomonas aeruginosa (P. aeru.)* culture, from American Type Culture Collection, 27853, is grown in tryptic soy broth. This broth will be centrifuged down, and the resulting pellet being washed and resuspended in 0.9% saline. Plate counts should be

performed to determine the concentration of the bacteria; the solution may be adjusted to give the desired concentration. Once prepared, samples of the bacterial solution will be repeated to confirm the concentration of the bacteria.

2. Administration of the test organism is intravenously (iv), in order to cause septicemia. Based on experimental data, a dosage of 2.3 CFU (colony-forming units) $\times$ 10^8/kg should be expected to challenge the immune system of the guinea pig and provide a minimally lethal response. Each animal should receive a single exposure. They should be lightly anesthetized with ether and the inoculum should be administered into an ear vein. The dose volume should be 1 ml/kg of body weight.

3. The concentration (determined upon solution preparation) of the *P. aeru.* is confirmed by the replating of the samples taken after preparation.

4. Once prepared, *P. aeru.* cultures should be stored in a refrigerator for no more than 3 days.

5. All materials that come into contact with the organism should be placed in plastic bags, marked as a biohazard, and incinerated as soon as possible.

Study Design

Group	#/Group	Test material (mg/kg/day)	P. aeru.
1	10	—	Yes
2	10	—	Yes
3	10	—	No

The guinea pig should be treated by the appropriate route with test material daily for 7 days. Guinea pigs should receive an intravenous dosage of *P. aeru.* on day 8 at a dosage of approximately 2.3 CFU $\times$ 10^8/kg. The experiment is then terminated on day 15.

Observations

1. Prior to *P. aeru.* challenge guinea pigs are observed at least twice daily. On the day of challenge, they should be observed periodically during the first 4 hr after challenge and then at least 3 times daily for the next 7 days for obvious signs of treatment, including death. Body weights of all animals will be determined prior to dosing on study days –3, 1, 8, and 15. Rectal temperatures are determined on days –1, 1 (2 hr postdosing), 2, 3, and 4, after *P. aeru.* challenge.

2. Animals found dead should be discarded. Necropsies are not conducted. Animals killed by design should be asphyxiated with carbon dioxide and discarded. Sacrifice schedule: Surviving animals are killed on study day 15 (7 days after dosing of *P. aeru.*).

Analysis and Interpretation

1. Mortality data will be analyzed by probit analysis or minimum normit chi-square analysis. Means and standard deviations are prepared for survival time body weights and rectal temperatures. Time-to-death analysis is also done.

2. A significant increase in mortality should be interpreted as a positive finding in this test system.

METABOLISM

The objective behind the use of any animal model in toxicology is almost always to predict what will happen in humans. A necessary and essential part of this is knowing the reasons for any differences in response between the model and the human. A major component of such differences is undoubtedly variations (qualitative and quantitative) in metabolism. Table 14 summarizes some key factors about guinea pig metabolism of xenobiotics.

Species Peculiarities

As is the case with all other animal models that have been studied for some time, a number of responses to potentially toxic xenobiotics have been identified in the guinea pig which are different from humans or other model species. This section will seek to overview these differences.

Guinea pigs are remarkable in their requirements for vitamin C. The animal maintained on a vitamin C–deficient diet develops scurvylike symptoms. Before the chemical methods were developed, guinea pigs were used for vitamin C assay in nutritional studies. The guinea pig is highly susceptible to human and bovine tuberculosis, and it may be used for the diagnosis of human mycobacteriosis. The guinea pig is an excellent model for anaphylaxis and other immunological procedures, but this excellence is founded on the fact that the immune responses in the guinea pig (both cellular and humoral) are exaggerated compared to humans.

Antibiotic Toxicity

Guinea pigs are highly sensitive to antibiotics, particularly those specific for gram-positive organisms. The normal intestinal flora of guinea pigs is predominantly gram-positive. Administration of antibiotics specific for gram-positive bacteria destroys the normal flora of the intestinal tract and permits an overgrowth of gram-negative organisms. Until recently, complications following antibiotic administration were attributed primarily

Table 14   Major Metabolic Characterictics of the Guinea Pig

Characteristics	Reference
Has high sulfotransferase and glucuronosyl-transferase form 1 in the jejunum than in the liver	Schwenk and Locher (1985)
Has higher substrate specificity for mono-oxygenases (benzo[a]pyrene hydroxylase and N-demethylase) in intestines than in liver	Gregus et al. (1983) Laitinen and Watkins (1986)
Liver size is proportionately (to body size) greater than in the human (2% of total body weight in the human, 3.5% in the guinea pig)	Experimental data
Does not have aromatic hydroxylation capability for amphetamines.	Caldwell (1981)
While rat and dog have more efficient biliary excretion than man, the guinea pig is comparable to man.	Levine, 1978

to *Escherichia coli;* but current evidence suggests that *Clostridium difficile* plays an important role in the enterotoxemia that follows antibiotic treatment. These antibiotics are not directly toxic and are not harmful when administered in therapeutic dosages to germ-free animals. Tetracycline, cephaloridine, chloramphenicol, and the sulfonamides are among the less hazardous antimicrobials, but all should be administered with caution, using the minimal effective dosage.

Response to Anti-inflammatories

The area of anti-inflammatories is (and had been for at least 15 years) a very active one in pharmaceutical research. These efforts have been hampered by the lack of good models for assessing the safety of such compounds, particularly in terms of potential gastrointestinal and renal toxicity.

Many of the anti-inflammatories (particularly the nonsteroidal anti-inflammatory drugs, or NSAIDs) act at least in part by inhibiting prostaglandin synthesis. Some of the standard models used for screening for potentially effective compounds include (1) assaying homogenates of the stomach of dosed guinea pigs for prostaglandin synthesis, and (2) inhibition of ultraviolet-induced erythema in the skin of dosed guinea pigs (Birnbaum et al., 1982).

The guinea pig, though still more sensitive than the human to the gastrointestinal ulceration induced by NSAIDs, is less so than the dog or rat for a range of NSAIDs (Mariani and Bonanomi, 1978; Birnbaum et al., 1982). The most common toxic effect reported for anti-inflammatories in the guinea pigs is gastrointestinal ulceration, however, and they are generally more sensitive than humans.

Cardiotoxic Effects of Catecholamines

Waldenstrom et al. (1987) have performed extensive evaluations of the cardiotoxicity of catecholamines in both the rat and guinea pig, and have found the guinea pig to be less sensitive than the rat to the local anoxia caused damage induced by catecholamines.

Table 15 summarizes a range of multispecies comparisons of susceptibility to toxic lesions.

STRAINS

There are three naturally occurring strains of guinea pigs, which can be distinguished from each other by differences in the length, texture, and direction of their hair growth. These are the (1) short-haired, smooth, and coarse-coated English, (2) the long-haired Abyssinian, which has its hair arranged in whirls, and (3) the long, fine-haired Peruvian.

The English, guinea pig, which comes as an albino, bi-, or tricolored animals and as outbred and inbred strains, is the commonest and the most often strain used in the laboratory. They are alert and well fleshed with smooth, shiny skin. The albino Hartley strain is the variety most familiar to toxicologists, and it is considered *the* standard animal for skin sensitization studies.

Recently, Charles River Breeding Laboratories has developed and made commercially available a hairless form of the Hartley guinea pig, designated the Crl:IAF/HA(hr/hr)BR). This is fertile, euthymic animal. There are also athymic/hypothymic varieties available.

Table 15 Comparisons of Species Differences in Toxic Lesions

Agent	Toxicity compared	Species								Reference
		rat	dog	mouse	rabbit	monkey	guinea pig	hamster	human	
BL-4162	Thrombocytopenia	(−)	(−)	(−)	(−)	(+)	(−)		(+)	Hottendorf (1985)
Benzylpenicillin	Delayed enterotoxemia	(−)	(−)	(−)	(−)		(+)	(+)	(−)	Boyd and Fulford (1961)
Capreomycin	Nephrotoxicity	(+)	(−)	(−)	(−)	(−)	(−)	(−)	(+)	Muraoka et al. (1968)
Decalin	Nephrotoxicity	(+)	(−)	(−)			(−)			Alden (1985)
Dimethylhydrazine	Colonic tumors	(+)	(−)	(+)			(−)	(+)		Wilson (1976)
Indomethacin	Ulcerogenesis	(+)	(+)	(+)			(−)		(+)	Wilhelmi (1974); Mariani and Bonamomi (1978)
Mepirizole	Ulcerogenesis	(+)	(−)	(−)	(+)		(+)			Ishihara et al. (1983)
Minoxidil	Cardiomyopathy	(−)	(+)	(−)	(−)	(−)	(−)		(−)	Carlson and Feenstra (1977); Sobota et al. (1980)

Pathology   **John C. Peckham**

USEFULNESS: STRENGTHS AND WEAKNESSES

Respiratory System

The well-known sensitivity of the respiratory system of the guinea pig has provided a basis for studies of inhalation phenomena, including bronchospasms, asthma, and reactions to dust and other air pollutants.

Digestive System

Guinea pigs are fastidious eaters. As they mature they develop rigid habit patterns that must be accommodated if the animal is to thrive. Any changes in feed (taste, odor, texture, form), water, feeder, or waterer may cause the guinea pig to stop eating or drinking (Harkness and Wagner, 1983). Starvation with clinical or subclinical illness from vitamin deficiencies may result.

The behavior of coprophagy and anatomical structure of a glandular stomach with a large cecum may modify the effects of experiments involving nutritional factors (Navia and Hunt, 1976).

Urogenital System and Fetal Tissues

Although the guinea pig has been employed infrequently in the past, it is unique among the animals available for reproductive and teratological studies. It occupies a position intermediate between the laboratory rodents, rats and mice, and the more evolved subhuman primates and man. For example, the endocrine control of its reproduction is similar to that of humans, even to the trimesteric characteristics, yet pregnancy is preceded by a well-defined estrus. Its placenta appears to be capable of endocrine activity, but it is labyrinthine, and its transfer functions are supplemented by an everted yolk sac exposed to uterine secretions. The elements of the reproductive cycle that precede pregnancy, i.e., estrus, ovulation, and fertilization, can be accurately determined as with all rodents, but its relatively long gestation allows the assessment of the effect of potentially harmful agents applied late in development upon organ functions or behavior patterns that develop after birth in other rodents (Hoar, 1976b, c). Their long gestation period of 68 days provides an opportunity for separating toxic or teratogenic effects on the embryo from those upon the fetus and allows investigation of a fetus with an essentially mature central nervous system prior to delivery (Hoar, 1976b). In many instances, pregnancy is maintained following ovariectomy at 25 or more days. The guinea pig is, therefore, an animal of choice for studying the effects of hormones and endocrine glands on pregnancy (Harkness and Wagner, 1989).

Malformations have been induced in guinea pigs by a variety of agents, including drugs, dyes, pesticides, vitamin excess, hyperthermia, adrenocortical hormone excess, synthetic steroids, ionizing radiation, and mineral deficient diets. Spontaneous malformations of genetic and unknown origin also occur (Hoar, 1976b, c).

Nervous System and Special Sense Organs

Because of the anatomy of the guinea pig ear and associated structures, it is an important animal model for ototoxicity studies. A postauricular surgical approach to the middle ear presents no major blood vessels or muscles. The petrous bone (otic capsule) is easily entered and dissected away without drilling to expose the inner ear structures in much less time than the cat and monkey. The guinea pig has been used to elucidate the pathophysiology of drugs which cause deafness and vestibular disorders, including the aminoglycosidic antibiotics such as neomycin, gentamicin, and other members of the streptomycin family, the diuretic ethacrynic acid, quinine, and salicylates (McCormick and Nuttall, 1976).

Integumentary System and Soft Tissues

Guinea pigs have been used extensively for the study of immunological and inflammatory reactions involving the skin and subcutis. They are frequently used to test the safety of skin lotions and ointments. The dermal response of the guinea pig to irritation by test materials has been shown in many instances to be more like that of man than the rabbit; therefore, the guinea pig is the species of choice for dermal irritation tests (Gilman, 1982). In addition, physiological characteristics of its skin are similar to those of humans, which has led to other areas of investigation such as that of wounds and burns (Hoar, 1976a).

The capability of chemical compounds to cause skin sensitization was first demonstrated in guinea pigs by Landsteiner and Jacobs (1935, 1936). Using substituted benzene compounds, they demonstrated development of a true allergic reaction following sensitization of the skin. Subsequently, experiments proved that skin could be sensitized by the administration of a chemical either topically, intradermally, or intraperitoneally. Skin sensitization tests are designed to determine if a chemical compound will cause an allergic reaction after there has been a previous contact to the same or a similar compound. The Hartley strain of guinea pig is the laboratory animal most commonly used for these tests (Gilman, 1982). Individual guinea pigs have been demonstrated to inherit differing skin susceptibilities to some compounds such as 2,4-dinitrochlorobenzene and poison ivy (Chase, 1941).

The female has one pair of inguinal mammary glands. Despite the apparent shortage of nipples, adult females have successfully raised litters of three, four, and more offspring (Harkness and Wagner, 1989).

Hematopoietic and Lymphoid Systems

The bone marrow of the guinea pig has been studied extensively because of its similarity to that of humans, its ease of dispersion to give uniform cell suspensions, and the ease of staining and identification of its cells (Sisk, 1976). Also, hormonally and immunologically the guinea pig more nearly resembles the human than do rats and mice (Ernstrom, 1970). Unlike many species which are very immature at birth, the neonatal guinea pig possesses very mature myeloid and lymphoid tissues. There is considerable data on cellular elements, physiological properties, and biochemical characteristics of circulating blood and bone marrow (Sisk, 1976). As a corticosteroid-resistant species, treatment with steroids does not markedly affect thymic physiology or peripheral lymphocyte counts (Sisk, 1976).

Mature females are an excellent source of serum complement used in a variety of immune and endotoxin serological reactions. Guinea pigs produce antibodies to specific proteins and are used to test for the presence or absence of small amounts of antigens by the production of anaphylaxis. Unlike the rabbit or chicken, injected antibodies protect the guinea pig from anaphylaxis (Harkness and Wagner, 1989).

Nutrition and Metabolic Diseases

The guinea pig is uniquely susceptible to vitamin C (ascorbic acid) deficiency, which results in bone/collagen disease and increased susceptibility to infections with inflammation, especially of the lungs and cervical lymph nodes.

The vitamin C requirement makes the guinea pig a useful model for (1) nutritional studies pertaining to vitamin C metabolism, (2) collagen studies, (3) skin studies, (4) bone studies, (5) atherosclerosis studies, (6) adrenal-pituitary studies, and (7) hydroxylating reactions where ascorbic acid seems to play a role (Navia and Hunt, 1976). The guinea pig was used for the biological assay of vitamin C before the chemical assays were developed (Fenner, 1986).

Bacterial, Viral, and Rickettsial Diseases

Guinea pigs were once used extensively for disease diagnosis and isolation of pathogenic agents such as in tuberculosis but their use in this field has declined (Jolly and Heywood, 1979). Guinea pigs are highly susceptible to both human- and bovine-type tubercle bacilli and long filled an important place in tuberculosis research and diagnosis. They are also susceptible to rickettsial infections, and a number of rickettsiae pathogenic to humans were first studied in the guinea pig (Fenner, 1986).

Neoplastic Diseases

Although guinea pigs have been used in large numbers as experimental laboratory animals, they have not been used as frequently in carcinogenesis studies. This has been in part because of a prevailing view that guinea pigs are particularly resistant to induced neoplasia.

Guinea pigs were considered to be resistant to chemical carcinogens until 1962 because exposure to chemicals known to be carcinogenic in rats failed to produce tumors (Mosinger, 1961; Argus, 1971). This observation led to investigation of tumor-resistant factors in guinea pigs. Guinea pig serum was found to have a factor which inhibited the growth of several lymphomas in mice. This factor was termed tumor inhibitory principle (TIP), but it could not be isolated. The existence of this principle is still uncertain (Manning, 1976). Since 1962, guinea pigs have been shown to be susceptible to the carcinogenic activity of a variety of agents, including physical and chemical irritants, hydrocarbons, nitrosamines, and hormones, particularly estrogens (Manning, 1976).

The refractoriness of the guinea pig to the carcinogenic action of aromatic amines and amino azo dyes possibly resides in its limited ability to metabolize these agents to their N-hydroxy derivatives. Miller et al. (1964) showed that N-hydroxy-2-acetylaminofluorene in guinea pigs induced adenocarcinomas of the small intestine (upon feeding) and sarcomas (upon injection), whereas 2-acetylaminofluorene is inactive. Very rapid elimination of N-hydroxy derivatives from guinea pig tissues has been proposed as another mechanism (Kiese and Wiedemann, 1968). Berenblum (1949) found that increasing the dosage of 9,10-dimethyl-1,2-benzanthracene to 20-fold that of the rat resulted in tumors in guinea pigs. Rogers and Blumenthal (1960) induced tumors in 57% of 735 guinea pigs with methylcholanthrene injected subcutaneously and intramuscularly.

Guinea pigs are susceptible to many different chemical carcinogens, including ethyl carbamate, polycylic hydrocarbons (7, 12-dimethylbenz [a] anthracene, 3-methylcholanthrene, benzopyrene, 1,2,5,6-dibenzanthracene and others), nitrosamine-type alkylating agents (diethylnitrosamine, dimethylnitrosamine, N-methyl-N-nitrosourea, nitrosomethyldodecyclamine, nitroso-2,6-dimethylmorpholine, dinitroso-2,6-dimethylpiperazine, di-N-butylnitrosamine), methylazomethanol, aflatoxin, and dioxan (Argus, 1971; Squire et al., 1978).

Animals used in carcinogenicity studies must be reasonable in cost to allow adequate numbers of both test and control animals, have a life span within both the financial capabilities of the sponsor to maintain them and the public health and political time constraints for determining an answer, and be well adapted to the laboratory environment without serious interfering infectious diseases. Although mice and rats meet the first two requirements better than guinea pigs, guinea pigs should be considered if the metabolism of the compound and its availability at the expected target site are similar to that in humans, and if the value or extended use of the test product warrants the extra cost (Robens et al., 1982).

It is important for the testing laboratory to establish the background tumor incidence and other lesions of aging guinea pigs to help determine if the incidence of tumors among the controls in any specific test is representative. The laboratory incidence should be compared with reported tumor incidence when the latter are available (Robens et al., 1982).

ORGAN WEIGHTS AND RATIOS

Organ weights have rarely been reported by investigators because of the infrequency of guinea pigs to be used in acute, subchronic, and chronic toxicity tests by the chemical, cosmetic, and pharmaceutical industries. The following organ/body weights were calculated based on data reported by Breazile and Brown (1976).

Organ	Weight (g)	Organ/Body weight ratio[a] (X adjustment factor)		Organ/brain ratio
Brain	4.300	4.778	(x1000)	—
Spinal cord	14.500	1.611	(x100)	3.372
Pituitary	0.022	0.024	(x1000)	0.005
Thyroid	0.134	0.149	(x1000)	0.031
Adrenal	0.725	0.806	(x1000)	0.169
Liver	42.500	4.722	(x100)	9.884
Lung	5.000	5.556	(x1000)	1.163
Kidneys	6.120	6.800	(x1000)	1.423
Pancreas	2.500	2.778	(x1000)	0.581
Testes	4.300	4.778	(x1000)	1.000
Epididymis	0.660	0.733	(x1000)	0.153
Ovaries	0.192	0.213	(x1000)	0.045
Stomach	0.420	0.467	(x1000)	0.098
Intestine	28.000	3.111	(x100)	6.512
Urinary bladder	4.250	4.722	(x1000)	0.988
Stomach and intestine (with contents)	120.000			
Eyes	1.250			
Skeleton and ligaments	64.000			
Musculature	320.000			

[a]Based on 900 - g guinea pig.

For additional information see the other portions of this chapter, and see Turton et al. (1977a,b)

SPONTANEOUS LESIONS: NONNEOPLASTIC AND NEOPLASTIC

Considering only animals of comparative ages, guinea pigs have a lower incidence of spontaneous neoplasms than rats or mice (Morgan, 1969). Accurate estimates of the incidence of spontaneous neoplasia in any species must be based on complete necropsies and thorough microscopic examination of tissues from animals allowed to live one-half or more of the natural life span (Manning, 1976; Peckham, 1980). The breeding life of laboratory guinea pigs is from 18 months to 4 years, and they have been known to live 8 years; however, they rarely survive in the home longer than 5 years (Harkness and Wagner, 1983; Ruf, 1984). The life span of the laboratory guinea pig is 4–6 years (Wallach and Boever, 1983). An occasional animal may reach 9.0 or 9.5 years of age (Kunstyr and Naumann, 1984). There are few definitive reports in the literature which meet the criteria of complete necropsy examinations with histopathology and full life spans. Shimkin and Mider (1941) reported no neoplasms in 15,000 guinea pigs of inbred strains born and observed for up to 5 years between 1916 and 1937. Papanicolaou and Olcott (1942) observed about 100 tumors in over 7000 guinea pig necropsies for an incidence of 1.4%; tumors were rare in animals less than 4–5 years of age.

Rogers and Blumenthal (1960) examined 6000 guinea pigs of two inbred strains over a 10-year period. These animals, which had not been used for experimental purposes, had a spontaneous tumor incidence of 0.4% for all ages and 14.4% (14 of 97) for animals surviving 3 years or more. All 14 tumors occurred in the R9 strain. The incidence of tumors in random-bred Hartley strain guinea pigs from necropsies of 8400 animals (estimated male and female ratio 1:3) at ages of less than 27 months was 0.75% and of 34 retired breeders (six males and 28 females) greater than 27 months of age was 29.4%.

Cardiovascular system

Generalized cardiovascular system septicemias sometimes occur with bacterial infections such as staphylococcosis and those caused by *Pseudomonas aeruginosa, Pasteurella multocida,* and *P. haemolytica.*

Heart

Nonneoplastic Lesions—Spontaneous. Cardiac "rhabdomyomas" are commonly observed circumscribed accumulations of glycogen which might be confused with neoplastic lesions. The rhabdomyomas may be congenital in origin (Manning, 1976; Vink, 1969).

Spontaneous interstitial lymphocytic myocarditis of unknown pathogenesis has been observed as an incidental finding in guinea pigs which is similar to that described in mice, rats, and rabbits (Miller, 1924). Vegetative endocarditis can be caused by *Streptococcus* spp. infections.

Neoplastic Lesions—Spontaneous. Spontaneous cardiovascular tumors are uncommon. Benign mesenchymal mixed tumors (mesenchymomas) have been observed in the heart of 12 females of the Hartley strain (McConnell and Ediger, 1968; Manning, 1976). Also, a fibrosarcoma of the heart and a cavernous hemangioma of the liver have been reported (Rogers and Blumenthal, 1960; Manning, 1976).

Aorta and Arteries

Nonneoplastic Lesions—Induced. Medial calcification of the major elastic arteries and soft tissue calcification have been associated with hypervitaminosis D (Wallach and Boever, 1983).

Respiratory System

Lung

Nonneoplastic Lesions—Spontaneous. Susceptibility to acute anaphylaxis is related to the quantity of histamine available for release in the lung. In highly susceptible Hartley animals, this amount can be more than 10 times greater than in the resistant strain 2. Strain 2 and Hartley guinea pigs are equally susceptible to histamine toxicity (Stone et al., 1964).

Adenomatosis or alveolar epithelial hyperplasia is a frequent lung lesion in guinea pigs which must be differentiated from alveolar or bronchogenic adenomas (Hoch-Ligeti et al., 1982). Proliferations of alveolar epithelium diagnosed as tumors were often associated with interstitial pneumonia, foreign bodies, or other inflammatory changes, which suggest many of these lesions are in reality hyperplasia (Manning, 1976).

Pneumonia is caused by one of several bacteria or viruses in guinea pigs. The most important of these bacteria include *Bordetella bronchiseptica, Klebsiella pneumoniae, Pasteurella multocida* or *P. pneumotropica,* and *Streptococcus (Diplococcus) pneumoniae.* Other microorganisms associated with pneumonia in guinea pigs are *Streptobacillus moniliformis, Corynebacterium kutscheri,* other *Streptococcus* spp., *Pseudomonas aeruginosa,* and *Mycoplasma pulmonis.* Signs in affected guinea pigs include rough hair coat, anorexia, emaciation, hunched posture, dyspnea, abdominal breathing, rales, sneezing, and sometimes a mucosanguineous to purulent discharge from the eyes and nose. At necropsy, *B. bronchiseptica* has been shown to cause partial consolidation of the lungs. Histologically, a marked purulent bronchitis and bronchiolitis or fibrinous bronchopneumonia can be observed. *S. pneumoniae* commonly causes a fibrinopurulent pleuritis or peritonitis (Parker et al., 1977). *S. zooepidemicus* may cause septicemia and pneumonia. *P. aeruginosa* may cause a focal necrotizing and granulomatous pneumonia with "sulfur" granules or green exudate. Pneumonias caused by *Escherichia coli* and *Klebsiella pneumoniae* are usually secondary and accompanied by pleuritis, pericarditis, and peritonitis (Ganaway, 1976; Wagner, 1979; Wallach and Boever, 1983; Ruf, 1984).

Guinea pigs that are latent carriers of *Streptococcus (Diplococcus) pneumoniae* frequently die of fibrinopurulent peritonitis, pericarditis, pleuritis, pneumonia, or meningitis following the injection of irritating substances into or removal of fluids from body cavities (Wagner, 1976). Vitamin C deficiency results in an increased susceptibility to pneumonia and pleuritis from bacterial infections.

Adenoviral pneumonia was fatal to 11 of 1600 preadult guinea pigs. The only clinical sign was dyspnea. Grossly partial consolidation of the anterior lobes was observed in the lungs. Lesions were limited to the respiratory system, and included emphysema, petechiation, hydrothorax, bronchiolitis, bronchial epithelial sloughing, and focal parenchymal necrosis and inflammation. The desquamated bronchial epithelium frequently contained large basophilic intranuclear inclusion bodies. Numerous viral particles of an adenovirus were found (Naumann et al., 1981; Brennecke et al., 1983; Kaup et al., 1984; Kunstyr et al., 1984; Richter, 1986).

Adiaspiromycosis caused by *Emmonsia parva* and *E. crescens* has been reported in guinea pigs. It is a benign self-limiting granulomatous pulmonary disease (Wallach and Boever, 1983).

Perivascular lymphoid nodules in the lungs of guinea pigs occur around smaller branches of the pulmonary arteries and veins. They have been reported as occurring in for 14–85% of guinea pigs of both sexes and all ages from seven strains, including a germ-free animal (Thompson et al., 1962). The nodules appear to enlarge with age and may be visible grossly as pinpoint, subpleural foci. Bony spicules have been observed in the interstitium of alveolar septa of the lungs of guinea pigs fed commercial diets (Kaufmann, 1970).

Nonneoplastic Lesions—Induced.   Histamine administration results in lethal bronchiolar smooth muscle contraction. When prostaglandin IR-PGF20 generation was studied, the peripheral lung responses closely resembled those of the peripheral human lung to histamine H_1 stimulation (Steel et al., 1979).

Experimental airborne tuberculosis in the guinea pig provides a useful model of human tuberculosis with a naturally occurring bacillemia and cavitary stages of the disease (Smith and Harding, 1977).

Neoplastic Lesions—Spontaneous.   Spontaneous lung tumors constitute some of the most important tumor types in guinea pigs and have been the most frequently reported solid tumors. The tumors included a number of alveologenic tumors; an adenoma, papillary or bronchogenic adenomas, and bronchogenic adenocarcinomas (Manning, 1976) as well as hemangiosarcoma, lymphangioma, and intrabronchial papilloma (Hoch-Ligeti et al., 1982).

Rogers and Blumenthal (1960) found that 64 papillary adenomas (2.6%) and one adenocarcinoma of the lungs had been reported in the literature. Eighteen adenomas and 17 adenocarcinomas were reported by Mosinger (1961). These bronchoalveolar or alveologenic tumors are common in animals over 3 years of age. In some studies, the proliferations of alveolar epithelium which were considered to be tumors were associated with interstitial pneumonia, foreign bodies, or other inflammatory changes, which suggest that some of these lesions were hyperplastic, not neoplastic (Manning, 1976).

Neoplastic Lesions—Induced.   Irradiation resulted in the earlier occurrence of alveologenic tumors and an increased number of tumor nodules than in untreated controls. The number of alveogenic tumors in guinea pigs which survived over 20 months was not statistically significantly different between irradiated and untreated groups. The tumors observed in the lungs were alveologenic tumors (synonyms: papillary adenomas, alveolar adenomas, adenomas), hemangiosarcomas, lymphangiomas, intrabronchial papillomas, and adenomatosis (Hoch-Ligeti et al., 1982).

Of 111 strains 2 and 13 guinea pigs injected intravenously with either 20-methylcholanthrene or 1,2,5,6-dibenzathracene, pulmonary tumors occurred in 32 animals with a similar frequency in both strains (Heston and Deringer, 1952).

Digestive System

Guinea pigs have a long colon (60% of the length of the small intestine vs only 16% in the rat) with a characteristic large, thin-walled cecum with numerous lateral pouches which occupies the left side of the abdominal cavity. The tenia coli has served as a preferred source of smooth muscle for physiologists (Breazile and Brown, 1976).

Teeth

Nonneoplastic Lesions—Spontaneous. Malocclusion and loss of opposing teeth lead to overgrowth of the teeth. Since all guinea pig teeth are open-rooted and erupt continuously, all teeth have a tendency to overgrow, especially the premolars or the anterior cheek teeth (Ediger et al., 1975; Harkness and Wagner, 1989). Calcium deficiencies can cause soft maxillary and mandibular bone with misalignment of the teeth and overgrowth of the incisors and molars. Soft foods aggravate the problem of malocclusion. Clinical signs include salivation (slobbers), loss of weight, anorexia (the animal is usually hungry but cannot eat), licking movements, and loss of the ability to close the mouth (Wallach and Boever, 1983).

Salivary Gland

Nonneoplastic Lesions—Spontaneous. Cytomegalovirus is a well-described salivary gland disease of guinea pigs. It is characterized by eosinophilic intranuclear and rarely by intracytoplasmic inclusion bodies in ductal epithelium of the salivary glands and the epithelium of the proximal and distal convoluted tubules of the kidneys. In the salivary glands, affected cells are markedly enlarged (Cook, 1958, Van Hoosier and Robinette, 1976). Disseminated cytomegalovirus disease has been reported (Van Hoosier et al., 1985).

Neoplastic Lesions—Spontaneous. A benign mixed tumor of a sublingual salivary gland was reported in a 1.5-year-old guinea pig (Koestner and Buerger, 1965).

Esophagus

Neoplastic Lesions—Induced. Spontaneous tumors of the esophagus are apparently extremely rare; however, a squamous cell papilloma and carcinomas were produced by methylcholanthrene and nitrosopiperidine, respectively (Squire et al., 1978).

Stomach

Nonneoplastic Lesions—Spontaneous. Gastric bloat occurs in guinea pigs when excesses of fresh green forage are fed. The clinical signs of bloat include distended abdomen, abdominal pain, depression, and cyanosis (Wallach and Boever, 1983). Acute gastric dilatation has been associated with gastric volvulus (Lee et al., 1977). Gastric ulcers are fairly common; most are secondary to other diseases, especially ketosis (Wagner, 1979).

Neoplastic Lesions—Spontaneous. Papanicolaou and Olcott (1940, 1942) reported five benign mesenchymal neoplasms in the stomach of guinea pigs. The tumors were a fibromyoma, three leiomyomas, and a lipoma.

Neoplastic Lesions—Induced. Adenocarcinomas and sarcomas of the glandular stomach have produced by methylcholanthrene (Squire et al., 1978).

Intestine

Nonneoplastic Lesions—Spontaneous. Guinea pigs are particularly prone to acute enteritis, although peracute, subacute, and chronic forms also occur. Diarrhea may or may not be present. Nonspecific signs include anorexia, weight loss, depression, and conjunctivitis. Latent forms of the disease may be precipitated by stressful environmental changes such as shipping, pregnancy, and research procedures. Acute enteritis has been also associated with subclinical scurvy (Clarke et al., 1980).

Enterocolitis, acute necrotic cecitis, or typhlocolitis is a highly lethal disease which resembles antibiotic "toxicity." It is characterized by sudden death and acute necrolysis of the intestinal mucosa, especially in the cecum, associated with a thermolabile toxin (Wagner, 1976, 1979).

Among the most common forms of enteritis are those of salmonellosis and the fatal necrolytic enterocolitis. The *Salmonella* spp. most commonly found are *S. typhimurium* and *S. enteritidis*; however, other salmonellae including *S. dublin* and *S. limete* have been isolated. Other bacteria associated with enteritis include pseudotuberculosis caused by *Yersinia* (*Pasteurella*) *pseudotuberculosis* and *Y. enterocolitica*; colibacillosis caused by *Escherichia coli*, *Klebsiella pneumoniae*, and *Arizona* spp.; Tyzzer's disease caused by *Bacillus piliformis* (Waggie et al., 1986); and *Pseudomonas* spp. Common necropsy findings of salmonellosis include an enlarged red spleen, sometimes with pale foci of necrosis; enlarged liver with necrotic foci; enlarged lymph nodes; and congested intestines (Habermann and Williams, 1958; Wagner, 1979; Wallach and Boever, 1983; Jayasheela et al., 1985; John et al., 1988). In a young guinea pig with Tyzzer's disease, the *B. piliformis* bacilli were associated with cryptosporidiosis and unclassified intestinal spirochetes (McLeod et al., 1977).

Segmental duodenal hyperplasia associated with an intracellular bacteria proliferation was observed in a female guinea pig, one of 140 obtained from a commercial colony. Two cagemates died with acute enteritis without the mucosal hyperplasia (Elwell et al., 1981).

Although a large number of protozoan parasites are observed in guinea pigs, protozoan diseases are rare. The most important protozoan disease is coccidiosis, which is caused by *Eimeria caviae*. Coccidia are sometimes seen in histological sections of cecum and colon, but rarely causes clinical disease. The clinical signs are anorexia, diarrhea, emaciation, dry hair coat, and rarely death. *Cryptosporidium wrairi,* a small coccidium of the small intestine, may be associated with chronic enteritis. Numerous other protozoa, including *Balantidium coli,* have been observed in the intestinal tract of guinea pigs with little evidence of clinical disease (Vetterling, 1976; Wagner, 1979).

The only intestinal nematodiasis reported in guinea pigs with any degree of frequency is the cecal worm *Paraspidodera uncincata*. It rarely causes clinical disease (Westcott, 1976; Wagner, 1979). Infections can result in diarrhea, lethargy, and anorexia (Wallach and Boever, 1983). No lesions are associated with these infections (Habermann and Williams, 1958).

Nonneoplastic Lesions—Induced.   Antibiotics should be used with caution. The abrupt changes in intestinal microflora following the use of several antibiotics, especially those with broad-spectrum activity, causes high mortality rates from enteritis and what is thought to be endotoxic shock due to overgrowth of gram-negative bacteria, with their accompanying toxins, in the large intestine (Wagner, 1979; Wallach and Boever, 1983). Therefore, penicillin "toxicity" is a well-recognized fatal disease in guinea pigs. Other antibiotics, including bacitracin, chlortetracycline, oxytetracycline, streptomycin, aureomycin, lincomycin, methicillin, erythromycin, and chloromycetin, have been also reported to be toxic to guinea pigs. Penicillin was not toxic for germ-free guinea pigs. The toxicity of intramuscular injections of chloromycetin was attributed to glycols used as vehicles (Altemeier et al., 1950; Hoar, 1976b).

Hartley guinea pigs infected with *Entamoeba histolytica* provide an animal model for enteric amebiasis, with the same type flora found in the original human host. The infection was produced by introducing *E. histolytica* trophozoites and the accompanying enteric flora obtained from humans into germ-free guinea pigs (Jervis and Takeuchi, 1979).

Inflammatory bowel disease (ulcerative colitis and Crohn's disease) can be induced by feeding degraded carrageenan (Anver and Cohen, 1976), or by immunization with an initial sensitization by dinitrochlorobenzene followed with multiple intrarectal instillations of this same chemical (Rabin, 1980). Grossly, multiple pinpoint ulcers and hemorrhages were present in the cecal and colonic mucosae. Cecal and colonic lymphoid tissues were enlarged. Microscopically, the colonic and cecal mucosae have multiple crypt abscesses, superficial mucosal ulcerations, depletion of mucus in cells lining the crypts, edema, infiltration of the lamina propria by a variety of inflammatory cells, mucosal distortion, craterous ulcers, and mucosal and submucosal granulation tissue resembling features of the human ulcerative disease (Anver and Cohen, 1976; Rabin, 1980).

Neoplastic Lesions—Spontaneous.   Spontaneous tumors of the intestine are apparently infrequent. Two tumors have been reported, a fibroid and a liposarcoma of the intestine (Rogers and Blumenthal, 1960, Manning, 1976).

Abdominal Cavity

Nonneoplastic Lesions—Spontaneous.   Abscesses in the visceral organs and peritonitis have been observed with staphylococcosis, *Pseudomonas* spp. (green exudate), and *Corynebacterium* spp. infections including *C. pyogenes*, *C. krutscheri*, and *C. pseudotuberculosis* (grayish and caseous exudate).

Neoplastic Lesions—Spontaneous.   One tumor, a fibrosarcoma, was observed in the peritoneal cavity (Manning, 1976).

Pancreas

Neoplastic Lesions—Spontaneous.   Adenomas or nodules of acinar cells are frequently observed in older animals (Squire et al., 1978).

Liver and Gallbladder

Nonneoplastic Lesions—Spontaneous.   Multifocal hepatic necrosis and enteritis occur together in a variety of conditions. These include salmonellosis, Tyzzer's disease *(Bacillus piliformis)*, pseudotuberculosis *(Yersinia pseudotuberculosis* and *Y. enterocolitica)*, listeriosis *(Listeria monocytogenes)*, and toxoplasmosis *(Toxoplasma gondii)* (Sparrow, and Naylor, 1978; Zwicker et al., 1978; Boot and Walvoort, 1984). Hepatic multifocal necrosis is often accompanied by similar lesions in the spleen. Hepatic necrosis also has been observed focally in clinically normal guinea pigs (Cuba-caparo et al., 1977) and produced by repeated administration of halothane (Hughes and Lang, 1972). A markedly fatty liver can result from ketosis.

Nonneoplastic Lesions—Induced.   Liver lesions have been produced by ingestion of pyrrolizidine alkaloids in *Crotalaris spectabilis* seeds. Clinical signs include ascites, distended abdomen, hepatic necrosis, thrombosis of portal veins, and focal hepatic fibrosis (Carlton, 1967; Chesney and Allen, 1973).

Neoplastic Lesions—Spontaneous.   Spontaneous hepatobiliary neoplasms in the guinea pig are very rare. Reports have included a hepatocellular adenoma, a hepatic cavernous hemangioma, and a papilloma of the gallbladder (Manning, 1976).

Adenocarcinomas of the gallbladder developed in 17 of 68 guinea pigs of strains 2 and 13 over 20 months of age, but none developed in nine noninbred guinea pigs. Significantly more females than males developed tumors (Hoch-Ligeti et al., 1979).

Nonneoplastic Lesions—Induced.   The biliary system of guinea pigs is exquisitely susceptible to hyperplastic or neoplastic stimuli. Benign and malignant neoplasms of the biliary tract were readily induced in guinea pigs by placement of foreign bodies (choleliths, pebbles, string sutures) in the gallbladder and by administration of chemical irritants (Pityrol, lanolin, pitch pellets) (Manning, 1976). Whole body exposure to γ- or x-ray irradiation increased both the number of adenocarcinomas and metastases in male inbred guinea pigs, but not in females (Hoch-Ligeti et al., 1979).

Hepatocellular carcinomas were produced by oral administration of diethylnitrosamine in 14 of 15 guinea pigs (Argus and Hoch-Ligeti, 1963). Hepatocellular tumors were also induced by N-nitroso-N-methylurea (Yoshida et al., 1977).

Urogenital System and Fetal Tissues

Kidney

Nonneoplastic Lesions—Spontaneous. Chronic interstitial nephritis is a commonly observed lesion of aged guinea pigs and ascribed to be the cause of wasting disease in old pet guinea pigs (Wagner, 1976). In this disease, the animal seems to waste away. It drinks a lot of water, loses weight, hunches up, loses condition, and gradually becomes weaker until death. Its mouth often has a strong odor (Ruf, 1984). Nephrosclerosis with increased blood pressure, resembling that in hypertensive humans, has been described in Abyssinian and Hartley guinea pigs (Takeda and Grollman, 1970).

Kidneys heavily infected by *Klossiella cobayae* may have an irregular surface with gray mottling, but in most cases, gross lesions are inapparent. Finding sporocysts in the kidney tubules is diagnostic. Subacute nephritis may accompany the protozoan infection (Vetterling, 1976). Pyelonephritis has been associated with *Corynebacterium* spp. infections, including *C. pyogenes*, *C. krutscheri*, and *C. pseudotuberculosis*.

Nonneoplastic Lesions—Induced. Studies with lead acetate have shown kidney lesions with aminoaciduria that are typical of lead poisoning (Bielecka, 1972).

Autoimmune tubulointerstitial nephritis can be induced by rabbit tubular basement membrane in both strains 2 and strain 13, but the nephropathy develops more quickly in strain 13 (Migrom et al., 1979). NIH Hartley strain guinea pigs are also susceptible to experimental autoimmune tubulointerstitial nephritis. (Hyman et al., 1976; Steblay, 1979).

Neoplastic Lesions—Spontaneous. Only four renal tumors have been reported; two adenocarcinomas (Mosinger, 1961), a round cell sarcoma (lymphosarcoma?) (Ball and Pagnon, 1935), and an osteogenic sarcoma (Twort and Twort, 1932).

Urinary Bladder and Urethra

Nonneoplastic Lesions—Spontaneous. The most common urinary problem in guinea pigs is cystitis, evidenced by pus and blood passed when the animal's bladder is pressed (Roach, 1983). Cystitis in males is sometimes secondary to occlusion of the penile urethra by coagulum from the vesicular glands (Wagner, 1979). Obstruction of the urethra with proteinaceous concretions, probably of seminal vesicular origin, is a contributing cause of death in aged males (Wagner, 1976).

Neoplastic Lesions—Spontaneous. Prior to 1976, five urinary bladder tumors, four of which were malignant, had been reported. These included two transitional cell carcinomas, a epidermoid papilloma, a epidermoid carcinoma, and an anaplastic tumor (Heston and Deringer, 1952; Manning, 1976). In 1980, an additional seven tumors were described in untreated control animals; two were hemangiopericytomas and the others were not specifically identified (Hoch-Ligeti et al., 1980).

Neoplastic Lesions—Induced. Evans (1968) reported an unspecified number of guinea pigs fed bracken fern developed transitional cell, glandular, and squamous cell tumors. A single animal developed an unspecified urinary bladder tumor after 26 guinea pigs received a single injection of 7,12-dimethylbenz(a)anthracene (Toth, 1970). Hemangiopericytomas, transitional cell carcinomas, squamous cell carcinomas, and adenosquamous carcinomas developed in untreated controls and guinea pigs exposed to γ- and x-ray irradiation. Irradiation was associated with significantly earlier tumors, but the increase in numbers of tumor-bearing animals was not statistically significant (Hoch-Ligeti et al., 1980).

Ovary

Nonneoplastic Lesions—Spontaneous. Ovarian and paraovarian cysts are very common in older breeding females. Cystic ovaries were found at necropsy in 54 of 71 (76%) female guinea pigs between 18 and 60 months of age. Fertility was markedly reduced in affected females over the age of 15 months. Cystic endometrial hyperplasia, mucometra, endometritis, inappropriate placental tissue, or fibroleiomyomas frequently accompanied the cystic ovaries (Keller et al., 1987).

Nonneoplastic embryonal malformations within the ovary were described by Loeb (1932). These structures could be misinterpreted as neoplasms. They represent parthenogenetic development of ova within the ovary, resulting in the formation of placental and embryonal structures, and are thought to occur frequently in guinea pigs. They were seen in females less than 6 months of age and most were in guinea pigs less than 4 months of age (Loeb, 1932). Estrogens appear to enhance their development (Mosinger, 1961).

Neoplastic Lesions—Spontaneous. True tumors of the ovary are rare and most (80%) of those reported are teratomas (Frisk et al., 1978). Nineteen of these tumors had been reported as of 1970 (Vink, 1970). The low incidence is indicated by finding only three in 4200 necropsied animals of the R9 strain (Blumenthal and Rogers, 1965) and 10 in 13,000 random-bred animals (Vink, 1970). A malignant ovarian teratoma was described by Gupta and Sarmah (1985). Five cystadenomas and a granulosa cell tumor have been reported (Jain, 1970; Manning, 1976; Squire et al., 1978).

Oviduct, Uterus, and Vagina

The adult female has an intact, epithelial vaginal closure membrane except for the few days of estrus and at parturition. Both these events are signaled by the perforation of this membrane.

Nonneoplastic Lesions—Spontaneous. Guinea pigs appear to be predisposed to high perinatal mortality (Eveleigh et al., 1987). These deaths are often associated with dystocia and subclinical ketosis.

Dystocia is a common problem in guinea pigs and usually occurs either in young females because of a relatively large fetus or in older females because of delayed breeding (Wallach and Boever, 1983). If the first breeding of female guinea pigs is delayed past 7 or 8 months, the pubic symphysis separates with increased difficulty at parturition and fat pads occlude the pelvic canal, which lead to dystocia and death (Harkness and Wagner, 1989). Also, dystocias, appear to be common sequelae of subclinical ketosis. Vaginal prolapse is occasionally associated with parturition (Wagner, 1976).

Metritis, or pyometra, and pyosalpinx can be caused by a variety of organisms, including *Staphylococcus* spp., *Streptococcus* spp., *Corynebacterium pyogenes*, *C. kruts-*

cheri, C. pseudotuberculosis, and *Escherichia coli*. The clinical signs are a mucopurulent to sanguinopurulent discharge from the vulva and a distended abdomen (Wallach and Boever, 1983).

The first deciduoma in a laboratory animal was reported in the guinea pig (Loeb, 1908). These lesions consist of proliferating decidual tissue of the uterus, and were originally regarded as tumors.

Simple cysts are common in the female reproductive tract of guinea pigs. They probably represent remnants of the Wolffian duct system (Squire et al., 1978). Cystic endometrial hyperplasia, mucometra, endometritis, inappropriate placental tissue, or fibroleiomyomas were seen in 21 of 54 (39%) guinea pigs with cystic ovaries, but in only one of 17 (6%) guinea pigs without cystic ovaries (Keller et al., 1987). Cystic endometrial hyperplasia has been described by Ong (1987).

Nonneoplastic Lesions—Induced. Clinical and pathological features of the acute and recurrent genital herpes disease, which are similar to those seen in human genital disease, can be produced in females by inoculation with low dosages of herpes simplex virus type 2. This includes complete healing of genital lesions, histological changes in the genital epithelium and nerve tissues, latent viral infection in the dorsal root ganglia, and transmission of the virus from mother to newborn through an infected birth canal. The cervical dysplasia seen in guinea pigs is similar to that seen in humans, but none of the guinea pigs has been kept long enough for cancer to develop (Lucia and Hsiung, 1981).

Neoplastic Lesions—Spontaneous. One oviduct tumor, an adenoma, and a variety of benign and malignant tumors in the uterus have been observed (Manning, 1976). Seven tumors were described in the uterus of R9 strain animals by Rogers and Blumenthal (1960). These included two leiomyomas, an adenomyoma, a leiomyosarcoma, a fibrosarcoma, a myxosarcoma, and a mixed mesenchymal tumor. Other tumors reported include a sarcoma, a fibromyoma, a myxofibroma, a fibroma, and two adenocarcinomas (Manning, 1976).

Neoplastic Lesions—Induced. Prolonged estrogen administration has induced benign tumors in the uterus of guinea pigs, including fibromas, fibromyomas, and leiomyomas (Manning, 1976).

Prepuce

Nonneoplastic Lesions—Spontaneous. Wood shavings or sawdust used for bedding can become lodged in the prepuce or around the anus in the male guinea pig and form a hard mass that prevents erection (Harkness and Wagner, 1989). Male guinea pigs occasionally develop infections due to these foreign materials in the prepucial folds. Long-standing infections may cause adhesions and infertility (Wagner, 1976).

Vesicular Glands

Nonneoplastic Lesions—Spontaneous. The vesicular glands of the adult male are bilateral, smooth, and transparent and extend approximately 10 cm into the abdominal cavity from their origin in the accessory sex glands. They can be confused with the uterus by an unexperienced observer (Harkness and Wagner, 1989). Their large size and the normal presence of open inguinal canals contributes to their herniation into the scrotum.

Testes

Nonneoplastic Lesions—Induced. Strain 13 guinea pigs are susceptible to the development of experimental autoimmune orchitis by immunization with isogenic and allogenic spermatozoa and with sperm autoantigens (Carlo et al., 1976; Toullet and Voisin, 1979).

Isoimmunization with testicular material in Freund's complete adjuvant resulted in acute and subsequent chronic orchitis (Parsonson et al., 1971).

Neoplastic Lesions—Spontaneous. Testicular tumors of any type are extremely rare in the guinea pig (Squire et al., 1978). There has been a single report of an embryonal carcinoma of the testis (Blumenthal and Rogers, 1965).

Musculoskeletal System

Bone and Joints

Nonneoplastic Lesions—Spontaneous. Broken limbs often occur when guinea pigs not raised in wire-bottomed cages are placed in such cages (Harkness and Wagner, 1983), or are incorrectly handled (Roach, 1983). Bone lesions of scurvy (vitamin C deficiency) include hemorrhage of the epiphyseal plate accompanied by subcutaneous and periarticular hemorrhages (Gleiser, 1974). Spontaneous cartilage degeneration, osteoarthrosis, or osteoarthritis of the femorotibial joint resembles that of osteoarthritis in humans (Gupta et al., 1972; Bendele and Hulman, 1988; Bendele et al., 1989). Septic arthritis has been associated with *Streptococcus* spp., *Corynebacterium* spp., including *C. pyogenes*, *C. krutscheri*, and *C. pseudotuberculosis*, and *Streptobacillus moniliformis*.

Metastatic calcification with calcium deposits in joints, muscles, and various internal organs, including the heart, aorta, lungs, kidneys, stomach, and colon, occurs most often in adult males over the age of 1 year. The guinea pig loses weight, has stiff joints, and usually dies. The causes are considered imbalances of magnesium, potassium, calcium, and phosphorus, aggravated by too much vitamin D (Ruf, 1984), It is believed that hyperphosphatemia results from the inability of the guinea pig to conserve fixed bases by excreting ammonia in the urine; thus, the low-base reserve impairs normal urinary excretion of phosphorus (Fraser et al., 1986).

Nonneoplastic Lesions—Induced. Progressive chronic osteoarthritis has been induced experimentally in the femorotibial joints of guinea pigs by partial medial meniscectomy (Bendele, 1987; Bendele and White, 1987).

Neoplastic Lesions—Spontaneous. Spontaneous tumors of bones are also rare. Manning (1976) cited five tumors which included an enchondroma, an osteogenic sarcoma (osteosarcoma), a chondrosarcoma, an osteochondrosarcoma, and a neurogenic fibrosarcoma. An osteosarcoma was described by Jolivet (1988). Multiple extraskeletal osteogenic sarcomas were reported in a 2-year old female (Cook et al., 1982).

Neoplastic Lesions—Induced. A few osteo- and chondrosarcomas were produced at injection sites by methylcholanthrene in the subcutaneous and muscular tissues (Blumenthal and Rogers, 1965).

Skeletal Muscle

Nonneoplastic Lesions—Spontaneous. Muscular dystrophy is characterized by lameness, stiffness, and refusal to move due to vitamin E deficiency (Ruf, 1984). In a colony of 150 animals, 54 were affected with a myopathy resembling nutritional muscular dystrophy. Fifty percent of those affected died. Major clinical signs were depression, conjunctivitis, and reluctance to move. Lesions were widespread throughout skeletal and cardiac musculature. There was pallor or pale longitudinal streaks in otherwise normal muscle. Microscopically, the lesions were characterized by widespread degeneration and coagulation necrosis with myositis and regeneration in various muscle groups (Ward et al., 1977).

Many cases of myopathy have been observed and reported in guinea pigs in a number of different experimental regimens which have no apparent common etiology. The large muscles of the rear legs are most involved. The lesions are characterized by general muscle degeneration having a varied degree of swelling, loss of cross striations, fragmentation of fibers, and vacuolation. (Wagner, 1976)

Myositis was characterized clinically by swelling and pain in the large muscle groups of the hind legs, followed by front leg involvement, prostration, and death in newly purchased animals. Gross ecchymotic hemorrhages and edema were observed in affected muscles. Microscopically, hemorrhage and edema of the skeletal muscles were the prominent changes with infiltration by acute- to subacute-type inflammatory cells. A virus was suspected but could not be isolated (Saunders, 1958). Guinea pig poxlike virus was isolated from young guinea pigs which spontaneously developed a fibrovascular proliferation in the thigh muscles (Van Hoosier and Robinette, 1976).

Spontaneous arthrogryposis has been reported in a guinea pig. The disease was tetramelic and apparently due to the reduced size of skeletal muscles and their individual fibers. There was an associated myelodysplasia characterized by focal duplication of the spinal canal and no central canal in other areas of the cord (Doige and Olfert, 1974).

Neoplastic Lesions—Spontaneous. Primary tumors of the skeletal muscle are very rare. Kroning and Wepler (1938) reported a lipomyxofibroma invading the psoas muscle in a 3-year-old male guinea pig.

Nervous System and Special Sense Organs

Brain, Spinal Cord, and Nerves

Nonneoplastic Lesions—Spontaneous. Lymphocytic choriomeningitis is a naturally occurring viral disease of the nervous system. The clinical signs include ruffled fur, huddled posture, palpebral edema, conjunctivitis, tremors, convulsions, and hind leg paralysis. Gross findings may be minimal or consist of interstitial pneumonia, pulmonary edema, pleural exudate, fatty liver, and enlarged spleen. Microscopically, marked lymphocytic infiltrations are observed in the meninges, especially at the base of the brain and in the choroid plexus, as well as the liver, adrenals, kidneys, and lungs (Van Hoosier and Robinette, 1976).

A polioviruslike disease, called guinea pig lameness, was associated with a flaccid paralysis and loss of weight. Microscopic changes consisted of a meningomyeloencephalitis affecting the lumbar spinal cord and medulla oblongata.

Spontaneous encephalomyelitis caused by *Encephalitozoon* (*Nosema*) *cuniculi*, a microsporidian organism (Moffatt and Schiefer, 1973) and encephalitis caused by *Toxoplasma gondii*, the tissue form of the feline coccidia, have been observed in guinea pigs (Vetterling, 1976). Meningoencephalitis is sometimes associated with *Streptococcus* (*Diplococcus*) *pneumoniae*.

Nonneoplastic Lesions—Induced. NIH Hartley strain guinea pigs were susceptible to experimental allergic encephalomyelitis (Lisak et al., 1975). Chronic demyelinating optic neuritis can be produced in juvenile strain 13 guinea pigs by intradermal injections of the spinal cord emulsified with Freund's adjuvant. After several months, the optic neuritis is followed by encephalomyelitis. Injections of adult strain 13 animals resulted in acute optic neuritis and allergic encephalomyelitis with death within 4–6 weeks (Rao et al., 1979).

Segmental demyelination and axonal degeneration of the peripheral and cranial nerves in guinea pigs have been produced by lead acetate (Gozdzik-Zolnierkiewicz and Moszynski, 1969; Fullerton, 1966). Asphyxia neonatorum in fetal animals resulted in signs of neural damage and a variety of histopathological changes (Windle and Becker, 1943).

Neoplastic Lesions—Spontaneous. Tumors of the nervous system are apparently very rare (Squire et al., 1978). Only one tumor was reported in the central nervous system, a teratoma of the pons (Lutz, 1910). Interestingly, no gliomas, which are the main type in most other species, were observed (Squire et al., 1978).

Three tumors of the nerve sheaths were described. All three appeared to be neurilem-momas, although one of the inner abdominal wall had a diagnosis of glioma. The other two occurred in the mesentery (Manning, 1976).

Ear

Nonneoplastic Lesions—Spontaneous. Suppurative ear infections (otitis media) are seen occasionally with torticollis, incoordination, and circling behavior if the infection extends to the inner ear. A number of bacterial agents can be involved. Among the most common are those which are also capable of causing respiratory disease such as *Streptococcus zooepidemicus*, *S. pneumoniae*, and *Bordetella bronchiseptica* (Wagner et al., 1976; Wagner, 1979; Roach, 1983; Boot and Walvoort, 1986).

The waltzer strain of guinea pig is characterized by a tendency to "waltz" or whirl and loss of hearing. Rotation does not elicit a nystagmus response and tilting does not evoke counter-rolling of the eyes. There is a loss of the Preyer reflex by 4–6 weeks. They have an impaired swimming ability and righting reflexes. The hearing loss, which affects the high frequency range first, is complete by 42 days. Vestibular capacity is decreased at birth and progresses to complete loss of function. The hair cells of the organ of Corti degenerated, followed by supporting cell degeneration and depopulation of neurons in the spiral ganglion (Ernston, 1970, 1971a,b, 1972a,b,c).

Eye

Nonneoplastic Lesions—Spontaneous. The most common eye disorders in guinea pigs are conjunctivitis, corneal ulcers, and keratitis (Roach, 1983). A wide variety of microorganisms have been isolated from eye lesions, including coliforms, *Streptococcus zooepidemicus*, hemolytic *Streptococcus* spp., *Micrococcus* spp., *Staphylococcus aureus*, *Pasteurella multocida*, *P. hemolytica*, *Salmonella typhimurium*, *S. enteritidis*, *S. dublin*, *Mycoplasma pulmonis*, and *Proteus* spp. (Wagner, 1976). Guinea pig inclusion conjunctivitis is caused by *Chlamydia psittaci* and usually is a mild, self-limiting ocular disease in animals 4–8 weeks old (Deeb et al., 1989).

Cataracts are occasionally seen in young and adult animals as incidental findings, irrespective of the diet. (Wagner, 1976). Senile cataracts develop in old pet guinea pigs at ages 6–8 years (Ruf, 1984).

Bilateral osseous choristomas of the ciliary body were observed in three guinea pigs of a research colony of about 200 animals. One of these animals had also bilateral cataracts (Griffith et al., 1988).

Nonneoplastic Lesions—Induced. Optic disk swelling, a protrusion of the optic nerve head into the vitreous with varying degrees of vascular and peripapillary retinal changes, can be produced in guinea pigs with β, β-iminodipropionitrile (IDPN) (Parhad et al., 1986). Optic disk swelling is seen also in association with optic neuritis and papilledema induced by the intradermal injection of the spinal cord emulsified with Freund's adjuvant (Rao et al., 1979). NIH Hartley strain guinea pigs were susceptible to experimental autoimmune uveitis. (McMaster et al., 1976).

Neoplastic Lesions—Spontaneous. A lymphosarcoma of the choroid and two intraocular reticulosarcomas were reported in guinea pigs by Congdon and Lorenz (1954). Widespread systemic involvement in malignant lymphoma can accompany or precede recognizable intraocular lesions. Scleral dermoids have been observed in four animals (Gupta, 1972).

Endocrine System

Pancreas

Nonneoplastic Lesions—Spontaneous. Acute spontaneous diabetes mellitus was characterized by polydipsia, polyuria, hyperglycemia, glycosuria, elevated glucose tolerance tests, and elevated plasma triglycerides in Abyssinian guinea pigs. It resembled human juvenile diabetes mellitus and spread from animal-to-animal (Munger and Lang, 1973; Lang et al., 1977).

Fatty deposits in the pancreas increase markedly with age. This increase is associated with a proportional increase in islet tissue and a decrease in exocrine pancreatic tissue (Wagner, 1976).

Neoplastic Lesions—Spontaneous. Very few endocrine tumors have been reported. The most frequent were islet cell adenomas. These benign pancreatic islet cell tumors were found in 0.7% of animals of the N:Hart NIH Hartley strain guinea pigs and in 3.5% of strain 13 animals which survived longer than 2 years (Yoshida et al., 1979).

Neoplastic Lesions—Induced. Pancreatic adenocarcinomas have been induced by N-methyl-N-nitrosourea (Reddy et al., 1974; Reddy and Rao, 1975).

Adrenal

Guinea pigs have normally large prominent adrenal glands, which must be considered when evaluating this organ at necropsy.

Nonneoplastic Lesions—Spontaneous. Occasional cortical adenomas or hyperplastic nodules are seen in older guinea pigs (Squire et al., 1978). A number of these lesions were reported in male guinea pigs some years after castration. Manning (1976) considered these lesions most likely to be castration-induced hyperplastic nodules. Enlarged adrenal glands with hemorrhage and cortical necrosis can result from ketosis.

Neoplastic Lesions—Spontaneous. Occasional cortical adenomas or hyperplastic nodules are seen in older guinea pigs (Squire et al., 1978). A number of these lesions were reported in male guinea pigs some years after castration. Manning (1976) considered these lesions to most likely to be castration-induced hyperplastic nodules. Other reports included three cortical adenomas, a cortical carcinoma, and an unclassified tumor (Manning, 1976).

Thyroid

Nonneoplastic Lesions—Induced. NIH Hartley strain guinea pigs (McMaster and Lerner, 1967; McMaster et al, 1967) and strain 2 (Braley-Mullen et al., 1975) guinea pigs are highly susceptible to experimental autoimmune thyroiditis.

Neoplastic Lesions—Spontaneous. Spontaneous thyroid tumors are also rare. One adenoma was observed in a Hartley strain animal. One carcinoma, possibly of parafollicular origin, was described by Zarrin (1974). No parathyroid tumors were reported (Manning, 1976).

Neoplastic Lesions—Induced. Spontaneous pituitary tumors are very rare, if they occur. None have been reported (Manning, 1976; Squire et al., 1978).

Integumentary System and Soft Tissues

Skin

Nonneoplastic lesions—Spontaneous. Guinea pigs born in wire-bottom cages learn to walk without mishap, but naive animals placed in such cages often fall through the mesh and break or lacerate their limbs. The latter animals may also exhibit hair loss, foot pad ulcers, decreased reproduction, and effects from stress (Harkness and Wagner, 1983).

The most common foot problem is peeling of the skin and thickening of the hock with or without ulceration. It seems to be associated with unsuitable bedding and the presence of moisture. Hard damp straw will cause the problem (Roach, 1983). Marked hyperkeratosis of the foot pads is occasionally observed. In some cases, the horny growths approached 2 cm in length. All cases were aged animals confined to laboratory cages (Wagner, 1976).

Abscesses are most commonly found around the jaw, neck, and feet. Abscesses near the throat are of two types. One type is the result of streptococcal infections, and usually involves the cervical lymph nodes. The other type results from inflammation around food materials caught in little pockets or indentations in the cheeks (Ruf, 1984). Abscesses of the skin and feet are often associated with *Staphylococcus aureus* infections (Taylor et al., 1971). A chronic ulcerative pododermatitis can result in which the foot lesions persist indefinitely, periodically ulcerating and bleeding and producing abscesses in draining lymph nodes, osteoarthritis, and generalized amyloidosis (Gleiser, 1974). Wounds and abscesses on the back may be the results of fighting between boars with a group of sows or overcrowding (Roach, 1983).

Dermatitis occurs as result of a variety of conditions in guinea pigs, and can be caused by vitamin C deficiency, bacterial infections, external parasites, or ringworm. External parasites include fleas, ticks, lice (*Gliricola porcelli*, *Gyropus ovalis*, *Tremenopon hispidium* [*jenningsi*]), and mites (*Chirodiscoides caviae*). Heavily louse-infested animals may have a rough, dry hair coat, and may scratch excessively. The signs of ringworm include patchy loss of hair and scaling of the hair or dark spots around the eyes and other parts of the body. Usually there is mild to severe itching, often leading to secondary scabbing and bleeding. The most common causes of ringworm are *Trichophyton mentagrophytes* and *Microsporum gypseum* (Wagner, 1979; Roach, 1983; Ruf, 1984; Fraser et al., 1986).

Alopecia is a manifestation of several conditions. It develops to a degree in all guinea pigs in late pregnancy and is considered a normal phenomenon in aged breeding females. The condition appears to be due to reduced anabolism of maternal skin associated with fetal growth. Adequate zinc levels in the diet are required for hair growth (Wallach and Boever, 1983). Thinning of the hair around the time of weaning is common in young guinea pigs during the period of transition as the baby fur is lost and the coarse guard hairs of adult fur appears (Wagner, 1976; 1979).

Loss of hair from stripping, barbering, or hair chewing occurs in some colonies, especially in animals reared in wire cages. It is thought to be mainly due to boredom. It can be self-inflicted or mutually inflicted (Roach, 1983).

Ear chewing occurs as vice associated with excessive aggressiveness of one or more individuals in a cage or primary enclosure (Wagner, 1976). This practice can lead to skin infections as well as to serious interference in the identification of individual animals from loss of ear notches or ear tags.

Dense populations of sebaceous glands, marking glands, are located circumanally and on the rump. Activity of these glands can result in excessive accumulation of sebaceous secretions in the folds of the circumanal and genital region of adult male guinea pigs. These folds must be cleaned periodically in older males to preclude infections and unpleasant odors.

Nonneoplastic Lesions—Induced. Injections of a mixture of droperidol and fentanyl citrate (Innovar-Vet) have resulted in self-mutilation, distal necrosis at the injection site, and amputation of the leg (Leach et al., 1973; Thayer et al., 1974; Newton et al., 1975; Wagner, 1979).

Neoplastic Lesions—Spontaneous. Prior to 1965, spontaneous skin tumors were considered rare in guinea pigs (Blumenthal and Rogers, 1965); however, examinations of Hartley strain animals at Fort Detrick, Maryland have revealed 29 trichofolliculomas (Manning, 1976). Twenty-one trichofolliculomas were noted at necropsy of 7670 guinea pigs (Ediger et al., 1971). Other skin and subcutaneous tumors reported were trichoepitheliomas, sebaceous adenomas, an undifferentiated adenocarcinoma, an undifferentiated carcinoma, a fibroma, a fibrolipoma, lipomas, fibrosarcomas, a schwannoma, and an undifferentiated sarcoma (Manning, 1976).

Neoplastic Lesions—Induced. Epidermal neoplasms have proven very difficult to induce by topical application. The few that have been reported required a minimum of 2 years of application and large doses of carcinogen (Stenbeck, 1970).

Mammary Gland

Nonneoplastic Lesions—Spontaneous. Bacterial mastitis is a fairly common disease of guinea pigs. It is caused by infections from a variety of organisms, including *Staphylococcus* spp., *Streptococcus* spp., and *Corynebacterium* spp. (Kinkler et al., 1976; Wagner, 1979).

Neoplastic Lesions—Spontaneous. Tumors of the mammary gland are relatively common. Blumenthal and Rogers (1965) reported 12 of the 140 tumors reported in guinea pigs were mammary gland lesions. Tumors that have been described are adenomas, a cystadenoma, fibroadenomas, an adenofibroma, fibrocytadenomas, papillary adenomas, papillary cystadenomas, adenocarcinomas, a liposarcoma, a carcinosarcoma, and a malignant mixed tumor. The adenomas were presumably of ductal or lobular origin. The most common mammary tumors are adenocarcinomas; several of which have been reported in males. Nearly all the carcinomas were believed to be of ductal origin. (Andrews, 1976; Manning, 1976; Squire et al., 1978).

Subcutis

Nonneoplastic lesions—Spontaneous. Subcutaneous abscesses are common lesions in guinea pigs from a variety of injuries. The microorganisms involved vary considerably, but may include *Staphylococcus* spp., *Streptococcus* spp., *Corynebacterium* spp., *Sphaerophorus necrophorus*, and *Escherichia coli* (Wallach and Boever, 1983).

Soft tissue calcification is a disease of nutritional origin characterized by metastatic calcification in various soft tissues, including the muscles, myocardium, joints, stomach, aorta, lungs, kidneys, and, most striking, at the colonic flexure. Microscopically, mineralization may be seen in almost any organ. The condition occurs when there is an imbalance in magnesium, calcium, and phosphorus interrelationships and is corrected by providing an adequate amount of magnesium (Lane-Petter et al., 1967).

Nonneoplastic Lesions—Induced. Soft tissue calcification is a toxic effect of the Argentinian plant *Solanum malacoxylon* (Camberos et al., 1970).

Neoplastic Lesions—Induced. Subcutaneous sarcomas, including fibrosarcomas, a fibromyxoliposarcoma, and liposarcomas, were produced at the site of injection by methyl-cholanthrene (Shimkin and Mider, 1941).

Hematopoietic and Lymphoid Systems

The thymus in immature animals is located subcutaneously in the neck on either side of the trachea, where it is easily removed by surgery (Harkness and Wagner, 1989).

Kurloff cells are mononuclear leukocytes containing intracytoplasmic inclusions of a glycoprotein composition. These cells proliferate during estrogenic stimulation and are found in highest numbers in the placenta, where they may have a function protecting fetal antigens from sensitized maternal lymphocytes and immune globulins. These cells are most prominent during late pregnancy. They are commonly seen in histological sections of the thymus, spleen, and placenta and may originate from the thymus gland (Wagner, 1979; Harkness and Wagner, 1989).

Lymphoid Tissues and Spleen

Nonneoplastic Lesions—Spontaneous. Cervical lymphadenitis primarily caused by β-hemolytic group C *Streptococcus zooepidemicus* results in abscesses of the cervical lymph nodes and occasionally other nodes. The lymph nodes are enlarged and full of pus, from which the organisms can readily be isolated. Other organisms which have been isolated are *Yersinia (Pasteurella) pseudotuberculosis*, *Streptobacillus moniliformis*, and *Sphaerophorus necrophorus*.

Sick guinea pigs should be palpated for enlarged mesenteric lymph nodes, which may indicate mesenteric lymphadenitis resulting from infections caused by *Yersinia pseudotuberculosis* or phycomycosis caused by a fungus in hay. Pseudotuberculosis can spread through the blood to the liver and spleen. Young guinea pigs with swollen mesenteric lymph nodes should be held for 30 days before being discarded, since phycomycosis usually resolves within a month of infection with no ill-effects (Hime and O'Donoghue, 1979). Phycomycosis (mucormycosis) is caused by *Mucor* spp. and *Absidia* spp., and results in a characteristic lymphadenitis and granulomatous inflammation of the viscera. This mycotic infection of the mesenteric lymph nodes must be differentiated microscopically from pseudotuberculosis. Other causes of lymphadenitis in various parts of the body include *Staphylococcus* spp.; *Pasteurella* spp.; *Pseudomonas* spp.; and *Corynebacterium* spp. infections, including *C. pyogenes*, *C. krutscheri*, and *C. pseudotuberculosis*, and toxoplasmosis.

Enlargement and focal necrosis of the spleen often accompanies bacterial diseases such as salmonellosis (*Salmonella typhimurium*, *S. enteritidis*, *S. dublin*, and *S. limete*) and pseudotuberculosis (*Yersinia pseudotuberculosis* and *Y. enterocolitica*).

Nonneoplastic Lesions—Induced. Feeding dried plant material of *Swainsona galegifolia* produces vacuolation of circulating lymphocytes as well as vacuolar lesions in the kidneys, liver, and neurons of the central nervous system. This vacuolation results from a mannoside storage disease caused by the indolizidine alkaloid swainsonine, a potent inhibitor of lysosomal α-D-mannosidase (Huxtable, 1969; Huxtable and Gibson, 1970; Huxtable and Dorling, 1982).

Neoplastic Lesions—Spontaneous. Disseminated lymphomas and lymphocytic leukemias are common in middle-aged to old guinea pigs (Blumenthal and Rogers, 1965). Blumenthal and Rogers (1965) reported an incidence of 7%, including the cases found in the literature. Lymphatic leukemia had an occurrence of 3.6% in the strain 2 guinea pig and an occurrence of 6.7% in strain 13 (Congdon and Lorenz, 1954). The clinical signs are anemia, anorexia, and enlargement of peripheral lymph nodes. On necropsy, grossly enlarged lymph nodes, spleen, and liver are usually present. Microscopically, lympho-blastic cells infiltrate many tissues, especially perivascularly. The spleen, cervical and mesenteric lymph nodes, Peyer's patches, and bone marrow are all heavily infiltrated (Van Hoosier and Robinette, 1976).

A virus has been isolated which produces acute lymphoblastic or stem cell leukemia in strain 2 or F_1 hybrid guinea pigs (Kaplow and Nadel, 1979). Four distinct morphological types of tumors developed in animals injected with the Snijders transplantable leukemia: (1) lymphoblastic leukemia, (2) aleukemic leukemia, (3) lymphosarcoma, and (4) "lym-phosarcoma resembling that of man" (Manning, 1976). Similarities of strain 2 leukemias to human leukemias include origin from bone marrow, rapidly fulminating course with lymphocyte counts of 25,000–100,000, frequent infiltration of practically all organ systems, and response to therapeutic agents (Opler, 1971, Kaplow and Nadel, 1979).

A histiocytic lymphosarcoma was reported by Kitchen et al. (1975). Robinson (1976) reported two primary spleen tumors; a splenoma and a sarcoma. An additional eight primary splenic tumors were reported in untreated control animals of both sexes. They were three glomerate vascular tumors, three sinusoidal hemangioendothelioma, one hemangiosarcoma, and a chrondromatous tumor (Hoch-Ligeti et al., 1981).

Neoplastic Lesions—Induced. Whole body irradiation with x-rays or γ-rays increased the rate of occurrence and number of splenic tumors after the age of 30 months. Lipomatous tumors occurred in addition to the types observed in untreated control animals. A significantly greater number of tumors occurred in inbred strains than in the noninbred strains (Hoch-Ligeti et al., 1981).

Nutrition and Metabolic Diseases

Nonneoplastic Lesions—Spontaneous

Vitamin C (Ascorbic Acid). Guinea pigs, like primates, are genetically deficient in the enzyme L-gulonolactone oxidase in the glucose to vitamin C pathway. They are unable to convert L-gulonolactone to L-ascorbic acid. Also, ascorbic acid turnover is rapid and tissue storage is insufficient for periods of inadequate intake. Therefore, they require adequate dietary ascorbic acid, which is approximately 10 mg/kg body weight per day for maintenance and 30 mg/kg body weight per day during pregnancy. The ascorbic acid can be supplied in the feed, added to the water, or by fresh vegetables such as cabbage, kale, or oranges. Carrots and lettuce are not good sources of vitamin C. Ascorbic acid should be placed in water daily because of the loss of the vitamin's activity. Feed containing ascorbic acid should be properly stored and used within 90 days of milling. Guinea pigs should not be fed diets indicated for other species. Rabbit food, for example, contains no ascorbic acid, and for guinea pigs, excess levels of vitamin D (Navia and Hunt, 1976; Harkness and Wagner, 1989). Guinea pigs fed feed accidentally autoclaved which destroyed the vitamin C have developed scurvy. Vitamin C (ascorbic acid) deficiency results in increased susceptibility to infectious agents such as *Streptococcus zooepidemi-cus*, *S. pneumoniae*, *Bordetella bronchiseptica*, and *Klebsiella pneumoniae* with in-flammation especially of the lungs and cervical lymph nodes.

Signs of vitamin C deficiency are unsteady gait, painful locomotion, hemorrhage from gums, swelling of costochondral junctions, and emaciation. Deaths are common. Lesions include serosal, subcutaneous, and periarticular hemorrhages. Microscopically, there are hemorrhages of the epiphyseal plate, disarray of the cartilage columns, and fibrosis of the marrow in areas of active osteogenesis (Navia and Hunt, 1976; Fraser et al., 1986). Many guinea pigs die of acute bacterial infections before they can die of classic scurvy (Gleiser, 1974).

Nine episodes of subclinical scurvy were observed in 28 guinea pigs. The clinical signs were diarrhea, weight loss, and dehydration. The classic lesions of hemorrhage in the subperiosteum, skeletal muscles, joints, and intestine were not seen. Microscopically, the epiphyses were attenuated and irregular. The amount of osteoid was less than normal. Many guinea pigs had acute enteritis. All episodes were associated with either autoclaving food without adequate supplementation or other inadequate feed management practices (Clarke et al., 1980).

Vitamin D.   Hypervitaminosis D is characterized by medial calcification of the major elastic arteries and soft tissue calcification.

Vitamin E.   Guinea pigs are very sensitive to α-tocopherol deficiency. The clinical signs are stiff and reluctant movements. Microscopically, the skeletal muscle has coagulation necrosis (Wagner, 1979).

Vitamin A.   Hypervitaminosis A is characterized by a high incidence of gross structural malformations in fetuses and newborn animals (Shenefelt, 1972).

Zinc.   Zinc deficiency results in alopecia, especially in female guinea pigs at about the fiftieth day of gestation. The hair will usually regrow in 2 or 3 weeks following parturition if the animals are on an adequate zinc diet (Wallach and Boever, 1983).

Ketosis.   Pregnancy ketosis (toxemia) is a common disease affecting mainly animals in late pregnancy fed low-energy diets, and it can be induced in obese virgin females. Ketosis is characterized clinically by rapid onset, inappetence, depression, and death within 2 to 5 days. Other features include hypoglycemia, lipemia, ketonemia, ketouria, aciduria, and proteinuria. Lesions are nonspecific and include usually a markedly fatty liver and enlarged adrenal glands. Some adrenals have hemorrhages and cortical necrosis. Obesity and stress, especially fasting, in late pregnancy may induce the syndrome (Navia and Hunt, 1976).

Starvation and Water Deprivation.   Starvation and water deprivation should not be underestimated as causes of death in guinea pigs. They are notoriously fixed in their eating habits and do not readily adapt to diets different from those to which they are accustomed. Likewise, they are quite inadept at finding new sources of drinking water in their environment (Wagner, 1979).

Bacterial, Viral, and Rickettsial Diseases

Guinea pigs scatter their bedding into feeders and water crocks. They are notorious for chewing on and otherwise blocking sipper-tubed waterers. They mix dry feed and water in their mouths and pass the slurry into the sipper tube, thereby blocking the tube or causing it to drip. They will also defecate into their feed and water crocks if the feeders and crocks are not suspended above the bedding (Harkness and Wagner, 1983). Because of these behavioral characteristics, infectious agents can become problems in research studies. Good general husbandry and disease prevention procedures are essential when using guinea pigs.

Bacterial Diseases

Infections—Spontaneous.   Guinea pigs are susceptible to a wide variety of microorganisms. At least 19 genera of bacteria, mycoplasmas, and rickettsialike agents have been recovered from laboratory guinea pigs with spontaneous diseases. The most frequently reported bacterial infections causing epizootic disease were *Salmonella* spp., *Bordetella bronchiseptica*, *Streptococcus* spp. (Lancefield group C), and *Yersinia pseudotuberculosis*. These infections have been associated often with high mortality in the guinea pig colony. Less frequently reported causes of epizootic disease have been *Streptococcus pneumoniae*, *Klebsiella pneuomoniae*, *Pasteurella multocida*, *Actinobacillus* spp., and *Pseudomonas* spp. After the epizootic disease subsides, carriers persist, resulting in enzootic disease. Predisposing factors that contribute to the severity of the illness or deaths in the colony are poor husbandry practices such as unhealthy sanitation, over-crowding, mixing of animal species in the same room, improper ventilation, incorrect temperature and humidity control, inadequate diet, transporting the guinea pigs, and experimental procedures (Ganaway, 1976; Boot et al., 1983).

Because they are susceptible to *Bordetella* pneumonia, guinea pigs should not be housed with rabbits, cats, dogs, and other species which carry *Bordetella* subclinically (Harkness and Wagner, 1989). *Campylobacter jejuni* was isolated from the intestines of guinea pigs with no clinical disease (Meanger and Marshall, 1989).

Infections—Induced. *Salmonella typhi* introduced into the gallbladder was recovered from bile and feces of infected, but apparently normal, animals of the NIH Hartley strain for up to 5 months. These animals provide a model for the asymptomatic human typhoid carrier (Lavergne et al., 1977).

Viral, Rickettsial, and Chlamydial Diseases

Infections—Spontaneous. Evidence of more than 16 viral and chlamydial agents have been reported in guinea pigs. These agents belong to a variety of groups including enterovirus (poliovirus), reovirus, paramyxovirus (Sendai virus, simian virus, parain-fluenza type 1), leukovirus (leukemia), arenavirus (lymphocytic choriomeningitis virus), herpesvirus, poxvirus, and psittacosis–lymphogranuloma venereum–trachoma (*Chlamydia*). Serological tests revealed antibodies against poliovirus (16%), reovirus type 3 (4%), pneumonia virus mice (23%), simian virus (25%), and Sendai virus (9%). Leukemia, lymphocytic choriomeningitis, cytomegalovirus (salivary gland), guinea pig herpeslike virus (Connelly et al., 1987), guinea pig poxlike virus, and guinea pig inclusion con-junctivitis chlamydiae have been isolated and described. Viruses are suspected to be involved in myositis (Saunders, 1958) wasting disease, hepatoenteritis, and pneumonia. Viral, rickettsial, and chlamydial diseases and their agents are described in more detail by Van Hoosier and Robinette (1976).

Infections—Induced. In addition to the naturally occurring or spontaneous diseases, the guinea pig has been proven to be a valuable experimental animal in the study of a wide variety of viral, rickettsial, and chlamydial diseases (Van Hoosier and Robinette, 1976). An example is the adaptation of Pichinde virus, an arenavirus, to strain 13 guinea pigs to produce infections similar by virological, pathological, and clinical features of the human disease Lassa fever (Moe and Jahrling, 1984).

Mycotic Diseases

The vast majority of spontaneous fungal diseases in guinea pigs are dermatophytoses limited to the skin. Systemic mycoses such as caused by *Mucor* spp. and *Absidia* spp. are sporadic and described in detail by Sprouse (1976).

Parasitic (Protozoan and Metazoan) Diseases

Protozoan Infection—Spontaneous

Although a large number of protozoan parasites are observed in guinea pigs, protozoan diseases are rare. The most important protozoan diseases are intestinal coccidosis caused by *Eimeria caviae* and renal coccidosis caused by *Klossiella cobayae* (Vetterling, 1976). Three protozoa can cause generalized infections during their acute phases: *Toxoplasma gondii*, the tissue form of the feline coccidia; *Sarcocystis caviae*; and *Encephalitozoon* (*Nosema*) *cuniculi*. *Toxoplasma* infections may produce encephalitis, visceral granulomas, lymphadenitis, splenomegaly, or myocarditis (Wallach and Boever, 1983). *Sarcocystis* is found in skeletal muscle, and *Encephalitozoon* has been reported in the brain (Yost, 1958). Protozoan parasites of guinea pigs have been reviewed in detail by Vetterling (1976).

Metazoan Infection—Spontaneous

The guinea pig may become infested with several different arthropod ectoparasites. Most of these are specific for the guinea pig and well adapted to their host with minimal disease (Ronald and Wagner, 1976).

The only helminth of importance reported in guinea pigs is the cecal worm, *Paraspidodera uncincata*. This intestinal nematode rarely causes clinical disease (Wescott, 1976).

Immunological Disease

Spontaneous Conditions

An inbred strain of complement 4–deficiency guinea pigs has a total deficiency of the C4 component of complement with no evidence of a C4 inhibitor in the serum (Ellman and Green, 1970). Passive anaphylaxis, contact and delayed hypersensitivity, and cellular exudative response to a foreign body are normal indicating the presence of an alternate complement pathway (Ellman et al., 1971a; Frank et al., 1971).

The NIH Hartley strain of guinea pig is susceptible to acute systemic anaphylaxis (Stone et al., 1964). Amyloidosis of multiple organs, particularly the kidneys, liver, spleen, and adrenal glands is rather commonly found in guinea pigs (Wagner, 1976).

Induced Conditions

Strain 2 guinea pigs develop an immune response to bovine serum albumin, 2,4-DNP protamine, human serum albumin, potassium dichromate, beryllium fluoride, hydralazine, insulin, human fibrinopeptide B β 1–14, GA, DNP-PLL, PLL, and DNP-PLA (Ellman et al., 1971; Ellman et al., 1971b; Barcinski and Rosenthal, 1977; Geczy and DeWeck, 1977; Rose et al., 1979; Thomas et al., 1979a; 1979b).

The strain 13 guinea pigs develop an immune response to benzyl-penicilloyl bovine γ-globulin, DNP guinea pig skin protein conjugates, 2,4-DNP guinea pig albumin, mercuric chloride, aspirin, poly(TGAG), GT, insulin, and human fibrinopeptide B β 1–14 (Geczy and DeWeck, 1977).

CONCLUSIONS

The guinea pig has great usefulness as an animal model in toxicology for a broad variety of experimental diseases and test systems in several organ systems. There are relatively few infectious, nutritional, and metabolic diseases which might interfere with toxicology studies. The majority of spontaneous diseases are well described and can be controlled by appropriate husbandry practices.

More information on husbandry, pathology, and diseases, including treatment, are given in the works of Melby and Altman (1974), Wagner and Manning (1976), Benirschke et al., (1978), Hime and O'Donoghue (1979), Wallach and Boever (1983), Rowsell (1984), Manning et al., (1984), Fraser et al., (1986), Anderson (1987), Poole (1987), and Harkness and Wagner (1989). Necropsy of the guinea pig is described by Feldman and Seely (1988). The detailed anatomy is presented by Cooper and Schiller (1975).

ACKNOWLEDGMENTS

The encouragement and assistance of Suzanne B. Neuenschwander, Pamela B. Luther, and Jerry F. Hardisty are profoundly appreciated. The technical assistance of Ann Marie Motley and Lorraine Turner is gratefully acknowledged.

Metabolism   **Christopher P. Chengelis**

XENOBIOTIC METABOLISM

The guinea pig is frequently used for various acute toxicological and pharmacological procedures, but is not often used for chronic systemic toxicity testing. While it has been studied, xenobiotic metabolism is not as well characterized in guinea pigs as in other rodent species. Very few article have been published in which in vivo pharmacokinetics for a particular drug or chemical were examined in guinea pig. Interestingly, despite the common use of the guinea pig in tests for contact sensitization, little work on dermal xenobiotic metabolism has been reported in guinea pigs.

The relatively long gastrointestinal tract, especially the large cecum, tends to make chemicals more bioavailable in the guinea pig than in other species. Other physiological considerations that may play a role in absorption and distribution, such as the extent of the enterohepatic circulation or the imperviousness of the blood/brain or blood/testis barriers have not been well characterized. Hence, the emphasis of this section will be on the biochemical parameters of xenobiotic metabolism in the guinea pig. As a point of reference, comparisons will be made to the rat.

As in other species, the liver is the main organ in the metabolism of xenobiotics in guinea pigs. The liver in the unfasted guinea pig has been reported to be 3.4–3.8% of body weight (Pitrolo et al., 1978). Others have reported a somewhat higher value, up to 4.5% (Smith et al., 1986; Oecsh et al., 1988). The reasons for this slight variability are not clear, but they may be due to age- and/or strain-related differences. In our hands, the mean liver weight of fasted, young adult male Hartley guinea pigs ranges from 2.5 to 3.0% of body weight, which is the same range we generally obtain for Sprague-Dawley rats. The ranges for some common hepatic parameters associated with xenobiotic metabolism are summarized in Table 16.

Table 16 Summary of Hepatic Xenobiotic Metabolizing Enzymes in Guinea Pigs

Enzyme	Concentration or activity	Comments and references
Cytochrome P-450	0.40–1.30 nmol/mg-m 8.0–26.0 nmol/g liver (est.)	Higher concentrations tended to be found in the Hartley strain. Astrom et al. (1986), Peterson et al. (1983), Pitrolo et al. (1978), Smith et al. (1986), Souhaili-el Amri et al. (1986), Ton and Fong (1984)
Cytochrome b_5	0.30–0.83 nmole/mg 6.0–17 nmol/g liver (est.)	Smith et al. (1986), Souhaili-el Amri et al. (1986), Ton and Fong (1984), Zannoni and Lynch (1973)
NADPH: Cytochrome P-450 reductase	24–290 nmol/min/mg-m	Higher activities more common. Amri et al. (1986), Litterest et al. (1975), Pitrolo et al. (1978), Smith et al. (1986), Souhaili-el Amri et al. (1986), Ton and Fong (1984), Zannoni and Lynch (1973)

MMFO activities
  aminopyrene
  aniline
  benzphetamine
  benzo[a]pyrene
	
	4–15 nmol/min/mg-m
	4.0–1.6 nmol/min/mg-m
	1.0–4.5 nmol/min/mg-m
	0.3–1.9 nmol/min/mg-m
		Determined under saturating conditions.
		Astrom et al. (1986), Litterest et al. (1975), Peterson et al. (1983), Pitrolo et al. (1978), Smith et al. (1986), Sikic et al. (1977), Zannoni and Lynch (1973)

Epoxide hydrolase (with styrene oxide)
  microsomal
  cytosolic
	
	5.0–35.0 nmol/min/mg-m
	6.0–300.0 nmol/min/mg-c
		Astrom et al. (1983), Thabrew and Emerole (1983), James et al. (1978), Oesch et al. (1988). Wide range of cytosolic activity probably due to GSH-transferase activity.

UDP-Glucuronosyl transferase
  1-naphthol
  4-aminophenol
  4-nitrophenol
  4-methylumbelliferone
	
	10–90 nmol/min/mg-m
	1.0–3.0 nmol/min/mg-m
	43 ± 2 nmol/min/mg-m
	112 ± 8 nmol/min/mg-m
		Astrom et al. (1987), Litterest et al. (1975), Sikic et al. (1977), Boutin et al. (1984), Ranges drawn from multiple papers, M ± SD from single source.

Glutathione S-transferase
  dinitrochlorobenzene
  dichloronitrobenzene
  4-nitrobenzyl chloride
	
	750–4900 nmol/min/mg-c
	15–60
	35–706
		Hayakawa et al. (1977), Gregus et al. (1985), James et al. (1977), Thabrew et al. (1983), Neal et al. (1987), Sikic et al. (1977)

Abbreviations:
mg-m = mg microsomal protein
mg-c = mg cytosolic protein

With regard to the microsomal mixed function oxidase (MMFO), cytochrome P-450 ranges from 0.40 to 1.30 nmol/mg protein, b_5 from 0.30 to 0.83 nmol/mg, and NAD-PH:cytochrome P-450 reductase from 24 to 290 nmol/min/mg. The broad range of the reductase activity is due the methodology used. While it may be assumed that cytochrome b_5 plays the the same role in MMFO activity in the guinea pig as it does in the mouse, this has not been experimentally established.

With regard to substrate specificity for the MMFO, no outstanding qualitative differences between rats and guinea pigs have been identified, as the guinea pig MMFO has been shown to be active with all substrates identified with activity in rats, but rates and K_ms are different. For example, the male guinea pig has 30 times the activity of benzphetamine N-demethylase, but comparable rates of p-nitroanisole N-demethylase (Souhaili-el Amri et al., 1986).

The guinea pig, however, does differ from the rat with regard to functional site specificity. Guinea pigs lack the ability of rats of N-hydroxylate aromatic amides, but do have a very active aminoalkyl-deamination pathway. It is not clear whether these differences are due to differences in the microsomal mixed function oxidase system, or whether they are due to differences in other enzyme systems. The relative importance of any one functional site on determining the spectrum of metabolites will also depend upon what other sites are available on a substrate. For example, both species have aromatic hydroxylating ability, as evidenced by aniline hydroxylase activity, but in the metabolism of amphetamine, the guinea pig produces no aromatic hydroxylated metabolites and the rat produces no deaminated products (Caldwell, 1981).

The sensitivity of the guinea pig MMFO to competitive inhibitors has not been well characterized. Lunam et al. (1985) demonstrated that 125 mg/kg (ip) SKF 525A inhibited the metabolism and hepatotoxicity (in vivo) of halothane in guinea pigs. Hayakawa et al. (1987) have reported data suggestive that metyrapone and n-octylamine inhibit the MMFO-mediated metabolism in vivo of at least one substrate (nicotine). As in rats, cadmium causes the destruction of cytochrome P-450, but not the reductase, as well as decreases in hexobarbital metabolism and increases in hexobarbital sleeping time (Iscan, 1988). One may accept, as a generalized working hypothesis, that chemicals that inhibit rat MMFO activity will also inhibit guinea pig MMFO activity. Depending on the nature of the experiment, one may need to do additional work to confirm this point.

The cytochrome P-450–dependent mixed function oxidase is not the only microsomal system involved in xenobiotic metabolism. There is also an independent FAD-containing mono-oxygenase system, more extensively described for pigs and rats, which is active in S-oxidation and N-oxidation. Little work has been reported on this enzyme from guinea pigs. Nakiyama et al. (1987) presented evidence that the FAD-containing oxidase is active in the metabolism of nicotine in guinea pigs. Thus, while one can assume that the guinea pig has an FAD-containing mono-oxygenase system, it remains to be fully characterized.

Like the rat, the guinea pig has epoxide hydrolase activity, which ranges from 5.0 to 35.0 nmol/min/mg microsomal protein. In fact, in the few papers that compared the activities in rats and guinea pigs, the latter had the higher activities (Astrom et al., 1987; Thabrew and Emerole, 1987). These studies were conducted with styrene oxide as the substrate; whether or not the differences between rats and guinea pigs also extends to other substrates remains to be established. A generalization that guinea pigs have higher epoxide hydrolase activity than rats would be premature. There is also evidence of a cytosolic epoxide hydrolase in guinea pigs. Great care should be taken in measuring this activity as cytosolic glutathione S-transferase will also metabolize styrene oxide. In fact, the activity of glutathione S-transferase against styrene oxide is much greater than that of cytosolic epoxide transferase. Hence, cytosolic epoxide hydrolase probably plays a relatively minor role in xenobiotic disposition in guinea pigs.

Like the rat, the guinea pig has the ability (Phase II) to conjugate the products of microsomal oxidation. A complete review of all conjugation reactions is outside of the purview of this section. It is assumed that the reader is familiar with the enzyme processes involved (see the introductory chapter, or Caldwell, 1982, for review). The guinea pig does have the ability to form amino acid conjugates, but glycine tends to be the preferred cosubstrate. For example, as presented by Caldwell (1981), the rat will convert 71% of administered 2-naphthylacetate to amino acid conjugates containing glycine, glutamine, and taurine. In the guinea pig, the glucuronide and amino acid conjugates are formed in equal percentage, and only the glycine amino acid conjugate was identified.

The guinea pig has the ability to form both sulfate and glucuronic acid conjugates. The sulfate pathway has been less extensively studied than the glucuronide pathway. Apparently, only one paper has been published in which the relative contributions of these two pathways to the disposition of a single chemical (4-hydroxy-3-methoxyphenyletha-nol) was studied in the guinea pig (Wong, 1976). This paper presents little data, but generally concludes that both processes are active in the guinea pig, but the "sulfate conjugation predominated in both species." Whether this generalization can also be applied to the conjugation of other substrates in the guinea pig remains to be established.

With regard to glucuronidation in the guinea pig, UDP-glucuronosyl transferase activity is generally of the same order of magnitude, but usually slightly higher than that of the rat. However, there can be exceptions to this generalization depending on substrate. The guinea pig has approximately double the activity of the rat in conjugating 1-naphthol (Atrom et al., 1987). In a comparison of different substrates, Boutin et al. (1984) reported that UDP-glucuronosyl transferase activity in guinea pigs was highest with 4-methylum-belliferone (112.4 nmol/min/mg microsomal protein as opposed to 41.6 for the rat) and nondetectable with serotonin (as opposed to 5.5 nmol/min/mg obtained in the rat). Like all species studied, inclusion of Triton X-100 in the in vitro enzyme assay results in activation or increased activity. Other factors that may govern the glucuronidation pathway, such as the availability (i.e., the in vivo "resting" concentration) or UDP-glucu-ronic acid, have not been characterized.

The guinea pig has glutathione S-transferase activity; the activity toward a few common substrates is summarized on Table 16. As with other species, the transferase is a spectrum of isozymes with broad and overlapping specificity, and generally high turnover numbers. Isozymes have been partially characterized. Hayakawa et al. (1977) isolated the isozyme with high activity toward styrene oxide and p-nitrobenzyl chloride. They con-cluded that glutathione S-transferase in guinea pigs does not distinguish between simple epoxides and arene oxides. Neal et al. (1987) characterized glutathione S-transferase in guinea pigs by isoelectric gel focusing on granular gels. For the guinea pig, they found three fractions, with almost all of the aflatoxin-conjugating ability in fraction B. the same system applied to rats yielded five fractions, four of which had significant activity with aflatoxin. When unfractionated cytosol was compared, the guinea pig had higher activity than the rat against three common substrates as well as "activated" aflatoxin. They hypothesized that the differences in sensitivity to aflatoxin between rats and guinea pigs is due to differences in glutathione S-transferase activity. This can not be generalized to all substrates, however. Gregus et al. (1985) have dcemonstrated that there can be consider-able differences in the reactivity of rats and guinea pigs to different substrates of the glutathione S-transferase. For example, guinea pigs have twice the activity toward DNBC than rats, but rats have 8 times the activity toward DCNB. Interestingly, while guinea pigs can form glutathione conjugates, they do not further metabolize these conjugates to mercapturic (N-acetyl-cystinyl conjugates) acids (Caldwell, 1982).

The process of induction refers to the ability of an animal to respond to chronic xenobiotic exposure by increasing the amounts and/or activities of the hepatic enzymes involved in xenobiotic metabolism. The increases in liver weight, microsomal protein, and activity of the MMFO in rats treated with phenobarbital is a well-established example of induction. The processes involved in induction have been well studied in the rat, but only recently examined in the guinea pig. Smith et al. (1986) examined the induction in the guinea pig by both phenobarbital (70 mg/kg/day ip for 4 days) and β-naphthaflavone (40 mg/kg/day ip for 4 days). Neither treatment caused increases in liver weight, but both caused increased cytochrome P-450 with no changes in NADPH:cytochrome P-450 reductase or cytochrome b_5. Phenobarbital, but not β-naphthaflavone, induced increases in aryl-hydrocarbon hydroxylase as well as ethoxyresorufin deethylase, ethoxycoumarin deethylase, and benzphetamine demethylase activities. β-Naphthaflavone increased activity only against ethoxycoumarin. These observations suggest that guinea pigs are less sensitive to induction by the aromatic hydrocarbon–type inducers; i.e., those that induce P-448 (also known as P_1-450). In general, this appears partially true. Thabrew and Emerole (1983) reported that both aniline hydroxylase and aminopyrene demethylase activity are induced by 3-methylcholanthrene and phenobarbital, but phenobarbital was more potent. Astrom et al. (1986) reported that 3-methylcholanthrene induced increases in cytochrome P-450 and ethoxyresorufin deethylase, but not aromatic hydrocarbon hydroxylase. 2-Acetylaminofluorene had no effects on guinea pig MMFO. Hence, not only is the guinea pig less sensitive to cytochrome P-448 type of induction, but the hallmark of this induction in the rat—increases in aromatic hydrocarbon hydroxylase activity—is absent in guinea pigs. Incidentally, the baseline (i.e. noninduced) activity of aromatic hydrocarbon hydroxylase in guinea pigs is much higher than that of rats (Astrom et al., 1986).

It is well established in rats that cytochrome P-450 exists as a family of isozymes and that different inducing agents induce different isozymes. Abe and Watanabe (1983) explored the isozymic nature of cytochrome P-450 and changes induced by 3-methylcholanthrene. It is one of the few papers in which the isozymic nature of cytochrome P-450 was examined. The purpose was to establish a molecular explanation for the refractoriness of guinea pig aromatic hydroxylase activity to 3-methylcholanthrene induction. Three isozymes were isolated and partially characterized with regard to molecular weight, absorption maximum, and substrate specificity. None had a absorption maximum at 448 nm or had distinctive specificity for benzo(a)pyrene. Hence, it would appear that guinea pig simply lacks cytochrome P-448, inducible or otherwise.

The microsomal mixed function oxidase system is not the only enzyme system that is inducible. For example, Atrom et al. (1987) have demonstrated that 3-methylcholanthrene induces increases in epoxide hydrolase, UDP-glucuronosyl transferase, and glutathione S-transferase activities in rats. Similar increases were not induced in guinea pigs. Thabrew and Emerole (1983) have also reported that the glutathione S-transferase and epoxide hydrolase activity in guinea pigs is less inducible (by both phenobarbital and 3-methylcholanthrene) than rats. Gregus et al. (1985) reported that phenobarbital did not induce increases in guinea pig glutathione S-transferase activity against a variety of substrates. Hence, unlike the rat, the phase II enzymes in the guinea pig, as a generalization, are poorly inducible.

Increases in liver weight are not always totally due to increases in microsomal enzymes. A distinct class of chemicals induce increases in peroxisomal enzymes in rats. In general, these are hypolipidemic agents and all are liver carcinogens in rats. Oesch et al. (1988) compared the response of rats and guinea pigs to three different hypolipidemic drugs. Only tiadenol had any effects in the guinea pig. For example, tiadenol (0.5 w/w in the diet for 4 weeks) induced a roughly twofold increase in peroxisomal β-oxidation and no increases in CoA hydrolase activity in guinea pigs, whereas in rats these activities were increased 16- to 18-fold. Hence, unlike the rat, the guinea pig is relatively refractory to the peroxisomal-inducing effect of clofibrate-type drugs. As such, the guinea pig may be good a species for exploring the potential hepatotoxicity of hypolipidemic agents in a model free of the overriding effects of peroxisomal induction.

There is no reported gender difference in guinea pigs with regard to either quantitative or qualitative differences in hepatic xenobiotic metabolism. In one of the few papers where this was investigated, Pitrolo et al., (1979) found no real differences between male and female guinea pigs with regard to cytochrome P-450 concentrations, and benzo-(a)pyrene hydroxylase or ethylmorphine demethylase activities.

The developmental aspects of xenobiotic metabolism has not been well explored. Pitrolo et al. (1977) have reported that hepatic MMFO activity in the guinea pig undergoes rapid perinatal development, reaching adult rates within 3 days after birth. Activity against ethylmorphine and benzo(a)pyrene remains fairly constant in guinea pigs between 25 and 75 days of age, but slowly declines thereafter. These declines occurred even though the total amounts of cytochrome P-450 and NADPH:cytochrome reductase re-mained constant. In contrast, James et al. (1977) reported that glutathione S-transferase and epoxide hydrolase developed somewhat differently, tending to start off low and increase steadily through the perinatal period, up to 27 days of age. Gregus et al. (1985) have demonstrate, however, that the perinatal development and maturational changes of glutathione S-transferase activity in guinea pigs. As a broad generalization, however, peak glutathione S-transferase activities occur in guinea pigs at 30 days of age.

Guinea pigs lack the ability to synthesize ascorbic acid. This has made them the animal model of choice for studying the effects of (deficiency or surplus) ascorbic acid on xenobiotic metabolism. Most of the work pertaining to the effects of ascorbic acid deficiency on MMFO activity in guinea pigs was completed in the 1960s and early 1970s, and is reviewed by Zannoni and Lynch (1973). The classic observation is that an ascorbic acid–deficient diet caused decreases in zoxazolamine metabolism and increases in zoxazo-lamine-induced time of paralysis. The extent to which MMFO activity is influenced by ascorbic acid deficiency depends upon the parameters examined and the time period of ascorbic acid denial. In general, pronounced decreases (e.g., 50% decreases in cyto-chrome P-450) can be obtained with a 21-day exposure period to an ascorbic acid–free diet, which results in hepatic ascorbate concentrations 75–80% less than those in control guinea pigs (Zannoni and Lynch, 1973). However, some changes can be detected in 12–14 days. The ascorbic acid–deficient guinea pigs can be used as a model to study MMFO-activated hepatotoxins. Ton and Fong (1984) reported that an scorbutigenic diet resulted in decreased MMFO activity and decreased N-nitrosodialkylamine clearance and the formation of deoxyribonucleic acid (DNA) adducts.

Given that ascorbic acid deficiency can cause decreases in MMFO activity, it was inevitable that the effects of ascorbic acid excess would also be examined. There was some debate on this issue in the literature (Sikic et al., 1977). Recent evidence suggests that MMFO activity is not altered to an appreciable extent by ascorbic acid excess. Sikic et al. (1977) examined the effect of three different ascorbic acid diets. The lowest (0.3 mg/kg diet) meet the minimum ascorbic acid requirement to prevent scurvy. The highest concentration was 7 mg/g diet. Eight weeks of treatment resulted in no differences between groups with regard to parameters of the MMFO or the UDP-glucuronosyl transferase activity. The guinea pigs on the lowest ascorbic acid diet had the lowest glutathione S-transferase activity. When Peterson et al. (1983) examined the effects of a high dosage of ascrobic acid (50 mg/kg/day by gavage for 10 weeks), they observed slight increases in cytochrome P-450, but not MMFO activity, when compared to "control" (low ascorbate, but not scorbutic) guinea pigs. There was also no effect on phenobarbital inducibility. Ton and Fong (1987) examined the effects of megadoses (400 mg/kg) on MMFO activity and concluded that the regimen did not cause increases in MMFO activity.

While the liver is the predominant organ, both in terms of size and enzyme activities, other organs may also have xenobiotic-metabolizing abilities. Such extrahepatic sites of xenobiotic metabolism may occasionally play a role in the disposition or specific target organ toxicity, and therefore deserve some mention. Litterest et al. (1975), in a now classic paper, examined MMFO and conjugative enzymes in the lung, liver, and kidney of various species, including the guinea pig. Except for the observation that kidney microsomes had undetectable aniline and biphenyl hydroxylase activity, the lung and kidneys tended to have low but measurable amounts of xenobiotic-metabolizing enzymes. For example, the concentrations of cytochrome P-450 were approximately 10-fold greater in the liver as compared to the concentrations in kidney and lung. Smith et al. (1986) confirmed that the renal concentrations of cytochrome P-450 and MMFO activity were much lower than those of the liver. Hietanen and Vanio (1973) reported that small intestine of the guinea pig has low but measurable aromatic hydrocarbon hydroxylase activity. In contrast, Pitrolo and co-workers (1979) reported that the adrenal, gland had higher concentrations of cytochrome P-450 and higher MMFO activity than those found in the liver.

James and co-workers (1977) examined the extrahepatic epoxide–metabolizing activity in the guinea pig. Measurable amounts of epoxide hydrolase and glutathione S-transferase were found in liver, lungs, intestine, and kidneys, but highest activities were found in the liver. For other organs, highest epoxide hydrolase activity was found in the intestine and highest glutathione S-transferase activity was found in kidney.

The flora of the gastrointestinal tract also play a role in xenobiotic metabolism. The gut bacteria tend to catalyze lytic or reductive reactions. In comparison to other rodent species, guinea pigs tend to have much larger cecal contents; roughly 20-fold that for a rat. On the other hand, guinea pigs have the lowest concentration of microflora-mediated enzyme activities, such as β-glucosidase, β-glucuronidase, azoreductase, and nitroreductases. Because of the higher cecal contents, however, total activity may be about the same between the two species. Only nitrate reductase has the activity similar in guinea pigs and rats (Rowland et al., 1986). Relative importance of hindgut microflora in the metabolism of any specific chemical needs to be established on a case-by-case basis.

Up to this point, this discussion has focused largely on quantitative difference between rats and guinea pigs. This last paragraph will briefly focus on qualitative differences; i.e., are there xenobiotic metabolizing systems in the guinea pig that do not exist in the rat? Steffenrud (1985) compared the metabolic profiles of prostaglandin E analogs in guinea pigs and rats. He observed that both species formed ω and ω-1 hydroxy metabolites. However, the guinea pig had prostaglandin hydroxylatory activity in the cytosol, whereas the rat did not. Kitamura et al. (1980) reported the discovery in guinea pigs of a cytosolic enzyme that reduces the sulfoxide moiety of sulindac. The actual implications of these two observations remain to be established. Finally, Lunam et al. (1985) reported that halothane-associated hepatotoxicity in the guinea pig, as in the rat, requires the metabolic activation of halothane by the MMFO; however, the lesion can be induced in the guinea pigs in the absence of enzyme induction and hypoxia. Hence, the guinea pig is a better model for the study of halothane-associated hepatotoxicity than the rat.

REFERENCES

Abe, T., and Watanabe, M. (1982) Purification and characterization of three forms of microsomal cytochrome P-450 in liver from 3-methylcholanthene-treated guinea pigs. *Mol. Pharmacology.* 23, 256–264.

Adrian, R. W., Walker, F. S., and Noel, P.R.B. (1976) Toxicological studies on azapropazone. *Curr. Med. Res. Opin.* 4, 17–34.

Alden, C. L. (1985) Species, sex and tissue specificity in toxicologic and proliferative responses. *Toxicol. Pathol.* 13, 135–140.

Alspaugh, M. A., and Van Hoosier, G. L., Jr. (1973) Naturally-occurring and experimentally-induced arthritides in rodents: A review of the literature. *Lab. Anim. Sci.* 23, 724–736.

Altemeier, W. A., McMurrin, J. A., and Alt, L. P. (1950) Chloromycetin and aureomycin in experimental gas gangrene. *Surgery* 28, 621–631.

Andersen, K. E. (1985) Sensitivity and subsequent "down regulation" of sensitivity induced by chromocresol in guinea pigs. *Arch. Dermatol. Res.* 277, 84–87.

Anderson, L. C. (1987) Guinea pig husbandry and medicine. *Vet. Clin. North Am.*, Small Anim. Pract. 17, 1045–1060.

Andrews, E. J. (1976) Mammary neoplasia in the guinea pig *(Cavia porcellus). Cornell Vet.* 66, 82–96.

Anonymous. (1987) *Animal Diet Reference Guide*, Purina Mills, Inc., Richmond, Indiana, p. 18.

Anver, M. R., and Cohen, B. J. (1976) Ulcerative colitis. *Am. J. Pathol.* 84, 481–484.

Arbab-Zadeh, von A. (1965) Tierversuche mit thalidomid und thalidomid-serum-mischung. *Med. Klin. (Munich)* 60, 1733–1736.

Argus, M. F. (1971) Susceptibility of the guinea pig to chemical carcinogenesis. *Cancer Res.* 31, 917–918.

Argus, M. F., and Hoch-Ligeti, C. (1963) Induction of malignant tumors in the guinea pig by oral administration of diethylnitrosamine. *J. Natl. Cancer Inst.* 30, 533–542.

Astrom, A., Maner, S., and DePierre, J. (1986) Induction of cytochrome P-450 and related drug-metabolizing activities in the livers of different rodent species by 2-acetylaminofluorene or by 3-methylcholanthrene. *Biochem. Pharmacol.* 35, 2703–2713.

Astrom, A., Maner, S., and DePierre, J. (1987) Induction of liver microsomal epoxide hydrolase, UDP-glucuronosyl transferase and cytosolic glutathione transferase in different rodent species by 2-acetylaminofluorene or 3-methylcholanthrene. *Xenobiotica* 17, 155–163.

Ayala, L. E., Alexandre, M. A., and Mora, L. Garcia (1988) Evaluation of different drugs in two models of immediate hypersensitivity. *J. Pharmacol.* 40, 188–191.

Ball, V., and Pagnon, F. (1935) Sarcome a cellules rondes du rein chez un cobave. *Bull. Soc. Sci. Vet. Med. Comp. Lyon* 38:40. Cited in Rogers, J. B. and Blumenthal, H. T. (1960) and Manning, P. J. (1976).

Barcinski, M. A., and Rosenthal, A. S. (1977) Immune response gene control of determinant selection. Intromolecular mapping of the immunogenic sites on insulin recognized by guinea pig T and B cells. *J. Exp. Med.* 145, 726–742.

Bartek, M. J., LaBudde, J. A., and Maibach, H. I. (1972) Skin permeability in vivo: Comparison in rat, rabbit, pig and man. *J. Invest. Dermatol.* 58, 114–123.

Bendele, A. M. (1987) Progressive chronic osteoarthritis in femorotibial joints of partial medial meniscectomized guinea pigs. *Vet. Pathol.* 24, 444–448.

Bendele, A. M., and Hulman, J. F. (1988) Spontaneous cartilage degeneration in guinea pigs. *Arthritis Rheum.* 31, 561–565.

Bendele, A. M., and White, S. L. (1987) Early histopathologic and ultrastructural alterations in femorotibial joints of partial medial meniscetomized guinea pigs. *Vet. Pathol.* 24, 436–443.

Bendele, A. M., White, S. L., and Hulman, J. F. (1989) Osteoarthrosis in guinea pigs: Histopathologic and scanning electron microscopic features. *Lab. Animal Sci.* 39, 115–121.

Benirschke, K., Garner, F. M., and Jones, T. C. (1978) *Pathology of Laboratory Animals.* Vols. 1 and 2. Springer-Verlag, New York.

Berenblum, I. (1949) The carcinogenic action of 9,10-dimethyl-1,2-benzanthracene of the skin and subcutaneous tissues of the mouse, rabbit, rat and guinea pig. *J. Natl. Cancer Inst.* 10, 167–174.

Bielecka, W. (1972) Urinary excretion of alanine, glycine, aspartic acid and glutamic acid of guinea pigs poisoned with lead. *Acta Pol. Pharm.* 29, 113–118. Cited by Hoar, R. B. (1976b), p. 272.

Birnbaum, J. E., Tolman, E. L., Slaboda, A. E., Sparano, B. M., and McClintock, D. K. (1982) Effects on gastric prostaglandin synthesis produced by fenbufen, a new nonsteroidal anti-inflammatory agent with low gastrointestinal toxicity. *Pharmacology* 25, 27–38.

Bivin, W. S., Bryan, J. R., Chang, J., Draper, D. D., Furrow, R. D., Nelson, L. R., and Rohde, N. D. (1969) Diseases of the guinea pig, in *An Outline of Diseases of Laboratory Animals,* Wescott, R. B., Ed. University of Missouri-Columbia, Columbia, Missouri, pp. 38–49.

Blumenthal, H. T., and Rogers, J. B. (1965) Spontaneous and induced tumors in the guinea pigs, in *Pathology of Laboratory Animals,* Ribelin, W. E., and McCoy, J. R., Eds. Thomas, Springfield, Illinois, pp. 183–209.

Boot, R., and Walvoort, H. C. (1984) Vertical transmission of *Bacillus piliformis* infection (Tyzzer's disease) in a guinea pig: Case report. *Lab. Anim.* 18, 195–199.

Boot, R., and Walvoort, H. C. (1986) Otitis media in guinea pigs: Pathology and bacteriology. *Lab. Anim.* 20, 242–248.

Boot, R., Oosterom, J., and Walvoort, H. C. (1983) Recovery of members of the *Pasteurella-Actinobacillus*-group from guinea pigs. *Lab. Anim.* 17, 285–289.

Boutin, J., Antoine, B., Batt, A., and Siest, G. (1984) Heterogeneity of hepatic microsomal UDP-glucuronyl-transferase activities: Comparison between human and mammalian species activities. *Chem. Bio. Int.* 52, 173–184.

Boyd, E. M. (1970) Testicular atrophy from analgesic drugs. *J. Clin. Pharmacol.* 222–227.

Boyd, E. M., and Fulford, R. A. (1961). The acute oral toxicity of benzylpenicillin potassium in guinea pigs. *Antibiot. Chemother.* 11, 276–283.

Braley-Mullen, H., Sharp, G. C., and Kyriakos, M. (1975) Differential susceptibility of strain 2 and strain 13 guinea pigs to induction of experimental autoimmune thyroiditis. *J. Immunol.* 114, 371–373.

Breazile, J. E., and Brown, E. M. (1976) Anatomy, in *The Biology of the Guinea Pig,* J. E. Wagner and P. J. Manning, eds. Academic Press, New York, pp. 115.

Brennecke, L. H., Dreier, T. M., and Stokes, W. S. (1983) Naturally occurring virus-associated respiratory disease in two guinea pigs. *Vet. Pathol.* 20, 488–491.

Bruce, H. M., and Parker, A. S. (1947) Feeding and breeding of laboratory animals. III. Observations on the feeding of guinea pigs. *J. Hyg.* 45, 70–78.

Brummett, R. E. (1983) Animal models of aminoglycoside antibiotic ototoxicity. *Rev. Infect. Dis.* 5, 5294–5303.

Buehler, E. V. (1964) A new method for detecting potential sensitizers using the guinea pig. *Toxicol. Appl. Pharmacol.* 6, 341.

Buehler, E. V. (1965) Delayed contact hypersensitivity in the guinea pig. *Arch. Dermatol.* 91, 171–177.

Burnette, J. C., Simpson, D. M., Chandler, D. C., Jr., and Bawden, J. W. (1968) Fetal blood calcium response to maternal parathyroid and vitamin D administration in guinea pigs. *J. Dent. Res.* 47, 444–446.

Calabrese, E. J. (1983) *Principles of Animal Extrapolation.* Wiley, New York.

Calabrese, E. J. (1988) Comparative biology of test species. *Environ. Health Perspect.* 77, 55–62.

Caldwell, J. (1981) The current status of attempts to predict species differences in drug metabolism. *Drug. Metab. Rev.* 12, 221–237.

Caldwell, J. (1982) Conjugation reactions in foreign-compound metabolism: definition, consequences, and species variations. *Drug Metab. Rev.* 13, 745–777.

Camberos, H. R., Davis, G. K., Djafar, M. I., and Simpson, C. G. (1970) Soft tissue calcification in guinea pigs fed the poisonous plant *Solanum malacoxylon. Am. J. Vet. Res.* 31, 685–696.

Campbell, R. L., and Bruce, R. D. (1981) Comparative dermatotoxicology. *Tox. Appl. Pharmacol.* 59, 555–563.

Cardy, R. H., and Lijinsky, W. (1980) Comparison of the carcinogenic effects of five nitrosamines in guinea pigs. *Cancer Res.* 40, 1879–1884.

Carlo, D. J., Hagopian, A., Jackson, J. J., Limjuco, G. A., and Eylar, E. H. (1976) Experimental allergic orchitis and aspermatogenesis. VI. Transfer of allergic orchitis with immune cells. *J. Immunol.* 116, 619–622.

Carlson, R. G., and Feenstra, E. S. (1977) Toxicologic studies with the hypotensive agent minoxidil. *Toxicol. Appl. Pharmacol.* 39, 1–11.

Carlton, W. W. (1967) Crotalaria intoxication in guinea pigs. *J. Am. Vet. Med. Ass.* 151, 845–855.

Cazals, Y., and Guilhaume, A. (1985) Otoconia and neural junctions of type I hair cells in amikacin-treated guinea pigs presenting saccular acoustic responses. *Arch. Otorhinolaryngol.* 242, 155–160.

Cazen, M. N. (1987) Retrospective evaluation of appropriate animal models based on metabolism studies in man, in *Human Risk Assessment: The Role of Animal Selection and Extrapolation.* Taylor and Francis, Philadelphia, pp. 99–112.

Chase, M. W. (1941) Inheritance in guinea pigs of the susceptibility to skin sensitization with simple chemical compounds. *J. Exp. Med.* 73, 711–726.

Chase, M. W. (1953) The inheritance of susceptibility to drug allergy in guinea pigs. *Trans. N.Y. Acad. Sci.* 15, 79–82.

Chesney, C. F., and Allen, J. R. (1973) Resistance of the guinea pig to pyrrolizidine alkaloid intoxication. *Toxicol. Applied Pharmacol.* 26, 385–392.

Christensen, O. B., Christensen, M. B., and Maibach, H. I. (1984) Flare-up reactions and desensitization from oral dosing in chromate sensitive guinea pigs. *Contact Dermatitis* 10, 277–279.

Chung, M., Parravicini, L., Assad, B. M., Cavanna, G., Radwanski, E., and Symchowicz, S. (1982) Comparative pharmacokinetics of aminoglycoside antibodies in guinea pigs. *Antimicrol. Agents Chemother.* 22, 1017–1021.

Clarke, G. L., Allen, A. M., Small, J. D., and Lock, A. (1980) Subclinical scurvy in the guinea pig. *Vet. Pathol.* 17, 40–44.

Collins, G. R. (1979) *Manual for Laboratory Animal Technicians,* Publication 67-3. American Association for Laboratory Animal Science, Joliet, Illinois.

Collins, M., and Elvehjem, C. A. (1958) Ascorbic acid requirement of the guinea pig using growth and tissue ascorbic acid concentrations as criteria. *J. Nutr.* 64, 503–511.

Congdon, C. C., and Lorenz, E. (1954) Leukemia in guinea pigs. *Am. J. Pathol.* 30, 337–359.

Connelly, B. L., Keller, G. L., and Myers, M. G. (1987) Epizootic guinea pig herpes-like virus infection in a breeding colony. *Intervirology* 28, 8–13.

Cook, J. E. (1958) Salivary gland virus disease of guinea pigs. *J. Natl. Cancer Inst.* 20, 905–910.

Cook, R. A., Burk, R. L., and Herron, A. L. (1982) Extraskeletal osteogenic sarcoma in a guinea pig. *J. Am. Vet. Med. Assoc.* 181, 1423–1424.

Cooper, G., and Schiller, A. L. (1975) *Anatomy of the Guinea Pig,* Harvard University Press, Cambridge, Massachusetts.

Cuba-caparo, A., Myers, D. M., and Germino, N. I. (1977) Focal hepatic necrosis in clinically normal guinea pigs: Bacteriological and pathological studies. *J. Comp. Pathol.* 87, 441–450.

D'Mello, G. D. (1986) Effects of sodium cyanide upon swimming performance in guinea pigs and the conferment of protection by pretreatment with p-aminopropiophenone. *Neurobehav. Toxicol. Teratol.* 8, 171–178.

Davitaya, M. D., and Nadirashvili, S. A. (1971) Method of recording blood pressure in the umbilical arteries of guinea pig fetuses with the placental circulation intact. *Bull. Exp. Biol. Med.* (U.S.S.R.) 71, 119–120.

Deeb, B. J., DiGiacomo, R. F., and Wang, S-P. (1989) Guinea pig inclusion conjunctivitis in a commercial colony. *Lab. Anim.* 23, 103–106.

Doige, C. E., and Olfert, E. D. (1974) Arthrogryposis and myelodysplasia in a guinea pig. *Lab. Animal Sci.* 24, 103–104.

Draize, J. H. (1959) *The Appraisal of Chemicals in Foods, Drugs and Cosmetics.* Association of Food and Drug Officials of the U.S., Austin, Texas, pp. 36–45.

Draize, J. H., Woodard, G., and Calvery, H. O. (1944) Methods for the study of irritation and toxicity of substances applied topically to the skin and mucus membranes. *J. Pharmacol. Exp. Ther.* 82, 377–390.

Ediger, R. D. (1976) Care and management, in *The Biology of the Guinea Pig,* Wagner, J. E., and Manning, P. J., Eds. Academic Press, New York, pp. 5–12.

Ediger, R. D., and Rabstein, N. (1968) Spontaneous leukemia in a Hartley strain guinea pig. *J. Am. Vet. Med. Ass.* 153, 954–956.

Ediger, R. D., Dill, G. S., and Kovatch, R. M. (1971) Trichofolliculoma of the guinea pig. *J. Natl. Cancer Inst.* 46, 517–523.

Ediger, R. D., Warnick, C. L., and Hong, C. C. (1975) Malocclusion of the premolar and molar teeth in the guinea pig. *Lab. Animal Sci.* 25, 760–762.

Edmondson, P. W., and Wyburn, J. R. (1963) The erythrocyte lifespan, red cell mass and plasma volume of normal guinea pigs as determined by the use of chromium, phosphorus labelled di-iso-propyl flurophosphonate and iodine labelled human serum Albumin. *Br. J. Exp. Pathol.* 44, 72–80.

Edwards, M. J. (1957) Congenital defects in guinea pigs, following induced hyperthermia during gestation. *Arch. Pathol.* 84, 42–48.

Edwards, M. J. (1969a) Congenital defects in guinea pigs: Fetal resorptions, abortions, and malformations following induced hyperthermia during early gestation. *Teratology* 2, 313–328.

Edwards, M. J. (1969b) Hyperthermia and congenital malformations in guinea pigs. *Aust. Vet. J.* 45, 189–193.

Edwards, M. J. (1969c) Congenital defects in guinea pigs: Prenatal retardation of brain growth of guinea pigs following hyperthermia during gestation. *Teratology* 2, 329–336.

Ellman, L., and Green, I. (1970) Genetically controlled total deficiency of the fourth component of complement in guinea pigs. *Science* 170, 74–75.

Ellman, L., and Green, I. (1971) L2C guinea pig leukemia: Immunoprotection and immunotherapy. *Cancer* 28, 645–654.

Ellman, L., Green, I., Judge, F., and Frank, M. M. (1971a) *In vivo* studies in C4-deficient guinea pigs. *J. Exp. Med.* 134, 162–175.

Ellman, L., Inman, J., and Green, I. (1971b) Strain differences in the immune response to hydralazine in inbred guinea pigs. *Clin. Exp. Immunol.* 9, 927–937.

Elwell, M. R., Chapman, A. L., and Frenkel, J. K. (1981) Duodenal hyperplasia in a guinea pig. *Vet. Pathol.* 18, 136–137.

Emerson, R. J. and Cole, P. J. (1983) Failure of macrophage activation to induce pulmonary fibrosis in asbestos-exposed guinea pigs. *Br. J. Exp. Pathol.* 64, 66–74.

Epstein, S. (1939) Photoallergy and primary photosensitization to sulfanilamide. *J. Invest. Dermatol.* 2, 43–51.

Ernston, S. (1970) Heredity in a strain of the waltzing guinea pig. *Acta Otolaryngol. (Stockh.)* 69, 358–62.

Ernston, S. (1971a) Cochlear morphology in a strain of the waltzing guinea pig. *Acta Otolaryngol. (Stock.)* 71, 469–482.

Ernston, S. (1971b) Vestibular physiology in a strain of the waltzing guinea pig. *Acta Otolarynggol. (Stockh.)* 72, 303–309.

Ernston, S. (1972a) *The Waltzing Guinea Pig*. A study on inherited inner-ear degeneration. Department of Otolaryngology, Karolinska Sjuhuset, and the King Gustaf V Research Institute, Stockholm, Sweden.

Ernston, S. (1972b) Cochlear physiology and hair cell population in a strain of the waltzing guinea pig. *Acta Otolaryngol.* (Suppl.) 297, 1–18.

Ernston, S. (1972c) *The Waltzing Guinea Pig*. A study on inherited inner-ear degeneration. Thule, Stockholm, pp. 1–15. Cited in Veterinary Resources Branch, 1981, p. 153.

Ernstrom, U. (1970) Hormonal influences on thymic release of lymphocytes into the blood. *Ciba Found. Study Group* 36, 53–65. Cited by Sisk, D. B. (1976).

Evans, I. A. (1968) The radiomimetic nature of bracken toxin. *Cancer Res.* 28, 2252–2261.

Eveleigh, J. R. (1988) The development of rabbit, guinea pig and mouse cages. *Anim. Technol.* 39, 107–116.

Eveleigh, J. R., McLaughlin, S. H., and Williams, H. L. (1987) Stillbirths and the Pirbright Dunkin Hartley guinea pig. *Anim. Technol.* 38, 191–200.

Fara, J. W., and Catlett, R. H. (1971) Cardiac response and social behavior in the guinea pig *(Cavia porcellus)*. *Anim. Behav.* 19, 514.

Feldman, D. B., and Seely, J. C. (1988) Necropsy of the guinea pig *(Cavia porcellus)*, in *Necropsy Guide: Rodents and the Rabbit*. Chemical Rubber Company Press, Boca Raton, Florida, pp. 105–131.

Fenner, F. (1986) The domestication and uses of laboratory rodents, in *Viral and Mycoplasmal Infections of Laboratory Rodents: Effects on Biomedical Research*, Bhatt, P. N., Jacoby, R. O., Morse, H. C., III, and New A. E. eds. Academic Press, Orlando, Florida, pp. 19–33.

Firpo, A., Godwin, T. A., Becker, G. C., Santos-Buch, C., Griffith, R. B., Thomas, M. A., and Davis, D. L. (1988) Pulmonary pathology in guinea pigs at 27 weeks of dose monitored cigarette smoke exposure. *F.A.S.E.B. J* 2, A578.

Flecknell, P. A. (1987) *Laboratory Animal Anaesthesia*. Academic Press, New York, pp. 95–97.

Frank, M. M., May, J., Gaither, T., and Ellman, L. (1971) *In vivo* studies of complement function in sera of C4-deficient guinea pigs. *J. Exp. Med.* 134, 176–187.

Fraser, C. M., Mays, A., and Huebner, R. A., (Eds.) (1986) *The Merck Veterinary Manual*. Merck and Co., Inc., Rahway, New Jersey, pp. 942–944.

Frisk, C. S., Wagner, J. E., and Doyle, R. E. (1978) An ovarian teratoma in a guinea pig. *Lab. Animal Sci.* 28, 199–201.

Fullerton, P. M. (1966) Chronic peripheral neuropathy produced by lead poisoning in guinea pigs. *J. Neuropathol. Exp. Neurol.* 25, 214–236.

Gad, S. C., and Chengelis, C. P. (1989) *Acute Toxicology*. Telford Press, Caldwell, New Jersey.

Ganaway, J. R. (1976) Bacterial, mycoplasma, and rickettsial diseases, in *The Biology of the Guinea Pig*, Wagner, J. E., and Manning, P. J., Eds. Academic Press, New York, pp. 121–135.

Geczy, A. F., and DeWeck, A. L. (1977) Molecular basis of T cell dependent genetic control of the immune response in the guinea pig. *Prog. Allergy* 24, 147–213.

Gibson, C. C., Hubbard, R., and Parke, D. V. (1983) *Immunotoxicology*. Academic Press, New York.

Gilman, N. (1982) Skin and eye testing in animals, in *Pathology of Laboratory Animals*. Vol. 2. Benirschke, K., Garner, F. M., and Jones, T. C., eds. Springer-Verlag, New York, pp. 210–216.

Giroud, A., and Martinet, M. (1959a) Teratogenese par hypervitaminosis A chez le rat, la souris, le cobaye et le lapin. *Arch. Fr. Pediatr.* 16, 971–975.

Giroud, A. and Martinet, M. (1959b) Extension a plusieurs éspèces de mammiferes des malformations embryonnaires par hypervitaminose A. *C.R. Soc. Biol.* 153, 201–202.

Gleiser, C. A. (1974) Diseases of laboratory animals-bacterial, in *Handbook of Laboratory Animal Science*. Vol II. Melby, E. C., and Altman, N. H., Eds. Chemical Rubber Company Press, Cleveland, Ohio, pp. 273–285.

Gorray, K. C., Baskin, D. G., and Fugimoto, W. Y. (1986) Physiological and morphological changes in islet B cells following treatment of the guinea pig with alloxan. *Diabetes Res.* 3, 187–191.

Gozdzik-Zolnierkiewicz, T., and Moszynski, B. (1969) VIII nerve in experimental lead poisoning. *Acta Oto-Laryngol.* 68, 85–89. Cited by Hoar, R. M. (1976).

Gregus, Z, Watkins, J. B., Thompson, T. N., Harvey, M. J., Rozman, K., and Klaassen, C. D. (1983) Hepatic phase I and phase II biotransformation in quail and trout: Comparison to other species commonly used in toxicity testing. *Toxicol. Appl. Pharmacol.* 67, 430–441.

Gregus, Z., Varga, F., and Schmelas, A. (1985) Age-development and inducibility of hepatic glutathione S-transfersase activities in mice, rats, rabbits and guinea-pigs. *Comp. Biochem. Physiol.* 80C, 85–90.

Griffith, J. F., and Buehler, E. V. (1977) Prediction of skin irritancy and sensitizing potential by testing with animals and man, in *Cutaneous Toxicity*, Drill, V. A., and Lazar, P., eds. Academic Press, New York, pp. 155–174.

Griffith, J. W., Sassani, J. W., Bowman, T. A., and Lang, C. M. (1988) Osseous choristoma of the ciliary body in guinea pigs. *Vet. Pathol.* 25, 100–102.

Guillot, J. P. and Gonnett, J. F. (1985) The epicutaneous maximization test. *Curr. Probl. Dermatol.* 14, 220–247.

Guillot, J. P., Gonnet, J. F., Loquene, J. F., Martini, M. C., Covert, P., and Cotte, J. (1985) A new method for the assessment of phototoxic and photoallergic potentials by topical applications in the albino guinea pig. *J. Toxicol. Cut. Ocular Toxicol.* 4(2), 112–133.

Gupta, B. N. (1972) Scleral dermoid in a guinea pig. *Lab. Anim. Sci.* 22, 919–921.

Gupta, B. N., Conner, G. H., and Meyer, D. B. (1972) Osteoarthritis in guinea pigs. *Lab. Anim. Sci.* 22, 362–368.

Gupta, P. P., and Sarmah, P. C. (1985) Malignant ovarian teratoma in a guinea pig. *Indian Vet. J.* 62, 906.

Gurll, N. J., and Denbesten, L. (1979) Gallstones, in *Spontaneous Animal Models of Human Disease*. Vol II, Anderews, E. J., Ward, B. C., and Altman, N. H., Eds. Academic Press, New York, pp. 57–58.

Habermann, R. T., and Williams, F. P., Jr. (1958) Salmonellosis in laboratory animals. *J. Natl. Cancer Inst.* 20, 933–948.

Harber, L. C. (1981) Current status of mammalian and human models for predicting drug photosensitivity. *J. Invest. Dermatol.* 77, 65–70.

Harber, L. C. and Shalita, A. R. (1975) The guinea pig as an effective model for the demonstration of immunologically-mediated contact photosensitivity, in *Animal Models in Dermatology*, Maibach, H., ed. Churchill Livingstone, New York, pp. 90–102.

Harkness, J. E., and Wagner, J. E. (1983) *The Biology and Medicine of Rabbits and Rodents*. 2nd ed. Lea & Febiger, Philadelphia.

Hayakawa, T., Myokei, Y., Yagi, H., and Jerina, H. (1977) Purification and some properties of glutathione-S-epoxide transferase from guinea pig liver. *J. Biochem* 82, 407–415.

Heston, W. E., and Deringer, M. K. (1952) Introduction of pulmonary tumors in guinea pigs by intravenous injection of methylcholanthrene and dibenzanthracene. *J. Natl. Cancer Inst.* 13, 705–718.

Hietanen, E., and Vainio, H. (1973) Interspecies variations in small intestinal and hepatic drug hydroxylation and Glucuronidation. *Acta Pharmacol. Toxicol.* 33, 57–64.

Hoar, R. M. (1969) Resorption in guinea pigs as estimated by counting corpora lutea: The problem of twinning. *Teratology* 2, 187–190.

Hoar, R. M. (1976a) Biomethodology, in *The Biology of the Guinea Pig,* Wagner, J. E., and Manning, P. J., Eds. Academic Press, New York, pp. 13–20.

Hoar, R. M. (1976b) Toxicology and teratology, in *The Biology of the Guinea Pig,* Wagner, J. E., and Manning, P. J., eds. Academic Press, New York, pp. 269–280.

Hoar, R. M. (1976c) Developmental abnormalities: Guinea pigs, in *Pathology of Laboratory Animal,* Vol. 2, Benirschke, K., Garner, F. M., and Jones, T. C., eds. Springer-Verlag, New York, pp. 1860–1866.

Hoar, R. M., and King, T. J. (1967) Further observations on resorption in guinea pigs following injections of trypan blue. *Anat. Rec.* 157, 617–620.

Hoar, R. M., and Salem, A. J. (1961) Time of teratogenic action of trypan blue in guinea pigs. *Anat. Rec.* 141, 173–182.

Hoch-Ligeti, C., and Argus, M. F. (1970) Effect of carcinogens on the lung of guinea pigs, in *morphology of Experimental Respiratory Carcinogenesis,* Nettlesheim P., Hanna, M. G., Jr., and Deatherage, J. W., Jr., Eds. United States Atomic Energy commission, Division of Technical Information, Washington, D.C., pp. 267–279.

Hoch-Ligeti, D., Congdon, C. C., Deringer, M. K., and Stewart, H. L. (1979) Adenocarcinoma of the gallbladder in guinea pigs. *J. Natl. Cancer Inst.* 62, 381–386.

Hoch-Ligeti, C., Congdon, C. C., Deringer, M. K., Strandberg, J. D., and Stewart, H. L. (1980) Hemangiopericytoma and other tumors of urinary tract of guinea pigs. *Toxicol. Pathol.* 8(1), 1–8.

Hoch-Ligeti, C., Congdon, C. C., Deringer, M. K., and Stewart, H. L. (1981) Primary tumors of the spleen in guinea pigs. *Toxicol. Pathol.* 9(1), 9–16.

Hoch-Ligeti, C., Congdon, D. C., Deringer, M. K., Strandberg, J. D., Sass, B., and Stewart, H. L. (1982) Primary tumors and adenomatosis of the lung and in irradiated guinea pigs. *Toxicol. Pathol.* 10(1), 1–11.

Holmes, D. D. (1984) *Clinical Laboratory Animal Medicine.* Iowa State University Press, Ames.

Hong, C. C. (1980) Spontaneous papillary cystadenocarcinoma of the ovary in Dunkin-Hartley guinea pigs. *Lab. Anim.* 14, 39–40.

Hong, C. C., and Lui, P. I. (1981) Osteogenic sarcoma in 2 guinea pigs. *Lab. Anim.* 15, 49–51.

Hong, C. C., Lui, P. I., and Poon, K. C. (1980) Naturally occurring lymphoblastic leukemia in guinea pigs. *Lab. Anim. Sci.* 30, 222–226.

Hottendorf, G. H. (1985) Carcinogenicity testing of antitumor agents. *Toxicol. Pathol.* 13, 192–199.

Hughes, R. E., Jr., and Lang, C. M. (1972) Hepatic necrosis produced by repeated administration halothane to guinea pigs. *Anesthesiology* 36, 466–471.

Hutchinson, P. (1983) *Howell Beginner's Guide to Guinea Pigs.* Howell Book House, New York.

Huxtable, C. R. (1969) Experimental reproduction and histopathology of *Swainsona galegifolia* poisoning in the guinea pig. *Aust. J. Exp. Biol. Med. Sci.* 47, 339–347.

Huxtable, C. R., and Dorling, R. (1982) Mannosidosis. *Am. J. Pathol.* 107, 124–126.

Huxtable, C. R., and Gibson, A. (1970) Vacuolation of circulating lymphocytes in guinea pigs and cattle ingesting *Swainsona galegifolia.* *Aust. J. Exp. Biol. Med. Sci.* 46, 446–448.

Hyman, L. R., Colvin, R. B., and Steinberg, A. D. (1976) Immunopathogenesis of autoimmune tibulointerstitial nephritis. I. Demonstration of differential susceptibility in strain 2 and strain 13 guinea pigs. *J. Immunol.* 116, 327–335.

Ichikawa, H., Armstrong, R. B. and Harber, L. C. (1981) Photoallergic contact dermatitis in guinea pigs: Improve induction technique using Freund's complete adjuvant. *J. Invest. Dermatol.* 76, 498–501.

Innes, J.R.M. (1965) Lesions of the respiratory tract of small laboratory animals, in *The Pathology of Laboratory Animals,* Ribelin, W. E., and McCoy, J. R., Eds. Thomas, Springfield, Illinois, pp. 49–59.

Ishihara, Y., Yamada, Y., Hata, Y. and Okabe, S. (1983a) Species and strain differences in mepirizole-induced duodenal and gastric lesions. *Dig. Dis. Sci.* 28, 552–558.

Ishihara, Y., Yoshiharu, Y., Hata, Y., and Susumu, O. (1983b) Species and strain differences in mepirizole-induced duodenal and gastric lesions. *Dig. Dis. Sci.* 28, 552–558.

Jain, S. K., Singh, D. K., and Rao, U.R.K. (1970) Granulosa cell tumor in a guinea pig. *Indian Vet. J.* 47, 563–564.

Jayasheela, M., Gowal, K. N., John, P. C., Mago, M. L., and Saxena, S. N. (1985) An outbreak of salmonellosis and guinea-pigs. *Indian Vet. J.* 62, 1009–1012.

Jervis, H. R., and Takeuchi, A. (1979) Animal model: Experimental *Entamoeba histolytica* infection in the germfree guinea pig. *Am. J. Pathol.* 94, 197–200.

John, P. C., Gowal, K. N., Jayasheela, M., and Saxena, S. N. (1988) Natural course of salmonellosis in a guinea pig colony. *Indian Vet. J.* 65, 200–204.

Jolivet, M. R. (1988) Osteosarcoma in a guinea pig. *Compan. Anim. Pract.* 2, 30–31.

Jolly, D. W., and Heywood, R. (1979) Disease prevention, in *Handbook of Diseases of Laboratory Animals,* Hime, J. M., and O'Donoghue, P. N., Eds. Heinemann Veterinary Books, London, pp. 1–16.

Kaplow, L. S., and Nadel, E. (1979) Acute lymphoblastic leukemia. *Am. J. Pathol.* 95, 273–276.

Kapusnik, J. E., and Sande, M. A. (1986) Novel approaches for the use of aminoglycosides: The value of experimental models. *J. Antimicrob. Chemother.* 17, 7–10.

Karol, M. H. (1980) Immunologic response of the respiratory system to industrial chemicals, in *Proceedings of the Inhalation Toxicology and Technology Symposium,* Leong, B.K.J., ed. Ann Arbor Science, Ann Arbor, Michigan, pp. 233–246.

Karol, M. H., Dixon, C., Brady, M., and Alarie, Y. (1980) Immunologic sensitization and pulmonary hypersensitivity by repeated inhalation of aromatic isocyanates. *Toxicol. Appl. Pharmacol.* 53, 260–270.

Kaufmann, A. F. (1970) Bony spicules in guinea pig lung. *Lab. Anim. Care* 20, 1002–1003.

Kaup, F. J., Naumann, S., Kunstyr, I., and Drommer, W. (1984) Experimental viral pneumonia in guinea pigs: An ultrastructural study. *Vet. Pathol.* 21, 521–527.

Keller, L.S.F., Griffith, J. W., and Lang, C. M. (1987) Reproductive failure associated with cystic rete ovarii in guinea pigs. *Vet. Pathol.* 24, 335–339.

Kibler, H. H., Brody, S., and Worstell, D. (1947) Surface area and metabolism of growing guinea pigs. *J. Nutr.* 33, 331.

Kiese, M., and Wiedemann, I. (1968) Elimination of N-hydroxy arylamines from the blood of guinea pigs. *Biochem. Pharmacol.* 17, 1151–1158.

Kinkler, R. J., Jr., Wagner, J. E., Doyle, R. E., and Owens, D. R. (1976) Bacterial mastitis in guinea pigs. *Lab. Anim. Sci.* 26, 214–217.

Kitchen, D. N., Carlton, W. W., and Bickford, A. A. (1975) A report of 14 spontaneous tumors of the guinea pig. *Lab. Anim. Sci.* 25, 92–102.

Klecak, G. (1983) Identification of contact allergens: Predictive tests in animals, in *Dermatotoxicology.* 2nd ed., Marzulli, F. N., and Maibach, H. I., eds. Hemisphere, New York.

Kligman, A. M. (1966) The identification of contact allergens by human assay. III. The maximization test. A procedure for screening and rating contact sensitizers. *J. Invest. Dermatol.* 47, 393–409.

Koestner, A., and Buerger, L. (1965) Primary neoplasms of the salivary glands in animals compared to similar tumors in man. *Vet. Pathol.* 2, 201–226.

Kohn, D. F. (1974) Bacterial otitis media in the guinea pig. *Lab. Anim. Sci.* 24, 823–825.

Komich, R. J. (1971) Anophthalmos: An inherited trait in a new stock of guinea pigs. *Am. J. Vet. Res.* 32, 2099–2105.

Kroning, F., and Wepler, W. (1938) Ein histologisch beachtenswerter tumor des meerschweinchens. *Z. Krebsforsch.* 48, 246–251. Cited in Manning, P. J. (1976).

Kunstyr, I. and Naumann, S. (1984) A contribution to guinea pig longevity data: Nine-and-half years old guinea pig. *Z. Versuchstierkunde* 26, 57–59.

Kunstyr, I., Maess, J., Naumann, S., Kaup, F. J., Kraft, V., and Knocke, K. W. (1984)

Adenovirus pneumonia in guinea-pigs, an experimental reproduction of the disease. *Lab. Anim.* 18, 55–60.

Laitinen, M. and Watkins, J. B., III (1986) Mucosal Biotransformations, in *Gastrointestinal Toxicology,* Rozman, K., and Hanninen, O., Eds. Elsevier, Amsterdam, pp. 169–192.

Landsteiner, K. and Chase, M. W. (1937) Studies on the sensitization of animals with simple chemical compounds. IV. Anaphylaxis induced by picrylchloride and 2:4 dinitrochlorobenzene. *J. Exp. Med.* 66, 337–351.

Landsteiner, K. and Chase, M. W. (1940) Studies on the sensitization of animals with simple chemical compounds. VII. Skin sensitization by intraperitoneal injection. *J. Exp. Med.* 71, 237–245.

Landsteiner, K., and Chase, M. W. (1941). Studies on the sensitization of animals with simple chemical compounds. IX. Skin sensitization induced by injection of conjugates. *J. Exp. Med.* 73, 431–438.

Landsteiner, K., and Chase, M. W. (1942). Experiments on transfer of cutaneous sensitivity to simple chemical compounds. *Proc. Soc. Exp. Biol. Med.* 49, 688.

Landsteiner, K., and DiSomma, A. A. (1938). Studies on the sensitization of animals with simple chemical compounds. V. Sensitization to diazomethane and mustard oil. *J. Exp. Med.* 68, 505–512.

Landsteiner, K., and Jacobs, J. (1935). Studies on the sensitization of animals with simple chemical compounds. *J. Exp. Med.* 61, 643–657.

Landsteiner, K., and Jacobs, J. (1936). Studies on the sensitization of animals with simple chemical compounds. II. *J. Exp. Med.* 64, 625–629.

Lane-Petter, W. (ed.) (1963). *Animals for Research: Principles of Breeding and Management.* Academic Press, New York.

Lane-Petter, W., Worden, A. N., Hill, B. F., Paterson, J. F., and Verzerf, H. G. (eds.) (1967). *The U.F.A.W. Handbook on Care and Management of Laboratory Animals.* Livingstone, Edinburgh.

Lang, C. M., Munger, B. L., and Rapp, F. (1977). The guinea pig as an animal model of diabetes mellitus. *Lab. Anim. Sci.* 27, 789–805.

LaRegina, M. C. (1979). Thyroid papillary adenoma in a guinea pig with signs of cervical lymphadenitis. *J. Am. Vet. Med. Ass.* 175, 969–971.

Lavergne, G. M., James H. F., Martineau, C., Diena, B. B., and Lior, H. (1977). The guinea pig as a model for the asymptomatic human typhoid carrier. *Lab. Animal Sci.* 27, 806–816.

Leach, A. M., Beyer, R. D., and Wilber, R. G. (1973). Self-mutilation following Innovar-Vet injection in the guinea pig. *Lab. Animal Sci.* 23, 720–721.

Lechat, P., Mudgett-Hunter, M. Margolies, M. N. Haber, E., and Smith, T. W. (1984) Reversal of lethal digoxin toxicity in guinea pigs using monoclonal antibodies and Fab fragments. *J.P.E.T.* 229, 210–213.

Lee, S. P. and Thomsen, L. L. (1982) Toxin-induced cell membrane injury in guinea pigs given lincomycin. *Pathology* 14, 317–322.

Lee, K. J., Johnston, W. D., and Lang, C. M. (1977) Acute gastric dilatation associated with gastric volvulus in the guinea pig. *Lab. Animal Sci.* 27, 685–686.

Lehr, D. (1965) Lesions of the cardiovascular system, in *The Pathology of Laboratory Animals,* Ribelin, W. E., and McCoy, J. R., eds. Thomas, Springfield, Illinois, p. 129.

Levine, W. G. (1978) Biliary excretion of drugs and other xenobiotics. *Ann. Rev. Pharmacol. Toxicol.* 18, 81–96.

Lisak, R. P., Zweiman, B., Kies, M. W., and Driscoll, B. (1975) Experimental allergic encephalomyelitis in resistant and susceptible guinea pigs: *In vivo* and *in vitro* correlates. *J. Immunol.* 114, 546–549.

Loeb, L. (1908) The production of deciduomata. *J. Am. Vet. Med. Assoc.* 50:1897–1901. Cited by Elcock, L. H., Stuart, B. P., Mueller, R. E., Hoss, H. E. (1987).

Loeb, L. (1932) The parthenogenetic development of eggs in the ovary of the guinea pig. *Anat. Rec.* 51, 373–408. Cited by Manning, P. J. (1976).

Loury, D. J., and Byard, J. L. (1985) Genotoxicity of the cooked-food mutagens IQ and MeIQ in primary cultures of rat, hamster and guinea pig hepatocytes. *Environ. Mutagen.* 7, 245–254.

Lunam, C. A., Cousins, M. J., and Hall, P. M. (1985) Guinea pig model of halothane-associated hepatotoxicity in the absence of enzyme induction and hypoxia. *J.P.E.T.* 232, 802–809.

Lucia, H. H., and Hsiung, D. D. (1981) Genital herpes model No. 238, in *Handbook: Animal Models of Human Disease,* Fasc. 22. Capen, C. C., Hackel, D. B., Jones, T. C., and Migaki, G., Eds. Registry of Comparative Pathology, Armed Forces Institute of Pathology, Washington, D.C.

Lutz, B. (1910) Ein teratom am Kleinhirnbruckenwinkel beim meerschwe inchen. *Arb. Neurol. Inst. Univ. Wien.* 18, 111–117. Cited by Mannig, P.L.J. (1976).

Magnusson, B. (1975) The relevance of results obtained with the guinea pig maximization test, in *Animal Models in Dermatology,* Maibach, H., ed. Churchill Livingstone, Edinburgh, pp. 76–83.

Magnusson, B., and Kligman, A. M. (1969) The identification of contact allergies by animal assay. The guinea pig maximization test. *J. Invest. Dermatol.* 52, 268–276.

Magnusson, B., and Kligman, A. M. (1970) Allergen contact dermatitis in the guinea pig, in *Identification of Contact Allergens,* Thomas, Springfield, Illinois.

Maguire, H. C. (1973a) Mechanism of Intensification by Freund's complete adjuvant of the acquisition of delayed hypersensitivity in the guinea pig. *Immunol. Commun.* 1, 239–246.

Maguire, H. C. (1973b) The bioassay of contact allergies in the guinea pig. *J. Soc. Cosmet. Chem.* 24, 151–162.

Maguire, H. C. (1975) Estimation of the allergenicity of prospective human contact sensitizers in the guinea pig, in *Animal Models in Dermatology,* Maibach, H., ed. Churchill Livingstone, Edinburgh, pp. 67–75.

Maguire, H. C., and Chase, M. W. (1967) Exaggerated Delayed-type hypersensitivity to simple chemical allergies in the guinea pig. *J. Invest. Dermatol.* 49, 460–468.

Maguire, H. C., and Chase, M. W. (1972) Studies on the sensitization of animals with simple chemical compounds. XIII. Sensitization of guinea pigs with picric acid. *J. Exp. Med.* 135, 357–374.

Manning, P. J., (1976) Neoplastic diseases, in *The Biology of the Guinea Pig,* Wagner, J. E., and Manning, P. J., eds. Academic Press, New York, pp. 211–225.

Manning, P. J., Wagner, J. E., and Harkness, J. E. (1984) Biology and diseases of guinea pigs, in *Laboratory Animal Medicine,* Fox, J. G., Cohen, B. J., and Loew, F. M. eds. Academic Press, New York, pp. 149–181.

Mariani, L., and Bonanomi, L. (1978) Resistance of the guinea pig to indomethasin ulcerogenesis. *Toxicol Appl. Pharmacol.* 45, 637–639.

Martin, F. N., and Maibach, H. L. (1988) *Dermatotoxicology.* 3rd ed. Hemisphere, Washington, D.C.

Maurer, T., Thomann, P. Weirich, E. G., and Hess, R. (1975) The optimization test in the guinea pig. *Agents Actions* 5, 174–179.

Maurer, T., Weirich, E. G., and Hess, R. (1980) The optimization test in the guinea pig in relation to other predictive sensitization methods. *Toxicology* 15, 163–171.

McConnell, R. F., and Ediger, R. D. (1968) Benign mesenchymoma of the heart in the guinea pig. *Pathol. Vet.* 5, 97–101.

McCormick, J. G., and Nuttall, A. L. (1976) Auditory research, in *The Biology of the Guinea Pig,* Wagner, J. E., and Manning, P. J., eds. Academic Press, New York, pp. 281–303.

McLeod, C. G., Stookey, J. L., Harrington, D. G., and White, J. D. (1977) Intestinal Tyzzer's disease and spirochetosis in a guinea pig. *Vet. Pathol.* 14, 229–235.

McMaster, P.R.B., and Lerner, E. M., II. (1967) The transfer of allergic thyroiditis in histocompatible guinea pigs by lymph node cells. *J. Immunol.* 99, 208–213.

McMaster, P.R.B., Lerner, E. M., II, Kyriakos, M., and Mueller, P. S. (1967) The influence of the dose of thyroid extract and mycobacteria upon experimental autoimmune thyroiditis in inbred histocompatible and random-bred guinea pigs. *J. Immunol.* 99, 201–207.

McMaster, P.R.B., Wong, V. G., and Owens, J. D. (1976) The propensity of different stains of guinea pigs to develop experimental autoimmune uveitis. *Mod. Probl. Ophthalmol.* 16, 62–71.

McMichael, R. F., Dipalma, J. R., Blumenstein, R., Amenta, P. S., Freedman, A. P. and Barbieri, E. J. (1983) A small animal model study of perlite and fir bark dust on guinea pig lungs. *J. Pharmacol. Meth.* 9, 209–217.

Meanger, J. D., and Marshall, R. B. (1989) *Campylobacter jejuni* infection within a laboratory animal production unit. *Lab. Anim.* 23, 126–132.

Melby, E. C., and Altman, N. H. (1974) *Handbook of Laboratory Animal Science.* Vols. I and II. Chemical Rubber Company Press, Cleveland, Ohio.

Melby, E. C., and Altman, N. H. (1976) *Handbook of Laboratory Animal Science.* Vol. III. Chemical Rubber Company Press, Cleveland, Ohio.

Melnikona, E. A., and Rodionov, G. A. (1979) Experimental pathology of the rabbit and guinea pig's eye caused by the antibiotic grisin. *Lab. Gig. Otsenki Biopreparet.* 6, 85–88.

Milgrom, M., Albini, B., and Noble, B. (1979) Antibodies in guinea pigs immunized with kidney and lung basement membranes. *Clin. Exp. Immunol.* 38, 249–258.

Miller, C. P., Jr. (1924) Attempts to transmit rheumatic fever to rabbits and guinea pigs. *J. Exp. Med.* 40, 525. Cited by Lehr, D. (1965).

Miller, E. C., Miller, J. A., and Enomoto, N. (1964) The comparative carcinogenicities of 2-acetylaminofluorene and its N-hydroxy metabolite in mice, hamster, and guinea pigs. *Cancer Res.* 24, 2018–2026.

Mitruka, B. M., Rawnsley, H. M., and Dharam, V. V. (1976) *Animals for Medical Research.* Wiley, New York.

Moe, J. B., and Jahrling, P. B. (1984) Fatal arenavirus infection. Model No. 301, in *Handbook: Animal Models of Human Disease.* Fasc. 13, Capen, C. C., Hackel, D. B., Jones, T. C., and Migaki, G., Eds. Registry of Comparative Pathology, Armed Forces Institute of Pathology, Washington, D.C.

Moffatt, R. E., and Schiefer, B. (1973) Microsporidiosis (encephalitozoonosis) in the guinea pig. *Lab. Anim. Sci.* 23, 282–284.

Morgan, G. (1969) Ocular tumors in animals. *J. Small Anim. Pract.* 10, 563–570.

Mosinger, M. (1961) Sur la canceroreistance du cobaye. Premiere partie. Les spontanees du cobaye. *Bull. Assoc. Fr. Etud. Cancer,* 48: 217–235. Cited by Manning, P. J. (1976).

Moto, T., Noguchi, Y., Suzuki, K., and Zaw, K. M. (1983) Adenomatous intestinal hyperplasia in guinea pigs associated with *Campylobacter*-like bacteria. *Jpn. J. Med. Sci. Biol.* 36, 337–342.

Munger, B. L., and Lang, C. M. (1973) Spontaneous diabetes mellitus in guinea pigs. *Lab. Invest.* 29, 685–702.

Muraoka, Y., Hayashi, Y., and Minesita, T. (1968) Studies on Capreomycin nephrotoxicity. *Toxicol. Appl. Pharmacol.* 12, 250–259.

Murphy, S. Y., and LoBuglin, H. F. (1977) L2C Leukemia: A model of human acute leukemia. *Fed. Proc.* 36, 2285–2289.

Nakayama, H., Fujihara, S., Nakashima, T., and Kurogochi, Y. (1987) Formation of two major nicotine metabolites in livers of guinea pigs. *Biochem. Pharmacol.* 36, 4313–4317.

NAS Publication 1138 (1977) *Principles and Procedures for Evaluating the Toxicity of Household Substances.* Prepared for the Consumer Product Safety Commission, National Academy of Sciences, Washington, D.C., pp. 36–39.

Naumann, S., Kunstyr, I., Langer, I., Maess, J., and Hoerning, R. (1981) Lethal pneumonia in guinea-pigs associated with a virus. *Lab. Anim.* 15, 235–242.

Navia, J. M. and Hunt, C. E. (1976) Nutrition, nutritional diseases and nutritional research applications, in *Biology of the Guinea Pig,* Wagner, J. E., and Manning, P. J., eds. Academic Press, New York, pp. 235–267.

Neal, G., Nielsch, U., Judah, D., and Hulbert, P. (1987) Conjugation of model substrates or mocrosomally-activated aflatoxin B1 with reduced glutathione, catalyzed by cytosolic glutathione-S-transferase in livers of rats, mice and guinea pigs. *Biochem. Pharmacol.* 36, 4269–4276.

Newton, W. M., Cusick, P. K., and Raffe, M. C. (1975) Innovar-Vet-induced pathologic changes in the guinea pig. *Lab. Anim. Sci.* 25, 597–601.

NIH (1985) *Guide for the Care and Use of Laboratory Animals.* NIH Publication No. 85-23, Bethesda, Maryland.

Nixon, G. A., Tyson, C. A., and Wertz, W. C. (1975) Interspecies comparisons of skin irritancy. *Toxicol. Appl. Pharmacol.* 31, 481–490.

Nungester, W. J., and Ames, A. M. (1948) The relationship between ascorbic acid and phagocytic activity. *J. Infect. Dis.* 83, 50–54.

Oecsh, F., Hartmann, R., Timms, C., Strolin-Benedetti, Dostert, M., Worner, W., and Schladt, L. (1988) Time-dependence and differential induction of rat and guinea pig peroxisomal β-oxidation, palmitoyl-CoA hydrolase, cytosolic and microsomal epoxide hydrolase after treatment with hypolipidemic drugs. *J. Cancer Res. Clin. Oncol.* 144, 341–346.

Olcott, C. T., and Papanicolaou, G. N. (1943) Studies of spontaneous tumors in guinea pigs. III. A chondrosarcoma of the iliac bone with metastasis to mammary region. *Cancer Res.* 3, 321–325.

Olson, L. C., and Anver, M. R. (1980) Ovarian stromal sarcoma in a guinea pig. *Vet. Pathol.* 17, 245–247.

Ong, C. D. (1987) Endometrial cystic hyperplasia in a guinea pig. *Mod. Vet. Pract.* 68, 368–369.

Opler, S. R., (1971) Defining the role of the guinea pig in cancer research: A new model for leukemia and cancer immunology studies, in *Defining the Laboratory Animal,* National Academy of Sciences, National Research, Council, Washington, D.C., pp. 435–449.

Papanicolaou, G. N., and Olcot, C. T. (1940) Studies of spontaneous tumors in guinea pigs. I. A fibromycoma of the stomach with adenoma (focal hyperplasia) of the right adrenal. *Am. J. Cancer* 40, 310–320.

Papanicolaou, G. N., and Olcott, G. T. (1942) Studies of spontaneous tumors in guinea pigs. II. Tumors of the stomach and intestine. *Arch. Pathol.* 34, 218–228.

Parhad, I. M., Griffin, J. W., and Miller, N. R., (1986) Optic disk swelling. Model No. 335, in *Handbook: Animal Models of Human Disease.* Fasc. 15, Capen, C. C., Jones, T. C., and Migaki, G. eds. Registry of Comparative Pathology, Armed Forces Institute of Pathology, Washington, D.C.

Parker, G. A., Russel, R. J., and Depaoli, A. (1977) Extrapulmonary lesions of Streptococcus pneumoniae infection in guinea pigs. *Vet. Pathol.* 14, 332–337.

Parker, D., and Turk, J. L. (1983) Contact sensitivity to acrylate compounds in guinea pigs. *Contact Dermatitis* 9, 55–60.

Parravicini, L., Forlani, A., Marzanatti, M., and Arpini, A. (1983) Comparative ototoxicity of dibekacin and netilmicin in Guinea Pigs. *Acta Pharmacol. Toxicol.* 53, 230–235.

Parsonson, I. M., Winter, A. J., and McEntee, K. (1971) Allergic epididymo-orchitis in guinea pigs and bulls. *Vet. Pathol.* 8, 333–351.

Peckham, J. C. (1980) Experimental oncology, in *The Laboratory Rat.* Vol II, Baker, H. J., Lindsey, J. R., and Weisbroth, S. J., Eds. Academic Press, New York, pp. 119–147.

Perez, R., Kriedemann, W. L., O'Donnell, R. W., and Cockerell, G. L. (1980) Endoscopic detection of experimentally induced colonic neoplasms in guinea pigs *(Cavia porcellus). Lab. Anim. Sci.* 30, 684–688.

Peterson, F., Holloway D., Duquette, P., and Rivers, J. (1983) Dietary ascorbic acid and hepatic mixed function oxidase activity in the guinea pig. *Biochem. Pharmacol.* 32, 91–96.

Petri, C. (1935) Die Entwicklung des Skeletts von Cavia. *Med. Dissert.* Zurich.

Pitrolo, D., Rumbaugh, C., and Colby, H. (1979) Maturational changes in adrenal xenobiotic metabolism in male and female guinea pigs. *Drug Metab. Dispos.* 7, 52–56.

Ponder, E. (1948) *Hemolysis and Related Phenomena.* Grune & Stratton, New York.

Poole, T. B. (1987) *The U.F.A.W. Handbook on the Care and Management of Laboratory Animals.* 6th ed. Churchill Livingstone, New York, pp. 393–410.

Quinn, G. P., Axelrod, J., and Brodie, B. B. (1958) Species, strain and sex-differences in metabolism of hexobarbitone, amidopyrine, antipyrine and aniline. *Biochem. Pharmacol.* 1, 152–159.

Rabin, B. S. (1980) Immunologic model of inflammatory bowel disease. *Am. J. Pathol.* 99, 253–256.

Rackemann, F. H., and Simon, F. A. (1934) The sensitization of guinea pigs to poison ivy. *Science* 79, 344.

Rao, V. R. (1979) Biological models for research in environmental toxicology. *Bull Haff. Janstt.* 7, 15–19.

Rao, N. A., Tang, R. A., and Irving, G. W., III (1979) Demyelinating optic neuritis. Model No. 166, in *Handbook: Animal Models of Human Disease*. Fasc. 8, Jones, T. C., Hackel, D. B., and Migaki, G., Eds. Registry of Comparative Pathology, Armed Forces Institute of Pathology, Washington, D.C.

Reddy, J. K., and Rao, M. S. (1975) Pancreatic adenocarcinoma in inbred guinea pigs induced by N-methyl-N-nitrosurea. *Cancer Res.* 35, 2269–2277.

Reddy, J. K., Svoboda, D. J., and Rao, M. S. (1974) Brief communication: Susceptibility of an inbred strain of guinea pig to the induction of pancreatic adenocarcinoma by N-methyl-N-nitrosurea. *J. Natl. Cancer Inst.* 52, 991–992.

Remmer, H., and Merker, H. (1963) Drug-induced changes in liver endoplasmic reticulum: Association with drug-metabolizing enzymes. *Science* 142, 1567–1568.

Rhim, J. S., and Green, I. (1977) Guinea pig L2C leukemia: Immunological, virological, and clinical aspects. *Fed. Proc.* 36, 2247–2332.

Rhim, J. S., Cho, H. Y., Kim, J. M., and Green, I. (1976) Characterization of virus-free guinea pig tumors *J. Natl. Cancer Inst.* 56, 1233–1236.

Richter, C. R. (1986) Mouse adenovirus, K virus, pneumonia virus of mice, in *Viral and Mycoplasmal Infections of Laboratory Rodents: Effects on Biomedical Research*, Bhatt, P. N., Jacoby, R. O., Morse, H. C., III, and New, A. E., eds. Academic Press, Orlando, Florida, pp. 19–33.

Roach, P. (1983) *The Complete Book of Pet Care*. Howell Book House, New York.

Robens, J. F. (1970) Teratogenic effects of hypervitaminosis A in the hamster and the guinea pig. *Toxicol. Appl. Pharmacol. 16*, 88–89.

Robens, J. F., Joiner, J. J., and Schueler, R. L. (1982) Methods in testing for carcinogenicity, in *Principles and Methods of Toxicology*, Hayes, A. W., Ed. Raven Press, pp. 80–81.

Robinson, F. R. (1976) Naturally occurring neoplastic disease. V. Guinea pig, in *Handbook of Laboratory Animal Science*. Vol. III, Melby, E. C., Jr., and Altman, N. H., eds. Chemical Rubber Press, Cleveland Ohio, pp. 309–323.

Rogers, J. B., and Blumenthal, H. T. (1960) Report of fourteen spontaneous guinea pig tumors with a review of the literature. *Cancer Res.* 20, 191–196.

Ronald, N. C., and Wagner, J. E. (1976). The arthropod parasites of the genus *Cavia*, in *The Biology of the Guinea Pig*, Wagner, J. E., and Manning, P. J., eds. Academic Press, New York, pp. 201–209.

Rose, S. M., Hahn, Y., and Schwartz, B. D. (1979) Tryptic-peptide identity of the GPLA-B.1 alloantigens derived from noncongenic inbred strain 2 and strain 13 guinea pigs. *J. Immunol.* 122, 2267–2271.

Rowland, I., Mallett, A., and Bearne C. (1986) Enzyme activities of the hindgut microflora of laboratory animals and man. *Xenobiotica* 16, 519–523.

Rowsell, H. C. (1984) Guinea pigs, in *The Guide to the Care and Use of Experimental Animals*. Vol. 2. Canadian Council on Animal Care, Ottawa, Ontario, Canada.

Ruebner, B. H., Lindsey, J. R., and Melby, E. C., Jr. (1965) Hepatitis and other spontaneous liver lesions of small experimental animals, in *The Pathology of Laboratory Animals*, Ribelin, W. E., and McCoy, J. R., eds. Thomas, Springfield, Illinois, pp. 160–181.

Ruf, C. (1984) Guinea pigs. T.F.H. Publications, Neptune City, New Jersey.

Saunders, L. Z. (1958) Myositis in guinea pigs. *J. Natl. Cancer Inst.* 20, 899–904.

Scarborough, R. A. (1931) The blood picture of normal laboratory animals. *Yale J. Biol. Med.* 3, 169–179.

Schinatarelli, P., Cadel, S., and Acerbi, D. (1984) A gastroprotective antiinflammatory agent: The β-morpholinoethye ester of niflumic acid (morniflumate). *Agents Actions* 14, 247–256.

Schlosser, M. J., Kapeghian, J. C., and Verlangieri, A. J. (1984) Effects of streptozetocin in the male guinea pig: A potential animal model for studying diabetes. *Life Sci.* 35, 649–655.

Schwenk, M., and Locher, M. (1985) 1-Naphthol conjugation in isolated cells from liver, jejunum, ileum, colon and kidney of the guinea pig. *Biochem. Pharmacol.* 34, 697–701.

Shenefelt, R. E. (1972) Gross congenital anomalies. *Am. J. Pathol.* 66, 589–592.

Shimkin, M. B., and Mider, G. B. (1941) Induction of tumors in guinea pigs with subcutaneously injected methylcholanthrene. *J. Natl. Cancer Inst.* 1, 707–725.

Sikic, B., Mimaugh, E., and Gram, T. (1977) Effects of dietary ascorbic acid supplementation on hepatic drug-metabolizing enzymes in the guinea pig. *Biochem. Pharmacol.* 26, 2037–2041.

Silverstein, E., and Sokoloff, L. (1958) Natural history of degenerative joint disease in small laboratory animals. 5. Osteoarthritis in guinea pigs. *Arthritis Rheum.* 1, 82–86.

Simon, F. A. (1936) Observations on poison ivy hypersensitiveness in guinea pigs. *J. Immunol.* 30, 275–286.

Simon, F. A., Simon, M. G., Rackemann, F. M. and Dienes, L. (1934) The sensitization of guinea pigs to poison ivy. *J. Immunol.* 27, 113–123.

Simpson, G. G. (1945) The principles of classification and a classification of mammals. *Bull. Am. Mus. Nat. Hist.* 85, 93–99.

Simpson, D. M., Burnette, J. C., and Bawden, J. W. (1967) Maternal-fetal blood tetracycline levels in guinea pigs. *J. Oral Ther. Pharmacol.* 3, 403–408.

Sisk, D. S. (1976) Physiology, in *The Biology of the Guinea Pig,* Wagner, J. E., and Manning, P. J., eds. Academic Press, New York, pp. 63–98.

Smith, D. W., and Harding, G. E. (1977) Pulmonary tuberculosis. *Am. J. Pathol.* 89, 273–276.

Smith, J., Rush, G., and Hook J. (1986) Induction of renal and hepatic mixed function oxidases in the hamster and guinea pig. *Toxicology* 38, 209–218.

Sobota, J. T., Martin, W. B., Carlson, R. G., and Feenstra, E. S. (1980) Minoxidil: Right atrial cardiac pathology in animals and man. *Circulation* 62, 376–387.

Souhaili-el amri, Batt, A., and Siest (1986) Comparison of cytochrome P-450 content and activities in liver microsomes of seven species including man. *Xenobiotica* 16, 351–358.

Sparrow, S., and Naylor, P. (1978) Naturally occurring Tyzzer's disease in guinea pigs. *Vet. Rec.* 102, 288.

Sprouse, R. F. (1976) Mycoses, in *The Biology of the Guinea Pig,* Wagner, J. E., and Manning, P. J., Eds. Academic Press, New York, pp. 153–161.

Squire, R. A., Goodman, D. G., Valerio, M. G., Fredrickson, T. N., Strandberg, J. D., Levitt, M. H., Lingeman, C. H., Harshbarger, J. C., and Dawe, C. J. (1978) Tumors, in *Pathology of Laboratory Animals,* Vol. 2, Benirschke, K., Garner, F. M., and Jones, T. C., eds. Springer-Verlag, New York, pp. 1051–1252.

Steblay, R. W. (1979) Anti-tubular-basement-membrane-antibody tubulointerstitial nephritis. *Am. J. Pathol.* 97, 649–652.

Steel, L., Platshon, L., and Kaliner, M. (1979) Prostaglandin generation by human and guinea pig lung tissue: Comparison of parenchymal and airway responses. *J. Allergy Clin. Immunol.* 64, 287–293.

Steffenrud, S. (1986) Metabolism of prostaglandin E analogs guinea pig and liver microsomes. *Eur. J. Drug Metab. Pharmacokinet.* 11, 39–50.

Stenbeck, F. (1970) Guinea pigs and carcinogens. *Acta Pathol. Microbiol. Scand.,* 78A, 192–204. Cited by Manning, P. J. (1976).

Stockard, C. R., and Papanicolaou, G. N. (1919) The vaginal closure membrane, copulation, and the vaginal plug in the guinea pig, with further consideration of estrus rhythm. *Biol. Bull.* 37, 222–245.

Stone, S. H. (1962) Differences in reactivity associated with sex or strain of inbred or random-bred guinea pigs in the massive hemorrhagic reaction and other manifestations of delayed hypersensitivity. *Int. Arch. Allergy Appl Immunol.* 20, 193–202.

Stone, S. H., Liacopoulos, P., Liacopoulos-Birot, M., Neveu, T., and Halpern, B. N. (1964) Histamine: Differences in amount available for release in lungs of guinea pigs susceptible and resistant to acute anaphylaxis. *Science* 146, 1061–1062.

Sulzberger, M. B. (1930) Arsphenamine hypersensitiveness in guinea pigs. *Arch. Dermatol.* 22, 839–848.

Takeda, T., and Grollman, A. (1970) Spontaneously occurring renal disease in the guinea pig. *Am. J. Pathol.* 60, 103–118.

Taylor, J. L., Wagner, J. E., Owens, D. R., and Stuhlman, R. A. (1971) Chronic pododermatitis in guinea pigs, a case report. *Lab. Anim. Sci.* 21, 944–945.

Thabrew, M., and Emerole, G. (1983) Variation in induction of drug metabolizing enzymes by trans-stilbene oxide in rodent species. *Biochem. Biophys. Acta* 756, 242–246.

Thayer, C. B., Wagner, J. E., Freund, B. S., and Tumbleson, M. E. (1974) Distal necrosis in guinea pigs due to Innovar-Vet injections. Nineteenth Annual Meeting of the Quad-Branch of the American Association for Laboratory Animal Science, abstract no. 2.

Thomas, D. W., Meltz, S. K., and Wilner, G. D. (1979a) Nature of T lymphocyte recognition of macrophage-associated antigens. I. Response of guinea pig T cells to human fibrinopeptide B. *J. Immunol.* 123, 759–764.

Thomas, D. W., Meltz, S. K., and Wilner, G. D. (1979b) Nature of T lymphocyte recognition of macrophage-associated antigens. II. Macrophage determination of guinea pig T cell responses to human fibrinopeptide B. *J. Immunol.* 123, 1299–1302.

Thompson, S. W., Hunt, R. D., Fox, M. A., and Davis, C. L. (1962) Perivascular nodules of lymphoid cells in the lungs of normal guinea pigs. *Am. J. Pathol.* 40, 507–517.

Thorne, P. S., Hillebrand, J. A., Lewis, G. R., and Karol, M. H. (1987) Contact Sensitivity by Diisocyanates: Potencies and cross-reactivities. *Toxicol. and Appl. Pharmacol.* 87, 155–165.

Ton, C., and Fong, L. (1984) The effects of ascorbic acid deficiency and excess on the metabolism and toxicity of N-nitrosodimethylamine and N-nitrosodiethylamine in the guinea pig. *Carcinogenesis* 5, 533–536.

Toth, B. (1970) Susceptibility of guinea pigs to chemical carcinogens: 7,12-Dimethylbenz(a)anthracene and urethan. *Cancer Res.* 30, 2583–2589.

Toullet, F., and Voisin, G. A. (1979) Induction of autoimmune aspermatogenic orchitis and of immune responses in inbred guinea pigs of strains 2 and 13 by immunization with isogeneic and allogenic spermatozoa and with sperm autoantigens. *Ann. Immunol. (Paris)* 130C, 373–384.

Tregear, K. T. (1966) Molecular movement, the permeability of skin, in *Physical Functions of Skin,* Academic Press, pp. 1–52.

Turton, J., Shaw, D., Bleby, J., Whiting, R., Williamson, J., and Tucker, D. (1977a) Organ weights, plasma electrolyte values, and blood parameters of three inbred strains of guinea-pigs (strains B, OM3, and R9). *Guinea Pig News Lett.* 11, 10–31.

Turton, J., Shaw, D., Tucker, D., Bleby, J., and Abolfathi, A. (1977b) Organ weights, plasma electrolyte values, and blood parameters of Dunkin Hartley strain specified pathogen free of guinea-pigs. *Guinea Pig News Lett.* 12, 11–22.

Twort, C. C., and Twort, J. M. (1932) Sarcoma and carcinoma in a guinea pig. *J. Pathol. Bacteriol.* 35, 976. Cited by Manning, P. J. (1976).

Van Hoosier, G. L., Jr., and Robinette, L. R. (1976) Viral and chlamydial diseases, in *The Biology of the Guinea Pig,* Wagner, J. E., and Manning, P. J., Eds. Academic Press, New York, pp. 137–152.

Van Hoosier, G. L., Jr., Giddens, W. E., Gillett, C. S., and Davis, H. (1985) Disseminated cytomegalovirus disease in the guinea pig. *Lab. Anim. Sci.* 35, 81–84.

Veterinary Resources Branch, Division of Research Services, National Institute of Health (1981) *NIH Rodents 1980: Catalogue Strains and Stocks of Laboratory Rodents Provided by the Genetic Resource.* Department of Health and Human Services, Public Health Service NIH Publication No. 81-606, National Institutes of Health, Bethesda, Maryland.

Vetterling, J. M. (1976) Protozoan parasites, in *The Biology of the Guinea Pig,* Wagner, J. E., and Manning, P. J., Eds. Academic Press, New York, pp. 163–196.

Vink, H. H. (1969) Rhabdomyomatosis (nodular glycogenic infiltration) of the heart in guinea pigs. *J. Pathol.* 97, 331–334.

Vink, H. H. (1970) Ovarian teratomas in guinea pigs: A report of ten cases. *J. Pathol.* 102, 180–182.

Waggie, K. S., Wagner, J. E., and Kelley, S. T. (1986) Naturally occurring *Bacillus piliformis* infection (Tyzzer's disease) in guinea pigs. *Lab. Anim. Sci.* 36, 504–506.

Wagner, J. E. (1976) Miscellaneous disease conditions of guinea pigs, in *The Biology of the Guinea Pig,* Wagner, J. E., and Manning, P. J., Eds. Academic Press, New York, pp. 228–234.

Wagner, J. E. (1979) Guinea pigs, in *Handbook of Diseases of Laboratory Animals,* Hime, J. M., and O'Donoghue, P. N., eds. Heinemann Veterinary Books, London, pp. 137–162.

Wagner, J. E., Owens, D. R., Kusewitt, D. F., and Corley, E. A. (1976) Otitis media of guinea pigs. *Lab. Animal Sci.* 26:902–907.

Wagner, J. and Manning, P. (ed.) (1979) *The Biology of the Guinea Pig.* Academic Press, New York.

Waldenstrom, A., Thornell, L. E., Hjalmarson, A., and Poupa, O. (1987) Cardiotoxic effects of catecholamines in guinea pigs *(Cavia porcellus)* and in albino rats *(Rattus norvegieus).* A comparative study. *Comp. Biochem. Physiol.* 87C, 269–274.

Wallach, J. D., and Boever, W. J., (1983) *Diseases of Exotic Animals.* Saunders, Philadelphia, p. 145.

Ward, G. S., Johnsen, D. O., Kovatch, R. M., and Peace, T. (1977) Myopathy in guinea pigs. *J. Am. Vet. Med. Assoc.* 171, 837–838.

Webb, J. N. (1970) Naturally occurring myopathy in guinea-pigs. *J. Pathol.* 100, 155–159.

Webster, J. (1986) Health and welfare of animals in modern laboratory systems—dairy cattle, in *Practice, Vet. Rec. Suppl.* 8, 85–89.

Wescott, R. B. (1976) Helminth parasites, in *The Biology of the Guinea Pig,* Wagner, J. E., and Manning, P. J., eds. Academic Press, New York, pp. 197–200.

Wilhelmi, G. (1974) Species differences in susceptibility to the gastro-ulcerogenic action of anti-inflammatory agents. *Pharmacology* 11, 220–230.

Willis, R. A. (1962) Ovarian tertomas in guinea pigs. *J. Pathol. Bacteriol.* 84, 237–239.

Wilson, R. B. (1976) Species variation in response to dimethylhydrazine. *Toxicol. Appl. Pharmacol.* 38, 647–650.

Wilson, T. M., and Brigman, G. (1982) Abdominal mesothelioma in an aged guinea pig. *Lab. Anim. Sci.* 32, 175–176.

Windle, W. F., and Becker, R. F. (1943) Asphyxia neonatarum. An experimental study in the guinea pig. *Am. J. Obstet. Gynecol.* 45, 183–200.

Wong, K. (1976) Species differences in the conjugation of 4-hydroxy-3-methoxypheylethanol. *Biochem. J.* 158, 33–37.

Yoshida, A., Iqbal, Z. M., and Epstein, S. S. (1977) Hepatocarcinogenic effects of N-nitroso-methylurea in guinea pigs. *Cancer Res.* 37, 4043–4048.

Yoshida, A., Iqbal, Z. M., and Epstein, S. S. (1979) Spontaneous pancreatic islet cell tumors in guinea pigs. *J. Comp. Pathol.* 89, 471–480.

Yost, D. H. (1958) Encephalitozoon infection in laboratory animals. *J. Natl. Cancer Inst.* 20, 957–963.

Zannoni, V., and Lynch, M. (1973) The role of ascorbic acid in drug metabolism. *Drug Metab. Rev.* 2, 57–69.

Zarrin, K. B. (1974) Thyroid carcinoma of a guinea pig: A case report. *Lab. Anim.* 8, 145–148.

Zwart, P., Vander Hage, M. H., Mullink, J.W.M.A., and Cooper, J. E. (1981) Cutaneous tumors in guinea pigs. *Lab. Anim.* 15, 375–377.

Zwicker, G. M., Dagle, G. E., and Adee, R. R. (1978) Naturally occurring Tyzzer's disease and intestinal spirochetosis in guinea pigs. *Lab. Anim. Sci.* 28, 193–198.

6

The Rabbit

Toxicology: **Clare M. Salamon**
               Hazleton Wisconsin, Inc.
               Madison, Wisconsin
               Karen M. MacKenzie
               RMT, Inc.
               Madison, Wisconsin

Pathology: **Robert R. Dahlgren**
               WIL Research Laboratories, Inc.
               Ashland, Ohio

Metabolism: **Chyung S. Cook**
               G. D. Searle and Company
               Skokie, Illinois

Toxicology   **Clare M. Salamon and Karen M. MacKenzie**

HISTORY

The domestic rabbit, *Oryctolagus cuniculus*, which belongs to the order Lagomorpha (and hence is referred to as a Lagomorph) and the family Leporidae (which also includes hares) is descended from the wild rabbits of western Europe and northwestern Africa, which were first discovered by the Phoenicians in 1100 B.C. (Fox, 1974). The rabbit is one of the most successful mammals of the world; it is both prolific and adaptable and appears to be equally at home on all the continents. Domestic rabbits are similar to rodents in many respects. The principal anatomical difference is that rabbits have two pairs of upper incisor teeth, whereas rodents have only one pair (Flatt, 1977). The additional pair of incisors in rabbits is smaller and located directly behind the other pair.

Domestication of the rabbit probably began in monasteries during the sixteenth century (Fox, 1974). By the middle of the seventeenth century, the rabbit was completely domesticated and rabbit raising was active in England and continental Europe. This is the only species of lagomorph that has been domesticated and, as such, the species has been introduced into every country of the world as a source of meat or fur, as a pet, or as a laboratory animal.

Early descriptions of research with rabbits date back to 1683 when Leewenhoeck first described the dominance of the wild-type coat ("normal" white-bellied agouti) over albinism, nonagouti, etc. (Sirks, 1959). Since then rabbits have been used extensively to investigate the genetics of coat color and hair morphology, and the rabbit is one of the most common species used for biomedical experimentation. In addition, their by-products are utilized for pharmaceutical and vaccine production.

CHOICE OF THE RABBIT IN TOXICOLOGICAL RESEARCH
Justification for Use

A number of size, shape, and color variations derived from centuries of selective breeding constitute the more than 50 well-established breeds recognized by the rabbit breeders' associations. Representatives of the small breeds (under 2 kg or 5 lb) include the American Dutch and Polish breeds, the medium-sized breeds (2–5 kg or 5–10 lb) are the California and New Zealand White (albino) rabbits, and the large breeds (5 kg or 10 lb and over) are the Flemish and Checkered Giants. The New Zealand White albino is the rabbit most commonly used for research purposes and is the focus for this chapter. However, other breeds, such as the American Dutch, Flemish Giant, and Polish, are also used as laboratory animals.

Compared to the high cost of cats, dogs, and monkeys and the problems associated with their proper care and maintenance, rabbits are relatively inexpensive, hardy, small, clean, and more easily housed and handled. Thus, they are readily used for a wide variety of experimental procedures and testing situations, including immunology (they are good antibody producers and blood is relatively easy to collect from their large and accessible ear veins), teratological, dermal, ocular, and implant studies. Specific study designs are discussed later in this chapter and are outlined in Tables 6–13.

Because the distribution of intestinal microflora within the gut (and hence, their potential metabolic activity) is more similar in rabbits to that of humans than that of the guinea pig, rat, or mouse (Williams, 1972), an orally administered compound is less likely to be metabolized, possibly into a toxic or active metabolite, in the rabbit than in these other laboratory species. However, since gastric emptying time for the rabbit can vary anywhere from 20 min to 20 hr in contrast to the human rate of 1.0–1.5 hr (Digens et al., 1977) the rabbit is a poor species for evaluating the absorption of orally administered compounds (Maeda et al., 1977).

Although rabbits are frequently used to study dermal toxicity, they may not be the best species. Because human skin has a thicker stratum corneum, it is more resistant to the dermal absorption of foreign substances and is penetrated much less easily by xenobiotics than the skin of the most widely used animal models, including the rabbit and the rat (Calabrese, 1984). In vitro, skin permeability to ionic and covalent substances in aqueous solution and organic solutes increases in the following order: human, pig, guinea pig, rat, and rabbit (Tregear, 1966). When Bartek et al. (1972) compared the in vivo skin permeability of several compounds, they also found that the absolute dermal absorption rate for the rabbit was higher than that of the rat, pig, or human (in a descending order). It appears that because the permeability of the skin of miniature swine is close to that of human skin, for studies in which dermal toxicity data are to be used to predict toxicity in humans, in some respects the miniature swine appears to be a more suitable test animal than the rabbit. However, despite the considerable species difference between rabbit and human skin, rabbits are routinely employed in dermal toxicity tests. Thus, when interpreting data generated using rabbits, the researcher must consider the following (Bartek et al. 1972). In general, for a single dermal dose, total exposure of the outer surface of the skin to the applied compound will be of shorter duration in the rabbit than in humans. However, because of the higher penetration rate in the rabbit, temporarily higher concentrations of compound might occur within the rabbit skin as compared to human skin. In addition, the time course of systemic exposure to the compound will also be markedly different in the two species.

Important Physical and Physiological Characteristics

Some general values for selected physical and physiological data in rabbits are in Table 1. More detailed information on these characteristics may be found under the appropriate subsection in this chapter.

Growth and Development

The New Zealand White rabbit grows very rapidly. At weaning these animals weigh 1.0–1.5 kg and the adult animal weighs 4–6 kg depending on sex. The life span of most strains of rabbits is 5–8 years, and some may live to 15 years (Harkness and Wagner, 1977). One index of age is the size and appearance of the claws. They do not project beyond the fur until the rabbit approaches maturity, and then they grow and curl with age.

Reproduction

The age at which rabbits reach puberty varies from 4 to 12 months and depends somewhat on breed and strain. It tends to be inversely related to size; i.e., smaller rabbits like Polish rabbits may be bred at 4 months, whereas heavier Flemish rabbits reach puberty between 9 and 12 months. The New Zealand White may be bred at 5–6 months (female) and 7–8 months (male). The male rabbit matures slower than the female. Motile spermatozoa appear in the ejaculate at 4 months and adult levels of sperm production are reached at about 7 or 8 months (Bivin and Timmons, 1974).

Although rabbits do not have a definite estrus cycle, there are short periods of 1–2 days every 2 weeks when the doe is not receptive to the male. Also, a doe may refuse to mate with one buck but may be receptive to another. Mating behavior consists of tail flagging and enurination, and sometimes chasing. In tail flagging, the buck elevates his hindquarters, walks stiff-legged, and lays his tail flat on his back, providing visual stimulus to the doe and olfactory stimulus from the inguinal glands. In enurination, the buck may turn his hindquarters toward the doe and emit a jet of urine in a display of sexual aggressiveness; sometimes this is followed by a circling of the cage. Enurination may also be directed toward bucks in adjacent cages. If the doe is receptive, she will elevate her hind quarters, permitting the buck to mount.

Rabbits are induced ovulators, which means the female remains in estrus until copulation, which triggers the induction of ovulation. Ovulation can also be induced by an injection of chorionic gonadotropin or other luteinizing hormone, which is done if the researcher wishes to employ artificial insemination. Ovulation occurs 10–13 hr after copulation or after the injection of a luteinizing hormone.

Rabbits have been used extensively for reproductive studies because of the precise timing that can be obtained for studies of egg maturation, fertilization, cleavage, and implantation. Pregnancy can be confirmed by palpation approximately 10–12 days after breeding. Fertile copulations result in pregnancy and a gestation of 30–35 days depending on the breed. Parturition is called kindling.

Clinical signs of pregnancy or pseudopregnancy are an increase in the size of the ruff, a large tuft of hair on the ventral neck and a subsequent increase in hair pulling, especially from the ruff to make a nest.

Pseudopregnancy, which lasts 16–17 days, is easily induced in the doe and can be caused by infertile mating, sexual excitement from a doe mounting another doe, injection

Table 1   Selected Normative Data for New Zealand White Rabbits

General
adult body weight
    male   4–5 kg
    female   4–6 kg
life span   5–13 years
surface area   2.5 kg: 1270 cm^2
                          4.8 kg: 3040 cm^2
chromosome number 44
  (diploid)
water consumption   50–100 mg/kg/day
food consumption   50g/kg/day
rectal temperature   102.0–103.5 °F
basal metabolism   110 cal/kg/day
GI transit time   4–5 hr

Reproduction
puberty   3–8 months
breeding age
    male   6–10 months
    female   5–9 months
breeding season   All year
                          (controlled conditions)
estrus cycle   Polyestrous, induced
breeding habits   Female brought to
                            male
time of ovulation   9.75–13.5 hr
                          Postcopulation
time of implantation Approximately 7 days
                          postcopulation
length of gestation   29–35 days
postpartum estrus   None
litter size   4–10
birth weight   30–100 g
weight at 3 days   400–700g
weaning age   4–6 weeks
weaning weight   1–2 kg

Cardiovascular
arterial blood pressure
  systolic   90–130 mm Hg
  diastolic   60–90 mm Hg
heart rate   100–300/min
blood volume   57–65 ml/kg

Respiratory
respiration rate   35–65/min
tidal volume   4–6 ml/kg
pattern   Obligate oral (mouth)
                      or nasal

Excretory
urine volume

day	40–100 ml
24 hr	20–350 mg/kg
urine specific gravity	1.003–1.036
urine pH	Alkaline, 8.2 (average)
feces excreted	15–60 g/day

Blood parameters

platelet count	250–750 (10^3/mm^3)
RBC	4–8 (10^6/mm^3)
hematocrit	36–46 (ml/100ml)
hemaglobin	8–13 (gm/100ml)
total WBC	3–10 (10^3/mm^3)
blood volume	45–70 (ml/kg)

Source: Data from Collins (1972), Harkness and Wagner (1983), Kaplan and Timmons (1979), and Kozmo et al. (1974).

of luteinizing hormone, or stress due to shipping or experimentation. During pseudopregnancy the doe is not receptive to mating.

Excretion

Rabbits have two types of feces: soft, moist nighttime feces and firm, dry daytime fecal pellets. The nighttime feces, which are covered with mucus and consist primarily of secretion from the cecum, are produced by the initial ingestion of food; hard feces are produced by reingestion of the soft feces. The soft feces are protein and vitamin rich, and their ingestion (coprophagy) directly from the anus improves the utilization of nitrogen (Thacker and Brandt, 1955), provides an abundance of certain B vitamins, plays an important role in the incorporation of sulfur in the soft tissues, and conserves water (Kulwich et al. 1953, 1954). Wild rabbits are able to survive up to a week without food because of reingestion of feces.

Because of their diet, rabbit urine is cloudy and ranges in color from light yellow to deep orange or red brown and may resemble purulent discharge. It contains carbonate and phosphate crystals, which cause a scale to accumulate on cage surfaces.

HUSBANDRY

As with other laboratory animals, the facilities, equipment, and husbandry procedures used for rabbits should be designed to afford maximum environmental control (i.e., minimal variation in temperature, humidity, and ventilation); optimal conditions for the animal's comfort, health, and welfare; and minimal exposure to injury and disease.

Facilities

Rabbits should be maintained in an area that is clean and dry, with adequate ventilation, away from excessive noise, and within a specified range of temperature and humidity.

Temperature, Relative Humidity, and Ventilation

Because the thermal environment can influence the severity, duration, and variability of toxic responses to chemicals by influencing the physiology of the animal and the metabolism and disposition of test materials (Fuhrman and Fuhrman, 1961; Weihe, 1973; Clough, 1982), the temperature, humidity, and ventilation of the animal facilities must be strictly controlled (Rao, 1986). The thermoneutral zone of resting laboratory animals (and humans) is very small (Weihe, 1973). When exposed to temperatures outside their thermoneutral zone, laboratory animals adapt behaviorally (unless they are prevented from doing so by experimentally enforced restrictions) and/or metabolically (by increasing or decreasing their metabolic rates). Thus, marked variations in the environmental conditions of the animal room may alter the animal's rate of metabolism, and, ultimately, the potential toxicity of a test material.

Ambient relative humidity is also a major factor in maintaining the heat balance of an animal (Clough, 1982). It is a very important consideration with dermal absorption studies, particularly when shaved animals are used. In these situations, the relative humidity will directly affect the rate of evaporation, the viscosity of the test material, and the animal's peripheral circulation, thus having a major impact on the potential toxicity of the applied material.

For rabbits, animal room temperatures should be maintained between 60 and 70°F (16 and 21°C) and relative humidity should be between 40 and 60% (ILAR, 1985). This temperature range is lower (vs 64.4–78.8 or 84.2 and 18 to 26 or 29°C) and the relative humidity range is narrower (vs 30–70%) than that required for other common laboratory animals (ILAR, 1985). With rabbits, elevated temperatures in particular can result in lower male fertility, lower conception rates for the does, and reduced litter sizes.

The recommended ventilation rate is 12 cu ft/min/animal (up to approximately 3.6 kg)/day (Runkle, 1964) or at least 10 complete air changes/hour (ILAR, 1985), preferably with 100% fresh air. Recirculation of air is not recommended. If the air is recirculated, more efficient filtration will be required to remove odors and contaminants.

Light and Noise

Most facilities maintain light cycles of 12 hr light and 12 hr dark. However, light cycles of 14–16 hr light for females are recommended when the rabbits are used in reproductive studies.

Situations that might result in elevated noise levels for extended periods of time, e.g., housing rabbits in the same area as dogs or in the vicinity of noisy equipment, should be regarded with caution and avoided if possible. Nayfield and Besch (1981) have reported indications of stress, i.e., increased spontaneous activity and adrenal weights and decreased spleen and thymus weights in rabbits that were exposed to elevated noise (1.5 hr of white noise at intensities of 107–112 dbls/day for 2 weeks). An auditory stimulus also appears to affect plasma cholesterol concentrations (Friedman et al., 1967) and initiates changes in the hypothalamus (Henkin and Knigge, 1963) of exposed rabbits.

Caging

Rabbit cages and racks should be constructed of a smooth, corrosion-resistant material, preferably stainless steel, that is impervious to liquids and moisture, and is easily sanitized and sterilized. The floor of the cage is usually made of steel grid or wire mesh with a recommended size of 1 in × ½ in or ⅝ in sq./1 × 2.5 cm. It should be smooth and free of sharp projections. The wire mesh floors allow excrement to fall to excreta trays below the cage. Some type of welded wire (1 in × 1 in or 1 in × 2 in) or solid metal walls with air vents are generally used on the sides, back, and top of the cage and wire grid is used on the front. Painting of cages and racks is not recommended. The racks and cages should be movable to facilitate transportation to a washing area.

The amount of floor space required/animal (or the cage size for individually housed animals) is determined by the weight of the rabbit. Current minimum space recommendations for rabbits are in Table 2 (ILAR, 1985). It is recommended that the racks holding the cages be placed at least 2 m apart to minimize the between-rack spread of airborne microorganisms due to convection currents (Teelman and Weihe, 1974).

Two standard sizes of cages that are available commercially and provide 3 and 4 sq ft of floor area have dimensions (width × depth × height) of 24 in × 18 in × 16 in and 24 in × 24 in × 15 in, respectively. Young immature rabbits may be group housed by sex, but rabbits that are sexually mature (over 4 months) often attack one another and should always be individually housed. Because wounding, pseudopregnancies, and infertility may occur in groups housed together, mature rabbits should be paired only at mating.

Nest boxes must be provided for does that are expected to deliver and nurse young. Suitable bedding used in nest boxes should be a nonedible material; e.g., wood shavings.

Dropping pans are lined with disposable absorbent liners that should be changed at least 3 times each week. The animals should be transferred to clean cages at least every 2 weeks. Facilities should be physically cleaned and sanitized at least 3 times a week.

Rabbit urine, with a pH of 8.2, is very alkaline and contains phosphate and carbonate crystals that accumulate on the cage surfaces and form a scale that is difficult to remove. Detergents, disinfectants, and lime-scale removers (acidic solutions such as vinegar or acid products at pH 2) may be applied with a stiff brush in routine cage cleaning. However, acidic materials, which may cause discoloration and damage the cages, should be used with caution. Flaming may also be necessary to remove hair and manure and kill coccidial oocysts.

Feed and Water

Feed and water systems should be clean and designed so that they cannot become easily contaminated. Metal feeders that attach to the front of the cage and can be filled outside without opening the cage door are commercially available and should be used in preference to crocks or other open containers. Likewise, water bottles (if an automatic water system is not available) are usually mounted on the outside on the front of the cage. Sipper-tube watering devices are preferred.

Table 2 Minimum Cage Sizes

Weight		Floor area/ rabbit	
kg	lb	ft^2	m^2
<2	5	1.5	0.14
2–4	5–10	3.0	0.28
4–5.3	10–12	4.0	0.37
>5.4	>12	5.0	0.46

Note: The cage height should be at least 14 in (25.56 cm). *Source:* ILAR (1985).

Rabbits should be provided ad libitum with a plentiful supply of fresh, clean water. Nonpregnant does drink approximately 10 ml/100 g of body weight per day, and lactating does may drink up to 90 ml/100 g/day (Harkness and Wagner, 1983). If water bottles are used, they should be filled with fresh water daily and sanitized at least once weekly.

Food hoppers should be constructed of durable material (other than wood) that is resistant to the gnawing of rabbits, is corrosion resistant, and is easily sanitized. They should be mounted 4 in from the floor of the cage and the design should permit easy access, but not allow the rabbit to enter. They should also be free of sharp edges that could cause cuts or scratches.

The preferred diet is a wholesome, nutritious, pelleted form of feed, free of drugs, hormones, pesticides, and animal and vermin contaminants. Because of the great variability in fiber and nutrient content in commercially available diets (Wise and Gilburt, 1980, 1981), and because of the potential presence of contaminants, it is recommended that only diets that have been analyzed for these materials be used. Recommended nutrient levels are presented in Table 3. The nutrient content of two commercially available diets, Purina Rabbit Chow #5322 and Purina High Fiber Rabbit Chow #5325 (Ralston Purina Co.), which are made of natural ingredients and purified, is presented in Table 4.

Fresh feed should be provided at least weekly. However, a once-daily feeding (limited feeding) of approximately 120 g (4 oz or ⅔ cup) of pellets is sufficient to maintain an adult, medium-sized rabbit at a constant weight; this is the amount of feed given to animals in our laboratory that are to be used for acute studies. For longer studies, the animals are provided with approximately 180 g (6 oz or 1 cup) of pellets each day. At peak lactation, a doe may consume up to 450 g (16 oz) of feed per day, and pregnant or lactating does should be provided with feed ad libitum. The feeders should be checked daily and any powdered feed removed.

The diet should contain 16–20% crude fiber and 14–18% crude protein (Harkness and Wagner, 1983). Rabbits have a higher requirement for fiber than other species. Fiber has an important role as bulk, but rabbits do not digest over 18% dietary fiber in a single passage. Diarrhea may result if the fiber concentration is below 6%, and fiber above 20% may lead to lowered feed efficiency (Harkness, 1987). The feeding of diets containing a high concentration of fiber (18–20%) is often utilized to reduce the occurrence of intestinal enteropathies.

Malnutrition is uncommon in rabbits. Other relatively uncommon nutritional problems include vitamin D, calcium, and phosphorus imbalances (atherosclerosis); vitamin A (hydrocephalus, prenatal death) and vitamin E (muscular dystrophy, prenatal mortality, seminiferous tubal degeneration) deficiencies; and some specific mineral or amino acid deficiencies.

Because feed and bedding are generally used in animal facilities without prior sanitization, they are potential sources of contamination for diseases, parasites, and hormones. Therefore, potential problems could occur and caution should be used in purchasing and storing feed and bedding.

Handling and Restraint

Rabbits must be picked up and held correctly to prevent both animal and human injuries. They should be handled firmly but gently. Because they are very shy animals and are easily frightened, they may often struggle and try to escape. With the exception of older bucks and primiparous does with strong territorial instincts, rabbits seldom bite people.

Table 3 Nutrient Requirements[a]

Energy and protein	
digestible energy (kcal)	2100–2500
TDN (%)	55–65
crude fiber (%)	16–20
fat (%)	2–4
crude protein (%)	14–18
Inorganic nutrients	
calcium (%)	0.4–0.5
phosphorus (%)	0.22–0.4
magnesium (mg)	300–400
potassium (%)	0.6
sodium (%)	0.2–0.5
chloride (%)	0.5
copper (mg)	3–10
iodine (mg)	0.2
iron (mg)	100
manganese (mg)	8.5–40
zinc (mg)	50
Vitamins	
vitamin A (mg)	0.33–0.44
vitamin A as carotene (mg)	0.83
vitamin E (mg)	20–40
vitamin K_3 (mg)	2
niacin (mg)	180e
pyridoxine (mg)	39
choline (g)	1.2[b]
Amino acids	
lysine	0.65
methionine + cystine	0.6
arginine	0.6
histidine	0.3[b]
leucine	1.1[b]
isoleucine	0.6[b]
phenylalanine + tyrosine	1.1[b]
threonine	0.6[a]
tryptophan	0.2[b]
valine	0.7[b]
glycine	—[c]

[a]Presented as percent (%) or mg/kg in the diet.
[b]May not be minimum but known to be adequate.
[c]Quantitative requirement not determined, but dietary need demonstrated.
Source: Data from Clarke et. al. (1977), Hunt and Harrington (1974), and National Academy of Sciences, 1977.

Table 4 Nutrient Contents of Purina Rabbit Chows #5322 and #5325 (High Fiber)

Nutrients	#5322	#5325
Energy and protein		
protein, min. (%)	16.0	14.0
fat, min. (%)	2.5	1.5
fiber, max. (%)	18.0	25.0
moisture, max. (%)	12.0	—
ash, max. (%)	8.0	10.0
added minerals, max. (%)	2.1	1.5
Nutrients		
protein (%)	16.2	14.5
fat (%)	2.5	1.7
cholesterol (ppm)	61.0	60.0
fiber, crude (%)	13.0	22.5
neutral detergent fiber (%)	27.4	40.9
acid detergent fiber 950	15.8	24.6
total digestible nutrients (%)	66.0	57.0
nitrogen-free extract, by difference (%)	52.0	42.4
gross energy (kcal/g)	4.0	3.9
physiological fuel (kcal/g)	2.95	2.43
ash (%)	7.3	8.9
calcium (%)	0.95	1.2
phosphorus (%)	0.50	0.5
potassium (%)	1.15	1.67
magnesium (%)	0.25	0.30
sodium (%)	0.25	0.32
chlorine (%)	0.50	0.79
iron (ppm)	276.2	315.9
zinc (ppm)	105.5	122.2
manganese (ppm)	107.2	127.5
copper (ppm)	27.8	25.8
cobalt (ppm)	0.38	0.46
iodine (ppm)	0.59	0.58
chromium (ppm)	4.5	5.0
selenium (ppm)	0.13	0.2
Vitamins		
vitamin A (IU/g)	20.0	20.0
carotene (ppm)	27.6	31.2
vitamin D (IU/g)	2.3	2.2
α-Tocopherol (IU/kg)	44.0	33.0
niacin (ppm)	33.0	33.4
pyridoxine (ppm)	4.5	4.5
pantothenic acid (ppm)	19.0	19.1
thiamine (ppm)	3.5	2.8
riboflavin (ppm)	5.0	8.6
choline (ppm $\times$ 100)	16.0	16.0
folic acid (ppm)	2.0	3.3
biotin (ppm)	0.12	0.14
B_{12} (μg/kg)	6.6	6.6

Amino acids (%)

lysine	0.78	0.61
methionine	0.35	0.30
arginine	0.90	0.68
histidine	0.40	0.32
leucine	1.3	1.06
isoleucine	0.82	0.79
phenylalanine	0.80	0.65
tyrosine	0.50	0.42
threonine	0.64	0.56
tryptophan	0.23	0.19
valine	0.84	0.68
glycine	0.77	0.70
cystine	0.25	0.20

Source: Ralston Purina Co.

However, a rabbit that is picked up incorrectly or is not held securely will kick violently with its hind legs and it is very easy to cause injury to the rabbit, particularly a broken back. In addition, while trying to escape, rabbits can inflict painful scratches on the handler with their powerful hind legs.

Rabbit ears are very fragile and they should never be used to pick up the animal or as a means for restraint. A safe method to handle or pick up rabbits is by firmly grasping the loose skin at the base of the skull (this area is commonly called the nape or the scruff) with one hand while supporting the rear legs with the other hand. A rabbit can also be held by encircling its body with one arm, with the sternum supported by the hand, while holding the scruff with the other hand. Or, it can be held with one arm holding the rabbit's hindquarters and pressing the animal toward the handler's body. The abdomen and sternum are then supported by the handler's forearm, with the other hand on the scruff. If the hindquarters are not supported, the rabbit may struggle. If the rabbit does struggle, it can easily be calmed by placing it on the forearm with the head concealed in the bend of the handler's elbow.

Various types of restraining devices are available for use with rabbits. They serve primarily to control the body of the rabbit while the head or ears are being manipulated. The most common devices are usually some variation of a restraint box or stocks. If the basic stocks/restraining box are used, the rabbit may need to be trained and calmed to avoid struggling, which may cause a broken back. A squeeze-cage stock is often used for intravenous injections and a cat bag may be used for gavage administration. The rabbit can also be manually restrained. If manual restraint is used, the rabbit should not be placed directly on a smooth surface because it may flail. Instead it should be placed on a towel or mat.

DOSING TECHNIQUES

Compounds may be administered to rabbits by a variety of routes. The more commonly used routes and specific techniques are described as follows.

Oral Administration

The simplest method of administering compounds orally is by incorporating them in the feed or water. However, as with other species, rabbits may not voluntarily consume the material if it has an unpleasant odor or taste, or if it is in a form that cannot be easily consumed. In addition, rabbits tend to spread their feed around and "play" with their water bottles. Thus, because of potential palatability problems, spillage, and wastage these methods may not be satisfactory if it is important that precise amounts of the material be administered.

Very small volumes of liquid materials may be administered by placing the tip of a ball-tipped syringe in the corner of the rabbit's mouth and slowly introducing the material. However, the most accurate method of administering compounds orally is to deliver the material by gavage. This may be done using a stainless steel ball-tipped needle (13 gauge) or a latex catheter (size 14 French, 16 in long). The needle is attached to a syringe with a locking end, the head and neck of the animal are manually restrained to avoid injury if the animal should struggle, and the needle is inserted into the back of the mouth and into the esophagus.

When using a latex catheter for gavage, the animal is also restrained. The animal may be manually restrained or a cat bag can be used for restraint. The mouth is held open and the catheter is inserted into the back of the throat, being careful to avoid the teeth, and then gently introduced into the esophagus and into the stomach. To establish that the catheter is in the stomach and not in the bronchi, there should be no air passage in the tube that corresponds to respiratory movements. If the animal struggles, the catheter should be removed and reinserted. After the catheter is inserted, a ball-tipped needle which is attached to a syringe is inserted into the open end of the catheter, and the plunger of the syringe is gently pushed to administer the dose. Depending on the nature of the material and the dose volume, it may be advisable to flush the catheter by leaving the catheter in place and affixing another syringe with water or the appropriate vehicle. The catheter, attached to the empty syringe, is then removed, again being careful to avoid the teeth. The volume of material administered is based on the vehicle used. In general, rabbits should not be given more than 2 ml/kg of corn oil; water or a water-based solution may be given at volumes up to 6 ml/kg.

Dermal Administration

Materials are applied topically on the dorsal area of the trunk. The fur is removed with an electric clipper before dosing and as needed thereafter. Care should be taken to avoid abrading the skin and only animals with healthy, intact skin should be used. If the dosing material is a liquid, it may be applied diluted or undiluted. If the dosing material is a solid, it should be slightly moistened with saline, deionized water, or another suitable vehicle before application to ensure good contact with the skin. The dosing material is then applied uniformly over the exposure area (from approximately 5 cm^2 to an area estimated to constitute approximately 20% of the total body surface area). The exposure area may be left uncovered or it may be held in contact with the skin by a gauze dressing secured with tape, covered with cellophane wrap, and overwrapped with elastic tape. The animals should be fitted with flexible "Elizabethan"-type plastic collars to prevent them from removing the dosing material or coverings (Barnett, 1958). At the end of the treatment period, the bindings and collar are removed and the exposure area may be washed with water and/or wiped clean with a towel moistened with water or a mild soap solution as thoroughly as possible without irritating the skin. The volume of material given is based on the size of the animal and the area of skin that is available for application.

Ocular Administration

Animals should be examined before the administration of the dose material and any that show prexisting ocular defects, irritation, or corneal injury should not be used. If a solid or granular material is to be administered, it should be finely ground into a dust or powder. The material is placed in the conjunctival sac and the upper and lower lids are then gently held together for a second before releasing to prevent loss of the dose material. The amount given should not exceed 10 μl or the equivalent weight.

Intravenous Administration

Materials are usually administered intravenously into the marginal ear vein (along the posterior edge on the outside of the ear). The animal is restrained, the hair is gently plucked from the area of the vein, and a disinfectant is applied. If the vein is not readily apparent, the area can be rubbed with alcohol, or the vein can be occluded by gently pressing on the base of the ear or by placing a paper clip at the base of the ear. For intravenous injections, the needle should be sharp (prepackaged, sterile, disposable needles are best) and should be the smallest size possible (1 in, 25 gauge, or smaller). The needle should first be inserted into the skin beside and parallel to the blood vessel, and then inserted into the vein with the beveled edge up. The syringe should only contain the dosing solution and no air. If there are signs of engorgement or swelling at the injection site, indicating that the needle is outside the vein, reposition the needle. After the material has been injected, withdraw the needle, and apply digital pressure to the puncture site for a short time to prevent bleeding.

Subcutaneous Administration

Subcutaneous injections are made under the skin of the neck or back, using a 1-in, 23- to 27-gauge needle. The skin is grasped with one hand and the material is injected into the tented skin. If large volumes are to be injected, the needle can be withdrawn slightly and redirected to spread the fluid over a wider area.

Intramuscular Administration

Intramuscular injections are made into the lateral aspects of the large muscles in the hindquarters; e.g., the gluteal or thigh muscles. Care must be taken to avoid hitting large blood vessels, nerves, and bone. First, the area of the injection site is immobilized, cleaned with disinfectant, and the needle is then inserted ½ to ¾ in perpendicularly, depending on the muscle thickness. After the needle is inserted, the plunger of the syringe should be withdrawn slightly to confirm that no blood can be aspirated; i.e., the needle has not inadvertently entered a blood vessel. If blood appears in the syringe, the needle should be carefully repositioned or withdrawn and reinserted. After the needle is placed properly, the fluid is injected slowly and the needle is withdrawn. The smallest gauge needle possible (1 in, 23–27 gauge) should be used for this procedure.

Intradermal Administration

Intradermal injections are given in the loin and flank areas where it is difficult for the rabbit to reach with its hind feet. The hair should first be removed from the site with clippers and depilatory cream. An antiseptic is then applied. The skin is stretched and the needle is inserted only into the dermis, forming a small bleb, and the injection is made using a 25-gauge needle attached to a syringe containing the dosing material. When the needle is removed, the site should be examined for seepage of the dosage material. If this occurs, the needle should be inserted further into the skin during the injection.

Intraperitoneal Administration

The rabbit is manually restrained with the hindquarters elevated and the needle (⅝ in, 23–25 gauge) is inserted bevel up into an area just lateral to the midline and just posterior to the area of the umbilicus at a steep angle toward the spine. The insertion is made with a quick thrust through the subcutaneous tissue and ventral abdominal muscles and abdominal wall, and into the peritoneal cavity. Using this procedure, up to 20 ml of fluid may be given in a single injection.

Vaginal Administration

The doe is placed in a restraining stock, and the tail is gently grasped between the thumb and forefinger while the rest of the hand is pressed firmly on the hip region of the animal. As the animal relaxes, the tail is pulled upward to expose the vaginal opening. A catheter (size 8 French, or a ball-tipped stainless steel 1 ½ in, 18-gauge needle) is gently inserted approximately 1 in into the vagina, the dose is administered, and the catheter or needle is withdrawn. The animal is kept in the restraining stock for 1–2 min after the procedure is complete to ensure that the dose material is retained.

COLLECTION TECHNIQUES

Blood Collection

Ear Vein

Blood is usually collected from the large, readily accessible marginal ear veins. To facilitate collection procedures, the animal is placed in a restraint box that allows access to the ears. A small amount of petroleum jelly is spread along the marginal vein. This causes the hair to lay flat in a natural direction toward the edge of the ear. A disinfectant such as 70% ethyl alcohol is applied and a paper clip may be applied as a tourniquet proximal to the intended bleeding site. Using a lamp as a heat source, the ear is warmed, which causes the vein to become engorged with blood. Slight digital irritation of the tip of the ear will also increase blood flow and facilitate blood collection. Although xylene is sometimes used for this purpose, it should not be used if the sample is to be used to determine white blood cell counts because of its severe inflammatory properties. While keeping the ear over the lamp, the vein is incised midway between the tourniquet and the tip of the ear, and blood is collected directly in appropriate tubes or containers. Alternatively, a needle attached to a syringe may be used and the blood drawn into the syringe by slow, steady manual pressure.

Auricular Artery

When larger blood samples are required, they may be collected from the centrally located auricular artery using a 20- or 23-gauge needle that is inserted into the artery toward the base of the ear.

Catheterization

Techniques for obtaining multiple blood samples from rabbits over short or extended periods of time, which are not traumatic, do not cause hematomas, and do not require anesthesia, invasive surgery, or sophisticated expertise involve implanting a flexible catheter into the auricular artery (Smith, et al., 1988; Heim, 1989). The site of the arterial puncture is depilated or the entire ear is shaved. A 2% nitroglycerin ointment may be applied over the artery to prevent arterial spasms, which can interfere with successful catheterization, and the area is stroked with the forefinger until the artery becomes engorged with blood. A 1-in, 22-gauge catheter is inserted into the artery approximately 3 cm from the tip of the ear with the needle at a 25-degree angle and the bevel up. The appearance of blood in the flash chamber confirms arterial entry. The catheter is then advanced into the arterial lumen until the hub meets the surface of the skin (the hub of the catheter should be below the tip of the ear) and an injection cap is attached to the hub of the catheter. Approximately 0.3 ml of heparinized (5 μ/ml) saline should be injected into the catheter to determine if the placement is correct. This is followed by rapidly infusing an additional 1 ml of heparinized saline and then aspirating blood until adequate blood flow is established. Tissue adhesive may be used to adhere the catheter hub to the skin surface. A piece of rolled gauze is placed inside the ear and then the ear and catheter hub are wrapped with adhesive tape, binding the ears together to prevent the rabbit from removing the injection cap and catheter. For longer sampling periods, gauze or bandaging tape should be used under the adhesive tape to prevent skin irritation.

For all these methods, blood flow from the puncture site is easily stopped by applying firm digital pressure at the site with a gauze pad. Alternatively, after the blood sample is collected, direct pressure may be applied to the incised area and a paper clip applied as a tourniquet to control bleeding until clotting takes place. The use of a surgical lubricant with the paper clip facilitates clotting.

Cardiac Puncture

Cardiac puncture may be used to collect larger quantities of blood or multiple blood samples from anesthetized or sedated rabbits. However, cardiac puncture is traumatic and can result in death. The rabbit should be anesthetized and placed in right lateral recumbency or dorsal recumbency on a restraining board. The heart beat may be used to directly locate the heart or the needle (1 ½ in, 18–21 gauge) is inserted at approximately a 30-degree angle immediately behind the xiphoid cartilage.

Posterior Vena Cava/Iliac Bifurcation

When large volumes of blood are needed at terminal sacrifice, and known enzyme alterations caused by cell trauma from other bleeding techniques are contraindicated, blood may be obtained from the posterior vena cava or iliac bifurcation of anesthetized animals.

The animal is placed on its back and a midline incision is made that exposes the abdominal viscera. The large intestine is moved laterally, away from the inguinal area, exposing the large abdominal vessels. The iliac vein is surgically isolated (cranial) just above the bifurcation of the internal iliac and femoral veins. If the posterior vena cava is to be used, it is isolated in a similar manner, just cranial to the common iliac vein and caudal to the renal vein. Because this is a terminal sampling procedure, a sterile surgical technique does not apply. Venipuncture is made using an appropriately sized flexible catheter and needle (the size depends on the size of the animal but will generally be between 20 and 25 gauge). After the needle is inserted into the vein, the flexible catheter is slid forward past the tip of the needle, further into the vein, and the needle is withdrawn. Blood will well up in the hub of the catheter and is collected using the syringe. Any bleeding around the venipuncture site may be controlled by digital pressure with a piece of gauze or cotton. Alternatively, a ligature can be positioned around the vessel before venipuncture and then firmly tied after the needle is inserted.

To obtain a blood sample, the injection cap and catheter are flushed with heparinized saline, approximately 0.3 ml is then aspirated to clear the saline from the catheter, and the required amount of blood is withdrawn. Patency is maintained by flushing the catheter and injection cap with a higher concentration of heparinized (100 μ/ml) saline and then leaving them filled with the solution between sampling intervals.

This technique has been used successfully to collect as many as eight blood samples from a single rabbit within a 2-hr period (with sampling intervals as short as 5 minutes) and for infusion periods that have lasted as long as 7 days (patency was maintained by daily flushing with heparinized saline). It is particularly applicable for studies to establish the pharmacokinetic properties of new drugs and for observing the reaction of rabbits to drug administration. It can also be used to obtain large (greater than 30 ml) amounts of blood.

Urine Collection

The most common method used to collect urine is by placing the animals in stainless steel metabolic cages, where the urine and feces are separated by a cone-shaped device (the urine drains off the collecting walls into a tube and the feces drop into an inverted cone). Food and water are provided in such a way that the urine will not be contaminated. However, some hair and fecal contamination of the urine may occur.

If contamination of the sample with fecal and other material is not acceptable, urine samples may be obtained by urethral catheterization (practicable in males only) or by direct puncture of the bladder (cystocentesis).

Catheterization

For this procedure, the catheters and any lubricating gels and speculums must be sterilized before use. The animal is sedated or anesthetized, restrained in dorsal recumbency, and the penis is extruded. The catheter (commercially available cat urethral catheter) is introduced into the urethral opening and gently advanced into the urethra and then the bladder. If the catheter is left partially in its container, it can be held without becoming contaminated. When urine flow begins, a syringe can be attached to the catheter and used to aspirate the urine remaining in the bladder.

Cystocentesis

For urine collection directly from the bladder through the body wall, the animal should be sedated and the skin shaved in the midline in the inguinal region. The bladder, located by palpation in the posterior abdomen, is held firmly through the body wall and the needle (1 or 1 ½ in, 23 gauge) is introduced through the body wall in the midline at approximately a 45-degree angle. The needle should be inserted in the posterior section of the bladder so it will remain in the bladder lumen as the urine is withdrawn. The urine may be expelled through the needle into a collection tube or by attaching a syringe to the needle.

SPECIAL PROCEDURES

Anesthesia

Because there is a great deal of interrabbit variability in sensitivity to anesthetics and because there is a narrow margin between anesthesia and death, a great deal of caution should be exercised in situations requiring anesthetization. The depth of anesthesia should be monitored by rate and depth of respiration and degree of jaw tension. Other indicators such as pedal reflexes, corneal reflex, and pupillary size are unreliable. Anesthetics that can be successfully used are ketamine (50 mg/kg) and paraldehyde (0.5 mg/kg), intramuscular; ketamine (20–40 mg/kg) and acepromazine (1 mg/kg), intramuscular; or methoxyflurane inhalation following premedication with acepromazine (1 mg/kg) or ketamine (20 mg/kg) intramuscular (Harkness and Wagner, 1983).

Euthanasia

Euthanasia may be accomplished by using an overdose of a barbituate such as sodium pentobarbital or a commercial euthanasia solution such as T-61.

Reproduction Procedures

To determine the sex of adult rabbits, the skin is gently pressed back from the genital opening. In males, the penis will be everted; females have an elongated vulva with a short slitlike opening. The mature male also has perineal, or inguinal, pouches lateral and anterior to the penis. In prepuberal rabbits, when pressure is applied against the genital orifice, the penis everts equally all the way around, whereas the vulva protrudes only laterally and ventrally; the posterior end that does not evert is attached near the anus.

Natural Mating

When breeding rabbits naturally, the doe must be taken to the male's cage. If the female is receptive, copulation will occur soon after introduction to the male. The buck mounts the doe and grasps the female's body with a foreleg on each flank. Intromission is usually accomplished after eight to 12 rapid copulatory movements and ejaculation follows on the first intromission. Immediately after ejaculation, the male may fall backward or off the side (both hind feet are off the ground during ejaculation) and emit a cry.

Artificial Insemination

For artificial insemination procedures, semen is collected in an artificial vagina. The buck is introduced to a teaser doe. When the buck begins to mount, the vagina is positioned so that the buck can ejaculate into it. Semen samples show considerable variation between individuals and for the same individual at different times. Therefore, the semen should be evaluated each time it is collected for amount (should have at least 0.5 ml) and color (if yellow/tan, it is probably contaminated with urine and should be discarded). To assess sperm viability, a small amount of semen is pipetted onto a glass slide and the sperm are observed using a 10× objective. Motility is graded as streaming (50–100% motility), waving, or shaking. Acceptable samples are streaming; waving or shaking samples should be discarded. The sample is then diluted 1:200, and a sperm count is done. The concentration of sperm should be at least of 40×10^6 sperm/ml. The semen preparation should be incubated at 37°C during the insemination procedure and must be used within 30 min of collection time.

Artificial insemination is done using methods similar to those for vaginal dosing. The doe is manually restrained, and the vaginal opening exposed. An insemination pipette (glass tubing approximately 18 cm in length with an inside diameter of 3 mm and an outside diameter of 4 mm) that is bent a a 45-degree angle approximately 4 cm from one end is warmed in 0.9% saline maintained at 37°C. A rubber bulb is attached to the longer end of the pipette and approximately 0.25 ml of diluted semen is gently drawn into it. The short end of the pipette is gently inserted into the vagina with the tip directed toward the dorsal wall to avoid the urethral orifice. After the pipette has been inserted as far as the angle, it is rotated 180 degrees so that the tip points toward the ventral wall and insertion is continued until slight resistence is felt. The bulb is gently squeezed to expel the semen while the pipette is slowly withdrawn. Ovulation is then induced by giving the doe an injection of 0.1 U/g of human chorionic gonadotropin into the marginal ear vein.

STUDY DESIGNS

The rabbit is used in numerous study designs to evaluate toxicological responses to pesticides, drugs, and industrial chemicals. Depending on the type of material to be evaluated, these tests are done according to the U.S. Food and Drug Administration (FDA), Environmental Protection Agency (EPA), Federal Hazardous Substances Act

Table 5 Scale for Scoring Skin Reaction

Erythema	
0	None
1.0	Slight
2.0	Moderate (well-defined)
3.0	Severe (beet red)
Edema	
0	None
1.0	Slight (barely perceptible to well-defined by definite raising)
2.0	Moderate (raised approximately 1 mm)
3.0	Severe (raised more than 1 mm)
Atonia	
0	None
1.0	Slight (slight impairment of elasticity)
2.0	Moderate (slow return to normal)
3.0	Severe (raised more than 1 mm)
Desquamation	
0	None
1.0	Slight (slight scaling)
2.0	Moderate (scaling and flaking)
3.0	Severe (pronounced scaling and denuding)
Fissuring	
0	None
1.0	Slight (definite cracks in epidermis)
3.0	Moderate (cracks in epidermis)
3.0	Severe (cracks with bleeding)

(FHSA), or the Organisation for the Economic Cooperation and Development (OECD) guidelines and range from short-term acute studies to 90-day toxicity studies.

The rabbit is also the nonrodent species most frequently used to evaluate developmental toxicity. (In the 1960s, the drug thalidomide was tested and shown to be safe in rats, but caused severe birth defects in humans. When given to pregnant rabbits, this drug caused fetal malformations, and now it is required that chemicals must be tested for developmental toxicity in both rodent and nonrodent species.)

Ocular and dermal irritation studies and dermal toxicity studies are types of acute studies that are routinely done using rabbits. Typical designs for these studies and other specialized acute studies such as photoirritation and USP pyrogen tests are presented in Tables 6–10.

Ocular Irritation

Eye, or ocular, irritation studies generally last from 72 hr to 7 days, but can be continued for 21 days if irritation persists. The guidelines that are followed indicate the number of animals tested and the number of test groups. Presently, the rabbits are given an examination to eliminate any animals with preexisting ocular defects, irritation, or corneal injury. The material is instilled in the conjunctival sac and the eye is examined at the specified intervals. If the pH of the test material evaluated is less than 3.0 or greater than 11.5, consideration should be given to not performing the test, since the material can be considered corrosive.

Dermal Irritation and Toxicity

Acute dermal irritation and toxicity studies last 14 days. The length of exposure is 24 hr and the numbers of animals and dose levels depend on the specific testing guidelines. Clinical observations and dermal irritation scores (Table 5) are recorded daily. As with the ocular study, if the pH of the material is less than 3.0 or greater than 11.5, consideration should be given to not performing the test, since the test material can be considered corrosive.

Dermal Toxicity

The rabbit is also used to evaluate the dermal toxicity of a test material. This study may be a short-term, 21-day study or may be 90 days in duration. The animals are clipped, treated, and wrapped like an acute dermal study, but the duration of treatment is daily, for 6 hr per day 5 (or 7) days per week. Clinical observations, body weights, and food consumptions are recorded weekly and dermal irritation scores are recorded daily. The animals are necropsied and microscopic examinations are done. Animals are bled before the terminal sacrifice and hematology and clinical chemistry data are obtained. Specific tissue lists, clinical pathology tests, and other specific requirements and tests for the 21-day and 90-day toxicity studies are listed in Table 11.

Teratogenicity

Rabbits are frequently used as the nonrodent species for teratogenicity studies (Table 12). In this study design, the pregnant doe is treated during fetal organogenesis, days 7–19 of gestation. The day of breeding or artificial insemination is gestation day 0. The doe is euthanatized prior to term (gestation day 29) and the uterine contents are examined for implantation sites, early and late resorption sites, and live or dead fetuses. The fetuses are weighed, sexed, and examined for external, soft-tissue, and skeletal development.

Table 6 Typical Study Designs for Acute Primary Eye Irritation Studies with Rabbits

Low-volume dose (unwashed)

duration	72 hr
dose level	10 μl or equivalent weight
number of animals	6, either sex
observations	Observe at 1, 24, 48, and 72 hr after instillation; if irritation persists, observe 96 hr, 7 days, 14 days, and 21 days after instillation or until irritation subsides (but not to continue past 21 days)
termination	Euthanatize and discard

Low-volume dose (unwashed and washed groups)

duration	72 hr
dose level	10 μl or equivalent wieght
number of animals	9 rabbits; 6 unwashed and 3 washed
dose administration	Washed at 4 sec after instillation (with 20 ml lukewarm water)
observations	Observe at 1, 24, 48, and 72 hr: if irritation persists, observe 96 hr, 7 days, 14 days, and 21 days after instillation or until irritation subsides (but not to continue past 21 days)
termination	Euthanatize and discard

FHSA and EPA (unwashed)

duration	72 hr
number of animals	6 rabbits
observations	Observe at 1, 24, 48, and 72 hr after instillation; if irritation persists, observe 96 hr, 7 days, 14 days, and 21 days after instillation or until irritation subsides (but not to continue past 21 days)
termination	Euthanatize and discard

EPA, 1978 (unwashed and washed groups)

duration	7 days
number of animals	9 rabbits; 6 unwashed and 3 washed
observations	Observe at 1, 24, 48, 72, and 96 hr and 7 days after instillation; if irritation persists, observe 14 days and 21 days after instillation or until irritation subsides (but not to continue past 21 days)
termination	Euthanatize and discard

OECD (unwashed)

duration	72 hr
number of animals	3 rabbits
observations	Observe at 1, 24, 48, and 72 hr after instillation; if irritation persists, observe 96 hr, 7 days, 14 days, and 21 days after instillation or until irritation subsides (but not to continue past 21 days)
termination	Euthanatize and discard

OECD (washed)

duration	72 hr
number of animals	6 rabbits; 3 washed for 5 min at 4 sec after instillation and 3 washed for 5 min at 30 sec after instillation
observations	Observe at 1, 24, 48, and 72 hr after instillation; if irritation persists, observe 96 hr, 7 days, 14 days, and 21 days after instillation or until irritation subsides (but not to continue past 21 days)
termination	Euthanatize and discard

Table 7 Typical Study Designs for Acute Primary Dermal Irritation Studies with Rabbits

DOT (corrosivity)

duration	48 hr
dose level	0.5 g(ml)/rabbit; 1 intact site per rabbit; 4-hr exposure
number of animals	6 rabbits
observations	Observe at 4, 24, and 48 hr after dosing
termination	Euthanatize and discard

FHSA

duration	72 hr
dose level	0.5 g(ml)/rabbit; 1 intact and 1 abraded site per rabbit
number of animals	6 rabbits
length of exposure	24 hr
Observations	Observe at 24 and 72 hr after dosing; if irritation persists, observe 96 hr, 7 days, and 14 days after dosing or until irritation subsides (but not to continue past 14 days)
termination	Euthanatize and discard

EPA

duration	72 hr
dose level	0.5 g(ml)/rabbit; 1 intact site per rabbit
number of animals	6 rabbits
length of exposure	4 hr
observations	Observe at 4, 24, 48, and 72 hr after dosing; if irritation persists, observe 96 hrs, 7 days, and 14 days after dosing or until irritation subsides (but not to continue past 14 days)
termination	Euthanatize and discard

PARASITES, DISEASES, AND PHYSICAL ANOMALIES

Because it is very difficult and expensive to obtain pathogen-free rabbits, the identification of common diseases and parasites is important to the investigator. In some instances, these conditions may cause an animal to be unsuitable for a study or may require euthanasia of a specific animal or an entire shipment of animals. This section includes a brief discussion of some of the more frequent conditions observed with rabbits, common clinical signs to aid in identification, and suggested treatments.

Mites

Ear Mites

Ear mange (otitis externa) is a condition caused by psoroptid mites which are nonburrowing parasites that chew the epidermal layers of the skin and produce a tan or brown crusty exudate on the inner surface of the ear. Clinical signs are the rabbit shaking its head or scratching its ears. Although ear mites are nonpathogenic, they can spread from rabbit-to-rabbit, and, if left untreated, can result in a secondary bacterial infection. Treatment is simple: The ear canal should be cleansed and treated with a few drops of plain mineral oil or mineral oil with a miticide added. A high standard of hygiene should be maintained (Kraus, 1974).

Table 8 Typical Study Designs for Acute Dermal Toxicity Studies with Rabbits

OECD
duration	72 hr
dose level	0.5 g(ml)/rabbit; 1 intact site per rabbit
number of animals	3 rabbits
length of exposure	4 hr
observations	Observe at 4, 24, 48, and 72 hr after dosing; if irritation persists, observe 96 hr, 7 days, and 14 days after dosing or until irritation subsides (but not to continue past 14 days)
termination	Euthanatize and discard

FHSA limit test
duration	14 days
dose level	2 g/kg
number of animals	5 males and 5 females
skin preparation	Half abraded, half nonabraded
length of exposure	24 hr
observations	Clinical observations daily
	Dermal irritation scored daily (Table 5)
necropsy	Necropsy all rabbits found dead
termination	Euthanatize and discard after 14 days

FHSA estimation of lethal dose
duration	14 days
dose levels	3 dose levels; determined by limit test
number of animals	5 males and 5 females/dose level
skin preparation	Half abraded, half nonabraded
length of exposure	24 hr
observations	Clinical observations daily
	Dermal irritation scored daily (Table 5)
necropsy	Necropsy all rabbits found dead
termination	Euthanatize and discard after 14 days

EPA/OECD limit test
duration	14 days
dose level	2 g/kg
number of animals	5 male and 5 females
length of exposure	24 hr
observations	Clinical observations daily
	Dermal irritation scored daily (Table 5)
necropsy	Necropsy all rabbits found dead
termination	Euthanatize and discard after 14 days

EPA/OECD estimation of lethal dose
duration	14 days
dose levels	3 dose levels; determined by on limit test
number of animals	5 males and 5 females/dose level
length of exposure	24 hr
observations	Clinical observations daily
	Dermal irritation scored daily (Table 5)
necropsy	Necropsy all rabbits found dead
termination	Euthanatize and discard after 14 days

Table 9 Typical Study Designs for Dermal Studies with Rabbits

Photoirritation/toxicity	
duration	72 hr
dose level	0.5 g(ml)/rabbit; 2 intact sites per rabbit
number of animals	6 rabbits
length of exposure	2-hr occluded exposure 10 J/cm^2 UVA to 1 site
observations	Observe at 24 and 72 hr
termination	Euthanatize and discard

Fur Mites

There are two types of fur mites that are commonly seen in laboratory rabbits, the cheyletid and sarcoptid mites. The cheyletid fur mite is seen mainly on the dorsal trunk in the scapular area. Often there are no clinical signs except for partial alopecia and a grayish white skin surface; generally there is no scratching by the rabbit. This mite is nonburrowing and ingests the keratin layer of the epidermis. Treatment for this mite consists of the application of a topical gel acaricide (Holmes, 1984).

Mange Mites

Another mite that can be seen in groups of laboratory rabbits is the sarcoptid mange mite. Unlike the noninvasive cheyletid fur mite, the sarcoptid mite tunnels through the skin, ingests epithelial cells, and may suck lymph. Clinical signs are rubbing and alopecia and a whitish yellow crust. The rubbing may lead to skin lesions and secondary bacterial infections. This condition is contagious and can become severe, leading to emaciation and death (Holmes, 1984). The recommended treatment is elimination of affected animals and clean, sanitary conditions.

Protozoan Infections

Coccidiosis

One of the most important diseases in rabbits is coccidiosis, which is caused by protozoan organisms of the genus *Eimeria*. There are two major types of coccidiosis that are detrimental to rabbits; one affects the liver and the other affects the intestine. Transmission is by ingestion of sporulated oocysts that are in the feces (Harkness, 1987).

Encephalitozoonosis

Encephalitozoonosis is a chronic disease seen in rabbits and is caused by the protozoan *Encephalitozoon cuniculi*. It is usually latent and actually prevalent in many colonies (estimates range from 15 to 78% affected). However, it is extremely difficult to diagnose

Table 10 Typical Study Designs for Biological Safety Tests with Rabbits

Pyrogen test	
duration	3 hr
dose level	1 dose level; single intravenous injection
number of animals	3 or 8 rabbits
observations	Record rectal temperatures at 1, 2, and 3 hr after injection

Table 11 Typical Study Design for Dermal Toxicity Studies with Rabbits

21-day toxicity	
duration	21 Days
dose levels	4 groups of 10 males and 10 females each; dose ml/kg based on most recently recorded weight
number/age of animals	80 (40 males and 40 females) rabbits; 10–12 weeks of age
area of exposure	Approximately 10% of total body surface
length of exposure	6 hr/day, 5 days per week
dose administration	Applied uniformly over exposure area
body weights	Weekly and at sacrifice
food consumption	Monitor quantitatively or qualitatively, depending on specific guidelines
observations	At least twice daily for signs of moribundity, mortality, toxicity, and abnormal behavior or poor health
dermal irritation	Scored daily, before each application of test material and on the day of necropsy
	Score using scale presented in Table 5
clinical pathology	Before terminal sacrifice
hematology	Red blood cell count, hemoglobin, hematocrit, mean corpuscular volume, mean corpuscular hemoglobin, mean corpuscular hemoglobin concentration, platelet count, white blood cell count, differential blood cell count, blood cell morphology, reticulocyte count smear
clinical chemistry	Glucose, urea nitrogen, creatinine, total protein, albumin, globulin, total bilirubin, cholesterol, aspartate, aminotransferase, alanine aminotransferase, γ glutamyl transferase, calcium, inorganic phosphorus, sodium, potassium, calcium
moribund sacrifices/deaths	Gross necropsy, save tissues
scheduled sacrifice	Gross necropsy, record organ weights, save tissues
tissues weighed	Brain, kidneys, liver, ovaries, or testes
tissues saved	Skin (treated and untreated); target organs; lesions
microscopic examination	Tissues saved from control and high-dose rabbits and macroscopic lesions from all rabbits
90-day toxicity	
duration	90 days
dose levels	4 groups of 10 males and 10 females each; additional rabbits (10/sex) may be added to the control and high-dose groups and used as recovery animals; dose ml/kg based on most recently recorded weight
number/age of animals	80 (40 males and 40 females) rabbits; 10–12 weeks of age
age of exposure	Approximately 10% of total body surface
length of exposure	6 hr/day, 5 days per week
dose administration	Applied uniformly over exposure area
body weights	Weekly and at sacrifice
food consumption	Monitor quantitatively or qualitatively, depending on specific guidelines
observations	At least twice daily for signs of moribundity, mortality, toxicity, and abnormal behavior or poor health

dermal irritation	Scored daily, before each application of test material and on the day of necropsy
	Score using scale presented in Table 5
ophthalmic examination	Before initiation of treatment and before terminal necropsy
clinical pathology	Before terminal sacrifice
hematology	Red blood cell count, hemoglobin, hematocrit, mean corpuscular volume, mean corpuscular hemoglobin, mean corpuscular, hemoglobin concentration, platelet count, white blood cell count, differential blood cell count, blood cell morphology, reticulocyte count smear
clinical chemistry	Glucose, urea nitrogen, creatinine, total protein, albumin, globulin, total bilirubin, cholesterol, aspartate, aminotransferase, γ-glutamyl transferase, calcium, inorganic phosphorus, sodium, potassium, calcium
moribund sacrifices/deaths	Gross necropsy, save tissues
scheduled sacrifice	Gross necropsy, record organ weights, save tissues
tissues weighed	Brain, kidneys, liver, ovaries, or testes
tissues saved	Adrenals, aorta, bone marrow smear, brains, cecum, colon, duodenum, epididymides, esophagus, eyes, femur and bone marrow, gallbladder, heart, ileum, jejunum, kidneys, lacrimal gland, liver, lungs, mammary gland, mesenteric lymph node, muscle, ovaries or testes, pancreas, pituitary, prostate, rectum, sciatic nerve, seminal vesicles, skin (both treated and untreated), spinal cord, spleen, sternum and bone marrow, stomach, submandibular salivary glands, thymus, thyroid with parathyroid, trachea, urinary bladder, uterus, and lesions
microscopic examination	Tissues saved from control and high-dose rabbits and macroscopic lesions from all rabbits

because clinical signs are only occasional neurological signs such as convulsions, tremors, and torticollis (Harkness, 1987). Transmission is thought to be via infectious urine. Pathologically, lesions are noted in the kidney and the brain. There is no known treatment (Holmes, 1984). The disease is important because it may interfere with and complicate the interpretation of experimental data.

Hepatic Coccidiosis

Eimeria stiedae is the organism that affects the liver. Clinical signs such as diarrhea and weight loss are often seen only in young animals; adults usually show no physical change. Pathologically this organism affects the bile duct epithelium and causes an enlarged or irregularly shaped liver (Pakes, 1974).

Intestinal Coccidiosis

Eimeria irresidua, E. magna, E. media, and E. perforans are the organisms responsible for intestinal coccidiosis. Clinical signs vary depending on the extent of infection and the age of the animal. In cases of mild infections, there are no clinical signs; severe infections result in weight loss, diarrhea, dehydration, and secondary bacterial infections (Holmes, 1984). Prevention and control of coccidiosis is by strict sanitization practices and elimination of infected animals.

Table 12 Typical Study Design for Teratology Studies with Rabbits

Range-find	
duration	Days 0–29 of gestation
dose levels	5 groups/5 inseminated females/group; dose ml/kg based on daily weight, most recently recorded weight, or day 7 weight
number of animals	25 young adult females, 5–6 months of age
length of exposure	Days 7–19 of gestation
body weights	Days 0, 7, 10, 13, 16, 20, 24, and 29 of gestation
observations	At least twice daily for signs of moribundity, mortality, toxicity, and abnormal behavior or poor health
moribund sacrifices/deaths/abortions	Necropsy, examine uterus for implantation sites, resorption sites, and fetuses, if possible.
C-section	Day 29 of gestation, gross necropsy, remove and weigh uterus then examine for corpora lutea, implantation sites, resorption sites, live and dead fetuses
	Options: expose uterine contents and examine fetuses for external malformations; or expose uterine contents, remove fetuses, examine for external development, and weigh
Definitive	
duration	Days 0–29 of gestation
dose levels	4 groups/16 inseminated females/group (must have 12 pregnant does per group; dose ml/kg based on daily weight, most recently recorded weight, or day 7 weight
number of animals	64 young adult females, 5–6 months of age
length of exposure	Days 7–19 of gestation
body weights	Days 0, 7, 10, 13, 16, 20, 24, and 29 of gestation
food consumption	Monitor quantitatively or qualitatively, depending on specific guidelines
observations	At least twice daily for signs of moribundity, mortality, toxicity, and abnormal behavior or poor health
moribund sacrifices/deaths/abortions	Gross necropsy, examine uterus for implantation sites, resorption sites, and fetuses, if possible
C-section	Day 29 of gestation, gross necropsy, remove and weigh uterus then examine for corpora lutea, implantation sites, resorption sites, live and dead fetuses
	Expose uterine contents, remove fetuses
fetal development	Examine for external development, and weigh. Euthanatize fetuses, examine internally (modification of **Staples** technique), and sex. Mid-coronal slice of head and brain, examine brain; remove eyes and examine; eviscerate fetuses and fix in alcohol. Mascerate fetuses with potassium hydroxide, stain skeletons with calcium-positive alizarine red s, and evaluate skeletal structures for development.

Bacterial Infections

Pasteurella Multocida

Pasteurella multocida is a frequent cause of bacterial disease in rabbits. It causes a multitude of clinical diseases such as snuffles, pneumonia, otitis media, abscesses and conjunctivitis, metritis, or pyometra, and orchitis. Many rabbits carry the organism without any clinical signs of infection until they are stressed as a result of experimental procedures.

Snuffles. This disease is also referred to as rhinitis or sinusitis. It occurs when *P. multocida* is found in the nasal cavities (Flatt, 1974). It is quite common for rabbits to have this infection without any clinical signs. When stressed, sneezing, coughing, and a nasal discharge may develop. The disease may persist as snuffles or it may progress to other clinical forms.

Pneumonia. *P. multocida* may cause pneumonia in young rabbits 4–6 weeks of age. It can progress to cause consolidation in the lungs or pleuritis, or in the case of acute pneumonia, may result in death without any clinical signs (Holmes, 1984).

Septicemia. Septicemia has often been associated with snuffles and pneumonia. Clinical signs for septicemia are not observed because, once infected, the animal dies quickly (Holmes, 1984).

Otitis. *P. multocida* may spread from the nasal cavities to the inner ear and cause torticollis or otitis interna (Holmes, 1984). This should not be confused with otitis externa, which is caused by mites. Rather, it is an infection of the inner ear that is often characterized by a head tilt or wry neck, and may be so severe that the head is upside down.

Metritus and Orchitis. Another condition caused by *P. multocida* is metritis, or pyometra, in the doe and orchitis or epididymitis in the buck. Genital infections occur more in the doe, although they also are observed in young rabbits and adult bucks. Clinical signs of the acute or subacute infection in the doe are seldom seen except for a vaginal discharge. This condition can cause a reduction in fertility either by a failure of the does to conceive or the buck may have enlarged testes (Flatt, 1974).

Abscesses and Conjunctivitis. These conditions are frequently seen in rabbits that have been exposed to *P. multocida* (Flatt, 1974). The abscess swellings contain a thick, tan or white creamy exudate and may be surrounded by a fibrous capsule. Conjunctivitis, possibly caused by the bacteria entering the conjunctival sac via the nasolacrimal duct, may occur in both young and mature rabbits. Clinical signs of conjunctivitis are reddened conjunctivae, moderately swollen or closed eyelids, and a mucus exudate (Flatt, 1974).

P. multocida is easily transmitted from rabbit-to-rabbit. It can be spread from dam to young by the respiratory route. It can have venereal transmission when genital infections are present. Since rabbits are infected with the disease without any clinical signs, it can be transmitted when new stock are introduced into an established colony. The bacteria is sensitive to a number of antibiotics such as chlortetracycline, oxytetracycline, penicillin, ampicillin, and chloramphenicol (Holmes, 1984). However, rarely do these treatments provide a complete cure. More often, remission occurs and infection is reestablished when treatment is ceased or when the rabbit is stressed. The best cure is elimination of the disease by euthanasia of affected animals and stringent sanitation practices. Also, it is recommended that investigators purchase rabbits from commercial colonies that provide rabbits that were cesarian derived and maintained in isolation (Holmes, 1984).

Tyzzer's Disease

Bacillus piliformis causes a bacterial disease commonly referred to as Tyzzer's disease. There is not a lot of information available on Tyzzer's disease; however, it is thought to be widespread. It is often diagnosed as mucoid enteritis because of the watery diarrhea, stained hindquarters, and dehydration that are seen clinically and very few animals survive (Flatt, 1974). This disease generally affects young rabbits, 10–12 weeks of age, but can occur in adults and preweanlings. It is transmitted through ingestion of the feces of infected animals. Then, if the rabbit is stressed because of overcrowding, heat, or experimentation, the organisms multiply. Treatment of infected animals rarely results in complete elimination of the bacteria. The best remedy is to eliminate infected animals and apply good sanitation practices (Holmes, 1984).

Staphylococcal Infections

There is little data concerning the incidences of staphylococcal infections; however, *Staphylococcosis aureus* is the most commonly identified pathogen. Clinical identification of the disease is difficult and is dependent on the site and duration of infection. These infections may range from dermatitis and slight subcutaneous swellings to septicemia and death (Flatt, 1974). Staphylococcal infections can be treated with systemic antibiotics, but they are best controlled by maintaining the animals in a clean, sanitary environment.

One of the more common staphylococcal infections is mastitis, or "blue breast." It is most prevalent in does that are heavy milk producers, or that have sustained an injury and are maintained in unsanitary conditions. Clinical signs are fever, decreased appetite, and inflammed mammary glands. These infections are not limited to lactating does and may also be seen in pseudopregnant does that are maintained in unsanitary conditions (Holmes, 1984). The disease is contagious and infected does should be isolated.

Escherichia Coli

Clinical signs of *Escherichia coli* infections are similar to other bacterial infections; i.e., diarrhea and death. This type of infection is thought to be a result of changes in the intestinal flora due to changes in environmental conditions. Although this organism is the predominant bacteria cultured, it is also thought to be a secondary infection rather than the primary cause of death (Flatt, 1974).

Treponematosis

Treponematosis, or rabbit syphilis, is characterized by inflammation of the face, genitalia, or regional lymph nodes. It is caused by a bacterium, *Treponema cuniculi*. Although it is not commonly seen clinically, the disease often observed serologically. Treponematosis has been confused with hutch burn, and the lesion may look like that seen with ear mites or sarcoptic mange. The lesions are primarily seen on the external genitalia, but they are also found on the chin, lips, nose, and eyelids. Treponematosis is transmitted by direct contact and is easily treated by isolation of infected individuals and penicillin (Flatt, 1974).

Mucoid Enteropathy

Mucoid enteropathy is probably one of the most common diseases affecting rabbits and at the same time is the least understood. It has been called bloat, enteritis, mucoid enteritis, mucoid diarrhea, and scours. It is most prevalent among young rabbits, 7–10 weeks of age, and is associated with the change in nutrition and feed of the suckling rabbit and the weanling. It is not certain if mucoid enteropathy is a disease in itself or just occurs in conjunction with other diseases. It is one of the most common causes of death in young rabbits. Clinical signs are diarrhea, depressed food consumption, hypothermia, bloated abdomen, depression, hunched posture, and the perineal region stained with yellow to brown colored fecal material. Macroscopic examinations frequently show stomach and sections of the intestines distended with gas or a watery fluid, gelatinous contents in the colon, and noninflammatory lesions in the intestinal mucosa. Microscopic examinations of the intestinal lesions support the noninflammatory condition and indicate an increase in the production of goblet cells (Flatt et al., 1974). The most productive treatment of mucoid enteropathy is management by prevention, practice good sanitation, reduce stress, and eliminate animals with clinical signs. Maintaining the animals on restricted feed rations is sometimes effective, or if that is not possible, restricting feed for the first few days postarrival and then gradually increasing to ad libitum. Also, feeding a high fiber diet has been shown to be effective in reducing the incidence of mucoid enteropathy.

Ulcerative Pododermatitis

Ulcerative pododermatitis is often seen among groups of older rabbits that have been maintained in wire cages for long periods of time. It is a pressure necrosis of the skin and is considered the result of heavy body weight on wire cage floors. It has mistakenly been called sore hocks, but this is an inaccurate term, since the affected area is the entire metatarsal region and is not restricted to the hocks (Flatt et al., 1974). The lesions vary in size and are well defined, ulcerated areas in the skin that are covered by a crusty scab. Secondary bacterial infections and abscesses may occur in the adjacent dermis (Holmes, 1984). The affected animal may appear clinically healthy, or it may show a weight loss, hunched appearance, and shifting of weight. The lesion can be treated and the reoccurrence reduced by housing the animal in solid-bottom cages with soft bedding material.

Fractures

The rabbit skeleton is very fragile and is only about 8% of its body weight (compared to a cat skeleton, which is 13% of its body weight) (Harkness and Wagner, 1983). Because the long bones and lumbar spine are surrounded by powerful muscle masses, the rabbit is particularly susceptible to fractures of the legs and back. Thus, although not a disease, the identification and diagnosis of the severity of a traumatic vertebral fracture is important. It is a posterior paralysis resulting from a vertebral fracture and damage to the spinal cord (Flatt et al., 1974). The onset is sudden, and often the fracture is the result of a struggle during restraint or improper support of the hindquarters when handled. Diagnosis is by clinical examination or radiography. Depending on the location of the lesion and the severity of the fracture, clinical signs are motor paralysis, loss of control of the anal sphincter and urinary bladder, and edema at the site. After a few weeks, function may return and the rabbit may not show any obvious signs of a previous injury (Flatt et al., 1974). However, if the injury is serious enough, it may be necessary to euthanatize the animal.

Moist Dermatitis

Moist dermatitis, also known as sore dewlap or hutch burn, is the result of constant wetting of the fur. It is a chronic, progressive disease and there may be various degrees of bacterial involvement. It may be caused from drooling because of malocclusion; drinking from open pans; cold, damp contact bedding; or continuous wetting of the fur because of experimental design (Holmes, 1984). Treatment is by the elimination or reduction of the causes; i.e., by using water bottles and sipper tubes or automatic watering systems instead of open pans, good sanitation, and by assuring that the fur is kept clean and dry.

Trichobezoar

Hair that has been ingested can accumulate in the stomach in the form of a ball, or trichobezoar. It generally does not cause any problems and is only noted at necropsy unless the mass becomes very large in size and obstruction can occur. If without apparent reason, an animal suddenly stops eating and drinking, a hair ball might be the cause. Hair balls can be detected by palpation or radiography. Successful treatment consists of giving mineral oil by a stomach tube if the hair ball is not too large.

Buphthalmia

Congenital or infantile glaucoma, buphthalmia, is a relatively common disease in laboratory rabbits. It is an increase in the size of the anterior chamber of the eye and may progress to cloudiness in the cornea, flattening of the cornea, and increased prominence of the eyeball. The condition progressively worsens over time and there is no treatment (Lindsey and Fox, 1974).

Heat Prostration

Rabbits are very sensitive to heat and husbandry practices should assure controlled temperatures. Clinical signs of heat prostration include rapid respiration, cyanosis, and prostration. Does near kindling and young rabbits in nesting boxes are particularly prone to temperature extremes. Hyperthermia can also cause abortion and a reduction of male fertility.

Malocclusion

Another clincial finding that is not necessarily life threatening but could have an adverse effect on an investigation is malocculusion. Rabbit teeth grow continuously and malocclusions occur when the incisors do not properly occlude and, therefore, are not worn away. Causes could either be a genetic shortening of the upper jaw or the result of an injury. This condition can be easily managed by clipping the teeth on a regular basis.

Pathology   **Robert R. Dahlgren**

Within the broad category of veterinary pathology, there are certain subspecialties which must deal, almost on a daily basis, with toxicological pathology. In many cases, changes or lesions observed in various organs or organ systems are related to the effects of specific compounds. The incidence and severity of these lesions may well be associated with the frequency of application and certainly with the dose range of these compounds. A further complication within this subspecialty of toxicological pathology deals with those lesions or changes which may be considered normal "abnormalities" or anatomical variations. The application of these experimental compounds may well exacerbate the severity and/or incidence of what might be considered normal abnormalities. No attempt here will be made to discuss all of the various specific tissue or specific organ system changes which are associated with various application routes as well as the use of experimental compounds. An attempt will be made, however, to discuss these so-called normal abnormalities which may be present and should be recorded during the examination of the rabbit both at gross and at microscopic examination. In certain cases, these lesions are age specific, or in some cases are associated with the length of time that animals have been present within a specific facility.

EFFECTS OF TRANSPORTATION STRESS

There is a general trend today for laboratories using a large number of animals to purchase animals at 8–10 weeks of age from major suppliers. Many of these suppliers provide specific pathogen–free animals, particularly animals free of *Pasteurella* and *Coccidia*. Young animals moving into a testing or research facility are under stress which is associated with transportation of the animal from the production site to the utilization site. During this process of transportation, animals usually experience numerous unfamiliar environmental influences such as temperature variations, unusual noise, and unfamiliar handling. The shipping and early utilization can be regarded as stressful. The stress has been shown in numerous species to cause marked variation in hematological and physiological parameters that may well predispose these young animals to numerous infectious agents which may be encountered in the new environment as well as agents which were carried from a production facility. Toth and January (1990) have shown the affect of shipment on various hematological and physiological parameters effecting adult male New Zealand White rabbits.

ENTEROTOXEMIA

Enterotoxemia is diarrheal disease of rabbits which presents generally within the first 24–96 hr after shipment. This diarrheal disease is generally seen in the quarantine period and rarely, if ever, diagnosed in animals that are placed on study or kept as stock animals after they have been removed from the quarantine regimen. Clinically, these animals are observed to be somewhat depressed and inactive and upon examination often a greenish brown discoloration is present in the perineal area. These animals are generally dehydrated, but death occurs before dehydration becomes a clinical manifestation. The cause is thought to be associated with a "iota" toxin which is produced by *Clostridium spiroforme*. In most cases, treatment is not effective, primarily because animals die with few clinical observations.

COLIBACILLOSIS

Colibacillosis is an acute diarrheal disease which often produces a high mortality rate in young rabbits in the 10- to 20-week age group. In most cases, *Escherichia coli* is presumed to be the etiological agent responsible for the outbreak of this disease. It is usually assumed that the *E. coli* causes the clinical disease when there is a rapid shift from predominantly gram-positive to a gram-negative bacterial flora. The most consistent lesions observed are mucosal and/or subserosal hemorrhages in the cecum or colon. Because of the etiology, colibacillosis is infrequently observed in those laboratories that provide good care and adequate diet. However, in animals used in studies with compounds which may affect the bacterial flora of either the small or large bowel, an outbreak of explosive diarrhea is possible.

TYZZER'S DISEASE

While colibacillosis and enterotoxemia are characterized in young rabbits by a florid, acute diarrhea and the presence of hemorrhage in the cecum and colon, the presence of multiple foci of liver necrosis which is characterized microscopically by hepatocelluar necrosis and a conspicuous absence of peripheral inflammatory cell involvement should cause one to be suspicious of Tyzzer's disease. This disease is caused by *Bacillus piliformis*. Long filamentous organisms can often be found in or near the areas of hepatic necrosis, but isolation of the bacteria in the laboratory has proven difficult.

PASTEURELLOSIS

Even though it is possible to obtain rabbits which are *Pasteurella* free, pasteurellosis remains a severe bacterial disease which can have several distinct clinical manifestations with little or no overlap between these clincal syndromes. Pasteurellosis comprises several diseases, including snuffles, septicemia, and other conditions. *Pasteurella multocida* stands as the unchallenged etiological agent for snuffles, enzootic pneumonia, otitis media, genital infection and abscesses, conjunctivitis, and septicemia. It has been assumed that *P. multocida* is spread from the dam to the offspring by the respiratory route shortly after birth. The introduction and spread of this organism within the rabbit colony may occur when new animals are brought into that colony. It is unusual to recognize clinical disease in suspected carrier animals, and this may allow for the introduction of asymptomatic carrier rabbits into a colony. Since asymptomatic rabbits carry the organism in the nasal cavity, it is assumed that some sort of stress compromises the host, thus allowing the bacteria to multiply. These initiating eposidoes of the rapid multiplication of the organism may allow the development of the various clinical syndromes depending on the route of infection or extent of dissemination.

Snuffles

Snuffles is characterized clinically by a mucous or mucopurulent nasal discharge which stimulates the animal to rub the nares with the medial surface of the front limbs and paws. The resulting wetness of the paws may be visible even though the nasal area exudation is dry. Sneezing, coughing, and respiratory "snuffling" are common symptoms. The gross and microscopic lesions are usually limited to the nasal cavity. Purulent exudate is present on the surface of the cavity or the turbinates with heterophils (neutrophils) and edema present within the submucosa or on the mucosal surface. Gram-negative bacterial rods may be found within the exudate with the aid of special stains. The incidence varies from 20 to 80%, but with the establishment of breeding colonies free of *P. multocida* the current incidence may well be below 10%.

Enzootic Pneumonia

Enzootic pneumonia is an acute fibrinous pneumonia. Extension to the pleural surface is a common secondary complication. Animals may present with acute death, pneumonia, or septicemia. This syndrome may occur after an outbreak of snuffles. The mortality rates are thought to vary between 5 and 40%; however, this is misleading because animals rarely show signs or symptoms which can be correlated with pneumonia unless other stressful mechanisms are present such as pregnancy or lactation. Perhaps the only helpful signs of pneumonia are anorexia and depression. The gross lesions in the lungs are typical of an acute fibrinous pneumonia, and involve the anteroventral areas most consistently. Microscopically, the bronchioles and alveoli are filled with heterophils, fibrin, and necrotic debris.

Otitis Media

Otitis media is generally recognized because of the head tilt or torticollis. Lesions are found in the tympanic cavities and consist of inflammatory exudate. Occasionally there may be extension to the ventral surface of the brain or the cerebellum in particular.

Metritis and Orchitis

Genital infection and abscesses may include metritis, or pyometra, in the female and onchitis and epididymitis in the male. These lesions are usually found at the termination of reproductive or teratology studies. It is possible that the male serves as a means of venereal transmission.

Conjunctivitis

Conjunctivitis caused by *P. multocida* is a poorly understood disease. This disease syndrome presents as swollen eyelids with mucoid exudate. The organism may be present in grossly normal eyes. Subsequent occular irritation studies may be compromised by the development of the inflammatory response to this organism.

Septicemia

Septicemia is usually a sequela to any of the other clinical syndromes caused by *P. multocida*. Animals may die peracutely with no evidence of clinical disease and few if any gross or microscopic changes.

By and large no treatment is attempted in any of the above clinical syndromes. Quarantine and sanitation procedures should be reexamined if these syndromes develop. Breeding sources must be reevaluated if snuffles or enzootic pneumonia is rediagnosed.

The following discussion will cover organ systems from the perspective of trying to include those changes which can be considered normal abnormalities in animals used for eye and skin irritation studies and animals used in reproductive or teratological studies. Both gross and microscopic changes will be discussed where relevant.

RESPIRATORY SYSTEM

Nasal Cavity

The nasal cavity presents no unusual anatomical structures. The respiratory surface may contain multifocal areas of mucoid material. The submucosa may contain individual or small aggregates of lymphocytes but no lymphoid follicles have been recognized.

TRACHEA AND LUNG

The trachea is similar in structure to the rat. The lung consists of apical, cardiac, and diaphragmatic lobes with the right diaphragmatic lobe divided into a large lateral and a smaller intermediate lobe. The left diaphragmatic lobe is not divided. There are peribronchiolar lymphoid foci which tend to increase in size with age. Several of the barbital-based anesthetic agents cause petechial homorrhages on the pulmonary surface which disappear with fixation. The presence of microphagelike cells with foamy-appearing cytoplasm can be found within the alveolar spaces. The alveolar wall surrounding these cells shows no evidence of damage at the light microscopic level.

DIGESTIVE SYSTEM

Tongue

The large tongue contains many, often paired papillae on the dorsal surface, which are occasionally mistaken for papillomatous growths. Microscopically, the papillae are shown to contain taste buds.

Stomach

The stomach appears thin walled, but the mucosal surface contains a glandular epithelium which varies in thickness as one approaches the pylorus. The submucosal areas often contain heterophils and lymphocytes. Grossly, the mucosa often appears to contain red foci which are not apparent microscopically. These areas are assumed to be areas of hyperemia which bleach out during fixation. Hair balls, (trichobezoars) are common in the stomach, especially in older adult animals which lick or pull their own fur. Hair balls rarely cause symptoms and are found incidentally at necropsy.

Small Bowel

The small bowel consists of a long duodenum and a relatively short jejunum and ileum. The terminal ileum is thin walled and dilated to form a rounded sacculus rotundus. Lymphoid patches (Peyer's patches) are found throughout the jejunum and ileum with the honeycomblike appearance of the sacculus being due to these lymphoid follicles.

Large Bowel

The large bowel consists of a spiral cecum, a sacculated colon, and the rectum. The proximal colon is similar in structure to the cecum, but it is located within the pelvic cavity. This location can be used to obtain accurate sections of the colon for microscopic examination. Lymphoid patches can be found throughout the submucosa of the cecum and colon. Sections of the rectum often contain submucosal lymphocytes which do not form aggregates or focci.

Liver

The liver presents four lobes. A deep median fissure divides the organ into right and left lobes. The right lobe is further divided into a posterior lobe. The quadrate lobe is a subdivision of the right lobe and is adjacent to the gallbladder. The caudate lobe is small and often found in the groove for the vena cava. The primary nonspecific microscopic changes consist of lymphocyte infiltration in the periportal area and varying degrees of hepatocyte cytoplasmic vacuolation or fatty change. The incidence of lymphoid infiltration varies with age and is more common in females. The severity is generally minimal to mild. Vacuolation of the cytoplasm is nonspecific but appears to be more common in females (Wells et al., 1988), and is greatly affected by ad libitum feeding of standard diets and fasting prior to blood collection (Weisbrode et al., 1990). Pregnancy toxemia, which can develop in pregnant, pseudopregnant, and post parturient females, causes extreme cytoplasmic vacuolation and hepatic necrosis. Even though the cause of this disease is complex, animals which are obese and lactating may develop extreme fatty livers and die with few clinical symptoms. Hill et al. (1988) have described a spontaneous storagelike disease in which hepatocytes have expanded, foamy cytoplasm and distinct cell borders. These lesions occurred singularly or as multifocal aggregates. Necrosis of individual or small groups of hepatocytes with no zonal distribution is not uncommon. It is assumed that the etiology is circulatory in origin.

Gallbladder

The gallbladder often contains echymotic serosal hemorrahges. These hemorrhages rarely extend the full thickness of the wall. Mucosal hyperplasia with frondlike papillary projections have been observed in animals which were being fed 40–50% of a normal ad libitum diet. It is assumed that this hyperplasia is in response to cholestasis or bladder distention.

Pancreas

The pancreas often contains foci of lymphocyte infiltration within the acinar area. There is no apparent acinar necrosis. Individual acinar necrosis or granular depletion of the cytoplasm can be found in animals which have undergone prior fasting for 12–16 hr. The islets are microscopically similar to other species.

CIRCULATORY SYSTEM

The heart is similar to other species except that the right atroventricular valve is bicuspid rather than tricuspid. Grossly, pale streaks running parallel to the long axis of the ventricle are often seen in obese females and in females late in gestation (26–30 days). These streaks are on the epicardial surface and can be confused with pericardial fat unless the pericardial sac is removed. Microscopically, these streaks may contain areas of fiber mineralization or loss of fiber staining but no evidence of inflammation. The etiology is unknown.

NERVOUS SYSTEM

Sections of the brain, in particular, the cerebrum may contain granulomas from animals which displayed no clinical signs of a central nervous system (CNS) disease. The etiology is considered to be a protozoan, *Encephalitozoon cuniculi* (often considered to belong to the family Nosematidae in the older literature). The protozoan is also known to infect the renal tubular cells (Shadduck and Pakes, 1971; Flatt and Jackson, 1970). Vertical transmission is strongly suspected. Focal meningeal aggregates of lymphocytes are often found in routine sections of the brain and the spinal cord. No known significance has been put forth, although viral causes have been suspected. Similar aggregates have been observed in the optic nerve as it leaves the globe.

EYE

The eye is a specific target organ in many toxicological studies; however, in many cases only gross or clinical observations are recorded. Microscopic changes often involve the conjunctiva and cornea and consist of multifocal areas of cellular infiltrates and necrosis of the superficial and deep corneal epithelium. Lymphoid infiltration is more common in the conjunctiva. The cellular infiltrates are an admixture of heterophils and macrophages. Corneal erosion of frank ulceration may be the final stage of many eye lesions. Sections of the globe may reveal anterior and/or posterior synechiae. The filtration angle is often difficult to visualize with H&E-stained section; however, the presence of inflammatory cells in the ciliary body or the base of the iris may contribute to the misconception of increased ocular tension. While the choroid lacks pigment, it is not unusual to find foci of melaninlike pigment which appears to extend into the layer of rods and cones of the retina. There is no evidence that this pigment is associated with inflammation.

SKIN

The skin is a common target system in toxicological studies. Gross observations range from erythema to ulcer formation. The severity of these lesions may depend on the application site and duration and frequency of application in addition to the chemical nature of the material involved. Microscopically, these lesions range from mild hyperemia and edema to extensive ulceration. Morgan et al. (1985) have described skin lesions including epidermal necrosis, hyperkeratosis, and inflammation which became complicated by dermal mucormycosis. The development of fungal dissemination may require more time than the usual 7- to 21–day studies. Multifocal aggregates of lymphocytes can be found surrounding hair follicles or the aggregates may be present in the deep dermal areas. The etiology is unknown.

UROGENITAL SYSTEM

The kidney is similar in structure to other laboratory species. This organ is bean shaped and on longitudinal section a single papilla projects into the renal calyx. The microscopic anatomy presents no unusual findings in young animals; however, aging changes should be recognized.

Glomerular changes begin to be apparent by 1 year of age. These changes consist of mesangial proliferation with a multifocal distribution. Progression to a more diffuse distribution and extension into the capillary loops is the end stage of this mesangial poliferation. The capillary wall appears to thicken with age, but the exact nature of this thickening has not been well documented. Numerous experimental studies exploring the histological and ultrastructural changes in immune complex glomerulonephritis have shown a deposition of immune complexes at varying locations along the capillary wall. It is not known if such immune complex disease(s) occur in the rabbit in a natural setting.

It is not unusual to find obsolete glomeruli or glomeruli which contain peripheral capillary loops that are collapsed or adherent to each other. There are no other changes and clinical chemistry and urinalysis values do not suggest renal disease. Perhaps ultrastructural changes occur, but such reports have not been forthcoming. Amyloid and hyaline material containing lipid has been found within capillary configurations. These deposits have been found in animals fed high lipid diets and used in cholesterol-related studies.

Tubular and interstitial changes consist of the deposition of pigments or lipids and lymphoid and macrophage infiltration. Lipid droplets are often found in the cytoplasm of the convoluted tubular epithelium in animals which have been fasted prior to sacrifice. Other pigments have been found in the convoluted and/or collecting tubules and usually represent products associated with red cell destruction or hepatic failure. Focal or multifocal areas of interstitial mononuclear cell infiltration are common findings. Usually, there is no evidence of tubular damage nor evidence of specific infectious agents. However, leptospirosis has been suggested as a possible etiological agent, but there has been no documented case in the recent English literature. The cause of these mononuclear infiltrates remains undetermined.

Female

Adult pregnant females may develop urinary retention due to the position of the uterus. Occasionally microscopic examination of the urinary bladder will reveal acute suppurative inflammation of the mucosa. Extension into the ureter and renal pelvis is to be expected.

The female genital organs present no unusual features as to location within the abdominal or pelvic cavities. It is not unusual to find oviductal "cysts" on one or both oviducts. Microscopic examination of these cysts suggest ductal origin. According to Avery (1965), the cranial portion of the mesonephric duct persists as the duct of the epoophoron and its tip becomes the cystic vesicular appendage. It appears that the most acceptable term for these cysts would be mesonephric or Wolffian duct cysts.

The right and left uteri are separate structures and unite to form a vagina and a cervical opening. The ovaries are slightly elongated but otherwise anatomically similar to other species.

Male

The male secondary sex glands, i.e., seminal vesicle, vesicular gland, prostate, and bulbourethral gland, are not separable except in general terms. Spontaneous vesicular and prostatic epithelial squamous metaplasia, hyperplasia, and keratinized nodules have been described by Zwicker et al. (1980). Interstitial perivascular mononuclear cell infiltration is a common observation in the epididymis and the secondary sex organs.

The testes may contain similar perivascular lesions, or in some cases there is evidence of vascular damage and inflammation; i.e. periarteritis. It is not uncommon to find peripheral seminiferous tubules on section of the testes which appear aspermatogenic or necrotic. This is most likely a fixation and handling artifact.

ENDOCRINE SYSTEM

Pituitary Gland

The pituitary often contains multiple endothelium-lined spaces at the junction between the pars distalis and intermedia. True cystic spaces or hyperplasia are not common in this species.

Adrenal Gland

The adrenal gland contains the usual cortex areas and a distinct medulla. The cortex often contains vacuolated cytoplasmic areas in cells which compromise the zona fascicularis. Accessary cortical nodules are found beneath the cortical capsule or embedded within the adipose tissue adjacent to the capsule. The adrenal medulla may contain areas of hyperplasia involving small groups of cells. While these foci may suggest preneoplasia, there is no reported evidence that pheochromocytomas develop from these hyperplastic foci.

Thyroid and Parathyroid Glands

The bilobed thyroid gland is located in the usual lateral aspect of the trachea, distal to the cricoid cartilage. Microscopically, the parathyroid is often embedded within the body of the thyroid. The thyroid contains follicles of various sizes which contain colloid. Typical C cells are difficult to identify by standard light microscopy. Thyroids of adult animals often contain lymphoid aggregates within the interstitial areas. Ectopic thymic tissue can be identified within the capsule of the thyroid. The parathyroid presents no unusual changes with advancing age.

NEOPLASTIC DISEASES

Weisbrode (1974b) has presented an excellent review of current literature through the early 1970s. The reported overall incidence of neoplasia is 2–3%. It must be understood that age is the predominant factor in determining neoplastic incidence. Benign and malignant tumors of the female reproductive tract and especially the uterus are the most common observed "spontaneous" neoplasms. Benign and malignant tumors of the mammary gland represent a close second system with regard to overall incidence. Based on the author's experience, rabbits used in "typical" toxicological or teratological studies present with few spontaneous neoplasms until these animals reach an age over 36 months, then previously mentioned tumors will be observed.

Metabolism   **Chyung S. Cook**

The hepatic microsomal cytochrome P-450 content in the rabbit has been studied and compared with those in other laboratory animals such as the mouse, rat, hamster, and guinea pig (Davis et al., 1969; Chhabra et al., 1974; Litterst et al., 1975, 1976). The cytochrome P-450 content (1.05–1.09 nmol/mg) and the activity of NADP:cytochrome c reductase (130–150 nmol/min/mg) in the rabbit were similar to those in the other species examined (Table 13). However, cytochrome P-450 reductase activity was much lower in the rabbit (3.0–3.4 nmol/min/mg) compared with that in the mouse and rat.

Souhaili-El Amri et al. (1986) conducted a similar study in six laboratory animal species and humans. Although the values for the cytochrome P-450 concentrations were somewhat lower in this study compared with those in the previous studies, the value in the rabbit (0.67 nmol/mg) was generally similar to those in the other animals, which is consistent with earlier findings. The cytochrome P-450 content in the rabbit was somewhat higher than the value in humans (0.31 ± 0.09 nmol/mg). The activity of NADPH:cytochrome c reductase and cytochrome b_5 contents in the rabbit were similar to those values in humans and the other animals examined.

Studies of rabbit cytochrome P-450 using SDS-acrylamide gel electrophoresis have demonstrated at least nine separable forms from liver microsomes (Lu and West, 1980; Coon and Koop, 1983). The PB-induced form, P-450 LM_2, and BNF/3-MC–induced form, P-450 LM_4, are the most active, although all of the P-450 isozymes displayed enzymatic activities. P-450 LM_2 was most effective in the metabolism of benzphetamine, whereas P-450 LM_4 was specific for acetanilide hydroxylation. However, they displayed comparable activity toward p-nitrophenetole, p-nitroanisole, and 7-ethoxycoumarin. The isozyme LM3, which is similar to cytochrome P-450$_p$ in the rat, was also found in the rabbit treated with macrolide antibiotics such as erythromycin and triacetyloleandomycin (Bertault-Peres et al., 1987; Fabre et al., 1988). This isozyme specifically mediates metabolism of cyclosporin. The isozymes LM_5 and LM_6 exclusively mediate the metabolism of 2-aminolfluorene and 7-ethocyresorufin, respectively.

The distribution pattern of mixed function oxidases for xenobiotics between smooth and rough microsomal membrane is known to be highly species dependent. In the rabbit, concentrations of all components of the mixed function oxidase system were 4–5 times higher in the smooth endoplasmic reticulum than in the rough endoplasmic reticulum of the hepatic microsomal fractions (Gram et al., 1971), whereas some animal (e.g., mouse) showed fairly even distribution between the smooth and rough membranes.

As reported for other species, the drug-metabolizing enzymes in newborn rabbits are not fully developed. For example, phenobarbital was more toxic to newborn than to adult rabbits and produced longer loss of the righting reflex in newborn rabbits (Weatherall, 1960).

The content of cytochrome P-450 and other electron transport chain components were highest in the rabbit liver among the organs examined. The content of cytochrome P-450 and cytochrome b_5 were approximately 2.5- to 5.0 fold higher than those in the lung and kidney (Uheleke, 1969; Oppelt et al., 1970). However, comparison of mono-oxygenase activity toward various substrates undergoing the same route of metabolism shows considerable variation in the ratio of lung to liver. For example, the activity of methylaniline ring hydroxylase, methylaniline N-demethylase, and 4-aminophenyl N-hydroxylase in the lung were about 10–25% of the liver activity, whereas the activity of biphenyl

Table 13 Summary of Hepatic Xenobiotic Drug Metabolizing Enzymes in the Rabbit

Enzyme	Concentration or activity	Comments and references
Cytochrome P-450 (nmol/ mg protein)	1.1[a], 0.779[b], 1.05 for M and 1.09 for F[c], 0.720[d], 0.67[e], 0.81[f,g]	[a]Chhabra et al. (1974), [b]Oppelt et al (1970), [c]Davies et al. (1969), [d]Gregus et al. (1983), [e]Souhaili-el Amri et al. (1986), [f]Atlas (1975), [g]Thorgeirssonet al. (1979)
Cytochrome b_5 (nmol/mg Protein	0.3[e], 0.84[b]	[e]Souhaili-el Amri et al. (1986), [b]Oppelt et al. (1970)
NADPH: cytochrome c Reductase (nmol/mg Protein)	185[a], 152[g], 130 for M and 150 for F[c]	[a]Chhabra et al. (1974), [g]Litterst et al. (1975), [c]Davies et al. (1969)
NADPH: cytochrome P-450 reductase (nmol/mg Protein)	3.0 for M and 3.4 for F[c]	[c]Davies et al. (1969)
Hydroxylase (nmol/min/mg) aniline hydroxylase	0.65[a], 0.542[b] 0.6[g], 0.72[h]	[a]Chhabra et al. (1974), [b]Oppelt et al. (1970), [g]Litterst et al. (1975), [h]Kato et al. (1979)
benzo(a)pyrene hydroxylase	0.061[d], 0.11[i]	[d]Gregus et al. (1983), [i]Thorgeirsson (1979)
biphenyl 4-hydroxylase	3.9[a], 1.7[g], 1.1[f], 2.0[i]	[a]Chhabra et al. (1974), [g]Litterest et al. (1975) [f]Atlas et al. (1975), [i]Thorgeirsson (1979)
Styrene oxide hydrolase	5.6[j], 5.8–6.4[k], 4.2[l], 2.3[m], 10.1[n]	[j]James et al. (1976), [k]James et al. (1977), [l]Pacifici et al. (1981), [m]Oesch (1973), [n]Oesch and Wolf (1989)
O-Dealkylase (nmol/min/mg) ethoxycoumarin O-demethylase	2.3[f]	[f]Atlas et al. (1975)
p-nitroanisole O-demethylase	5.4[f]	[f]Atlas et al. (1975)
N-Demethylase (nmol/min/ mg Aminopyrene N-demthylase	15.0[b] 9.8[g], 8.0[h]	[b]Oppelt et al. (1970), [g]Litterst et al. (1975), [h]Kato (1979)

Ethylmorphine N-demethylase	4.0[a], 4.0 for M & 4.3 for F[c] 2.0–2.2[o]	[a]Chhabra et al. (1974), [c]Davies et al. (1969) [o]Nerland et al. (1978)
N-hydroxylase (nmol/min/mg) dibenzylamine N-hydroxylase	2.9[p]	[p]Beckett and Gibson (1975)
2-acetylaminofluorene N-hydroxylase	0.2[f], 0.1[i]	[f]Atlas et al. (1975), [i]Thorgeirsson (1979)
Glutathion S-transferase (nmol/min/mg) 1-chloro-2,4-dinitrobenzene	4091[n] (cytosol), 81[n] (microsomes) 156[q] (microsomes)	[n]Oesch and Wolf (1989), [q]Morgenstern et al. (1984)
hexachloro-1,3-butadiene	0.14[n] (microsomes)	[n]Oesch and Wolf (1989)
ethacrynic acid	5.81[r]	[r]Gregus et al. (1985)
styrene oxide	30.5[j], 21.3–26.9[k], 36[l]	[j]James et al. (1976), [k]James et al. (1977), [l]Pacifici et al. (1981)
Protein estimates Microsoamal (mg/g)	24.1[g], 13.8–22.8[k], 18.1[d]	[g]Litterst et al. (1975), [k]James et al. (1977), [d]Gregus et al. (1983)
Cytosolic (mg/g)	72.7–82.0[k], 86.5[d]	[k]James et al. (1977), [d]Gregus et al. (1983)

hydroxylase, benzphetamine N-demethylase, and methylaniline N-hydroxylase in the lung were comparable to those in the liver. Therefore, lower cytochrome P-450 in the lung may not be rate limiting for some substrates.

Distribution of mono-oxygenase activities among the tissues varied depending on the substrates. For example, when benzypyrene hydroxylase activity was examined in the small intestinal mucosa preparations of the rabbit, mouse, cat, guinea pig, and rat, the rabbit had medium benzypyrene hydroxylase activity in the small intestine, although the hydroxylase activity in the liver microsomes was least active in the rabbit (Hietanen and Vainio, 1973). The UDP-glucuronyl transferase measured using p-nitrophenol as a substrate was highest in the small intestinal mucosa of the rabbit, although the transferase activity of the rabbit liver was intermediate and similar to the activity of rat and mouse liver.

Despite the large sex variations in the metabolism of many substrates by rats and some substrates by mice, investigation of sex difference in the rabbit have so far not revealed similar differences. The contents of cytochrome P-450 and the activities of cytochrome P-450 reductase and NADPH:cytochrome c reductase were similar between the male and the female rabbit (Davies et al., 1969). Furthermore, there was no sex difference in the N-demethylation of ethylmorphine and aminopyrine or hydroxylation of phenobarbital (Davies et al., 1969; Testa and Jenner, 1976).

Strain differences in drug-metabolizing ability could account for varying biological responses to such compounds as hexobarbital, adrenal cortex hormones, and 2-naphthylamine. In contrast to two- to three-fold variation in drug-metabolizing ability seen in the mouse and rat strains, up to 20-fold variations were observed between various rabbit strains. California rabbits, wild cottontails, and jack rabbits exhibited the most striking difference, each being fairly deficient in some enzymes. For example, the in vitro hepatic microsomal metabolism rate of hexobarbital and amphetamine was 19 and 8 nmol/mg protein/hr, respectively, in the Cottontail rabbit, whereas the metabolism rate of hexobarbital in the New Zealand rabbit was 254 nmol/mg/hr and the metabolism rate of amphetamine in the Dutch rabbit was 154 nmol/mg/hr (Cram et al., 1965).

The capacity for aromatic hydroxylation in the rabbit appears to be medium to high in general as illustrated with aniline, biphenyl, and coumarin. After intravenous administration of aniline, about 50% of the dose was excreted as p-aminophenol (Parke, 1960). While 4-hydroxylation of biphenyl was observed in the rabbit as in humans, 2-hydroxylation was not observed. Biphenyl 2-hydroxylation was limited to a few species such as the mouse and hamster. When the in vitro metabolism of N-benzyl-4–substituted anilines were studied using the rabbit, mouse, hamster, and guinea pig, ring hydroxylation was the major pathway in the rabbit and guinea pig, whereas in the mouse and hamster, N-debenzylation was the major pathway (Gorrod and Gooderham, 1987). The rat used both pathways to an equal extent. Coumarin 7-hydroxylase was present in rabbit hepatic preparations but absent in the rat and mouse preparations (Kulkarni and Hodgson, 1980).

In contrast to the above examples, the aromatic hydroxylation activity in the rabbit was low with benzpyrene, amphetamine, and ethyl biscoumacetate. The hepatic benzpyrene hydroxylase activity of the rabbit was two- to fivefold lower compared with that of the rat and mouse (Hietanen and Vainio, 1973; Gregus et al., 1983) and also somewhat lower than that in humans with a variation of about sixfold (Pelkonen et al., 1975). The range of aryl hydrocarbon hydroxylase activity in humans was approximately 20 to 320 pmol/g liver/min with no sex difference. In the rabbit, ethyl biscoumacetate, an anticoagulant drug, was exclusively deesterified and no aryl hydroxylation was observed whereas in humans and dogs, aryl hydroxylation of the drug was observed.

In the metabolism of amphetamines, aromatic hydroxylation was minor and deamination was the major pathway in the rabbit (Caldwell, 1976, 1981). Only small amounts were excreted as the unchanged drugs. In humans, deamination and unchanged drug excretion were equally important. In addition, substantial amounts of aromatic hydroxylated metabolites were excreted. N-Dealkylation of amphetamines was a minor pathway in humans as observed in the rabbit (Brodie, 1962). Green et al. (1986) have studied amphetamine metabolism using isolated hepatocyte suspension from the rabbit, rat, dog, squirrel monkey, and human livers. As observed in the in vivo studies, rabbit hepatocytes metabolized amphetamine almost exclusively to the products of the oxidative deamination pathway, whereas rat hepatocytes primarily metabolized by aromatic hydroxylation. Metabolism of the drug by the hepatocytes from three other species (dog, monkey, and human) was mixed but oxidative deamination was somewhat more active than aromatic hydroxylation.

N-Dealkylating activity in the rabbit was highly variable, ranging from low to high depending on the substrate. For example, N-demethylation of benzphetamine by the rabbit was about twofold higher than that in the rat and mouse, about fourfold higher than that in the dog (Gregus et al., 1983), and more than 10-fold higher than that in humans (Souhaili-El Amri et al., 1986). The maximum velocity (V_{max}) of N-dealkylase activity for aminopyrine in the rabbit was slightly lower compared with the mouse and male rat (SD strain), similar to that of the monkey and female rat, and about twofold higher than that of humans (Souhaili-El Amri et al., 1986). N-Demethylase activity of ethylmorphine in the rabbit was less than half that of the mouse and male rat, similar to that in the dog and female rat, and about twofold higher than that in humans (Gregus et al., 1983; Souhaili-El Amri et al., 1986). In contrast, N-dealkylation of benzylaniline in the rabbit was minor and ring hydroxylation was the major pathway. Similar results were also observed with tolbutamide, an antidiabetic drug. Tolbutamide is metabolized via methyl hydroxylation and N-dealkylation pathways. In rabbits as well as in humans, monkeys, and rats, the methyl hydroxylation was the major pathway (Thomas and Ikeda, 1966; Tagg et al., 1967; Gee and Green, 1984). In dogs, N-dealkylation was the major pathway (Remmer et al., 1964).

N-Hydroxylase activity is predominately mediated via the polycyclic hydrocarbon-inducible cytochrome P1-450 (Felton et al., 1976) and is of great importance for toxicity evaluation. For example, acetaminophen-induced hepatic injury was found to be related to the rates of N-hydroxylation of the drug by the hepatic microsomes (Davis et al., 1974). In the rabbit, N-hydroxylation activity was medium to high as illustrated with 4-aminobiphenyl and 2-acetylaminofluorene (2AAF). The major metabolic pathway of 4-aminobiphenyl was N-hydroxylation in the rabbit, mouse, guinea pig, and hamster (McMahon et al., 1980). Interestingly, the N-hydroxylase activity in the rabbit was not induced by methylcholanthrene or Aroclor 1254, a potent cytochrome P1-450 inducer, although it was induced by phenobarbital. N-Hydroxylation of 4-aminophenyl in the rat, mouse, and guinea pig was enhanced more than fivefold by Aroclor 1254.

The N-hydroxylase activity of 2-acetylaminofluorene in rabbit liver microsomes was higher than that in the mouse, rat, and guinea pig (Lotlikar et al., 1967). The N-hydroxy metabolite was practically undetectable in the guinea pig, which explains resistance of the guinea pig to hepatoma induction by 2-acetylaminofluorene. When in vitro metabolism of dibenzylamine was studied using hepatic microsomes of the rabbit, rat, mouse, hamster, guinea pig, chick, and cat, N-oxidase activity in rabbit microsomes was highest (86.9 nmol/mg/30 min) and approximately 5 and 7 times greater than the activity of mouse and rat microsomes (Beckett and Gibson, 1975). In vitro metabolism of N-benzyl-4-substituted anilines were studied using rabbit, rat, mouse, hamster, and guinea pig liver homogenates (Gorrod and Gooderham, 1987). In contrast to the findings with dibenzylamine, the rabbit had the lowest N-oxidase activity, which was followed by the rat, mouse, guinea pig, and hamster in increasing order. In the rabbit, ring hydroxylation was the major pathway.

Hepatic microsomal levels of epoxide hydrolase activity in rabbits have been compared with those of humans and several commonly used animal models, including the mouse, rat, guinea pig, and rhesus monkey (Oesch, 1973, 1980). With benzo(a)pyrene 1,1-oxide as a substrate, the hydrolase activity in the rabbit was similar to that in the rat but approximately half that in humans and guinea pigs. The monkey had the highest activity and the mouse had the least activity. When the activity of epoxide hydrolase was measured with styrene oxide as a substrate, the enzyme activity in rabbit liver (4.2–10.1 nmol/min/mg) was similar to that in rat liver as observed with benzo(a)pyrene 1,1-oxide but three- to sixfold lower than that in human liver (Pacifici et al., 1981; Gregus et al., 1983; Oesch and Wolf, 1989). As observed with other enzyme activities, the styrene oxide hydrolase activity in the rabbit kidney and lung (1.5 and 0.4 nmol/min/mg) was lower compared with that in the liver.

The N-acetyltransferase enzyme system is important in understanding the toxicity induced by arylamines. This enzyme system can be viewed as a component of activation pathways with respect to arylamine hepatocarcinogenesis and as a component of detoxification pathways with respect to arylamine bladder carcinogenesis, whereas N-hydroxylating enzyme systems can be viewed as components of activation pathways with respect to both arylamine bladder carcinogenesis and arylacetamide hepatocarcinogenesis. The rabbit is known as the best acetylator of aromatic amines and sulfonamide with low arylacetamide deacetylase activity. For example, consistently high levels of N-acetyl transferase activity were observed in the rabbit toward p-aminobenzoic acid, isoniazid, sulfamethazine, 2-aminofluorene, and β-naphthalylamine, whereas the rat and mouse showed markedly different activity depending on substrate (Gregus et al., 1983). When acetylase activity was studied with sulfanilamide (Williams, 1967) and various mono- and dimethoxy-6-sulfanilamidopyrimidines (Bridges et al., 1969) in various species (such as rabbit, human, monkey, and rat) the major metabolites in the rabbit urine were N^4-acetyl derivatives except in the case of the 2,5-dimethoxy compound, which was excreted largely unchanged. The rat also favored the formation of N^4-acetyl derivatives, but overall excreted more unchanged drug than the rabbit. Comparable results were apparent in humans with a lesser degree of N^4-acetylation compared with the rabbit. Rabbits display a genetic polymorphism with respect to acetylation, as do humans. This leads to speculation that the rabbit may be a predictive animal model for population-based acetylation of aromatic amines (Calabrese, 1988).

Glowinski et al. (1978) compared rates of acetylation in both fast and slow acetylator phenotypes in rabbits and humans for seven compounds, sulfamethazine, p-aminobenzoic acid, and five arylamine carcinogens (α-naphthylamine, β-naphthylamine, benzidine, 2-aminofluorene, and methylene-bis-2-chloroaniline). In general, the fast acetylator rabbits displayed a 10- to 50-fold greater rate of activity than the fast acetylator humans. For all compounds except p-aminobenzoic acid, the acetylation activity for the fast acetylator rabbits was 90- to 580-fold higher than that of the slow acetylator rabbits, whereas in humans the activity in fast acetylators was approximately four- to 13-fold higher. Therefore, for some compounds, the levels of acetylation activity in the slow acetylator rabbits were in the range of the fast or slow acetylator humans. For example, the slow acetylator rabbits were very similar to the slow acetylator humans for 2-aminofluorene (0.013 vs 0.021 μmol/mg/hr) and benzidine (0.016 vs 0.019 μmol/mg/hr), but more closely comparable to the fast acetylator human for β-naphthylamine (0.28 vs 0.23 μmol/mg/hr).

Many studies have been conducted to determine UDP-glucuronyltransferase activity in the rabbit. However, the enzyme activity appears to be highly substrate specific and no general conclusion could be drawn. For example, the transferase activity in the rabbit was high toward 1-naphthol, p-nitrophenol, estrone, morphine, and chloramphenicol when compared to the activity in other species such as the mouse, rat, guinea pig, and cat (Gregus et al., 1983). The transferase activity was medium or low toward phenolphthalein, diethylstilbestrol, testosterone, digitoxigenin, valproic acid, and bilirubin. In the rabbit, the concentration of hepatic UDP-glucuronic acid, which is required in the glucoronidation reaction as a glucuronic acid donor, was about half the values of the rat and guinea pig and similar to that of the dog. Therefore, UDP-glucuronic acid did not appear to be a limiting factor for glucuronidation metabolic pathway.

Emudianughe et al. (1978, 1987) studied glucuronidation and other conjugation reactions of radiolabeled naphthylacetic acids. Following 1-naphthylacetic acid administration, the majority of urinary radioactivity (88%) was accounted for by a glucuronide conjugate, whereas only a small amount (6%) of glycine conjugate was present in the rabbit. However, with 2-naphthylacetic acid the majority of urinary radioactivity was accounted for by amino acid conjugates (glycine, glutamine, and taurine), whereas the glucuronide conjugate represented about 24% of the urinary radioactivity. This was explained by the steric hindrance of 1-naphthylacetic acid for activation in amino acid conjugation (Caldwell, 1981). The amino acid conjugations require that the carboxylic group of the xenobiotic acid should be readily accessible for activation to the essential acyl CoA intermediate.

Interestingly, solubilized rabbit liver microsomes had relatively high UDP-glucuronyl transferase activity toward estrone and β-estradiol but not testosterone (Falany et al., 1983). Glucuronidation observed at the 3-OH position of β-estradiol is 20-fold greater than at the 17-OH position. In contrast, solubilized liver microsomes from female rats possessed approximately fourfold more activity toward testosterone (17-OH) than estrone (3-OH). Rat liver microsomes formed 2.5-fold more β-estradiol 17-glucuronide than 3-glucuronide. The highly substrate- and species-specific UDP-glucuronyltransferase appears to be due to, at least in part, multiple forms of the enzyme.

Sisenwine et al. (1982) studied in vivo and in vitro stereoselective effects in the glucuronidation of oxazepam in various species. They reported that conjugation of S-(+)-oxazepam was favored in rabbits as well as in humans, dogs, rats, and miniature swine. In rhesus monkeys, conjugation of R-(−) isomer was favored. In contrast to oxazepam, glucuronidation of propranolol was stereoselective for (R)-propranolol in the rabbit and for (S)-propranolol in humans and dogs (Yost et al., 1981; Von Bahr et al., 1982). These workers also found that glucuronic acid conjugation of 4-hydroxypropranolol, a metabolite of propranolol, was not stereoselective. After administration of racemic 2-arylpropionic acid, the formation of the glucuronide was enantioselective for the S(−) isomer in the rat and mouse but showed no stereoselectivity in the rabbit (Fournel and Caldwell, 1987). These findings as a whole demonstrated complex stereoselectivity of UDP-glucuronyl transferases among different species and broad generalization could not be made for the suitability of animal models for evaluating stereoselectivity of the enzyme.

Hydrolysis of glucuronide conjugates is carried out by the lysosomal enzyme β-glucuronidase, which is present in most tissues, particulary liver, kidney, spleen, intestinal tract, and endocrine and reproductive organs. The level of β-glucuronidase in multiple tissues has been studied in a variety of animal species as well as in humans. When β-glucuronidase activity was measured with phenolphthalein glucuronide, the enzyme activity in the rabbit liver (5000 μg/g liver/hr) was about 1.7-fold higher than that of human liver, similar to that of guinea pig and hamster liver, and three- to sixfold lower than that of rat liver (Calabrese, 1988). In contrast to liver enzyme activity, the enzyme activity in the kidney was lower in the rabbit (300 μg/g liver/hr) than in humans (2000 μg/g liver/hr).

Gastrointestinal tract levels of β-glucuronidase activity may markedly affect the response to some carcinogenic agents. Many carcinogenic agents such as benzo(a)pyrene are conjugated with glucuronic acid and excreted via the bile. Low β-glucuronidase activity in the small intestine is expected to reduce enterohepatic circulation, thereby reducing the residence time of the carcinogens in the body. Rabbits are estimated to have approximately 120- and 50-fold higher β-glucuronidase activity in the proximal and distal small intestine, respectively, compared with humans (Calabrese, 1988). Mice and rats are estimated to have approximately 60,000- and 15,000-fold, respectively, higher β-glucuronidase activity in the proximal small intestine than humans. Such findings suggest that the rabbit model may offer a closer approximation to the human even though the rabbit far exceeded the human values.

Glutathione transferase activity in rabbit liver was highly variable depending on the substrate. For example, glutathione transferase activity toward 1-chloro-2,4-dinitroben-zene was approximately five- and twofold higher in the rabbit than in the rat and mouse, respectively (Gregus et al., 1983; Igarashi et al., 1986). However, toward 1,2-dichloro-4-nitrobenzene, the enzyme activity in the rabbit was less than one-sixth of the activity in the rat and mouse. Gregus et al. (1985) studied glutathione transferase activities in the 60-day-old rabbit and other commonly used laboratory animals, such as rat, mouse, and guinea pig, toward seven substrates. The rabbit was the least active in the conjugation of six substrates (3,4-dichloronitro-benzene, sulfobromophthalein, p-nitrobenzyl chloride, ethacrynic acid, trans-4-phenyl-3-butene-2-one, and 1,2-epoxy-3-(p-nitrophenoxy pro-pane) out of seven, yet it was the most active in the conjugation of 1-chloro-3,4-dinitro-benzene. The transferase activity toward styrene oxide in rabbit liver (36 nmol/min/mg) was two- and fourfold lower than that in rat and mouse liver, but about 1.9 and 1.4 times higher than that in dog and human liver (Pacifici et al., 1981). This high variation of the enzyme activity appears to be in part due to different substrate specificities and subunit composition of the enzymes among the different species (Igarashi et al., 1986). The glutathione transferase activities toward styrene oxide in the rabbit kidney and lung (18.0 and 6.5 nmol/min/mg, respectively) were lower than that in the liver (Pacifici, 1981).

Oesch and Wolf (1989) determined glutathione transferase activity in liver microsomes and cytosol from various species, including rabbits and humans. The glutathione trans-ferase activity toward the microsomal specific compound, hexachloro-1,3-butadiene in rabbit liver microsomes (0.14 nmol/min/mg) was about one-tenth of that in human liver microsomes. The transferase activity toward the cytosol enzyme-specific compound, 1-chloro-2,4-dinitrobenzene, in rabbit liver cytosol fractions (4091 nmol/min/mg) was more than twofold higher than that in human liver cytosol fractions.

When perinatal development of glutathione S-transferase and epoxide hydrolase was studied in rabbit liver and extrahepataic organs, activity of glutathione S-transferases toward 1,2-dichloro-4-nitrobenzene and styrene oxide was different in liver, intestine, lung, and kidney (James et al., 1977). In the liver, which has higher activity compared with the other organs, the transferase activity toward both substrates was within the adult range at 70 days after birth. The transferase activity toward styrene oxide in fetal rabbit liver was 1–2 nmol/mg/min. This activity increased sharply and reached about 50% of the adult value between 1 and 6 days after birth. However, the age development of glu-tathione transferase activities in rabbits was highly substrate specific (Gregus et al., 1985). For example, the glutathione transferase activity in rabbit liver for ethacrynic acid increased only 1.8-fold from the neonatal value during the first 120 days after birth, whereas the enzyme activity toward 1,2-epoxy-3-(p-nitrophenoxy)-propane increased about 18-fold.

Depletion of glutathione in the liver was found to be directly correlated with acetamin-ophen hepatotoxicity (Green et al., 1984). After treatment of acetaminophen, hepatocytes of acetaminophen-resistant species such as the rabbit retained higher amounts of glu-tathione, produced no detectable covalent adducts, and metabolized more extensively to polar metabolites compared to hepatocytes from other species. In contrast, hepatocytes of acetaminophen-susceptible species such as the hamster were depleted of glutathione more rapidly, produced more covalent adducts of acetaminophen, and formed polar metabolites at a slower rate than the rabbit hepatocytes.

Although information on S-methyl reactions in the rabbit is limited, a membrane-bound enzymatic activity has been found in rabbit liver microsomes which catalyzes the transmethylation from S-adenosylmethionine to a series of C1-C3 alkane thiol (Holloway, 1979). Methane and ethane thiols are known to be endogenous toxins, which may play an important role in the pathogenesis of hepatic coma, and methylation could provide an important pathway for metabolic detoxification through neutralization of the highly reactive sulfhydryl group.

The rabbit appears to have low to moderate sulfate conjugation capability. After administration of dopamine about 1% of the dose was excreted as sulfate conjugate in the 0 to 72-hr rabbit urine, whereas about 61, 5.3, and 7.0% of the dose were excreted as sulfate conjugates in the dog, rat, and mouse urine, respectively, over the same time periods. Following administration of phenacetin, the sulfate conjugate was a minor metabolite (4–9%) and N-acetyl-p-aminophenylglucuronide was the major metabolite in the rabbit, whereas in humans glucuronide and sulfate conjugates were about equally important (36–42 and 23–31%, respectively) (Smith and Timbrell, 1974). However, with phenol, the percentage of the total sulfate conjugate excreted in rabbit urine was 54% of the administered dose (Capel et al., 1972). This value is comparable to those in the rat (55%) and mouse (51%) but somewhat lower than that in humans (78%).

The formation of arylsulfoconjugates is known to be rate limited by the endogenous sulfate ion, and thus the extent of conjugation is dose dependent. Liver concentrations of adenosine 3'-phosphate-5'-phosphosulfate (PAPS), which is required for sulfation reactions as the sulfate donor, was 32.7 nmol/g of tissue in the rabbit. This concentration was about half the value in the rat, similar to that in the hamster and mouse, but about twofold higher than that in the dog (16.1–17.3 nmol/g). The concentrations of PAPS in the rabbit kidney, lung, and intestine were approximately one-third of the value in the rabbit liver.

The rabbit utilizes the glycine conjugation pathway in the metabolism of many arylacetic acid compounds, such as phenylacetic acid, indoleacetic acid, and phenylcysteine. In contrast, humans did not form any substantial amount of glycine conjugate with these compounds. Interestingly, 1-naphthylacetic acid was conjugated only with glycine in addition to glucuronic acid in the rabbit, whereas 2-naphthylacetic acid formed conjugated metabolites with glycine, glutamine, and taurine as well as glucuronic acid (Emudianughe et al., 1978, 1979).

The drug-metabolizing enzymes in the rabbit are generally induced or inhibited with the known enzyme inducers or inhibitors in the other species, respectively. However, the effects of some inducers and inhibitors have been reported to differ in rabbits from those in the other species. When differential inductive effects in the rabbit liver were studied after treatment with phenobarbital, β-naphtho-flavone (BNF), 2,3,7,8-tetrachlorodibenzo-p-dioxin (TCDD), and 3-methylcholanthrene (3-MC), metabolism of 2-AAF to the mutagenic metabolite N-hydroxy 2-AAF was increased from seven- to 13-fold after treatment with 3-MC, BNF, or TCDD (Atlas et al., 1975). The N-hydroxylation of 2-AAF increased twofold with phenobarbital in the rabbit but not in the rat, mouse, hamster, and guinea pig. A more detailed study revealed that in the rabbit, a significant portion of the microsomal metabolism of 2-AAF to the mutagenic metabolite was initiated by deacetylation to aminofluorene followed by N-hydroxylation, which was catalyzed by phenobarbital-inducible cytochrome P-450 LM_5 as well as by 3-MC–inducible cytochrome P-450 LM_4.

Acetanilide hydroxylation in the rabbit was induced from 2.4- to 3.9-fold with BNF, TCDD, 3-MC, and phenobartital (Atlas et al., 1975). However, arylhydrocarbon hydroxylase (AHH) activity toward benzo(a)pyrene was increased only by phenobarbital but not by any of the other inducers in this study. Furthermore, Aroclor 1254 and methylcholanthrene, which were potent inducers of N-hydroxylation of 4-aminophenyl in the rat and guinea pig, were not inducers in the rabbit (McMahon et al., 1980). Interestingly, TCDD stimulated the demethylase activity for p-nitroanisole in the rabbit after 3 days of treatment, but the effect was lost after 6 days.

Cytochrome P-450 LM_5, which is found in rabbit liver and extrahepatic tissues, does not appear to be similar in all properties to any cytochrome P-450 isozymes isolated from other species. Although phenobarbital induces the synthesis of both isozyme LM_5 and LM_2 in rabbit liver, the relationship between these isozymes is not comparable to that between P-450$_b$ and P-450$_e$, highly related isozymes that are induced by phenobarbital in rat liver.

Vanderslice et al. (1987) examined the presence of homologs of rabbit cytochrome P-450 LM_5 in pulmonary and hepatic preparations from the rat, mouse, hamster, guinea pig, and monkey. Homologs of isozyme LM_5 were detected in pulmonary preparations from all five species. However, only hepatic preparations from the hamster, in addition to those from the rabbit, contained detectable levels of this isozyme. Although LM_5 isozyme in rabbit liver was induced by phenobarbital, treatment of other animals with phenobarbital did not increase the hepatic or pulmonary content of isozyme LM_5 homologs or the amount of 2-aminofluorene metabolism which was inhibited by antibodies to isozyme LM_5. Subchronic treatment of phenobarbital induced renal cortical microsomal monooxygenase and arylhydrocarbon hydroxylase and cytochrome P-450 content in rabbits but did not induce these renal enzyme systems in the rat (Kuo et al., 1982).

In addition to cytochrome LM_5 isozyme, rabbit pulmonary cytochrome P-450 comprises two other isozymes, LM_2 and LM_6. In the untreated rabbit lung, cytochrome LM_2 and LM_5 isozymes are present in approximately equal proportions. However, the isozyme LM_6 has been identified only after treatment with TCDD. In the liver, the isozymes LM_2 and LM_5 make up a small fraction of the total complement, which comprises at least nine forms. Phenobarbital, an inducer of forms 2 and 5 in liver, has no inductive effect in the lung. Induction of form 4 by aromatic hydrocarbons occurs in the liver but not in lung, except perhaps in the neonate. Pulmonary concentrations of isozyme 2 were decreased to trace levels by the administration of Aroclor 1260 (Ueng et al., 1980, 1981; Serabjit-Singh et al., 1983). The pulmonary content of isozyme 6 was also decreased twofold by treatment with phenobarbital but increased five- and 10-fold by administration of Aroclor 1260 and TCDD, respectively.

It has been reported that metabolism of stereoisomers was selectively induced by pretreatment with different inducing agents. For example, when the stereoselective glucuronidation of oxazepam was studied using rabbit liver microsomes with a series of inducing agents, the ratio of diastereomeric products produced varied dramatically relative to noninduced animals (Yost and Finley, 1985). The R/S enantiomer ratio for noninduced rabbits was 0.76, but this was reversed to 1.41 after treatment with β-naphthaflavone. These data clearly suggest that various forms of glucuronyltransferase with different stereoselectivities were present in rabbit liver.

α-Naphthoflavone has been reported to be a potent inhibitor of reconstituted rabbit liver P-450 IA2 (LM_4) biphenyl 4-hydroxylation ($IC_{50} = 27$ nM) and 7-ethoxy-resorufin-0-demethylation ($IC_{50} = 10$ nM) (Johnson et al., 1979). In contrast, P-450 IIB4–dependent activity (rabbit LM_2) was only inhibited to a minor extent at an α-naphthoflavone concentration of 240 nM. Thorgeirsson et al. (1979) also studied the in vitro effect of α-naphthoflavone on four hepatic mono-oxygenase activities (aryl hydrocarbon hydroxylase, 2-acetylaminofluorene N-hydroxylase, biphenyl 2-hydroxylase, and biphenyl 4-hydroxylase) before and after methylcholanthrene treatment of the rabbit and other laboratory animals (mice, rat, hamster, and guinea pig). In vitro addition of α-naphthoflavone selectively inhibited 2-AAF N-hydroxylase and biphenyl 4-hydroxylase activity in the methylcholanthrene-treated rabbit, which is consistent with the findings of Johnson et al. (1979). However, in vitro addition of α-naphthoflavone enhanced the activities of aryl hyhdrocarbon hydroxylase and biphenyl 2-hydroxylase in liver microsomes from both control and methylcholanthrene-treated rabbit. The enhancement of mono-oxygenase activities by the in vitro addition of α-naphthoflavone may be caused by an interaction with the allosteric binding site(s) on the heme proteins. In contrast to the rabbit, in vitro addition of α-naphthoflavone selectively inhibited all four mono-oxygenase activities from the 3-MC–treated rat, mouse (C57BL/6N strain), and hamster.

Species differences in toxicity of a compound may be due to factors other than differences in its metabolism. Some of these factors include protein binding and biliary excretion in addition to absorption and renal elimination of drugs. When protein binding of some drugs (clofibric acid, etodolac, tolrestat, perrinone, benoxaprofen) was examined in the rabbit and other laboratory animals (rat, mouse, dog, rhesus monkey) as well as in humans, the binding in the rabbit appeared to be medium. In general, the binding was highest in human serum and weakest in the mouse. However, when the protein binding of prednisolone was studied in serum from rabbits, dogs, rats, and humans, the binding characteristics of the drug in rabbit serum were most similar to those in human serum (Rocci et al., 1980). A similar phenomenon was observed with a new cephalosporin, CL284635 (Bialer et al., 1986).

Enterohepatic circulation as a result of biliary excretion of a drug may have pronounced toxicologial implications. For example, the intestinal toxicity of indomethacin in laboratory animals (rabbit, rat, dog, monkey, and guinea pig) is reported to be inversely proportional to the exposure of the intestinal mucosa to the drug as a consequence of enterohepatic circulation. In general, the rabbit is relatively inefficient in biliary excretion, and appears to be similar to the human. The bile flow in the rabbit (65.2 μl/min/kg) was lower compared to that in the mouse (83.9 μl/min/kg), rat (101 μl/min/kg), hamster (111 μl/min/kg), and guinea pig (151 μl/min/kg) (Stein et al., 1988). There is a minimum molecular weight at which the elimination of compounds in the bile is appreciable (10% or more of the administered dose). For organic anions such as conjugates produced by phase II biotransformation, this value in the rabbit was 475 $\pm$ 50 (Hirom et al., 1976), whereas in man the value was approximately 500 (Millburn, 1970). The threshold molecular weights for biliary excretion were about 325 and 400 in the rat and guinea pig, respectively. The biliary excretion rate of methyl mercury was very low in the rabbit (0.03 nmol/min/kg) compared to the guinea pig (0.15 nmol/min/kg) and the rodents such as the rat, mouse, and hamster (approximately 0.8 nmol/min/kg) (Stein et al., 1988).

REFERENCES

Arey, L. D. (1965) *Developmental Anatomy*. Saunders, Philadelphia, p. 295.

Atlas, S. A., Thorgeirsson, S. S., Boobis, A. R., Kumaki, K., and Nebert, D. W. (1975) Differential induction of murine Ah locus-associated monooxygenase activities in rabbit liver and kidney. *Biochem. Pharmacol.* 24, 2111–2116.

Barnett, M. (1958) The use of polythene for "Elizabethan" collars. *J. Anim. Tech. Assoc.* 9, 50–52.

Bartek, M. J., LaBudee, J. A., and Maibach, H. I. (1972) Skin permeability *in vivo:* Comparison in rat, rabbit, pig, and man. *J. Invest. Dermatol.* 58, 114–123.

Beckett, A. H., and Gibson, G. G. (1975) Microsomal N-hydroxylation of dibenzylamine. *Xenobiotica* 5, 677–686.

Bertault-Peres P., Bonfils C., Fabre, G., Just, S., Cano, J. P., and Maurel, P (1987) Metabolism of cyclosporin A. II., Implication of the macrolide antibiotic inducible cytochrome P-450 3c. *Drug Metab. Dispos.* 15, 391–398.

Bialer, M., Tonelli, A. P., Kantrowitz, J. D., Yacobi, A. (1986) Serum protein binding of a new oral cephalosporin, CL284635, in various species. *Drug Metab. Dispos.* 14, 132–136.

Bivin, W. S., and Timmons, E. H. (1974) Basic methodology, in *The Biology of the Laboratory Rabbit.*, Weisbroth, S. H., Flatt, R. E., and Kraus, A. L., eds. Academic Press, New York, pp. 194–236.

Bridges, J. W., Kirby, M. R., Walker, S. R., and Williams, R. T. (1969) Structure and species as factors affecting the metabolism of some methoxy-6-sulfanilamido-pyrimidines. *Biochem. J.* 111, 67–172.

Brodie, B. B. (1962) Difficulties in extrapolating data on metabolism of drugs from animal to man. *Clin. Pharmacol. Ther.* 3, 374–380.

Calabrese, E. J. (1984) Suitability of animal models for predictive toxicology: Theoretical and practical considerations. *Drug Metabol. Rev.* 15, 505–523.

Calabrese, E. J. (1988) Comparative biology of test species. *Environ. Health Perspect.* 77, 55–62.

Caldwell, J. (1976) The metabolism of amphetamines in mammals. *Drug. Metab. Rev.* 5, 219–280.

Caldwell, J. (1981) The current status of attempts to predict species differences in drug metabolism. *Drug Metab. Rev.* 12, 221–237.

Capel, D., French, M. R., Milburn, P., Smith, R. L., and Williams, R. T. (1972) The fate of [14C]phenol in various species. *Xenobiotica* 2, 25–34.

Chhabra, R. S., Pohl, R. J., and Fouts, J. R. (1974) A comparative study of xenobiotic-metabolizing enzymes in liver and intestine of various animal species. *Drug Metab. Dispos.* 2, 443–447.

Clarke, H. E., Coates, M. E., Eva, J. K., Ford, D. J., Milner, C. K., O'Donoghue, P. N., Scott, P. P., and Ward, R. J. (1977) Dietary standards for laboratory animals: Report of the laboratory animals center diets advisory committee. *Lab. Anim.* 11, 1–28

Clough, G. (1982) Environmental effects on animals used in biomedical research. *Biol. Rev.* 57, 487–523.

Collins, G. R. (1972) Syllabus for the laboratory animal technologist, in *American Association for Laboratory Animal Science.* Jolliet, Illinois. Publ. 72-2, 440–445.

Coon, M. J., Koop, D. R. (1983) *The Enzymes,* Vol. 16, Boyer, P. D. Academic Press, New York

Cram, R. L., Juchau, M. R., and Fouts, J. R. (1965) Differences in hepatic drug metabolism in various rabbit strains before and after pretreatment with phenobarbital. *Proc. Soc. Exp. Biol. Med.* 118, 872–875.

Davies, D. S., Gigon, P. L., and Gillette, J. R. (1969) Species and sex differences in electron transport system in liver microsomes and the relationship to ethylmorphine demethylation. *Life Sci.* 8, 85.

Davis, C. D., Potter, W. Z., Jollow, D. J. and Mitchell, J. R. (1974) Species differences in hepatic glutathione depletion, covalent binding and hepatic necrosis after acetaminophen. *Life Sci.* 14, 2099–2109.

Digens, G., Gerlin, R., Thodorakis, M., and Shamfu, M. (1980) In application of pharmacokinetics and biopharmaceutics in the design of toxicological studies. *Toxicol. Appl. Pharmacol.* 53, 179–180.

Emudianughe, T. S., J. Caldwell, P. A. F. Dixon, and Smith, R. L. (1978) Studies on the metabolism of arylacetic acids 5. The metabolic fate of 2-naphthylacetic acid in the rat, rabbit and ferret. *Xenobiotica* 8, 525–534.

Emudianughe, T. S., Caldwell, J., and Smith, R. L. (1979) Aminoacid conjugation responses to 2-naphthylacetic acid in rodents. *Biochem. Soc. Trans.* 7, 522–524.

Emudianughe, T. S., J. Caldwell, and R. L. Smith (1987) Studies on the metabolism of arylacetic acids, 6., Comparative metabolic conjugation of 1- and 2-naphthylacetic acid in the guinea pig, mouse, hamster and gerbil. *Xenobiotica* 17, 815–821.

Fabre, G., Crevat-Pisano, P., Dragna, S., Covo, J., Barra, Y., and Cano, J. P. (1988) Involvement of the macrolide antibiotic inducible cytochrome P-450 LM3c in the metabolism of midazolam by microsomal fractions prepared from rabbit liver. *Biochem. Pharmacol.* 37, 1947–53.

Falany, C. N., Chowdhury, J. R., Chowdhury, N. R., Tephly, T. R. (1983) Steroid 3- and 17-OH UDP-glucoronosyltransferase activities in rat and rabbit liver microsomes. *Drug. Metab. Dispos.* 11, 426–432.

Feldman, D. B. (1977) Simplified gastric intubation in the rabbit. *Lab. Anim. Sci.* 27, 1037.

Felton, J. S., Nebert, D. W., and Thorgeirsson, S. S. (1976) Genetic difference in 2-acetylaminofluorene mutagenicity *in vitro* associated with mouse hepatic aryl hydrocarbon hydroxylase activity induced by polycyclic aromatic compounds. *Mol. Pharmacol.* 12, 225.

Flatt, R. E. (1974) Bacterial diseases, in *The Biology of the Laboratory Rabbit*, Weisbroth, S. H., Flatt, R. E., and Kraus, A. L., eds. Academic Press, New York, pp. 194–236.

Flatt, R. E. (1977) Introduction and biology., in *The Rabbit*, ACLAM Laboratory Animal Medicine and Science Series, Van Hoosier, G. L., Jr., Coord. University of Washington, Seattle, pp. 1–6.

Flatt, R. E., and Jackson, S. J. (1970) Renal nosematosis in young rabbits. *Pathol. Vet.* 7, 492–497.

Flatt, R. E., Weisbroth, S. H., Kraus, A. L. (1974) Metabolic, traumatic, mycotic, and miscellaneous diseases of rabbits., in *The Biology of the Laboratory Rabbit.*, Weisbroth, S. H., Flatt, R. E., and Kraus, A. L., eds. Academic Press, New York, pp. 435–451.

Fournel, S. and Caldell, J. (1986) The metabolic chiral inversion of 2-phenylpropionic acid in rat, mouse and rabbit. *Biochem. Pharmacol.*, 35, 4153–9. Erratum, *Biochem. Pharmacol.* 36, 405 (1987).

Fox, R. R. (1974) Taxonomy and genetics., in *The Biology of the Laboratory Rabbit*, Weisbroth, S. H., Flatt, R. E., and Kraus, A. L., eds. Academic Prses, New York, pp. 1–22.

Friedman, M., Byers, S. O., and Brown, A. E. (1967) Plasma lipid responses of rats and rabbits to an auditory stimulus. *Am. J. Physiol.* 212, 1174–1178.

Fuhrman, G. J., and Fuhrman, F. A. (1961) Effects of temperature on the action of drugs. *Ann. Rev. Pharmacol.* 1, 65–78.

Gee, S. J. and Green, C. E. (1984) Comparative metabolism of tolbutamide by isolated hepatocytes from rat, rabbit, dog, and squirrel monkey. *Drug Metab. Dispos.* 12, 174–178.

Glowinski, I. R., Radtke, E. H., and Weber, W. W. (1978) Genetic variation in N-acetylation of carcinogenic arylamines by human and rabbit liver. *Mol. Pharmacol.* 14, 940–949.

Gorrod, J. W. and Gooderham, N. J. (1987) The metabolism of N-benzyl-4-substituted anilines: Factors influencing *in vitro* C- and N-oxidation. *Xenobiotica* 17, 165–177.

Gram, T. E., Schroeder, D. H., Davis, D. C., Regan, R. L. and Guarino, A. M. (1971) Enzymic and biochemical composition of smooth and rough microsomal membranes from monkey, guinea pig and mouse liver. *Biochem. Pharmacol.* 20, 1371–1381.

Green, C. E., Dabbs, J. E., and Tyson, C. A. (1984) Metabolism and cytotoxicity of acetaminophen in hepatocytes isolated from resistent and susceptible species. *Toxicol. Appl. Pharmacol.* 76, 139–149.

Green, C. E., LeValleyl S. E., and Tyson, C. A. (1986) Comparison of amphetamine metabolism using isolated hepatocytes from five species including human. *J. Pharmacol. Exp. Ther.* 237, 931–6.

Gregus, Z., Watkins, J. B., Thompson, T. N., Harvey, M. J., Rozman, K., and Klaassen, C. D. (1983) Hepatic phase I and II biotransformations in quail and trout in comparison to other species commonly used in toxicity testing. *Toxicol. Appl. Pharmacol.* 67, 430–441.

Gregus, Z., Varga, F., and Schemelas, A. (1985) Age-development and inducibility of hepatic glutathione S-transferae activities in mice, rats, rabbits and guinea-pigs. *Comp. Biochem. Physiol.* 80C, 83–90.

Harkness, J. E. (1987) Rabbit husbandry and medicine. *Vet. Clin. North Am., Small Anim. Pract.* 17, 1019–1044.

Harkness, J. E., and Wagner, J. E. (1983) *The Biology and Medicine of Rabbits and Rodents.* Lea & Febiger, Philadelphia.

Heim, R. A. (1989) A Practical technique for obtaining multiple blood samples from rabbits. *Lab. Anim. Sci.* Jan./Feb., 32–33.

Henkin, R. I., and Knigge, K. M. (1963) Effect of sound on the hypothalamic-pituitary-adrenal axis. *Am. J. Physiol.* 204, 710–714.

Hietanen, E. and Vainio, H. (1973) Interspecies variations in small intestinal and hepatic drug hydroxylation and glucuronidation. *Acta Pharmacol. Toxicol.* 33, 57–64.

Hill, J. E., Long, R. H., Rowland, G. N., and Procter, J. E. (1988) Spontaneous storage-like disease in a rabbit. *Vet. Pathol.* 25, 91–92.

Hirom, P. C., Millburn, P., and Smith, R. L. (1976) Bile and urine as complementary pathways for the excretion of foreign compounds. *Xenobiotica* 6, 55.

Hollaway, C. J., Husmann-Hollaway, S. H., and Brunner, G. (1979) Enzymatic methylation of alkane thiols. *Enzyme* 24, 307–312.

Holmes, D. D. (1984) *Clinical Laboratory Animal Medicine, An Introduction.* Iowa State University Press, Ames.

Hunt, C. E., and Harrington, D. D. (1974) Nutrition and nutritional diseases of the rabbit, in *The Biology of the Laboratory Rabbit,* S. H. Weisbroth, S. H., Flatt, R. E., and Kraus, A. L., eds. Academic Press, New York, pp. 287–315.

Igarashi, T., Tomihari, N., Ohmori, S., Ueno, Koichi, Kitagawa, H., and Satoh, T. (1986) Comparison of glutathione S-transferases in mouse, guinea pig, rabbit, and hamster liver cytosol to those in rat liver. *Biochem. Int.* 13, 641–648.

Institute of Laboratory Animal Resources (ILAR), National Regulatory Commission (1985) *Guide for the Care and Use of Laboratory Animals.* NIH Publication No. 85-23. Bethesda, Maryland, 18–20.

James, M. O., Foureman, G. L., Law, F. C., and Bend, J. R. (1977) The perinatal development of epoxide metabolizing enzyme activities in liver and extrahepatic organs of guinea pig and rabbit. *Drug Metab. Dispos.* 5, 19–28.

James, M. O., Fouts, J. R., and Bend, J. R. (1976) Hepatic and extrahepatic metabolism, in vitro of an epoxide (8-^{14}C-styrene oxide) in the rabbit. *Biochem. Pharmacol.* 25, 187–193.

Johnson, E. F., Schwab, G. E., and Muller-Eberhard, U. (1979) Multiple forms of cytochrome P-450: Catalytic differences exhibited by two homogeneous forms of rabbit cytochrome P-450. *Mol. Pharmacol.* 15, 708–718.

Kaplan, H. M., and Timmons, E. H. (1979) *The Rabbit, A Model for the Principles of Mammalian Physiology and Surgery.* Academic Press, New York.

Kato, R. (1979) Characteristics and differences in the hepatic mixed function oxidases of different species. *Pharmac. Ther.* 6, 41–78.

Kozma, C., Macklin, W., Cummins, L. M., and Mauer, R. (1974) The anatomy, physiology, and the biochemistry of the rabbit, in *The Biology of the Laboratory Rabbit,* Weisbroth, S. H., Flatt, R. E., and Kraus, A. L., eds. Academic Press, New York, pp. 50–72.

Kraus, A. L. (1974) Arthropod parasites, in *The Biology of the Laboratory Rabbit,* Weisbroth, S. H., Flatt, R. E., and Kraus, A. L., eds. Academic Press, New York, pp. 287–315.

Kraus, A. L., Weisbroth, S. H., Flatt, R. E., and Brewer, N. (1984) Biology and disease of rabbits., in *Laboratory Animal Medicine,* Fox, J. G., Cohen, B. J., and Loew, F. M., ed. Academic Press, Orlando, Florida.

Kulkarni, A. P., and Hodgson, E. (1980) Comparative toxicology., in *Introduction to Biochemical Toxicology,* Hodgson, E., and Guthrie, F. E., eds. Elsevier, New York, pp. 106–132.

Kulwich, R., Struglia, L., and Pearson, P. B. (1953) The effect of coprophagy on the excretion of B vitamins by the rabbit. *J. Nutr.* 49, 639–645.

Kulwich, R., Pearson, P. B., and Lankenau, A. H. (1954) Effect of coprophagy on S25 uptake by rabbits after ingestion of labeled sodium sulfate. *Arch. Biochem.* 50, 180–187.

Kuo, C. H., Rush, G. F., and Hook, J. B. (1982) Renal cortical accumulation of phenobarbital in rats and rabbits: Lack of correlation with induction of renal microsomal monooxygenases. *J. Pharmacol. Exp. Ther.* 220, 547–51.

Lindsey, J. R., and Fox, R. R. (1974) Inherited diseases and variations, in *The Biology of the Laboratory Rabbit.*, Weisbroth, S. H., Flatt, R. E., and Kraus, A. L., eds. Academic Press, New York, pp. 377–401.

Litterst, C. L., Mimnaugh, E. G., Regan, R. L., and Gram. T. E. (1975) Comparison of *in vitro* drug metabolism by lung, liver and kidney of several common laboratory species. *Drug Metab. Dispos.* 3, 259–265.

Litterst, C. L., Gram. T. E., Mimnaugh, E. G., Leber, P., Emmerling, D., and Freudenthal, R. I. (1976) A comprehensive study of *in vitro* drug metabolism in several laboratory species. *Drug. Metab. Disp.* 4, 203–207.

Lotlikar, P. D., Enomoto, M., Miller, J. A. and Miller E. C. (1967) Species variations in the N- and ring-hydroxylation of 2-acetylaminofluorene and effects of 3-methylcholanthrene pretreatment. *Proc. Soc. Exp. Biol. Med.* 125, 341–346.

Lu, A. Y. H., and West, S. B. (1980) Multiplicity of mammalian microsomal cytochrome P-450. *Pharmacol. Rev.* 31, 277–295.

Maeda, T., Takenaka, H., Yamahira, Y., and Noguchi, T. (1977) In *Application of Pharmacokinetics and Biopharmeceutics in the Design of Toxicological Studies*, R. D., Smyth, and G. H., Hottendorf, eds. (1980). *Toxicol. Appl. Pharmacol.* 53, 179–180.

Matsui, T. S., Taugchi-Ochi, Takano, M., Kuroda, S., Taniyama, H., and Ono, T. (1985) Pulmonary aspergillosis in apparently healthy young rabbits. *Vet. Pathol.* 22, 200–205.

McMahon, R. E., Turner, J. C., and Whitaker, G. W. (1980) The N-hydroxylation and ring-hydroxylation of 4-aminobiphenyl *in vitro* By hepatic mono-oxygenases from rat, mouse, hamster, rabbit and guinea-pig. *Xenobiotica* 10, 469–481.

Millburn, P. (1970) Factors in the biliary excretion of organic compounds, in *Metabolic Conjugation and Metabolic Hydrolysis*. Vol. 2, Fisherman, W. H., ed. Academy Press, New York, pp. 1–77.

Morgan, R. L., Castles, T. R., Zeicker, G. M., and Taylor D. (1985) Skin irritation testing in rabbits complicated by dermal mucormycosis. *Toxicol. Pathol.* 13(3), 185–191.

Morgenstern, R., Lundqvist, G., Andersson, G. L., Balk, L., and DePierre, J. (1984) The distribution of microsomal glutathione transferase among different organelles, different organs, and different organisms. *Biochem. Pharmacol.* 33, 3609–3614.

National Academy of Sciences (1977) *Nutrient Requirements of Rabbits.* 2nd ed. rev. Washington, D.C.

Nayfield, K. C., and Besch, E. L. (1981) Comparative responses of rabbits and rats to elevated noise. *Lab. Anim. Sci.* 31, 386–390.

Nerland, D. E., and Mannering, G. J. (1978) Species, sex, and developmental differences in the O- and N-dealkylation of ethylmorphine by hepatic microsomes. *Drug Metab. Dispos.* 6, 150–153.

Oesch, F. (1973) Mammalian epoxide hydrases: Inducible enzymes calalysing the inactivation of carcinogenic and cytotoxic metabolites derived from aromatic and olefinic compounds. *Xenobiotica* 3, 305–340.

Oesch, F. (1980) Microsomal epoxide hydrolase, in *Enzymatic Basis of Detoxification*, Vol. II, Jacoby, W. B., ed. Academic Press, New York, pp. 277–290.

Oesch, F., and Wolf, C. R. (1989) Properties of the microsomal and cytosolic glutathione transferases involved in hexachloro-1:3-butadiene conjugation. *Biochem. Pharmacol.* 38, 353–359.

Oppelt, W. W., Zange, M., Ross, W. E., and Remmer, H. (1970) Comparison of microsomal drug hydroxylation in lung and liver of various species. *Res. Commun. Chem. Pathol. Pharmacol.* 1, 43–56.

Pacifici, G. M., Boobis, A. R., Brodie, M. J., McManus, M. E. and Davies, D. S. (1981) Tissue and species differences in enzymes of epoxide metabolism. *Xenobiotica* 11, 73–79.

Pakes, S. P. (1974) Protozoal diseases, in *The Biology of the Laboratory Rabbit,* Weisbroth, S. H., Flatt, R. E., and Kraus, A. L., eds. Academic Press, New York, pp. 332–275.

Parke, D. V. (1960) The metabolism of [^{14}C]aniline in the rabbit and other animals. *Biochem. J.* 77, 493–503.

Pelkonen, O., Kaltiala, E. H., Karki, N. T., Jalonen, K., and Pyrola, K. (1975) Properties of benzpyrene hydroxylase from human liver and comparison of the rat, rabbit and guinea pig enzymes. *Xenobiotica* 5, 501–509.

Port, C. D., and Dodd, D. C. (1983) Two cases of corneal epithelial dystrophy in rabbits. *Lab. An. Sci.* 33, 587–88.

Ralston Purina Co. *Certified Rabbit Chow #5322*. Checkerboard Square. St. Louis, Missouri.

Ralston Purina Co. *Certified High Fiber Rabbit Chow #5325*. Checkerboard Square. St. Louis, Missouri.

Rao, G. N. (1986) Significance of environmental factors on the test system, in *Managing Conduct and Data Quality of Toxicology Studies,* Hoover, B. K., Baldwin, J. K., Uelner, A. F., Witmire, C. E., Davies, C. L., and Bristol, D. W., eds. Princeton Scientific, pp. 173–186.

Remmer, H., Siegerrt, M., Merker, H. J., Naunyn-Schmiedebergs, (1964) Vermehrung arzneimit-teloxydierender enzyme durich tolbutamid. *Arch. Exp. Path. Pharmak.,* 249, 71–84.

Ribelin, W. E., and McCoy, J. R. (1965) *The Pathology of Laboratory Animals.* Thomas, Springfield, Illinois.

Rocci, M. L., Johnson, N. F., and Jusko, W. J. (1980) Serum protein binding of prednisolone in four species, *J. Pharm. Sci.* 69, 977–778.

Runkle, R. S. (1964) Laboratory animal housing. Part II. *Am. Inst. Archit. J.* 41, 77–80.

Serabjit-Singh, C. J., Albro, P. W., Robertson, I. G. C., and Philpot, R. M. (1983) Interactions between xenobiotics that increase or decrease the levels of cytochrome P-450 isozymes in rabbit and liver. *J. Biol. Chem.* 258, 12827–12834.

Shaddock, J. A., and Pakes, S. P. (1971) Encephalitozoonosis (nosematosis) and toxoplasmosis. *Am. J. Pathol.* 64, 657–674.

Sirks, M. J. (1959) Leeuwenhoek on dominance in rabbits. *Genetica* 30, 292.

Sisenwine, S., Tio, C., Hadley, F., Liu, A., Kimmel, H., Ruelius, H. S. (1982) Species differences in the stereoselective glucuronidation of oxazepam. *Drug. Metab. Dispos.* 10, 605–8.

Smith, R. L. and Timbrell, J. A. (1974) Factors affecting the metabolism of phenacetin I. Influence of dose, chronic dosage, route of administration and species on the metabolism of [1-^{14}C-acetyl]phenacetin. *Xenobiotica* 4, 489–501.

Smith, P. A., Prieskorn, D. M., Knutsen, C. A., and Ensminger, W. D. (1988) A method for frequent blood sampling in rabbits. *Lab. Anim. Sci.* 38, 623–625.

Souhaili-el Amri, H., Batt, A. M., and Siest, G. (1986) Comparison of cytochrome P-450 content and activities in liver microsomes of seven animal species, including man. *Xenobiotica* 16, 351–358.

Stein, A. F., Greguds, Z., and Klaassen, C. D. (1988) Species variations in biliary excretion of glutathione-related thiols and methyl mercury. *Toxicol. Appl. Pharmacol.* 93, 351–359.

Tagg, J., Yasuda, D. M., Tanabe, M., and Mitoma, C., (1967) Metabolic studies of tolbutmide in the rat. *Biochem. Pharmacol.* 16, 143–153.

Teelman, K., and Weihe, W. H. (1974) Microorganism counts and distribution patterns in air conditioned animal laboratories. *Lab. Anim.* 8, 109–118.

Testa, B. and Jenner, P. (1976) *Drug Metabolism, Chemical and Biochemical Aspects.* Marcel Dekker, New York, pp. 395–397.

Thacker, E. M., and Brandt, C. S. (1955) Coprophagy in the rabbit. *J. Nutr.* 55, 375–386.

Thomas, R. and C., Iketa, G. J. (1966) The metabolic fate of tolbutamide in man and in the rat. *J. Med. Chem.* 9, 507–510.

Thorgeirsson, S. S., Atlas, S. A., Boobis, A. R., and Felton, J. S. (1979) Species differences in the substrate specificity of hepatic cytochrome P-448 from polycyclic hydrocarbon-treated animals. *Biochem. Pharmacol.* 28, 217–216

Toth, L. A., and January, B. (1990) Physiological stabilization of rabbits after shipping. *Lab. An. Sci.* 40(4), 384–387.

Tregear, R. T. (1966) Physical functions of Skin. Academic Press, New York, pp. 6–13.

Ueheleke, H. (1969) Extrahepatic microsomal drug metabolism. *Proc. Eur. Soc., Study Drug Toxic.* 10, 94.

Ueng, T. H., and Alvares, A. P. (1981) Selective loss of pulmonary cytochrome P-450 in rabbits pretreated with polychlorinated biphenyls. *J. Biol. Chem.* 256, 7536–7542.

Ueng, T. H., Eiseman, J. L., and Alvares, A. P., (1980). Inhibition of pulmonary cytochrome P-450 and benzo(a)pyrene hydroxylase rabbits by polychlorinated-biphenyls (PCBS). *Biochem. Biophys. Res. Commun.* 95, 1743–1749.

Vanderslice, R. R., Domin, B. A., Carver, G. T., and Philpot, R. M., (1987) Species-dependent expression and induction of homologues of rabbit cytochrome P-450 isozyme 5 in liver and lung. *Mol. Pharmacol.* 31, 320–325.

von Bahr, C., Hermansson, J., and Magreta, L., (1982) Oxidation of (R)- and (S)-propranolol in human and dog liver microsomes, species differences in stereoselectivity, *J. Pharmacol. Exp.* 222, 456–462.

Weatherall, J. A. C. (1960) Anesthesia in new-born animals. *Br. J. Pharmacol.* 15, 454–457.

Weihe, W. H. (1973) The effect of temperature on the action of drugs. *Ann. Rev. Pharmacol.* 13, 409–425.

Weisbroth, S. H. (1974a) in *The Biology of the Laboratory Rabbit*. Weisbroth, S. H., Flatt, R. E., Kraus, A. L., ed. Academic Press, Orlando, Florida, pp. 331–375.

Weisbroth, S. H., (1974b) Neoplastic diseases, in *The Biology of the Laboratory Rabbit*, Weisbroth, S. H., Flatt, R. E., and Kraus, A. L., eds. Academic Press, New York, pp. 332–375.

Wiesbroth, S. H., Flatt, R. E., and Kraus, A. L. (1974) *Biology of the Laboratory Rabbit*. Academic Press, Orlando, Florida.

Weisbroth, S. H., Mauer, J. K., Bennett, F. B., Capen, C. C., and Bruce, R. D. (1990) Hepatocellular vacuolization in rabbits: Effects of feed restriction orchiectomy and ovariectomy. *Toxicol. Pathol.* 18, 56–60.

Wells, M. Y., Weisbroth, S. H., Mauere, J. K., Capen, C. C., and Bruce, R. D. (1988) Variable hepatocellular vacuolization associated with glycogen in rabbits. *Toxicol. Pathol.* 16, 360–365.

Williams, R. T. (1967) Comparative patterns of drug metabolism. *Fed. Proc.* 26, 1029–1039.

Williams, R. T. (1972) Toxicologic implications of biotransformation by intestinal microflora. *Toxicol. Appl. Pharmacol.* 23, 769–781.

Williams, C. S. F. (1976) *Practical Guide to Laboratory Animals*. Mosby, St. Louis.

Williams, C. S. F. (1979) Guinea pigs and rabbits. *Small Anim. Pract.* 93, 487–497.

Wise, A., and Gilburt, D. J. (1980) The variability of dietary fibre in laboratory animal diets and its relevance to the control of experimental conditions. *Food Cosmet. Toxicol.* 18, 643–648.

Wise, A., and Gilburt, D. J. (1981) Variation of minerals and trace elements in laboratory animal diets. *Lab. Anim.* 15, 299–303.

Yost, G., and Finley, B. (1985) Stereoselective glucuronidation as a probe of induced forms of UDP-glucuronyltransferase in rabbits. *Drug Metab. Dispos.* 13, 5–8.

Yost, G. S., Johnson, L. E., Pallante, S., Colvin, M., and Fenselau, C. (1981) Glucuronyltransferase stereoselectivity. *Fed. Proc.* 40, 650.

Zwicker, G. M., Killinger, J. M., and McConnel, R. F. (1985) Spontaneous vesicular and prostatic gland epithelial squamous metaplasia, hyperplasia and keratinized nodule formation in rabbits. *Toxicol. Pathol.* 13(2), 222–228.

7

The Ferret

Toxicology: **Daniel E. McLain**
                Searle European Development Centre
                Mont-Saint-Guibert, Belgium
                Richard M. Hoar
                Argus International, Inc.
                Horsham, Pennsylvania

Pathology: **Glen K. Miller**
                G. D. Searle and Company
                Skokie, Illinois

Metabolism: **Christopher P. Chengelis**
                WIL Research Laboratories, Inc.
                Ashland, Ohio

Toxicology   **Daniel E. McLain and Richard M. Hoar**

Interest in the ferret as a laboratory animal has grown in direct concordance with the escalating public opposition to the use of "domestic" animals in scientific research and, conversely, with the more recently identified need for a smaller nonrodent species to be used as a surrogate for the canine. To this end, conventional nonrodents such as the canine are being increasingly excluded from the testing of genetically engineered human biologics (for example) because a sufficient quantity of test material may simply not be available. The search for a surrogate nonrodent has, therefore, been focused primarily on smaller contemporary species considered more accommodating to the task at hand. One such small laboratory-adapted carnivore that has found increasing application in this present environment is the ferret (Fig. 1).

SCIENTIFIC APPLICATIONS OF THE FERRET AND THE EXTENT OF ITS USE IN TOXICOLOGY

Research with the ferret falls into two main categories: that directed toward gaining basic knowledge applicable to human health, and the more recent efforts directed toward ensuring the safety of humans (and their environment) exposed to a multitude of chemical and biological agents. Much of the knowledge gained from the basic biomedical research studies with ferrets has, quite fortunately, found application in studies of the problems

497

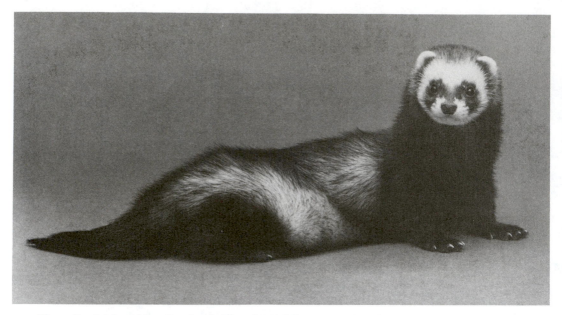

Figure 1 Adult, sable-colored male ferret (*Mustela putorius*). (Courtesy of Marshall Farms, Inc., North Rose, NY)

related to human toxicity assessment. In this respect, Thornton et al. (1979), Beach (1982), Hoar (1984), and Hart (1986) have previously described the applicability of ferrets in the toxicology laboratory, and several symposia devoted to an analysis of uses of the ferret in preclinical safety studies and biomedical research highlighted important contributions (Haddad, 1981; Fox, 1987; Greener, 1987). The use of ferrets in such diverse biomedical research areas as cardiology (Breisch, 1980; Marino et al., 1981; Marino and Severdia, 1983), ophthalmology (Thorpe and Herbert, 1976; Braekevelt, 1982; Wen et al., 1985; McLain and Lin, 1989a), pulmonary physiology and pathology (Sweet et al., 1981; Vinegar et al., 1982, 1985), virology (Chevance, 1978; Kauffman et al, 1982; Bird et al., 1983), bacteriology (Fox et al., 1982, 1983; Koshimizu et al, 1982), toxicology (Brantom et al., 1977; McLain et al., 1987), and developmental toxicology (Beck, et al, 1978; Beck, 1981; McLain and Roe, 1984; McLain et al., 1985) has become frequent and important.

The extent of the research effort with ferrets is further indicated by a recent survey of the scientific literature accessed through the BIOSIS and MEDLINE computerized database search systems, which cover entries from over 8000 journals from over 70 different countries. This selected list of references on the use of ferrets in biomedical research was published by Frederick and Babish (1985), and includes more than 569 entries of papers issued from 1977 to 1984. Earlier compendia of similar scientific literature were published by Hahn and Wester (1969), Marshall and Marshall (1973), and Shump et al. (1974), which span the years 1866–1974. As indicated by these literature reviews, the number of scientific publications specifically mentioning the ferret in their title or as a keyword prior to 1974 averaged approximately five per year, whereas from 1977 to 1983 the number increased to approximately 113 per year. Although only 23% of these latter citations were toxicological in content, they may be viewed as an indication of the ferret's increasingly important role in the area of toxicology research.

The increasing number of scientific applications of the ferret and the unprecedented growth of the biotechnology industry correlate highly with commercial sales of the animal over the last 10 years. Therefore, whether used as a surrogate nonrodent for testing the efficacy and safety of limitedly available human biologics, or as a simple alternative to more conventional laboratory carnivores, the present usage rate of ferrets suggests that information delineating the species' applications and restrictions in the toxicology laboratory is duly warranted. This chapter, therefore, is an attempt to consolidate current information on the ferret which may be applicable to preclinical safety evaluations.

HISTORY

Taxonomy and Origin

The present-day domesticated ferret, *Mustela putorius furo* (see Table 1 for taxonomic classification), is believed to have originated in North Africa over 5000 years ago (Miller, 1933; Hagedoorn, 1947; Thomson, 1951). Some accounts credit the Egyptians with the domestication of ferrets (ca. 3000 B.C.) and their subsequent introduction to Europe, Asia, and Great Britain (Pyle, 1940; Owen, 1969). Most historical reviews describe the modern laboratory ferret as descending from the wild European ferret or polecat (*M. putorius* or *M. furo*) or the steppe polecat *(M. eversmanni),* with which they may breed and produce offspring (Pocock, 1932; Fox, 1988). The black-footed ferret *(M. nigripes),* an endangered species native to the western United States, is a distinctly different strain and is not used for research purposes (Clark, 1978; Boggess et al., 1980; Moody et al, 1985).

The Mustelidae family of the ferret is considered to be the most primitive living group of terrestrial carnivores, with a total of some 70 different species in 25 genera. Genera such as *Lutra* (river otter), *Pteronura* (giant otter), *Aonyx* (small-clawed, or clawless, otter) and *Enhydra* (sea otter) are aquatic, whereas most other members of the Mustelid family are land dwelling (fissipedia). In the widely distributed Mustilinae subfamily in particular, there are approximately 11 genera and 33 recent species. The more familiar relatives of the ferret include the weasel (ermine, sable), mink, marten, polecat, fisher,

Table 1 Taxonomic
Classification of Ferrets

Kingdom	Animal
Subkingdom	Metazoa
Phylum	Chordata
Subphylum	Vertebrata
Class	Mammalia
Subclass	Eutheria
Order	Carnivora
Suborder	Fissipedia
Family	Mustilidae
Subfamily	Mustelinae
Genus	*Mustela*
Species	*Putorius*
Subspecies	*Furo*

skunk, wolverine, otter, and badger. Less commonly known relatives include the zorille and ratel (honey badger). In Europe and Great Britain, the wild ferret is also known as a fitch, fitchew, fitchet, foul marten, or foumart.

Most mustilids have well-developed anal scent glands. The skunks, zorille, marbled polecat, stink badger, and ratel can forcibly eject the vile-smelling fluid as a spray or fluid. In contrast, the laboratory ferret is incapable of projecting its anal gland fluid, which many researchers also rate low on the odoriferous discomfort scale.

Economic Applications

Early Greek Ferreting and Falconry

Early Greek literature indicates that ferrets made their first social impact as hunters of rabbits (Thomson, 1951). Similar to the use of grisons to flush chinchillas from their burrows, "ferreting" for rabbits consists of muzzling a ferret and placing it into one entrance of a rabbit burrow. The characteristic musk odor of the ferret would cause the burrow's occupants to flee by a rear entrance, whereupon they were duly dispatched by the hunter. The Greeks were probably the first to employ falconry as a method of capture for rabbits flushed from their burrow in this manner. However, many hunters simply held a net or cloth sack over the rear entrance to the burrow, hoping that their strength could match the speed and force by which the rabbits exited the hole. Ferreting (or "rabbiting") with firearms is viewed as unsportsmanlike and is prohibited in many parts of the United States.

English Ferret-Legging

The English are credited with popularizing the notable sport of "ferret-legging," which has seen a resurgence in recent years. In this contest, a competitor's trousers are tied off at the ankles and a ferret is inserted. After tightening the belt, the contestant proceeds to tolerate the ferret's repeated escape attempts. Katz (1987) described the "ideal" ferret for ferret-legging as . . ."having claws like hypodermic needles and teeth like number 16 carpet tacks." Accordingly, the current record for ferret-legging is 5 hr and 26 minutes, a mark held by a 72-year-old Yorkshire man.

Use of the Ferret as a Rodent Exterminator

In the early part of the twentieth century ferrets were popular as rodent exterminators in the United States and England. However, with the advent of chemical rodenticides, this specific application of the species has waned.

Pet Ferrets and Their Legal Restrictions

Currently there are an estimated 4–5 million ferrets in the United States, with approximately 1,000,000 in the state of California alone. Some states such as Georgia, Massachusetts, New Hampshire, and South Carolina, however, have banned the ownership of ferrets completely, and other states such as California, Minnesota (Minneapolis), and New York have restricted ownership by requiring licensing, neutering, or leashing. Some localities, such as Carson City, Nevada, have gone as far as to prohibit the sale of ferrets to households that have children under the age of 3 years. These various restrictions have apparently resulted from controversial issues such as whether the ferret may be considered a truly domesticated species, media accounts of instances when young infants have been bitten, and the present lack of an FDA-approved rabies vaccine. Proponents of ferrets have, nevertheless, successfully argued their cause in the courts of Alaska, Maine,

Pennsylvania, and West Virginia, and have had restrictions reversed or overruled in these states. Based on scientific information presented by lobbyists to individual state legislatures, the ferret is being increasingly categorized as a domesticated animal, thus exempt from control by the individual State Game Commissions. Moreover, a recent trade journal survey indicated that ferret bites are much less frequent (and severe) than dog bites when expressed relative to species population size, and laboratory researchers have found the ferret to be accommodatingly docile and predictable.

Early Biomedical Research Studies with the Ferret

Pioneering biomedical research studies utilized the ferret in experiments concerned with the pathogenesis of human influenza virus (Smith et al., 1933; Pyle, 1940; Moody et al., 1985; Pearson and Gorham, 1988), and because of its sensitive pulmonary vasculature, the species continues to be viewed as a valuable model for investigating pulmonary hypotension in humans (Vinegar et al., 1982; Andrews, 1988). Similarly, ferrets have also been used quite successfully in assessments of reproductive toxicity (Mould et al., 1973; Beck et al., 1976, 1978; Gulamhusein et al., 1980; Beck, 1981; McLain and Roe, 1983) and a Stanford University symposium (1981) and several review articles (Beck, 1975; Haddad and Rabe, 1980; Gulamhusein and Beck, 1977) have highlighted the species' many advantages and contributions to this specific scientific discipline. Beck (1978, 1981) and Hoar (1984), for example, contrasted human, rat, and ferret placentas and concluded that the latter was most similar in structure and function to the human. Literature reports continue to demonstrate that similar reproductive responses in humans and ferrets (Elizan and Fabiyi, 1969; Beck et al., 1974; Collie et al., 1978; Gulamhusein et al., 1980; McLain and Roe, 1984).

HUSBANDRY

Specific husbandry practices for the ferret are summarized in Table 2. Details of selected parameters are outlined in the following sections.

Caging and Bedding

The staff veterinarian or designee should be responsible for determining suitable housing for newly arriving ferrets. In addition, rooms in which ferrets are housed should be of adequate space, clean, ventilated, and environmentally controlled in accordance with government regulations and guidelines established for the care and use of laboratory animals, and in accordance with applicable facility standard procedures. Before modifying details of an established animal care program, the staff veterinarian (or designee) should notify the research scientist whose animals are affected by the proposed change.

The recognition that ferrets adapt readily to the various types of caging routinely found in the small animal vivarium has undoubtedly contributed to the success of the species in the biomedical research laboratory. Stainless steel rabbit cages (2' L × 2' W × 1' 3" H), for example, will house one or two ferrets quite comfortably. Cat cages (2' L × 2' W × 2' H) are quite adequate when group housing is preferred. The most recent issue of the National Institute of Health (NIH) *Guide for the Care and Use of Laboratory Animals* (1985) did not specify standards for the size of ferret caging, but it is likely that either of the dimensions just discussed will more than satisfy any potentially forthcoming criteria. Both cage types described are low stress, providing for sufficient lateral (horizontal) and vertical (rearing) motion. In addition, they exceed the dimensions specified by Wilson and

Table 2 Recommended Husbandry Practices for Ferrets Maintained Under Controlled Environmental Conditions

Parameter	Units	Value
Cage dimensions (L × W × H)		
Breeding (2 adults)	cm	60 × 60 × 40
Growing (1–8 kits)	cm	40 × 40 × 30
Experimental	cm	Varies
Cage bar spacing	cm	<2.5
Area temperature	°C	15 ± 5
Area humidity	%	50 ± 20
Room air changes	no./hr	10–15
Lighting (incandescent or fluorescent)		
sexually inactive	hr/day	8 ± 2
sexually active	hr/day	14 ± 2
Nest material (other than ⅜″ grid flooring)		
all ages	—	Shavings
pregnant females	—	Nest box
Food intake (not accounting for spillage)		
energy (maint.)	kcal/kg/day	200–300
dry matter	g/day	50–70
Solid food, age at	weeks	1–2
Diet peculiarities		
growing	—	ad libitum
breeding, lactating	—	ad libitum
adult	low body fat	limit feed
Water requirements	ml/24 hr	75–100 or ad libitum

Donnoghue (1982), and by the Royal Society of England (Andrews and Illman, 1987). Wilson and O'Donoghue (1982) have described a mobile rack of cages for ferrets.

Group housing and opportunity for interaction suitable to ferrets should be provided whenever possible, but it should also be recognized that group housing of mature adults is frequently impractical (see below). Therefore, wherever possible, caging should be provided which permits easy viewing of neighboring cages and their occupants.

Limitations of Cage Bar Dimensions

A variety of cage dimensions may be satisfactory for housing ferrets, as long as the interior dimensions provide for uninhibited movement and the cage bar spacing of the unit is <2.5 cm, or modified appropriately. With respect to cage height, behavioral observations indicate a natural rearing motion of this species (similar to cats and dogs), which is probably related to a strong dependency on smell when hunting and the need to extend their head above tall grasses to examine the upper air currents. Observations have also indicated that ferrets with body weights ≤700 g will escape through any cage bars spaced ≥2.5 cm apart, as well as through the popular J-type gravity feeder. Therefore, containment should be assured by employing commercially available stainless steel grid door inserts (Lab Products, Inc., Maywood, New Jersey, ¼″ grid) and by locating feed dishes inside the cage bars. It is also possible to insert an appropriately shaped section of stainless steel grid (spacing approximately ¾″ H × 1 ½″ L) inside the J-type gravity feeder, which prevents escape and reduces the digging and scattering of feed (see below).

Excretory Habits of Caged Ferrets

Ferrets are accommodating in that they characteristically deposit their wastes in distinct corners of the cage. Thus, cage floor grids should be large enough to allow excreta to fall through to the catch pans below, yet small enough so as not to cause the animal discomfort when walking, or to allow escape. Commercially available wash-down rabbit caging with ⅜″ grid flooring fits these criteria and requires little maintenance time for hygiene control. Alternatively, direct-contact bedding material (wood chips, paper strips, etc.) may be used with similar success, with soiled corner material removed daily and complete changes occurring as needed. For short-term housing or transportation, some investigators have employed the large polycarbonate rat breeding cage (9″ H × 9″ W × 16″ L), covering the bottom with wood chips to facilitate cleaning. As indicated, however, these units should not be used for any extended housing period because of their small size. Moreover, the units should be dedicated to ferrets because they will tend to retain the musk odor, causing considerable consternation for the next small rodent inhabitant.

Nest Boxes for Pregnant Ferrets

A nest box (approximately 6″ H × 6″ W × 12″ L) constructed of either metal or plastic, partially filled with wood chip or paper strip bedding material, and containing a 2-3-in diameter entrance hole is a valuable cage addition for the pregnant jill and for increasing the comfort of animals subjected to chronic treatment protocols. Nontransparent nest boxes such as metal, however, are not conducive to recording detailed daily clinical observations because the animals will tend to spend a disproportionate amount of time inside them. The smaller sized polycarbonate rat and mouse cages have been employed with greatest success. Entrance holes should be cut approximately 2 in above floor level, which prevents the newborn kits from falling out while permitting easy access for the jill.

Individual Caging Requirements of Adult Ferrets

Littermates of both sexes may be group housed until sexual play or aggressive behavior becomes too violent. Thereafter, individualized caging is required, especially during periods of peak sexual activity and pregnancy, or when suppression of estrus is desired. Sexually active male ferrets, and to a lesser extent females, will fight when housed with others of the same sex. Similarly, although the species is not prone to cannibalism, jills who have just whelped should be allowed to recover and nurse their litter of kits undisturbed. Segregating by sex and by room will generally help to suppress the incidence and onset of estrus in females. Conversely, desegregation may promote the onset of sexual activity, and the sexual play of females may elicit ovulation or a pseudopregnancy.

For breeding purposes, it is recommended that receptive females be transferred to the sexually active male's home cage. When coitus is completed, the female should be returned to her own cage.

Reproductive sterilization apparently reduces aggressive behavior sufficiently such that animals may be group housed. However, a pecking order or individual domination may still become manifest.

Lighting

Similar to the effects of altered photoperiodism documented for mink, the light/dark cycle employed in the ferret vivarium may be manipulated to control the breeding cycle. Ferrets are seasonal breeders and will become conditioned for breeding with exposure to longer day lengths or periods of artificial illumination. To prevent the onset of sexual activity (or first estrus) in younger animals arriving at the vivarium during the natural breeding season (January–March), or to maintain a colony of stock animals in a sexually inactive state, lighting is optimally set between 6:18–10:14 light/dark to simulate the early winter (nonbreeding) months (Ryland and Gorham, 1978; Moody et al., 1985). Conversely, increasing the period of illumination to between 12 and 16 hr may stimulate sexual activity in this species (Donovan, 1967). Detailed discussions of the effects of day length on the coat-shedding cycles, body weight, and reproduction of the ferret have been published by Harvey and MacFarlane (1958) and Donovan (1966, 1967). Earlier but equally informative studies were reported by Bissonnette (1932), Hart (1951), and Hammond (1952).

It is noteworthy that loss of hair, which may proceed to the development of alopecia, is observed in ferrets (especially marked in estrus females) subjected to long exposure of 16 hr of light daily. Conversely, marked growth of hair takes place under short-day conditions. Since marked hair growth can help to confirm that animals are being maintained in a sexually inactive state, as opposed to pregnancy or pseudopregnancy (marked by hair loss), the condition of the coat should be monitored and included as part of the clinical observations protocol. A classic study of the molting and fur growth pattern in the adult mink, which applies to the ferret, was published by Bassett and Llewellyn (1949).

Temperature and Humidity

Because of their thick fur, ferrets will tolerate low environmental temperatures and, in fact, many commercial producers began their businesses by group housing their sexually inactive animals in outdoor sheds throughout the year. Freezing winter temperatures were evident when the high moisture diets fed to these animals froze on the cage floor pallets. Prolonged cold spells simply caused these animals to mold together into a single, continuous ball of fur buried deep beneath the straw bedding. This natural tolerance for cold temperature may be extrapolated to the vivarium.

For maximum thriftiness of mature, individually housed animals, environmentally controlled rooms should maintain an optimal temperature of $15 \pm 5°C$. Thickly furred adults will benefit from the lower end of this temperature range. Conversely, lactating jills and their unweaned litters may require the slightly warmer temperatures at the upper end of this temperature range.

As with most other species, high relative humidity is apparently not an important factor in ferret performance, except when accompanied by prolonged elevation in temperature. The recommended relative humidity for the vivarium is $50 \pm 20\%$.

Clinical Signs of Heat Stress

Ferrets are particularly vulnerable to heat stress, and special care is necessary when moving them from one area to another during hot weather. Adult ferrets and breeding stock are especially sensitive owing to their subcutaneous fat cover and their inability to dissipate heat by sweating. Clinical signs of hyperthermia include panting and mouth breathing, prostration followed by eventual flaccidity, and emesis. When a tiered caging system is used, particular attention should be paid to animals housed in the tier closest to the ceiling, where the warmer air may concentrate.

Room Air Changes

Regardless of species, most modern vivariums are designed to maintain a range of 10–15 complete exchanges of room air (nonrecirculated) per hour. Ferrets do well under these conditions, but because of their musky odor and suseptibility to respiratory pathogens, the higher end of the range is frequently indicated. In the authors' experience, environmentally controlled animal rooms measuring $14' \times 22'$, employing nine racks of nine cages per rack of wash-down caging (cleaned with water once daily), nonabsorbable wall and floor surfaces, and 15 air exchanges per hour will not retain an odor even when ferrets are housed two per cage at maximum room density.

Diet and Water

Natural Ingredient and Purified Diet Formulations

A recent survey (McLain et al., 1985) of a large commercial ferret colony (Marshall Farms, North Rose, New York) detailed a successful natural ingredient diet for ferrets (Table 3). Reproduction data reported in this survey demonstrated that primiparous females fed this natural ingredient diet whelped an average of 10.3 ± 0.2 kits per litter (range: 1–18), successfully weaned 80% of these, and frequently produced three to four litters per year. Subsequently, the Marshall Farms natural ingredient ferret diet was analyzed and reproduced as a purified formulation (McLain and Roe, 1983; McLain et al., 1988). Moreover, when prepared with animal fat and ≥50% moisture (using 2% agar), adequate weight gain is demonstrated for animals consuming this purified formulation.

Commercial Diets

Two large commercial producers of animal feed presently market least-cost formulation ferret diets that also promote adequate weight gain. Ralston-Purina (St. Louis, Missouri) offers the Purina 5280 ferret chow, which is pelleted and available as a certified ration. Agway, Inc. (Ithaca, New York) also offers a pelleted ration that closely parallels the nutrient composition of the Marshall Farms natural ingredient diet.

Consumption Patterns and Acclimation of Ferrets to Commercial Rations. For maintenance of body weight, ferrets will require between 200 and 300 kcal/kg body weight daily. This translates to between 50 and 70 g/day of the pelleted commercial rations described previously, not accounting for spillage (McLain and Roe, 1983; McLain et al.,

Table 3 Composition of a Successful Natural Ingredient Ferret Diet[a]

Ingredient	Approx. Wt. per batch[a]
Wayne dog food cereal	100
Agway dog food cereal	50
Beef tripe	100
Beef lung	50
Beef liver	10
Fortified cod liver oil	1
Water	(varies)

[a]Total batch weight is approximately 1000 lb. Dry ingredients are added to a mechanical mixer from bags or cans; water is added until desired consistency is achieved.
Source: Courtesy of Mr. Gilman Marshall, Marshall Farms, North Rose, New York.

1988). Bleavins and Aulerich (1981) reported food consumption to average 43 g/kg body weight in the ferret, and mean food passage time (as measured by a dye marker in the feed) was reported to average approximately 3 hr, indicating a relatively short digestive tract.

The study of food habits of ferrets living in the wild has resulted in several interesting and informative behavioral publications (Roser and Lavers, 1976; Kaufman, 1980). However, nothing has been published which will prepare the naive investigator for an unacclimated ferret's first encounter with a pelleted diet offered in a stainless steel or glass bowl. Initially, new arrivals will appear to immensely enjoy the sound of digging in metal or glass food dishes and subsequently spilling their daily allotment of food. To cure this habit, replenish the food only during designated feeding times. By approximately the third day, the animal will have lost body weight and be sufficiently hungry so that food pellets moistened slightly with water will be ravenously consumed. Gradually decrease the amount of water added to the pellets until dry food is consumed exclusively. This process may have to be repeated. Fortunately, the burden of pelleted diet acclimation has been assumed by the more conscientious animal vendors.

On rare occasion, an individual animal may appear to have chosen starvation rather than consume a dry food ration. In these cases, canned (moist) cat or dog food or fresh organ meats may have to be fed to ensure survival. Although animals receiving these diets and special considerations may have to be excluded from controlled protocol studies, they may still be used subsequently for technical training purposes or exploratory protocols.

Automatic Watering Systems

Many commercial ferret producers use automatic watering systems in their facilities. Consequently, ferrets will readily adapt to the demand-controlled automatic systems present in the newer caging units, or to water bottles attached to the cage. As with other species, the valves of automatic watering systems must be checked on a routine basis to ensure that they are functional, and water bottles should be changed daily.

Acclimation and Quarantine Procedures

Special Attention for New Arrivals to the Vivarium

It would be naive to assume that newly arriving ferrets will tolerate the type of handling that is afforded the more "conditioned" animals of this or any other species. In reality, ferrets arriving from most commercial breeders will have been selectively bred for an even disposition, but memories of pecking order and perhaps competition for food and water during shipping may still be fresh in their mind. Many of the new animals will be confused and frightened by the unfamiliar sights and sounds experienced during shipping. A small percentage of ferrets may, in fact, have become overly stressed and understandably resist (hiss, scream, back away from the hand) any initial attempts to handle them. To reduce the risk of injury to either animal or technician, therefore, shipping crates containing newly arriving animals should be unpacked cautiously (preferably away from bright light or loud noise) and animals offered fresh food and water and dim lighting as soon as possible. Additionally, a qualified animal health technician or laboratory veterinarian should be available to assist in the identification and treatment of any animals having succumbed to heat or shipping stress. Ferrets will generally respond rapidly to this initial attention paid to them by allowing handling and petting within only hours of arrival. Slower responding animals will require more patience, but will usually assume a more even disposition with additional efforts during acclimation.

Initial Physical Examination Parameters and the Observations Recorded During the Period of Quarantine

All animals should be subjected to a complete physical examination within 1–2 days of arrival. Examination should include inspection for disorders of the skin and fur (ectoparasites), nose and throat, eyes and ears, obvious physical impairments which would preclude the use of the animal in scientific research, fecal and urine screening (see later section on urinalysis), and the presence and condition of vendor-applied ear tags. The quarantine period for ferrets should be long enough to allow an evaluation of daily clinical observations, body weight change, and food and water consumption patterns for their individual contribution to the animals' physical health. Routine clinical observations and body weight changes by themselves, when recorded over a 1- to 2-week period, will usually enable the identification of animals infected with either respiratory or intestinal pathogens. Optimum prophylaxis requires that diseased animals be culled or isolated from healthy animals and administered appropriate professional health care.

Depending upon the scientific application, blood samples may or may not be collected from animals during the quarantine period (see later section on blood sampling techniques).

A typical animal history chart for use during the quarantine periods of ferrets is shown in Figure 2.

Veterinary Procedures and Common Diseases

General veterinary care of the ferret is similar in many aspects to that provided the feline and canine species. Approximate drug dosages, when required for specific veterinary procedures or prophylaxis, are listed in Tables 4 and 5. Confirmation of these dosages is recommended for each laboratory before routine use.

Anesthetics and Drug Dosages

Anesthesia, sedation, or tranquilization, although not mandatory, will frequently facilitate initial, detailed physical examinations of the ferret and significantly reduce the potential for inadvertant injury to the examiner or animal. In addition, mild tranquilization will also facilitate examination of the eyes and have an indirect calming effect on the ophthalmologist as well. The following sections, therefore, provide general information concerning recommended agents, routes of administration, and doses of anesthetics, tranquilizers, and other various drugs frequently used in the ferret. These guidelines are intended to comply with appropriate sections of the Animal Welfare Act.

General Anesthetics. General anesthetics used successfully in ferrets include those drugs which produce controllable and reversible loss of consciousness with analgesia. The same general anesthesia principles apply to ferrets as would be practiced with most other species. For example, when possible, withhold food from ferrets prior to anesthetic administration. In addition, give a general physical examination immediately prior to treatment to evaluate the general condition of the animals in terms of anesthetic risk. Once anesthesia is induced, monitor the animals every 15 min for heart and respiration rate, mucous membrane color, capillary refill time, and plane of anesthesia. During recovery from anesthetics, isolate the animal, place it in sternal recumbency until swallowing and jaw reflex return, and provide for maintenance of body temperature. Ferrets should be turned to the opposite side every 30 min during prolonged recovery to prevent hypostatic congestion of the lungs.

The various ketamine (KET) mixtures listed in Table 4 are apparently the most

Facilities:
Address: **ANIMAL HISTORY**

DATE RECEIVED	:	VENDOR	:	U.S.D.A. NO.	:	INITIAL WGT.	:	SCALE NO.
	:		:		:		:	
	:		:		:		:	
DATE OF BIRTH	:	BREED/DESCRIPTION			:	SEX	:	HISTORY
	:				:		:	
	:				:		:	

		DATE	BY	REVIEW	:	LAB
PHYSICAL EXAMINATION					:	

NA : GENERAL APPEARANCE: :
   :   :
NA : INTEGUMANT: ( ) ECTOPARASITES   ( ) ALOPECIA
   :
NA : DIGESTIVE: ( ) ORAL ( ) STOOL ( ) AUSCULTATE ( ) PALPATE
   :
NA : CV - RESPIRATORY: ( ) AUSCULTATE   ( ) NASAL DISCHARGE
   :
NA : LYMPH NODES: ( ) CERVICAL   ( ) AXILLARY   ( ) INGUINAL
   :
NA : MUSCULOSKELETAL:
   :
NA : UROGENITAL: ( ) VULVAL SWELLING   ( ) DESCENDED TESTICLES
   :
NA : EYES: ( ) NUCLEAR OPACIFICATION ( ) CONJUNCTIVITIES
   :
NA : EARS: ( ) OTITIS   ( ) ACARIASIS
   :

	ASSIGNMENT HISTORY		:	**FINAL DISPOSITION**	:	DATE
			:	(CIRCLE ONE)	:	
DATE :	PROJ. NO. :	STUDY DIR.	:	DIED EUTHANIZED	:	
:	:	:	:	CAUSE/METHOD		
:	:	:	:	COMMENTS	:	INITIALS
:	:	:	:		:	

COMMENTS:

VACCINATIONS (TYPE/DATES)
_____
SPAYING/NEUTERING (DATE)   : DESCENTING (DATE)
                                    :
POSTQUARANTINE BODY WGT./SCALE NO. : FOOD HABITS/DIET FED
                                    :
I.D. NUMBER   : OTHER I.D.
                                    :

Figure 2 Quarantine information chart for ferrets. Additional physical examination data should be
added as required by each facility.

frequently used anesthetics for minor surgical and noninvasive procedures, with a 25–35
mg/kg dosage inducing a desirable limpness and flacidity to the animal body for approximately 30–45 min. Limited observations by one of the present authors (D.E.M.) suggest
that the albino strain of ferret may be slightly more sensitive to KET-Acepromazine
(ACE) than the more common sable strain. Several informative discussions of ferret
tranquilization, preanesthesia, and anesthesia have been published (Moreland and Glaser,
1985; Moody et al., 1985; Johnson, 1987; Fox, 1988). Unfortunately, very little discussion is afforded to KET-ACE, a mixture with which one of us (D.E.M.) has had great
success.

Table 4 Guidelines for Sedative, Preanesthetic and Anesthetic Dosages in the Ferret[a]

Sedatives	
acepromazine (ACE)	0.2–0.5 mg/kg im, sc
ketamine (KET)	10–20, mg/kg im
xylazine (XYL)	1.0 mg/kg im, sc
diazepam (DZP)	1.0–2.0 mg/kg im
Preanesthetics	
acepromazine	0.1–0.25 mg/kg im, sc
atropine	0.05 mg/kg im, sc
Anesthetics	
KET	30–60 mg/kg im
KET + ACE	KET: 20–35 mg/kg
(100:1 Mixture)	ACE: 0.2–0.35 mg/kg im
KET + Valium	KET: 25 mg/kg
(10:1 Mixture)	VAL: 2.5 mg/kg im
XYL (followed by KET)	XYL: 2–3 mg/kg sc
	KET: 20–30 mg/kg im
DZP (followed by KET)	DZP: 2.0–3.5 mg/kg sc
	KET: 20–35 mg/kg im
pentobarbital	25–35 mg/kg ip

[a]Dosages should be confirmed in each laboratory before application.

Table 5 Guidelines for Antibiotic, Hormone and Steroid Dosages in the Ferret[a]

Antibiotics	
Albon (oral, inject)	Feline dose
Albon (coccidia Rx)	Feline dose
amoxicillin (oral)	25–35 mg/kg bid
ampicillin	10 mg/kg bid sc
gentamicin	5 mg/kg im
griseofulvin tabs	25 mg/kg
ivermectin	1 mg/kg
neomycin	10–20 mg/kg
penicillin (Flo-Cillin)	Feline dose
piperazine salts	Feline dose
tetracycline (oral)	25 mg/kg bid
Hormones and steroids	
dexamethasone	0.25 mg/kg
GnRH	20 ug
HCG	100 IU im
insulin	1–2 units/kg
oxytocin	0.2–3 U/kg SC im
prednisone (oral)	0.5–2 mg/kg
	Feline schedule

[a]Dosages should be confirmed in each laboratory before application.

Preanesthetics.   Preanesthetics include those drugs which facilitate effective anesthesia in the ferret. Atropine sulfate and acepromazine (Table 4) are used effectively and are indicated to reduce excessive upper respiratory secretions associated with some anesthetics, and to decrease bradycardia (vagal effects). Atropine sulfate, for example, should be administered approximately 15–30 min prior to anesthesia, and has a duration of action of approximately 15–30 min. It may cause dilation of the pupils and decreased lacrimation; therefore, use of ophthalmic ointments may be indicated.

Tranquilizers and Sedatives.   These agents are frequently used to facilitate restraint for nonpainful procedures such as bandaging, radiology, parenteral injections, venipuncture, or examination (including ophthalmic); to decrease excitment in nervous or frightened animals; and, as preanesthetics, to decrease the dose of anesthetic required. *Note:* These agents are not analgesic or anesthetic in nature and should not be used as pain relievers.

The tranquilizing effect of acepromazine (Table 4) may last several hours in the ferret. Moreover, when combined with ketamine, it is excellent for analgesia, sedation, and minor surgical procedures. However, since it may cause peripheral vasodilation, thermoregulation should be maintained.

Prophylaxis aand Vaccination Schedules

Most commercial suppliers of ferrets routinely vaccinate kits against canine distemper virus (CDV) at approximately 6–8 weeks of age (2 weeks earlier if the jill has not been recently vaccinated), with boosters administered approximately 4 weeks later and every 3 years thereafter. A modified-live distemper virus of chick embryo tissue culture origin has been used successfully, as has the modified-live virus of canine origin. Killed vaccines may be ineffective (Ott and Svehag, 1959) and unattenuated viral vaccines derived from ferret cell culture may be too virulent. Pregnant ferrets are routinely vaccinated by commercial breeders without harm to the fetus (Hagan et al., 1970). Unvaccinated ferrets exposed to the canine distemper virus for only 15 min will acquire the disease, and close to 100% of these animals will die (Hahn and Wester, 1969). Since there is no cure for the disease once it is acquired, it is strongly recommended that the initial vaccination and subsequent booster be a prerequisite of animal purchase. A detailed clinical description of the disease in ferrets was published by Ryland and Gorham (1978).

The incidence of rabies in domestic ferrets is very slight. The Centers for Disease Control (CDC) in Atlanta, Georgia, reports only five cases in the United States over a period from 1958 through 1983, and no recent cases have been confirmed. The U.S. Food and Drug Administration (FDA) has not yet approved a rabies vaccine, but the Canadian Council on Animal Care clearly states in its *Guide to Care and Use of Experimental Animals*, Vol. 2, that inactive ("killed") rabies vaccine is effective for ferrets. More recently, according to McBride (1989), Norden Laboratories of Lincoln, Nebraska, has finished preliminary testing on an inactivated ferret rabies vaccine and has begun the challange test. Consequently, it is anticipated that an approved (licensed) ferret rabies vaccine will be available in late 1989 or early 1990. Testing has shown a slight difference in serological response from males to females, which could mean ferrets may require a two-dose initial vaccination (recommended vaccination age will be 12 weeks), with boosters (dosage = 1 cc) given every 12 months thereafter.

Surgical Sterilization Procedures and Anal Musk Gland Removal

Reproductive sterilization of laboratory ferrets is accomplished using surgical procedures and conditions typically described for the feline and canine species (Randolph, 1986).

Moreover, removal of the ferret's anal musk glands is similar to that documented for other mustelids (Creed and Kainer, 1981). These procedures (spaying, castration, and descenting) are typically performed by vendors (upon request) on animals as young as 8 weeks of age, apparently with minimal blood loss or tissue trauma when the proper anesthesia and surgical techniques are employed. When allowed by scientific protocol, these procedures are recommended for the chronic (repeated), restrained, intravenous (caudal vein) treatment of the stronger smelling and more aggressive male ferrets especially, and to preclude estrous cycling of females.

Most Frequently Observed Diseases of Ferrets Maintained Under Controlled Laboratory Conditions

Although they are probably 10 breeding years behind the current virus-free and specific pathogen–free (SPF) rats, laboratory ferrets maintained under controlled conditions manifest a relatively low incidence of debilitating diseases. On the contrary, very few diseases with unique clinical signs which would enable early detection for prophylaxis have been documented in ferrets. Moreover, underlying pathological conditions appear to be rarely evidenced by more than a reduction in body weight and a diminution of appetite and food intake. Literature reviews of the various diseases observed in this species have been published by Ryland and Gorham (1978), Hammond and Chesterman (1972), Seamer and Chesterman (1967), and Andrews and Illman (1987) as well as the very extensive review by Fox (1988).

Influenza and Pneumonitis. As demonstrated by earlier classic studies (Smith et al., 1933; Shope, 1934; Smith and Stuart-Harris, 1936; Fisher and Scott, 1944; Bell and Dudgeon, 1948) the human influenza virus can be readily transmitted from human-to-ferret, ferret-to-ferret, and ferret-to-human by way of aerosolized droplets containing infective viral particles. Infection is characterized by lethargy, elevated rectal temperature (40–41°C, lasting 1 day and then returning on the third day), and bouts of sneezing accompanied by a mucoserous nasal discharge. Some animals may also manifest a conjunctivitis and/or otitis. Clinical signs may persist for up to 2 weeks, with resistance to the same strain of influenza virus demonstrated upon subsequent exposure. Congestion may be relieved by antihisamines suitable for other species.

Preventive measures include the wearing of face masks by personnel exposed to outbreaks of the viral infection, and the isolation of infected animals. Limited prophylaxis has been reported with 6 mg/kg bid aerosolized amantadine hydrochloride (Cochran et al., 1965; Cusumano et al, 1965; Fenton et al., 1977) and to a lesser extent with 100 mg/kg ribavarin (Fenton and Potter, 1977). An additional influenzalike disease includes the respiratory syncytial virus (RSV) infection of infant ferrets (Tyrrell and Hoorn, 1965; Prince and Porter, 1976).

Bacterial pneumonias affecting ferrets are similar to those seen in other species. The list of reported strains includes *Bordetella* sp. (McLain, 1989) and *Streptococcus* sp. (Andrews et al., 1979), as well as the various gram-negative bacteria *(E. coli, K. pneumoniae, P. aeruginosa)*.

Interstitial pneumonitis in conjunction with focal mononuclear cell infiltrates may be caused by bacterial, viral, or protozoan infections, including *Pneumocystis carinii*. The latter protozoan parasite is known to inhabit the lungs of various domestic and laboratory animals with compromised immune systems (Farrow et al., 1972; Milder et al., 1980; Long et al., 1986). Recently, Stokes et al. (1987) studied the disease in ferrets by immunosuppressing the animals with cortisone acetate (10–20 mg/kg sc for 9–10 weeks).

Aleutian Disease. Aleutian disease, a persistent and frequently fatal parvovirus infection first reported to be common in the Aleutian mink (Obel, 1959; Henson et al., 1961) also occurs in the ferret (Kenyon et al., 1966, 1967; Ohshima et al., 1978). However, the strain of parvovirus infecting ferrets, while resulting in similar pathological lesions (e.g., hypergammaglobulinemia and plasma cell dyscrasia), is rarely fatal to them. Reviews have been published for Aleutian disease in mink (Porter et al., 1980) and in ferrets (Porter et al., 1982). Mild to moderate lymphocytic infiltrates of the liver (periportal localization), lung (pneumonitis), and kidney (polynephritis/glomerulonephropathy) are the predominant histological finding in ferrets with Aleutian disease. Occasionally, an animal will become anorexic and thin, and pass black tarry feces.

Kenyon et al. (1967) have defined the hypergammaglobulinemia associated with Aleutian disease in ferrets as greater than 20% of total serum protein as γ-globulin. Moreover, Porter et al. (1982) demonstrated that ferrets with the highest Aleutian disease virus antibody titer also had the greatest increase in serum gamma globulin levels and the most severe tissue lesions. Since ferrets infected with Aleutian disease are generally asymptomatic, and the corresponding changes associated with the disease have potential for misinterpretation, McLain and Lin (1989) developed a method for predicting the degree of periportal lymphocytic infiltrates from routine blood samples. When both pretreatment and posttreatment blood samples are used in the "liver lymphocyte index" (LvLI) equation, the prediction/correlation was shown to have a 92–96% success rate (see below).

Proliferative Colitis. Fox et al. (1982) described proliferative colitis in ferrets and addressed the histopathological and bacteriological features of this disease entity which, according to the authors, is fatal or requires euthanasia in almost all of the affected animals. The etiological agent is probably a *Campylobacter* sp., with fecal-oral spread and food- and waterborne transmission apparently the principal avenues for infection.

Clinical signs of proliferative colitis include diarrhea, anorexia, and marked weight loss ($\geq$10–15%/week). Significant elevations in urine pH ($\geq$8.0) and urobilinogen ($\geq$2.0) may occur, compared with normal values of approximately 6.0–6.5 and 0.1, repectively. In the experience of one of the authors (D.E.M.), the incidence of the disease has been three in approximately 1000 animals (newly arriving only), with mortality occurring in only one of these. Antemortem fibrinogen was 442 mg/dl in the single fatality, compared with a normal value of 189 $\pm$ 78 mg/dl (95% uper tolerance limit=387 mg/dl). It is noteworthy that in the same author's experience, no cases of proliferative colitis have occurred in resident animals released from quarantine.

Treatment for proliferative colitis should be instituted immediately upon noting diarrhea and anorexia. Amoxicillin (oral suspension, 250 mg/5 cc), Pepto Bismol, and water should be given orally twice a day for 5–7 dys in a dosage containing 1 cc amoxicillin, 1 cc Pepto Bismol and 1 cc water (personal observation/recommendation, R.M.H.).

Bone Marrow Hypoplasia and Estrogen-Induced Anemia. Aplastic anemia has been associated with prolonged estrus in the female ferret (Kociba and Caputo, 1981). Similarly, bone marrow hypoplasia in estrous ferrets has been attributed to prolonged exposure to estrogens (Bernard et al., 1983). Since unbred female ferrets will remain in estrus for the duration of the normal breeding season (March–August), the potential for this pathological condition to occur would seem high.

Clinical signs of bone marrow hypoplasia include cutaneous petechiae and ecchymoses, gastrointestinal hemorrhages, systemic bacterial infections, and pale mucous membranes (Kociba and Caputo, 1981; Bernard et al., 1983). Hematological findings include initial thrombocytosis and leukocytosis followd by thrombocytopenia, leukopenia, and anemia. Decreased platelets ($<50,000/\mu l$), hemorrhagic anemia, and death may occur in 40–50% of affected animals. Histopathological findings include bone marrow hypoplasia affecting all cell lines and decreased splenic extramedullary hematopoiesis (Sherrill and Gorham, 1985). Prevention of the condition requires sterilization or breeding of estrus females, a controlled lighting regimen to preclude estrus cycling, or an intramuscular injection of human chronic gonadotropin (HCG, 100 IU) (Table 5) administered at the peak of vulval swelling (diameter ≥ 15 mm) and repeated in 7–10 days if vulval regression does not occur.

DOSING

The ferret is a seemingly very forgiving and forgetting creature, rarely holding a grudge following dosing by any route. In fact, first-time ferret users are usually amazed at the rapidity in which these animals recover from the physical restraint and various degrees of mechanical trauma possible with some forms of test article dosing. The desirability of this particular trait contributes immensely to the ferret's growing popularity as an animal model.

Most of the conventional methods of dosing employed with other laboratory animals are applicable to ferrets. Special techniques and considerations are outlined below.

Oral Dosing

Gastric intubation is accomplished in fully conscious ferrets with a 10-16-gauge $\times$ 6-in straight, stainless steel dosing needle with a 6.4-mm stainless steel ball on the end (EJAY International, Inc., Glendora, California) or, alternatively, with an appropriate diameter plastic tubing or French catheter. Because of the required length of the intubation needle or tubing, the animal should be held and treated in a vertical position. This is most easily accomplished by holding or resting the animal vertically across one's chest, allowing the intubation tube a straight, downward motion.

As with other test species, placement of the intubation tube within the stomach of the ferret is confirmed by visual examination of aspirate. McLain and Roe (1984) described the successful, daily intubation of approximately 40 pregnant female ferrets (20 doses/animal, 800 doses) without incident using this procedure.

Gag Reflex and Emesis in the Ferret

Similar to the dog and cat, the ferret is capable of a gag or vomit reflex and has received considerable attention as an alternative animal model for the study of the physiology of emesis (Florczyk et al., 1981). Oral dosing of nausea-producing agents will elicit characteristic behavior, including licking, chin rubbing, walking backward, and slit eyes.

Gut Physiology and Microflora

Poddar and colleagues (Poddar and Murgatroyd, 1976; Poddar, 1977; Poddar and Jacob, 1977) and Pfeiffer (1970a, b) have published rather extensively on the morphological and histological similarities of the gastrointestinal tract of the human, ferret, and monkey.

Recent efforts have failed to identify any anaerobic gut microflora in the ferret (Gad, 1989). Identified enteric organisms include *Salmonella, Campylobacter* sp., *Cryptosporidia* sp., and *Eimeria* sp.

Intravenous Dosing

Moody et al. (1985) concluded that the intravenous administration of a test article to ferrets is virtually impossible without an indwelling catheter because the species lacks easily accessible veins. More recently, Fox (1988) reiterated this and suggested that venous access (jugular, cephalic, and/or femoral) in the ferret may require sedation, local anesthesia, and a surgical skin incision for placement of a catheter for short-term drug of fluid administration.

However, McLain et al. (1987) have reported on the subchronic (90 day, thrice weekly), intravenous administration protocol in ferrets without the use of an indwelling catheter. Moreover, these authors routinely administer intravenous fluids repeatedly, and large volumes have been administered daily with prolonged infusion times by using either a 23 ga. × 1 in. needle, Angio- or Quik-Cath catheter. These procedures are possible with either mechanical or physical restraint of test animals (Figure 3A–C) and by access of the caudal vein.

The caudal veins of the ferret cannot be palpated, nor are they visible to the naked eye. To access these veins, view the dorsal surface of the shaved tail as the 12 o'clock position. Turn the tail in a clockwise or counterclockwise direction so that either of the large veins residing at the 10 o'clock or 2 o'clock position now assumes the 12 o'clock position. Insert a 23-gauge × 1-in needle (or Quik-Cath catheter, for example) at a depth and angle similar to that which would be used for rodents. The caudal artery assumes a 6 o'clock position when the animal is viewed dorsally. A diagram of a transverse section of the ferret tail, showing location of caudal artery and veins, was published by Bleakley (1980).

Typical intravenous infusion volumes and rates employed for ferrets depend, as with other species, upon the glomerular filtration rate (GFR) and the physical characteristics of the specific test article. Ferrets can probably receive between 2 and 4 ml/kg/hr of intravenous fluids without a notable increase in urine volume or frequency. This compares with an approximate continuous infusion rate of 0.5 ml/kg/hr for dogs, and 8 ml/kg/hr for rats. Using the aforementioned ratios and "reference" body weights of 0.25, 1.5, and 10.0 kg for rat, ferret, and dog, respectively, the approximate total daily (24 hr) fluid volume that may be delivered to these test species without notable increases in the urine volume or frequency is, therefore, 50 ml (rat), 70–140 ml (ferret), and 120 ml (dog). Humans (70 kg) typically may recieve volumes up to 3000 ml/day, or approximately 2 ml/kg/hr (Plumer, 1975). Increased fluid administration rates and volumes will generally be accommodated by all test species in direct relation to their individual GFRs.

Restraining Tube for Intravenous Dosing

Limited or initial intravenous dosing success may be possible with the crude ferret restraining device originally proposed by Curl and Curl (1985) for serial blood sampling. However, as the intravenous access capabilities of the laboratory improve, and more prolonged and frequent infusions are required in animals of different sizes, a more sophisticated restraint system will be necessary.

The device shown in Figure 3A was designed for the purpose of accommodating the increasing skills of the laboratory's technical staff. Four different sized restrainers have been developed and are proposed to accommodate the sexual dimorphism of ferrets, the seasonal deposition of body fat, and the various ages used in different research investigations. The inside diameters (ID) of the restraining tubes, and the corresponding weight ranges that they have accommodated include: 6.4 cm, 400–700 g; 7.9 cm, 650–1100 g; 8.8 cm, 1000–1750 g; 10.1 cm, 1500–2300 g. Details of construction have been reported by McLain and McGrain-Dutson (1989).

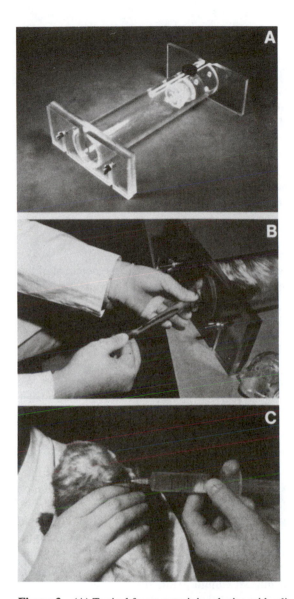

Figure 3 (A) Typical ferret restraining device with adjustable nose cone. The unit was designed to allow access to the caudal vessels, and for acute or chronic administration of test agents via indwelling catheters (see text for literature reference for restrainer construction). (B) Immobilized ferret with caudal vein marked on shaved tail. When multiple intravenous administrations are required, injections should commence at the tip of the tail and proceed caudad. (C) Physically restrained ferret with test agent being administered via an indwelling jugular catheter (see text for reference for construction and placement of indwelling venous catheters).

Surgical Implantation and Maintenance of Indwelling Intravenous Catheters in Ferrets

Indwelling intravenous catheters may be implanted in ferrets when it is necessary to administer solutions at a very slow or constant rate using an infusion pump, or for chronic studies requiring many consecutive days of treatment.

Greener and Gillies (1985) have developed a method to ensure catheter patency throughout the course or acute of chronic studies without the use of heparin. These authors fill the catheter lumen with saline solution, and clamp the catheter with a rubber-shod hemostat at the end of each infusion. They then remove the syringe containing a blunt needle from the lumen of the tubing, insert an appropriately sized stainless steel blocking pin, then remove the rubber-shod hemostat. When the stainless steel pin is pushed slightly further into the catheter, the saline fluid is forced to fill the lumen tip at the venous end, discouraging clot formation. A detailed description of catheter implantation and maintenance in ferrets was published by Greener and Gillies (1985). An earlier method for the chronic jugular catheterization of the ferret was published by Florczyk and Schurig (1981). Animals may be treated in the restraining tubes shown in Figure 3A and B (exciting catheter from the top of the tube) or hand-held and treated as shown in Figure 3C.

Inhalation Exposure of Ferrets

The pulmonary mechanics and physiology of the ferret lung as well as the potential of the species as an animal model for inhalation toxicology have been described quite thoroughly by Vinegar et al. (1979, 1982, 1985) and by Boyd and Mangos (1981). Noteworthy advantages to the use of ferrets in inhalation toxicology include the fact that since the ferret has more submucosal glands in bronchial wall and an additional generation of terminal bronchioles, it is closer to the human lung than is the dog lung. Moreover, the disportionately large lungs of the species may provide a useful tool for the studies of uptake, clearance, and deposition of aerosols, pulmonary blood flow, and diffusion. As suggested by Vinegar et al. (1985), they may also be good candidates for an isolated perfused lung preparation for metabolic studies and for regional lavage to look for markers of lung injury.

Physiological Measurements of the Ferret Lung

Physiological measurements were made by Vinegar et al. (1985) on anesthetized, tracheotomized, supine male ferrets. Six animals weighing 576 ± 12 g had tidal volumes (V_t) of 6.06 ± 0.30 ml, respiratory frequencies (f) of 26.7 ± 3.9/min, minute volume of 157.0 ± 14.8 ml/min., dynamic lung compliance (C-dyn) of 2.48 ± 0.21 ml/cmH$_2$O, pulmonary resistance (R) of 22.56 ± 1.61 ml/cmH$_2$O/L/sec. Measurements on nine ferrets (including the six above) revealed a total lung capacity (TLC) of 89 ± 5 ml, vital capacity (VC) of 87 ± 5 ml, expiratory reserve volume of 16 ± 2, and a functional residual capacity (FRC) of 17.8 ± 2.0 ml. Maximum expiratory flow-volume curves showed peak flows of 10.1 VC/sec at 75% VC and flows of 8.4 and 5.4 VC/sec at 50% and 25% VC.

The total lung capacity of ferrets was estimated to be approximately 297% of what would be predicted for an animal of its size.

Miscellaneous Dosing Routes

Intramuscular (im), subcutaneous (sc), intradermal (id), dermal, or intraperitoneal (ip) dosing procedures in the ferret are essentially no different than what would be practiced for other test species. Intramuscular administration, for example, is most easily given in the lateral aspect of the upper leg using a 28-gauge × ⅝-in needle. Subcutaneous or intradermal administration can be given just above the shoulders on the dorsal aspect of the neck, taking care not to deposit lipophilic test materials in subcutaneous fat pads as they will be poorly absorbed. A dermal application site (for an uncovered test material) which is inaccessible to the ferret is the dorsal aspect of the neck, immediately above the shoulders.

Intraperitoneal administration to ferrets is generally easier when performed by two people. One person should restrain the animal by securing the neck, shoulders, and front limbs with one hand while using the other hand to secure the hind limbs and position the animal on its back or against the holder's chest. The injection may be administered with an appropriate gauge needle through an elevated, pinched portion of skin located around mid-abdomen. Since ferret skin is very thick, care should be taken to assure that the test material is not deposited subcutaneously or intradermally.

Less frequently used routes of administration in the ferret might include intracerebral, intraduodenal, intrapleural, intranasal, intratracheal, intrathoracic, intravaginal, and rectal. Apparently, there are no unique anatomical features of the ferret which would preclude the use of any of these routes when the appropriate procedures are employed.

IMPORTANT PHYSICAL PARAMETERS

Developmental Milestones

At birth, ferret kits weigh between 7 and 10 g (Willis and Barrow, 1971; Shump and Shump, 1978). The deciduous teeth begin to erupt at approximately 2 weeks of age, and emerge completely through the gums at 18 days of age (Fox, 1988). Young ferrets will begin to consume moistened solid food as early as 2–3 weeks of age. They will begin to hear sound at approximately 32 days of age, and the eyes begin to open at approximately 34 days. The permanent canine teeth begin to appear at 47–52 days of age, and the deciduous canines are shed at approximately 56–70 days. Young ferrets are weaned at approximately 6–8 weeks postnatally.

Growth Curves and Typical Body Weight Ranges

At approximately 6–8 weeks of age a marked sexual dimorphism becomes apparent (Fig. 4), with adult male body weights (reached at approximately 4–5 months) eventually exceeding approximately twice that of adult females. Under optimum controlled environmental conditions, sexually inactive adult male ferrets, or hobs, will generally weigh between 1–2 kg at 5–7 months of age. In contrast, anestrous females (jills) will generally weigh between 0.5 and 1.0 kg at this same age. The observed range in body weight of sexually inactive animals maintained under controlled conditions is largely dependent upon the specific husbandry practiced, although the strain and source of supply (specific vendor) may also contribute.

Marked, seasonal body weight fluctuations as high as 30–40% are commonly observed in both sexes and coincide with the natural breeding season of the species (March–August). Hobs and jills as young as 4–5 months of age will generally begin to deposit subcutaneous body fat in the fall (under natural lighting conditions) in preparation for the spring breeding season. Teleologically speaking, this conformational change probably evolved to facilitate propagation and survival of the species. Under natural conditions, for example, sexually active male ferrets may ignore food for extended periods in their concentrated search for receptive females. In addition, the prolonged coitus (several hours) of the species and the frequently fatal exchange following the chance encounter of

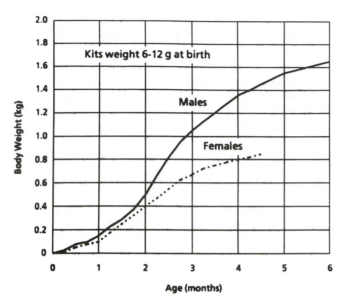

Figure 4   Growth curve for ferrets. A newborn kit's bodyweight will range between 6–12 grams at birth. At approximately eight weeks the sexual dimorphism of the species begins, with male ferrets eventually attaining an adult body weight approximately twice that of females.

two sexually active, territorial males can require tremendous amounts of energy. Males will generally return to, or remain at, a sexually inactive (undescended testicles) body weight under controlled lighting conditions. Females, on the other hand, because they are induced ovulators, may manifest a prolonged estrus with diminutive apetite and subsequent marked body weight loss. Optimum environmental lighting (see above) and hormonal injections (see above) will preclude the onset of bone marrow hypoplasia or pyometra associated with prolonged estrus in this species (Sherrill and Gorham, 1985).

Age at Maturation

Male and female ferrets are generally assumed to be sexually mature at 6–8 months of age. However, this will depend to a great extent on the photoperiodicity to which the individual animals are exposed (natural vs controlled), or to the month (season) in which they are born. It is possible, for example, for animals as young as 4 months of age to conceive and produce viable offspring.

Although rats are sexually (i.e., physiologically) mature at 50–60 days of age (Rowett, 1965), they are not routinely first-mated until approximately 100–120 days of age so that reproductive performance is maximized. McLain et al. (1985) has demonstrated that reproductive performance in primiparous ferrets is maximized at approximately 7–10 months of age, and decreases thereafter. Consequently, although physiological sexual maturity may occur earlier, 7–10 months is probably an optimum breeding age for ferrets.

Weight and Appearance of Testes

The male ferret's potential breeding season under natural lighting conditions extends from December to July, which precedes the female's breeding season of approximately March through August. Ryland and Gorham (1978) attribute this earlier sexual maturation of the male to a functional adaptation to allow for adequate sperm maturation.

Ishida (1968) and Basrur and Gilman (1968) also described the age and seasonal changes in the testis of the ferret. In ferrets born in June (natural lighting), bilateral testicular development started in December and reached maturity by February. The functional period lasting from March until July; the period of quiescence being from August until December.

Infantile ferret testes are characterized by the lack of a germinal cycle, by undifferentiated precursors of Sertoli cells, by the absence of a tubular lumen, and by small interstitial cells. The prepubertal testes become large as a result of the development of the germinal epithelium and tubular lumen, and by virtue of the growth of the Sertoli and interstitial cells (Ishida, 1968; Boissin and Boissin, 1979). The testes may range in weight from 0.8 to 3.8 g/kg, with a mean weight of approximately 2.02 g/kg (Fox, 1988).

The male ferret lacks seminal vesicles and bulbourethral glands. Moreover, the presence of a prostate gland in the ferret has been a subject of debate and, as in the majority of male mustelids, it has been classified as poorly developed (see Mead, 1970, and Allanson, 1932, for reviews). However, during the first several months of postnatal development of the male ferret and during its sexual quiescence, prostatic tissue is difficult to locate except through histological examination. The prostate of the adult, sexually active ferret, on the other hand, is visible at gross autopsy.

The ventrally located os penis is large for the animal's size, with the distal section curving dorsally so that it ends in a hook (Moody et al., 1985). The testes are located in the subcutaneous tissue of the caudoventral abdomen and descend into the scrotum only during the breeding season.

Frequency of Estrus

Female ferrets are seasonally polyestrous and will generally reach sexual maturation at approximately the same age as males. Estrus is induced by increased day length, or by manipulation of the photoperiod with artificial illumination (see above). The onset of estrus in female ferrets is recognized by a continuous vulval swelling occurring over an approximate 2-3-week period. The vulva will increase in size approximately 10-fold, measuring approximately 1.0–1.5 cm diameter in primiparous females, and aproximately 1.5–2.0 cm diameter in multiparous animals at peak receptivity. Mating should occur at the peak of vulval swelling (approximately 2 weeks after the onset), when it has a slightly pink and mucous-covered appearance. Ovulation is induced in the ferret approximately 30–36 hr after coitus, with implantation occurring approximately 12–13 days postcoitus. The vulva will begin to regress approximately 3–4 days after mating, regaining its preestrus size in approximately 2–3 weeks.

As indicated previously, female ferrets are induced ovulators and will remain in estrus for as long as 6 months if not mated. Prolonged estrus in this species may precipitate pyometra and/or complications of bone marrow hypoplasia and estrogen-induced anemia (see above). Females will generally return to estrus approximately 2 weeks after weaning of the litter (McLain et al., 1985). Occasionally, a lactation estrus will occur in females with less than five suckling young (Fox, 1988).

Gestational Period and Litter Size

McLain et al. (1985) analyzed demographic data for 945 female ferrets from a commercial breeding colony for the effects of various maternal characteristics on subsequent reproductive performance. In general, litter size (mean ± SEM) was found to be greatest for young, primiparous females (10.3 ± 0.2) and decreased with advanced maternal age and parity to a cohort mean of 8.1 ± 0.1 for third-parity females 16 months of age. Gestational length (mean ± SD) was 41.3 ± 1.1 days and appeared to decrease with increasing day length and total litter size. The gestation period in this cohort ranged from 39 days (observed in 32 primiparous jills) to 46 days (observed in four multiparous females). Reproductive data for ferrets are summarized in Table 6.

Normative Physiological Data

Studies of the effects and mechanisms of experimental treatments require that substantial normative physiological data for the species be established. Thus, as a contemporary animal model, the ferret continues to benefit from ongoing investigations contributing to this monumental task. Normative physiological data also aid in test species selection because in addition to its particular similarities with man, toxicologists will frequently select an animal model because the system of interest may be externally manipulated, or adapted to operate under extreme conditions. In this respect, much of the normative physiological data generated for ferrets has proven rewarding in that several potentially

Table 6 Typical Parameters of Reproduction in Ferrets Maintained Under Controlled Environmental Conditions

Parameter	Units	Value
Age at pairing, M/F	Months	8–10
Breeding life, M/F	Years	2–5
Breeding season, M/F	By photoperiod	All year
Type of estrus cycle	—	Monoestrus
Duration of estrus	Days	Prolonged
Copulation time	Hours	Up to 3
Sperm deposition site	—	Posterior cervix
Sperm capacitation	Hours	3–11
Sperm viability	Hours in tract	36–48
Mechanism of ovulation	—	Induced
Time of ovulation	Hours, postcoitus	30–36
No. of ova	Average	12, range: 5–18
Ovum transit time	Days, postcoitus	5–6
Time of implantation	Days, postcoitus	12–13
Length of gestation	Days	41, range: 39–46
Litter size	Average	8–10, range: 1–18
Wt. at birth	g	8, range: 6–12
Age at weaning	Weeks	6
Wt. at weaning	kg	0.2–0.4
Rebreeding	—	Immediately

Source: Data from Fox (1988), Marshall and Marshall, (1973); McLain et al. (1985), and Moody et al. (1985).

superior systems have been identified. On the other hand, the same contemporaries of ferrets continues to leave many questions unanswered.

Table 7 provides available normal cardiopulmonary data for the ferret.

Cardiovascular Parameters. Earlier discussions of the ferret's cardiovascular system were offered by Kempf and Chang (1949, macroscopic) and Borelli and Filho (1971, microscopic). Later reviews include those by Andrews et al. (1979), Baskin et al. (1981), and Andrews (1988).

Heart rate and blood pressure measurements have been made in both anesthetized and unanesthetized ferrets, but considerably more data have been generated for anesthetized animals. An apparent anesthetic effect on the heart rate is evident by the differences reported by Andrews et al. (1979) for animals under urethane anesthesia (387 ± 54 beats/min), and that reported by Thornton et al. (1979) for animals under barbituate anesthesia (230 ± 26 beats/min). In the unanesthetized animal, heart rates have been reported to range from 341 ± 39 beats/min (Andrews et al., 1979) to 200–255 beats/min (Thornton et al. 1979). Smith and Bishop (1985) have reported similar disparities in the heart rate (beats/min) of anesthetized (sodium pentobarbital) adult control ferrets (309, r.

Table 7 Selected Normative Cardiopulmonary Data for Ferrets Maintained Under Controlled Environmental Conditions

Parameter	Units	Value
Cardiovascular		
blood volume	ml/kg	60–70
blood pressure		
systolic	mmHg	140–164
diastolic	mmHg	110–125
cardiac output	ml/min	139 (r. 82–200)
circulation time		
fluorescein	sec	6.8 ± 1.2
cyanide	sec	4.5 ± 0.7
heart rate		
barbituate	beats/min	230 ± 26
halothane	beats/min	387 ± 54
conscious, active	beats/min	341 ± 39
conscious, inactive	beats/min	200–255
Pulmonary		
tidal volume	ml	6.06 ± 0.30
respiration rate		
conscious	bpm	33–36
pentabarbital	bpm	26.7 ± 3.9
dynamic compliance	ml/cmH$_2$O	2.48 ± 0.21
pulmonary resistance	cmH20/L/sec	22.56 ± 1.61
total capacity	ml	89 ± 5
functional resid. cap.	ml	17.8 ± 2.0

Source: Data from Andrews et al. (1979), Thornton et al. (1979), Kempf and Chang (1949), Andrews (1988), and Vinegar et al. (1985).

250–380), anesthetized (sodium pentobarbital) adult ferrets with right ventricular hyper-trophy (300, r. 245–380) and anesthetized (ketamine) weanling ferrets (280, r. 210–360). Andrews and Illman (1987) have suggested that the problem of variations in the heart rate of the ferret could be resolved by recording the animal's activity level and by viewing the results under different anesthetics as two ends of a spectrum, between which the heart rate of the unanesthetized animal would operate according to the animal's activity level.

Apparently, Kempf and Chang (1949) have provided the only measurement of cardiac output and circulation time in ferrets. In their study of barbituate-anesthetized animals, cardiac output measured 139 ml/min (range 82–200 ml/min) and circulation time meas-ured 6.8 ± 1.2 sec (fluorescein) and 4.5 ± 0.7 sec (cyanide). Under urethane or barbituate anesthesia, mean systolic blood pressure values between 140–164 mmHg have been reported for the ferret, with diastolic values of 110–125 mmHg (Kempf and Chang, 1949; Andrews et al., 1979). In the conscious animal, systolic values have been reported as 161 mmHg (males) and 133 (females), with some animals presenting with blood pressure values as high as 190 mmHg (Thornton et al., 1979).

The electrocardiogram (ECG) of normal ferrets and ferrets with right ventricular hypertrophy has been reported by Smith and Bishop (1985). These authors concluded that the normal ferret has a mean electrical axis of +86 degrees $\pm$ 6.6 (SD), with a narrow range between +69 and +97 degrees. All animals in their study exhibited a normal sinus rhythm, composed of the expected P wave, QRS complex, and T wave.

Experience from our (D.E.M.) laboratory has indicated that a maximum of approx-imately 50–60% of a ferret's total blood volume be removed by cardiac puncture technique (exsanguination). Therefore, estimates suggest that the ferret's total blood volume is 6–7% of the body weight, or approximately 60–70 ml/kg.

Pulmonary Parameters. An early study by Barer et al. (1979) and a species comparison study by Peake et al. (1981) investigated the response of the blood-perfused ferret lung to hypoxia. Both groups of authors concluded that of several species investigated, the ferret has the most marked pulmonary vasoconstriction in response to hypoxia, with a maximum response occurring at approximately 25 mmHg. Vinegar et al. (1982) have postulated that the sensitivity to hypoxia in the ferret may be an adaptation to burrowing. The sensitivity of the ferret's pulmonary vasculature to hypoxia makes it a valuable model for the study of pulmonary hypertension in humans.

In addition to the extensive data generated by Vinegar et al. (1985), which was discussed previously, various other investigators have examined the respiratory rate of ferrets. For example, Pyle (1940) reported the rate to be 33–36 breaths/min in the conscious ferret as compared to values of 31 ± 6 breaths/min in urethane-anesthetized animals (Andrews et al., 1979) and 43.5 ± 4.6 breaths/min in pentobarbital-anesthetized animals (Boyd and Mangos, 1981). Similar to the results in the cardiovascular system, the disparity in reported repiration rates of the ferret may be the result of differences in type or dosage of anesthesia, or the age of the animals. Scientific protocols should, therefore, include requirements for documentation of these variables.

Normative pulmonary and cardiovascular values for ferrets are summarized in Table 7.

CLINICAL LABORATORY PARAMETERS

Data for hematological and serum chemistry determinations in ferrets have been reported by Thornton et al. (1979), Lee et al. (1982), Moody et al. (1985), and Fox (1988).

However, all of these studies used small numbers of animals, and only Lee and colleagues described the variability in their sample of five females and eight males (three intact, five castrated). Fox (1988) contrasted the analytical results obtained in his laboratory from both orbital plexus and cardiac blood sample sites in ferrets. However, the data were not expressed statistically and an estimation of variability was not provided. To date, therefore, no studies have satisfactorily described the hemogram of laboratory ferrets with respect to sample variability and the distribution around the mean. Moreover, since Neptun et al. (1985, 1986) concluded that both sampling site and collection method are a major source of variation in clinical laboratory measurements of homogeneous laboratory rats, the potential for sample site and collection method differences must be adequately evaluated in ferrets. Obviously, when differences can be demonstrated, selection of an appropriate collection method and sampling site should include a consideration of which parameters are likely to be of major interest. For heterogeneous species such as the ferret, this would seem especially important.

In our (D.E.M.) experience, a significant amount of clinical laboratory data have been personally accumulated from ferrets used in acute and subacute GLP testing protocols. Moreover, the experimental results generated with these animals have been submitted to the FDA in fulfillment of the requirement for test data generated in a second species. In all probability, the sound statistical treatment of the data generated in these studies (McLain and Lin, 1989c), which is deemed necessary and appropriate for normalization of any heterogeneous species, was well received by the FDA reviewers and contributed significantly to the success of each submission process. Therefore, these data and discussion of their statistical treatment are summarized in the following sections.

Blood Sample Collection

Blood samples for clinical laboratory determinations in ferrets may be collected by several routes. Cardiac puncture and orbital plexus sampling of anesthetized animals may be the most rapid and efficient method when large numbers of samples are to be processed. However, alternative sites include toenail clipping, jugular venipuncture, and tail vein and artery for repeated sampling such as in pharmacokinetic analyses (McLain et al., 1985a).

Hematological Parameters

In construction of the following database, blood for clinical pathology was collected in tubes containing either sodium citrate (3.8%) or potassium ethylenediaminetetraacetate (EDTA). Blood collected in tubes containing sodium citrate was used for the determination of prothrombin time (PT), activated partial thromboplastin time (APTT), and fibrinogen level. Blood collected in tubes containing EDTA was used for determination of all other hematological parameters.

Hematological determinations collected before experimental treatment in 370 adult (6–10 months) ferrets (187 males, 183 females) are summarized in Tables 8 to 9. Reference values for the clotting factors (APTT, PT) were determined after intravenous saline treatment (single dose) of 64 animals (32 males, 32 females) from the above cohort, and from 32 additional animals (16 males, 16 females) who served as untreated controls in the above cohort. All ferrets were obtained from the same vendor. Fasted blood samples were collected from anesthetized animals (KET-ACE, 10:1, 35 mg/kg im) via cardiac puncture and assayed by conventional methods. Approximately 1.3% of the samples collected for hematology were not analyzed for various reasons. Approximately 13.5% of

Table 8 Hematology Values for Adult Ferrets Maintained Under Controlled Environmental Conditions

Parameter	Sex	Mean	STD	N	MIN	MAX	Central tendency	Tolerance limit			Sex effect	Transformation
								lower	upper	method		
Hemoglobin (g/dl)	F	16.2	1.3	180	10.9	19.0	16.2	13.5	18.9	P	P<0.001	None
	M	16.8	1.2	185	13.3	20.0	16.8	14.3	19.3			
Hematocrit (%)	F	48.4	4.0	180	33.2	57.8	48.4	40.0	56.8	P	P<0.01	None
	M	49.8	3.7	185	39.6	62.0	49.8	42.0	57.5			
RBC (mil/mm³)	F	9.30	0.84	180	5.77	11.52	9.30	7.52	11.08	P	P<0.001	None
	M	9.69	0.71	185	7.95	11.86	9.69	8.18	11.19			
MCV (µ³)	F	52.2	2.0	180	42.5	60.3	52.2	48.0	56.4	P	P<0.001	None
	M	51.4	1.4	185	47.9	54.9	51.4	48.4	54.4			
MCH (pg)	F	17.5	0.7	180	14.8	20.5	17.5	16.0	19.0	P	NS	None
	M	17.3	0.7	185	15.6	19.2	17.3	15.9	18.7			
MCHC (%)	F	33.5	0.9	180	30.5	36.7	33.5	31.6	35.4	P	P<0.05	None
	M	33.8	0.9	185	31.5	36.1	33.8	31.8	35.8			
Platelet (10³/mm³)	F	764	246	157	330	1520	726	364	1447	P	NS	Ln(X)
	M	766	196	163	315	1525	742	438	1256			
Fibrinogen (mg/dl)	F	184	66	182	83	548	170	99	376	P	NS	Ln(X-63)
	M	189	28	187	93	657	173	101	387			
WBC (10³/mm³)	F	7.6	3.2	180	2.9	23.1	7.0	3.0	16.3	P	P<0.001	Ln(X)
	M	9.2	2.7	185	3.7	18.2	8.8	4.6	16.6			
Lymphocytes (10³/mm³)	F	3.4	1.8	180	1.0	11.1	3.0	1.1	8.2	P	P<0.001	Ln(X)
	M	4.2	1.6	185	1.2	8.3	3.9	1.7	9.0			
PMN (10³/mm³)	F	3.8	2.0	180	1.2	13.3	3.4	1.2	9.4	P	P<0.001	Ln(X)
	M	4.5	2.0	185	1.4	13.0	4.1	1.7	9.9			
EOS (10³/mm³)	F	0.25	0.22	180	0.00	1.39	0.18	0.00	0.78	N	P<0.01	NA
	M	0.33	0.28	185	0.00	2.13	0.25	0.00	0.92			
MONO (10³/mm³)	F	0.09	0.13	180	0.00	0.86	0.05	0.00	0.48	N	NS	NA
	M	0.11	0.13	185	0.00	0.84	0.09	0.00	0.37			
BASO (10³/mm³)	F	0.03	0.07	180	0.00	0.46	0.00	0.00	0.23	N	P<0.05	NA
	M	0.04	0.08	185	0.00	0.49	0.00	0.00	0.25			
STAB (10³/mm³)	F	0.01	0.03	180	0.00	0.22	0.00	0.00	0.13	N	NS	NA
	M	0.01	0.05	185	0.00	0.40	0.00	0.00	0.14			

P = parametric; N = nonparametric; NS = not significant; NA = not applicable; Ln = natural logarithm.

Table 9 Whole Blood Clotting Factors, Serum Electrolytes, and Serum Enzyme Levels for Adult Ferrets Maintained Under Controlled Environmental Conditions

Parameter	Sex	Mean	STD	N	MIN	MAX	Central Tendency	Tolerance limit Lower	Upper	Method	Sex effect	Transformation
Blood clotting factors												
PT (sec)	M+F	11.1	0.4	94	10.3	12.4	11.0	10.3	12.1	P	NS	Ln(X-9)
APTT (sec)	M+F	20.9	24.5	94	13.9	200.0	17.1	14.8	21.2	P	NS	Ln(X-11.8)
Serum Electrolytes												
Na (mEq/L)	M+F	150	4	96	135	159	150	141	159	P	NS	None
K (mEq/L)	M+F	4.76	0.5	96	3.90	6.80	4.70	4.09	5.97	P	NS	Ln (X-3.5)
Cl (mEq/L)	M+F	114	3	96	96	124	114	108	120	P	NS	None
Serum enzymes												
Alk. Phos.	F	40	18	183	13	106	35	18	92	P	NS	Ln(X-10)
(IU/L)	M	37	18	187	15	99	33	17	88			
LDH	F	621	407	183	174	2030	476	177	2341	P	NS	Ln(X-120)
(IU/L)	M	595	505	187	143	3030	426	163	2309			
SGOT	F	97	48	183	34	271	82	41	282	P	NS	Ln(X-30)
(IU/L)	M	92	56	187	36	442	78	41	236			
SGPT	F	210	226	183	47	1710	146	55	765	P	NS	Ln(X-40)
(IU/L)	M	205	207	187	45	1850	153	60	670			

P = parametric; N = nonparametric; NS = not significant; NA = not applicable; Ln = natural logarithm.

the platelet samples were "clumped" and not suitable for analysis. Only one of 370 fibrogen samples collected was not reported. Mortality associated with this blood collection procedure was generally low (approximately 2%), occurred largely in females, and was apparently correlated with the quantity of blood withdrawn from the animal (10 ml/animal, or approximately 10 and 20% of the total blood volume of males and females, respectively).

Methodological procedures used on the Coulter hemoglobinometer, Coulter ZBI, MLA 700, or by microscope for determination of hematology reference values included: APTT (clotting time, cephaloplastin), PT (clotting time, thromboplastin), hemoglobin (HGB, Coulter Hemoterge II), hematocrit (HCT, calculated), erythrocytes (RBC, electrical resistance), mean corpuscular volume (MCV, electrical resistance), mean corpuscular hemoglobin (MCH, calculated), mean corpuscular hemoglobin concentration (MCHC, calculated), platelet count (Unopette, manual), fibrinogen (optics), leukocytes (WBC, electrical resistance), and lymphocyte count, PMN count, eosinophils (EOS), monocytes (MONO), basophils (BASO), and band neutrophils (STAB) by Wright-Giemsa stain.

Noteworthy observations in sample collection included the fact that many citrate tubes were hemolyzed and a large percentage of platelet samples were clumped. Additionally, a manual method, which takes three times longer than the automated method, was necessary for analysis of platelets because of their large size. Finally, relative to other species, ferrets have many RBCs and blood samples will require a dilution before running on the Coulter ZBI. An additional 20–80% may require further dilution.

Table 8 lists the calculated reference values for selected hematology measurements of the ferret. The first column lists the various parameters and their units. The third through seventh columns list the descriptive statistics, which include the mean, standard deviation (STD), number of observations (N), minimum value (MIN), and maximum value (MAX). These descriptive statistics were based on the original units (scale) and were not affected by the transformation, if needed. The last column lists the transformation, if needed, for skewed distributions of measurement to become approximately normally (Gausian) distributed. The eighth column lists the central tendency of each parameter. The central tendency is the antitransformation of the transformed mean. For example, it is the geometrical mean if a logarithmic transformation is applied. If a transformation is needed, the central tendency better represents the norm of the population than the mean would. The next two columns list the tolerance limits. The tolerance limits contain 95% of the measurements (in the original scale) of untreated ferrets with 90% confidence. The next to the last column lists the test on the difference between means of males and females. Finally, the eleventh column explains whether the tolerance limits and the sex effect were determined by parametric (P) or nonparametric (N) methods.

Reference values for the clotting factors (PT, APTT) are listed separately with the electrolytes and serum proteins (Table 9). Unlike the values in Table 8, these reference values are listed combining males and females. This was done because the database was much smaller, and no sex differences were detected for any of the parameters.

By comparison, the variance observed in ferret hematology is approximately one-half of that reported for humans (Conn, 1963), minimally greater than the beagle dog, and considerably greater than the inbred SPF and virus-free rat (see specific chapters). Notable exceptions (increases or decreases) in mean values for hematological parameters in ferrets relative to humans include (males only, ferret/human): RBC (million/mm^3), 9.69 $\pm$ 0.71/5.4 $\pm$ 0.8; MCV (μ^3), 51.4 $\pm$ 1.4/87 $\pm$ 5; MCH (pg), 17.3 $\pm$ 0.7/29 $\pm$ 2; and, platelets (range, mm^3), 438–1236/150–450. Thornton et al. (1979) observed a higher

HCT (and RBCs) in ferrets relative to rats and dogs and recommended a 20% longer spin time (due to a negligible RBC sedimentation rate of the ferret) for blood samples used for microhematocrit determination. These authors also reported a higher HGB level in males (55.4, n = 28) relative to females (49.2, n = 11), and no sex difference in number of WBCs (or differential). The present database confirmed a high HCT and HGB in ferrets. However, the sex difference in HGB, although still significant, is apparently not as large when cardiac blood samples are used or when the sample size is increased. Furthermore, the observation in the present study that male ferrets have significantly greater numbers of WBCs (including lymphocytes, polymorphonuclear neutrophils, eosinophils, and basophils) than females is in contrast to what Thornton et al. (1979) have reported and in agreement with Lee et al. (1982).

Serum Chemistry Parameters

Reference serum chemistry values obtained from the same population of animals are listed in Table 10. The blood collection procedure and table format are the same as described above. Serum electrolytes and enzymes have been included in Table 9 with the clotting factors.

Methodological procedures used on the Hitachi 705 Chemistry Analyzer for determination of reference values included: albumin (bromcresol green), alkaline phosphatase (modified Bowers/McComb), SGOT and SGPT (modified Henry), BUN (urease), calcim (CPC), chloride (Beckman E4), cholesterol (esterase/oxidase), creatinine (Jaffe), glucose (hexokinase) LDH (modified Wacker), Na and K (Beckman E4), phosphorus (molybdate), total bilirubin (DPD), total globulin and A/G ratio (calculated), total protein (Biuret), uric acid (uricase).

Similar to the hematological findings, the variance observed in ferret clinical chemistry is minimally greater than the beagle dog and considerably greater than the inbred SPF and virus-free rat (see specific chapters). Notable exceptions (increases or decreases) in the range in values for serum chemistry parameters in ferrets relative to humans (Conn, 1963) include (males only, ferret/human): glucose (fasting, mg/dl), 81–142/60–100; BUN (mg/dL), 13–37/10–20; uric acid (mg/dl), 0.4–2.8/3.0–6.0; creatinine (mg/dl), 0.20–0.70/0.7–1.5; SGOT (IU/dl), 41–236/5–40; SGPT (IU/dl), 60–670/5–35; LDH (IU/dl), 163–2309/200–680; and, alkaline phosphatase (IU/dl), 17–88/5–13. The considerable range in clinical chemistry parameters of the ferret, especially the liver enzymes, obviates the need for an analysis of the "change from baseline" rather than any particular absolute value in this species. Moreover, appropriate transformations should be applied whenever possible to all posttreatment values adjusted for pretreatment measurements.

Effect of Sampling Site on Variations in Baseline Clinical Pathology Parameters of the Ferret

Tables 11 and 12 describe the influence of sample collection site on the variance of certain blood parameters of the ferret. In this analysis, the variances of select parameters of samples collected by the cardiac puncture technique described previously (n = 370) were compared to the variation in pretreatment blood samples, collected by orbital plexus technique, from 58 additional ferrets. The sex effect was removed in this comparison (i.e., the variance was pooled across sexes). The p value in Tables 11 and 12 is for comparing variances between collection sites.

For all of the hematology parameters listed in Table 11, except WBCs and basophils,

Table 10 Serum Chemistry Values for Adult Ferrets Maintained in a Controlled Environment

Parameter	Sex	Mean	STD	N	MIN	MAX	Central Tendency	Tolerance Limit			Sex Effect	Transformation
								Lower	Upper	Method		
Calcium	F	9.6	0.9	183	5.0	11.0	9.6	8.0	11.2	P	NS	None
(mg/dl)	M	9.5	0.7	187	6.9	11.2	9.5	8.0	11.1			
Phosphorus	F	6.5	1.0	183	4.0	8.7	6.5	4.4	8.5	P	p<0.001	None
(mg/dl)	M	7.0	1.0	187	4.9	9.5	7.0	5.0	9.0			
Glucose	F	118	25	183	62	387	116	85	152	P	p<0.001	Ln(X+96)
(mg/dl)	M	110	15	187	28	164	110	81	142			
BUN	F	27	14	183	5	76	23	12	71	P	p<0.001	Ln(X-9)
(mg/dl)	M	21	7	187	12	76	20	13	37			
Uric acid	F	1.8	0.5	183	0.5	3.5	1.7	0.8	3.2	P	p<0.001	Ln(X+0.74)
(mg/dl)	M	1.3	0.6	187	0.2	3.0	1.3	0.4	2.8			
Cholesterol	F	183	33	183	96	269	183	112	254	P	p<0.001	None
(mg/dl)	M	162	25	187	107	238	162	108	215			
Bilirubin	F	0.2	0.1	183	0.0	0.4	0.2	0.0	0.3	N	NS	NA
(mg/dl)	M	0.2	0.1	187	0.0	0.4	0.2	0.0	0.3			
Creatinine	F	0.44	0.12	183	0.30	1.00	0.40	0.20	0.70	N	p<0.001	NA
(mg/dl)	M	0.48	0.10	187	0.20	1.00	0.50	0.20	0.70			
Total protein	F	5.9	0.8	183	3.5	9.7	5.9	4.3	7.6	P	NS	None
(g/dl)	M	6.0	0.8	187	3.9	11.2	6.0	4.6	7.4			
Albumin	F	3.4	0.5	183	1.8	5.7	3.4	2.4	4.4	P	NS	None
(g/dl)	M	3.5	0.4	187	2.2	4.5	3.5	2.6	4.4			
Globulin	F	2.5	0.5	183	1.2	5.5	2.4	1.8	3.8	P	NS	Ln(X-1.23)
(g/dl)	M	2.6	0.7	187	1.7	8.4	2.4	1.8	3.8			
A/G ratio	F	1.39	0.28	183	0.56	3.25	1.40	0.80	1.82	P	NS	X^2
	M	1.42	0.29	187	0.33	2.05	1.45	0.72	1.92			
Bilirubin	F	0.2	0.1	183	0.0	0.4	0.2	0.0	0.3	N	NS	NA
(mg/dl)	M	0.2	0.1	187	0.0	0.4	0.2	0.0	0.3			

P = parametric; N = nonparametric; NS = not significant; NA = not applicable; Ln = natural logarithm

Table 11 Effect of Sampling Site on Variations in Baseline Hematology Parameters of Ferrets

Parameter[a]	No. of samples[b]	Cardiac puncture mean	STD	Orbital plexus mean	STD	p value
Hemoglobin, g/dl	365/37	16.50	1.46	17.90	1.79	0.00000
Hematocrit, %	365/37	49.10	3.82	54.80	6.39	0.00000
RBC, 10^6/mm^3	365/37	9.50	0.78	10.53	1.01	0.00000
MCV, mm^3	365/37	51.80	1.73	52.00	3.02	0.00000
MCH, pg	365/37	17.40	0.71	17.00	0.77	0.02304
MCHC, %	365/37	33.70	0.95	32.80	1.10	0.00088
Platelet, 10^3/mm^3	320/27	6.60	0.28	6.30	0.37	0.00000
WBC, 10^3/mm^3	365/37	2.06	0.36	2.48	0.28	0.04223
lymphocytes, %	365/37	45.90	12.15	47.80	14.07	0.00274
STAB, %	365/37	0.14	0.44	0.34	0.95	0.00000
MONO, %	365/37	1.16	1.31	2.66	1.83	0.00000
EOS, %	365/37	3.41	2.42	2.90	2.59	0.08827
BASO, %	365/37	0.41	0.74	0.05	0.23	0.00000
POLY, %	365/37	49.10	12.28	46.50	13.57	0.02803

[a]Transformed values include: platelet = Ln(X) and WBC = Ln(X).
[b]No. of samples = cardiac puncture/orbital plexus.

the sample variance was significantly increased when collected by the orbital plexus relative to cardiac puncture. Moreover, when the critical level of significance is set at $\alpha = 0.05$, only eosinophils collected by each technique did not differ. Based upon the number of clotted hematology samples in this analysis (12/58), however, as well as the personal (D.E.M.) observations, it is recommended that each laboratory confirm their collection proficiency by this route in this species before protocol collection is initiated. In addition, the acceptability of each sample should be confirmed before an animal is returned to the home cage.

For 16 clinical chemistry parameters in Table 12, eight parameters (uric acid, calcium, total protein, albumin, globulin, alkaline phosphatase, LDH, and SGPT), especially the liver enzymes, showed significantly smaller variances when collected from the orbital plexus. Conversely, five parameters (BUN, creatinine, bilirubin, glucose, and phosphorus) showed significantly larger variance, and cholesterol, SGOT, and A/G showed no significant difference.

Although reference to previously published mean values for this species is inappropriate, it is noted that the orbital plexus appears to provide hematological and clinical chemistry mean values similar to those reported by Thornton et al. (1979) for samples collected form the abdominal aorta. A much larger database would, however, have to be examined to confirm this.

Data from the foregoing analyses indicate that if protocols specify that blood samples are to be collected from multiple sites (i.e., cardiac puncture for hematology and orbital plexus for clinical chemistry), reductions in sample variance can be expected in most parameters, especially the liver enzymes. Alternatively, one can choose to opti-

Table 12 Effect of Sampling Site on Variations in Baseline Serum Chemistry Parameters of Ferrets

Parameter[a]	No. of samples[b]	Cardiac puncture		Orbital plexus		p Value
		mean	STD	mean	STD	
Calcium, mg/dl	368/57	9.59	0.74	9.90	0.55	0.00329
Phosphorus, mg/dl	370/57	6.72	0.97	8.60	1.12	0.00346
Glucose, mg/dl	369/57	5.35	0.10	5.33	0.17	0.00000
Cholesterol, mg/dl	370/57	173	29.7	185	30.6	0.28056
BUN, mg/dl	369/57	2.51	0.59	2.53	0.69	0.00169
Uric acid, mg/dl	370/56	0.80	0.25	1.17	0.18	0.00222
Bilirubin, mg/dl	370/58	0.17	0.10	0.06	0.13	0.00001
Creatinine, mg/dl	370/57	0.46	0.11	0.51	0.13	0.00012
Total protein, mg/dl	369/57	5.96	0.73	6.20	0.40	0.00000
Albumin, mg/dl	370/57	3.44	0.46	3.69	0.30	0.00014
Globulin, mg/dl	368/57	0.19	0.36	0.24	0.26	0.00241
A/G ratio	368/57	2.04	0.69	2.33	0.64	0.24671
Alk. phos., IU/l	370/58	3.18	0.57	3.32	0.30	0.00000
LDH, IU/l	370/58	5.80	0.90	6.67	0.62	0.00064
SGOT, IU/l	370/58	3.91	0.72	4.24	0.52	0.00158
SGPT, IU/l	370/58	4.70	0.87	4.61	0.60	0.00053

[a]Transformed values include: glucose = $Ln(X+69)$; BUN = $Ln(X-9)$; uric acid = $Ln(X+0.74)$; globulim = $Ln(X-1.23)$; A/G Ratio = X^2, alk. phos. $Ln(X-10)$; LDH = $Ln(X-120)$; SGOT = $Ln(X-30)$; SGPT = $Ln(X-40)$.
[b]No. of samples = cardiac puncture/orbital plexus.

mize the ability to detect subtle changes in a select parameter by collecting a blood sample from the site affording the least variability.

Estimation of Ferret Sample Size Requirements for Optimum Statistical Power

McLain and Lin (1989c) demonstrated that, when it is desired to achieve a statistical power in ferrets similar to that enjoyed with the less heterogeneous beagle dog, the needed sample size to detect a prespecified difference with prespecified statistical power and type I error is proportional to the pure variance (random error). Therefore, the ferret's sample size requirement for any select parameter relative to the beagle dog's is, for practical purposes, the ratio of their pure variances adjusted (optimally) for pretreatment measurements using ANCOVA. When there is no a priori knowledge of target organ, or of a specific parameter's potential for change in response to experimental treatment, then a weighted average of parameter variances can be used to estimate sample size requirements. The correlation coefficient between a parameter's posttreatment and pretreatment value should be used to assign weights, and the geometrical mean should be calculated. When the variance by cardiac puncture sample site is employed, the weighted geometrical mean of the sample size ratio of ferret/dog (based on the author's data) can be calculated to be 1.8, or approximately two ferrets for each beagle dog. When the variance and correlation coefficient calculations incorporate the effect of sample site, then the weighted geometrical mean of the sample size of ferret/dog is reduced to 1.3, or aproximately three ferrets for every two dogs. Table 13 and Figure 5 illustrate the calculated variance ratios (ferret/dog) for serum chemistry and the various liver enzymes by different sample sizes and sampling sites. These data demonstrate that when a single ferret is used for each dog, the variance ratio for alkaline phosphatase, for example, is approximately 2.5; i.e., it can be concluded that 2.5 times more ferrets are necessary to achieve a parameter variance which is approximately equal to that of the dog. Conversely, when alkaline phosphatase is calculated from an orbital plexus blood sample, the variance ratio drops to approximately 0.75; i.e., it is now concluded that 1.25 dogs are necessary to achieve a parameter variance which is approximately equal to that of the ferret.

Urinalysis

Urinalysis is a good general screening procedure for ferrets that can provide a wide variety of useful clinical information regarding an individual ferret's kidneys and the systemic diseases that may affect this excretory organ. Collection procedures are similar to what would be performed for rodents, with a special emphasis placed upon minimizing fecal contamination of the sample. Prestudy samples will help to identify pathological conditions which would justify eliminating an animal from consideration for testing. Additionally, prestudy urine samples can be subtracted from posttreatment samples to more precisely evaluate the response to experimental treatment.

Table 13 Effects of Sample Size and Sample Method on the Adjusted (ANCOVA) Variance Ratios for Serum Chemistry Parameters of Ferrets and Dogs

	Variance Ratio (ferret/dog)			
	Cardiac puncture		Orbital plexus	
Sampling method: Sample size Ratio:	1:1	2:1	1:1	2:1
Parameter				
calcium	1.353	0.677	0.735	0.368
glucose	4.272	2.136	—	—
BUN	2.777	1.389	—	—
uric acid	0.640	0.320	0.419	0.210
bilirubin	0.614	0.307	0.389	0.195
creatinine	0.802	0.401	—	—
total protein	1.864	0.932	0.568	0.284
albumin	2.492	1.246	1.079	0.540
globulin	1.091	0.546	0.631	0.316
A/G ratio	0.899	0.450	0.749	0.375
Alk. phos.	2.514	1.257	0.760	0.380
LDH	1.647	0.824	1.070	0.535
SGOT	4.244	2.122	3.395	1.698
SGPT	3.992	1.996	2.016	1.008

Missing values show no improvement with orbital plexus collection.

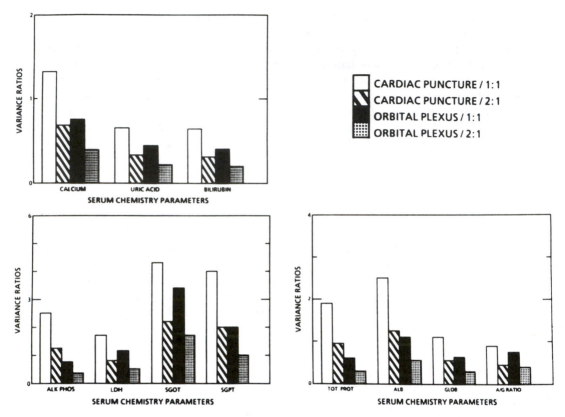

Figure 5   Serum chemistry parameter variance ratios for ferrets relative to beagle dogs (ferret/dog) as a function of sample site (cardiac puncture or orbital plexus) and sample size (ferret : dog = 1 : 1 or 2 : 1). Ratios less than one favor the ferret.

Thornton et al. (1979) published the means and ranges for volume (ml), sodium (mmol), potassium (mmol), and chloride (mmol) for "feces-free" urine samples collected over a 24-hr period from 40 male and 24 female ferrets. In addition, they analyzed the urine samples for protein, ketones, blood, and bilirubin using reagent strips (Ames Bililabstix), and discussed the results of these findings.

The following database of macroscopic (Table 15) and microscopic (Table 16) urine parameters of the ferret was compiled in our (D.E.M.) laboratory from ferrets used in the GLP studies discussed previously. All of the ferrets were obtained from the same supplier (Marshall Farms, North Rose, New York) and were approximately the same age. Animals were placed in rodent metabolism cages for overnight urine collection. The particular type of metabolism cage employed minimized (but probably did not totally eliminate) urine-feces contact and precluded drinking water dilution of the urine samples.

Statistical Treatment of Urine Data

Analysis of variance (ANOVA, $\alpha = 0.05$) techniques were used in the following macroscopic and microscopic urine parameter databases to test for a sex effect for the continuous parameters (specific gravity and total volume). Sex differences were detected for total volume. Therefore, reference values must be considered separately for males and females for this parameter.

Scores were assigned to the responses for the catagorical parameters. These scores are summarized in Table 14. The assignment of scores was necessary to test for a sex effect and for calculating summary statistics. Table 14 must be used to interpret the categorical parameters in Tables 15 and 16. The scoring method of Grizzle et al. (1969) was applied to test for a sex effect ($\alpha = 0.05$). Sex differences were detected with respect to pH, blood, epithelial cells, WBCs, RBCs, and bacteria. Therefore, reference values must be considered separately for males and females for these parameters. The parameters of urobilinogen, glucose, ketone, and crystals were constant.

The reference values were calculated as statistical tolerance limits (90% confidence for 95% of the ferret population). These are expressed as a low and high value and are interpreted as follows: 95% of normal ferrets will have a parameter response between the low value and high value (with 90% confidence).

Nonparametric tolerance intervals were calculated for the categorical parameters. Categorical parameters are not normally distributed. The lower and upper limits for nonparametric intervals are of the form of "order statistics" of the categorical data. examples of order statistics are: lowest value, highest value, third highest value, or sixth highest value. The selection of the order statistic depends on the sample size, the confidence level and the proportion of the population which the interval is to include.

Tolerance limits based on the normal distribution were calculated for the continuous, normally distributed parameters. The lower and upper limits for normal tolerance limits are of the form: mean $\pm$ factor $\times$ standard deviation. The selection of the factor depends on the sample size, the confidence level, and the proportion of the population which the interval is to include.

If a continuous parameter was skewed, an appropriate transformation was determined to normalize the distribution. The normal tolerance limits were then calculated for the

Table 14 Scores Assigned to Categorical Responses in Ferret Urinalysis

Parameter	Assigned score				
	0	1	2	3	4
Color	Pale Yellow	Yellow	Light Amber	Amber	Brown
Turbidity	Clear	Sl. Cloudy	Cloudy	Turbid	—
Protein, glucose, ketone, blood	Neg.	Trace	1+	2+	3+
Bilirubin	Neg.	Pos.	1+	2+	—
Mucous, epithelial cells, crystals, triple PO4, Ca oxalate, bacteria, sperm	None	Rare	Few	Mod.	Many
Casts	None	Rare	1–4	5–9	—

Assigned scores for WBC and RBC									
0	1	2	3	4	5	6	7	8	9
None	Rare	1–4	5–9	10–14	15–19	20–29	30–49	50+	TNTC

TNTC = too numerous to count.

Table 15   Reference Semiquantitative Macroscopic Urine Profiles of Adult Male and Female Ferrets Maintained Under Controlled Environmental Conditions

Parameter	Sex	Mean	STD	N	MIN	MAX	Median	Tolerance limit		method	Sex effect	Transformation
								lower	upper			
Volume (ml)	F	21.4	11.9	94	1	59	19.0	4.0	58.0	P	$p<0.05$	Ln $(X+5.27)$
	M	31.8	21.0	98	6	114	27.4	6.1	88.5			
Color	F	1.0	0.4	94	0	3	1	0	3	P	NS	None
	M	1.0	0.4	98	0	4	1	0	2			
Turbidity	F	1.2	1.1	95	0	3		0	3	P	NS	None
	M	1.2	0.9	98	0	3	1	0	3			
Spec. Grav.	F	1.043	0.016	94	1.013	1.080	1.042	1.007	1.078	P	NS	None
	M	1.047	0.016	98	1.013	1.084	1.047	1.012	1.082			
pH	F	6.2	0.3	94	6.0	7.5	6.0	6.0	7.5	P	$p<0.05$	None
	M	6.1	0.2	98	6.0	7.0	6.0	6.0	6.5			
Protein	F	1.0	1.0	94	0	4	1	0	3	P	NS	None
	M	0.9	0.9	98	0	4	1	0	3			
Glucose	F	0	—	94	0	0	0	0	0	P	NS	None
	M	0	—	98	0	0	0	0				
Ketone	F	0	—	94	0	0	0	0	0	P	NS	None
	M	0	—	98	0	0	0	0				
Bilirubin	F	0.1	0.4	94	0	3	0	0	2	P	NS	None
	M	0.1	0.4	98	0	2	0	0	2			
Blood	F	1.2	1.3	94	0	4	1	0	4	P	$p<0.05$	None
	M	0.3	0.7	98	0	4	0	0	3			
Urobilinogen	F	0.1	—	94	0.1	0.1	0.1	0.1	0.1	P	NS	None
	M	0.1	—	98	0.1	0.1	0.1	0.1	0.1			

P = parametric; N = nonparametric; NS = not significant; Ln = natural logarithm.
The Central Tendency for urine volume: males, 27.4 ml; females, 19.0 ml.

Table 16 Reference Microscopic Urine Profiles of Adult Male and Female Ferrets Maintained Under Controlled Environmental Conditions

| Parameter | Sex | Mean | STD | N | MIN | MAX | Median | Tolerance limit | | | Sex effect | Transformation |
								lower	upper	method		
Mucous	F	1.3	1.3	94	0	4	2	0	4	P	NS	None
	M	1.5	1.3	98	0	4	2	0	4			
Epith. cells	F	1.7	1.2	94	0	4	2	0	4	P	p<0.05	None
	M	2.5	1.1	98	0	4	2	0	4			
Crystals	F	0	—	94	0	0	0	0	0	P	NS	None
	M	0	—	98	0	0	0	0	0			
Triple PO4	F	0.2	0.8	94	0	4	0	0	4	P	NS	None
	M	0.1	0.4	98	0	3	0	0	2			
Ca oxalate	F	0.02	0.2	94	0	2	0	0	0	P	NS	None
	M	0.1	0.5	98	0	4	0	0	2			
Casts	F	0.1	0.5	94	0	3	0	0	2	P	NS	None
	M	0.2	0.6	98	0	2	0	0	2			
WBC	F	3.5	2.4	94	0	9	3	0	8	P	p<0.05	None
	M	1.3	1.2	98	0	4	2	0	4			
RBC	F	1.7	1.6	94	0	8	2	0	6	P	p<0.05	None
	M	1.0	1.3	98	0	6	1	0	5			
Bacteria	F	2.1	1.3	94	0	4	2	0	4	P	p<0.05	None
	M	1.1	1.2	98	0	4	0	0	4			
Sperm	M	1.2	1.5	98	0	4	0	0	4	NA	—	—

P = parametric; NS = not significant; Ln = natural logarithm.

normalized data. These limits and the mean of the normalized data were then expressed back in the original units. For example, the transformation for total urine volume (X) was found to be $Ln(X+5.27)$. The mean, standard deviation and normal tolerance limits (TL) for total urine volume of male ferrets, for example, was determined to be: mean (3.48553), STD (0.485852), lower TL (2.430259), upper TL (4.540801). To express these in the original units of total volume, the inverse of $Ln(X+5.27)$ is applied. The inverse is to exponentiate then subtract 5.27. The resulting central tendency (CT), low and high limits for male ferret total urine volume are: CT (27.4), low (6.1), high (88.5). The standard deviation of the normalized data cannot be expressed in the original units of total volume meaningfully.

Semiquantitative Macroscopic Urine Parameters

Thornton et al. (1979) reported that the mean 24-hr urine volume and range in volume was greatest in female ferrets (mean = 28 ml, range = 8–140 ml) as opposed to males (mean = 26 ml, range = 8–48 ml). In contrast, data listed in Table 15 suggests that the opposite is true for overnight urine collection in ferrets, and that the distribution is skewed. Collection vessels employed during urine collection should be able to contain approximately 150 ml.

The color of normal ferret urine collected by ureter catheterization varies widely from colorless to deep yellow (unpublished observation from D.E.M.'s laboratory). However, when metabolism cages are employed, the color may be altered by fecal chromogen contamination. Animals consuming the Ralston Purina Ferret Chow 5280, for example, produce a semisoft, dark green colored stool which is difficult to separate completely from urine and results in a yellow-green to yellow-green-brown appearance. The fecal pellets, food pellets, and the greenish tinged urine samples will all give a maximum positive response for blood, protein, and bilirubin with the Ames Multistix test strip. Consequently, when these parameters are key issues of a protocol, urine samples should probably be taken directly from the bladder by catheterization at or before necropsy.

Thornton et al. (1979) reported ketones in 50% of male urines, proteinuria in the majority of animals, and blood in larger amounts in females (attributed to estrus) than in males. In the present database, no ketones were detected in either males or females with the Ames Multistix. However, bilirubin was detected in some samples collected by metabolism cage (confirmed by bladder catheterization), and positive results were found for blood and protein in a number of animals. The presence of urine blood was significantly greater in females than in males and may, as indicated above, be associated with estrus. Alternatively, the propensity for urine to be contaminated with feces would seem greater in female ferrets because of their shorter anal-genital space.

Similar to the evaluation of different blood sampling sites, macroscopic urine data collected for ferrets suggests that a comparative study is warranted. This evaluation should include parameter values (by sex) obtained from bladder specimens, immediate versus delayed analysis, the contribution of various diets, and a comparison of estrus and anestrus females.

Reference Microscopic Urine Profiles

Significantly greater amounts of leukocytes, erythrocytes, and bacteria are observed in overnight urine samples of female ferrets when compared with males. However, the levels reported in Table 16 are probably well below those which may be considered clinically important in this or any other species. Conn (1963) has indicated that normal human urine, for example, may contain a large range in leukocytes (0–650,000/24 hr) and erythrocytes (0–130,000/24 hr) when measured by the Addis count. Moreover, the presence of bacteria (in association with WBC) in the overnight urine samples described in Table 16 is probably related more to storage conditions and time than to a manifestation of pyuria.

The mean number of RBCs observed in female ferrets corresponds to a Table 14 classification range of between "rare" to "1–4" (per magnification field). To evaluate the contribution of estrus to this measurement, however, catheterization of the bladder would be required.

ORGAN WEIGHTS AND HISTOLOGY FOR ASSESSMENT OF TOXICITY

Prolonged toxicity testing (as opposed to acute testing) frequently involves the evaluation of all animals (or at least high-dose animals) for gross pathological and histological effects at least at the end of the experiment, but also for moribund animals sacrificed prematurely. The weight of various organs are usually included in this evaluation. Details of ferret organ weights are listed in Tables 17 through 20. Common histological findings are detailed in Table 21.

Organ Weights and Transformations

The absolute organ weights of the ferret (Table 17), when divided by the body weight at necropsy, are routinely expressed as relative organ weights (Table 18). This calculation assumes, however, that the organ weight increases in proportion to the body weight. This assumption is approximately valid for the liver weight and kidney weight but (as can be demonstrated in most species) is grossly violated for the brain weight. Consequently, a revised relative organ weight must be calculated (Table 19) such that the calculation becomes independent of the body weight. Figure 6 demonstrates how ferret brain weight, for example, varies with respect to sex and body weight, and is then made proportional to body weight when the appropriate transformation is applied.

A species comparison of revised relative organ weights is listed in Table 20. This particular control animal database includes 94 male and 87 female rats, 24 male and 24 female beagle dogs, and 48 male and 48 female ferrets. Table 20 demonstrates that (since the exponents are all less than 1) the ratio of organ weight (especially the brain) to body weight (unrevised) would be larger for smaller animals than for larger animals. The revised organ weight formulas remove the effect of body weight entirely and provide a valuable addition to the statistical protocol.

Common Histological Findings in Ferret Tissues

The histological findings detailed in Table 21 provide a summary of what has been reported by two independent pathologists for 40 untreated control animals and 64 intravenously saline-treated control animals. Most noteworthy in this database is the fact that what one pathologist may consider reportable, another pathologist may consider normal for the species (and thus not reportable). This is evident by the contrasting frequency of histological citations for specific organs, with extramedullary hematopoiesis of the spleen being the most extreme example.

Mononuclear cell infiltration is apparently the most frequently observed histological

Table 17 Reference Absolute Organ Weights (g) of Adult Male and Female Ferrets Maintained Under Controlled Environmental Conditions

Organ	Sex	Mean	STD	N	MIN	MAX	Central tendency	Tolerance limit			Sex effect	Transformation
								lower	upper	method		
Brain	F	5.95	0.41	48	4.57	6.83	5.95	5.00	6.90	P	p<0.001	None
	M	7.35	0.62	48	5.70	8.94	7.34	5.92	8.76			
Heart	F	4.02	0.52	48	3.01	5.80	4.04	2.84	P	p<0.001	None	
	M	6.62	0.81	48	3.88	8.25	6.62	4.76	8.48			
Lung	F	5.70	0.78	48	4.03	7.57	5.71	3.89	7.53	P	p<0.001	None
	M	9.08	1.09	48	6.61	13.03	9.11	6.64	11.58			
Liver	F	21.9	4.5	48	12.5	35.8	22.1	12.1	32.2	P	p<0.001	None
	M	37.8	5.0	48	19.7	44.8	37.8	26.4	49.2			
Spleen	F	4.73	1.63	48	1.99	8.62	4.77	1.03	8.50	P	p<0.001	None
	M	7.92	1.73	48	3.26	12.06	7.92	3.92	11.91			
L Kidney	F	2.07	0.27	48	1.58	2.84	2.08	1.47	2.69	P	p<0.001	None
	M	3.40	0.37	48	2.45	4.24	3.40	2.55	4.25			
R Kidney	F	1.99	0.27	48	1.46	2.62	2.00	1.38	2.63	P	p<0.001	None
	M	3.27	0.36	48	2.26	4.23	3.27	2.44	4.10			

P = parametric.

Table 18 Reference Relative Organ Weights (g/kg) of Adult Male and Female Ferrets Maintained Under Controlled Environmental Conditions

Organ	Sex	Mean	STD	N	MIN	MAX	Central tendency	Tolerance limit lower	Tolerance limit upper	method	Sex effect	Transformation
Brain	F	7.03	1.04	48	4.34	10.12	7.09	4.86	9.31	P	p<0.001	g/kg
	M	4.75	1.21	48	3.39	11.60	4.60	3.06	6.15			
Heart	F	4.73	0.68	48	2.42	6.03	4.78	3.41	6.15	P	p<0.001	g/kg
	M	4.19	0.49	48	3.51	5.78	4.19	3.05	5.33			
Lung	F	6.68	0.91	48	3.83	8.49	6.74	4.86	8.63	P	p<0.001	g/kg
	M	5.80	1.10	48	4.27	10.81	5.69	3.80	7.58			
Liver	F	25.6	4.3	48	10.4	36.3	25.9	17.4	34.5	P	p<0.001	g/kg
	M	23.9	2.6	48	19.5	30.3	23.9	17.9	29.8			
Spleen	F	5.56	1.92	48	2.34	10.1	5.61	1.21	10.0	P	p<0.001	g/kg
	M	5.01	1.09	48	2.06	7.63	5.01	2.48	7.54			
L kidney	F	2.44	0.35	48	1.30	3.32	2.46	1.74	3.18	P	p<0.001	g/kg
	M	2.18	0.38	48	1.57	3.54	2.18	1.29	3.06			
R kidney	F	2.34	0.34	48	1.19	3.14	2.37	1.68	3.06	P	p<0.001	g/kg
	M	2.09	0.35	48	1.65	3.27	2.09	1.28	2.89			

P = parametric.

Table 19 Reference Revised Relative Organ Weights (g/kg^{power}) of Adult Male and Female Ferrets Maintained Under Controlled Environmental Conditions

Organ	Sex	Mean	STD	N	MIN	MAX	Central tendency	Tolerance limit			Sex effect	Transformation
								lower	upper	method		
Brain	M+F	6.35	0.58	96	4.65	8.90	6.33	5.22	7.45	P	NS	g/kg$^{0.28}$
Heart	M+F	4.61	0.52	96	2.61	6.32	4.63	3.59	5.67	P	NS	g/kg$^{0.75}$
Lung	M+F	6.52	0.87	96	4.25	9.54	6.52	4.81	8.22	P	NS	g/kg$^{0.66}$
Liver	M+F	25.3	3.5	96	10.9	36.2	25.5	18.6	32.3	P	NS	g/kg$^{0.83}$
Spleen	M+F	5.40	1.45	96	2.36	9.66	5.44	2.34	8.53	P	NS	g/kg$^{0.79}$
L kidney	M+F	2.41	0.32	96	1.44	3.15	2.42	1.75	3.08	P	p<0.05	g/kg$^{0.68}$
R kidney	M+F	2.31	0.30	96	1.31	3.05	2.32	1.69	2.95	P	p<0.05	g/kg$^{0.68}$

P = parametric.

Table 20 Revised Relative Organ Weight for Rats, Beagle Dogs, and Ferrets (Revised Relative Organ Weight = Organ Weight/[Body Weight]^{power})

Organ	Power factor (exponent)		
	rat	beagle dog	ferret
Brain	0.17	0.18	0.28
Lung	0.44	0.71	0.66
Heart	0.72	0.81	0.75
Liver	0.82	0.95	0.83
Spleen	0.40	0.97	0.79
Kidney	0.76	0.94	0.68

finding in ferret tissues. This particular microscopic finding occurred in 100% of the livers examined and to a lesser and more variable degree in various other organs. The mean severity grade of "slight" assigned (by both pathologists) to the degree of mononuclear cell infiltration of the liver implies that "moderate" or greater infiltrations could have occurred in approximately one-third of the animals examined. Therefore, to minimize the number of "moderate" infiltrations and decrease the overall mean score, McLain and Lin (1989b) devised an index method of severity prediction based on pre-and posttreatment blood samples (see later section). Use of this index to predict the degree of lymphocyte infiltration enables the culling of animals with unacceptable scores (defined by the investigator). Alternatively, the index may be used as a blocking factor to randomize animals into test groups such that lymphocyte infiltration scores between groups are similar.

Although the severity is slightly greater, the incidence of pneumonitis reported in Table 21 for ferrets is not markedly different from what has been observed for beagle dogs (unpublished observations). On the other hand, the minimal to slight cardiac fibrosis observed, which is apparently a residual effect of the blood sampling procedure, is not a common finding in the beagle dog. The pathology section of this chapter provides a more detailed evaluation and overview of the toxicological histopathology of the ferret.

Derivation and Application of the Liver Lymphocyte Index (LvLI)

When using ferrets as a nonrodent animal model for safety assessment studies, the preexisting histological lesions of the species must be addressed. Obviously, improved hygiene and breeding efforts by the vendor will reduce the frequency of some lesions. Preceding this, however, statistical control can be used to accommodate and/or minimize their effects.

To control existing liver lesions common to the ferret, a database was constructed from pre- and posttreatment hematology and clinical chemistry measurements obtained by cardiac puncture from 152 male and 152 female ferrets. Tissues from all animals were evaluated microscopically for the presence and severity of lymphocyte infiltration in

Table 21 Microscopic Findings of the Intravenous Saline-Treated (ST) and Un-treated (UT) Male and Female Ferret's Major Organs as Reported by Two Independent Pathologists (Incidence [%], Severity[a])

Organ/microscopic finding	Pathologist		
	A(ST)	B(ST)	B(UT)
Brain			
mononuclear cell infiltration, choroid plexus	15/32	0/32	0/40
	(46.9)	(0.0)	(0.0)
	NG	—	—
mononuclear cell infiltration, meninges	2/32	0.32	0/40
	(6.3)	(0.0)	(0.0)
	1.0	—	—
Lungs			
pneumonitis	26/32	26/32	33/40
	(81.3)	(81.3)	(82.5)
	1.7	1.5	1.5
Heart			
fibrosis	0/32	4.32	5/40
	(0.0)	(12.5)	(12.5)
	—	1.2	1.2
Liver			
mononuclear cell infiltration, portal or periportal	32/32	32/32	40/40
	(100)	(100)	(100)
	2.0	2.0	2.2
Kidney			
mononuclear cell infiltration, interstital	3/32	0.32	0/40
	(9.4)	(0.0)	(0.0)
	1.3	—	—
nephritis, glomerulo- or interstitial	1/32	13/32	13/40
	(3.1)	(40.6)	(32.5)
	1.0	1.2	1.2
Spleen			
extramedullary hematopoiesis	0/32	32/32	40/40
	(0.0)	(100)	(100)
	—	2.5	2.4
Stomach			
mononuclear cell infiltration	1/32	1/32	2/40
	(3.1)	(3.1)	(5.0)
	3.0	2.0	1.5

[a]Severity: 1 = minimal; 2 = slight; 3 = moderate; 4 = moderately severe/high; 5 = severe/high; NG = not graded.

various organs. Organs evaluated included (but were not limited to) liver, lung, kidney, thyroid, stomach, colon, and brain. The histology scoring system used was 0 = none, 1 = minimal, 2 = slight, 3 = moderate, 4 = high, and 5 = severe. Attempts were made to predict the pathologist's score for liver lymphocyte infiltration, for example, by quantitative lesion indices based on: (1) pretreatment clinical chemistry and hematology measure-

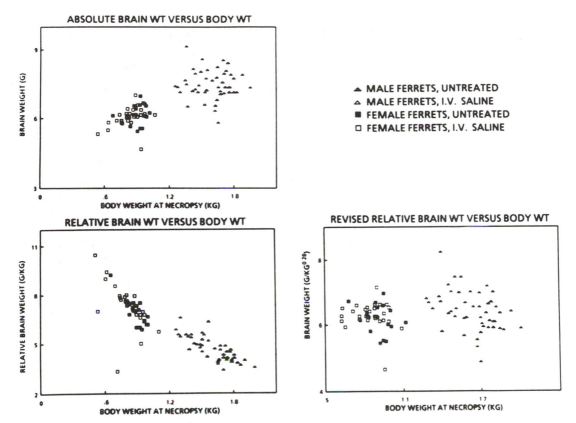

Figure 6 Scattergram of ferret brain weight expressed as the absolute weight (top left), relative weight (bottom left), and revised relative weight (bottom right). By applying the power transformation to body weight (i.e. revised relative organ weight) the effect of sexual dimorphism is eliminated, thus sample size (N) is increased accordingly.

ments of individual animals (pretreatment lesion index), and (2) all pre- and posttreatment measurements (including organ weights) of these same animals (final lesion index).

The benefits of using pretreatment lesion indices for prediction of lesion severity and/or presence include the following: (1) Since an animal's organ tissue cannot be examined until the animal is sacrificed, the index may be used to screen for healthy animals based on measurements of their pretreatment blood samples, (2) the index may be used as a blocking factor to randomize animals such that all treatment groups (including the control group) contain animals with similar lesions, and, (3) the index may be used as a covariable in the statistical analysis to control for variation due to preexisting lesions. Similarly, the benefits of using the final index include the fact that it is an objective, quantitative, and continuous score instead of a subjective and ordinal score (pathologist score). In addition, it is statistically more powerful and easier to be evaluated when comparing organ lesions across treatment groups.

The lesion index is the linear combination of all parameters that yield the best geometric separation between "less than moderate" and "moderate or higher" lymphocyte infiltration conditions. In other words, it is the weighted average of all paremeters that yield the most power (or the least error) to predict a "moderate or higher" lymphocyte infiltration of an animal. The weight (coefficient) that is assigned to each parameter depends on how much that parameter contributes to the prediction power.

Table 22 lists the liver lymphocyte infiltrate index based on pretreatment parameters (LvLI-pre). The first column of Table 22 presents all parameters listed in order of decreasing importance of their contribution in prediction power. The third column lists the coefficient (weight) that was assigned to each parameter. The fourth column shows how each parameter correlated with the index. For this index, globulin is the strongest predictor, with a correlation coefficient of 0.583. After knowing the globulin level, the lymphocyte count provides more additional predictive power than any other parameter. Similarly, mean corpuscular hemoglobin concentration (MCHC) is the third highest predictor after we know the globulin and lymphocyte count. Total protein has a higher correlation (0.478) with the index than does MCHC in this example, but it is given a lower priority because it is highly correlated with globulin. In other words, the joint information from globulin, lymphocyte count, and MCHC is more predictive than the joint information from globulin, lymphocyte count, and total protein. The same arguement can be used for the rest of the information in Table 22.

Table 22 Prestudy Parameters Used for the Calculation of a Liver Lymphocyte Infiltrate Index

$$\left(\text{LvLI-pre} = 6.2335 + \sum_{I=1}^{18} C_I Y_I\right)$$

Parameter (X)[a]	Transformation (Y)	Weight coefficient (C)	Correlation coef. (rank)[b]
Globulin	Ln(X−1.23)	1.11690	0.583 (1)
Lymphocyte count	Ln(X)	0.78835	0.476 (3)
MCHC	X	0.25618	0.218 (7)
LDH	Ln(X−120)	−0.47096	−0.311 (5)
SGPT	Ln(X−40)	0.88691	0.361 (4)
Uric acid	Ln(X+0.74)	−0.94505	−0.093 (13)
RBC	X	−0.30556	−0.225 (6)
Basophil count	Ln(X+0.001)	0.13193	0.156 (10)
Alk. phos.	Ln(X−10)	−0.64420	−0.055 (17)
Cholesterol	X	0.01485	0.092 (14)
Glucose	Ln(X+96)	−1.83530	−0.158 (9)
Monocyte count	Ln(X+0.001)	0.06817	0.178 (8)
STAB count	Ln(X+0.001)	−0.11888	−0.088 (15)
Albumin	X	−0.85864	−0.029 (18)
Total protein	X	0.41570	0.478 (2)
BUN	Ln(X−9)	−0.44574	−0.106 (11)
Creatinine	X	1.80620	0.095 (12)
Fibrinogen	Ln(X−63)	−0.21236	−0.056 (16)

[a]Parameters are listed in order (top to bottom) of additional predicting power.
[b]The correlation coefficient explains the predicting power of the parameter if all other parameters are unknown.

Table 23 lists the liver lymphocyte infiltrate index (LvLI) based on all information collected, including the organ weights at necropsy and all pretreatment data. The LvLI-pre explains 72% (0.846) of this index. The posttreatment SGPT is a strong predictor. The posttreatment globulin is a weak predictor because it is highly correlated with LvLI-pre.

Success Rate of LvLI-pre and LvLI

Table 24 shows the success rate of LvLI-pre and LvLI. For those ferrets with LvLI-pre greater or equal to 3, we would expect a moderate or high severity score (degree of lymphocyte infiltration) when their liver tissue is evaluated by the pathologist at sacrifice (2–3 weeks later). Among the 74 ferrets in the present database that were judged to have a "moderate or high" severity score by the pathologist, 65 were judged to have "moderate or high" with the LvLI-pre. Therefore, we have 88% confidence that the index (based on pretreatment blood samples) would agree with the pathologist's opinion 2–3 weeks later. Similarly, among the 224 ferrets that were judged to have a "slight or less" severity score by the pathologist, 196 (88%) were judged the same by the LvLI-pre.

LvLI is shown to have a 92% (68/74) success rate in predicting "moderate or high"

Table 23 Poststudy Parameters Used for the Calculation of a Liver Lymphocyte Infiltrate Index

$$(LvLI = 8.5207 + \sum_{I=1}^{21} C_I Y_I)$$

Parameter (X)[a]	Transformation (Y)	Weight coefficient (C)	Correlation coef. (rank)[b]
LvLI-pre	X	0.44589	0.846 (1)
SGPT	Ln(X–40)	0.72639	0.630 (2)
A/G ratio	X^2	0.06011	–0.409 (5)
Creatinine	X	0.85106	0.192 (11)
Potassium	Ln(X–3.5)	–0.49440	–0.196 (10)
Heart, rev.-rel.	X	0.38091	0.096 (15)
Kidney, rev.-rel.	X	–0.47868	0.004 (21)
Spleen, rev.-rel.	X	0.08443	0.388 (6)
A/G ratio-pre	X^2	0.15299	–0.381 (7)
MCV	X	–0.07150	–0.081 (16)
Glucose	Ln(X+96)	–1.05990	–0.151 (12)
Hct-pre	X	–0.03010	–0.226 (9)
STAB count–pre	Ln(X+0.001)	–0.06265	–0.081 (17)
Phosphorus-pre	X	0.09743	0.138 (13)
Lung, rev.-rel.	X	–0.05949	–0.044 (19)
Cholesterol-pre	X	0.00204	0.076 (18)
EOS count	Ln(X+0.001)	–1.05796	0.008 (20)
Liver, rev.-rel.	X	0.01964	0.356 (8)
BASO count–pre	Ln(X+0.001)	0.02406	0.126 (14)
Globulin	Ln(X–1.23)	1.48610	0.551 (3)
Total protein	X	–0.51067	0.479 (4)

[a]Parameters are listed in order (top to bottom) of additional predicting power.
[b]The correlation coefficient explains the predicting power of the parameter if all other parameters are unknown.

Table 24 Performance Measurements of LvLI-pre and LvLI

	Scored by Pathologist	
	slight or less	moderate or high
Based on LvLI-pre		
Slight or less, LvLI[3	196	9
Moderate or high, LvLI]3	28	65
Total	224	74
Based on LvLI (final)		
Slight or less, LvLI[3	212	6
Moderate or high, LvLI]3	9	68
Total	221	74

liver lymphocyte infiltrate severity scores and has a 96% (212/221) success rate in predicting "slight or moderate" scores as judged by a pathologist.

TYPICAL PROTOCOLS

Acute Toxicity Testing

Traditionally, the single test that is conducted on essentially all chemicals that are of any biological interest is the acute toxicity test. In the classical sense, the test consists of administering the compound to the animals on one occasion, for a time period which is usually less than 24 hr. The purpose of the test is to determine the symptomology consequent to administration of the compound and, as it is used less frequently today, to determine the order of lethality of the compound. Essentially all initial, acute toxicity tests are performed in rodents because of their small size, availability, and the abundance of reference toxicological data generated for the species. Subsequent testing using similar procedures is performed in other species such as the ferret for the purpose of contrast and confirmation.

The ferret has proven especially useful in the screening type of acute toxicity study. These studies aid in identifying compounds of such low toxicity that, when considered in relation to a proposed use of low exposure, extensive investigations to make a judgement of safety are not justified. In the screening type of acute toxicity study the amount of test agent to which an animal is exposed is usually so massive that it generally bears no practical relationship to the expected human exposure.

Acute Oral Testing

Acute oral toxicity testing in ferrets, commonly performed subsequent to rodent testing, is designed to elicit the qualitative and quantitative nature of the toxic effects from a one-time oral exposure to a large dose of a chemical or test agent. Whether the puspose of testing is to provide data for estimating the lethal dose for 50% of a group of animals, or for demonstration that some large multiple of the potential human dose does not result in an irreversible manifestation of toxicity, the number of animals employed should be sufficient for a sound statistical evaluation. Typically, six to eight adult ferrets/sex/group are sufficient when there is no a priori knowledge of the type of effects resulting from exposure to the test agent. Procedures for testing would be similar to that prescribed for rodents, with the exception that emesis should be included in the physical and observational examination protocol. In addition, phonation should be monitored as it is more common in the ferret than it is in rodents.

Acute Dermal Testing

The ability of some chemicals to penetrate intact and abraded skin and produce systemic toxicity is well known, and steps should therefore be taken to evaluate this possibility when appropriate. The albino rabbit is, of course, the animal most frequently used in assessing dermal toxicity. However, the mouse, rat, guinea pig, and dog have also been used. The ferret would most likely parallel the dog in this type of evaluation, with its thick skin severalfold less permeable than the rat or rabbit (thus closer to human skin).

An ideal dermal application site in the ferret is the dorsal surface just above or at the level of the shoulders. Large "rat jackets" or vests may be fitted to the animals when it is necessary to cover a test material. After an appropriate exposure period, excess material is removed, and the local changes and any gross signs of toxicity are noted. Animals should be observed for an appropriate period of time and postmortem studies performed.

Acute Inhalation Toxicity

Test article exposure by inhalation is probably the most time consuming and expensive of all toxicological dosing procedures. Vinegar et al. (1985) have convincingly argued, however, that the ferret is a less expensive substitute for the dog in acute inhalation toxicity testing. Moreover, because the ferret has more submucosal glands in bronchial walls and an additional generation of terminal bronchioles, these authors have stated that the ferret lung is closer anatomically to the human lung than is the dog lung (see above). Protocols for acute inhalation toxicity in ferrets should parallel those used for rodents, with the possible exception of perhaps increasing the ferret sample size to accommodate the increased heterogeneity of the species. In addition, since pulmonary changes are likely manifestations of response to experimental treatment, ferrets selected for study should be thoroughly screened during quarantine for the absence of respiratory disease. Application of a lung lymphocyte infiltrate index (LuLI), as described previously for the liver, can detect ferrets with "moderate or higher" infiltrates with an 88% success rate when using LuLI-pre, and a 94% success rate when all variables are used in the calculation.

Subchronic Toxicity Testing

Subchronic toxicity procedures are designed to determine the adverse effects that may occur during repeated exposure over a period of a few days to usually 3 months (90 days). The subchronic procedures usually include the routes of exposure expected for man, with exposure levels lower than in the acute toxicity protocols. A high exposure level that is judged to be sufficiently large to produce adverse effects and at least one lower exposure level that is not expected to produce adverse effects are used. Intermediate exposure levels should be introduced when they are considered necessary. The number of ferrets used should be sufficient for statistical confidence (usually six to eight adult ferrets/sex/group). Observations should include over signs of toxicity, food consumption (when appropriate), and body weight change, hematology, clinical chemistry, urinalysis, organ weights, and gross and microscopic pathology. To increase the statistical power, clinical pathology should be evaluated as the change from baseline (i.e., pretreatment samples must be collected from all animals).

Clinical observations of test animals should include daily cageside evaluations as well as detailed examinations performed at least once per week. The detailed physical examination can be scheduled with the body weight measurement. Standard procedures employed for other test species are acceptable. Additional clinical notations should include inspections for excessive fur/hair under the cage, swelling of the vulva in females, and testicular prominance in males. To maintain all animals in a sexually inactive state, they should be segregaged by sex (when possible) and subjected to shortened photoperiods. Recovery studies can be included if the changes observed indicate that this type of procedure is necessary. As with the other types of toxicity procedures, subchronic toxicity data generated with ferrets are most complementary when expressed as a contrast to subchronic rodent data.

Long-Term Bioassays for Chronic Toxicity and Carcinogenesis

The classic approach to the study of chronic toxicity and the carcinogenic potential of test substances involves studies in two or more species of animals (one of which should ideally be a nonrodent) for periods of time ranging from many months to several years. Rats and mice have, of course, been the predominate test species for these protocols. However, long-term testing with ferrets would seem to be a plausible and welcomed alternative.

Irrespective of the variability observed in the normal ferret's clinical or microscopic profile, with increasing dosage in the continuum of the dose-response relationship, a region is generally entered where the effects are clearly adverse.

The detection of adverse effects in chronic toxicity protocols begins with gross observations of the intact animal in terms of growth, appearance, and activity. The next point of discrimination is at the organ-system level, wherein changes of a biochemical and physiological nature are assessed. These are followed by an examination of morphological changes at the gross and cellular levels in sacrificed animals or biopsy material. Clearly, adverse effects which occur in ferrets or any other species are those which result in impairment of functional capacity (as determined by anatomical, physiological, and biochemical or behavioral parameters), or in a decrement of the ability to compensate for additional stress; are irreversible during exposure or following cessation of exposure; and enhance the susceptability of the individual to the deleterious effects of other environmental influences.

Developmental Toxicity Assessment

It is evident that there is no one animal species that can be considered ideal for evaluating human developmental toxicity. Ferrets are no exception to this dilemma, of course, and provide just a higher level of evaluation for embryotoxicity than what is offered with rodents. The ferret's chief advantage in reproductive toxicity assessment is its small size and the fact that it does not have the atypical yolk-sac placenta which is common to the rat.

Protocols for evaluation of developmental toxicity in the ferret follow guidelines similar to that which would be used for rodents, with the exception that animals obtained from a reputable supplier should be vaccinated for distemper and subjected to a thorough veterinary examination upon arrival at the vivarium. Estrous females at their peak of vulval swelling should be placed with sexually active males of proven fertility and observed for successful coitus on several successive occasions. The first successful coitus is considered day 0 of pregnancy because ovulation generally occurs approximately 30 hr postcoitus. The examination of vaginal lavage for motile sperm after observed mating would be helpful in determining successful insemination. Presumed-mated jills may also be shipped from the supplier (Marshall Farms, North Rose, New York) the day following coitus (day 1 of gestation) with no apparent effect upon reproductive parameters if transportation is completed on gestation day 1. Acclimatization to the vivarium is easily accomplished between arrival and day 12 of gestation when dosing should begin (personal observations, R.M.H.). Vulval regression and obvious weight gain would indicate successful conception. The critical period in the ferret is generally accepted as days 12–30, with implantation occurring on approximately day 12.

Litters should be taken by cesarean section on gestation day 35 and subjected to the same examination procedures used for rats and rabbits. That is, living fetuses should be weighed, sexed, and examined externally and internally by gross dissection of all cavity organs or by the Wilson or Staples techniques. Skeletal visualization by KOH clearing should be done on a predetermined number of fetuses. Other parameter evaluations and reporting are similar to what would be done for rodents.

Routine acceptance of the ferret in developmental toxicity studies is still to be established within the various governmental agencies. It is recommended, therefore, that a positive control group (15 mg/kg all-*trans* retinoic acid on day 14 of gestation) be included with every study (personal observations/recommendation, R.M.H.).

Figure 7 depicts morphological changes occurring in the ferret embryo/fetus between gestation days 16 and 27.

SUMMARY

Review of Advantages and Disadvantages

The most obvious advantages to the use of the ferret as an animal model in toxicology include the relatively low cost, small body size, ease of handling (mild disposition) and maintenance, and their ability to adapt to most existing facilities and laboratory equipment. Less obvious advantages include the current lack of opposition to their use (traditionally voiced by antivivisectionists), and their apparent physiological and/or biochemical similarities with humans. The increasing popularity of ferrets in biomedical research correlates highly with growth of the biotechnology industry. In this respect, the ferret requires only about one-tenth of the limited test article which would be needed for the more conventional beagle dog.

Disadvantages of the ferret include their large relative heterogeneity, their current lack of extensive databases, the lack (temporary) of an approved rabies vaccine, the lack of "virus-free" ferrets, their limited availability, and the small number of vendors selling the animal.

Steps that Can Be Taken to Minimize Disadvantages

A significant portion of the current book chapter was devoted to the presentation and discussion of material which could be viewed as a beginning database for the ferret. In addition, novel methods for decreasing the level of heterogeneity in this species (or any other species) and eliminating undesirable animals from testing consideration have been proposed. New information has been presented with respect to the pending approval of a rabies vaccine for ferrets. However, only the continued use and demand for ferrets will cause the number of vendors available to increase, and only concentrated research and breeding efforts will provide the scientific community with a virus-free ferret.

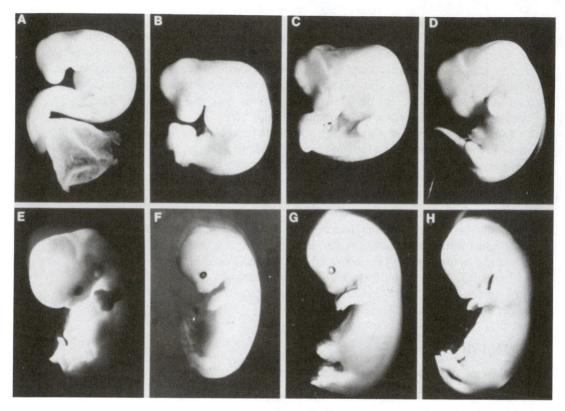

Figure 7 Various developmental stages of the ferret corresponding to the following days of gestation and developmental milestones: (A) d. 16, ten somites, anterior neuropore closed, three branchial arches, (B) d. 18, lower limb bud appears, (C) d. 19, (D) d. 21, (E) d. 22, digital rays in upper extremities, (F) d. 24, crown-rump length >10 mm, (G) d. 26, ossification begins, heart septation complete, d. 25–26, (H) d. 27, palate closed completely.

Pathology   **Glen K. Miller**

Domestic ferrets are becoming more popular as pets but also have received wider applications in biomedical research programs. The successful use and application of this animal model necessitates an understanding of the common maladies of this species. Although a wide variety of spontaneous or sporadic diseases are documented in ferrets, our purpose is to highlight only the more common disorders which are likely to be encountered in conventionally derived ferrets used for subacute or chronic toxicity studies. The reader is referred to more exhaustive commentaries and sources for the less common disorders or for in-depth discussion of individual diseases (Jubb, et al. 1985; Fox, 1988).

Currently, the ferret is likely to present with more background diseases having the potential to complicate interpretations of adverse findings in toxicology studies than when using more traditional laboratory species. Improvements in husbandry and identification of pathogen-free stock will enhance the suitability of the ferret in the foreseeable future.

MORE COMMON DISORDERS IN FERRETS

Parvoviral Infection

Ferrets are susceptible to a strain of parvovirus that causes persistent infection, hypergammaglobulinemia, and a spectrum of histopathological lesions. This disorder of ferrets, sometimes referred to as Aleutian disease, or hypergammaglobulinemia of ferrets, shares some similarities to the Aleutian disease in mink (Jones, 1983), except renal complications are not as frequently reported in ferrets (Ohshima, 1978). Whether the virus in ferrets is identical to that causing Aleutian disease in mink is unclear, since ferret Aleutian disease virus (ADV) will persistently infect mink but fails to elicit histopathological lesions in mink (Ohshima 1978; Porter 1982). However, serological and experimental transmission studies indicate that the two virus strains are related antigenically, but are biologically distinct (Porter, 1982, 1987). Ferrets are not naturally susceptible to other parvoviruses found in domestic animals or certain feral species (Parrish, 1987).

Various clinical syndromes attributable to persistent parvoviral infection have been documented in ferrets. Asymptomatic animals may remain carriers for up to 180 days prior to onset of clinical signs (Porter, 1982). Some animals subsequently exhibit a slowly progressive wasting syndrome, with abnormal stools, episodic fevers, posterior paresis, splenomegaly, and death. On occasion, afflicted animals may demonstrate sudden behavioral changes, such as aggressiveness and hyperactivity prior to weight loss and the wasting syndrome. These latter changes in behavior patterns have been attributed to lymphocytic thyroiditis and subsequent endocrine imbalances (Fox, 1988).

Experimental studies and studies of natural outbreaks indicate that the most frequent and probably one of the earliest histopathological observation is periportal (periacinar) accumulation of lymphoid cells within the liver (Ohshima, 1978). The extent and severity of infiltrates can be variable, but in more severe cases, germinal center formation is not uncommon and compression or disruption of the limiting hepatic plate with destruction of adjacent hepatic plates can be observed. Mild elevations of serum alanine aminotransferase and asparatate aminotransferase may accompany the more advanced instances of hepatic infiltration (Miller, unpublished observation).

Prominent lymphoid hyperplasia of the lymph nodes and the spleen can be observed during the early stages of the disease, whereas immune complex–mediated lesions are less common in the kidney, liver, or vasculature and are only observed with more advanced, protracted disease (Kenyon, 1966, 1967; Fox, 1988). Infiltration of lymphocytes and plasma cells can also be found in a variety of organs, including the leptomeninges and brain (Ohshima, 1978). However, most references indicate that advanced lesions are not as common in the ferret as in the mink (Ohshima, 1978; Porter, 1982).

The virus elicits an immunological response in the host, resulting in hypergammaglobulinemia. Gamma globulins in excess of 20% of total protein is considered diagnostic for the disease by some reports (Ohshima, 1978). However, serology is recommended for more definitive confirmation. Information regarding the incidence of confirmed parvoviral infections is fragmentary. The incidence of hepatic lymphoid infiltrates is relatively high (>90%), although the incidence of hepatitis suspected to be due to parvoviral infection is approximately 15% (Miller, unpublished observation).

Pneumocystis carinii Infection

Pneumocystis carinii, a protozoan parasite, is a commensal inhabitant of the lungs of many domestic and laboratory species (Dungworth, 1985). This organism is normally kept in check by alveolar macrophages, but it is not unusual to encounter sporadic, subclinical infections as demonstrated by microscopic collections of foamy macrophages admixed with lymphocytes or plasma cells within the lungs of ferrets. Although the organism may be demonstrated in these foci, minimal pathology is usually associated with them. However, *P. carinii* demonstrates pathogenicity in animals which receive long-term immunosuppressive treatment or secondary to viral infections that compromise the integrity of the immune system (Stokes, 1987; Fox, 1988).

Gross pathological lesions including patchy or diffuse discoloration of the lung with areas of firmness or consolidation can be observed in more advanced forms of pneumocystis pneumonia. Histologically, focal and diffuse interstitial pneumonia with a characteristic accumulation of foamy, pale acidophilic material within alveoli is observed (Dungworth, 1985). The severity of inflammation is variable, consisting of accumulation of lymphocytes, plasma cells, macrophages, and a variable degree of type II epithelial hyperplasia. The latter occurs owing to the fact that the organism infects the type I alveolar cells, resulting in their necrosis and replacement by type II cells. *P. carinii* is poorly stained with hematoxylin and eosin and is better demonstrated using Grocott's methenamine silver nitrate (Vacca, 1985). An important etiological differential diagnosis when finding interstitial pneumonia is that caused by *Toxoplasma gondii* (Dungworth, 1985).

Cryptosporidiosis

Cryptosporidium, a small protozoan parasite having a typical coccidian life cycle, infects the intestinal epithelium of the lower small intestine and the large intestine of most mammals (Barker, 1985). This organism frequently inhabits the gastrointestinal tract of ferrets and is capable of causing enteric disease in them (Rehg, 1988). Unlike most coccidia, which are host specific, cryptospordia lack species specificity, and therefore pose a zoonotic threat to laboratory workers. The pathogenicity of crystosporidia is variable, since infection in ferrets in most instances is asymptomatic. One survey indicates that subclinical cryptosporidiosis was present in approximately 50% of young laboratory ferrets between the ages of 4 and 6 months, and higher percentages (70) of new arrivals at 3 months of age had fecal oocysts (Regh, 1988). However, *Cryptosporidium* has been incriminated more frequently as a primary pathogen in immunosuppressed animals (Barker, 1985).

Histologically, intestinal cryptosporidiosis may be associated with mild to moderate degrees of villus atrophy, blunting or fusion of villi, and hypertrophy of the crypts of Lieberkühn. Varying numbers of cryptosporidium are usually visible on routine H&E stains within the microvillus border of surface epithelial cells, predominantly in the ileum, but in the large intestine as well (Barker, 1985). However, it is not uncommon to encounter an occasional ferret having low numbers of intestinal cryptosporidium unassociated with histopathological alteration of the mucosa. Some citations indicate that intestinal cryptosporidiosis is associated with eosinophilic infiltrates within the lamina propria (Fox, 1988), but in our experience, eosinophils are commonly observed in the gut of ferrets unassociated with cryptosporidiosis or other enteric pathogens (Miller, unpublished observations). Most infections in ferrets by *Cryptosporidium* are thought to be self-limiting (Fox, 1988).

Granulomatous Inflammatory Disorders

Granulomatous inflammatory disorders of uncertain etiology have been observed occasionally in ferrets, none of which are likely to produce clinical signs, but nonetheless may complicate histopathological interpretations in routine toxicology studies. Grossly observable lesions are usually lacking, but microscopically are confined to any of the lymph nodes draining the small and large intestines and to the submucosa or smooth muscle wall of the intestine. These foci comprise an admixture of lymphocytes, plasma cells, and large, swollen macrophages, with some foci resembling granulomas with or without the presence of multinucleated giant cells. Special stains for fungi and microorganisms have been unrewarding (Miller, unpublished observations).

An important differential diagnosis when such foci are encountered includes tuberculosis, especially that due to *Mycobacterium bovis,* which reportedly can cause nodular lesions in the intestines and associated lymph nodes, but also may result in hepatosplenomegaly (Fox, 1988). Another differential diagnosis includes enzootic granulomatosis (Momberg-Jorgensen, 1951), a rare disorder of unknown etiology that has been described only once in Europe in 1951. In this latter disorder, lesions are not confined to the gastrointestinal system, but usually also involve the spleen and liver. This latter disease bears some resemblance to a variant (dry form) of feline infectious peritonitis caused by the feline picornavirus; however, it is uncertain whether ferrets are susceptible to the feline picornavirus.

Cardiomyopathy

Cardiomyopathy is being recognized as an important cause of congestive heart disease in ferrets, especially in those animals over 3 years of age, and in males more than in females. The definition of cardiomyopathy as applied in this instance refers to disease of the heart muscle of unknown cause and does not apply to heart disease which is secondary to known or established etiologies (Robbins, 1988). Cardiomyopathies are classified according to their pathophysiological characteristics into three types: dilated or congestive, hypertrophic, and restrictive or obliterative (Robinson, 1985). Hypertrophic and dilated forms are more common in ferrets (Lipman, 1987).

Hypertrophic cardiomyopathy, usually of the left ventricle, is probably the more common form, at least in the early stages of the disease. Dilated or congestive cardiomyopathy, on the other hand, has grossly dilated ventricles and atria with thinning of the interventricular septum and ventricular walls. In both forms, enlargement of cardiac contours can be demonstrated radiographically, with some degree of hydrothorax or pleural effusion, lung densities reflecting pulmonary edema, and generalized edema in advanced cases. Hepatosplenomegaly usually accompanies congestive heart failure. Cardiomyopathies in ferrets are associated with a variety of ECG changes (Greenlee, 1984; Lipman, 1987).

Histopathology may reveal little or no significant changes or a spectrum of relatively mild, nonspecific changes such as myocardial degeneration, loss of staining intensity of myofibers, and low-grade inflammation or endocardial thickening (Robinson, 1985).

Proliferative Colitis

A relatively less common disorder in young laboratory ferrets is proliferative colitis associated with *Campylobacter* sp. *Campylobacter* also poses a potential zoonotic hazard for laboratory workers and animal handlers. Signs are usually observed in younger (4–6 months old) animals and includes either an acute onset of bloody diarrhea and death in 3 to 4 days, or more commonly, chronic disease with weight loss, intermittent soft stools and mucoid or bloody diarrhea, tenesmus, and vocalization during defecation (Fox 1982, 1986, 1987). Abdominal palpation may reveal an enlarged, thickened colon and prominent abdominal lymph nodes.

Histologically, colonic mucosa is thickened owing to hyperplasia of the crypt epithelium, with prominent inflammatory cell infiltrates within the lamina propria, and thickening of the smooth muscle wall (Fox 1982; Barker 1985). The lamina propria typically contains numerous lymphocytes with fewer plasma cells, macrophages, and neutrophils with inflammation extending into the muscularis mucosa. In protracted cases, crypt epithelium penetrates the submucosa and the tunica muscularis of the colon. Warthin-Starry stains or other silver stains are necessary to demonstrate the organism in tissue sections, and modified acid fast techniques can be applied to colonic mucosal scrapings (Barker 1985; Vacca 1985).

Aplastic Anemia

The reproductive physiology of the ferret presents a unique laboratory mangement problem in that the female ferret (jill) is seasonally polyestrous usually from March through August. Jills which have not been mated can remain in estrus for up to 180 days, and prolonged estrus can lead to fatal consequences. Hyperestrogenism associated with prolonged estrus is responsible for a syndrome of marrow failure, termed aplastic anemia. Although use of the term aplastic anemia is a misnomer in that it implies deficient production of the erythroid series, contemporary use of the term refers to a syndrome of pancytopenia due to deficient production of all marrow lineages (e.g., myeloid, lymphoid, megakaryocytic, and erythroid lineages).

Females that have been in heat for 1 month or longer develop anorexia, depression, posterior limb paresis, and lethargy. Animals frequently have vulvar enlargement, pale mucous membranes, subcutaneous hemorrhages, and may present with bilaterally symmetrical alopecia (Fox, 1988). Animals with early stages of the disorder may have a low-grade normocytic, normochromic anemia, neutrophilia with a left shift, and variable platelet numbers. However, leukopenia and thrombocytopenia usually precede overt anemia, since the neutrophils and platelets have shorter life spans than the erythrocytes (Duncan, 1986). Peripheral blood changes become more pronounced over time, and are characterized by profound nonregenerative anemia with packed cell volume as low as 12–15% in severe cases, or lower in fatal cases. Marrow aspirates are extremely hypocellular or nearly acellular.

Hemorrhages or complications thereof are common causes of death from this syndrome. Coagulopathy, related to hepatic dysfunction and thrombocytopenia, is the cause for the subcutaneous hemorrhages observed clinically and the internal hemorrhages observed in fatal cases. The extent of the hemorrhage also tends to accentuate the anemia. Hemosiderosis is usually observed microscopically in the lymph nodes, spleen, and marrow, along with a marked reduction in marrow cellularity and replacement with mature fat. Hydrometra or pyometra accompanied by microscopic evidence of cystic endometrial hyperplasia is another sequela of hyperestrogenism.

Metabolism   **Christopher P. Chengelis**

The ferret is a relatively new species in toxicological and pharmacological research. The last 15 years have seen increased interest in this species (Hoar, 1984), more so in Europe than in the North America. Interestingly, however, the pace of research specifically on xenobiotic metabolism in this species has declined from a relative flurry of papers published in the late 1970s to relatively few papers published in the late 1980s. As a result, xenobiotic metabolism has not been very well characterized. For example, with regard to disposition, there is no published information on the blood-brain barrier, the blood-testis barrier or plasma protein binding in the ferret. One has to assume that the ferret is not radically different from other species with regard to these parameters. This review will concentrate on the published literature, which tends to fall into three main groups, (1) Characterizations of the microsomal mixed function oxidase (MMFO) system, (2) studies to characterize in vivo pharmacokinetics of various chemicals, and (3) studies on species-related differences in conjugation reactions.

Peculiarities of oral absorption in the ferret should be mentioned. The ferret has no cecum, and the transition from small to large intestine can only be detected by histological examination (Hoar, 1984). The intestine is a relatively short tube, and recent work has failed to isolate any anaerobic gastrointestinal bacteria. Hence, oral bioavailability of chemicals tends to be less in the ferret than in rodents.

Some indices of xenobiotic metabolism in the ferret are summarized on Table 25. Ioannides et al. published the first, and one of the few, extensive examinations of the microsomal mixed function oxidase system in 1977. They established that there were definite age (day 0–56)–related increases in, for example, cytochrome P-450 and aniline hydroxylase activity. Hence, the data given in Table 25 are drawn from adult animals of the age and or size that most investigators report using. Ioannides et al. (1977) also reported on slight quantitative strain differences between the polecat ferret and the albino ferret for various parameters. For example, both strains had essentially the same activity

Table 25   Summary of Hepatic Xenobiotic Metabolizing Enzymes in Ferrets

Enzyme	Concentration or activity	Comments and references
Cytochrome P-450	0.16–0.73 nmol/mg-m	Ioannides et al., 1977; Lake et al., 1979; Shull et al., 1982. Strain, sex, and sex variability identified. Costello and Chengelis, 1989.
Cytochrome b$_5$	0.15–0.22 nmol/mg-m	Ioannides et al., 1977; Shull et al., 1982; Costello and Chengelis, 1989.
NADPH: Cytochrome C reductase	60–113 nmol/min/mg-m	Ioannides et al., 1977; Lake et al., 1979; Costello and Chengelis, 1989.
MMFO activities		Ioannides et al., 1977; Lake et al., 1979; Shull et al., 1982. Good agreement between papers. Costello and Chengelis, 1989.
ethylmorphine demethylase	1.2–3.3 nmol/min/mg-m	
aniline hydroxylase	0.3–1.3 nmol/min/mg-m	
benzo(a)pyrene hydroxylase	0.95 ± 0.13 nmol/min/mg-m	
Epoxide hydrolase	No data identified	No applicable publications identified
UDP-glucuronosyl transferase	Limited data available using these substrates	Lake et al., 1979; Shull et al., 1982. Available papers use conflicting data presentations, making comparisons difficult.
1-naphthol		
4-methylumbelliferone		
Glutathione S-transferase		
p-nitrobenzyl chloride	18.2 ± 4.6 nmol/min/mg-c	Costello and Chengelis, 1989.
chlorodinitrobenzene	485 ± 107 nmol/min/mg-c	
Protein content estimaes		
microsomal	10–30 mg/g tissue	Ioannides et al., 1977, Costello and Chengelis, 1989; Lake et al., 1977.
cytosolic	110–150 mg/g tissue	

mg-m = mg microsomal protein; mg-c = mg cytosolic protein.

toward biphenyl as a substrate, but the albino had much greater activity toward ethylmorphine. Sexual dimorphism was also identified only for the albino ferret, the males having higher amounts of microsomal protein, cytochrome P-450, and ethylmorphine N-demethylase activity (Ioannides et al., 1977). In contrast, Shull et al. (1982) reported that while the concentrations of cytochrome P-450 were not different, females had higher microsomal activity toward benzo(a)pyrene, hexobarbital, ethoxycourmarin, and ethylmorphine. Given this information, one should assume that there is the potential for strain- and sex-related differences in xenobiotic metabolism in the ferret, and one should consider establishing baseline data for the ferrets being used in specific studies. This is further reenforced by the variability displayed in the sets of clinical chemistry data reported elsewhere in this chapter.

Depending on the age, sex, and strain of the ferret, relative liver weight ranges from

3.0 to 5.0% of body weight. There is also some variability in microsomal protein from adult animals: values as high as 33.8 mg/g liver (Lake et al., 1977) and as low as 12.1 mg/g (Ioannides et al., 1977) have been reported. Concentrations of P-450 are likewise varied, ranging from 0.19 nmol/mg microsomal protein to 0.73 nmol/mg (values inferred from data presented by Lake et al., 1977, and Ioannides et al., 1977, respectively). However, the values of 0.29 (Lake et al., 1979) and 0.19 nmol/mg microsomal protein (Shull et al., 1982) would appear to be better estimates. Ferrets tend to have less microsomal protein and less cytochrome P-450/mg protein than rats. Hence, on a gram liver basis, ferrets have considerably less cytochrome P-450 than rats. In general, however, ferret cytochrome P-450 has a higher rate of substrate turnover.

The activity on a microsomal protein basis toward common model substrates, such as aniline and ethylmorphine, has been reported to be about the same (Ioannides et al., 1977) or somewhat less (Lake et al., 1979) than the rat. The exception to this observation is that Ionnides et al. reported that the male albino ferret had much higher activities than the rat toward ethylmorphine. This high activity toward ethylmorphine was not confirmed by Lake et al. (1979) or Shull et al. (1982), and the reason for this difference is not clear. These observations again underscore the potential variability in xenobiotic metabolism in the ferret and the importance of establishing baseline values in one's own laboratory.

Only Ioannides et al. (1977) have discussed the developmental aspects of the microsomal mixed function oxidase. At birth, the hepatic content and concentration of the microsomal mixed function oxidase are very low. Different enzyme activities develop differently thereafter. Biphenyl 4-hydroxylation parallels the activity of NADPH reductase, and reaches adult levels (on a gram liver basis) in 14 days. Other activities tend to follow the development of cytochrome P-450, reaching adult levels approximately 2 months after birth. The largest increases in the components of the mixed function oxidase occur after weaning (4–6 weeks of age). Unlike the rat, the mature adult ferret retains measurable biphenyl 2-hydroxylation and p-nitrobenzaote reduction activities.

Few in-depth studies on the inducibility of the ferret microsomal mixed function oxidase system have been reported. There are no reports on the effects of phenobarbital on xenobiotic metabolism in the ferret. Lake et al. (1979) have demonstrated, however, that Aroclor 1254 (single ip dose, 500 mg/kg) will cause large increases in microsomal protein, the content of cytochrome P-450, and the specific activity toward aminopyrine, benzphetamine, ethylmorphine, and aniline. In contrast, Shull et al. (1982) have reported that Aroclor 1016 and 1242 (by dietary admix, 20 ppm, for 28 days) caused increases in relative liver weight without increases in the microsomal concentration of cytochrome P-450. In a shorter term experiment, two doses of Aroclor 1242 (100 mg/kg on day 0, 200 mg/kg ip on day 5, and sacrifice on day 10) caused fivefold increases in cytochrome P-450, with a shift in the absorbance maximum toward 448 nm. These authors (Shull et al., 1982) concluded that the ferret is weakly inducible. The ferret differs from the rat in that the polychlorinated biphenyl (PCB) induction results in large increases in cytochrome P-450 with only modes increases in benzo(a)pyrene hydroxylase.

Lake et al. (1977) reported that a phthalate ester ([di-(2-ethylhexyl)phthalate]) caused increases in liver weight in the ferret, but no increases in microsomal protein. The concentration of cytochrome P-450 and microsomal mixed function oxidase activity actually decreased. Here is an example of how an increase in liver weight does not necessarily mean microsomal induction. It has since been established that phthalate esters induced peroxisome proliferation (Reddy and Lalwani, 1983). Lake *et al.* (1977) did not examine the more common peroxisomal marker enzymes. Hence, the suitability of the ferret as a model for studying peroxisomal proliferation, or in examining toxicity in the absence thereof, remains to be established.

Very few, if any, papers have been published on the activities of epoxide hydrolase or glutathione S-transferase in the ferret. Traditionally, these enzymes are considered protective in that they react with and deactivate reactive potentially toxic metabolites. Early data discussed by Williams (1972) would suggest that the ferret is capable of forming mercapturic acids in a fashion similar to rodents, at least with chlorobenzene. Preliminary data from our laboratory would suggest that ferret glutathione 5-transferase activity with p-nitrobenzyl chloride and chlorodinitrobenzene (Table 25) are less than those seen in rats. An interesting paper by Frederick and Babish (1981) may provide some clues as to the activities of these enzymes relative to those of the rat. These investigators compared the mutagenic activity of uninduced rat and ferret S-9 liver fractions in the Ames assay. Ferret liver fraction had more mutagenic activity (with 2-acetylamidofluorene, cyclophosphamide, and 7,12-dimethylbenzanthracene) than that of the rat. When calculated on a cytochrome P-450 basis, ferret S-9 has 5 to 10 times the activity. The higher mutagenic activity in ferrets could be due to lower detoxification activity, but this remains to be established.

While glutathione S-transferase reactions have not been extensively studied in the ferret, other conjugative processes have been examined. These include glucuronide, sulfate, glycine, and taurine conjugate formation. In general, as a carnivore, the ferret is more likely to form amino acid conjugates (glycine and taurine) whereas rodents are more likely to form glucuronide and sulfate conjugates. This area was extensively reviewed by Hiram et al., in 1977. With regard to the ferret, there has been limited activity in this field since. In general, these investigations were of similar design in that model chemicals, usually an aromatic acetic acid, were administered to a variety of species and the different conjugates identified. For example, Emudianaughe et al. (1978) examined the metabolism of 2-naphthyl-acetic acid. In the ferret, the main urinary metabolite was the taurine conjugate, whereas this was undetectable in the rat where the glucuronide was the main metabolite. There was also a large species difference in the percentage of dose excreted in the urine, 3% in the rat vs 30% in the ferret. This is not surprising as glucuronides in the rat tend to be actively excreted in the bile. Idle et al. (1978) compared the metabolism of 10 aromatic acids in the rat and ferret. The ferret generated substantial (greater than 5%) amounts of taurine metabolites with seven of the test chemicals, whereas the rat did so only with one (2-naphtylacetic acid). Qualitatively, both species had essentially equivalent ability to elaborate glycine conjugates, although the rat tended to have higher activity for any specific chemical. In contrast, the rat produced little glucuronide with benzoic acid, whereas this was the major pathway for benzoic acid metabolism in the ferret. In their studies on phenoxybenzoic acid, Huckle et al. (1981) reported that the glycine and taurine conjugates were the major metabolites in ferrets, whereas the rat produced no detectable taurine conjugate and the sulfate was the major metabolite. These investigators have further shown that the majority of the glycine conjugative ability lies in the kidney, not the liver (Huckle et al., 1981). Therefore, as a general rule of thumb in working with ferrets, one should expect that amino acid conjugates will be the main metabolites of aromatic acids, and that these will be primarily excreted in the urine.

The conclusion of the previous paragraph not withstanding, the ferret does have the ability to form glucuronides with aromatic alcohols (phenol, naphthols, etc.). Conjugation with this class of substrates simply has not been well studied. Ioannides (1977) examined glucuronide formation using 4-methyl-umbelliferone, and detected relatively low activity.

Lake et al., detected much higher activities with 1-naphthol as the substrate. For both these substrates, the reported activity is less than that reported for rats. As in other species, glucuronosyl transferase is largely a hepatic enzyme, and is inducible by treatment with Aroclor 1254 (Lake et al., 1979). Hence, glucuronosyl transferase activity in the ferret has been established, but in-depth study remains to be completed.

While hepatic metabolism normally accounts for the majority of xenobiotic metabolism, extrahepatic pathways can sometimes be substantially involved in certain pathways. For example, the importance of the kidney in glycine conjugation has been mentioned. Extrahepatic pathways can sometimes be important with regard to toxicological mechanisms. Extrahepatic metabolism has been only marginally explored in the ferret. Lake et al. (1979) reported measurable amounts of benzo(a)pyrene hydroxylase, 7-ethoxycoumarin O-deethylase, and 1-naphthol glucuronyl transferase activities in the intestinal mucosa, kidney, lung, and testes of ferrets. As with the rat, these activities were present at much lower (2 to 3 orders of magnitude) concentrations than in the liver. Extrahepatic activities of benzo(a)pyrene hydroxylase and 7-ethoxycoumarin O-deethylase tended to be similar between the rat and ferret, but rats had 10-fold higher benzo(a)pyrene hydroxylase in the kidney. Rats consistently had higher 1-naphthol glucuronyl transferase activities. Extrahepatic benzo(a)pyrene hydroxylase, 7-ethoxycoumarin O-deethylase activities were induced by Aroclor 1254. Hence, extrahepatic metabolism in the ferret is not dissimilar to that in the rat, and the potential involvement of these enzymes in metabolism and disposition and toxicity should be kept in mind.

The disposition and metabolism of a specific chemical in the ferret has been examined in a few papers. Bleavins et al. (1982) compared the disposition of hexachlorobenzene in pregnant and nonpregnant ferrets. Clearance was greatly accelerated in the pregnant and nursing dams. This was attributed to a high degree of placental and mammary transfer of the chemical to pups. This could suggest that the ferret would be a good nonrodent model for multigenerational studies.

Gorrod and Damani (1980) examined the in vivo N-oxidation of 3-substituted pyridines in various animal species. Interestingly, the ferret more closely resembled the other species examined, with regard to N-oxide formation, than the rat. The ferret excreted approximately 34% of the dose as the N-oxide, whereas this figure was only 10% in the rat. Treatment with 3-methylcholanthrene radically changed this relationship, decreasing the amount of N-oxide to 0.43% in the ferret but increasing it to 4.2% in the rat. This is an example of not only species differences in metabolism, but species differences in response to hepatic MMFO induction.

Ioannides et al. (1982) examined glyceryl trinitrate (GTN) metabolism in the ferret as part of a broader examination on the effects of species, sex, age, and route of administration on the elimination of this chemical. They observed that there was an excellent correlation between body weight and plasma half-life of GTN (the higher the weight, the higher the half life). The results from the ferret were in line with this conclusion. Ferrets, however, had lower than expected volumes of distribution, which the authors attributed to the smaller proportion of body fat in the ferret in comparison to other species.

Ideally, one would like to know or be able to compare xenobiotic metabolism in the model species to that in humans. Predictive comparisons between humans and the ferret, however, are particularly difficult because xenobiotic metabolism in the ferret is not as well characterized as that for other species. Very few papers have been published comparing the disposition of specific chemicals in both species. In general, there are few hard rules in anticipating species similarities in metabolism. For example, Williams

(1972), in a classic work, noted that the human more closely resembled the rat than the ferret in the metabolism of phenol and benzoic acid. In contrast, the rabbit resembles the ferret in the metabolism of phenol, but the human in the metabolism of benzoic acid.

Perhaps, as the MMFO of the ferret becomes better characterized, out ability to predict similarities in xenobiotic metabolism between human subjects and ferrets will also improve.

REFERENCES

Andrews, P.L.R. (1988) The physiology of the ferret, in *Biology and Diseases of the Ferret*, Fox, J. G., ed. Lea & Febiger, Philadelphia, pp. 100–134.

Andrews, P.L.R., Bower, A.J., and Illman, D. (1979) Some aspects of the physiology and anatomy of the cardiovascular system of the ferret (Mustela putorius furo). *Lab. Anim.* 13, 215–220.

Andrews, P.L.R., and Illman, O. (1987) The ferret, in *UFAW Handbook on the Care and Management of Laboratory Animals*. 6th ed., Poole, T., ed. Longman's Scientific and Technical, London.

Barker, I.K., and Van Dreumel, A.A. (1985) The Alimentary System, in *Pathology of Domestic Animals*. Vol. 2. 3rd ed., Jubb, K.V.F., Kennedy, P.C., and Palmer, N., eds. Academic Press, New York, pp. 1–237.

Barer, G.R., Mohammed, F., Suggett, A., and Twelves, C.L. (1978) Hypoxic pulmonary vasconstriction in the ferret. *J. Physiol.* (Lond.) 281, 40P–41P.

Baskin, S.I., Finnegan, J.O., Garvin, L.C., et al. (1981) The utilization of the isolated ferret heart to study the effects in cardioplegia solutions. *Teratology* 24, 9A–10A.

Basrur, P.K., and Gilman, J.P.W. (1968) Synaptinema-like complex in spermatids of some Mustelids. *Can. J. Genet. Cytol.* 10(2), 426–432.

Bassett, C.F., and Llewellyn, L.M. (1949) The molting and fur growth pattern in the adult mink. *Am. Midland Naturalist* 42(3), 751–756.

Beach, J.E. (1982) The ferret for nonrodent toxicity studies—A pathologist's view. *Arch. Toxicol.* (Suppl.), 5:279–282.

Beck, F. (1975) The ferret as a teratological model, in *New Approaches to the Evaluation to Abnormal Embryonic Development*, Neubert, D., and Merker, H.-J., eds. Publishing Sciences Group, Acton, Massachusetts, pp. 8–20.

Beck, F., Swidzinska, P., and Gulamhusein, A. (1978) The effect of trypan blue on the development of the ferret and rat. *Teratology* 18, 187–192.

Bird, R.A., Sweet, C., Husseini, R.H., and Smith, H. (1983) The similar interaction of ferret alveolar macrophages with influenza virus strains of differing virulence at normal and pyrexial temperatures. *J. Gen. Virol.* 64, 1807–1810.

Bissonnette, T.H. (1932) Modification of mammalian sexual cycles: Reactions of ferrets of both sexes to electric light added after dark in November and December. *Proc. Roy. Soc. B* 110, 322–336.

Bell, F.R., and Dudgeon, J.A. (1948) An epizootic of influenza in a ferret colony. *J. Comp. Pathol.* 58, 167–171.

Bleakley, S.P. (1980) Simple technique for bleeding ferrets (Mustela putorius). *Lab. Anim.* 14, 59–60.

Bleavins, M.R., and Aulerich, R.J. (1981) Feed consumption and food passage time in mink (Mustela vison) and European ferrets (Mustela putorius furo). *Lab. Anim. Sci.* 31, 268–269.

Bleavins, M., Breslin, W., Aulerich, R., and Ringer, R. (1982) Excretion and placental and mammary transfer of hexachlorobenzene in the European ferret (mustela putorius furo) *J. Toxicol. Environ. Health* 10, 929–940.

Boggess, E. K., Henderson, F. R., and Choate, J. R. (1980) A Black-footed ferret (*Mustela nigripes*) from Kansas. *J. Mammal.* 61(3), 571.

Boissin-Agasse, L., and Boissin, J. (1979) Seasonal changes of testicular function, volume and plasma testosterone in two Mustelids: ferret, Mustela furo, and mink, Mustela vision. *J. Physiol. (Paris)* 75, 227–232.

Borelli, V., and Filho, A.F. (1971) Contribution to the study of the topography, morphology, and arterial irrigation of the sinusal node of the ferret (Mustela putorius furo) heart. *Mammalia* 35(3), 501–503.

Boyd, R.L., and Mangos, J.A. (1981) Pulmonary mechanics of the normal ferret. *J. Appl. Physiol. Respir. Environ. Exerc. Physiol.* 50(4), 799–804.

Braekevelt, C.R. (1982) Fine structure of the retinal epithelium, Bruch's membrane (Complexis Basalis) and choriocapillaris in the domestic ferret. *Acta Anat.* 113, 117–127.

Brantom, P.G., Gaunt, I.F., and Hardy, J. (1977) One-year toxicity study of Orange G in the ferret. *Food Cosmet. Toxicol.* 15, 379–382.

Breisch, E. (1980) A quantitative ultrastructural study of cardiac hypertrophy and regression. *Anat. Rec.* 190, 347.

Chevance, L.G., Simon-Lavoine, N., Valancogne-Grosjean, S., et al. (1978) Scanning and transmission electron microscopy study of ferret respiratory mucosa infected with influenza A virus. *Ann. Microbiol. (Paris)* 129, 177–206.

Clark, T.W. (1978) Current status of the black-footed ferret in Wyoming. *J. Wildl. Manage.* 42(1), 128–134.

Cochran, K.W., Maassab, H. F., Tsunoda, A., and Berlin, B.S. (1965) Studies on the antiviral activity of amantadine hydrochloride. *Ann. N.Y. Acad. Sci.* 130, 432–439.

Costello, A., and Chengelis, C. (1989) Previously unpublished data.

Conn, R.B. (1963) Normal laboratory values of clinical importance, in *Textbook of Medicine,* Beeson, P. B., and McDermott, W., eds. Saunders, Philadelphia, pp. 1826–1835.

Curl, J.L., and Curl, J.S. (1985) Restraint device for serial blood sampling of ferrets. *Lab. Anim. Sci.* 35(3), 296–297.

Cusumano, C.L., Sever, J.L., Schiff, G.M., and Huebner, R.J. (1965) Effect of amantadine hydrochloride on Rubella virus in tissue culture and in ferrets. *Abstr. Bact. Proc.* p. 119.

Donovan, B.T. (1966) The effect of light upon reproductive mechanisms as illustrated by the ferret, in *Ciba Foundation Study Group on the Effects of External Stimuli on Reproduction,* 27 July 1966. Little, Brown, Boston, Ciba Foundation Study Group, 26:43–52.

Donovan, B.T. (1967) Light and control of the estrous cycle in the ferret. *J. Endocrinol.* 39(1), 105–113.

Duncan, R.J., and Prasse, K.W. (1986) *Veterinary Laboratory Medicine, Clinical Pathology.* 2nd ed. Iowa State University Press, Ames.

Dungworth, D.L., (1985) The respiratory system, in *Pathology of Domestic Animals.* Vol. 2. 3rd ed. Jubb, K.V.F., Kennedy, P.C., and Palmer, N., eds., Academic Press, New York, pp. 413–556.

Emudainughe, T., Caldwell, J., Dixon, P., and Smith, R. (1978) Studies on the metabolism of arylacetic acids. 5. The metabolic fate of 2-naphthylacetic acid in the rat, rabbit and ferret. *Xenobiotica* 8, 525–534.

Farrow, B.R.H., et al. (1972) Pneumocystic pneumonia in the dog. *J. Comp. Pathol.* 82, 447.

Fenton, R.J., and Potter, C.W. (1977) Dose-response activity of ribavirin against influenza virus infection in ferrets. *J. Antimicrob. Chemother.* 3, 263.

Fenton, R.J., Bessell, C., Spilling, C.R., and Potter, C.W. (1977) The effects of oral or local aerosol administration of 1-aminoadamantane hydrochloride (amantadine hydrochloride) on influenza infections of the ferret. *J. Antimicrob. Chemother.* 3, 463.

Fisher, J.W., and Scott, P. (1944) An epizootic of influenza A in a ferret colony. *Can. J. Publ. Health* 35, 364–366.

Florczyk, A.P., Schurig, J.E., and Bradner, W.T. (1981) Cisplatin-induced emesis in the ferret (Mustela putorius furo), a new animal model. *Cancer Treat. Rep.* 66, 187–194.

Florczyk, A.P., and Schurig, J. E. (1981) A technique for chronic jugular catheterization in the ferret (Mustela putorius furo). *Pharmacol. Biochem. Behav.* 14, 255–258.

Fox, J.G. (1987) Symposium: The Biology and Diseases of Ferrets. J.G. Fox (Chairman). *J. Am. Vet. Med. Assoc.* 190, 1610.

Fox, J.G. (1988) *Biology and Diseases of the Ferret*. Lea & Febiger, Philadelphia.

Fox, J.G., Murphy, J.C., Ackerman, J.I., Prostak, M.S., Gallagher, C.A., Rambow, V.J. (1982) Proliferative colitis in ferrets. *Am. J. Vet. Res.* 43:858–864.

Fox, J.G., Ackerman, J.I., and Newcomer, C.E. (1983) Ferret as a potential reservoir for human campylobacteriosis. *Am. J. Vet. Res.* 44, 1049–1052.

Fox, J.G., Ackerman, J.I., Taylor, N., Claps, M., and Murphy, J.C. (1987) *Campylobacter jejuni* infection in the ferret: An animal model of human campylobacteriosis. *Am. J. Vet. Res.* 48, 85–90.

Fox, J.G., Edrise, B.M., Cabot, E.B., Beaucage, C., Murphy, J.C., and Prostak, K.S. (1986) *Campytobacker*-like organisms isolated from gastric mucosa of ferrets. *Am. J. Vet. Res.* 47:236–239.

Fox, J.G., Pearson, R.C., and Gorham, J.R. (1988) Viral and chlamydial disease, in, *Biology and Diseases of the Ferret*, Fox, J.G., ed. Lea & Febiger, Philadelphia, pp. 217–234.

Frederick, K., and Babish, J. (1984) *In vitro* activation of the promutagens 2-acetylamidofluorene, cyclophosphamide, and 7, 12-dimethylbenzanthracene by constitutive ferret and rat heptic S-9 fractions. *Toxicology* 21, 73–84.

Frederick, K.A., and Babish, J.G. (1985) Compendium of recent literature on the ferret. *Lab. Anim. Sci.* 35(3),298–318.

Gad, S.C. (1989) Personal communication to D. McLain (August, 1989).

Gorrod, J., and Damani, L. (1980) The metabolic N-oxidation of 3-substituted pyridines in various animal species *in vivo*. *Eur. J. of Drug Metab. Pharmacokinet.* 5, 53–57.

Greener, Y. (1987) Symposium: The Use of Ferrets as an Animal Model in Preclinical Safety Studies and Biomedical Research. Y. Greener (Chairman). Twenty-sixth Annual Meeting of the Society of Toxicology. February 23–27, Washington, D.C.

Greener, Y., and Gillies, B. (1985) Intravenous infusion in ferrets. *Lab. Anim.* Sept.: 41–44.

Greenlee, P.G., and Stephens, E. (1984) Meningeal cryptococcosis and congestive cardiomyopathy in a ferret. *J. Am. Vet. Med. Assoc.* 184, 840–841.

Gulamhusein, A., and Beck, F. (1971) The value of the ferret as an experimental animal in teratology, in *Methods in Prenatal Toxicology: Evaluation of Embryotoxic Effects in Experimental Animals*, Neubert, D., Merker, H.-J., and Kwasigroch, T.E., eds. Publishing Sciences Group, Acton, Massachusetts, pp. 44–51.

Haddad, R.K., and Hoar, R.M. (1981) Symposium: Conference on the Ferret as an Alternative Species in Teratology and Toxicology. R.K. Haddad and R.M. Hoar (Chairmen). Teratology Society and Behavioral Teratology Society (Sponsors). Stanford University, Stanford, California, June 25–26.

Haddad, R.K., and Rabe, A. (1980) Use of the ferret in experimental neuroteratology: Cerebral, cerebellar and retinal dysplasias induced by methylazoxymethanol acetate, in *Advances in the Study of Birth Defects. Neural and Behavioral Teratology*, Persaud, T.V.N., ed. MTP Press, Lancaster, England: 45–62.

Hagedoorn, A.L. (1947) The waltzing ferret and its origin. *Genetics* 24, 1–10.

Hagen, K.W., Goto, H., and Gorham, J.R. (1970) Distemper vaccine in pregnant ferrets and mink. *Res. Vet. Sci.* 11, 458–460.

Hammond, J. Jr. (1952) Control of reproduction and pelt changes in ferrets: Some experiments with animals kept entirely upon artificial light. *J. Agric. Sci.* 42, 293–303.

Hammond, J., and Chesterman, F.C. (1972) The ferret, in *UFAW Handbook on the Care and Management of Laboratory Animals*. 4th ed. Churchill Livingstone, London.

Hart, D.S. (1951) Photoperiodicity in the female ferret. *J. Exp. Biol.* 28:1–12.

Harvey, N.E., and MacFarlane, W.V. (1958) The effect of day length on the coat shedding cycles, body weight, and reproduction of the ferret. *Austral. J. Biol. Sci.* 11, 187–199.

Henson, J.B., Leader, R.W., and Gorham, J.R. (1961) Hypergammablobulinemia in mink. *Proc. Soc. Exp. Biol. Med.* 107, 919–920.

Hirom, P., Idle, J., and Milburne, P. (1977) Comparative aspects of the biosynthesis and excretion of xenobiotic conjugates by non primate mammals, in *Drug Metabolism: From Microbes to Man*. Purke, D. V., and Smith, R. L., eds. Crane, Russak, New York, pp. 299–329.

Hoar, R.M. (1984) Use of ferrets in toxicity testing. *J. Am. Coll. Toxicol.* 3(6), 325–330.

Huckle, K., Hutson, D., Millburn, P., (1981) Species variations in the renal and hepatic conjugation of 3-phenoxybenzoic acid with glycine. *Xenobiotica* 11, 635–644.

Idle, J., Milburn, P., and Williams, R. (1978) Taurine conjugates as metabolites of arylacetic acids in the ferret. *Xenobiotica* 8, 253–264.

Ioannides, C., Sweatman, B., Richards, R., and Parke, D. (1977) Drug metabolism in the ferret. Effects of sex, age and strain. *Gen. Pharmacol.* 8, 243.

Ioannides, C., Parke, D., and Taylor, I. (1982) Elimination of glyceryl trinitrate: Effects of sex, age, species and route of administration. *Br. J. Pharmacol.* 77, 83–88.

Ishida, K. (1968) Age and seasonal changes in the testis of the ferret. *Arch. Histol. Jpn.* 29(2), 193–205.

Jubb, K.V.F., Kennedy, P.C., and Palmer, N. (1985) *Pathology of Domestic Animals*. 3rd ed. Academic Press, New York.

Katz, D.R. (1987) Ferret legging. *Outdoors*, Feb/Mar, 73.

Kaufman, L.W. (1980) Foraging costs and meal patterns in ferrets (Mustela putorius furo). *Physiol. Behav.* 25, 139–142.

Kauffman, C.A., Bergman, A.G., and O'Conner, R.P. (1982) Distemper virus infection in ferrets: An animal model of measles-induced immunosuppression. *Clin. Exp. Immunol.* 47, 617–625.

Kempf, J.E., and Chang, H.T. (1949) The cardiac output and circulation time of ferrets. *Proc. Soc. Exp. Biol. Med.* 72, 711–714.

Kenyon, A.J., Magnano, T., Helmboldt, C.F., and Buko, L. (1966) Aleutian disease in the ferret. *J. Am. Vet. Med. Assoc.* 149, 920–923.

Kenyon, A.J., Howard, E., and Buko, L. (1967) Hypergammaglobulinemia in ferrets with lymphoproliferative lesions (Aleutian disease). *Am. J. Vet. Res.* 28, 1167–1172.

Koshimizu, K., Kotani, H., and Syukuda, Y. (1982) Isolation of mycoplasmas from experimental ferrets (Mustela putorius). *Jikken Dobutsu* 31, 299–302.

Lake, G., Brantom, P., Gangolli, S., Butterworth, K., Grasso, P., and Lloyd, A. (1977) The hepatic effects of orally administered di-(2-ethylhexyl) phthalate in the ferret. *Biochem. Soc. Trans.* 5, 310–311.

Lake, B., Collins, M., Harris, R., and Gangolli, S. (1979) The induction of hepatic and extrahepatic xenobiotic metabolism in the rat and ferret by a polychlorinated byphenyl mixture (Aroclor 1254). *Xenobiotica* 9, 723–731.

Lee, E.J., Moore, W.E., Fryer, H.C., and Minocha, H.C. (1982) Haematological and serum chemistry profiles of ferrets (Mustela putorius furo). *Lab. Anim.* 16, 133–137.

Lipman, N., and Fox, J. G., (1987) Clinical, preclinical, and pathologic changes associated with a case of dilatative cardiomyopathy in a ferret. *Lab. An. Sci.* 37, 210–212.

Long, E.G., Smith, J.S., and Meier, J.L. (1986) Attachment of Pneumocystis carinii to rat pneumocytes. *Lab. Invest.* 54(6), 609–615.

Marino, T.A., Biberstein, D., and Severdia, J.B. (1981) The ultrastructure of the atrio-ventricular junctional tissues in the newborn ferret heart. *Am. J. Anat.* 161, 383–392.

Marshall, K.R., and Marshall, G.W. (1973) *The Biomedical Use of Ferrets in Research*. Supplement 1. Published by Marshall Research Animals, Inc., North Rose, New York.

McBride, A.R. (1989) PSIN training guide: An update on ferrets. *Pet Supplies Marketing* 43(8), 64.

McLain, D.E. (1989) Bacterial/viral infection of the pregnant ferret and neonate and the response to various prophylactic treatments. In preparation.

McLain, D.E., and Lin, L. (1989a) Spontaneous eye lesions in the laboratory ferret: Genetic distribution in relation to age and sex. In preparation.

McLain, D.E., and McGrain-Dutson, S. (1989) An adjustable restraint device for accessing the venous and arterial systems of the ferret. In preparation.

McLain, D.E., and Roe, D.A. (1983) Nutrient composition of a natural ferret diet and the reproductive response to several purified formulations. *Fed. Proc.* 43, 1318.

McLain, D.E., Babish, J.G., and Roe, D.A. (1985a) Pharmacokinetics of ethanol in the ferret. *Alcohol. Clin. Exp. Res.* 9(2), 138–142.

McLain, D.E., Harper, S.M., Roe, D.A., Babish, J.G., and Wilkinson, C.F. (1985b) Congenital malformations and variations in reproductive performance in the ferret: Effects of maternal age, color and parity. *Lab. Anim. Sci.* 35(3), 251–255.

McLain, D.E., McCartney, M., Giovanetto, S., Martis, L., Greener, Y., and Youkilis, E. (1987a) Assessment of the subchronic intravenous toxicity and disposition of ($^{14}C^-$) acrolein in the rat and the acute and subchronic toxicity in ferrets. *Toxicologist* 7(1), 208.

McLain, D.E., Lin, L., Greener, Y., and Youkilis, E. (1987b) Required sample sizes for increasing the statistical power of hematologic-biochemical evaluations in a heterogeneous population. *Toxicologist* 7(1), 211.

McLain, D.E., Thomas, J.A., and Fox, J.G. (1988). Nutrition, in *Biology and Diseases of the Ferret*, Fox, J.G., ed. Lea & Febiger, Philadelphia, pp. 135–152.

Milder, J.E., et al. (1980) Comparison of histological and immunological techniques for the detection of Pneumocystis carinii in rat bronchial lavage fluid. *J. Clin. Microbiol* 2, 409.

Miller, G.S. (1933) The origin of the ferret. *Scot. Nat. Edin.* 153–154.

Momberg-Jorgensen, H.C., (1951) Enzootic malignant granulomatosis in ferrets. *Ach. Pathol.* 29, 297–306.

Moody, K.D., Bowman, T.A., and Lang, C.M. (1985) Laboratory management of the ferret for biomedical research. *Lab. Anim. Sci.* 35(3), 272–279.

Moreland, A.F., and Glaser, C. (1985) Evaluation of ketamine, ketamine-xylazine and ketamine-diazepam anesthesia in the ferret. *Lab. Anim. Sci.* 35(3), 287–290.

Neptun, D.A., Smith, C.N., and Irons, R.D. (1985) Effect of sampling site and collection method on variations in baseline clinical pathology parameters in Fischer-344 rats: 1. Clinical chemistry. *Funk. Appl. Toxicol.* 5, 1180–1185.

Neptun, D.A., Smith, C.N., and Irons, R.D. (1986) Effect of sampling site and collection method on variations in baseline clinical pathology parameters in Fischer-344 rats: 2. Clinical hematology. *Fund. Appl. Toxicol.* 7, 658–663.

Obel, A.L. (1959) Studies on a disease in mink with systemic proliferation of plasma cells. *Am. J. Vet. Res.* 20, 384–393.

Ohshima, K., Shen, D.T., Henson, J.B., et al. (1978) Comparison of the lesions of Aleutian disease in mink and hypergammaglobulinemia in ferrets. *Am. J. Vet. Res.* 39, 653–657.

Ott, R.L., and Svehag, S.E. (1959) Resistance to experimental distemper in ferrets following the use of killed tissue vaccine. *West. Vet.* 6, 107–111.

Owen, C. (1969) The domestication of the ferret, in *The Domestication and Exploitation of Plants and Animals,* Ucko, P.J., and Dimbleby, G.W., eds. Gerald Duckworth, London, pp. 489–493.

Parrish, C.R., Leathers, C.W., Pearson, R., and Gorham, J.R., (1987) Comparisons of feline panleukopenia virus, canine parvovirus, raccoon parvovirus, and mink enteritis virus and their pathogencity for mink and ferret. *Am. J. Vet. Res.* 48, 1429–1435.

Peake, M.D., Harabin, A.L., Brennan, N.J., and Sylvester, J.T. (1981) Steady-state vascular responses to graded hypoxia in isolated lungs of five species. *Am. J. Physiol.* 51, 1214–1219.

Pfeiffer, C.J. (1970a) Surface topology of the stomach in man and the laboratory ferret. *J. Ultrastruct. Res.* 33(3/4), 252–262.

Pfeiffer, C.J. (1970b) Gastric surface morphology in man, monkey and ferret: Evidence for *in situ* surface cell degeneration. *Exp. Mol. Pathol.* 13(3), 319–328.

Pocock, R.I. (1932) Is the ferret a domesticated polecat? *Field (Lond.)* 159(4134), 410.

Poddar, S. (1977) Gross and microscopic anatomy of the biliary tract of the ferret. *Acta Anat.* 97, 121–131.

Poddar, S., and Jacob, S. (1977) Gross and microscopic anatomy of the major salivary glands of the ferret. *Acta Anat.* 98, 434–443.

Poddar, S., and Murgatroyd, L. (1976) Morphological and histological study of the gastrointestinal tract of the ferret. *Acta Anat.* 96, 321–334.

Porter, D.D., Larsen, A.E., and Porter, H.G. (1980) Aleutian disease of mink. *Adv. Immunol.*, 29:261–268.

Porter, H.G., Porter, D.D. and Larsen, A.E., (1981) Aleutian disease in the ferret. *Fed. Proc.* 40:(3 Pt. 2), 1120.

Porter, H.G., Porter, D.D., and Larsen, A.E. (1982) Aleutian disease in ferrets (Mustela putorius). *Infect. Immunol.* 36(1), 379–386.

Porter, D.D., Porter, H.G., Larsen, A.E., Bloom, M.E. (1987) Restricted viral antibody specificity in many ferrets infected with the ferret Aleutian Disease parvovirus. *Arch. Virol.* 93(1–2), 155–161.

Prince, G.A., and Porter, D.D. (1976) The pathogenesis of respiratory synctial virus infection in infant ferrets. *Am. J. Pathol.* 82, 337.

Pyle, N.J. (1940) Use of ferrets in laboratory work and research investigations. *Am. J. Pub. Health* 30, 787–796.

Randolph, R.W. (1986) Preventive medical care for the pet ferret in *Current Veterinary Therapy*. Kirk, R.W., ed. Saunders, Philadelphia, pp. 772.

Reddy, J., and Lalwani, N. (1983) Carcinogenesis by hepatic peroxisomal proliferators; evaluation of the risk of hypolipidemic drugs and industrial plasticizers to humans. *CRC Crit. Rev. Toxicol.* 12, 1–58.

Rehg, J.E., Gigliotti, F. and Stokes, D.C., (1988) Cryptosporidiosis in Ferrets. *Lab. Anim. Sci.* 38, 155–158.

Robbins, S.L., Cotran, R.S. and Kumar, V., (1984) The heart, in *Pathologic Basis of Disease*. 3rd ed. Saunders, Philadelphia, pp. 547–609.

Robinson, W.F., and Maxie, M.G., (1985). The cardiovascular system, in *Pathology of Domestic Animals*. Vol. 3, 3rd ed., Jubb, K.V.F, Kennedy, P.C., and Palmer, N., eds. Academic Press, New York, pp. 1–81.

Roser, R.J., and Lavers, R.B. (1976) Food habits of the ferret (Mustela putorius furo) at Pukepuke Lagoon, New Zealand. *N.Z.J. Zool.* 3, 269–275.

Rowett, H.G.Q. (1965) *The Rat as a Small Mammal*. John Murray, London.

Ryland, L.M., and Gorham, J.R. (1978) The ferret and its diseases. *J. Am. Vet. Med. Assoc.* 173(9); 1154–1158.

Seamer, J., and Chesterman, F.C. (1967) A survey of diseases in laboratory animals. *Lab. Anim.* 1, 117–139.

Sherrill, A., and Gorham, J. (1985) Bone marrow hypoplasia associated with estrus in ferrets. *Lab. Anim. Sci.* 35(3), 280–286.

Shull, L., Bleavins, M., Olson, B., and Aulerich, R. (1982) Polychlorinated biphenyls (Aroclors 1016 and 1242): Effect on hepatic microsomal mixed function oxidases in mink and ferret. *Arch. Environ. Contam. Toxicol.* 11, 313–321.

Shump, A.U., and Shump, K.A. (1978) Growth and development of the European ferret (Mustela putorius). *Lab. Anim. Sci.* 28(1), 89–91.

Smith, S.H., and Bishop, S.P. (1985) The electrocardiogram of normal ferrets and ferrets with right ventricular hypertrophy. *Lab. Anim. Sci.* 35(3), 268–271.

Smith, W., and Stuart-Harris, C.H. (1936) Influenza infection of man from the ferret. *Lancet 2*, 121.

Smith, R. and Timbrell, J. (1974) Factors affecting the metabolism of phenacetin-1. Influence of dose, chronic dosage, route of administration and species on the metabolism of (1-14C-acetyl)-phenacetin. *Xenobiotica 4*, 489.

Smith, W., Andrews, C.H., and Laidlow, P.O. (1933) The virus obtained from human influenza patients. *Lancet 2*, 66.

Stokes, D.C., Gigliotti, F., Rehg, J.E., Snellgrove, R.L., and Hughes, W.T., (1987) Experimental *Pneumocystis carinii* pneumonia in the ferret. *Br. J. Exp. Pathol.* 68, 267–276.

Sweet, C., MacCartney, J.C., Bird, R.A., et al. (1981) Differential distribution of virus and histological damage in the lower respiratory tract of ferrets infected with influenza viruses of differing virulence. *J. Gen. Virol.* 54, 103–114.

Thompson, A.P.D. (1951) A history of the ferret. *J. Hist. Med. Allied Sci.* 6, 471–480.

Thornton, P.C., Wright, P.A., Sacra, P.J., and Goodier, T.E.W. (1979) The ferret, Mustela putorius furo, as a new species in toxicology. *Lab. Anim.* 13, 119–124.

Thorpe, P.A., and Herbert, J. (1976) The accessory optic system of the ferret. *J. Comp. Neurol.* 170, 295–309.

Vacca, L.L., (1985) *Laboratory Manual of Histochemistry*. Raven Press, New York, pp. 355–392.

Vinegar, A., Sinnett, E. E., and Kosch, P.C. (1979) Respiratory mechanics of a small carnivore: The ferret. *Physiologist* 22(4):127.

Vinegar, A., Sinnett, E.E., and Kosch, P.C. (1982) Respiratory mechanics of a small carnivore: The ferret. *J. Appl. Physiol. Respir. Environ. Exerc. Physiol.* 52(4), 832–837.

Vinegar, A., Sinnett, E.E., Kosch, P.C., and Miller, M.L. (1985) Pulmonary physiology of the ferret and its potential as a model for inhalation toxicology. *Lab. Anim. Sci.* 35(3), 246–250.

Wen, G.Y., Sturman, J.A., and Shek, J.W. (1985) A comparative study of the tapetum, retina and skull of the ferret, dog and cat. *Lab. Anim. Sci.* 35, 200–210.

Williams, R. (1972) Species variations in drug biotransformation, in *Fundamentals of Drug Metabolism and Drug Disposition*, LaDa, B., Mandel, H., and Way, E. L. eds. Williams & Wilkins, Baltimore, pp. 187–205.

Willis, L.S., and Barrow, M.V. (1971) The ferret (Mustela putorius furo L.) as a laboratory animal. *Lab. Anim. Sci.* 21(5), 712–716.

Wilson, M.S., and O'Donoghue, P.N. (1982) A mobile rack of cages for ferrets (Mustela putorius furo). *Lab. Anim.* 16, 278–280.

8

The Dog

Toxicology: **Gillian C. Haggerty**
G. D. Searle and Company
Skokie, Illinois

Pathology: **Robert W. Thomassen**
G. D. Searle and Company
Skokie, Illinois

Metabolism: **Christopher P. Chengelis**
WIL Research Laboratories, Inc.
Ashland, Ohio

Toxicology **Gillian C. Haggerty**

The canine model in biomedical research has served a dual role by helping to provide information on biomedical problems in humans as well as fundamental knowledge of benefit to dogs themselves. Advantages of using the dog in the laboratory were recognized by researchers as early as the seventeenth century. The dog's internal system, organs, and muscles are similiar to those of man, a fact which has stimulated the development of canine models in numerous areas such as circulation and cardiovascular research. The relatively large size and longevity of the dog and the high incidence of malignancies inherent in the species makes the dog advantageous for sequential studies in individual animals related to the etiology, pathogenesis, and therapy of malignancies (Shifrine and Wilson, 1980). Also, the extensive database available on canine immunohematological parameters has made the dog an extremely valuable animal model for organ transplantation studies, especially in the areas of kidney preservation and the evaluation of immunosuppressant drugs (Shifrine and Wilson, 1980).

HISTORY

The history of the domestic dog *(Canis familiaris)* is obscure. While the genus *Canis* also includes wolves, jackals, dingos, coyotes, and more distant relatives such as various foxes *(Alopex, Vulpes,* and *Urocyon)* and the Cape Hunting dog *(Lycaon)*, there is no wild species from which the dog is definitely known to derive. The wolf and the jackal have been considered as likely ancestors, although an alternative suggestion has been made that the dog as a species may have arisen as a result of a hybridization between some doglike ancestor and the wolf (Fox, 1965b).

The dog is thought to be the oldest of domesticated animals, a fact which has contributed to the difficulty in attempting to identify its wild ancestors. Skeletal remains place its domestication as far back as 8000 B.C. (Andersen, 1970). It is likely that for many centuries the early dog remained of one general type which was similiar to the modern-day Australian dingo (Andersen, 1970). The ability to selectively breed dogs through several generations for specific traits is believed to have been a relatively early human discovery, and was probably triggered by the recognized benefit of using the dog for hunting and scavenging activities. Examples of early breeding efforts include a Pekingese type which has existed in China for about 4000 years, a mastiff breed depicted in Assyrian sculpture about 600 B.C., a greyhound type in Egypt of similiar antiquity, and the powerful hunting dogs of early Britain and Gaul.

The division into a multiplicity of breeds is a more recent development of the last 300 years. Great Britain has historically been the country most active in the selective breeding of a great variety of dogs; by the nineteenth century, a full complement of breeds was developed for a variety of tasks, including sporting (setter, pointer, spaniel, and the smaller bull and fox terriers), coursing (greyhound), shepherding (Old English and Scottish collie), sight and smell hunting (including wolfhound, foxhound, and beagle), guarding (mastiff), and for use as pets (King Charles spaniel, pug, and Pomeranian).

The use of animals that have an unknown history and are of questionable health is a major concern for many researchers. From a clinicopathological standpoint, heterogeneous populations of mongrel dogs do not appear to be more variable than homogeneous populations; however, laboratory bred animals generally show less clinical, gross, and microscopic evidence of disease (Pick and Eubanks, 1965). Because of such concerns, researchers have moved in the direction of using laboratory bred dogs.

Of the many breeds available, only a limited number possess the qualities (such as moderate size, even temperament, and ease of handling) desired in an experimental dog. Specific breeds that have been used in biomedical research include the greyhound for its well-defined muscles and nerves and large chest cavity, the Dalmation for its human-like excretory functions, and the German Shepherd for its good bone and joint configuration.

In the general area of toxicological research, the beagle is probably the most frequently used species of dog, although the Pembrokshire corgi has been advocated as a satisfactory alternative (Noel, 1970). Because of this, much of the following discussion will specifically refer to the beagle.

NORMAL PARAMETERS

In toxicological research, determining whether a statistically significant change is biologically relevant can often be difficult. Establishing the existance of an adverse effect is in great part accomplished by making comparisons between treatment and control groups. A great deal of reliance is placed on control data, which in the case of most nonrodent toxicology studies, are often collected from a relatively limited number of animals (usually four to six for a 2- or 4-week study). On this basis, it is extremely important to have a well-established database of normal physiological parameters with a good estimate of the expected magnitude of variability.

Growth Curves and Feed Consumption

Table 1 and Figure 1, respectively, show beagle feed consumption and growth weight data over a 1-year period starting at approximately 5 months of age. The biggest relative increase in feed consumption is seen between 4.5 and 6 months of age (Noel, 1970). A slower rate of increase is observed over the following 3–4 months, and by about 10 months of age, feed consumption levels off and remains stationary thereafter. This pattern coincides fairly well with the rapid fall in the rate of body weight gain which begins between 6.5 and 7.0 months of age (see Fig. 1). By about 12 months of age, animals have almost attained full adult weight. In the beagle, there appears to be an increase in the variability in body weight with increasing age. The average male gains more weight with age than the average female; by puberty, males are about 2 kg heavier than females.

Reproductive and Physiological Parameters

Normal physiological and reproductive parameters are shown in Tables 2 and 3, respectively. The four phases of the estrus cycle are proestrus, a preparatory phase which leads to estrus; metestrus, which is dominated by the influence of the corpus luteum; and anestrus, a period of sexual quiesence (Christie and Bell, 1971). While most mammals can be classified as seasonal or continuous breeders, the dog fits neither category. The observations of cyclical ovarian events and accompanying behavioral and morphological changes in genitalia at one heat period that continue until the next suggest that the bitch has an extended estrous cycle (Engle, 1946; Jochle and Andersen, 1977).

In the male beagle dog, the reproductive organs appear to reach a peak of development at about 32 weeks of age (Tsutsui et al., 1986). This sexual maturation is preceded by the rapid development of the anterior pituitary gland, which in turn stimulates testicular development by gonadotropin release.

Table 1 Feed Consumption in Beagles

Approximate age range (months)	Mean feed consumption (95% CL) (kg dry diet/dog/week)	
	Males[a]	Females[a]
4.5–5.0	2.27	2.05
	(1.6–2.8)	(1.4–2.7)
5.5–6.0	2.62	2.39
	(2.1–2.8)	(1.8–2.8)
6.5–7.0	2.68	2.45
	(2.3–2.8)	(1.9–2.8)
7.5–8.0	2.73	2.55
	(2.4–2.8)	(2.0–2.8)
9.5–10.0	2.76	2.60
	(2.7–2.8)	(2.2–2.8)
10.5–16.0	2.77	2.59
	(2.6–2.8)	(2.1–2.8)

[a]N = 130

Source: From Noel (1970); used with permission.

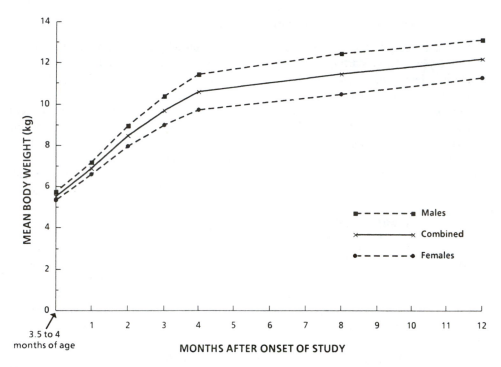

Figure 1 Growth weight curves in the beagle. (Adapted from Noel, 1970.)

Table 2 Normal Physiological Parameters

Average life span	12.5 years[a]
Daily food consumption	25–40 g/kg body weight
Daily water consumption	Ad libitum; approximately 600 ml
Rectal temperature	37.8°C ±0.13 (SD)[c]
Respiration rate	20/min (10–30)[b]
Oxygen consumption	0.36 ml O_2/g/hr[b]
Tidal volume	24 ml/kg (18–35)[b]
Minute volume	4.5 L ±0.2[c]
Functional residual capacity	367 ml (248–540)[b]
Lung compliance	117 ml ±5.6 (5 cm H_2O)
PO_2	73.7 mmHg (61–87)[b]
PCO_2	36 mmHg (29–46)[b]
pH	7.44 (7.37–7.51)[b]
Basal metabolism	2 cal/kg/hr[d]

[a]In dogs raised under "protected" environmental conditions (Andersen and Rosenblatt, 1974).
[b]Measured in beagles weighing from 6.8–11.5 kg (Pickrell et al., 1970).
[c]Measured in beagles weighing 13 kg (Andersen, 1970).
[d]Michaud and Elvehjem, 1944.

Table 3 Reproductive Parameters

Puberty	6–12 months of age
Breeding age:	
males	10–12 months
females	9–12 months
Gestation	60–65 days
Estrus Cycle:[a]	
proestrus	5–15 days
estrus	5–15 days
metestrus	60–65 days
anestrus	Length variable
Weaning age	5–8 weeks
Litter size	1–11 pups; 5–6 average
Breeding age (males)	10–12 months
Peak testis development	32 weeks[a]
Peak testis weight	8.6 g[a]
Peak epididymis and deferens gland, penis, and prostate development	32 weeks[a]

[a]Tsutsui et al., 1986.

HUSBANDRY

Proper handling and care of the experimental dog is essential for its general physical and psychological well-being. While dogs have many of the same general requirements as other experimental animals, special consideration must be given to factors such as space adequacy and degree of socialization

Housing

Housing is one of the most important features in the physical environment of the laboratory animal and usually consists of a microenvironment, or primary enclosure (the cage or pen), and the macroenvironment, or secondary enclosure (the room containing the cage or pen). The housing system employed should allow adequate space for freedom of movement and postural adjustment and provide a comfortable resting area for the animal. It should also be escape proof, provide adequate ventilation and access to feed and water, keep the animal dry and clean, and meet biological needs. Ideal housing can be turned into metabolism cages by the addition of trays and movable partitions, thus causing minimal disturbance during feces and urine collection. The most common types of housing for experimental dogs are cages and pens (or runs). The current space recommendations of the National Research Council (NRC) for laboratory dogs, as published in the 1985 revision of the *Guide for the Care and Use of Laboratory Animals* (NIH, 1985), are shown in Table 4.

Indoor Pens

Indoor pens are excellent for the maintenance of dogs over an extended period of time under controlled conditions. Such kennels are usually constructed with concrete flooring and a drain gutter outside the runs. Typical dimensions for pens that can house up to four dogs are 3' 8" wide, 8' high, and 10' long. Care needs to be taken to ensure that the

Table 4 Minimum Space Requirements for Laboratory Dogs[a]

Weight	Type of housing	Floor area/animal (cm²)	Height[b] (cm)
<15 kg	Pen/run	0.74	—
15–30 kg	Pen/run	1.12	—
<15 kg	Cage	0.74	81.28
15–30 kg	Cage	1.12	91.44

[a]These recommendations may require modification according to the body conformation of individual animals and breeds.
[b]From the resting floor to the cage top.
Source: Adapted from the NIH Publication, 1985

surface is not so rough that it abrades the dog's footpads, nor so smooth that the floor becomes slippery when wet (due to water or urine) and causes injury to the animals or handlers.

Caging

When purchasing caging, special attention needs to be given to provisions for cage ventilation, drainage, and durability. The most commonly used and recommended materials for dog cages are fiberglass or stainless steel, both of which are durable and easy to clean. Most cages used in research facilities are equipped with automatic watering systems and modified doors with feed bowl holders as well as mobile bases to allow easy movement of the cage racks in and out of animal rooms (Fig. 2).

In general, the current standard size cages (generally 35" × 30.5" × 33.75" or 35" × 40.5" × 33.75" for larger dogs) used in most research facilities should only be used to maintain dogs for limited periods of time. An alternate to the use of pen/runs are modular and expandable stainless steel dog kennels, which allow the investigator to increase the cage floor space as needed (Fig. 3).

Exercise

While the dog can adapt to a wide variety of environments, the question has repeatedly arisen as to whether the degree of physical activity possible in a standard laboratory cage is sufficient for maintenance of normal physiological activity. It is likely that future amendments to the Animal Welfare Act will require that an exercise program be established for dogs maintained in a laboratory environment. The difficulty arises, however, in establishing a program that will be of most benefit to the dogs.

There are several reports in the literature that indicate there are no differences in clinical laboratory determinations, growth weight, and immunological, electro-cardiographic and ophthalmic parameters for dogs housed continuously in standard sized cages, large cages, or those released for exercise (Namand et al., 1975; Hite et al., 1977; Campbell et al., 1988). Newton (1972) has also demonstrated that, in terms of the musculoskeletal system, the physiological well-being of cage-confined dogs (relative to dogs housed in pens or those cage confined with access to a pen) is unaffected.

Analysis of activity patterns of dogs confined in cages of different sizes indicates that cage size has no effect on the amount of time spent sitting, standing or lying down (Campbell et al., 1988). Regardless of the size of the cage, dogs do not exercise unless humans are in the room. The most beneficial effects are seen when dogs are released and

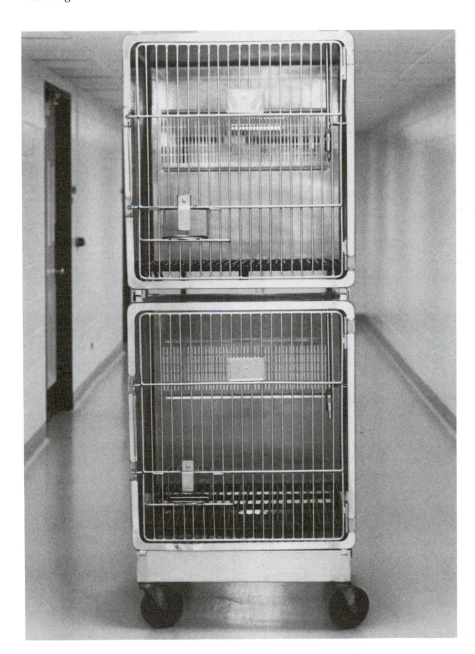

Figure 2 Stainless steel caging.

exercised as a group rather than alone. Dogs released alone tend to spend most of their time walking or investigating the area rather than running and jumping.

Socialization

Whatever the kennel design or exercise program used by a research facility, the needs of the confined laboratory dog for a certain level of socialization should be recognized. Both

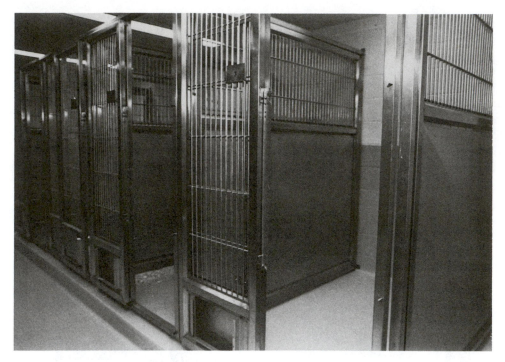

Figure 3 Modular stainless steel kennel.

dog-dog and human-dog contact is important. Generally, laboratory dogs are more content if they can share a cage with a companion. One approach adopted by some facilities has been to allow two dogs of the same sex and treatment group daily access to each other's cage from early evening to early morning. This approach, however, is not always logistically possible or scientifically feasible. In situations where experimental design dictates that animals be housed separately, normal behavior can be maintained by permitting visual, auditory, and olefactory access to roommates by appropriate spatial cage arrangement. Early handling of young animals to familiarize them with the laboratory environment is extremely important, since lack of early socialization can result in abnormal behavior later in life (Fox, 1965a). One of the most effective measures to prevent such problems in dogs is frequent human contact, which should continue throughout the animals' adult life.

Sanitation

Good sanitation is essential in an animal facility. The macroenvironment as well as the microenvironment need to kept free of dirt, debris, and contamination. Bacterial, viral, and parasitic problems can be magnified by an improperly maintained facility. Special attention should be given to cracks, rough areas, and depressions which can harbor moisture and provide shelter for parasite ova and other infectious agents (Bebiak et al., 1987).

Animal rooms, corridors, and storage areas should be routinely cleaned and sanitized. Pens and caging should be mopped or hosed out daily to prevent accumulation of fecal material and general debris. Cages and pens should be scrubbed down with a sanitizing solution about every 2 weeks; cages are rotated and thoroughly sanitized (e.g., soaking the cage in a 5% acid solution for about 20 min and then passing them through a 170°F cage wash). Watering systems also need to be cleaned regularly, either through flushing with water or cleansing with an antibacterial agent.

Another area of special attention is feed storage. While most laboratory chow is of good quality and contamination free when it leaves the manufacturer, biological and chemical spoilage can result during transit or by improper use. A dry, cool environment is recommended for feed storage to prevent mold formation and insect infestation. Feed should be stored off the floor either in unopened bags or in waterproof, cleanable containers after opening.

Temperature, Relative Humidity, and Ventilation

Special attention must be given to regulation of the macroenvironment as well as the microenvironment in which the laboratory animal resides. Environmental stress in humans and animals has been shown to affect physiological status, which in turn can alter susceptibility to infections and toxic chemicals (Baetjier, 1968; NIH, 1985).

Recommended dry-bulb temperatures and relative humidity ranges for dogs are 64.4–84.2°F (16–27°C) and 30–70%, respectively (NIH, 1985). Fluctuations in temperature and humidity can affect factors such as behavior and metabolic rate in dogs (Lusk, 1931). Increases in temperature and high humidity are a particular concern because of the dog's limited capacity to dissipate heat (Norris et al., 1968). Sweat glands in the dog are confined to the foot pads, and the animal primarily responds to high temperatures by panting and, to a lesser extent, by radiation and conduction. It has been shown that a stress zone for dogs, defined as a 1.1° increase in rectal temperature for all subjects tested, can be created at dry bulb temperatures greater than 32.6°C (Besch et al., 1984). Norris et al. (1968) have noted that the dog probably cannot survive for extended periods of time in environments appreciably in excess of 40°C and 40% relative humidity. Exposure to higher temperatures may lead to decreases in feed consumption in normal animals, and it is possible that exposing animals to toxic agents in the presence of elevated ambient temperatures may result in an increase in the incidence or severity of toxicity.

Temperature and humidity are also considered to be coincident factors in many diseases caused by chemicals and infectious agents in contact with the skin and can alter cutaneous absorption of compounds, local reaction of the skin to irritants, and reaction to sensitizing agents.

Ventilation control is necessary in order to minimize variations due to climatic conditions, provide adequate oxygen, remove thermal loads, and dilute gaseous and particulate contaminants. The necessary volume of air change per room will depend on its maximum holding capacity (i.e., number of animals in the room and room size). The number of air changes per hour are normally between 10 and 20 (Munkeldt, 1948; Runkle, 1964). It has been suggested that recirculated room air can be utilized as long as all airborne contaminants have been removed (NIH, 1985); however, this concept has not proven to be successful, in part because of improper or insufficient maintenance of recirculation systems (Gorton, 1978). Special care should also be paid to the positioning of the room inlet and outlet grills so that air is evenly distributed around the room and to each cage irrespective of its position.

Diet

While the dog is classed as a carnivore, it readily adapts to an omnivorous diet. The digestive tract of the dog is relatively short (compared to other mammalian species), which facilitates the rapid passage of food. Dogs also lack intestinal diverticula or bacterial harboring sacs which prevent foods that require microbial breakdown (prior to absorption) from being used effectively. Holding times of food in the beagle stomach, small intestine, and large intestine have been reported to be about 3–5 hr, 1 hr, and 10 or more hours, respectively; total passage time throughout the gastrointestinal tract is 24 hr (Andersen, 1970).

Dogs require dietary sources of energy, amino acids, glucose precursors, fatty acids, minerals, vitamins, and water. A summary of nutrient requirements for dogs (based on the recommendations of the National Research Council, 1985) is presented in Table 5. Dogs do not appear to have a specific requirement for carbohydrates; however, in a well-balanced diet, they can utilize large amounts of carbohydrates (up to 70%, dry basis) (Andersen, 1970).

Adult laboratory beagles maintained in a laboratory environment function well with one feeding of standard laboratory chow per day. Dogs tend to bolt their food, and animals on a once-a-day feeding regimen will often eat all their food within a 30- to 45-min period. In order to ensure that the slow eaters have sufficient opportunity to finish most of their food, most laboratories allocate a longer period (2–4 hr) for access to feed.

Although commercially available dog chows provide sufficient amounts of all necessary nutrients, some test compounds may induce deficiencies through loss of appetite, malabsorption, or vomiting that can complicate interpretation of toxic effects. Protein deficiency in the dog results in depressed food intake, growth retardation, hypoprotein-emia (associated with edema), and a rough, dull hair coat. Deficiencies in any of the essential amino acids can result in similar clinical signs. Diets low in fat can cause dry, coarse hair and flaky dermatitis (Michaud and Elvehjem, 1944). Inadequate intake or loss of essential minerals (e.g., calcium, phosphorus, potassium, and sodium chloride) can result in problems such as spontaneous fractures, bone loss, osteoporosis, and osteomalacia (calcium and phosphorus); restlessness, muscular paralysis, and lesions of the heart and kidney (potassium); and fatigue exhaustion, inability to maintain water balance, dryness of the skin and loss of hair (sodium chloride). Vitamin deficiencies, exacerbated by test compound effects, can also induce significant pathology.

Water

The body of the adult dog contains about 60% water and has a limited capacity to store water (Gaebler and Choitz, 1964). The dog can normally cope with a large fluid intake owing to a readily adjustable urine volume, but the unsalvagable water losses of the body dictate the minimum water intake. Average daily water intake in adult dogs has been determined to be approximately 600 ml (Richter, 1938), and the amount consumed daily has been shown to closely approximate total daily water loss (Gaebler and Choitz, 1964). The individual dog's requirements for water appear to be self-regulated and depends on factors such as the type of feed consumed, ambient temperature, amount of exercise, physiological state, and temperament. For these reasons, in most cases dogs should be permitted free access to water at all times.

Drinking devices for dogs include pans, water bottles, and, most commonly, automatic watering devices. The water source is usually either tap water or a filtered/sterilized water. As with other species, if an automatic watering system is used, the water lines and valves need to be routinely checked to ensure they are working properly and the animal has an uninterrupted supply of water. Whatever the water delivery system used, dogs need

Table 5 Nutrient Requirements for Dogs

Nutrient	Unit	Growth requirements	Adult maintenance requirements
Fat	g	2.7	1
Linoleic acid	mg	540	200
Protein			
arginine	mg	274	21
histidine	mg	98	22
isoleucine	mg	196	48
leucine	mg	318	84
lysine	mg	280	50
methionine cystine	mg	212	30
phenyalanine-tyrosine	mg	390	86
threonine	mg	254	44
tryptophan	mg	82	13
valine	mg	210	60
dispensable amino acids	mg	3414	1266
Carbohydrate			
Minerals			
calcium	mg	320	119
phosphorus	mg	240	89
potassium	mg	240	89
sodium	mg	30	11
chloride	mg	46	17
magnesium	mg	22	8.2
iron	mg	1.74	0.65
copper	mg	0.16	0.06
manganese	mg	0.28	0.10
zinc	mg	1.94	0.72
iodine	μg	0.032	0.012
selenium	μg	6	2.2
Vitamins			
A	IU	202	75
D	IU	22	8
E	IU	1.2	0.5
K			
thiamin	mg	54	20
riboflavin	mg	100	50
pantothenic acid	μg	400	200
niacin	mg	450	225
pyridoxine	mg	60	22
folic acid	mg	8	4
biotin[a]	mg	—	—
B_{12}	mg	1	0.5
choline	mg	50	25

[a]Dogs have a metabolic requirement, but a dietary requirement was demonstrated when foods from natural ingredients were fed.
Source: Adapted from National Research Council Recommendations, 1985.

to be observed on a daily basis for signs of dehydration so that prompt steps can be taken toward rehydration. Dehydration can usually be detected by checking the elasticity of the skin at the back of the neck. A common rehydration procedure is to subcutaneously administer lactated Ringer's solution (200–400 ml, depending on the size of the animal).

Disease

The four diseases of most concern in maintaining a dog colony are canine distemper, infectious canine hepatitis, leptospirosis, and rabies. While various immunization programs can be undertaken, the most common approach is to administer a single multigenic vaccine.

Some of the most common infectious and parasitic diseases observed in dogs are listed in Table 6. The most common ectoparasites include fleas, lice, ticks, and mites. Otodectic mites especially can be a problem if neglected; however, treatment can easily be effected by the use of an oil containing a nonirritating insecticide. The most serious mange mite is *Demodex follicularum*, which in some colonies has been detected as a facultative pathogen in about 80% of the animals (Greve and Gaatar, 1964).

Of the endoparasites found in dogs, whipworm is of most concern because of its location in the cecum and colon, which makes treatment difficult.

Coccidiosis (*Isospora* spp.) is a common cause of diarrhea and even death in dogs. Most species of coccidia are self-limiting and nonpathogenic; diffuse hemmorhage of the intestinal mucosa, however, can be seen in dogs infected with *Isospora bigemina* (Andersen, 1970). In dogs, as in many other species, adults are generally more resistant to this disease than young animals.

Giardia species are flagellate protozoa that inhibit the small intestine of a wide range of vertebrates. In dogs (usually young animals), the main sign is intermittent or chronic diarrhea. The disease can often be difficult to detect because animals may harbor the organism and not shed it in the feces until triggered by a factor such as stress, diet/environmental change, or treatment with a test article.

Heartworm *(Dirofilaria immitis)* can be hazardous in dog colonies because of the toxic side effects associated with administering filaricides. This disease is endemic to the eastern and southern states, and dogs entering a facility should be tested for the presence of microfilaria in the blood. It has been suggested that microfilaria counts about 25/ml of blood warrant euthanasia (Andersen, 1970).

Finally, it should be noted that susceptibility to disease can be enhanced in dogs by factors such as poor sanitation, improper environmental control, number of animals in the primary enclosure and the animal room, and/or inadequate or poor quality diet and insufficient water intake. Personnel who handle dogs must also be trained in proper handling techniques to avoid cage-to-cage or dog-to-handler transmissions of infections.

Quarantine and Veterinary Care

Procedures conducted upon arrival of dogs at a research facility should include the performance of a gross physical examination to look for signs of disease or physical defects, measurement of body weight and rectal temperature, and blood collection for hematological (including microfilaria testing) and clinical chemistry analysis. While colony-bred animals should be fully vaccinated by the breeder, random-source animals will likely need to be vaccinated at the receiving facility. If animals are intended for long-term studies (of more than 1 year duration), they will need to be annually vaccinated for rabies. Most facilities will also prophylactically treat dogs for ear mites. Depending on

Table 6 Some Common Parasitic and Infectious Diseases of the Dog

Disease	Pathogenic Agent	Clinical Picture	Common Source of Infection
Coccidiosis	*Isospora*	Primarily a disease of young animals. Diarrhea and dehydration.	Ingestion of sporulated oocysts.
Campylobacter Enteritis	*Camphylobacter fetus* subsp. *jejuni* and *intestinalis*	Watery diarrhea (puppies).	Direct contact with infected animals, ingestion of contaminated food, placental transfer, exposure at delivery.
Giarrdia	*Giarrdia trophozoites*	Disease most important in young dogs. Intermittent or chronic diarrhea which may persist for several months. Signs associated with malabsorption of nutrients (reduced growth rate, weight loss, dull coat, etc.)	Direct contact with feces.
Brucellosis	*Brucella canis*	Females—Abortion in third trimester. Generalized lymphadenitis and persistent bacteremia. Males—orchitis, epididymitis, and prostatis	Contact with the urine of infected animals.
Leptospirosis	*Leptospira interrogans*	Often a sudden onset with anorexia, vomiting, fever, and conjunctivitis followed in a few days by hypothermia, depression, dypsnea, muscle soreness, and oral mucosa hemorrhagic areas. Death (10% of cases) usually related to nephritis.	Direct contact with urine of infected animals.
Listeriosis	*Listeria monocytogenes*	Abortion, perinatal infections with CNS signs.	Unknown.
Tuberculosis	*Mycobacterium bovis* *M. tuberculosis*	1. Coughs of long duration. 2. Lung and pleural lesions almost exclusively exudative in nature.	Exposure to bovine or human tuberculosis.

Table 6   *(continued)*

Disease	Pathogenic Agent	Clinical Picture	Common Source of Infection
Dermatomycosis (ringworm)	*Microsporum canis M. distortum* (most common agents)	Frequently no clinical signs. If lesions occur, commonly seen as circular alopecic areas surrounded by vesicles, pastules, erythema, or scaling.	Direct contact with the lesions of affected animals.
Demodicosis (demodectic mange, red mange)	*Demodex mites*	Most common in dogs 3–5 months old. Pruritic, alopecia, red lesions around eyes or muzzle. Immune deficiency. Severe infestation can become systemic and prove fatal.	Direct contact with infected animals.
Heartworm (canine filariasis)	*Dirofilaria immitis*	Early and moderate heartworm disease—early tiring on exercise. Advanced disease—Lungs exhibit large emboli, thrombi, and pneumonia, and right heart is enlarged and worm filled. Signs consistent with right heart failure.	Exposure to infected mosquitoes.
Cutaneous larval migrans (creeping eruption)	*Ancylostoma braziliense A. caninum A. duodenale Necator americanus*	Normally the parasite is hookworms in dogs. Generally young dogs show clinical disease. Pale gums, weight loss, failure to grow properly. Tarry feces in heavy infections.	
Dipylidium caninum infection	*Dipylidium caninum* (common tapeworm of dogs)	Generally asymptomatic. In clinically recognized cases, diarrhea and pruritus around anal area.	Infection through direct contact with feces of an infected animal or contaminated sand or soil. Ingestion of infected fleas.

Table 6 *(continued)*

Disease	Pathogenic Agent	Clinical Picture	Common Source of Infection
Leishmaniases	*Leishmania donovani* *L. tropica* *L. brasiliensis*	May be harbored in bone marrow, liver, or spleen, resulting in macrophages containing the parasite. In more advanced cases, dermal lesions, emaciation, alopecia, keratitis, and seborrhea. Fatality is common.	Animal bitten by infected sandflies.
Salmonellosis	*Salmonella* sp. (many serotypes)	Acute gastroenteritis with diarrhea, vomiting, and resultant dehydration.	Ingestion of contaminated foods or water.
North American blastomycosis	*Blastomyces dermatitidis*	A chronic disease in dogs. Depression, fever, anorexia, leading to chronic weight loss, and nonproductive dry coughs. Nodules and abscesses through the lung. Dissemination by hematogenous route leads to destruction of peripheral lymph nodes, bones, and meninges.	Unknown.
Rabies	Rabies virus	Two clinical forms in dog: (1) paralytic form characterized by paralysis of the muscles of the throat and masseter region. (2) Furious form in animals will attack humans, moving or inert objects, or other dogs. Death usually follows within 5 days of these signs.	Contamination of bite wounds by saliva of infected animal in the terminal stages of the disease.

Source: Adapted from Bekaert, 1982.

animal health status, newly acquired dogs are generally maintained in quarantine for at least 2–3 weeks for colony-bred animals and 3–4 weeks for random-source animals. Random-source animals should be well separated from colony-bred animals. All dogs should be regularly examined during the quarantine period and observed frequently for signs of any potential health problems.

DOSING TECHNIQUES

It is essential that personnel who are responsible for the dosing of dogs be confident in the handling and manipulation of the animals. The first step is to establish a sense of confidence and security between the dog and its handler. During this conditioning period, the handler should crouch down to reduce his or her height and slowly bring his hand toward the muzzle so that the dog can sniff it. Next, the hand should move along the neck and hindquarters, and the response of the dog assessed. Most dogs, especially beagles, respond well to such handling.

If possible, it is better during a study to use the same team of people who were involved in the conditioning process. Efforts should be made to distinguish potential "fear biters" prior to selection of dogs for a study. To remove a dog from its cage or pen, the handler should hold the animal by the nape of the neck while keeping the forearm in line with the spine and supporting the animal under the abdomen with the other hand.

Oral

The two oral dosing procedures most commonly used with the dog are gavage and capsule administration. Dietary administration, as commonly used with rodents, is another possible oral route; however, this is not an optimal route of administration in dogs for several reasons. The increased activity of the dog, especially when humans enter or are present in the animal room, can result in a continual problem with feed spillage. Another concern is that dogs are often finicky eaters and sometimes will consume little or nothing during the course of a day while compensating by eating more the next day, which can result in erratic blood levels of test compound.

Capsule

The general approach in the administration of a gelatin capsule to a dog is to first wet the capsule with water, open the animal's mouth, and then place the capsule as far back on the animal's tongue as possible (Fig. 4). The muzzle is held closed, the head lifted, and the throat stroked until the animal swallows the capsule. The person dosing the animals should look for evidence of swallowing; almost all dogs will lick their lips after swallowing a capsule. After animals have been dosed, cages should be checked for spit-out capsules and any undamaged capsules readministered. Many facilities include a 1- to 2-week prestudy conditioning period in which dogs are dosed daily with empty capsules in order to help the animals become familiarized with the dosing procedure. It is not uncommon for dogs treated with certain test compounds to exhibit salivation prior to daily capsule dosing; this is probably a conditioned response in which capsule dosing is related to adverse systemic and/or local effects of the test article.

Gavage

The first step in gavaging a dog is to place a wooden bit between the teeth (Fig. 5). A flexible intubation tube is then inserted through the hole in the bit into the mouth, back

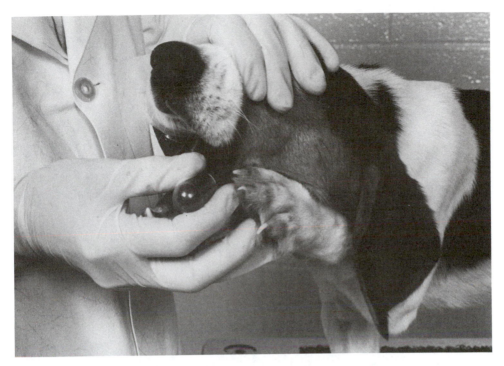

Figure 4 Dosing by capsule.

into the esophagus, and down toward the stomach. Correct placement of the tube can be ascertained by inserting the free end of the gavage tube into a beaker of water and checking for the absence of bubbles. Dosing volumes for gavage are generally in the range of 5–10 ml/kg, and fluid should be slowly administered in order to prevent gastric reflux.

Capsule administration is generally the preferred method of oral administration in dog studies. Gavaging is more labor intensive and there is always the chance of gavage error or aspiration. One approach in dealing with compounds that cause extensive vomiting in fasted dogs either by capsule or gavage administration is to allow the dogs access to feed for a few hours prior to dosing. Since the incidence of daily vomiting in control dogs can be as high as 50% (see Species Peculiarities below), it is often useful to sham dose animals with a water solution for several days before actually starting a gavage study. This will frequently accomodate animals to dosing and reduce emesis during the study.

Subcutaneous

For subcutaneous dosing, the skin over the side of the neck anterior to the scapula is picked up in a triangular fold and a needle (usually 21 gauge) is inserted into the base of the skin fold parallel to the body wall (Fig. 6). The plunger of the syringe is then pulled back gently to ensure that the needle has not gone through both sides of the skin fold or that a blood vessel has not been penetrated. In either case, the needle should be repositioned. The volume administered should generally be in the range of 5–10 ml/kg. In general, the irritation produced by subcutaneous administration is relatively moderate, and the route can be used for limited repeated dose studies. The site of injection can be

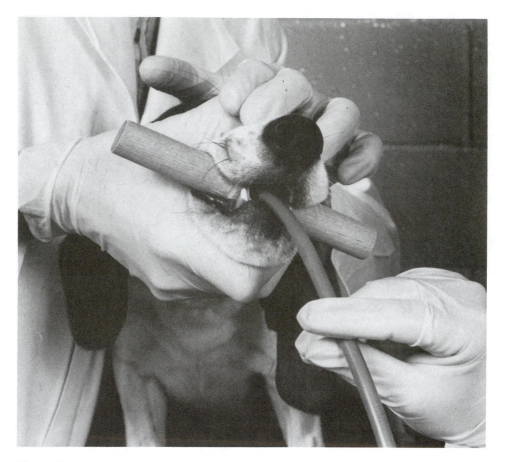

Figure 5 Dosing by gavage.

regularly moved from left to right and front to back in a predetermined pattern of injection (e.g., either side of the neck, either side of the midback, and on either side of the far back close to the rump).

Intramuscular

For intramuscular administration, the injection area (usually the meaty part of the hindleg) is swabbed with alcohol. The injection is made with a 20- or 21-gauge needle, and the maximum volume used should be in the range of 2–5 ml. It is important not to insert the needle too deeply in order to avoid hitting the sciatic nerve. The plunger of the needle is pulled back to ensure that a blood vessel has not been penetrated; if blood is present, the needle should be repositioned. The site of injection should be rotated during a repeated dose study. An important consideration is the potential for a test compound to induce intramuscular irritation. Because of this, it is advised that muscle irritation studies be conducted prior to initiating a repeated dose study.

Intraperitoneal

For intraperitoneal injection, the dog is usually held in a lateral position, and a small needle (usually a 23-gauge, ¾-in needle) is inserted about ¼ in into the lower right

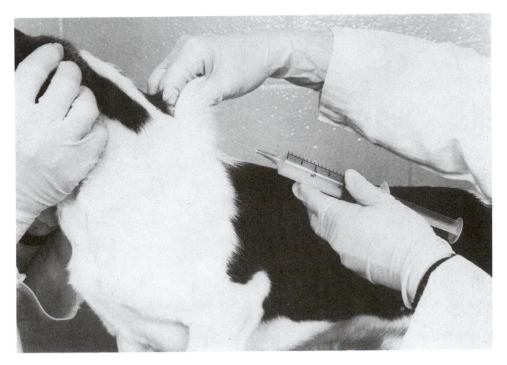

Figure 6 Dosing by the subcutaneous route.

quadrant of the belly, taking care to avoid damage to the internal organs. The midline should be avoided, so as to reduce the risk of penetrating the bladder. If necessary, the needle should be checked for proper placement and repositioned. The volume given should be in the range of 3–5 ml/kg of body weight.

Intravenous

Bolus

The femoral, cephalic, and saphenous veins are commonly used for intravenous administration in the dog. With the dog restrained by a second person, the hair over the vein is shaved (or clipped), swabbed with an alcohol solution, and the vein dilated (by pressure or heat) proximal to the injection site. Usually a 21- or 22-gauge needle is used, and the maximum volume for an adult dog should be about 3–5 ml/kg. For repeated dose bolus or infusion studies, injections should be kept as low on the vein as possible throughout the study so as to prevent the formation of scar tissue.

The use of a butterfly catheter (Fig. 7), to which the syringe is attached, is recommended to help avoid slippage of the needle from the vein in case of movement by the animal. The needle should be inserted in the direction of the blood flow and checked for proper placement by pulling back gently on the plunger of the syringe. The contents of the syringe are slowly injected (over 2–4 min). As with intrasmuscular administration, the potential for intravenous irritation should be determined prior to starting intravenous toxicity studies.

Infusion

For intravenous infusions lasting up to 2 hr, the dog should be restrained by the use of a device such as a sling, and a jacket and tether should be used for infusions of 2 or more

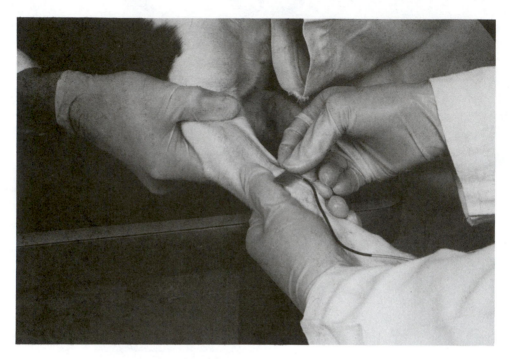

Figure 7 Dosing by the intravenous route.

hours duration. As with bolus injections, the vein to be infused is dilated by the application of pressure or heat, and an infusion catheter (usually 23 gauge) is inserted into the vein. The needle is withdrawn when blood flows out (thus, ensuring proper placement of the catheter), the catheter and tubing are loosely anchored to the leg with tape, and the catheter is connected to the tubing from the prepared syringe. The flow control valve is then opened and the infusion pump turned on. During the infusion, the limb being infused should be periodically checked for the presence of a swelling or bulge. If this occurs, the infusion should be stopped, the catheter repositioned higher on the vein (or another leg used), and the infusion recommenced. Sufficient slack should be maintained in the catheter so that if an animal moves during the infusion, the catheter will not be pulled out.

For continuous intravenous infusions, one approach is the use of a vascular access port system. A subcutaneously placed rigid multipuncturable reservoir with an indwelling catheter is inserted into the jugular vein. The test compound is accessed via catheter tubing encased in a swivel/tether apparatus connected to a jacket harness. The advantage of such a system is that it allows the animal greater freedom of movement during the infusion procedure.

Rectal and Vaginal

Compounds administered rectally to dogs can be delivered in the form of suppositories (emulsion and suspension types), rectal gelatin capsules (solutions and suspensions), or microenemas; the most frequently used dosage form, however, is the suspension suppository (De Boer et al., 1982). Microenemas are generally prepared as either a gelatin/saline solution or a simple physiological saline solution and administered in a volume of 0.5–1.0

ml. Suppositories are commonly in the weight range of 0.5–1.0 g, should be short and blunted in shape, and are inserted about 4 cm from the outer rectal sphincter. Liversidge et al. (1986) have also described a device for delivery of suppositories which consists of a stainless steel tube (95 × 2.7 mm) with a plunger to eject the suppository; the use of this device allows the suppository to be maintained in the proper position.

Compounds administered vaginally are usually in the form of suppositories or creams. Creams are usually placed in the vagina by means of an applicator. The vaginal opening is then closed with a plastic alligator clip for a specified period of time. Suppositories and tablets can be inserted vaginally with a plastic tamponlike applicator (Fulper et al., 1987).

DATA COLLECTION

Observations and Physical Examinations

Clinical observations and routine physical examinations are integral parts of safety assessment studies. Daily clinical observations in dogs are usually conducted both pretreatment and postreatment and consist of a home-cage observation to record any signs indicative of poor health status or abnormal behavior (such as motor incoordination/ reduced motor activity, tremors, salivation, abnormal feces, etc.). Before making such observations, it is important to be familiar with the spectrum of clinical signs that can be seen in a normal population of dogs. Some examples of clinical signs that are occasionally observed in untreated dogs are shown in Table 7.

Physical examinations are conducted less frequently during a study than are clinical observations. Some of the activities of a typical physical examination in dogs are depicted in Figure 8. The animal is first allowed to move around freely on the floor, and exploratory behavior, motor activity, gait, and general demeanor is evaluated. Next, the animal is moved to a table for examination of the head, including the eyes, ears, nose, mouth, teeth, gums, and tongue (for signs of swellings, abnormal nasal, eye, or ear discharges, tension of facial musculature, salivation, swallowing difficulties, etc.). The animal's body is then palpated for signs of masses and nodal swellings (Fig. 8A), the urogenital and anal region is examined, and rectal temperature is recorded. Pupillary light (Fig. 8B), corneal, patellar (Fig. 8C), wheelbarrowing (Fig. 8D), and hopping reflexes are usually tested, and righting and auditory responses are recorded.

Table 7 Occasional Clinical Observations in Normal Dogs

Vomitus: Usually clear or brown in color
Soft stool: Loosely formed stool
Mucoid stool: Yellowish or dark in color
Diarrhea: liquid feces
Nasal discharge: Usually slight runny nose
Injected sclera: Slightly blood shot eyes
Protruding nictitating membrane (cherry eye)
Hair loss: Slight to severe focal or generalized hair loss
Cage sores: Usually between the digits of the paws
Signs associated with females "in heat"
    vulval bleeding
    vulval turgidity
    restless behavior

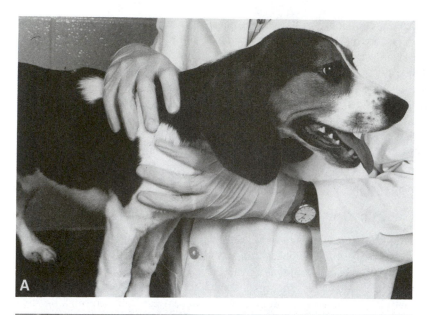

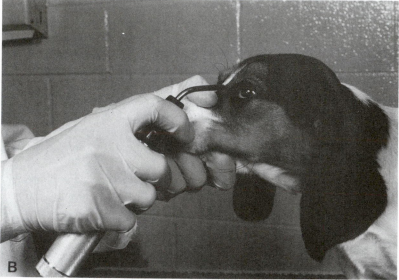

Figure 8 Typical features of a physical examination. (A) Palpation for masses and nodal swellings; (B) examination of pupillary light reflex; (C) patellar reflex testing; (D) wheelbar-
row reflex testing.

Cardiovascular Parameters

Blood Pressure

Blood pressure can be determined in dogs by either indirect (noninvasive) methods or by
direct determination. An example of a noninvasive method has been described by Weiser
et al. (1977). The method requires the placement of an inflatable cuff over the cranial

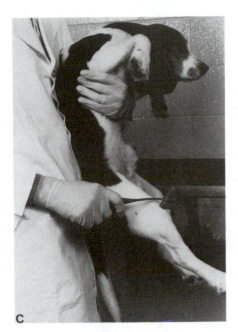

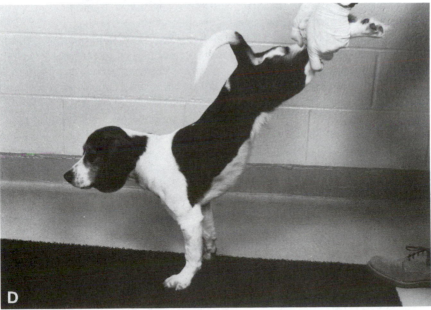

Figure 8 *(continued)*

tibial artery and the use of an ultrasonic Doppler sensing device to detect arterial wall motion. Direct determination of blood pressure can be accomplished by cannulation of an artery (such as the femoral artery) with a 22-gauge hypodermic needle that is connected to fluid-filled polyethylene tubing that leads to a pressure transducer (Weiser et al., 1977; Tabaru et al., 1987). Transducer activity can then be monitored on an oscilloscope equipped with a paper recorder.

Blood pressure measurements in unanesthetized dogs can vary widely owing to variables such as exercise, anxiety, and excitement. For this reason, all recordings from conscious dogs should always be performed in a quiet, environmentally controlled room with the animals placed in a comfortable position. Some investigators find it of value to condition the dogs for several days prior to recording blood pressure to lay or sit in a given position. At least three readings are usually made and the average blood pressure determined. Andersen (1970) has reported mean systolic/diastolic values of $98 \pm 28/46 \pm 16$, $121 \pm 40/65 \pm 27$, and $130 \pm 29/67 \pm 8$ for beagles in the age ranges of 2–8, 7–10, and 28–59 months, respectively.

Electrocardiography

Procedure for Taking ECGs.   While over the last 30 years the use of serial electrocardiograms (ECGs) has become routine in toxicity studies, generally accepted standards for adequate lead systems, recording techniques, frequency of taking samples, and principles for interpretation have not been established (Detweiller, 1980). A 10-lead system, consisting of the bipolar leads (I, II, III), the augmented unipolar leads (aVR, aVL, and aV6), and the unipolar precordial leads [V10, CV6LL (V2), CV6LU (V4), CV5RL (rV2)], has been recommended for dogs (Detweiler et al., 1979). There is some debate as to what is the most suitable body posture for the dog. The right lateral recumbent position (dog restrained on right side with the head and neck held flat and in line with the long axis of the trunk) has been the position of choice in many facilities. The sternal recumbent, "sphynx" position (Fig. 9) and the standing position have been also found to work well. Use of a standardized body position, however, is essential during recording, and the most critical factor is consistent positioning of the forelimbs and scapula in order to prevent alterations in the amplitudes of ECG waves in the various leads and resultant vectors (Detweiler, 1980). Whatever the position used, complete reproducibility in any position is unattainable, probably because of the impossibility of being able to maneuver the heart into the same position each time (Katz et al., 1934; Eckenfels and Trieb, 1979).

For recording purposes, animals should be kept on a warm insulating nonconductive surface, such as a table covered with a rubber mat or blanket. The procedure normally requires two people; one to hold and calm the dog and ensure correct positioning during the recording and one to attach the electrodes and take the ECG. Electrode clips are attached directly to the animal's skin. Stainless steel or copper alligator clips (with the teeth filed down to prevent pinching) are commonly used as electrodes, and the total area of contact should be about 1 cm^2. Suitable electrode contact materials include electrode paste, water, and alcohol. Prior to taking an ECG, the thermal pens for each channel should be checked for correction positioning and to ensure the elimination of extraneous noise due to improperly attached electrodes. It has been recommended that ECGs be recorded for a total period of 60 sec (Detweiler, 1980). For a programmed three-channel 10-lead electrocardiograph, a rhythm strip of any three selected leads should be taken to complete the 1 min of recording.

Many cardiologists prefer to record ECGs at a chart speed of 50 mm/sec (rather than 25 mm/sec) because the faster speed will "stretch out" the electrocardiogram, and the time intervals can be measured with greater accuracy (Tilley, 1985). It has been noted, however, by Detweiler (1980) that 25 mm/sec is a satisfactory chart speed for dog electrocardiograms, and adequate accuracy can be achieved.

For toxicity studies, ECG records are usually taken by technical personnel on groups of dogs and read at a later time by a cardiologist. The quality of the tracings and decision as to whether to rerun any ECGs will be determined by evaluation of instrument performance, technician error (such as incorrect body positioning or electrode placement), and the presence or absence of artifacts (such as 50- to 60-Hz interference, muscle tremor, and

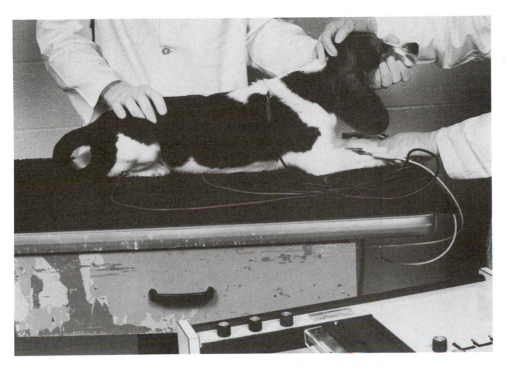

Figure 9 The sternal recumbent "sphynx" position for electrocardiographic examination.

baseline drift). An acceptable quality tracing should have no errors present, a minimum of two complexes in each lead free of artifact (except minor variations in amplitude), and artifacts present in no more than 1/5 or 2/10 leads (Detweiler, 1980).

Normal ECG Pattern.   Normal values for untreated dogs with aging are shown in Table 8. The data show that by about 7–8 months of age, most of the ECG parameters have reached adult values.

Dog ECGs can be highly variable, and it is important to take this factor into account when interpretating ECG findings. Electrocardiographic variations that occur relatively frequently in dogs include changes in direction and amplitude (in the same lead) of P-waves, which appear to be related to nervousness and excitation; changes in the amplitude and reversal of direction of T waves; and changes in the amplitude or disappearance of Q- and S-waves in all leads (Lalich et al., 1940). Positive T waves are found more frequently in sitting dogs than those standing or lying down and are more common in Lead I and less common in lead II. Variations in the direction of the cardiac vector have been shown even when the same animal position is held correctly (Eckenfels and Trieb, 1979). Eckenfeld (1979) noted that in serial ECG measurements, individual variability appears to be less than that between (or among) animals.

Heart Rate.   The heart rate (number of beats per minute) is usually measured from the R-R interval over a specified period of time. The heart rate has been shown to change during the growing period. At 6 months of age, the heart rate is about 150 beats/min, but it progressively falls over the next 12 months to a value of about 120 beats/min (Noel, 1970). The heart rate is often extremely variable in the dog; values can range from 45–220 beats/min in the conscious mature Beagle (Eckenfels and Trieb, 1979). For this reason,

Table 8 Effects of Aging on Electrocardiographic Parameters in Beagle Dogs[a]

		0–2 months	3–4 months	4–5 months	7–8 months	9–10 months	11–12 months	2–3 years	4–5 years	6 years
HR (/min)	Mean	189.1	165.9	146.9	136.5	129.6	130.8	135.8	134.2	134.4
	SD	23.1	24.9	26.0	30.0	28.7	25.7	25.3	22.1	19.3
	Range	153–228	120–202	94–182	80–186	76–178	79–175	76–176	90–174	94–163
	N	131	272	248	118	114	95	56	71	34
PR (msec)	Mean	73.0	83.8	93.7	94.7	98.7	99.7	98.8	104.1	104.4
	SD	8.3	10.4	11.4	12.0	14.4	12.1	11.3	11.4	9.1
	Range	60–84	66–100	74–112	72–114	74–122	78–114	78–116	84–124	82–120
	N	131	271	248	118	114	93	56	71	34
QRS (msec)	Mean	41.8	43.1	44.9	46.7	46.1	47.1	48.4	49.1	50.2
	SD	3.6	4.2	3.9	4.7	3.8	4.7	4.4	3.9	5.0
	Range	36–48	36–48	36–50	36–54	38–50	38–56	40–56	42–56	42–56
	N	130	272	247	117	114	92	56	71	34
QT (msec)	Mean	161.6	156.4	171.1	177.3	181.5	180.1	184.4	184.9	187.6
	SD	13.5	31.2	16.6	15.7	14.9	13.7	13.5	13.6	10.7
	Rance	140–190	138–178	150–194	150–202	145–204	154–202	160–202	160–206	158–204
	N	130	270	233	114	109	90	54	68	33
QTc	Mean	285.7	259.3	265.5	263.1	263.3	263.0	273.6	274.0	278.8
	SD	20.0	50.8	26.1	21.5	20.9	23.4	23.4	17.5	18.7
	Range	258–317	228–292	229–293	224–298	222–292	209–296	227–302	244–294	232–308
	N	130	270	233	114	109	90	54	68	33
AXIS (°)	Mean	66.2	74.5	74.3	68.5	70.9	69.3	64.8	68.5	64.7
	SD	36.8	29.3	22.5	27.2	34.0	24.9	32.0	15.8	21.5
	Range	6–105	28–103	32–96	16–92	36–89	33–87	4–88	41–87	3–84
	N	130	271	247	116	113	95	54	71	33

Source: Adapted from Shimizu et al., 1986.

ECGs should always be measured in a quiet unstressful setting. There is also the concern that keeping an animal in a fixed position while taking an ECG will cause stress and lead to an increase in the heart rate and an exhibition of other excitement-induced ECG anomalies. The unrestrained standing and the intermediate sitting positions have been found to induce less excitation in the animals than other positions (Eckenfels and Trieb, 1979). It is also recommended that a conditioning period be established prior to study start during which the electrodes are attached and the animals positioned for ECG recording.

Frequent Anomalies in Control Animals. A frequent finding in normal dogs is respiratory-influenced sinus arrhythmia, which is an irregular sinus rhythm that originates in the sinoatrial (SA) node. It is a vagally mediated event and represented by alternating periods of a slower and more rapid heart rate; the heart rate increases with inspiration and decreases with expiration (Eckenfels, 1979; Tilley, 1985). These cyclical changes in the heart rate are often accompanied by cyclic alterations in the amplitude of ECG waves. This type of sinus arrhythmia is well differentiated from nonrespiratory sinus arrhythmia because of the positive correlation with the phases of respiration.

Sinus tachycardia, with a heart rate above 160 beats/min (above 180 in toy breeds and above 220 in puppies) is the most common arrhythmia in dogs. It can most often be explained by nervousness (fear or aggression). Sinus bradycardia is normally vagus dependent and often occurs in calm dogs and those accustomed to the investigator (Eckenfelds and Trieb, 1979).

A wandering pacemaker consists of a shift of the pacemaker from within the SA node or from the SA to the atrioventricular (AV) node (Tilley, 1985). This is a variant of sinus arrhythmia and is a frequent finding in normal dogs. The shifting of the pacemaker within the SA node causes a gradual change in configuration of the P-wave without it becoming negative, whereas shifting of the pacemaker between the SA node and AV junction results in a gradual change in the configuration of the P-wave, which can become positive, biphasic, isoelectric, and negative.

Another ECG finding that can be found in normal healthy dogs is incomplete right bundle branch block (IRBBB), characterized by the presence of a right axis deviation and a large wide S-wave in leads I, II, III, aVF, CV6LL(V2), and CV6LU(V4). It has been found in the beagle as a genetically determined localized variation in right ventricular wall thickness, or just as focal hypertrophy of the right ventricle (Tilley, 1985). Studies conducted in this laboratory have indicated the presence of IRBBB in about 20–25% of a population of young adult beagles in the absence of accompanying cardiac pathology (unpublished data).

CLINICAL LABORATORY SAMPLE COLLECTION

Blood Collection

The most commonly used site of blood collection in the dog is the jugular vein; other veins used less frequently are the femoral, brachial and saphenous. The advantage of the jugular vein is that it is large and easy to access, and therefore suitable for serial sampling in a toxicity study. The collection site is shaved and swabbed with an ethanolic solution, and a 20- or 21-gauge needle is used to collect the sample. The vein is occluded, and the needle is inserted (bevel upward) pointing toward the animal's head (Fig. 10); usually one person restrains the dog and occludes the vein while a second person collects the sample. Once the desired volume of blood has been collected (usually a total of 5–6 ml for clinical laboratory determinations and 1–2 ml at each pharmacokinetic collection time), the needle

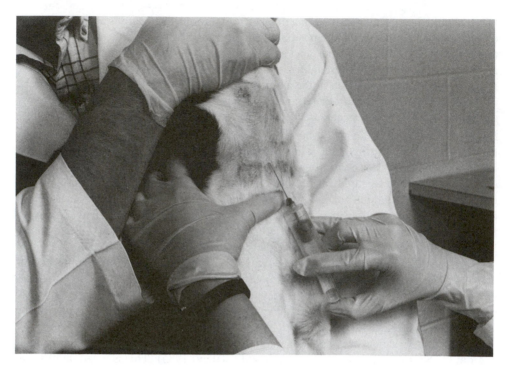

Figure 10 Blood collection from the jugular vein.

is withdrawn, and dry gauze applied (with pressure) to the site until the bleeding stops. Because of the potential for commercial diets to affect clinical parameters such as blood urea, glucose, and cholesterol, it is recommended that animals be fasted overnight prior to blood collection (Street et al., 1968).

Urine Collection

In many laboratories, urine collection from dogs is conducted overnight (approximately a 15-hr period) because of the difficulty in consistently obtaining sufficient volumes of urine in some dogs during shorter collection periods. There are problems, however, associated with such a protracted collection time. Urine casts can dissolve, bacterial activity increase, and bilirubin break down to biliverdin with exposure of the sample to light. Since only a small sample is needed for urinalysis, it is recommended that one be collected from each dog as soon as possible during the collection period. Collection containers should also be protected from light. Common urine collection systems for dogs are metabolism cages (Fig. 11) or stainless steel troughs that attach to the home cage. When collecting samples, care should be taken to avoid males being housed in cages directly above those of females because of the possibility of the males urinating along the side of the cage and contaminating the sample being collected in the lower cages.

Ad libitum access to water can also be a problem because of accidental dilution of the urine sample. Consequently, it is common for the dogs not to have access to water during the overnight collection period. It is recommended, however, that dogs have free access to water on the following day prior to dosing. Work done in this laboratory to examine the effects of water rehydration on erythrocyte parameters has shown that 30–60 min is a sufficient rehydration period (Guy, 1989).

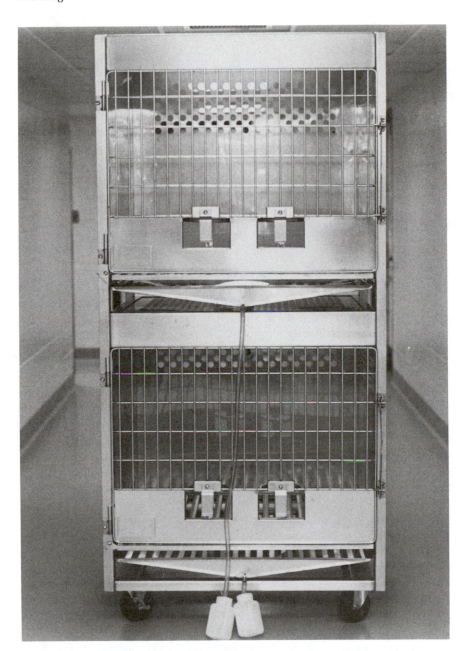

Figure 11 Metabolism cages for urine collection.

COMMON STUDY PROTOCOLS AND ASSOCIATED CONSIDERATIONS

Because of the large amount of background data available on the dog, in particular the beagle, it is a commonly used nonrodent species in acute, limited repeated dose (2- or 4-week studies), subchronic (up to 13 weeks of duration), or chronic (26 weeks or longer) toxicology studies. Examples of experimental designs and suggested timing of various study activities for 4- and 13-week toxicity studies are shown in Tables 9 and 10, respectively.

For teratology studies, the dog does not appear to be as sensitive an indicator of teratogens as other nonrodent animal models such as primates (Earl et al., 1973) and ferrets (Gulamhusein et al., 1980). Likewise, for studies aimed at evaluating reproductive function, the dog is not the species of choice, primarily because fertility testing is virtually impossible to conduct owing to prolonged anestrus and the inability to predict the onset of proestrus. Also, there is no reliable procedure for the induction of estrus or ovulation. Although semen is relatively easy to collect from the dog, the number of sperm in an ejaculate can vary widely owing to factors such as age, testicular size, and season (Amann, 1982).

Selection of Study Animals

Age

It has been recommended that, depending on the age of the human population projected to be exposed to a given compound, dogs should be at least 4–6 months and no more than 9 months of age at study start (Mosberg and Hayes, 1989). For many laboratories, dogs are usually in the age range of 7–9 months at study start; however, for short-term studies (acute 2 or 4 weeks), there is usually no problem with using older animals (up to 12 months of age).

Pretreatment Evaluation

It is imperative that dogs be properly screened prior to assignment to a study. Animals should be selected on the basis of acceptable findings from body weight, physical, ophthalmic, and electrocardiographic examinations as well as urinalysis, clinical chemistry, and hematological evaluations. Pretreatment evaluation should take place within 3 to 4 weeks of study start, and it is recommended that clinical laboratory determinations be made close to the start of the study. Additionally, it is advisable to limit the number of siblings that are assigned to a study to no more than one per sex per treatment group.

Table 9 4-Week Toxicity Study

Experimental Design
  4/sex/group; 4 dosage groups + 1 control
  Dose daily for 29 or 30 days
  Sacrifice days 29, 30, or 31

Study activities
  Daily observations: Pretreatment and twice daily during the study period
  Physical examination: Pretreatment and after dosing during weeks 2 and 4
  ECG: Pretreatment and after dosing during weeks 2 and 4
  Ophthalmic examination: Pretreatment and during week 4
  Body weight: Pretreatment and weekly, for moribund animals, and the day of scheduled
              sacrifice
  Feed consumption: Pretreatment and weekly
  Clinical lab: Twice before the first dosing day, before dosing on day 2, during week 2, and prior
              to sacrifice
  Urine collection: Pretreatment and during weeks 2 and 4
  Pharmacokinetic sample: Blood collected at specified times after dosing on days 1 and 28

Table 10 13-Week Dog Toxicity Study

Experimental design
  8/sex/group; 3 dosage groups + control
  Dose daily for 91, 92, or 93 days
  Sacrifice main group (6/sex/group), week 14
  Sacrifice reversal group (2/sex/group), week 18

Study activities
  Daily observations: Pretreatment, twice daily during treatment phase, and once daily during
      reversal
  Physical examination: Pretreatment, after dosing during weeks 4, 8, and 13 of treatment, and
      during week 4 of reversal
  ECG: Pretreatment, after dosing during Weeks 4, 8, and 13 of treatment, and during week 4 of
      reversal
  Ophthalmic examination: Pretreatment, during weeks 6 and 13 of treatment, and during week 4
      of reversal
  Body weight: Pretreatment (3 times), weekly during the treatment and reversal periods, for
      moribund animals, and at scheduled sacrifice
  Feed consumption: Pretreatment, weekly through first month, bimonthly during the remainder
      of the treatment period, and weekly during reversal
  Clinical lab: Pretreatment, during weeks 4 and 8 of treatment, day 1 of reversal, for moribund
      animals, and prior to scheduled sacrifice
  Urine collection: Pretreatment, monthly during treatment, and during week 4 of reversal
  Pharmacokinetic samples: Blood collected at specified times after dosing on days 1 and during
      weeks 6 and 12

Numbers of Animals and Experimental Design Considerations

The number of animals assigned to a treatment group will depend on the duration of the
study (see Tables 9 and 10). In general, fewer animals are used for a 2- or 4-week study
(suggested "N" is 4 animals per sex per group; no reversal group) than for a 26-week or
1-year study (suggested "N" is nine animals per sex per group; includes two to three dogs
per sex per group for reversal). Whichever type of study is conducted, the number of
animals should be equal across sexes for any given treatment group.

Often there is little information on repeated dose toxicity of a test compound at the time
2- or 4-week dog toxicity studies are conducted, yet findings from these studies are often
the main basis for dose selection for the more long-term studies. Thus, it is recommended
that four (rather than three) dosage groups be used in these studies in order to obtain a
more complete toxicity profile of the compound.

Randomization

Dogs are usually randomly assigned to treatment groups using a blocking procedure with
blocks defined from stratified body weights. Because of possible inherited susceptibility
or resistance to toxic effects induced by a test compound, the distribution of siblings needs
to taken into account when reviewing the final randomization. A general rule is to limit
the number of siblings to one per sex per group. This can be achieved by placing a limit on
the number of siblings (i.e., not to exceed the number of groups in the study) that will be
accepted from the animal supplier. Random assignment of reversal animals is usually

done prior to study start; however, if any adverse findings are detected during the treatment phase, the study director may want to include some of the affected animals in the reversal group.

Study Activities

When scheduling activities for dog studies it should always be taken into consideration that most, if not all, activities will generally be conducted in all animals. The repeated manipulation of dogs for blood collection as well as for ECG, ophthalmic, and physical examinations will likely induce some stress in the animals. For shorter-term studies, this can be a concern, especially at the beginning and end of a study where there are multiple study activities to be conducted in a relatively short period of time (see Table 9). Efforts should be made to separate the various study activities so that no more than two activities are scheduled on the same day.

SPECIES PECULIARITIES

Emesis

Dogs have a natural tendency to vomit. While this may be easier to explain in the pet dog which has a greater chance of ingesting foreign materials and spoiled foods, emesis is often seen in the laboratory dog living in a controlled environment. For a given study, the incidence of vomitus in control animals on a single day can be as high as 40–50% (unpublished data). The cause of this emesis is unclear, but it is probably related to the inherent excitability of the dog. Vomiting can be a particular problem when a drug is given orally, since a portion of the dose may be lost.

Shedding and Alopecia

Shedding is frequently seen in beagles. This is in part seasonal in that it occurs in both sexes primarily in the spring and is in part estrous related (Al-Bagdadi et al., 1977). A more serious problem arises when dogs develop pruritic alopecia, which occurs at a greater frequency in the summer and appears to be more common in females. Clinical signs include bilateral alopecia of increasing severity, pruritic ears progressing to thickening of the skin around the ears, face, and neck, and skin inflammation in severe cases.

Polysorbate-Induced Histamine Reaction

Intravenous administration of polysorbates (Tweens) 20, 40, 60, and 80 in dogs have been found to cause a release of histamine or a histaminelike substance which results in a profound cutaneous response (includes reddening of the muzzle, inside of the ears, and sometimes of the general body as well as swollen and bloodshot eyes), scratching, vomiting, signs of weakness and postural difficulties, and hypotension (Krantz et al., 1948). These effects have been seen in this laboratory after administration of a 0.1% aqueous polysorbate 80 solution at a volume of 5 ml/kg (unpublished data). Polysorbate 80 has also been demonstrated to be a potent cardiac depressant in dogs. This allergic depressor response is not seen in the guinea pig, cat, rat, rabbit, or humans (Krantz et al., 1948).

Table 11 Use of the Beagle in Safety Assessment Studies

Advantages
  medium size
  moderate length of hair coat
  even temperament and friendly disposition (easy to handle)
  adaptability to living in groups
  easy to work with (e.g., dosing, blood collection, ECG)
  satellite animals not needed for serial blood collection

Disadvantages
  variation in size and body weight
  loud, penetrating bark
  cost of acquisition and maintenance
  greater test compound requirements than smaller species
  availability
  exercise and housing requirements

ADVANTAGES AND DISADVANTAGES OF THE DOG

There are well-defined advantages and disadvantages in working with the beagle (Table 11). The suitability of the beagle as an experimental model arises from factors such as its medium size and even temperament. The relative ease of handling the beagle makes it possible to be able to perform many routine study-related activities (such as serial collection of blood and electrocardiographic examination) in the conscious animal.

Disadvantages in the use of the beagle can include an often wide variation in size and body weight and a loud penetrating bark, which can be controlled by partial ventriculocordectomy, a procedure which usually gives permanent results but does not affect the well-being of the dog (Andersen, 1970). Housing and exercise requirements for the laboratory dog can be a disadvantage in terms of the large amount of laboratory space and additional personnel needed to maintain and exercise animals on study. This is particularly relevant in light of revisions in the Animal Welfare Laws of many countries (e.g., U.S. Department of Agriculture) which have resulted in increased space requirements for dogs and/or a specified periods of daily exercise. Additionally, test compound requirements are higher for the dog (relative to the rat, guinea pig, ferret, and monkey), which can often be a major disadvantage when only limited quantities of test compound are available. As mentioned in the section on species peculiarities, the high incidence of vomiting and the histamine release reaction to intravenous injection of Tweens can also be disadvantages. Finally, it should be recognized that experiments using large numbers of beagles usually cannot be set up quickly, and careful advance planning is needed to ensure that animals of the right age range and number can be obtained and housed in time to meet projected deadlines.

Pathology   **Robert W. Thomassen**

This section on the pathology of the laboratory dog is not intended to be a comprehensive treatise on canine pathology, but rather a source of information on spontaneous gross and microscopic changes seen in young adult beagle dogs in the context of short-term safety studies. Limiting the discussion to young dogs is reasonable, for few safety studies exceed 12 months and most are of shorter duration. Hopefully, the information will be useful not only to study pathologists, but to those who assist them in the postmortem laboratory and also to toxicologists and students of pathology and toxicology. To this end, the material is presented on an organ system basis, which includes a review of gross and microscopic anatomy, suggested necropsy procedures, and a summary of reported spontaneous pathology augmented by the writer's own experience.

INTEGUMENTARY SYSTEM

Anatomy and Histology

The entire body of the dog is covered by an organ known as the integument, or skin (integumentary system), which includes epidermis, dermis, hair, hair follicles, sweat and sebaceous glands, digital pads, claws, and mammary glands (Calhoun and Stinson, 1976). The integument is bound to underlying fascia and skeletal muscles by a sub-cutaneous, or hypodermal, layer (subcutis, hypodermis) of loose and adipose connective tissue that is not part of the integument but which is often removed with it during dissection. The integument is continuous at all natural body openings with the mucous membranes of the digestive, respiratory, and urogenital systems. At the margins of the eyelids, the stratified squamous ectoderm of the skin becomes the mucous membrane (conjunctiva) of the eye. The outer layer of the tympanic membrane (stratum cutaneum) is very thin without hair or glands (Breazile, 1976). The integument is a large organ. In the newborn puppy, the skin, hair, and subcutis represent 24% of the total body weight (Lovell and Getty, 1967). At maturity, the same tissues represent 12% of the body weight. The principal function of the skin is to separate and protect the body from the environment. Additional functions include temperature regulation, sensory perception, blood pressure control, secretion, storage, and synthesis of vitamin D (Muller et al., 1983). Although the functions of the integument are similar in various laboratory animals, significant morphological differences exist between animals and significant regional differences exist within an animal. Adam and co-authors (1970) have illustrated many of the regional differences in the beagle. Some regional differences are subtle and are best recognized utilizing carefully collected age-, sex-, and site-matched specimens.

Epidermis, Dermis, and Hair Coat

The thickness of the skin (epidermis and dermis) and density of the hair coat (pelage) vary in a consistent way over the body. Both skin and pelage are thickest over the dorsal and lateral surfaces of the trunk and lateral surfaces of the limbs, and are thinnest on the ventral surface of the trunk and medial surfaces of the limbs (Calhoun and Stinson, 1976). As a separate layer, the epidermis is generally the thinnest in well-haired areas and the thickest in hairless areas. In contrast, the dermis is usually thickest in well-haired areas and thinnest in hairless areas. In the beagle, the thinnest epidermis is found in the cheek and thinnest dermis is found in the scrotum (Warner and McFarland, 1970).

The hair coat of the beagle is typically tricolored; consisting of black, white, and shades of brown (Warner and McFarland, 1970). Individual variation is great and some beagles are bicolored. Beagles tend to shed hair throughout the year and some have seasonal molts.

Dogs have three general types of hair: tactile, coarse, and fine. Tactile hairs include sinus hairs (vibrissae, whiskers) and tylotrich hairs. Sinus hairs function as slow-adapting mechanoreceptors and are located on the muzzle, upper and lower lips, chin, intermandibular space, near the oral commissures, and above the eyes (Warner and McFarland, 1970). Eyelashes (cilia) are large hairs but are not sinus hairs. Sinus hairs have large follicles containing an endothelial-lined blood sinus between the two sheaths of the follicle (Calhoun and Stinson, 1976).

Tylotrich hairs are stout hairs scattered among ordinary hairs and function as rapid-responding mechanoreceptors (Yager and Scott, 1985). Tylotrich follicles are large, contain a single tylotrich hair and have a ring of neurovascular tissue at the level of the sebaceous gland. The tylotrich follicle is associated with a focal area of epidermal thickening (tylotrich pad) resting upon a layer of well-vascularized and innervated connective tissue (Yager and Scott, 1985).

Ordinary coarse (primary, guard) and fine (secondary) hairs comprise the bulk of the pelage and grow in compound follicles in the dog with a single long coarse hair and several fine hairs emerging from a single opening in the skin. As many as 15 hairs may grow in one follicle (Calhoun and Stinson, 1976).

Sebaceous and apocrine sweat glands are the two principal skin glands in the dog (and mammary gland in the female).

Sebaceous Sweat Glands

Sebaceous glands are simple alveolar glands whose oily secretion (sebum) results from complete disruption of cells (holocrine secretion). Sebaceous glands are located in the superficial dermis where each gland empties into the upper part of a hair follicle or onto the surface of the skin in hairless areas. Each primary hair has its own sebaceous gland. Secondary hairs usually share sebaceous glands. A ring of sebaceous glands opens into the follicle of tactile hairs (Muller et al., 1983). Where hair is dense, sebaceous glands tend to be long and narrow. Sebaceous glands are larger where hair is sparse and are the largest where associated with small hairs and at mucocutaneous junctions such as the lips and prepuce.

Special Sebaceous Glands. The dog has several special sebaceous glands. Two types are found in the eyelids. Meibomian glands lie within the tarsal plates of the upper and lower lids. Secretion from Meibomian glands seals the lid margins when the eyelids are closed and prevents overflow of tears when the eyelids are open (Kuwabara and Cogan, 1977). Sebaceous glands associated with the eyelashes are known as the glands of Zeis.

A complex arrangement of glands is found in the anal region of the dog.

Circumanal Glands.   The largest and most widely distributed glands in the subcutaneous perianal region are known as circumanal, or perianal, glands. Circumanal glands are bipartite glands with a typical sebaceous gland superficial portion and a larger, deeper nonsebaceous portion. The sebaceous portion is functional and empties into hair follicles through patent ducts. The nonsebaceous portion is apparently nonfunctional and is connected to the sebaceous portion by nonpatent "ducts" (Calhoun and Stinson, 1976). The nonfunctional portion comprises large cells which resemble hepatocytes, causing them to be referred to as hepatoid cells (Yager and Scott, 1985). Circumanal glands have been found ectopically in a number of sites, including the tail, flank, back, prepuce, and chin (Yager and Scott, 1985) and walls of anal sac ducts (Miller et al., 1967). Circumanal glands continue to grow throughout the life of the noncastrated male.

Tail Gland.   Large, well-developed sebaceous glands are also found in a circumscribed oval area of skin on the dorsum of the tail, a short distance from its base. This gland complex is known as the tail, or supracaudal, gland (Calhoun and Stinson, 1976). Large apocrine glands are also present in this area. The tail gland is marked grossly by stiff hairs and a yellow, waxy appearance to the skin surface (Lovell and Getty, 1967).

Apocrine Sweat Glands

Apocrine sweat glands, as with sebaceous glands, are located throughout the skin of the dog, mainly in connection with hair follicles. The bodies of apocrine sweat glands are located deeper in the dermis than sebaceous glands; however, their ducts enter follicles above the ducts of sebaceous glands. Only one sweat gland is associated with each hair follicle complex. Apocrine sweat gland secretions are scant and rarely perceptible in the dog (Calhoun and Stinson, 1976).

Specialized apocrine sweat glands are found in the eyelids, external ear canal, and anal region. In the eyelid, rudimentary sweat glands are associated with the eyelashes and are know as the glands of Moll (Getty, 1967).

The apocrine sweat glands of the external ear canal are known as ceruminous glands, but are apparently only partly responsible for the waxy secretion known as cerumen (ear wax). Cerumen appears to be a product of sebaceous and apocrine sweat glands with desquamated epithelial cells as an additional ingredient (Warner and McFarland, 1970).

Large apocrine sweat glands are present within the walls of the anal sacs. The ducts of anal sacs also contain sebaceous glands making the anal sac contents a mixture of sebaceous and apocrine gland secretions. Apocrine sweat glands, known as anal glands, also open directly into the intermediate zone of the anal mucosa (Warner and McFarland, 1970).

Eccrine Sweat Glands

Eccrine (merocrine) sweat glands are limited to the footpads of dogs. They have no thermoregulatory function (Muller et al., 1983).

Mammary Glands

Mammary glands are compound tubuloalveolar glands located in the ventral thoracic, abdominal, and inguinal skin of female dogs. The secretory product, milk, is produced by both apocrine and merocrine secretion (Calhoun and Stinson, 1976). The bitch typically has 10 mammary glands arranged in two symmetrical rows. Teats indicate the location of the glands in the male and immature female. One or more glands may be missing. Nine is the usual number of functional glands in the beagle (Sekhri and Faulkin, 1970). Supernumary teats are common. Mammary glands usually show a size gradient from small (thin) anterior glands to large (thick) posterior ones. The cranial two pairs of glands are the cranial and caudal thoracic glands or simply, glands 1 and 2. The next two pairs are the cranial and caudal abdominal glands, or glands 3 and 4. The most caudal pair are the inguinal, or pubic, glands, or gland 5.

The mammary glands are under hormonal control, which regulates development at puberty, sequential changes during the estrous cycle, and growth during pregnancy. Not all parts of active glands are necessarily in synchrony and there may be substantial variation in the size of ducts and alveoli, luminal content, and the character of lining cells.

Detailed descriptions of the mammary glands during all stages of the estrous cycle have been published (Sekhri and Faulkin, 1970; Nelson and Kelly, 1974).

The selection of mammary gland specimens for microscopic examination should be consistent not only for the purpose of group comparisons, but also for correlation of mammary gland and reproductive tract histology. Nelson and Kelly based their observations on specimens from the inguinal glands. Sixty to 65% of mammary tumors are found in the caudal abdominal and inguinal mammary glands (Crow, 1980; Moulton, 1990), a fact to consider in the design of long-term studies.

Necropsy and Laboratory Techniques

In anesthetized animals, a general examination of the skin should be done prior to exsanguination. All of the body surface, including the mammae, should be palpated to locate masses and to evaluate the texture, elasticity, and thickness of the skin. The luster and texture of the hair should be noted. Abnormal coloration (pallor, erythema, jaundice) should be looked for in lightly pigmented and sparsely haired regions such as the axillae and inguina. The perineal region should be examined as well as the surfaces of the pinnae, visible portions of the ear canal, interdigital spaces and footpads.

If no significant abnormality is revealed by the general examination, a single specimen of inguinal or posterior abdominal skin that includes the mammary gland may be collected as a representative sample of the epidermis, dermis, and glandular adnexa. If specimens of diseased skin are taken, adequate margins of normal skin should be included. Generally, hair should be removed from skin samples to facilitate processing and sectioning. Hair is preferably removed prior to exsanguination. Whether hair is removed by clippers or scissors, the work should be done carefully so as not to disturb or remove surface pathology or create artifacts.

Skin specimens should be flattened prior to fixation. This may be accomplished by carefully stapling the specimen, with the subcutaneous surface down, to small pieces of cardboard or corkboard. The boards may be labeled to identify multiple specimens. Fixation in a flattened position allows proper anatomical orientation and prevents artifacts associated with curling and folding. Three- to four-millimeter wide blocks of tissue may be excised from the fixed tissue for embedding, leaving a largely intact and labeled specimen for archival storage.

Ten-percent buffered formalin is the preferred fixative for skin specimens (Muller et al., 1983; Hargis, 1988). Hematoxylin and eosin (H&E) is the most widely used stain but acid orcein–Giemsa is also recommended as a routine stain for skin biopsies (Muller et al., 1983). The latter authors list several special stains that are useful in dermatopathology.

Special investigations, such as those utilizing the bitch as a test animal in which to study the effects of contraceptives on mammary tissue, may require a detailed examination of the mammary glands. An approach reported by El Etreby and Wrobel (1978) utilized the right mammary system as a whole mount for gross examination and the left mammary system for microscopic examination. Utilizing a modified technique of Cameron and Faulkin (1971), the entire right mammary system was fixed in Tellyesniczky's solution. After removal of the skin and additional fixation, the mammary complex was defatted in acetone, stained with hematoxylin, and cleared with methyl salicylate. The whole mount was weighed and examined by dissecting microscope and photographed utilizing transmitted light. Specimens of the left mammary system were fixed in Carnoy's, Bouin's, or paraformaldehyde solutions and stained by a variety of stains for histomorphology and histochemistry. Frozen sections were also utilized to demonstrate lipids and enzymes. Other approaches to examining the entire mammary system include slicing formalin-fixed glands at 5-mm intervals and examining each slice for gross abnormalities (Nelson et al., 1973) or obtaining specimens from palpable nodules in addition to routine sampling of normal glandular tissue (Giles et al., 1978).

Microscopic examination of lymph nodes draining the mammary glands is rarely indicated in short-term, routine studies. Nevertheless, a knowledge of the usual lymphatic drainage pattern is desirable. The following information was obtained from Christensen (1967) and Moulton (1990). Mammary glands 1 through 3 drain to the axillary lymph nodes on the same side. Glands 4 and 5 drain to the superficial inguinal nodes on the same side. The lymphatics of glands 3 and 4 sometimes connect, allowing both anterior and posterior flow of lymph. Lymphatics may cross the midline and may pass directly through the thoracic wall to the sternal lymph nodes.

Pathology

Several authors have reported on the character and incidence of spontaneous disease in the laboratory beagle (Pick and Eubanks, 1965; Fritz et al., 1966, 1967; Andersen, 1970; Hottendorf and Hirth, 1974; Maita et al., 1977; Oghiso et al., 1982; Glaister, 1986). Disease of the skin or the mammary gland is rarely cited, which probably reflects a true absence of pathology and a failure to sample and diagnose minor or incidental lesions.

Oghiso et al. (1982) reported alopecia of unknown cause associated with atrophy of hair follicles, hyperkeratosis, and necrosis of the epidermis. Alopecia (the complete or partial, diffuse, or circumscribed loss of hair) without underlying skin changes is seen in laboratory dogs over bony pressure points such as the elbow and hock. Continued trauma to such areas may result in a localized hyperkeratotic lesion known as a callus (callosity). Calluses may be ulcerated and infected and become pressure point granulomas.

Circumscribed, erythematous, scaly areas of alopecia near the eyes, commissures of the mouth, or on the forelegs may be a sign of demodectic mange. The presence of demodectic mites in the skin of laboratory beagles has been reported (Hottendorf and Hirth, 1974). *Demodex canis* is a normal resident of the skin of the dog and inhabits hair follicles and sebaceous glands (Muller et al., 1983; Yager and Scott, 1985). The mites are transmitted by direct contact from dam to nursing puppies. A disease state (demodicosis) develops when the favorable equilibrium between dog and parasite is altered, allowing excessive proliferation of the mite. Microscopic examination of demodectic lesions reveals varying degrees of perifolliculitis, folliculitis, and furunculosis (penetrating or perforating folliculitis) in the presence of a large mite population (Muller et al., 1983).

Multiple irregular, soft tan nodules may be seen on the margin of the pinnae. Microscopically, the lesion consists of orthokeratotic (anuclear) and/or parakeratotic (nucleated) hyperkeratosis and is consistent with a condition in pendulous-eared dogs known as ear margin dermatosis (Muller et al., 1983).

Dermatohistopathology has developed a specialized vocabulary based largely on human disease. Some of the diagnostic criteria and terminology are not applicable to veterinary pathology and their use may be confusing if not misleading. The reader is referred to the excellent discussions and illustrations in Hargis (1988), Muller et al. (1983), and Yager and Scott (1985) for guidance in the recognition and diagnosis of conditions that may be encountered in the integument of laboratory dogs.

The peak age of neoplasia in the dog is between 6 and 14 years (Muller et al., 1983); however, tumors do occur in young dogs including laboratory beagles. The following skin tumors were reported in beagles under 2 years of age: histiocytoma (Hottendorf and Hirth, 1974) and sarcoma and mast cell sarcoma, (Fritz et al., 1966).

Apparently, mammary gland inflammation is rare; a single case of mastitis was found in 499 young beagle bitches (Hottendorf and Hirth, 1974). Although mammary tumors are the most common tumor in bitches, they are rarely encountered in dogs less than 2 years old (Moulton, 1990). A survey of reports on the effects of oral or injectable contraceptives in the beagle revealed that mammary nodules rarely developed in nontreated (control) bitches. In a 7-year study, a total of 40 mammary nodules were palpated in 7 of 18 control bitches (Giles et al., 1978). Most of the nodules were transient and only nine remained in six bitches at the time of necropsy. Histopathological examination of the nine nodules revealed five lobular or intraductal hyperplasias, two benign mixed mammary tumors, and two nonmammary nodules (benign soft tissue tumors, epidermal cysts, lymph nodes, or inflammatory nodules). In a 4-year study, nodules were palpable in 4 of 20 control beagle bitches at 21–24 months (Nelson et al., 1973), but all nodules had disappeared by the time of necropsy. The reader is referred to Moulton (1990) for a description and classification of tumor and tumorlike lesions of the canine mammary gland.

MUSCULOSKELETAL SYSTEM

Anatomy and Histology

Bones

The vertebrate skeleton supports the body, provides rigid attachment for muscles of locomotion and respiration, protects internal organs, stores minerals, and is the site of blood cell formation (Miller et al., 1967; Wasserman, 1977). The skeleton consists of many bones varying in size, shape, and function. Long bones such as the femur, tibia, humerus, radius, ulna, metacarpals, metatarsals, and phalanges make up most of the appendicular skeleton and serve primarily as levers. The limbs also contain many short bones (carpal and tarsal) that provide flexibility to their respective joints and sesamoid bones that alter the course of tendons and protect tendons at points of greatest friction (Miller et al., 1967). Flat bones are found in both the appendicular skeleton (scapula) and axial skeleton (ribs, sternum, calvarium). The calvarium protects the brain, whereas the ribs and sternum assist in respiration as well as protect the thoracic organs. Irregular bones are characterized by jutting processes. Much of the axial skeleton comprises irregular bones, including the vertebrae, bones of the base of the skull, and the fused hip bones (Miller et al., 1967). The processes of irregular bones are mostly for muscular and ligamentous attachments; however, some are for articulation. The os penis is the single bone of the heteroptropic skeleton of the dog and forms the skeleton of the penis.

Bones are entirely of mesodermal origin and develop either by direct transformation of connective tissue to bone (intramembranous osteogenesis), by replacement of previously formed cartilage by bone (endochondral osteogenesis), or by a combination of the two processes (Wasserman, 1977). Intramembranous osteogenesis is exemplified by the formation of flat bones of the skull and subperiosteal bone in the shafts of long bones. Endochondral osteogenesis is exemplified by the longitudinal growth of long bones. Bones contain many cell types: endothelial, fat, hemopoietic, chrondoblasts, chondrocytes, osteoblasts, osteocytes, and osteoclasts. Of these, osteoblasts, osteocytes, and osteoclasts have specific bone-related functions. The three types of cells are derived from a common ancestor in the bone marrow (Doige, 1988).

Osteoblasts. These arise from bone marrow stromal stem cells to produce and mineralize an organic matrix called osteoid. Osteoblasts are readily observed during the formation of new bone where they appear as epithelial-like sheets of plump, basophilic cells aligned along bone-forming surfaces. As subsequent rows of osteoblasts differentiate, new osteoblasts begin secreting and osteoblasts of the first row become embedded in bone matrix.

Osteocytes. Osteoblasts buried in mineralized matrix are known as osteocytes. Only about 10% of osteoblasts become osteocytes, the rest apparently die (Jubb et al., 1985). Osteocytes generally appear as single, flat or oval cells in spaces called lacunae. Although surrounded by bone, osteocytes are not isolated, but maintain contact with other osteocytes and osteoblasts by means of a vast network of cytoplasmic processes contained within minute channels called canaliculi (Doige, 1988). Osteocytes play a role in calcium homeostasis by demineralization and remineralization of perilacunar bone. The demineralizing process is known as osteocytic osteolysis. Osteocytes also retain some capacity for bone formation (Doige, 1988).

Osteoclasts. The typical osteoclast is a large, multinuclear cell with abundant eosinophilic cytoplasm. Osteoclasts arise by fusion of mononuclear phagocytes whose precursors are derived from bone marrow hemopoietic stem cells (Doige, 1988). The principal function of osteoclasts is removal of bone, both matrix and mineral. When active, osteoclasts are located in bone structure concavities known as Howship's lacunae. Osteoclasts are highly mobile, capable of migrating along surfaces of bone, and also of entering the bloodstream (Wasserman, 1977). The work of osteoclasts is the basis of the resorption phase of all bone modeling and remodeling (Jubb et al., 1985).

Bone Modeling and Remodeling. Bone modeling refers to the formation and reformation of bone required in the shaping of a growing skeleton (Doige, 1988). Modeling allows the overall shape of bones to be maintained while the skeleton is growing and depends on cellular activity in all parts of the bone. Bone remodeling is the turnover of tissues in mature bones and is the process by which the skeleton renews itself throughout life (Jubb et al., 1985). Remodeling occurs on three surfaces: periosteal, endosteal and intracortical. Since various bones stop growing at different times, the changeover from modeling to remodeling will vary from site-to-site in the skeleton.

Modeling and remodeling occur in both cancellous (trabecular, spongy) and compact (dense, cortical, Haversian) bones.

Cancellous Bone. This is elaborated in the extremities of long bones (epiphysis and metaphysis), forms the internal substance of short and irregular bones, and is interposed between the cortices of most flat bones (Miller et al., 1967). The trabeculae of cancellous bone vary in form from densely packed plates to interconnecting rods to a delicate filigree (Jee et al., 1970). No cancellous bone is present in the middle region of long bones and the space thus formed is known as the medullary cavity. The medullary cavity in adult animals is largely filled with yellow bone marrow.

Compact Bone. This comprises mostly long, bony rods with a central vascular canal. This structure is known as the osteon, or Haversian system, and is the classic structural unit of diaphyseal bone. Osteons form between trabeculae of cancellous bone, eventually filling in the intertrabecular space and converting cancellous bone to compact bone (Jubb et al., 1985). The remaining intertices of cancellous bone are occupied by red marrow.

The cancellous bone of ribs and vertebrae and many short and flat bones is filled with red marrow throughout life (Miller et al., 1967).

Joints

Joints, or articulations, are structures that join two or more bones in unions that may or may not be movable. Three main types of joints are recognized: fibrous, cartilaginous, and synovial.

Fibrous Joints.
These are simple unions that provide for little movement. Examples are sutures of the skull and unions of long bones such as the tibia and fibula (tibiofibular syndesmosis).

Cartilaginous Joints.   Two types of cartilaginous joints are recognized: hyaline and fibrocartilaginous.

Hyaline Cartilaginous Joints.   The site of endochrondral osteogenesis in long bones (physis) is a temporary hyaline cartilage joint that is eventually replaced by bone. The unions between ribs and costal cartilages are permanent hyaline cartilage joints, although they may be partially ossified with age (Miller et al., 1967).

Fibrocartilaginous Joints.   The unions between the right and left mandibular bodies (mandibular symphysis) and right and left os coxae (pelvic symphysis) are examples of fibrocartilaginous joints. The mandibular symphysis persists throughout life, but the pelvic symphysis ossifies in the adult (Miller et al., 1967).

The unions of vertebrae (intervertebral disks) are special fibrocartilaginous joints consisting of a collagenous ring (annulus fibrosus) surrounding a space filled with semifluid material (nucleus pulposus).

Synovial Joints.   These joints are the truly movable articulations. All synovial joints feature a capsule, cartilaginous articular surfaces, joint cavity, and a lubricating fluid. A few synovial joints also possess intra-articular ligaments, fibrocartilaginous plates (menisci), and fat pads (Miller et al., 1967). The fibrous joint capsule is continuous with the periosteum of the bone ends and encloses the joint cavity. The inner layer (intima) of the joint capsule lines the cavity except on the surfaces of the cartilage and is responsible for the production and turnover of the fluid (synovia) that lubricates the joint and nourishes the articular surfaces (Jubb et al., 1985). The articular surfaces of all principal synovial joints are covered with typical hyaline cartilate that is thickest in the young animal and at sites of maximum weight bearing. The normal capsule is strong but not rigid. Normal intima is smooth and glistening. The articular cartilage in young and healthy animals is smooth, white or somewhat bluish, semitransparent, and moist. The normal synovia is viscous, clear, colorless, or slightly yellow (Jubb et al., 1985; Doige, 1988).

Muscle

Muscles are specialized collections of cells that produce directed movement through strong organized contractions (Venable and Dellmann, 1976). Muscles are customarily classified as smooth, cardiac, and skeletal.

Smooth Muscle.   This type of muscle is found in the walls of the digestive, respiratory, urinary, and reproductive tracts, blood vessels, spleen, and eyeball, and it is also associated with glands and hair follicles (Miller et al., 1967; Goll et al., 1977). Smooth muscle has a simple appearance consisting of spindle-shaped (tapered) cells without cytoplasmic cross striations and a single, centrally placed nucleus. Smooth muscle is commonly referred to as visceral muscle (by its location) or involuntary muscle (by its innervation), and has also been called plain, or unstriated, muscle (Miller et al., 1967).

Cardiac Muscle.   This type of muscle forms the bulk of the heart and combines the features of smooth and skeletal muscles. As in smooth muscle, the nuclei are centrally placed and the fibers are under involunatry nervous control. As in skeletal muscle, the fibers are cross-striated and multinucleated. Cardiac muscle has also been called involuntary striated muscle.

Skeletal Muscle.   This type of muscle is so named because of its relationship to the skeleton. Skeletal muscle comprises the single largest tissue mass in the body; 40% of the body weight for mammals in general (Goll et al., 1977) and from 35 to 54% of the body weight of beagles (Andersen and Goldman, 1970). Skeletal muscles range in size from the minute stapedius muscle of the middle ear to the massive muscles of the rump (Miller et al., 1967).

Individual muscles are surrounded by and separated from other muscles by a sheet of connective tissue known as the epimysium (Greek *epi* = upon, above, beside). The epimysium may be fairly thick and tough and is the site of intermuscular fat deposits.

At irregular intervals, thinner sheets of connective tissue, called perimysium (Greek *peri* = around), pass into the muscle and divide it into bundles (fasciculi). The perimysium also envelopes blood vessels and nerves and is the site of intramuscular fat deposits (Goll et al., 1977).

Very delicate sheets of connective tissue, called endomysium (Greek *endo* = within), extend from the perimysium and surround individual muscle fibers. The endomysium lies immediately adjacent to the muscle cell outer membrane (sarcolemma). The endomysium carries a longitudinally oriented capillary network.

Skeletal muscle fibers are striated and multinucleated, with the majority of nuclei located peripherally. Skeletal muscle is under control of the somatic or voluntary nervous system, and hence is also called somatic, or voluntary, muscle.

Muscle Fibers.   Not all normal skeletal muscles have the same depth of color. Color variation depends upon a number of factors, but is in part due to the relative percentages of type I and type II fibers. Histochemical techniques have allowed the division of skeletal muscle fibers into two major groups: type I fibers, which are rich in oxidative enzymes, darker in color, and show a slow twitch response; and type II fibers, which are rich in glycogen, paler in color, and show a fast-twitch response (Hulland, 1985). The ratio of the two fiber types varies widely from muscle-to-muscle. In the dog, type I fibers comprise less than 15% of the extensor carpi radialis and over 90% of the vastus intermedius (Armstrong et al., 1982).

Necropsy and Laboratory Techniques

A "complete" postmortem examination rarely includes a complete examination of bones, joints, and muscles. While a complete dissection of the musculoskeletal system is neither practical nor necessary, something more than a cursory examination is in order. Antemortem clinical findings, including clinical laboratory results, should be known.

A brief visual examination and palpation of the body before exsanguination or skinning should reveal swollen or stiff joints, muscle wasting, and skeletal deformities and asymmetry. Certain bones, joints, and muscles should be routinely examined to provide completeness to the necropsy and to establish normal baseline values for color, hardness, size, volume, etc. The prosector should be alert to general changes in the musculoskeletal system during the course of the postmortem examination.

Ventral and lateral muscles of the neck and trunk are exposed during the primary ventral midline incision and reflection of the skin. Skin should also be reflected from the inner aspect of the limbs to expose the shoulder, elbow, and knee joints and major muscles of the legs. Several of the large medial muscles of the limbs must be cut to fully extend the legs and in the process large cross-sectional areas of muscle are brought to view. Several large synovial joints should be opened completely.

The hindlimbs can be extended fully only by disarticulating the coxofemoral joints; however, in the process the joints are usually contaminated with blood from the femoral vessels. With practice the shoulder, elbow, and knee joints may be opened without contamination, but the disarticulation must be done carefully to avoid slicing articular cartilage. Joints should be examined immediately upon opening because articular cartilage rapidly dehydrates and discolors when exposed to air (Doige, 1988). It is helpful to compare contralateral joints; however, the prosector should realize that under normal circumstances the synovial fluid may have a different appearance from joint-to-joint within an animal and in the same joint between animals (Jubb et al., 1985). An additional opportunity to examine a large synovial joint arises when the atlanto-occipital joint is disarticulated to remove the head.

During removal of the spinal cord (as a whole or in segments) the surface of the spinal canal overlying intervertebral disks should be examined. The ventral surface of the vertebral column should be palpated following removal of the thoracic, abdominal, and pelvic viscera.

Bone strength may be assessed as the ribs, calvarium, and os coxae are cut while opening the thoracic, cranial, and pelvic cavities. Jaws and teeth should be examined during removal of the tongue and larynx. At least one long bone (preferably a femur) should be examined in detail and fixed for microscopic evaluation. The femur should be cut in a standardized, midline longitudinal plane to establish a baseline for normal width of cortical bone, density of cancellous bone, width and uniformity of physes, curvature of articular surfaces, and relative proportion of red and yellow marrow. The marrow contents may be flushed away by a jet of water from one of the halves for better exposure of bony structure.

For good fixation, bone slabs should be no wider than 5 mm; therefore, additional bone will need to be cut from the proximal and distal ends of the femur. The femur is collected primarily for the study of osseous, cartilaginous, and articular tissues.

An additional bone, preferably a flat bone such as a sternebra, should be collected specifically for bone marrow cytology. The sternebrae of young dogs may be cut with a stout sharp knife, thus avoiding the problem of the marrow surface being filled with bone and muscle debris from a saw.

Skeletal muscle is usually one of the last tissues collected at necropsy. Delay in fixation is not a concern, for muscle is one tissue that may appear worse histologically when fixed immediately than when fixed hours, even days, after death (McGavin, 1983). Artifacts are the problem. Fresh muscle is very sensitive and will vigorously contract when pinched, crushed, cut, stretched, and placed in most fixatives. The resulting artifacts (severe contraction bands; sarcoplasmic masses; shredded, cracked, and rounded and hyalinized fibers) will mask and even mimic pathological change (McGavin, 1983).

Another problem in interpretation confronts the microscopist when the histological sections contain mostly tangentially sectioned fibers. Both transverse and longitudinal sections of muscle are required for the proper interpretation of many pathological processes. Transverse and longitudinal sections can be obtained only from muscles in which the majority of the fibers are oriented parallel to each other. Three hindlimb muscles (biceps femoris, semitendinosus, semimembranosus) have such an orientation of fibers and are also large (for ease of sampling) and easily identified. In addition, each of the above muscles presents a fairly good representation of type I and type II fibers. The following percentages of type I fibers were found by Armstrong et al. (1982): biceps femoris (32±8), semitendinosus (27±11), and semimembranosus (28±5). Once selected, the same muscle should be the site from which all samples are taken.

To minimize the problem of artifacts, the muscle must be handled gently; but, most importantly, the muscle must be prevented from contracting during removal and fixation. McGavin (1983) recommends the following relatively simple procedure: make two parallel incisions, 3 to 6 mm apart, into the belly of the muscle and in the same direction as the muscle fibers, suture each end of the isolated strap of muscle to a narrow, flat wooden stick, undercut the muscle, sever the muscle beyond the sutures, remove the stick and muscle together, and place in fixative.

Paraffin embedded, H&E stained sections of bone and muscle meet the needs of most toxicology studies. There are, however, a number of special laboratory techniques to study both bone and muscle. Many of the bone procedures have been used extensively in the beagle and include the measurement of bone ash, volume and specific gravity; labeling sites of mineralization by fluorescent markers; and microscopic and microradiographic examination of undemineralized sections (Saville and Krook, 1969; Jee et al., 1970; Anderson and Danylchuk, 1978, 1979a–c; Jorch and Anderson, 1980; Kunkle et al., 1982; Martin et al., 1981; Norrdin and Shih, 1983; Snow et al., 1986). Bone specimens for routine H&E staining should be well-fixed, free of debris from the bone saw, not overly decalcified, and represent both cancellous and cortical bone, an articular surface, and a physis. McGavin (1983) lists special stains and enzyme histochemical procedures to study muscle. As mentioned, H&E stained specimens of muscle should always include transverse and longitudinal sections.

Pathology

Little is mentioned about disease of the musculoskeletal system in the review articles. Hottendorf and Hirth (1974) report fracture of the rib and chondrodystrophic change in costochondral junctions. Hottendorf and Hirth also report congenital hernias (digestive system). In the writer's experience, these are usually small umbilical hernias containing only omental fat. Barron and Saunders (1966) report the fortuitous finding of *Toxocara* granulomas in skeletal muscle.

DIGESTIVE SYSTEM

Anatomy and Histology

The digestive system consists of a series of connecting, mostly tubular, hollow structures that includes the mouth, pharynx, esophagus, stomach, small and large intestines; and a group of accessory organs that includes the teeth, tongue, salivary glands, liver, gallbladder and pancreas. The tubular portion from the esophagus distally is the alimentary canal.

Mouth

The mouth (oral cavity) is the most anterior opening and cavity of the digestive system. Its limits anteriorly and anterolaterally are the upper and lower lips, posterolaterally the right and left cheeks, dorsally the palate, and ventrally the floor of the mouth and tongue.

Anteriorly, the palate has a bony core, and is termed the hard palate. Posteriorly, the palate has a muscular core, and is termed the soft palate. The soft palate is unusually long in the dog and may extend to or beyond the epiglottis (Miller et al., 1967). Gingiva is the keratinized epithelial membrane that covers the alveolar processes of the jaws and attaches to the teeth. The gingival tissue adjacent to the tooth surface is known as the free gingival margin.

The dog usually has 42 permanent teeth (Miller et al., 1967), whose names and placement in the upper and lower dental arcades are shown in the following formula (I = incisor, C = canine, PM = premolar and M = molar):

$$I \tfrac{3}{3} \ C \tfrac{1}{1} \ PM \tfrac{4}{4} \ M \tfrac{2}{3} \ X \ 2 = 42$$

According to their location, the incisors are known as central, intermediate, or corner; the premolars as first, second, third, or fourth; and the molars as first, second, or third. Deciduous (temporary) teeth immediately replace permanent teeth in the dog (Miller et al., 1967). In the beagle, the average age of eruption (in months) for permanent teeth is as follows (Bartley et al., 1970):

	Central	Intermediate	Corner	
Incisor	3.8	4.1	4.4	
	3.9	4.1	4.1	

	Central
Canine	4.7
	4.7

	First	Second	Third	Fourth
Premolar	3.5	5.0	5.1	4.5
	4.3	5.0	5.2	5.2

	First	Second	Third	Fourth
Molar	4.4	5.2	—	—
	4.3	5.0	5.8	—

Permanent dentition should be complete in most beagles by the age they are placed on study.

The tongue forms most of the floor of the mouth. The posterior one-third of the tongue is the root and the slender anterior two-thirds is the body. A long mucosal fold (frenulum) connects the body of the tongue to the floor of the mouth.

Pharynx

The mouth is continuous posteriorly with the pharynx, a funnel-shaped connection between the mouth and the esophagus and between the nasal cavity and the larynx. The pharynx serves both digestive and respiratory functions. An exclusively respiratory portion (nasal pharynx) lies above the soft palate. The portion below the soft palate (oral pharynx), serves a mixed digestive/respiratory function, being respiratory during panting.

The nasal and oral pharynges unite just posterior to the soft palate to form the pharyngeal isthmus, where the digestive and respiratory tracts change relationships. The respiratory tract continues ventrally as the larynx and thereafter as the trachea. The digestive system continues dorsally as the laryngeal pharynx and thereafter as the esophagus. The lateral walls of the nasal pharynx are obliquely pierced by two slit-like openings, the pharyngeal ostia of the auditory tubes. The lateral walls of the nasal pharynx are indented by two crypts which contain long, thin lymphoid structures, the palatine tonsils.

Salivary Glands

Salivary glands are the first of the accessory organs to discharge secretions into the digestive tube. Salivary glands are classified by size (major, minor), by secretion (mucous, serous, mixed), and named by location. All major salivary glands are paired and include the parotid, mandibular, sublingual, and zygomatic glands (Miller et al., 1967).

Saliva. The individual and collective secretions of the salivary glands are discharged into both the dorsal and ventral parts of the mouth. Dorsally, most secretions come from the parotid and zygomatic glands and ventrally from the mandibular and sublingual glands. The saliva of the dog has no enzymatic activity of note (Harvey et al., 1983).

Parotid Gland. This is a coarsely lobulated and reddish V-shaped organ that closely embraces the base of the ear. It is predominantly serous, but occasional isolated mucous secretory units may be found (Stinson and Calhoun, 1976). The parotid duct opens into the mouth lateral to the upper fourth premolar tooth.

Mandibular Gland. This is a lightly lobulated and light tan ovoid body lying just caudal and ventral to the parotid gland. It is a mixed gland (Stinson and Calhoun, 1976) and its ducts open below the tongue near the frenulum.

Sublingual Gland. This gland consists of a series of two or more elongated, lobulated masses extending from the mandibular gland to the anterior margin of the frenulum. The most posterior portion of the sublingual gland is enveloped by the capsule of the mandibular gland (Miller et al., 1967). Grossly, the sublingual gland is distinguished from the mandibular gland by its darker color; however, its subcapsular location within the mandibular gland may puzzle the microscopist when first seen. The sublingual gland is a mixed gland (Stinson and Calhoun, 1976) whose ducts empty onto the floor of the mouth.

Zygomatic Gland. This gland is a moderately lobulated gland located beneath the zygomatic arch, ventral and posterior to the eye. The zygomatic gland is predominantly mucous, but a few serous demilunes are present (Stinson and Calhoun, 1976). Zygomatic gland secretions enter the mouth through several openings lateral to the upper moler teeth.

Minor Salivary Glands. These glands consist of clusters of serous, seromucous, or mucous elements found in various oral structures, including the tongue, lips, palate, and pharynx.

Esophagus

The esophagus is the first part of the alimentary canal and connects the laryngeal pharynx with the stomach. The esophagus may be divided into cervical, thoracic, and abdominal segments. The cervical esophagus extends from the pharynx to the thoracic inlet, the thoracic esophagus extends from the thoracic inlet to the diaphragm, and the abdominal esophagus is the short segment between the diaphragm and the stomach. The abdominal esophagus acts as a flutter valve and is important in preventing gastroesophageal reflux (Strombeck, 1979).

The esophagus is capable of great distention except at its beginning and end and as it passes through the thoracic inlet. The collapsed mucosa forms numerous longitudinal folds. In the dog, the entire length of the mucosa is covered by nonkeratinized stratified squamous epithelium. The submucosa contains numerous mucous glands with serous demilunes, and the tunica muscularis is comprised entirely of two oblique layers of striated muscle fibers (Miller et al., 1967).

Stomach

The stomach is the largest dilatation of the alimentary canal. A line drawn through the axis of the stomach appears somewhat like a letter C. The longer, outer convex surface of the organ is the greater curvature. The shorter, inner concave surface is the lesser curvature. The walls between the two curvatures are the dorsal and ventral walls. The inlet from the esophagus is the cardiac ostium and the outlet into the small intestine is the pyloric ostium.* For gross, microscopic, and functional purposes, the stomach may be divided into five, three, and two regions, respectively (Strombeck, 1979). Grossly, the regions consist of a narrow zone between the esophagus and body known as the cardiac region. The body is the large middle region, and the fundic region is the blind outpocketing of the body located to the side of the cardia on the greater curvature. The terminal, funnel-shaped, one-third of the stomach is the pyloric region. The pyloric region is subdivided into an initial thin-walled portion (pyloric antrum) and a terminal thick-walled portion (pyloric canal). The normal color of the cardiac, fundic, and body mucosa is pink to grayish red. The pyloric mucosa is a pale tan. The mucosa of an empty or even moderately distended stomach is thrown into numerous folds (gastric rugae).

Close examination of the gastric mucosa reveals that it is comprised of minute raised areas (areae gastricae) surrounded by narrow furrows. This blocklike subdivision of the gastric mucosa may be recognized in tissue section, especially in the pyloric region. The gastric mucosa in the dog is entirely glandular.

According to its glandular makeup, the stomach is histologically divided into cardiac, gastric gland proper, and pyloric regions (there is intermixing of glands between adjacent regions). The cardiac and pyloric regions comprise primarily mucous glands. Cardiac glands are characterized by deep gland openings (foveolae) and short gland bodies. Pyloric glands have foveolae and bodies of about equal length. The body and fundic regions are populated principally by gastric glands proper (sometimes erroneously called fundic glands), which have comparatively shallow foveolae and long bodies.

The gland bodies are lined by mucous neck, parietal (oxyntic), chief, and argentaffin cells. Small numbers of parietal and argentaffin cells are also found in the pyloric region and parietal cells also may be found in the cardiac region.

The submucosal mucous glands of the esophagus extend into the cardiac region (Stinson and Calhoun, 1976). Similarly, the submucosal glands of the duodenum (Brunner's glands) extend into the submucosa of the pyloric region.

Functionally, the proximal two-thirds of the stomach (body and fundus) adapts by expansion to serve as a storage reservoir and the caudal one-third (pyloric region) performs as a grinding mill and funnel to propel ingesta into the small intestine (Strombeck, 1979).

Studies of the rate at which digesta move through the gastrointestinal tract of the dog reveal that at 8 hr, roughly 90% of the meal is in the stomach and roughly 10% has entered the small intestine (Stevens, 1977). At 12 hours, approximately equal quantities are found in the stomach, small intestine, and colon. At 24 hours, roughly 30% remains in the stomach, 10% is in the small intestine and 30% each in the colon and feces. The bulk of the meal (90%) has been evacuated at 38 hr.

---

*The term *cardia* has not been used because it has variously referred to the cardiac region, ostium, and sphincter. Similarly, the term *pylorus* was not usd because it has variously referred to the pyloric region, antrum, canal, ostium, and sphincter.

Small Intestine

The small intestine extends from the stomach to the colon. It is the longest portion of the alimentary canal, representing about 85% of length of the entire intestine (Stevens, 1977). (A length of 225–290 cm has been reported for the small intestine of the adult beagle; Andersen, 1970). The small intestine represents only 23% of total capacity of gastrointestinal tract. The stomach, cecum, colon and rectum represent 62, 1, and 13%, respectively (Stevens, 1977).

There are no gross features to definitely separate the three segments of the small intestine and the beginning (duodenum), middle (jejunum), and end (ileum) must be set arbitrarily.

Duodenum. This is considered to be the proximal one-tenth, or 25 cm, of the small intestine (Miller et al., 1967). The duodenum is divided into cranial, descending, caudal, and ascending portions. Brunner's glands are limited primarily to a narrow region of the pyloric duodenal junction (Titkemeyer and Calhoun, 1955). Pancreatic and bile ducts discharge into the descending duodenum. The common bile and ventral pancreatic ducts share a small protuberance (major duodenal papilla) found 3–5 cm caudal to the pyloric ostium. The dorsal pancreatic duct opens on a smaller protuberance, (minor duodenal papilla) located about 5 cm caudal to the major papilla. To the uninitiated, the duodenal papillae may appear to be tumorous enlargements in the gut wall. While the pancreatic ducts penetrate the gut wall more or less at right angles, the common bile duct courses intramurally for a distance of 1.5–2.0 cm. The microscopist should be aware of the lengthy intramural placement of the bile duct and not misinterpret its presence as an anomaly or tumor.

Jejunum and Ileum. These comprise the bulk of the small intestine. Most veterinary anatomists consider the jejunum to be substantially longer than the ileum and generally regard only the short, usually contracted, terminal part of the small intestine as ileum (Miller et al., 1967). The circularly arranged folds (plicae circulares) that characterize the small intestine of humans and some domestic animals are absent in the dog. The intestinal glands (crypts of Lieberkuhn) are long in the dog, resulting in villus-length:crypt-depth ratios of 2:1, 1:1, or even less (compare to ratios of 4:1 or greater in species such as mice, rats, pigs, and humans). Dogs lack Paneth cells (Stinson and Calhoun, 1976).

Aggregated lymph follicles (Peyer's patches) are easily recognized in the dog from either the exterior or interior surface of the small intestine. Generally, the patches appear on either side of the mesenteric attachment. On the mucosal surface, Peyer's patches appear as ovoid elevations measuring about 1.5 by 2.0 cm. An average of 22 Peyer's patches have been reported for the dog (Titkemeyer and Calhoun, 1955). They exist throughout the length of the small intestine, but most are found in the duodenum and jejunum. Villi overlying Peyer's patches are generally short and oddly shaped, may even be entirely effaced, and in general are not representative of villi elsewhere in the gut. Peyer's patches, solitary lymph follicles, tonsils, and the diffuse lymphoreticular tissue of the digestive system comprise the gut-associated lymphoid tissue (GALT).

Large Intestine

The large intestine of the dog is short, representing about 13% of entire length of the intestine (Stevens, 1977), and it lacks special features such as sacculations, bands, and a vermiform appendix found in other species. The large intestine begins at the ileocolic orifice and ends at the anus, and includes the cecum, colon, rectum, and anal canal.

Colon. This is the most proximal segment of the large intestine. It is about 25 cm long and is divided into ascending, transverse, and descending portions. The cecum is a relatively short and small diverticulum of the ascending colon and communicates with the colon only through the cecocolic orifice. (Some authors erroneously refer to an ileocecal valve and orifice.)

The descending colon is the longest and straightest portion of the colon. The large intestine continues as the short (about 5 cm long), entirely intrapelvic portion known as the rectum.

The anal canal is the terminal 1 cm of the alimentary tube. For its length, the anal canal is very complex with three mucosal zones, two types of glands, and the site of drainage for the anal sacs.

Solitary lymph nodules are found throughout the mucosa of the entire large intestine; however, they tend to be particularly large in the rectum and often appear as raised nodules, 3 to 4 mm in diameter, with central craterlike depressions. The depressions are due to circular discontinuities in the muscularis mucosae, allowing intimate mixing of intestinal glands and submucosal lymphoid aggregates. Solitary lymph nodules are also found in the esophagus, stomach, small intestine, and gallbladder mucosae.

Liver

The liver is undoubtedly the digestive organ of greatest interest in toxicology studies. It is a large organ in keeping with its many functions. The liver represents about 7% of the body weight of 2- to 3-month-old pups and about 4% in adults (Andersen, 1970).

The liver is divided into four lobes: left, right, quadrate, and caudate. The left lobe is the largest, comprising up to one-half of the entire liver. Both the left and right lobes are divided into sublobes, which are called lobes nevertheless. On the left, the larger sublobe is the left lateral lobe. Medial to it lies the left medial lobe. The right hepatic lobe is divided into the right medial lobe and the right lateral lobe. The quadrate lobe lies between the right and left hepatic lobes. The gallbladder lies partially in a depression (fossa) on the right side of the base of the quadrate lobe. The left half of the fossa is formed by the base of the right medial lobe. The caudate lobe is the most irregularly shaped and most caudally placed lobe of the liver. Its most cranial portion is called the papillary process. The most caudal portion is the caudate process which is marked by a deep impression for the right kidney.

The fresh liver is reddish brown, firm to the touch, yet friable. Normally, the borders (margins) are sharp-edged and the cut surface does not bulge. The capsular surface is tightly covered by a thin, transparent membrane (peritoneum). Close inspection reveals about 1-mm sized subunits (hepatic lobules) that vary considerably in prominence according to the physiological and pathological state of the liver.

Gallbladder

The gallbladder is a pear-shaped vesicle that lies between the quadrate and right medial lobes of the liver. It has a capacity of 10–15 ml (Andersen, 1970). When fully distended, the gallbladder is visible on the diaphragmatic surface of the liver. The emptying of the gallbladder is related to gastric digestion; during fasting it remains distended. The gallbladder has a neck, body and a blind, rounded, cranial end known as the fundus.

Bile is formed in the liver and stored and concentrated in the gallbladder. The dog has a high concentrating ability (Stevens, 1977). Bile reaches the gallbladder by way of the hepatic and cystic ducts. The cystic duct extends from the neck of the gallbladder to the union with the first hepatic duct. The common bile duct extends from the junction of cystic and hepatic ducts to the major duodenal papilla. Bile may be watery to mucoid in consistency and greenish yellow to golden brown in color. Dark green flecks are not unusual. The gallbladder mucosa is normally smooth but solitary lymph follicles may cause a slight roughness.

Pancreas

The pancreas is a V-shaped gland formed by the fusion of a slim right lobe and a shorter, but thicker and wider left lobe. The left lobe lies in the greater omentum adjacent to the stomach. The right lobe lies in the mesoduodenum adjacent to the descending duodenum. Numerous variations in the pancreatic duct system have been described in the dog (Miller et al., 1967). Most commonly, the larger ventral pancreatic duct drains the right lobe and the smaller dorsal pancreatic duct drains the left lobe. The ventral pancreatic duct terminates as a slitlike opening adjacent to the common bile duct on the major duodenal papilla. The dorsal pancreatic duct opens upon the minor duodenal papilla.

The pancreas is soft, coarsely lobulated and has a pinkish gray coloration in life. The pancreatic islets of the dog usually are not visible to the naked eye.

Necropsy and Laboratory Techniques

Disease of the digestive system produces a wide variety of clinical signs. Some signs are nonspecific (anorexia, weight loss, pain, weakness, reluctance to move, generalized malaise, shivering, fever, dehydration, hemorrhage, anemia), and some signs are shared with disease of other organs (depression, coma, polydipsia, polyuria), but many signs indicate disease somewhere within the digestive system.

The most common signs associated with problems in the upper digestive tract (mouth, pharynx, esophagus, stomach, proximal small intestine) are vomiting (forcible expulsion of ingesta into the mouth), regurgitation (passive backward flow of ingesta into the mouth or nasal cavity), and dysphagia (difficulty in swallowing) (Strombeck, 1979). Additional signs of upper digestive tract disease are halitosis (offensive breath), excessive salivation, hematemesis (blood in the vomitus), melena (black feces, digested blood), abdominal pain, and bloating.

Diarrhea (an increase in the frequency, fluidity, or volume of feces) is the most consistent indicator of problems in the lower digestive tract (middle and distal small intestine, large intestine) (Strombeck, 1979). The character of the diarrhea (and other signs) often indicate what part of the intestine is diseased.

Signs of small intestine involvement include: large quantity of bulky or watery feces, undigested food in the feces, melena, weight loss, and generalized malaise (Sherding, 1983). Signs of large intestine involvement include: very frequent defecation, small volume of feces, urgency, tenesmus (painful straining), mucus in the feces, red-stained feces (fresh blood), and constipation.

Liver disease is also associated with numerous clinical signs, including abdominal pain, anorexia, ascites, coma, depression, dark brown urine, dark or light-colored stools, diarrhea, fever, hemorrhage, icterus, polydipsia (excessive thirst), polyuria (abnormally large volume of urine), pruritus, weakness, weight loss, and vomiting (Strombeck, 1979). Since the liver has a large functional reserve and an amazing capacity to regenerate, as much as 70–80% of the liver's mass must be impaired before signs of dysfunction are seen (Hardy, 1983).

The clinical signs of acute pancreatic disease include: vomiting, pain, anorexia, depression, fever, diarrhea, abdominal distress (aside from pain, dehydration, shock, and respiratory distress (Strombeck, 1979). Signs of chronic pancreatic disease (pancreatic atrophy) include diarrhea, steatorrhea (excessive amount of fat in the feces), and weight loss. With these signs in mind and all available clinical and laboratory data at hand, the prosector may undertake examination of the digestive system.

The oral cavity should always be examined, preferably after anesthesia and before exsanguination. The breath of a healthy dog is usually not unpleasant. The normal oral mucosa is pink, has a smooth and glistening surface, and shows little accumulation of saliva (Harvey, 1983). Normal free gingival margins may be slightly hyperemic. The oral cavity may be fully explored after removal of the tongue and pharynx. A cross-section of the body of the tongue is usually taken to represent the oral mucosa histologically. The parotid and mandibular salivary glands should be inspected. The mandibular gland is usually chosen to histologically represent the salivary gland system. The mandibular gland is a reasonable choice for it is readily accessible and contains both mucous and serous secretory units.

The initial examination of the thoracic and abdominal viscera should be done with all organs in place and natural relationships undisturbed. This is particularly true when a dilated, flaccid esophagus is found (megaesophagus), for one possible cause is a persistent right aortic arch. The tongue, pharynx, larynx, esophagus, and trachea are usually removed intact along with the heart, great vessels, thymus, and lungs. The esophagus should be completely opened, examined, and a midsection collected for histopathology. The pancreas is excised (after removal of the spleen and liver), examined, and a specimen taken (consistently from the right or left lobe) for histopathology. The gastrointestinal tract is removed. (The pelvic girdle must be cut through at the obturator foramina to excise the rectum and anal canal.) The suspensory ligaments, omenta, and mesentery may be stripped from the gastrointestinal tract as it is removed. The tract should be completely opened and the entire length examined. The stomach unfolds nicely when opened along the greater curvature. Bulk digesta and feces may be picked from the surface. Brief flushing with tap water may be required to remove adherent material. Sloshing a specimen in saline or fixative may be desirable for critical examination of lesions.

A complete sampling of the gastrointestinal tract would include two samples of the stomach (body and pyloric regions), cranial duodenum (to include Brunner's glands), jejunum (mid portion), ileum (a few centimeters from the ileocolic junction), entire cecum, and a segment of the descending colon and rectum. One of the jejunum/ileum specimens should include a Peyer's patch.

All of the specimens (except the cecum) are preferably fixed in a flattened position. This may be done by stapling the specimens (serosal surface down) to small pieces of corkboard. The boards may be labeled to identify the specimens. The gallbladder also should be fixed in a flattened position. All surfaces of the liver should be examined and multiple parallel slices made through each lobe. Slices of tissue (no wider than 5 mm) should be taken from at least two lobes for histopathology. The right and left lateral lobes are suggested.

Pathology

Numerous observations have been reported for the digestive system of young laboratory beagles. Most of the observations are of no clinical or experimental significance. A few may complicate interpretation of apparent treatment-related effects and the pathogenesis of several have never been explained.

Mouth and Salivary Glands

A number of minor dental abnormalities may be encountered: missing permanent teeth (usually upper and lower premolars), retained deciduous teeth (usually canine), imperfect apposition of teeth, dental plaque (soft bacterial masses), dental calculus or tartar (mineralized plaque, usually discolored, most abundant next to orifices of salivary ducts), and gingivitis (usually associated with plaque or tartar). Hottendorf and Hirth (1974) report oral papillomatosis and mild focal sialoadenitis. Oral papillomas (warts) are benign epithelial tumors caused by papovaviruses. They occur mainly in young dogs and spontaneously disappear. The warts may be found on the lips, inside the cheeks, and on the tongue, palate, and pharynx. The gums are usually not affected. Glaister (1986) reports glossitis.

Esophagus

Megaesophagus (grossly dilated and flaccid esophagus) may be seen. This is a congenital condition occasionally due to a persistent right aortic arch, but more commonly due to an apparent neuromuscular developmental disorder. A swollen, thick-walled esophagus suggests reflux esophagitis, an erosive and ulcerative lesion of the esophageal wall. Dogs with histories of repeated regurgitation or vomiting should be examined for the condition. Slight dilatation of esophageal gland ducts may be seen in an otherwise normal esophagus.

Stomach

Chronic gastritis and granuloma are reported by Hottendorf and Hirth (1974). Microscopic mineralization (microcalculi) of the gastric mucosa is reported by Glaister (1986). Lymphocytic nodules or follicles may be present within the lamina propria, particularly of the pyloric region. Gastric glands may be slightly dilated. Spirillumlike bacteria are frequently found within the lumina of gastric glands and within the intracellular canaliculi of parietal cells (Barker and Van Dreumel, 1985; Weber et al., 1958). The bacteria incite no inflammatory response, but may be associated with dilatation of the canaliculi and gland lumina and cytoplasmic vacuolation of the parietal cells. Henry et al. (1987) indicate that large numbers of gastric spirilla may induce lymphoreticular hyperplasia and premature senescence of parietal cells.

Intestine

Hottendorf and Hirth (1974) report the presence of ascarids, cestodes, and strongyloides, hernia, intussusception, granuloma, catarrhal enteritis, and mild focal cecitis and colitis. Fritz et al. (1967) report Meckel's diverticulum. Oghiso et al. (1982) report mucoepithelial cysts of the small intestine. Barron and Saunders (1966) report *Toxocara* granuloma. Glaister (1986) reports nematodes and granuloma. Pick and Eubanks (1965) report trichuriasis, ascariasis, and ancylostomiasis. Giardiasis may be diagnosed clinically on the basis of cysts or trophozoites found in fecal samples. Generally, there is no evidence for histopathological diagnosis of the disease. Mild hyperplasia of individual or aggregate lymph follicles in the lamina propria may be seen. Usually this correlates with an increased gross prominence of the nodules. Congestion of the capillary network of the gastrointestinal mucosa is common.

Liver

Of all the digestive organs, gross and microscopic findings are reported most frequently for the liver. Hottendorf and Hirth (1974) report small, light yellow foci in the caudate lobe near the porta hepatis, eosinophilic phlebitis and periphlebitis (suggestive of a hypersensitivity reaction to migrating parasites), focal necrosis and inflammation, mild bile duct hyperplasia with mild portal inflammation, mild portal inflammation without bile duct hyperplasia, granuloma, and intranuclear rhomboid inclusions. Oghiso et al. (1982) report granulomatous aggregation of mononuclear cells, vacuolar degeneration, fatty degeneration, lipofuscin deposition, acidophilic intranuclear inclusions, and necrosis. Maita et al. (1977) report small granulomas, cubic or rectangular intranuclear hyaline bodies, lipofuscin deposition, necrosis at the base of hepatic ligaments, and periodic acid–Schiff positive cytoplasmic inclusions. Andersen (1970) reports periodic acid–Schiff positive cytoplasmic inclusions and subcapsular cysts filled with serous fluid. Glaister (1986) reports leukocytic foci and granuloma. Barron and Saunders (1966) report *Toxocara* granuloma.

The most common histological "lesions" in the liver of young beagles are small focal collections of histiocytes, lymphocytes, and an occasional neutrophil, at times accompanied by a few degenerate hepatocytes. The foci are commonly referred to as microgranulomas. Their pathogenesis and significance appear to be unknown.

The focal subcapsular lipidosis and necrosis seen near the hilus of the liver is compatible with so-called tension lesions seen in other species.

Rectangular or cubic acidophilic inclusions in the nuclei of hepatocytes (and renal tubular cells) have been frequently seen in the beagle and other dogs (as well as wolves, foxes, and jackals) (Thompson et al., 1958a, b; Richter et al., 1965). These structures are commonly referred to as acidophilic intranuclear inclusions (ACN). They appear to be protein in nature. Their significance and origin remain obscure.

Hepatocytes of beagles also contain acidophilic, globular intracytoplasmic inclusions of equally obscure origin and significance (Murti and Borgmann, 1965; Holmes and Smith, 1969; Harleman et al., 1987). These structures are commonly referred to as periodic acid–Schiff (PAS) positive, nonglycogenic intracytoplasmic inclusions. Studies indicate they consist of proteinaceous material and bound lipids. Small brown pigment granules may be seen in both hepatocytes and Kupffer cells. In the absence of biliary stasis, the pigment is usually lipofuscin or hemosiderin or both. Lipofuscin ("wear-and-tear" pigment) is PAS- and oil red 0–positive. Hemosiderin is iron-positive. Individual hepatocytes and Kuppfer cells may contain both pigments. Glucose is normally stored within hepatocytes as glycogen. Large amounts of glycogen are expected after a meal; however, surprising degrees of cytoplasmic vacuolation due to glycogen may be seen in dogs fasted overnight.

Gallbladder

The early stages of cystic mucinous hyperplasia may be seen. Individual lymphoid follicles may be prominent. Fine brown or black crystalline gallstones were reported by Maita et al. (1977).

Pancreas

Hottendorf and Hirth (1974) report chronic focal pancreatitis. Maita et al. (1977) and Barron and Saunders (1966) report *Toxocara* granuloma. Oghiso et al. (1982) report alternative changes in acinar and islet cells (without elaboration), edema, and cellular infiltration. Ovoid, acidophilic intracytoplasmic inclusions (often containing basophilic particles and surrounded by halos) may be seen in acinar cells of the pancreas. Hartman et al. (1975) have shown the inclusions to consist of whirls of rough endoplasmic reticulum, vacuoles, and cytoplasmic organelles in various stages of decomposition and to be similar to dense ribosomal autophagic vacuoles.

RESPIRATORY SYSTEM

Anatomy and Histology

The respiratory system comprises the nasal cavity, paranasal sinuses, nasopharynx, larynx, trachea, and lungs. The principal function of the respiratory system is the exchange of gases (oxygen and carbon dioxide). Other functions include the warming, humidifying, and cleansing of incoming air; regulating airflow; olfaction; phonation; and temperature control of the whole organism (Dellman, 1976a). Important immunological and metabolic functions are also attributed to the respiratory system (Yates, 1988).

Nasal Cavity

The nasal cavity is the facial portion of the respiratory system, and is also known as the internal nose (Miller et al., 1967). The part of the head known as the nose consists of an internal nose (a mucosa-lined cavity) and an external nose comprising bones (incisive, maxillae, nasal) and movable cartilages (nasal cartilages). The bones give rise to an elaborate system of bony scrolls (turbinates) that are covered by mucous membranes of the nasal cavity. The nasal cartilages surround the nostrils and nasal vestibule and direct the flow of air into the various passages (meatuses) among the scrolls. On inspiration, air enters the nasal cavity through paired nostrils (nares, singular: naris) and is drawn over four types of epithelium (stratified squamous, transitional, respiratory, olfactory) (Adams and Hotchkiss, 1983) before it leaves via the paired choanae (internal nares) to enter the nasopharynx. The rostral (anterior) 20–35% of the nasal cavity is lined by thick stratified squamous epithelium. Transitional epithelium lines the next 15–20%. Ciliated pseudostratified columnar (respiratory) epithelium lines the next 40–50%, and olfactory epithelium lines the remainder of the cavity. The area lined by respiratory epithelium is the most vascular of the four regions. Nasal glands, scattered throughout the nasal mucosa, are present in greatest density in the olfactory region. Plasma cells are most abundant rostrally. Lymphocytes are present throughout the nasal mucosa, but frequently occur as nodular masses in the caudal portion, forming grossly visible nodules near the choanae (Adams and Hotchkiss, 1983).

The nasal and oral pharynges have been described with the digestive system.

Larynx

The laryngeal ostium is guarded by a cartilaginous valve (epiglottis) that prevents inspiration of food and water and controls the volume of air entering the lower respiratory system.

Trachea

The trachea is a flexible tubular connection between the larynx and lungs. Its flexibility is derived from a skeleton of C-shaped hyaline cartilages connected longitudinally by fibroelastic tissue and closed dorsally by smooth muscle and connective tissue (Miller et al., 1967). The tracheal mucosa is covered by respiratory epithelium in which the population of individual cell types (ciliated, preciliated, basal, secretory) varies significantly anteriorly and posteriorly and even dorsally and ventrally (Schwartz, 1987). Ciliated cells account for the bulk of the tracheal mucosal cells and are responsible for moving secretions. Glands of the tracheal mucosa are predominantly serous with occasional mucous acini (Dellman, 1976a).

Bronchi and Bronchioles. The trachea terminates by the formation of the right and left principal bronchi. The principal bronchi divide into lobar bronchi (secondary bronchi) which are named according to the lobe supplied. Lobar bronchi divide into segmental bronchi and the branching continues until respiratory bronchioles are formed. As bronchi penetrate into the lungs they become embedded in a sheath of loose connective tissue, which contains lymphatics, nerves, bronchial vessels, and pulmonary arteries. Bronchi are kept patent by overlapping curved cartilages. When terminal bronchioles reach a diameter of 1 mm or less, cartilages are no longer found (Miller et al., 1967).

Bronchi/bronchioles are lined by respiratory epithelium containing three general categories of secretory cells: serous, mucous, and nonciliated secretory bronchiolar (NBE or Clara) cells (Schwartz, 1987). Clara cells are present mainly in the peripheral airways. Clara cells have been shown to be the site of cytochrome P-450–dependent mixed function oxidase activity in the lung (Gill, 1982). Tubuloacinar mucous or mixed glands are located in the submucosa. Characteristically, glandular elements (and goblet cells) decrease as the bronchi decrease in size. In general, all bronchioles lack cartilage, the columnar epithelium gradually becomes cuboidal epithelium, and goblet cells are gradually replaced by Clara cells.

Respiratory bronchioles give rise to alveolar ducts, alveolar sacs, and pulmonary alveoli. Alveoli are lined by three types of epithelium: type 1 alveolar epithelial cell (squamous pneumocyte), type 2 alveolar epithelial cell (secretory pneumocyte), and type 3 pneumocytes (brush cells) (Schwartz, 1987). Type 1 cells appear to line the alveolus and type 2 to produce pulmonary surfactant. The function of Type 3 cells is unknown. Intra-alveolar macrophages are also important components of alveoli.

There appear to be permanent lymphoid structures beneath the bronchial mucosa (localized infiltrations of the lamina propria with lymphocytes have long been recognized) that are comparable to those that constitute the gut-associated lymphatic tissue (GALT) of the intestine. The lymphoid structures in the lung have been called bronchus-associated lymphoid tissue or BALT (Gill, 1982).

Lungs

The lungs (right and left) are divided into lobes. Each lung as an apical (cranial), cardiac (middle), and diaphragmatic (caudal) lobe. The right lung also has an intermediate (accessory) lobe. The pulmonary pleura is thin and adheres tightly to the surfaces of the lung and follows all its irregularities. The pleura is covered by a pavement of flat mesothelial cells and contains elastic, collagenous, and smooth muscle fibers. The subserosa of the pleura contains a superficial lymph vessel system that drains the pleura through the interlobular septa to the hilus of the lung.

A deep lymph vessel system is oriented around the bronchial tree. It too drains toward the interlobular septa. Distended portions of the superficial lymphatic system may be prominent enough to be seen grossly; usually as clear, interconnecting, threadlike tubules. Pulmonary lymphatics drain into the right, middle, and left tracheobronchial lymph nodes. Smaller, bronchopulmonary lymph nodes are occasionally seen. When present, they lie on the surface of primary bronchi.

The lung (in common with the liver) has two blood supplies: bronchial arteries which provide oxygen for the conducting airways, and pulmonary arteries which deliver blood to the alveoli for oxygen-carbon dioxide exchange. Bronchial arteries form plexuses in the bronchial wall. Pulmonary arteries branch more frequently than the airways and eventually supply the most peripheral parts of the alveoli with blood via a capillary network. The origin and relationships of veins are not as well defined as the arteries.

Necropsy and Laboratory Techniques

Disease of the respiratory system produces a wide variety of clinical signs. Some of the signs may indicate pathology within a specific portion of the system, others are less specific. Pathology of the nasal cavity may be indicated by nasal discharge, snorting, sneezing, and nasal rubbing. Disease of the larynx and trachea may be indicated by dyspnea (difficulty or distress in breathing), stridor (high-pitched noisy respiration), gagging or retching (striving to vomit), and coughing. Coughing and dyspnea may also indicate problems in the lower respiratory tract, as does tachypnea (very rapid respiration) or hyperpnea (deep and rapid respiration). Rales (abnormal respiratory sounds heard on auscultation) may be detected. Many varieties of rales are described. Cyanosis (bluish discoloration of the skin and mucous membranes) may indicate problems in either the respiratory or cardiovascular system. Pulmonary cyanosis is the result of poor oxygenation of blood in the lungs.

Many special procedures have been used in the morphological study of the respiratory system, including airway and vascular perfusion with a variety of fixatives, formalin vapor fixation of the lungs, whole lung sections (macrosections), thick and thin histological sections, vascular injection with colored latex, silicone rubber casts of airways, in vivo rapid freezing of the lung, stereology, and, of course, scanning and transmission electron microscopy (Dungworth et al., 1976). The complexities of the respiratory system dictate that a variety of techniques are required for adequate evaluation of toxic effects in inhalation studies. However, the basic necropsy and fixation procedures that are essential for inhalation studies are also recommended for general toxicology studies. The procedures add neither cost nor time to the postmortem examination.

The critical step is perfusion of the lungs (or one or more lobes) with fixative either by the trachea or primary bronchus at a pressure that is adequate to inflate the lungs to approximately normal full expansion. After perfusion, the trachea (or bronchus) is closed (clamped or ligated) and the lung is fixed in the expanded state. Simply immersing pieces of collapsed lung in fixative is not acceptable except when the lungs are massively consolidated, edematous, or contain large solid tumors (Dungworth et al., 1976). Even in the presence of such lesions, it is usually worthwhile to attempt to fix a portion of the lung by airway perfusion. Airway perfusion should be done at 30 cm of fluid (water) pressure. (Ideally, the lungs should be supported in a bath of fixative while being perfused.) Airway perfusion not only restores normal dimensions and configurations to the lung, it also provides a large volume of fixative in intimate contact with all surfaces of respiratory tree. The disadvantages of airway perfusion are the dislocation of exudates and distension of the tissue spaces around pulmonary vessels (so-called edema artifact) (Dungworth et al., 1976). The edema artifact is dealt with during the microscopic interpretation. Immersion fixation of an additional affected portion of lung can compensate for the displacement of exudates by perfusion.

The lungs should be in view as the thoracic cavity is opened. The customary approach is to catch a glimpse of the distended lungs as the diaphragm is incised close to its sternal and costal attachments. Healthy lungs collapse as air enters the thorax. Failure of the lungs to collapse should be noted by the prosector. The thoracic cavity is opened preferably by cutting the ribs just dorsal to costochondral junctions to give adequate exposure of the thoracic contents. As noted earlier, all of the thoracic organs should be examined in situ and the tongue, larynx, trachea, lungs, heart, great vessels, and thymus removed in toto. The larynx and trachea are incised along their dorsal surface (with the prosector being alert to unusual content) to the bifurcation of the trachea. The lumina of the primary and lobar bronchi are inspected. The extent to which major airways need to be opened depends upon the type and amount of gross pathology. At least two lobes of the lung should be left intact for intrabronchial perfusion. A compromise must be made between thoroughness and practicality in deciding upon the number of lobes to perfuse and the number of blocks to take from each lobe for microscopic examination. Perfusion of two lobes (one a cranial lobe, the other a caudal lobe) seems to be reasonable for general toxicology studies. After fixation, samples (blocks) should be taken from the dorsal (hilar) and ventral (peripheral) aspects of each lobe.

The trachea is usually represented by a segment taken from the midsection. If the nasal cavity needs to be examined at necropsy, it may be split sagittally. If specimens are required, one or both halves of the nasal cavity may be fixed and tissue blocks removed after decalcification. Nasal passages should be gently flushed with fixative to remove air and any material that would prevent intimate contact between the nasal epithelium and the fixative. The frontal sinus should be opened as a routine matter when the calvarium is removed to expose the brain.

Pathology

Most pathology of the respiratory system involves the lungs. Hottendorf and Hirth (1974) report perivasculitis, peribronchiolitis, subpleural fibrosis, endobronchiolitis, focal interstitial pneumonia, granuloma, vascular microgranuloma, and cholesterinic granuloma. They also report chronic tracheitis. Most of the pulmonary pathology was thought to be due to infection by a lung worm *(Filaroides hirthi)*. The vascular microgranulomas were attributed to emboli from intravenous injection sites. Pick and Eubanks (1965) report anthracosis, bronchopneumonia, granulomatous pneumonitis, pleuritis, pulmonary granuloma, pulmonary hyperemia, pulmonary helminthiasis, and pulmonary hemorrhage. Fibrous thickening of alveolar walls, atelectasis, and granulomatous nodules were reported by Oghiso et al. (1982). Glaister (1986) reports the following changes in the lung: leukocytic foci, bronchitis/bronchiolitis, pneumonitis, fibrosing alveolitis, granuloma, and nematodes. Barron and Saunders (1966) and Maita et al. (1977) report *Toxocara* granuloma in the lungs.

Pneumonia due to *F. hirthi* infection is probably the most common nontreatment-related respiratory pathology seen in the laboratory beagle. The true incidence of the disease in laboratory dogs (and the canine population at large) is unknown. Clinical signs of infection are rare. The diagnosis can usually be made at necropsy based on the finding of tan, green or gray subpleural nodules ranging from 1 to 5 mm (and larger) in diameter. A granulomatous response is evoked by dead or degenerating worms. Focal granulomatous interstitial pneumonitis is often seen when remnants of the parasite can no longer be identified. *F. hirthi* has a direct life cycle with infective first-stage larvae in the feces. Most pups are probably infected by their dams (Dungworth, 1985). Hirth and Hottendorf (1973) first reported the pathological changes associated with *F. hirthi* infection in the laboratory beagle. The parasite has been further characterized in subsequent articles (Georgi and Anderson, 1975; Georgi et al., 1975). Microscopists should not automatically conclude that all pulmonary granulomas are due to lungworm infection; some may be due to foreign body emboli from intravenous injection sites and others from *Toxacara canis* infection.

The anthracosis and bronchopneumonia reported by Pick and Eubanks are unusual, since most laboratory beagles are not exposed to dusty environments and are immune to canine distemper virus and its sequelae. Recently, bronchopneumonia apparently due to *Mycoplasma* spp. was reported in four laboratory beagles (Kirchner et al., 1990).

CARDIOVASCULAR SYSTEM

Anatomy and Histology

The cardiovascular system is a closed system of tubes (blood vessels) containing a liquid tissue (blood) that is circulated by a four-chambered, double pump (heart). Blood is a complex tissue that serves several functions, including respiratory (transport of oxygen from the air in the lungs to the tissues and carbon dioxide in the tissues to the lungs), nutritive (conveys food materials from the digestive tract to the tissues), excretory (transports waste products from tissues to organs of excretion), homeostasis (maintains a dynamic equilibrium of water, pH and electrolyte concentration), regulation of body temperature (functions in heat transport), chemical communication and protection (circulates hormones and antibodies) (Cronkite, 1973).

Blood Vessels

The blood vessels comprise an enormous network of tubes (vascular system) that serve as a distributing system (arteries), a diffusion and filtration system (microcirculation), and a collecting system (veins).

Arteries. The first arteries in the distributing system are elastic arteries (aorta, pulmonary artery, brachiocephalic trunk, etc.), which merge with muscular arteries that conduct blood to various organs and regions of the body. Elastic arteries have a high content of elastic fibers and are characterized by large lumina and relatively thin walls. Most arteries in the body are muscular arteries, named because of their abundant smooth muscle content. Muscular arteries have smaller lumina and thicker walls than elastic arteries. In most muscular arteries, the wall thickness represents one-fourth of the vessel diameter (Simionescu and Simionescu, 1977).

Microvasculature. The arterial circulation connects with the venous circulation by way of the microvasculature. The microvasculature consists of the arterioles, capillaries, and venules. Arterioles are the smallest arteries in which the media is reduced to a layer of one or two smooth muscle cells. Arteriole lumina are small (less than 300 μm), but the arteriole wall is relatively thick (about one-half the diameter of the vessel).

Capillaries. The term *capillary* is restricted to minute vessels that consist only of endothelium, basal lamina, and a few pericytes (Simionescu and Simionescu, 1977). The inner diameter of blood capillaries ranges from 5 to 10 μm. Three principal types of blood capillaries have been described: continuous capillaries, fenestrated capillaries, and discontinuous capillaries (sinusoids). Continous capillaries are characterized by a continuous endothelium and found in skeletal, cardiac, and smooth muscle; connective tissue; central nervous system; exocrine pancreas, and gonads.

Fenestrated capillaries have transcapillary openings (fenestrae) approximately 600–800 Å in diameter. Fenestrated capillaries are found in the mucosa of the gastrointestinal tract, endocrine glands, renal glomerular and peritubular capillaries, choroid plexus, and ciliary body.

Discontinuous capillaries are thin-walled vessels with large gaps (up to thousands of angstroms in diameter) in the endothelium and basal lamina. Discontinuous capillaries are found in the liver, spleen, and bone marrow.

Venules. These are similar to capillaires but are larger. The immediate postcapillary venules are characterized by the presence of pericytes (pericytic venules). Pericytic venules are drained by venules of increasing diameter whose media contain one or two thin layers of smooth muscle cells (muscular venules) (Simionescu and Simionescu, 1977).

Veins. From venules, the blood is collected in veins increasing in size, eventually becoming large veins such as the venae cavae and pulmonary vein. Blood vessels have three basic tunics: intima, media, and adventitia. The intima comprises (at most) the endothelium, basal lamina, subendothelial connective tissue, and the internal elastic lamina. The media is composed of muscular cells, elastic lamellae, and the external elastic lamina. The adventitia contains connective tissue and fine collagen and elastic fibers. As indicated above, the proportions and composition of the tunics vary with types of blood vessels.

Heart

The heart is basically a three-tunic segment of the vascular system with the middle layer (media) greatly developed. The outer tunic (adventitia) is called the epicardium. The media is termed the myocardium and the inner tunic (intima) the endocardium. The myocardium forms most of the mass of the heart. The heart is formed of four chambers: two atria and two ventricles.

Atria. The atria are the thin-walled, low pressure chambers of the heart. The right atrium receives blood from the systemic circulation and contains openings for the coronary vein, posterior vena cava, anterior vena cava, and the azygos vein. The right atrium opens into the right ventricle through the right atrioventricular orifice. The left atrium receives blood from the pulmonary circulation and contains several openings for the pulmonary veins. The left atrium opens into the left ventricle through the left atrioventricular orifice. The atria are sometimes incorrectly referred to as the auricles. The auricle (L. little ear) is the blind-ending, forward-directed outpouching from each atrium.

Atrioventricular Valves. The atrioventricular valves are intake valves to the ventricles. The right atrioventricular valve (known as the tricuspid valve in humans) consists basically of two cusps in the dog (Miller et al., 1967). The cusp adjacent to the interventricular septum is the septal, or dorsal, cusp. The cusp adjacent to the outer wall is the lateral, or ventral, cusp. The left atrioventricular valve (mitral valve in humans) is basically bicuspid in the dog also, but the subdivisions are indistinct. The cusp adjacent to the interventricular septum is the dorsal cusp. The cusp adjacent to the ventricular wall is the ventral cusp.

Ventricles. The right ventricle pumps systemic blood to the lungs by way of the pulmonary orifice. The left ventricle pumps oxygenated blood to the systemic circulation by way of the aortic orifice. The valves guarding the pulmonary and aortic orifices are similar, with each consisting of three semilunar cusps.

Both ventricles contain muscular projections known as papillary muscles. Papillary muscles are larger in the left ventricle. Thin fibromuscular cords (chordae tendinae) arise from the apices of the papillary muscles and attach to the atrioventricular valves. The chordae tendinae keep the atrioventricular valves from being pushed into the atria during contraction of the ventricles. The ventral portion of the thick wall of the left ventricle forms the apex of the heart.

The base of the heart is the dorsal portion where atria and ventricles join and valves are inserted into narrow fibrous rings.

Functionally, there are two general types of myocardial cells: muscle cells and impulse-formation and conduction cells. The cardiac muscle cells have been described with the musculoskeletal system. The impulse-formation and conduction cells form the sinoatrial node, atrioventricular node, and atrioventricular bundle.

Sinoatrial Node.   In the dog, the sinoatrial node is located in the right atrium in the terminal crest at the confluence of the anterior vena cava, sinus venarum cavarum, and auricular orifice (Miller et al., 1967).

Atrioventricular Node.   This node is also located in the right atrium, about 5 mm cranioventral to the opening of the coronary sinus and craniodorsal to the septal cusp of the right atrioventricular valve.

Atrioventricular Bundle.   This bundle runs forward and downward from the atrioventricular node. The bundle divides into right and left branches, which lie closely under the endocardium of the septal wall of the right and left ventricles. In the dog, the Purkinje fibers of atrioventricular bundle are readily identified by their large diameter, centrally located large spherical nucleus and scarce myofibrils (Dellman and Venable, 1976).

Pericardium.   The heart is enclosed in a fibroserous envelope (pericardium, heart sac). The pericardium is divided into an outer fibrous part and an inner serous part. The serous pericardium in turn is divided into two parts or layers. The visceral layer is the epicardium and is attached firmly to the heart except in the region of coronary grooves. The parietal layer is fused with the fibrous pericardium. The pericardial cavity is located between the two layers of the serous pericardium and typically contains a small quantity of clear, light yellow fluid (pericardial fluid). The fibrous pericardium forms the strong outer part of the heart sac.

Lymphatic Circulatory System

There is also a lymphatic circulatory system which is made up of a network of channels which originate in connective tissue spaces as anastomosing capillaries. Although called a circulatory system, the lymph flows in just one direction, toward the thorax. In the dog, the thoracic duct is the chief return channel for lymph. The thoracic duct generally joins the venous circulation near the junction of the left jugular vein with the anterior vena cava (Miller et al., 1967).

Necropsy and Laboratory Techniques

Clinical signs of cardiovascular disease include weakness, fatigue, syncope (fainting), reluctance to lie, cyanosis, ascites, subcutaneous edema, venous distension, dyspnea, polydipsia, abnormal pulse, and a wide range of abnormal auscultory sounds.

The initial examination of the heart and major vessels (pulmonary trunk, aorta, brachiocephalic trunk, left subclavian artery, and anterior and posterior venae cavae) is made with the thoracic organs in place. Abnormal location, size, shape, and proportion are looked for. The initial examination of the pericardial sac is also done in situ. The sac is grasped near the apex of the heart and a small incision made to access the volume and character of the pericardial fluid. If indicated, a sample of the contents may be taken at this time. The sac is then fully opened and both of its surfaces examined. The thoracic organs are removed. The aorta and posterior venae cavae are severed at the diaphragm. The remaining major vessels (or branches of them) are severed at the chest wall or thoracic inlet. In separating the heart from the lungs, the pulmonary veins are cut at the left atrium and the pulmonary trunk left attached to the heart. The pericardial sac is removed.

A routine should be followed in opening the heart. One that is easily mastered is to follow the flow of blood through the heart, beginning with the right atrium. The posterior vena cava is opened. The incision is continued into the wall of the right atrium just dorsal and parallel to the coronary groove and into the right auricle. The anterior vena cava is not incised to avoid disturbing the sinoatrial node. The right ventricle is opened by cutting along the junction of the right ventricular free wall and ventricular septum. The incision begins caudally at the right atrioventricular orifice and proceeds to the apex, conus arteriosus, and through the pulmonary orifice and pulmonary trunk. Most papillary muscles of the right ventricle arise from the apical portion of the interventricular septum. With care, the incision separating the wall from the septum will leave the papillary muscles attached to the septum.

The left atrium is opened through one of the pulmonary veins. The free atrial wall is cut just dorsal and parallel to the coronary groove with the cut continuing into the left auricle. An incision is then made caudally through the left atrioventricular orifice continuing between the posterior papillary muscle of the left ventricle and the ventricular septum. The incision is extended to the apex and into the anterior wall. Scissors are then inserted through the aortic outflow tract and an incision is made through the aortic orifice, wall of the aortic arch, and the aorta.

The brachiocephalic trunk and left subclavian arteries should also be opened. All chambers, surfaces, and valves of the heart are now exposed for detailed examination. It is suggested that the gross examination also be systematic, following the flow of blood through the heart.

The heart is usually weighed in toxicology studies. Heart weight is essentially a measure of the mass of the myocardium; therefore, as much of the nonmyocardial tissue as possible should be removed. The pericardial sac has been removed. The pulmonary trunk and aortic arch are severed just distal to their respective valves. Any great length of anterior or posterior vena cava should be removed. Fat within the coronary grooves accounts for a small fraction of heart weight and need not be removed; and, of course, the heart valves are left intact. If extracardiac tissues are removed in a consistent manner, the resulting heart weights should be representative. If the heart is opened in the manner described, it is easily subdivided into various components: right ventricular wall, left ventricular wall, interventricular septum, atrial walls, and interatrial septum. Weighing individual components was useful in documenting the cardiac hypertrophy of cor pulmonale in beagle pups (Brewster et al., 1983).

The prosector should be alert to lesions in the larger systemic vessels during the course of the postmortem examination. The abdominal aorta and external iliac entries should be examined in situ after the abdominal and pelvic viscera are removed.

Selection of tissues for histological study should be as standardized as the gross examination. A complete histological examination would include samples of the conducting system, each valvular region, walls, and septa of the atria and ventricles, and segments from the pulmonary trunk, and and thoracic and abdominal aortae. The entire heart of the average beagle may be fixed after the right and left ventricular walls are removed and subdivided into two or three segments. The atrial and ventricular septa should be subdivided by vertical cuts that leave the sinoatrial and atrioventricular nodes intact.

Pathology

A variety of gross and histological changes have been reported for the cardiovascular system of laboratory beagles. Hottendorf and Hirth (1974) report chronic valvular fibrosis, valvular telangiectasis, pulmonic stenosis, patent ductus arteriosus, myocarditis, focal myocardial fibrosis and calcification, granuloma, chronic focal pericarditis, focal medial degeneration of the aorta, and periarteritis of the coronary artery. Pick and Eubanks (1965) report myocardial fat infiltration. Glaister (1986) reports leukocytic foci in the myocardium, telangiectasis of atrioventricular valves, arteritis, and mineralization of the aorta. Barron and Saunders (1966) report *Toxocara* granuloma of the myocardium.

Valvular endocardiosis is probably the most frequently observed incidental finding in the heart. Endocardiosis chiefly affects the septal cusp of the right atrioventricular valve in young beagles. The cusp appears to be diffusely or irregularly swollen, soft, and glistening. The septal cusp of the right atrioventricular valve is also the most common site for valvular telangiectasis (hematocyst, congential hematoma). The lesion usually appears as a dark red cyst, 1–5 mm in diameter, that protrudes from the atrial surface of the cusp. Valvular telangiectasis appears to be a congenital malformation (Hubben et al., 1963). Neither the cysts nor the valvular endocardiosis appear to be of any functional significance.

Apparent degenerative changes within the myocardium must be interpreted with caution for, as with skeletal muscle, many artifacts may result from handling and from contraction of myofibrils during fixation, Muscular arteries may also undergo postmortem contraction and appear to be unusually thick walled. The contracted arteries are usually devoid of blood and their internal elastic lamina has a scalloped appearance in cross-section. Postmortem imbibition of hemoglobin produces a diffuse red staining of the intima of both the heart and blood vessels that simulates hemorrhage.

HEMOPOIETIC SYSTEM

Anatomy and Histology

The hemopoietic system consists of the blood, bone marrow, and lymphoreticular tissues. Blood is a liquid tissue comprised of a fluid portion (plasma), red cells (erythron), white cells (leukon), and platelets (thrombon) (Payne et al., 1976).

Erythron

The erythron consists of the erythrocytes and their precursors. The primary function of the erythrocyte is to mediate the exchange of oxygen and carbon dioxide. In the adult dog, red cell production (erythropoiesis) occurs predominantly in the bone marrow; however, other organs (spleen, liver, lymph nodes, adrenals, kidneys) retain the potential to produce erythrocytes (extramedullary hematopoiesis) in adult life (Valli, 1985). The average erythrocyte life span for the dog is 110 days (Duncan and Prasse, 1986).

Leukon

The leukon consists of granulocytes (neutrophils, eosinophils, basophils), monocytes, and lymphocytes. In the adult dog, virtually all granulocytes are produced in the bone marrow.

Granulocytes

Neutrophils.   Neutrophils are the most abundant of the circulating white blood cells (60–77% in the dog) (Duncan and Prasse, 1986). After a brief period of circulation, neutrophils migrate to tissues and remain there. Blood neutrophils are replaced about 2.5 times a day. The major function of neutrophils is to phagocytize and kill microbes.

Eosinophils: Like neutrophils, eosinophils are mobile phagocytes with antimicrobial properties, but they are not protective against bacterial infection. Two to 10% of the circulating white blood cells are eosinophils. Eosinophils are more numerous in tissues than in blood.

Basophils.   These are weakly motile phagocytes. Basophils and mast cells (related functionally but not by origin) contain mediators of inflammation, including histamine, heparin, eosinophil chemotactic factor of anaphylaxis, platelet activating factor and, other substances (Prasse, 1983). Basophils are rarely seen in the circulating blood.

Monocytes.   Produced in the bone marrow, monocytes migrate into the blood and quickly enter into tissues (lung, liver, spleen, bone marrow, pleura, peritoneum, lymph nodes) to become tissue macrophages (Valli, 1985). They are the Kupffer cells of the liver and the osteoclasts of the bone. Monocytes represent 3–10% of circulating white blood cells. The activities of the monocyte-macrophage system include phagocytosis, myeloproliferative control, antigen processing, and production of various cytokines.

Lymphocytes.   In early embryonic life, lymphoid precursors from the yolk sac colonize the bone marrow and thymus (primary lymphopoietic organs). Progeny from the primary lymphopoietic organs in turn populate lymph nodes, spleen, tonsils, gut, and lung (secondary lymphopoietic organs). The bone marrow is the larger and more active primary lymphopoietic organ. The fate of most bone marrow lymphocytes is unknown (Wintrobe et al., 1981), but some enter the circulation and migrate to the secondary lymphopoietic organs to become the source of antibody-producing cells (B lymphocytes, bone marrow–derived cells). Most thymic lymphocytes experience an intrathymic death, but some enter the blood and seed out in the thymus-dependent areas of secondary lymphopoietic organs, where they become progentors of cells involved in cell-mediated immunity (T lymphocytes, thymus-derived cells). Compared to other leukocytes, lymphocytes are long lived (weeks to years). They also are unique because they recirculate (Duncan and Prasse, 1986). The majority of permanently circulating lymphocytes are T cells. The majority of B cells remain in the lymphoid tissue. Lymphocytes comprise 12–30% of the circulating white blood cells.

Thrombon

The thrombon consists of the circulating blood platelets and the megakaryocytes and megakaryoblasts of the bone marrow (Payne et al., 1976).

Blood Platelets.   Extramedullary megakaryopoiesis does occur and is most common in the lung, but is also seen in the spleen, liver, kidney, and heart (Green, 1983). The normal blood platelet count in the dog is $2–9 \times 10^5/\mu l$ (Duncan and Prasse, 1986). The platelet number can be affected by splenic contraction (increases number of platelets) and congestion (decreases number). The circulating life span of platelets is approximately 10 days. The platelets' central role is in hemostasis. The major platelet reactions are adhesion to damaged endothelium, release of biochemical substances, causing vasoconstriction, and further platelet aggregation (Green, 1983).

Bone Marrow.   Bone marrow maintains an embryonic function throughout adult life. Bone marrow may be red (due to the hemoglobin contact of erythrocytes and their precursors) or yellow (due to fat cells). The bone marrow has two compartments: vascular and hematopoietic. The vascular compartment is supplied by nutrient arteries that divide and gradually narrow to capillaries and then open to large sinuses lined by discontinuous endothelium. The marrow lying between the sinuses is the hematopoietic compartment. The hematopoietic compartment of red marrow contains mostly hematopoietic cells and a few fat cells. Fat cells predominate in the hematopoietic compartment in yellow marrow.

Lymphoreticular Tissues

Lymphoreticular tissues include the thymus, spleen, lymph nodes, and lymphoid tissues of the digestive and respiratory systems.

Thymus.   This is a light gray, multilobulated organ that lies in the cranial ventral part of the thoracic cavity almost entirely covered by the precardial mediastinum. At birth, the thymus is large and continues to grow during the first 3 months of postnatal life in the beagle (Andersen and Goldman, 1970). Thereafter, the thymus involutes rapidly but never completely disappears (Miller et al., 1967).

The thymus is a composite of epithelial and lymphoid tissues. Each thymic lobule is comprised of a cortex that contains many lymphocytes (or cells that give rise to lympho- cytes) and a medulla that contains epithelial and myoid cells (Valli, 1985). The epithelial cells of the thymus provide a unique environment essential for T-lymphocyte develop- ment. Various subsets of T cells are formed that are released and undergo final maturation in the spleen or other secondary lymphoid organs. The medullary epithelial cells form morphologically distinct clusters of cells (thymic corpuscles, Hassall's corpuscles) whose function is unknown.

Lymph Nodes.   Lymph nodes are the most organized of the lymphatic organs. External lymph nodes are found in the protective environment of small fat pads. Internal nodes are found in the mediastinum, mesentery, near the angles of many larger vessels, and the hilus of organs. Lymph nodes are usually named according to their location. The capsules of lymph nodes are perforated at various points by afferent lymphatics that empty into subcapsular sinuses. Branches of the sinuses (medullary sinuses) extend into the node and terminate at the hilus, where the efferent lymphatics emerge. Lymph percolates into and out of the parenchyma through gaps in the sinus walls. The cortex is made up of lymphoid nodules (primary nodules) whose size and morphology vary greatly. The primary follicles represent B-cell areas. Upon antigenic stimulation, the primary follicles enlarge and develop pale-staining germinal centers. B-cell progeny leave the germinal centers to either migrate to medullary cords where they become plasma cells or enter the blood lymphocyte pool (Valli, 1985). The paracortex (outer cortical area not occupied by germinal centers) is largely occupied by T cells. Medullary cords are papillary like extensions of the paracortical cells toward the hilus of the node.

Spleen

The spleens of domestic animals vary in their blood-storage capacity and the relative amount of smooth muscle found in the capusle and trabeculae. The canine spleen has abundant venous sinuses capable of storing large amounts of blood and abundant smooth muscle in the capsule capable of considerable contraction (Brown and Dellmann, 1976). Splenic parenchyma is called pulp, most of which is red (red pulp) due to the presence of blood. The red pulp is almost entirely made up of splenic sinuses and thin plates of cells (splenic cords) lying between the sinuses. Scattered throughout the red pulp are lymphoid nodules (splenic nodules) and lymphoid perarterial sheaths. The lymphoid nodules and sheaths constitute the white pulp. The lymphoid nodules represent concentrations of B lymphocytes; the sheaths are predominantly T lymphocytes. The spleen has no afferent lymph supply, consequently all antigen reaches the spleen with the blood. The spleen filters unwanted elements from the blood (aged and damagaged erythrocytes, particulate matter), is a major secondary lymphoreticular organ, a secondary source of hematopoiesis, and a reserve pool of erythrocytes and platelets (Contran et al., 1989).

Necropsy and Laboratory Techniques

Anemia is defined as an absolute decrease in the packed cell volume, hemoglobin concentration, and red blood cell count (Duncan and Prasse, 1986). The clinical signs of anemia include pale mucous membranes, weakness, loss of stamina, dyspnea on exertion, tachycardia, and heart murmur. Icterus, hemoglobinuria, hemorrhage, and fever may also be seen depending upon the pathogenesis of the anemia. Enlarged superficial lymph nodes may indicate disease in the region being drained: parotid, mandibular, medial retropharyngeal lymph nodes (head and neck); superficial cervical lymph nodes (head, neck, thoracic limb, thoracic wall); axillary nodes (thoracic limb, thoracic wall, cranial and middle mammary glands); superficial inguinal nodes (abdominal wall, caudal mammary glands, penis, scrotum, entire pelvic limb); and popliteal (distal pelvic limb) (Miller et al., 1967).

Bone marrow specimens (for histology and cytology) should be obtained as soon after death as possible (second in priority only to the eyes). Specimens may be easily gotten from the sternum. For histology, one or two sternebrae may be cut longitudinally with a stout sharp knife. Segments are placed in fixative. One segment may be reserved for archival storage and the other decalcified and processed for paraffin embedding. Smears for marrow cytology and cell counting may be gotten from another sternebra. After removal of muscle, fat, and an intersternabral cartilage, pressure is applied by a sturdy pair of pliers to force marrow to the cut surface, where it is removed by means of a tapered artist's brush (moistened in fetal bovine calf serum) and applied in streaks upon a glass slide. The specimen is air dried.

The prosector should be alert to abnormalities in individual lymph nodes during the course of the general postmortem examination. Specimens of both external and internal lymph nodes are usually taken for microscopic examination. Commonly, these are a medial retropharyngeal lymph node (the largest node in the head and neck, readily identified and easily removed) and a mesenteric lymph node. The anterior pole of the medial retropharyngeal lymph node may be discolored (tattoo ink from the ear). Mesenteric lymph nodes are often reddened (congested). Lymph nodes should be handled carefully to minimize artifacts. Searcy (1988) recommends that lymph nodes be fixed for about 1 hr prior to slicing (lymph nodes cut in the fresh state bulge through the capsule). Touch imprints may be prepared from the cut surface of one pole before the node is placed in fixative.

The size of the thymus varies considerably in short-term toxicology studies. The thymic involution begun prior to sexual maturity (Andersen and Goldman, 1970) may be enhanced by the direct or indirect effect (malnutrition) of test compounds.

Congestion of the spleen is common at necropsy, and it especially follows euthanasia with barbiturates. Several parallel slices should be made through the spleen to examine the pulp. One or two narrow slices should be placed in fixative.

Pathology

A variety of incidental changes have been reported for the hemopoietic system of laboratory beagles. Hottendorf and Hirth (1974) report siderofibrotic nodules and hematoma for the spleen, accessory spleen, and granuloma in the mesenteric lymph node. They observed, but did not report as lesions, congestion of the mesenteric lymph nodes and mild hyperplasia of lymph follicles in the pylorus, small intestine, cecum, and gallbladder. Oghiso et al. (1982) report lymphoid hyperplasia and reticulosis in the spleen and lymphoid hyperplasia and plasmacytosis in the lymph nodes. Pick and Eubanks (1965) report splenic extramedullary hematopoiesis, fibrosis, hemorrhage, hemosiderosis, and hyperemia. Maita et al. (1977) report *Toxocara* granuloma in the spleen and lymph nodes and small Gandy-Gamna–like bodies in the splenic capsule. Glaister (1986) reports granuloma in the mesenteric lymph node, ectopic thyroid, cyst in the thymus, and telangiectasis of the spleen. Barron and Saunders (1966) report *Toxocara* granuloma in lymph nodes. Fritz et al. (1966) report lymphosarcoma in the spleen and lymph nodes of beagles under 1 year of age.

Gandy-Gamna bodies (an eponym from medical pathology) refers to firm, nodular discolorations seen on or within the spleen. In veterinary pathology, the lesions are commonly referred to as siderofibrotic nodules (Ishmael and Howell, 1967). In the dog, they may appear as small, irregular slightly raised nodules on the capsular surface to extensive irregular encrustations covering large areas of the capsule and as nodules within the pulp. The color of the nodules varies from yellow to grayish brown. The nodules are seen most frequently on the margins of the spleen with concentrations at the extremities and also on the visceral surface with concentrations at the attachment of the gastrosplenic omentum. Microscopically, the nodules are fibrotic foci that are commonly calcified and contain brown pigment (hemosiderin) and bright yellow pigment (hematoidin, bilirubin). Siderofibrotic nodules are probably the end result of hemorrhage or marginal telangiectasis, as noted by Glaister.

One or more masses of splenic tissue may be found in the gastrosplenic omentum in addition to the spleen itself. These are known as accessory spleens. They may be congenital, but apparently many are acquired through traumatic rupture of the spleen (Valli, 1985).

ENDOCRINE SYSTEM

Anatomy and Histology

Two systems have major coordinating responsibilities in the body. One is the nervous system, and the other is the endocrine system. Glands of the endocrine system communicate principally by way of the blood through which raw materials and special releasing and inhibiting factors (hormones) are received and into which the glands' own secretions (hormones) are discharged. Glands that are universally recognized as endocrine glands are the hypophysis (pituitary gland), thyroid, parathyroids, adrenals, pancreas (pancreatic islets, endocrine pancreas), testes, and ovaries. The endocrine function of other organs such as the pineal body, thymus, kidney, and gastrointestinal tract, are beyond the scope of this chapter.

Hypophysis

The hypophysis is structurally and functionally a part of a complex hypothalamohypophyseal system (Dellman, 1976b). Traditionally, only two divisions of this system (adenohypophysis and neurohypophysis) are included in a discussion of the hypophysis. The adenohypophysis consists of the pars tuberalis, pars intermedia (intermediate lobe), and pars distalis (anterior lobe). The neurohypophysis consists of the pars nervosa (posterior lobe) and the infundibulum.

The hypophysis has a dual embryological origin. The adenohypophysis arises as an upward evagination of the oropharyngeal ectoderm (the lining of the future oral cavity, Rathke's pouch). The neurohypophysis is a downward evagination of the brain (diencephalon).

The hypophysis of the dog is a slightly flattened ovoid body lying in a shallow concavity of the basisphenoid bone and attached to the base of the brain by a short hollow stalk (infundibulum). The hypophysis is partly surrounded by bone (sella turcica), which is prominent caudally as a well-developed ridge with two prominent lateral projections (dorsum sellae and clinoid processes). The dura mater (outer tough membrane of the meninges) is intimately associated with both the hypophysis and the sella turcica. The close association of gland, bone, and dura mater makes it difficult to remove the hypophysis without producing artifacts. In the dog, the adenohypophysis surrounds the neurohypophysis. Dorsally, the pars tuberalis surrounds the infundibulum and more ventrally, the pars distalis and pars intermedia surround the pars nervosa. The pars distalis is by far the largest part of the hypophysis.

The adenohypophysis produces a number of hormones: growth hormone (GH, somatotropin), luteotropic hormone (LTH, prolactin), luteinizing hormone (LH), follicle-stimulating hormone (FSH), thyrotropic hormone (TSH), adrenocorticotropic hormone (ACTH), and melanocyte-stimulating hormone (MSH). Hormones produced elsewhere in the neurohypophysis but released into the bloodstream in the pars nervosa include antidiuretic hormone (ADH, vasopressin) and oxytocin (Capen, 1985).

Thyroid

The thyroid is a single gland consisting of two lobes that lie lateral to the first five to eight carilaginous rings of the trachea (Miller et al., 1967). Occasionally, a glandular isthmus is found on the ventral surface of the trachea connecting the ventral poles of the two lobes. The thyroid is fairly loosely attached to the trachea. The size and shape of the lobes are not always identical.

The thyroid arises from pharyngeal epithelium in close association with the aortic sac (a relationship that accounts for deposits of thyroid parenchyma anywhere from the larynx to the diaphragm). The bud of thyroid epithelium expands and the attachment to the pharynx is narrowed to a slender stalk. A vestige of this stalk may persist on the midline as the thyroglossal duct. The thyroid expands laterally and fuses with the ultimobranchial bodies which arise from the fourth branchial pouch. The inclusion of parafollicular cells in the thyroid is the result of this fusion. Parafollicular cells (calcitonin-secreting cells, C cells) are of neural crest origin and migrate to the ultimobranchial body and from there to the thyroid.

The thyroid is unique among endocrine glands because the final assemblage of hormone occurs outside the cell, within the lumen of the thyroid follicle (Capen, 1985). The manufacture and release of thyroid hormones, therefore, has an exocrine phase (synthesis and secretion of the protein, thyroglobulin, into the follicular lumen) and an endocrine phase (absorption of colloid from the lumen, release of hormones from the thyroglobulin molecule, and secretion of the hormones into the blood stream). The thyroid hormones are triiodothyronine (T_3) and thyroxine (T_4).

Parathyroid Glands

The parathyroid glands are paired and usually four in number. The parathyroids are entodermal in origin and derived from the third and fourth pharyngeal pouches (Miller et al., 1967). Parathyroid III (commonly referred to as the external parathyroid) is a flattened oval body, two to five mm long, and most commonly found in the connective tissue about the cranial pole of a thyroid lobe. Its location may vary, but it is always external to the capsule of the thyroid. Parathyroid IV (commonly referred to as the internal parathyroid) is generally smaller than the external parathyroid. The internal parathyroid is usually found beneath the capsule on the tracheal surface of a lobe, but it is also found deep within the thyroid.

Accessory parathyroids may be found within the thyroid, in the region of the larynx, the carotid sheath, anterior mediastinum, and within or associated with the thymus (Miller et al., 1967).

The parathyroid glands contain a single basic type of secretory cell which secretes parathyroid hormone (parathormone, PTH).

Adrenal Glands

The adrenal glands are composed of two separate endocrine organs which differ in embryological origin, type of secretion, and function. The adrenal glands of the dog are generally flattened, bilobed, and located cranial and medial to the kidneys on either side of the aorta and posterior vena cava (Miller et al., 1967). The left adrenal lies further caudal than the right. The right adrenal is more irregular in shape, usually with a distinct hook or comma form. On section, the adrenal cortex is usually firm and yellow, the medulla is softer and is usually light red to brown.

The adrenal cortex develops from the cells of the celomic epithelium. The chromaffin tissue and sympathetic ganglion cells of the adrenal medulla are derived from the neural crest. Neural crest cells invade the already formed cortical primordium, frequently leaving islands of medullary cells in the cortex or carrying groups of cortical cells into the medulla (Miller et al., 1967). Some of the medullary cells may not be incorporated in the adrenal gland and develop to form paraganglia and aortic and carotid bodies. The adrenal cortex is traditionally divided into three zones: glomerulosa, fasciculata, and reticularis. The zones may not be distinct. The outer zona glomerulosa (zona arcuata) represents about 15% of the cortex, and is responsible for secretion of mineralocorticoid hormones. The middle zona fasciculata comprises about 70% of the cortex, and is responsible for secretion of glucocorticoid hormones. The inner zona reticularis accounts for the remaining 15% of the cortex and is responsible for the secretion of sex steroids (Capen, 1985). The widths of the three zones vary and the demarcation between them may not be distinct. The adrenal medulla secretes epinephrine and norepinephrine.

Pancreas

The gross anatomy of the pancreas has been described with the digestive system. The pancreas is both an exocrine and endocrine gland. Cells responsible for the exocrine (digestive) secretions are the acinar cells. The cells of the pancreas responsible for hormone secretion (insulin and glucagon) are present within small spherical or oval islands (islets of Langerhans) dispersed throughout the organ. Islet cells are derived in common with acinar cells and are thus of entodermal origin.

Testis and Ovary

The anatomy of the testis and ovary are described with the genitourinary system. Testosterone is produced by interstitial cells (cells of Leydig) of the testis. Estridial is produced by cells of the ovarian follicle. Progesterone is produced by cells of the corpus luteum.

Necropsy and Laboratory Techniques

A presentation of clinical signs of endocrine disease is beyond the scope of this chapter. The reader is referred to Ettinger (1989) as a source of clinical information.

The endocrine glands should be handled carefully during dissection and weighing to minimize the production of artifacts. The thyroid and parathyroids should be removed while the larynx, trachea, and esophagus are in place and anatomical landmarks are undisturbed. Having all structures in place is particularly helpful when the thyroid is small or outside its normal location. Parathyroid glands should be included with the thyroid. The adrenal glands should be removed before the kidneys. The hypophysis may be removed from the sella turcica with minimal damage by first, freeing the dorsum sellae by cutting through its base with small bone cutters. Second, grasp a clinoid process with fine forceps to support the hypophysis as the dura mater is cut with fine curved scissors to free the hypophysis from the basisphenoid bone. Third, remove the hypophysis from the cranial cavity attached to the dorsum sellae. Fourth, weigh the hypophysis by cutting the dura mater between the hypophysis and the bone to allow the hypophysis to drop upon a tared weighing boat.

Generally, a small strand of dura mater will be found on the hypophysis that may be grasped to transfer the gland to fixative or cassette. The hypophysis may be processed intact. If embedded with the dorsal (infundibular) surface down, three step sections of the gland will usually result in a good representation of the pars distalis, pars intermedia, and pars nervosa.

Cells of the pars distalis are traditionally classified as eosinophils, basophils, and chromophobes on the basis of their uptake of acidic or basic dyes. Immunocytochemical methods using specific hormonal antibodies now reliably distinguish the various cells responsible for secretion of each of the various hormones.

During the trimming process, attempts should be made to include at least one parathyroid gland with each lobe of the thyroid. Both lobes of the thyroid should be represented in stained sections. Adrenal glands should be cut parasagittally. The thicker segment from each gland is embedded. The block may be rough cut on the microtome to obtain nearly full width representations of the cortex and medulla in stained sections.

Pathology

Of all the endocrine glands, potentially significant lesions are most likely to be seen within the thyroid gland. Hottendorf and Hirth (1974) report cysts and granuloma in the pituitary; chronic lymphocytic thyroiditis, ultimobranchial cysts, atrophy and focal squamous metaplasia in the thyroid; hyperplasia in the parathyroid; and focal cortical hyperplasia and minor focal inflammation in the adrenal. Maita et al. (1977) report cysts in the anterior lobe of the hypophysis and follicular epithelial hyperplasia in the thyroid. Oghiso et al. (1982) report fatty degeneration and nodular hyperplasia of the adrenal cortex, cysts of the anterior lobe of the pituitary and follicular atrophy, interfollicular cellularity, and lymphocytic thyroiditis in the thyroid. Pick and Eubanks (1965) report pituitary cyst and thyroiditis. Glaister (1986) reports cyst in the pituitary and parathyroid and cyst, ectopic thymus, C-cell hyperplasia, and lymphoid hyperplasia of the thyroid. Barron and Saunders (1966) report *Toxocara* granuloma in the thyroid and pituitary.

Cysts are frequently found (less frequently reported) in the hypophysis, parathyroid, and thyroid. Cystic remnants of the craniopharyngeal duct are frequently found at the periphery of the pars tuberalis and pars distalis. Most of the cysts are microscopic, but a few are visible grossly. The cysts are lined by cuboidal to columnar epithelium, often ciliated, and contain mucin. Small cysts (apparently from remnants of the duct connecting thymic and parathyroid primordia) may be found within or near the parathyroid. Parathyroid cysts are usually multiloculated, lined by cuboidal to columnar epithelium, often ciliated, and contain densely eosinophilic material. Ultimobranchial duct cysts are frequently seen within the thyroid. They are derived from remnants of the ultimobranchial body and have a keratinized squamous epithelial lining (Capen, 1985).

Minor changes frequently seen within the thyroid include disassociation of follicular cells (probably artifactual), minute intrafollicular corpora amylaceae–like bodies, and the presence of brown pigment (lipofuscin) in follicular cells. Potentially significant changes seen in the thyroid include idiopathic follicular atrophy and lymphocytic thyroiditis. Idiopathatic follicular atrophy is a progressive loss of follicular epithelium and replacement by adipose cells. One lobe may be affected more than the other. Severely affected lobes are difficult to locate at necropsy. Parafollicular cells are not affected and remain in the adipose tissue.

Dogs with idiopathic thyroid atrophy may be hypothyroid. Hypothyroidism may also be seen in dogs with lymphocytic thyroiditis. Glands with lymphocytic thyroiditis may be enlarged, but they may also be normal or even reduced in size.

Lymphocytic thyroiditis in dogs appears to have an immunological basis and familial occurrence in beagles. Histological alterations consist of multifocal to diffuse infiltrates of lymphocytes, plasma cells, and macrophages. Lymphoid nodules may be present. Thyroid follicles are usually small and may be disrupted and contain degenerate follicle cells, lymphocytes, and plasma cells. Lymphocytic thyroiditis in the beagle has been extensively investigated (Tucker, 1962; Mawdesley-Thomas and Jolly, 1967; Mawdesley-Thomas, 1968; Beierwaltes and Nishiyama, 1968; Musser and Graham, 1968; Fritz et al., 1970; Mizejewski et al., 1971). The microscopist will encounter varying numbers of parafollicular cells in the thyroid of young beagles. Occasionally, the number or focal concentration appear adequate to justify a diagnosis of C-cell hyperplasia.

As noted earlier, the width of the various layers of the adrenal cortex may vary. The zona glomerulosa may be thin or seem to be absent for substantial distances. Also, there may be appreciable differences in cortical cell vacuolation from animal-to-animal. Cortical cells may be found in the medulla and medullary cells may be found in and on the cortex (all explainable in the embryological development of the gland).

UROGENITAL SYSTEM

Anatomy and Histology

The urogenital system is made up of the urinary organs (kidneys, ureters, urinary bladder, and urethra), the male genital organs (scrotum, testes, epididymides, deferent ducts, prostate, and penis) and the female genital organs (ovaries, oviducts, uterus, vagina, and vulva).

Kidneys

The kidney performs metabolic, humoral, and excretory functions. The excretory function produces a fluid (urine) that is conducted from the kidney by fibromuscular tubes (ureters) to a storage reservoir (urinary bladder), where the fluid accumulates and is periodically discharged through a single tube (urethra) to the exterior.

The kidneys are bean-shaped glands located in the sublumbar area, one on each side of the aorta and posterior vena cava. The right kidney is usually located slightly anterior to the left and is more firmly secured in its position. A whole kidney cut in a midsagittal plane has two distinct zones (cortex and medulla). The cortex is the darker outer zone lying beneath the renal capsule. The medulla is the remaining lighter zone shaped like an inverted pyramid. The apex of the pyramid is the papilla, which projects into the expanded end of the ureter (renal pelvis). The renal pelvis lies within an opening in the medial border of the kidney called the renal hilus (renal sinus). In addition to the renal pelvis, the hilus contains adipose tissue, branches of the renal artery, vein and lymphatics, and nerves. Since the dog has only one papilla, it is classified as a unilobular or unipyramidal kidney; however, the single pyramid is actually the result of several pyramids fusing during development (Brown, 1976).

The nephron is the functional unit of the kidney and has six morphologically distinct segments: renal corpuscle, convoluted and straight portions of the proximal tubule, thin segment, and straight and convoluted portions of the distal tubule. The distal tubules join collecting tubules. Collecting tubules join with other collecting tubules and finally converge into large collecting ducts (papillary ducts) that open onto the apex of the papilla. The renal corpuscles and convoluted portions of the proximal and distal tubules are located in the cortex. The thin segment and straight portions of the proximal and distal tubules are located in the medulla. The latter three segments form a loop called the loop of Henle. In unipyramidal kidneys, segments of Henle's loops are so regularly arranged that a separation of medulla into outer and inner zones is visible to the naked eye. The boundary between the zones is the junction of the ascending limb of the thin segment and the straight portion of the distal tubule. The junction of the straight portion of the proximal tubule with the descending thin limb subdivides the outer zone into inner and outer bands, which are also visible to the naked eye (Brown, 1976).

Ureters

The ureters are slightly flattened tubes that begin at the renal pelvis and enter the urinary bladder by separate orifices near the neck of the bladder.

Urinary Bladder

The urinary bladder is a hollow musculomembranous organ whose form, size, and position vary according to the volume of urine it contains. The near full capacity of the bladder in the beagle is about 150 ml (Andersen, 1970). The urinary bladder is divided into a neck region (connecting with the urethra), a blunt cranial end (fundus), and a body portion between the neck and fundus (Miller et al., 1967). Internally, a triangular area near the neck is termed the trigone. The base of the trigone is a line connecting the ureteral openings; the apex is the urethral orifice.

Urethra

The male urethra is the canal that carries urine and seminal secretions to the exterior. It is divided into prostatic, membranous, and penile portions.

The female urethra extends from the urinary bladder to enter the vulva just caudal to the vaginovulvar junction.

Scrotum

The scrotum is divided by a median septum into two cavities, each of which is occupied by a testis, its associated epididymis, and a distal part of the spermatic cord. The scrotum functions as a temperature regulator for the testes; made possible by its thin gland-rich skin, lack of subcutaneous fat, and an ability to contract toward the body (by means of the cremaster muscles) or relax away from the body.

Testis

The canine testis is oval and is thicker dorsoventrally than from side-to-side. The size (weight) of testes of young adult beagles varies so greatly as to be significant concern in short-term toxicology studies. James and Heywood (1979) demonstrated the magnitude of the weight variation in beagles on 13-, 26-, and 52-week (and longer) studies (Table 12). In their experience, male beagles attain full sexual maturity between 35 and 40 weeks of age (based on testicular size, semen evaluation, hormonal profiles, and quantitative histometric analysis of spermatogenesis).

The cut surface of a normal testis bulges. The color of the testis in young beagles is light pink to tan (depth of color increases with age due to increased pigmentation of the interstitial cells).

The testis is subdivided into numerous lobules by delicate connective tissue septa that extend from a core of connective tissue (mediastinum testis) to the capsule of the testis (tunica albuginea). Ducts, blood vessels, lymphatics, and nerves enter and leave the testis through the mediastinum. Each of the lobules contain one or more convoluted sperm-producing tubules (seminiferous tubules) that empty at both ends into straight tubules (tubuli recti) that connect with a series of epithelial lined channels (rete testis) in the mediastinum. Spermatozoa are swept out of the seminiferous tubules, through the rete testis, and into the epididymis in a fluid secreted by the sustentacular cells (Sertoli cells). The interstitial cells (Leydig cells) are the endocrine (testosterone-producing) cells of the testis.

Epididymis

The epididymis consists of the ductuli efferentes and the much longer and highly tortuous ductus epididymidis. The ductuli efferentes emerge from the mediastinum to connect the rete testis with the ductus epididymidis. The epididymis lies along the dorsolateral surface of the testis.

For descriptive purposes the epididymis is divided into three portions. The initial portion located near the cranial extremity of the testis and into which the ductuli efferentes empty is called the head of the epididymis (caput epididymis). The portion of the head with the ductuli efferentes is called the initial segment. The main length of the epididymis is the body (corpus epididymis), and the segment attached to the caudal extremity of the testis is the tail (cauda epididymis). The epididymis is the maturation and storage site for the spermatozoa. The ductus epididymidis is subdivided further, with each subdivision apparently fulfilling a specific function in the maturation process of the sperm.

Table 12 Testicular Weight in Beagles Under 2 Years of Age

Number of dogs	Mean age (weeks)	Mean body wt. (kg)	Mean testicular wt (g)	% of dogs with testicular wt in range (g)			
				<9.9	10.0–19.9	20.0–29.9	>30
42	37±4	11.9±1.8	20.7±6.1	4.8	35.7	52.4	7.1
38	46±2	15.6±2.0	23.6±5.0	0.0	26.3	63.2	10.5
41	73±4	12.4±2.0	25.0±6.6	2.4	17.1	56.1	24.4

Ductus Deferens

The ductus deferens (deferent duct) is a thick-walled tube that is continuous with the tail of the epididymis and extends to the prostatic urethra. Its initial portion is located within the spermatic cord and surrounded by the veins of the pampiniform plexus, arteries, lymph vessels, nerves, and smooth muscle.

Prostate Gland

The prostate gland (the only accessory male sex gland in the dog) is an ovoid musculo-glandular organ that completely surrounds the proximal portion of the ureter.

The prostate is composed of two portions: external and internal. The external portion forms most of the dog's prostate and consists of two large bilateral lobes. The internal portion consists of a few small glands scattered along the urethra. Trabeculae divide the two external lobes into lobules in which the glandular elements are most prevalent near the periphery. Secretion from prostate glands enters the urethra by way of numerous excretory ducts. The paired ductus deferens enter the dorsal surface of the prostate and run caudoventrally on either side of the median plane to open into the dorsal surface of the prostatic urethra. James and Heywood (1979) found incomplete prostate development in beagles 9–10 months of age and demonstrated a wide range of prostate weights in control beagles on short-term toxicity studies (Table 13).

Penis

The male copulatory organ (penis) is composed of three principal parts: root, body, and distal free part (glans penis). The glans penis is mostly enveloped in stratified squamous epithelium and, when not erect, is entirely withdrawn into a tubular sheath of integument (prepuce). The mucosa of the penile urethra is lined by transitional epithelium except near the external urethral opening, where it changes to stratified squamous epithelium similar to that covering the penis.

The female genital organs consist of the ovaries, oviducts, uterus, vagina, and vulva. The ovaries, oviducts, and uterus are attached to the walls of the abdominal and pelvic cavities by folds of peritoneum called broad ligaments. Each broad ligament contains an ovary, oviduct, and uterine horn (plus vessels, nerves, and fat).

Ovary

The ovary is an ovoid gland situated within a fossa of the peritoneum (ovarian bursa) and supported by the mesovarium (cranial portion of the broad ligament) and the suspensory ligament of the ovary. The ovary is completely enclosed by the ovarian bursa except for a narrow slit, 2 to 15 mm long, located on the medial side. The structure of the ovaries varies with age and the phase of the sexual cycle.

Table 13 Prostate Weight in Beagles Under 2 Years of Age

Number of dogs	Mean age (weeks)	Mean body wt. (kg)	Mean prostate wt (g)	% of dogs with prostate wt in range (g)			
				<5.0	5.1–10.0	10.1–20.0	>20
42	37±4	11.9±8	3.3±1.6	84.4	15.6	0.0	0.0
38	46±2	15.6±2.0	6.5±2.3	23.4	66.1	10.5	0.0
41	73±4	12.4±2.0	8.1±2.9	9.8	63.4	26.8	0.0

The ovary is composed of a cortex and medulla which contains a prominent rete ovarii. The cortex consists of a connective tissue stroma which contains blood vessels, lymphatics, follicles, and corpora lutea. The surface of the cortex is smooth in immature ovaries.

Oviducts

The oviducts (uterine tubes) are tortuous structures that extend from the region of the ovary to the uterine horns. In the bitch, the oviduct almost completely encircles the ovary. The large funnel-shaped ovarian end of the duct is called the infundibulum and is located near the slit in the ovarian bursa.

Uterus

The uterus is a Y-shaped tubular organ which communicates with the oviducts cranially and the vagina caudally. The uterus consists of a neck (cervix), body (corpus), and two horns (cornua).

In the bitch, the uterine body is short and the horns relatively long and straight. The right horn is usually longer than the left. The size and shape of the uterus varies according to age and the stage of the sexual cycle. The uterine horns unite at the body. The body extends from the point of convergence of the uterine horns to the cervix. The wall of the uterus consists of three layers: mucosa (endometrium), muscularis (myometrium), and serosa (perimetrium). The endometrium is the thickest of the three layers and consists of three zones: crypt, intermediate, and basal (McEntee, 1990). The crypt zone has numerous short, epithelial-lined recesses. The intermediate zone contains uterine glands, but it is predominantly connective tissue. The uterine glands branch, coil, and terminate in the basal zone.

Vagina

The vagina is the highly dilatable musculocutaneous canal extending from the uterus to the vulva. Cranially, the vagina is limited by the cervix, which may protrude up to 1 cm into the vagina. Caudally, the vagina ends just cranial to the urethral opening. Flat longitudinal folds extend throughout the length of the vagina. The tunica mucosa is nonglandular stratified squamous epithelium.

Vulva

The vulva is the external genitalia of the bitch and consists of the vestibule, clitoris, and labia. The vestibule is the space connecting the vagina with the external genital opening and is the largest part of the vulva. The vestibule is the common opening for the genital and urinary tracts. The clitoris (homologue of the male penis) is located in the extreme caudal region of the vestibule near the ventral commissure of the vulva. The labia (lips) form the external boundary of the vulva. The vestibule is lined by stratified squamous epithelium and contains small, mucus-producing vestibular glands. Numerous lymph follicles are present in the vestibular mucosa and may be large enough to be seen grossly. The labia are covered with stratified squamous epithelium and are rich in sebaceous and tubular sweat glands.

The Estrous Cycle

Puberty is the age at which first estrus occurs in the bitch and varies among breeds and within breeds. The range is usually given as 6–12 months. The average age for first estrus in the laboratory beagle appears to be about 12 months, with a range of 10–14 months (Andersen, 1970; Sekhri and Faulkin, 1970; Sokolowski, 1973). Most female beagles will be sexually immature when started on toxicology studies. At termination of short-term studies, they may still be sexually immature or be in any stage of their first estrous cycle. The sexual stage of the bitch at termination of a study impacts the gross and microscopic appearance of the sex organs (and mammary gland) and the weights of the ovaries, uterus, and conceivably the hypophysis and adrenal glands.

Traditionally, the cyclical changes occurring in the reproductive system of the bitch have been divided into four phases; proestrus, estrus, metestrus, and anestrus. This classification has deemphasized the important extended luteal phase of the cycle and obscured several events which occur during the estrus phase of the cycle. Recently, several workers (Cupps et al., 1969; McDonald, 1969; Holst and Phemister, 1974) have reexamined the traditional classification and suggested modification. Phemister (1974) summarizes the revised view.

> According to this revised view, proestrus remains the phase of rapid follicular growth and rising estrogen levels when there is swelling of the vulva, generalized congestion of the genital tract, and a sanguineous vaginal discharge. As a rule, proestrus lasts about 9 days. Estrus is the period of sexual receptivity, usually lasting 7 to 10 days. In most bitches the initial day of estrus coincides approximately with a surge of luteinizing hormone (LH) from the pituitary gland. The LH surge is followed by ovulation 2 days later, usually on about the 3rd day of estrus. Metestrus, as the term is used for other species, defines the brief period when the corpus luteum is being formed and becoming functional. In the bitch this phase lasts for about 4 days and occurs entirely within the period of acceptance (estrus). By 4 days after ovulation, the genital system is dominated by luteal progesterone. By definition this phase of progesterone dominance is diestrus. Its onset is signaled by an abrupt change in vaginal cytologic characteristics: from predominantly large cornified, superficial squamous cells to noncornified, small intermediate and parabasal cells. On an average, diestrus begins 2 to 3 days before the end of estrus, and based on hormonal data, lasts for 2 to 3 months, or even longer if morphologic data are used. Following diestrus, the bitch enters a period of reproductive quiescence, anestrus, which lasts for 3 months or more.

Metestrus in the revised classification describes the period more in accordance with its use in other species, and emphasizes the fact that corpora lutea form and function for comparable periods (2–3 months) in a bitch whether she is pregnant or not pregnant. In other words, every nonpregnant bitch experiences a period of pseudopregnancy (pseudocyesis) to some degree. When the bitch's appearance and behavior closely mimic pregnancy, the pseudopregnancy becomes a clinical problem.

Necropsy and Laboratory Techniques

Because of the large functional reserve of the kidney, renal diseases may or may not be associated with renal dysfunction. Two-thirds to three-fourths of the renal parenchyma must be functionally impaired before clinical signs develop in chronic renal failure (Osborne et al., 1983). Functional abnormalities of the kidney can be clinically manifested in a number of ways, including polyuria (formation and elimination of large quantities of urine), oliguria (decrease in the rate of formation and/or elimination of urine), anuria (lack of urine formation/lack of urine elimination), polydipsia (excessive thirst), weight loss, anorexia, vomiting, diarrhea, dehydration, edema, stomatitis, weakness, and depression. Cloudy urine or hematuria may indicate disease of the urinary bladder. It is unlikely that signs of a reproductive system disorder would be detected in short-term toxicology studies.

At postmortem, the initial examination of the urogenital system should be done with all organs of the system in place.

Kidney

The kidneys should be approximately equal in size. The normal cortex is brownish red and the medulla white to pink. The kidney should be cut in multiple transverse sections and the surfaces of each examined. One or two sections (4–5 mm thick) should be taken from the midpyramidal region and placed in fixative. Proximal tubular epithelium autolyzes rapidly and kidneys should be placed in fixative as early as possible. Both the immature and mature kidney of the beagle have been studied in detail and much is known about the normal morphology and morphometry of the organ (Stuart et al., 1975; Eisenbrandt and Phemister, 1977, 1978, 1979, 1980; Jaenke and Phemister, 1980).

Ureters and Urinary Bladder

Usually, the ureters need only be examined externally in situ. The urinary bladder should be removed, incised longitudinally, everted, and the mucosal surface examined. The entire bladder should be fixed. Usually, the bladder contains some urine at necropsy. Uncontaminated urine specimens may be gotten by puncturing the undisturbed bladder with a hypodermic needle (avoiding blood vessels) and withdrawing urine into a syringe.

Prostate, Scrotum, and Epididymis

The prostate should be removed and its internal surface examined by one or more transverse cuts (some prostates are so small that bisection is adequate). At least two sections should be fixed. The scrotum should be incised, the scrotal ligaments severed, the testes removed and the vaginal tunics surrounding the spermatic cords incised to the level of the abdominal wall. After examining the structures of the spermatic cord and the surfaces of the testis and epididymis, the testis and epididymis are freed. The epididymis should be dissected from the testis before the testis is weighed. The epididymides may be fixed intact. The testis should be sliced before fixation to verify that the cut surface bulges. (Failure to bulge indicates degeneration of seminiferous tubules.) McEntee (1990) recommends midsagittal bisection, followed by multiple transverse cuts into each half of the testis and examination of each cut surface. The incisions should be made with a very sharp knife. McEntee also recommends samples be taken from the head extremity, middle part, and caudal extremity. Bouin's solution is the recommended fixative for the testis.

Ovaries and Uterus

The ovaries and uterus are usually weighed in toxicology studies. As with the testis and prostate, the weight of the female organs varies according to sexual maturity, and, additionally, upon the phase of the estrous cycle. Reproductive organs should be examined in detail in studies of compounds with known or potential effects upon the repoductive system. Less attention may be paid to the reproductive tract in other studies; nevertheless, it seems appropriate that some observations be made to establish the probable sexual state of a bitch at necropsy and to have these observations to correlate with microscopic findings and organ weight data.

Gross and Microscopic Appearance of Female Genital Organs at Necropsy

The gross and microscopic appearance of the female genital organs of the beagle during the various phases of the estrous cycle have been described (Andersen, 1970; Sokolowski et al., 1973; Sokolowski, 1977).

Vulva.   The external genitalia swell and discharge a sanguineous fluid at the onset of proestrus. (The sanguineous discharge of proestrus and estrus is not due to mucosal hemorrhage but due to extravasation of erythrocytes by diapedesis through the endometrium and into the lumen of the uterus and vagina). The thickening of the labia and wall of the vestibule is due to congestion and edema that account for the warm feeling of the external genitalia from which the expression "in heat" is derived. The vestibular mucosa remains unwrinkled during proestrus and estrus, but lymph follicles may become prominent.

Vagina. The vaginal mucosa shows extensive wrinkling beginning at proestrus and continuing into estrus. (The normal longitudinal folds are exaggerated and in turn irregularly subdivided by numerous transverse wrinkles.) The wrinkling decreases later in estrus and by early metestrus (diestrus) the folds have lost their wrinkled appearance. The cervix protrudes prominently into the vagina during estrus, and its surface is marked by numerous folds. The cervical canal is patent throughout estrus and early diestrus. By the end of diestrus and throughout anestrus, the cervical canal is almost completely sealed.

Uterus. Enlarged blood vessels appear in the broad ligaments and in the perimetrium with proestrus and are present throughout estrus. The uterine wall thickens owing to congestion, edema, and proliferation of uterine glands. The uterus attains maximum nonpregnant size 20–30 days post ovulation and exhibits a characteristic "corkscrew" appearance. At 60 days postovulation, the uterus is about the same size as in proestrus. The uterus never returns to the size seen in immature bitches.

Oviduct. During estrus, a small mass of red tissue protrudes from the slitlike opening of the bursal sac. The tissue is hyperemic and edematous fimbriae which almost completely close the slit.

Ovary. The ovaries of immature bitches are small, smooth, and have no follicles larger than 1 mm in diameter. A definite cortex and medulla are present at 6 months. On the first day of proestrus, follicles may be up to 4 mm in diameter and up to 14 mm in diameter just prior to ovulation. Ovarian weight is greatest at approximately the time of ovulation (presumably due to the size of follicles and the luteinizing that is occurring). Luteinizing begins immediately after follicles rupture, and it is not unusual to find follicles of varying size and corpora lutea in the same ovary at estrus. Corpora lutea are most numerous and fully developed about 10 days after ovulation. Corpora lutea begin to degenerate at about 20 days postovulation and by 60 days postovulation have undergone fatty degeneration and appear nonfunctional. Corpora lutea are bright salmon pink from the time of ovulation until 10 days after ovulation. They then gradually yellow and are light tan about 60 days after ovulation. No remnants of corporea lutea (corpora albicantia) are seen in ovaries during the first estrous cycle.

Mammary Gland. Gross changes are imperceptible in the mammary gland until shortly after ovulation, when a bluish plaque can be observed at the base of each teat. Thereafter the mammary glands enlarge and regress during the metestrus (diestrus) stage of the estrous cycle.

Pathology

Many changes have been reported for the kidney and male genital organs. A few observations have been made for the female genitalia. Hottendorf and Hirth (1974) report the following for the kidney: hydronephrosis, unilateral renal agenesis, renal carcinoma, microcalculi of the renal medulla (found in almost 50% of males and females), minor focal inflammation, pyelitis-pyelonephritis, granuloma, chronic interstitial nephritis, glomerulitis-glomerulonephritis, and focal embolic nephritis. Calculi and cystitis were seen in the urinary bladder. Calculi were also seen in the urethra. They report focal atrophy, intratubular giant cells, and interstitial cell hyperplasia for the testis; epididymitis; and focal cystic hyperplasia and atrophy for the prostate. Catheterization may have been the cause of some prostatitis and cystitis. Calcification of the round ligament of the bladder (remnant of the umbilical artery of the fetus) was seen, but not listed as a significant finding. Parovarian cyst was reported for the ovary and myometrial cyst for the uterus.

Glaister (1986) reports the following for the kidney: leukocytic foci, mineralization of the renal papilla (males and females), focal interstitial nephritis, pyelitis (minor degrees of mononuclear infiltration of the lamina propria and epithelium of the renal pelvis) and *Toxocara* granuloma of the cortex. For the prostate, he reports minor accumulations of lymphocytes (leukocytic foci) to large lymphoid aggregates with germinal center formation accompanied by interstitial fibrosis and epithelial atrophy (prostatitis). Focal atrophy was reported for the testis and distention was reported for the uterus.

Pick and Eubanks (1965) refer only to the kidney and report pyelitis, pyelonephritis, collecting tubule calcification, and cortical granuloma.

Oghiso et al. (1982) found changes only in the kidney and report urinary cast (albuminous), calcification, acidophilic crystalline intranuclear inclusions, interstitial nephritis, and pyelonephritis. They mention degenerative changes of the glomeruli and tubules but do not elaborate.

Maita et al. (1977) report chronic inflammation of the prostate and *Toxocara* granuloma in the kidney.

Guttman (1970) reports a progressive alteration of the renal glomerulus called progressive intercapillary glomerulosclerosis (ISG). The change is seen as early as 6 months of age and consists of thickening of basement membranes and increase in the mesangial maxtrix. Barron and Saunders (1966) report the kidney as a common site for *Toxocara* granuloma.

James and Heywood (1979) report spermatocoele granuloma (spermatic granuloma) and inflammation for the epididymis and foci of chronic inflammation in the prostate.

Unilateral renal agenesis was seen in adult breeding colony beagles (Fritz et al., 1977). Since unilateral renal agenesis is not lethal and is not detected by routine physical examination, the condition is occasionally found in laboratory beagles (Robbins, 1965; Vymetal, 1965; Hottendorf and Hirth, 1974). The ureter may or may not be missing. The developed kidney is usually about twice normal size (weight) and histologically of normal appearance, suggesting that the increased size is due to an absolute increase in the number of nephrons. Postnatal nephrogenesis is a characteristic of the canine kidney. Eisenbrandt and Phemister (1979) have shown that nephrogenesis continues through the first 8–10 days of life in the beagle, a fact that probably accounts for the normal histological appearance of the single enlarged kidney seen in unilateral renal agenesis.

Local or diffuse mesangial proliferation and thickened and wrinkled glomerular basement membranes are not an unusual finding in clinically healthy, nonproteinuric laboratory beagles (Stuart et al., 1975). Periglomerular sclerosis may also be present. With time, the intercapillary sclerosis generally increases in severity and may be associated with intermittent or persistent proteinuria.

The majority of the review authors report mineralization in the kidney. Mineralization is very common in dogs and is usually seen in the form of clumps of basophilic granules adjacent to and in the lumen and lining of collecting tubules. The incidence is probably higher than the reported 50%. Acidophilic crystalline intranuclear inclusions (identical in appearance to those seen in hepatocytes) are also commonly found in nuclei of cells lining proximal and distal tubules. Occasionally, one or more lobules of the glomerular tuft will be filled with large foam cells, which with appropriate stains are shown to contain fat. The condition is known as glomerular lipidosis and has no known functional significance.

Subclinical prostatitis is common in the dog. The inflammation is usually minimal in young adult beagles. Testicular degeneration occurs naturally in the dog and may be focal of diffuse, unilateral, or bilateral. Early degenerative lesions consist of loss of primordial germ cells which may appear within the lumen of the seminiferous tubule as individual cells or as multinucleated giant cells. As the degeneration advances, more germinal cells are lost and tubules may be lined only by sustentacular cells. Lymphocytic orchitis occurs in beagle colonies and may be seen in laboratory beagles, usually associated with lymphocytic thyroiditis. The lymphocytic infiltration may be diffuse, aggregated, or nodular (with germinal centers) and is commonly associated with focal or diffuse degeneration and atrophy of seminiferous tubules (Fritz et al., 1976). The epididymis may be involved. It is normal to find intranuclear, eosinophilic, periodic acid–Schiff positive inclusions in the epididymal epithelium of the dog (McEntree, 1990). The significance of the inclusions is unknown. Normal epididymal cells also contain granular, yellow to yellow-brown pigment. Mild balanoposthitis (inflammation of the glans penis and prepuse) is common and may result in slight mucopurulent preputial discharge.

Occasionally, clear cysts may be found in the vicinity of the ovary. The cysts have one of several origins (McEntree, 1990) and parovarian cyst is not a specific diagnosis.

NERVOUS SYSTEM

Anatomy and Histology

The nervous system is the chief coordinating system of the body. The body's other major coordinating system, the endocrine system, is controlled by the nervous system and a major part of it (the hypothalamus) is also a major part of the nervous system. The overall function of the nervous system is to produce the proper reaction of the organism to changes in both the external and internal environment (Jenkens, 1978). This function depends directly on the neuron. Neurons, along with supportive cells (neuroglia), make up the nervous system. The nervous system is divided into the central nervous system (CNS) and the peripheral nervous system (PNS), more for discussional purposes than on the basis of structure or function. The CNS consists of the brain and spinal cord (neuraxis). The PNS consists of cranial and spinal nerves, sensory and motor ganglia, sensory and motor nerve endings, and the automatic nervous system.

The autonomic nervous system is that part of the nervous system concerned with motor innervation of smooth muscle, cardiac muscle, and glands. On anatomical, pharmacological, and functional bases the autonomic nervous system is divided into a sympathetic portion and a parasympathetic portion. The general function of the sympathetic portion is to prepare the body for a state of emergency. The general function of the parasympathetic portion is to restore the body to a normal state of quiescence. The hypothalamus is the key to autonomic regulation. The rostral hypothalamic area controls the parasympathetic function and the caudal hypothalamic area controls the sympathetic function.

Divisions of the Nervous System: Structure and Function

All divisions of the nervous system are structurally and functionally connected. The PNS transmits impulses toward the CNS by way of sensory (afferent) neurons and away from the CNS by way of motor (efferent) neurons. The typical spinal nerve and the majority of cranial nerves have both types of functional neurons and are referred to as mixed nerves.

A typical peripheral nerve consists of an outer connective tissue sheath (epineurium) enclosing bundles (fasciculi) of nerve fibers. Each fasciculus is surrounded by its own connective tissue sheath (perineurium) and is made up of individual nerve fibers (microscopic in size) surrounded by their connective tissue sheaths (endoneurium). Individual nerve fibers consist of an axon and an enclosing sheath formed by lemmocytes (Schwann cells).

The axon is the elongated cytoplasmic extension (process) of the nerve cell. The surface membrane of the axon is the axolemma. Most peripheral axons are surrounded by an insulating sheath of lipoprotein (myelin). Myelin is the nonnucleated plasma membrane of the Schwann cell. The nucleated portion of the Schwann cell is the neuilemma (regeneration of axons is possible in Wallerian degeneration owing to survival of the nucleated neurilemma). The terms *axolemma* and *neuilemma* are not synonymous, and neither *neurilemma* nor *myelin* is synonymous with the total *Schwann cell*. The terms *axon* and *axis cylinder* are synonymous. Unfortunately, the total nerve fiber is also referred to as the axon.

Nerves of the CNS

The nerves attached to the brain are referred to as cranial nerves. There are 12 pairs, and except for the first pair (olfactory), all are attached to the brain stem.

Nerves attached to the spinal cord are referred to as spinal nerves. There are usually 36 pairs of spinal nerves in the dog, derived from 36 spinal cord segments: 8 cervical, 13 thoracic, 7 lumbar, 3 sacral, and 5 coccygeal. With the exception of the first cervical nerve, all spinal nerves pass through intervertebral foramina. Because the spinal cord is shorter than the spinal column (in the embryo, the vertebral column grows more rapidly than the spinal cord, resulting in a relative caudal migration of vertebrae) there is not a one-to-one relationship between the spinal cord segments and the vertebrae. As a result, spinal nerves generally exit caudal to their segment of origin and vertebrae of one region may contain spinal cord segments of another region. The actual spinal cord segment/vertebral body correlations must be in mind when spinal cord segments are chosen for histological examination. The nerve distribution to the fore- and hindlimbs allows the spinal cord to be divided into functional units. The location of the units within vertebrae are shown in Table 14 (Bailey and Morgan, 1983):

The CNS is protected, supported, and nourished by three sheetlike connective tissue

Table 14 Vertebrae and Spinal Cord Segments

Cord segment	Nerve/tract distribution	Vertebrae
Cervical C_1–C_5	Nerve fiber tracts ascending from forelimbs and hindlimbs and descending from brain	C_1–C_4
Cervicothoracic, C_6–T_1/T_2	Origin of nerves to forelimbs	C_5–C_7
Thoracolumbar, T_2–L_3	Nerve fiber tracts ascending from hindlimbs and descending from brain	T_1–L_3
Caudal lumbar, L_4–L_7	Origin of nerves to hindlimbs except S_1 contribution to the sciatic nerve	L_3–L_4
Sacral, S_1–S_3	Origin of nerves to the anus, urinary bladder, and perineum. S_1 contribution to sciatic nerve	L_5
Coccygeal, C_1–C_5	Origin of nerves to tail	L_5 caudally

coverings called the meninges (singular: meninx). The outermost (and toughest) meninx is the dura mater. The dura mater of the cranial cavity serves a dual function: meningeal covering for the brain and endosteal (or periosteal) lining for the bones of the calvarium. The spinal dura mater is separated from the periosteum of the vertebrae by the epidural cavity.

The second meninx (arachnoid) is much thinner and more delicate than the dura mater. The arachnoid is separated from the dura mater by an almost nonexistent subdural cavity. The arachnoid connects with the pia mater (the third meninx) by delicate trabeculae, but it is separated from the pia mater by a large underlying space (subarachnoid space) filled with cerebrospinal fluid. The cerebrospinal fluid (CSF) pushes the arachnoid peripherally to contact the dura mater, forming a fluid envelope to cushion and protect the brain and spinal cord.

The pia mater is closely adherent to the brain and extends deeply into the sulci of the cerebral hemispheres and between the folia of the cerebellum. The pia mater is the vascular meninx and mainly concerned with the nutrition of the CNS. The pia mater and arteries combine to form the tela choroidea of the choroid plexuses, which produce the major portion of the CSF.

The cerebrospinal fluid is a clear, colorless fluid that fills the ventricular system of the brain, the subarachnoid space of both the brain and spinal cord, and the central canal of the spinal cord.

The ventricular system of the brain and the central canal of the spinal cord are lined by a layer of closely packed cuboidal or columnar epithelial cells known collectively as the ependyma. In the ventricles of the brain, the ependyma is modified to form the special secretory epithelium of the choroid plexus. There are four ventricles in the brain: two lateral and single midline third and fourth ventricles. The lateral ventricles communicate with the third, the third with the fourth, and the fourth with a dilatation of the subarachnoid space (cisterna magna) between the cerebellum and medulla oblongata.

Necropsy and Laboratory Techniques

As noted in preceding sections, disease in another organ system can directly or indirectly involve the nervous system. Some of the more prominent signs of neurological disease include depression (dull, lethargic, inattentive), disorientation (loss of proper bearings, mental confusion), stupor (partial unconsciousness, can arouse with stimulation), coma (unconsciousness from which animal cannot be aroused with powerful stimuli), hyperexcitable (excessive response to normal stimuli), tilting of head, twisting of body, tremors, paresis (incomplete loss of voluntary motor function) or paralysis (complete loss of voluntary motor function) of one or more limbs, ataxia (incoordination of gait), abnormal reflexes, loss of control of urination and defecation and hyperesthesia, among others (Greene and Oliver, 1983).

If in-life observations indicate that a neurological problem exists, thorough physical and neurological examinations should be done to fully characterize the clinical signs, to localize the disease process (brain, spinal cord, peripheral nervous system), and, if possible, to define more precisely where in the brain, spinal cord, or peripheral nervous system the problem may be. Based on these (and clinical laboratory) findings, the pathologist may modify the postmortem procedures as needed to assure that all appropriate areas are examined and all appropriate tissues are taken.

To minimize the handling of the brain, the head should be removed from the body. First, reflect the skin from the head and neck, sever neck muscles at their attachment to the posterior aspect of the skull, and cut completely through the spinal cord at the atlanto-occipital articulation. The cut is made by passing a thin narrow blade through the dorsal atlanto-occipital membrane into the cisterna magna and then through the spinal cord. As the cisterna magna is entered, a quick appraisal of the CSF should be made. Expose the calvarium by removing the temporalis muscles. Remove the head by completing the disarticulation of the atlanto-occipital joint. (The disarticulation can be done quickly, if the prosector is methodical in cutting the joint capsule and the various ligaments.) Three cuts are made through the calvarium. One cut is made transversely through the frontal bone at the anterior limit of the cranial cavity slightly rostral to the zygomatic processes. The incision includes the frontal sinuses. Two identical cuts are made on each side of the calvarium, just dorsal to the widest part of the brain case. The lateral cuts connect the transverse cut with the foramen magnum. The foramen magnum should be entered at its widest point slightly dorsal to the occipital condyles. The cuts through the calvarium require practice and a sense as to when the saw is about to leave bone and enter the brain. Pull the calvarium upward and backward. Generally, the dura mater will strip from the calvarium and remain with the brain.

After examining the dura mater, cut it (and the arachnoid) parallel to the bone incisions. Two large folds of the dura mater will also need to be freed from their insertions between parts of the brain. The falx cerebri is the midsagittal fold between the cerebral hemispheres. The tentorium cerebelli is the transverse fold between the occipital poles of the cerebral hemispheres and the cerebellum. Failure to completely remove these folds will interfere with removal of the brain. The brain is extremely fragile and should be removed from the skull mostly by gravitational force and a little gentle traction. This is accomplished by holding the head upside down in one hand and freeing the brain by severing the cranial nerves, posteriorly rostrally, as they come to view. In the process, the brain gradually falls into the palm of the supporting hand.

The hypophyseal stalk (infundibulum) is severed as soon as it is seen so that the hypophysis remains intact in the sella turcia. The optic nerves are cut and as much of the olfactory lobes are removed as possible. Examine the ventral surface of the brain as it lies in the palm of the hand. Place the brain in a weighing boat and examine the dorsal surface. The brain need not be grasped, but may be slid from weighing boat to weighing boat or weighing boat to fixative. The removal of the hypophysis has been described in the endocrine system. The inner surface of the calvarium and ventral surface of the cranial cavity should be examined.

The entire spinal cord, or segments of it, may be removed by either a ventral or dorsal approach. Before attempting to remove a segment, always completely transect the cord cranially and caudally to prevent stretching and twisting of the spinal cord as the spinal column is manipulated. The spinal cord should be removed by grasping the dura mater. If the entire spinal cord is to be collected, it should be fixed in a fully extended position in an adequately long container. Cervical and thoracolumbar segments of the spinal cord are easily removed from vertebrae C_1–C_4 and T_2–L_4, respectively. These segments sample ascending and descending tracts of all the limbs and the nerves of origination to the hindlimbs.

Traditionally, a portion of a sciatic nerve is collected as the representative sampling of the peripheral nervous system. The sciatic nerve can be removed with minimal trauma and is large enough to provide adequate samples (5 cm or longer). The sciatic nerve contains both afferent and efferent nerve fibers (mixed nerve). If a sensory nerve (afferent fibers) is required, a branch of the sciatic nerve, the caudal (lateral) cutaneous sural nerve, may be taken. The caudal cutaneous sural nerve has been studied in healthy adult beagles and morphometric and electrophysiological data exist for it (and the ulnar and saphenous nerves) (Illanes et al., 1988).

Artifacts in nervous tissue can be as troublesome as artifacts in muscle tissue. The makeup of nervous tissue makes it unusually sensitive to autolysis, rough handling, and the chemical effects of fixative. Primary fixation by whole body perfusion with buffered glutaraldehyde addresses most of the problems and can be performed as successfully in the dog as in smaller laboratory animals. However, whole body perfusion has practical application only in selected studies, leaving the problem of tissue artifacts in the brain, spinal cord, and peripheral nerves to be dealt with on a daily basis in routine studies.

With the brain, the choice is between the artifacts of handling and distortion from slicing a brain in an unfixed state and the artifacts of autolysis in brains fixed by immersion. The choice is usually to fix the brain in toto and examine for gross internal lesions when the brain is sectioned for processing. Full transverse (coronal) sections are preferred for microscopic examination.

Cross and longitudinal sections of the spinal cord should be prepared. Specimens of peripheral nerves should be at least 5 cm in length and removed with great care. Peripheral nerves should be fixed in a gently stretched state on cardboard or corkboard. Ten percent neutral buffered formalin is the traditional fixative for nervous tissue. Brains should be fixed in large volumes of fixative which should be changed frequently. The investigator may wish to treat peripheral nerve specimens as surgical specimens and follow a nerve biopsy protocol (Asbury and Johnson, 1978), which provides for plastic and/or paraffin embedding; routine, thick or thin sections; special stains and nerve fiber microdissection (nerve teasing, teased specimen).

Routine sections of peripheral nerves should always include transverse and longitudinal sections. Hematoxylin and eosin is the most universally used stain; however, it does not stain specific nerve components and special stains are required for myelin, Nissl substance, neurofibrils, neuroglia, etc. The writer fully agrees with Dr. Jenkins (1978): "Neurostaining is a special technique which ideally should be reserved only for the experienced histotechnician who has the time and interest to devote to the subject."

Microscopists who are unfamiliar with the artifacts commonly encountered in peripheral nerves are referred to Asbury and Johnson (1978). Readers interested in contemporary neuropathological methods in toxicology are referred to Spencer and Bischoff (1982).

Pathology

Hydrocephalus is the most frequently reported lesion of the nervous system. Hottendorf and Hirth (1974) reported hydrocephalus in 14% of their animals and in 15% of their studies. They also reported chronic focal meningitis and focal encephalitis for the brain and focal myelitis for the spinal cord. They observed, but did not report as lesions, the small subependymal collections of glial cells usually seen around the anterior parts of the lateral ventricles. Oghiso et al. (1982) also reported hydrocephalus (ventricular dilatation) associated with spongelike alteration in the surrounding brain tissue. Pick and Eubanks (1965) report brain hemorrhage without further elaboration. Barron and Saunders (1966) report *Toxocara* granuloma in the brain and spinal cord (cauda equina). Fritz et al. (1967) report several cases of hydrocephalus.

Hydrocephalus is the abnormal accumulation of CSF. It is usually manifested as dilatation of one or more ventricles of the brain (internal hydrocephalus), but ventricles may be unaffected and it is the subarachnoid space that is dilated with the excess CSF (external hydrocephalus). If excess CSF is present in both locations, the condition is referred to as communicating hydrocephalus (Sullivan, 1985). While hydrocephalus appears to be fairly common in laboratory beagles, it is likely that minor degrees of ventricular dilatation are unrecognized and the real incidence of the condition is greater than reported. Lateral ventricles of surprising size (some with thinning or rupture of the septum pellucidum) are found incidentally while trimming brains of dogs that showed no neurological signs. At necropsy, the ventral surface of the brain should be closely examined, for the piriform area will dimple under slight pressure even in mild hydrocephalus. Hydrocephalus in laboratory beagles is probably a congenital condition.

The attentive microscopist may find spherical, eosinophilic granular structures in the medulla oblongata, pons, or anterior cervical cord (the structures seem to be most common in the gracilis tract and nucleus). Niewberne et al. (1960) and Innes and Saunders (1962) believe the structures are degenerating axis cylinders. They apparently have no neurological or pathological significance.

During examination of the peripheral nerve, the microscopist may encounter cylindrical, loosely textured, whorled, cell-sparse structures within the nerve. These are Renaut bodies and were well known to histologists of the late nineteenth century, but they have gradually been forgotten (Asbury, 1973; Asbury and Johnson, 1978). Renaut bodies are particularly well developed in the horse and donkey, but are less conspicuous in the dog and humans. Their purpose is unknown. It is important that the microscopist recognize them as normal structures and not misdiagnose them as nerve infarction or necrotizing angiopathic neuropathy, as has been done in the past (Asbury, 1973).

Spontaneous degenerative lesions of the peripheral nerve may be seen in the beagle as they are other laboratory animals. While commonly considered an aging change, occasionally "digestion chambers" and "myelin bubbles" are seen in the sciatic nerves of young beagles.

EYE AND EAR

Anatomy and Histology

Eye

The eye is the organ of vision, and it is composed of the eyeball (globe), the optic nerve, and accessory structures including the eyelids, conjunctiva, lacrimal apparatus, and ocular muscles. The canine eye is relatively large for the size of the animal. The human eye is approximately 2.5 cm in diameter (Kuwabara and Cogan, 1977); the eye of an adult beagle is approximately 2.2 cm in diameter (Andersen, 1970). The canine eye is also placed well forward in the head, giving the dog a large field of binocular vision. The eyeball is roughly spherical in shape, with the rostral curvature of the cornea making the anterioposterior diameter the greatest diameter of the eye. To facilitate description and orientation of the eye, special designations as to side, direction, and position are used. Oculus dexter (OD) designates the right eye; oculus sinister (OS) designates the left eye; and oculus unitus (OU) designates both eyes. The side of the globe nearest the nose is the nasal, or medial, side; the opposite side is the temporal, or lateral, side. The dorsal side is superior; the ventral side is inferior. The corneal pole is distal, or anterior; the cerebral pole is proximal, or posterior. The line connecting the two poles is the anatomical or optic axis. The equator is the greatest expansion of the eyeball perpendicular to the anatomical axis. A horizontal plane through the poles divides the eyeball into an upper half and a lower half. A vertical plane through the poles divides the eyeball into a nasal half and a temporal half.

Eyeball. The eyeball consists of an inner coat, or tunic, of neural light-sensitive tissue (retina) held in shape by surrounding coats that protect it (corneoscleral coat, outer fibrous coat) and nourish it (uvea, middle vascular coat). The outer fibrous coat is subdivided into a larger, tough, white posterior portion (sclera) which covers about 0.75 of the globe and a smaller, transparent anterior portion (cornea). The transition from the opaque sclera to the transparent cornea is comparatively abrupt and occurs at the corneoscleral (sclerocorneal) junction, or limbus. The limbal area of the sclera is pigmented laterally and medially but not dorsally or ventrally.

Sclera. The thickness of the sclera varies. At the equator, it is so thin as to be semitransparent and the dark color of the uvea shows through. It is thick at the ciliary region where extraocular muscles insert and around the optic nerve.

Cornea. The cornea is transparent, colorless, and nonvascular; however, it possesses dense nerve fiber plexuses and is highly sensitive. Opposite to what exists in humans, the cornea of the dog is thicker in the center than at the periphery (Getty, 1967). The transparency of the cornea is due to a nonkeratinized and nonpigmented surface epithelium, lack of blood vessels and lymphatics, cell-poor stroma composed of thin collagen fibrils arranged in orderly lamellae, and a sodium-potassium pump in the cell membrane of the corneal endothelium that maintains a high degree of stromal dehydration (Wilcock, 1985).

The composition of the cornea is notably uniform and consists of six or seven layers (six in the dog). The outermost and often overlooked layer is the tear film (not seen in histological sections). The outer stratified squamous epithelium is a continuum of the conjunctival epithelium. The basement membrane of the epithelium is the third layer. According to Dellmann (1976c), the dog does not have an anterior limiting membrane (Bowman's membrane). However, Prince et al. (1960) indicate that an anterior limiting membrane is present, but that it is extremely thin (1.5 vs 30 μm in humans). Shively and Epling (1970), in their study of the fine structures of the beagle eye, found no consistent layer of randomly oriented collagen fibers that would constitute an anterior limiting membrane. The stroma constitutes the bulk of the cornea. Descemet's membrane is present (a required constituent, since it is the basement membrane of the innermost layer, the endothelium). The endothelial layer should probably be known as mesothelium based on its structural characteristics and its probable origin (Shively and Epling, 1970).

Uvea. The uvea is the highly pigmented and vascular coat of the eye. It consists of the iris, ciliary body, and choroid.

Iris. This the most anterior portion of the uveal tract and is the diaphragm of the eye.

Ciliary Body. This is a ring of tissue that extends from the base of the iris to the neurosensory retina posteriorly. The main components of the ciliary body are the ciliary processes and the ciliary muscle.

The ciliary processes are actually linear folds that when seen from the rear appear as multiple radiating ridges. The ciliary processes are highly vascular and are thought to be the main sites for formation of the aqueous humor (an arrangement comparable to the formation of CSF by the choroid plexuses of the brain).

In accommodating for near vision, the ciliary muscle contracts, pulling the ciliary body forward, which allows the supporting fibers (zonule fibers) of the lens to relax, leading to relaxation and an anteriorposterior thickening of the lens.

Choroid.   The bulk of the uvea is formed by the choroid, which consists mainly of blood vessels and melanocytes. Externally, it blends with the sclera; internally, it is bounded by a basal lamina called Bruch's membrane; and dorsally (above the optic disc) it displays a peculiar structure known as the tapetum lucidum.

Tapetum.   Many animals have one of two types of tapeta: tapetum lucidum fibrosum or tapetum lucidum cellulosum. The dog has a tapetum lucidum cellulosum. The tapetum lucidum is a light-reflecting layer (responsible for the luster of eyes) that is situated in the dorsal half of the choroid. The tapetum is triangular to semicircular in shape, extending about halfway to the periphery of the choroid and has a horizontal base that just contacts the top of the optic disc. Although the tapetum appears to be immediately adjacent to the pigment epithelium cells of the retina, there is a layer of capillaries (choriocapillaris) between the tapetum and Bruch's membrane. The tapetum is made up of flat cells varying in number from 9 to 10 layers centrally to 1 or 2 layers peripherally (Prince et al., 1960).

Retina.   The innermost tunic of the eye is the retina. It is divided into a sensory portion (pars optica) that rests upon the choroid and a nonsensory portion that rests upon the ciliary body (pars ciliaris) and the posterior surface of the iris (pars iridica). The sensory and nonsensory portions join posterior to the ciliary body at a scalloped border known as the ora serrata. The sensory retina is firmly attached at the ora serrata and optic disc, but it is loosely attached over the choroid. Under normal circumstances, the pressure of the vitreous is sufficient to hold the retina in contact with the choroid.

The nonsensory retina consists of a simple layer of pigmented cuboidal epithelial cells that continues at the ora serrata to form the outermost of the 10 layers of the sensory retina. Not all of the pigment epithelium is pigmented; the cells overlying the tapetum lucidum are not. According to Kuwabara and Cogan (1977), two pigments may be found in the pigment epithelium: melanin and lipofuscin. The pigment epithelium interdigitates with the overlying photoreceptors. Among other functions, the epithelial cells engulf and degrade obsolete rod and cone cell segments. The accumulation of lipofuscin appears to be a result of this phagocytic activity. In humans, the quantity of lipofuscin increases with age and the number of melanin granules decreases (Kuwabara and Cogan, 1977).

The inner transparent layer of the sensory retina comprises nine layers, named from within outward: internal limiting membrane, nerve fiber layer, ganglion cell layer, inner plexiform layer, inner nuclear layer, outer plexiform layer, outer nuclear layer, external limiting membrane, and the layer of rods and cones. The retinal receptors in the dog are predominantly rods. That feature (and others) indicates that the dog is predominantly a nocturnal animal (Prince et al., 1960).

To the ophthalmologist, the visible portion of the posterior globe is the ocular fundus, which for descriptive purposes is commonly divided into a dorsal tapetal fundus and a ventral nontapetal fundus (tapetum nigrum). The optic disc is usually at the junction of the two.

The optic disc (optic papilla) is the rounded, raised area where the optic nerve leaves the eye. Jenkins (1978) emphasizes the following important features relative to the optic nerve: since the optic nerve is a fiber tract of the brain, it has no neurilemmal sheath of Schwann and regeneration is not possible; it contains neuroglial elements; has a meningeal investment but no epi-, peri-, or endoneurium; and the individual nerve fibers are all myelinated. Wilcock (1985), points out that, in contrast to most domestic species, the fibers in the optic papilla of the dog are myelinated. Since the optic nerve is in direct contact with the eye and brain via neurons and CSF, it may be affected by diseases of both the eye and brain.

Branches of the ciliary and internal ophthalmic arteries and veins lie just along the optic nerve. When they reach the eye, some plunge into globe and others (medial and lateral long posterior ciliary arteries and veins) pass into the superficial layers of the sclera and are externally visible for a distance along the horizontal meridian of the eye. These vessels serve as landmarks in orienting the eye at trimming.

The transparent media of the eye include the cornea, aqueous humor, lens and vitreous body (the retina, excluding the pigment epithelium is also transparent). The aqueous humor is the water-clear fluid contained in a cavity bounded anteriorly by the cornea and posteriorly by the lens. The space between the cornea and the anterior surface of the iris is the anterior chamber and the space between the posterior surface of the iris and the lens is the posterior chamber. Aqueous humor is produced in the posterior chamber and drains from the anterior chamber into a meshwork of channels located at the junction of the cornea, sclera, and iris (iris angle, filtration angle).

The lens is composed entirely of epithelial cells whose basement membrane is the thick outermost capsule of the lens. The bulk of the lens is formed by layers of epithelial processes that cannot be shed, but are compacted with age to the center of the lens. The adult lens depends entirely upon the aqueous humor for delivery of nutrients and removal of wastes.

The vitreous body is the transparent gel that fills the inner portion of the eyeball between the lens and the retina. The vitreous shows considerable shrinkage with most fixatives (over 99% of the vitreous is water) and its normal, in-life distribution is not apparent in microscopic sections.

Third Eyelid. The dog has a third eyelid, or nictitating membrane, located at the medial angle of the palpebral aperture (medial canthus, nasal canthus). A T-shaped hyaline cartilage forms the skeleton of the third eyelid. The cross of the "T" supports the free margin of the lid. The lower shaft of the "T" is surrounded by a mixed lacrimal gland (superficial gland of the third eyelid, nictitans gland). According to Getty (1967), the dog does not have a Harder's gland (deep gland of the third eyelid). The inner conjunctival covering (bulbar conjunctiva) contains numerous lymphoid nodules.

Ear

The ear is the organ of hearing and equilibrium. It is composed of three connected divisions, each of which is referred to as an ear: external (outer) ear, middle ear, and internal (inner ear). The inner ear is the organ for both hearing and equilibrium. The external and middle ears are sound-collecting and -conducting apparatuses (Getty, 1967).

External Ear. This consists of the pinna (auricle) and the external auditory meatus (ear canal). The pinna is composed of a sheet of elastic cartilage (auricular cartilage) covered by skin on both sides. The auricular cartilage is pierced by many foramina which permit the passage of blood vessels. Histological sections that include foramina give the impression that the cartilaginous sheet is not continuous. The function of the pinna is to direct air vibrations into the funnel-like ear canal to the tympanic membrane (ear drum). The tympanic membrane is the partition between the external ear and the middle ear.

Middle Ear. This consists of the tympanic cavity, the auditory tube, and a chain of three small bones (auditory ossicles) that connect the tympanic membrane to the oval window of the inner ear. The tympanic cavity is air filled and communicates with the nasal pharynx by means of the auditory tube (eustachian tube).

Inner Ear. This is contained within the temporal bone and consists of the membranous labyrinth containing the organs of hearing and equilibrium and the bony labyrinth surrounding the membranous labyrinth. The inner ear is fluid filled. The bony labyrinth, which lodges the membranous labyrinth, contains a fluid, perilymph, and communicates with the cerebrospinal space by way of the vestibular aqueduct. The membranous labyrinth is filled with a fluid called endolymph.

Necropsy and Laboratory Techniques

Eye

Many lesions of the eyelids, conjunctiva, and cornea will be clinically apparent; however, most lesions within the globe will be hidden to the pathologist without the assistance of an ophthalmoscopic examination. Ideally, the pathologist will have the notes, drawings, or photographs of an ophthalmologist to direct him or her to pathology within the eye. Minute lesions can be difficult to find without directions and lesions involving the lens may be obscured or lost because of the difficulty in obtaining complete, artifact-free sections of the lens.

Autolytic changes can be detected in the canine retina within 5 min of death (Saunders and Rubin, 1975). Unless there are compelling reasons to do otherwise, the eyes should be the first organs removed at necropsy and both eyes should be in fixative well within the first 5 min of the necropsy. To meet the 5-min deadline, all preliminary procedures (weighing, external examination, clipping of hair) should be done prior to exsanguination. Good exsanguination limits the degree of hemorrhage into the orbit during dissection. The enucleation can be done by a single prosector, but the assistance of a second person is required to have both eyes removed, cleaned, and in fixative within the 5-min time frame.

A single incision through the lateral palpebral angle will free the upper and lower eyelids sufficiently to give access to the eye. With an assistant stabilizing the head and stretching the skin to spread the eyelids, the prosector grasps a lateral fold of palpebral conjunctiva with tissue forceps and with curved blunt scissors (the writer prefers Metzenbaum scissors) makes an initial incision in the conjunctiva behind the forceps. With gentle traction and well-directed cuts with the scissors, the prosector severs the conjunctiva and extraocular muscles on the lateral, dorsal, and ventral sides of the eye, working toward the cerebral pole where the optic nerve and remaining muscles are cut. The eye is pulled gently forward and remaining extraocular tissue is cut, including the third eyelid. The position of the forceps never need be changed. The globe is placed on a wet sponge to cushion it and the extraocular muscles, fat, and fascia are gently removed close to the sclera, using the convex surface of the scissors.

Although the left and right side identity of the eyes may be made using anatomical landmarks, it is easier to maintain the identity of the eyes by placing the globes in identified containers or to tie a piece of black thread to a bit of loose extraocular tissue on one of the eyes. The eyes are gently lowered by the thread or forceps into the fixative. At least 5 mm of optic nerve should be left attached to the eye. With proper cleaning, the eye will sink in fixative. The thorough cleaning is required to permit rapid penetration of fixative and to prevent retinal detachment because of the pressure exerted by contracting muscles. For the same reason, the globe should not be grasped by the fingers.

Usually, eyes are not weighed. Measuring the diameters of unfixed globes is time consuming and increases the likelihood of retinal detachment. The volume of an eye is easily determined by displacement. Choose a graduated cylinder with an inside diameter just great enough to accept an eye. Partially fill the cylinder with fixative, read the volume, lower the eye into the fixative, and read the new volume. The difference in the volume readings is the volume of the eye. Using an appropriate cylinder, the volume of a beagle eye can be measured to 0.2 ml. After measuring, the eye is poured into the primary container of fixative.

There appears to be no ideal fixative for the eye. Ten percent neutral buffered formalin generally gives good results for the cornea and lens but poor results for the retina. Rapidly penetrating fixatives such as Zenker's, Helly's, and Bouin's are generally good for the retina, but require strict attention to a fixation schedule to avoid over fixation. Many additional fixatives have been used. The author has had good results with 2.5% phosphate buffered glutaraldehyde. Dog eyes placed in this fixative may be "cut in" in 1.5–2.0 hr, allowing a gross examination while the tissues retain much of their original color and the lens is still relatively clear. Fixation is complete in about 72 hr. Davidson's fixative (Humason, 1972) is a simple, easy to use fixative that gives good results. Unless there is good reason to do otherwise, the canine eye should be trimmed perpendicular to the horizontal meridian (posterior ciliary vessels) to obtain a midsagittal block that includes the tapetal and nontapetal fundus and optic nerve. A complete sampling of the eye would include a transverse section of the optic nerve. Preparing top-quality eye sections requires special skill and (as with neurohistological technique) should be reserved for the experienced histotechnician with the time and interest to devote to the subject.

Ear

The middle and inner ears are not routinely examined in toxicology studies; however, it is not difficult to collect and prepare sections that include the tympanic membrane and middle and inner ears. The external ear is removed close to the tympanic membrane. After removal of the brain and disarticulation of the mandible, two transverse cuts are made through the base of the skull just anterior and posterior to the external acoustic meatus. One of these cuts will usually just enter the tympanic cavity of the middle ear. After ample fixation and decalcification (the temporal bone is very dense), the specimens may be trimmed and processed in a routine manner.

Pathology

Only Glaister (1986) reports ocular disease, and his observations are limited to sores and conjunctivitis (without elaboration). Oghiso et al. (1982) mention lymphoid cell infiltration of the third eyelid and gland of the third eyelid. Hottendorf and Hirth (1974) examined both eyes in 85% of their studies but report no ocular pathology. Rubin and Saunders (1965) report *Toxocara* granuloma in the retina or choroid in three young beagles.

Heywood et al. (1976) followed ocular changes in 86 laboratory beagles from 6 months to 8 years of age, at which time the animals were necropsied. Prominent posterior lens sutures were the only ophthalmological change seen in beagles under 3 years of age. From 3 to 8 years of age, ophthalmological changes included corneal opacities, asteroid bodies, and tapetal pigmentation. For the lens they reported prominent posterior sutures, nuclear opacities, and anterior, posterior, and peripheral capsular opacities. Histological findings at 8 years of age included: keratitis, cystoid degeneration of the retina (85% incidence), thinning, and absence of tapetal cells, pigment cells in rod and cone layer, scarring of the retina, and calcified body between the pigment epithelial layer and choroid.

Schiavo and Field (1974) examined 532 beagles of various ages ophthalmoscopically and biomicroscopically and reported the following in dogs between 6 and 12 months of age: superficial keratitis, deep keratitis, posterior polar opacities, posterior cortical opacities, prominent posterior lens sutures, lenticular sheen, vacuoles in lens cortex, persistent hyaloid vessel remnants, zones of discontinuity (lens), vitreous floaters/filaments, atapetal fundi, tigroid fundi, tapetal aberrations/pigment clumps, peripapillary reflectivity, and increased tapetal reflectivity. Lenticular sheen is a yellowish reflection from the lens media and is generally expected as a senile change. The hyaloid artery is responsible for development of the vitreous and for nourishment of the fetal lens. Normally, the vessel regresses shortly after birth, but sometimes remains to be seen in the adult. Zones of discontinuity reflect stratification of lens fibers and is thought of as a presenile change. Vitreous floaters are asteroid bodies (small calcium bodies). Vitreous filaments are fibrous strands from vitreous hemorrhage or remnants of the posterior vascular capsule. Tigroid fundi describes the appearance of choroidal vessels through areas of nonpigmented pigment epithelium. Tapetal aberrations include areas of hyperreflectivity and old hemorrhage or scars.

Bellhorn (1974) reports similar ocular findings in 8- to 10-month-old beagles plus prolapse of the third eyelid.

The abundance of ophthalmoscopic observations and the paucity of histological findings emphasize the comparative sensitivities of the two modes of examination. The discrepancy is easily understood for the ophthalmologist has the entire living cornea, iris, lens, and fundus to examine. On the other hand, the pathologist is limited to one or two thin sections of an organ that is both difficult to fix and difficult to section.

Peripheral retinal cystoid degeneration describes single or multiple microcysts within the retina at or near the ora serrata. This is a common change in older beagles, but it also occurs in young animals. The lesion has no apparent functional significance. Focal retinal dysplasia manifested as retinal folds, retinal rosettes, focal absence of retinal cells, and blending of nuclear layers is not an infrequent finding. Protrusion of the third eyelid may be seen in young beagles. Histological findings include inflammation of the bulbar conjunctiva and stroma of the superficial gland. The ducts of the gland may be dilated and contain leukocytes. The conjunctival lymphoid tissue is usually hyperplastic.

There is no mention of ear pathology in the review articles. Cutaneous lesions of the external ear were discussed with the integumentary system.

Metabolism   **Christopher P. Chengelis**

Among the nonrodent species, the dog has been the best characterized with regard to xenobiotic metabolism. This is probably because the dog has been extensively used in biomedical research for almost 100 years. Its relatively large size also provides the advantage of allowing repeat serial sampling of large amounts of biological fluids for time-course analyses. Data on the dog is a staple in numerous review articles and book chapters published on species comparisons elsewhere (see Chap. 1). The focus here will not only be on species differences, but also on other items (e.g., inducibility) that have not necessarily been covered in detail elsewhere. Insofar as the beagle dog is the more common breed used in toxicity testing, this chapter will focus on data from beagles, and discuss data from other breeds where available.

As reported by Gregus et al. (1978), the dog has a somewhat smaller liver to body weight ratio than the rat (2.3 vs 4.0%) and somewhat less microsomal protein (20.5 vs 25.7 mg/g liver). Some of the more common parameters of hepatic xenobiotic metabolism in the dog are summarized in Table 2. Concentrations of cytochrome P-450 range from about 0.30 to 0.80 nmol/mg protein. Using HPLC and other techniques, Amacher and Smith (1987) characterized the cytochrome P-450 isozymic "fingerprint" of naive beagle dogs. Their results suggested that cytochrome P-450 exits as three distinct isozymic groups in female dogs, and two main groups and two to three subgroups in male dogs. Further, they identified sex-related differences in chromatographic behavior between the major isozymic groups. This is an interesting finding because few, if any, sex-related differences in the activity of the microsomal mixed function oxidase (MMFO) have been identified in dogs.

Ohta, et al. (1989) has identified two PCB-inducible isozymes (P-450-D2 and P-450-D3), which are immunologically similar to rat cytochrome P-450d. In a reconstituted MMFO system, these isozymes activated aflatoxin and benzo(a)pyrene in the Ames assay. This group (Ohta et al., 1989b) has also compared the activation by dog, monkey, and human microsomes of four representative mutagens in the Ames assay. As could be expected, there were species differences. The dog produced the highest number of revertants with 3-aminio-1-methyl-5H-pyrido-[4,3-b]indole acetate, which was inhibited (approximately 50%) by antibodies to rat cytochrome P-448.

McKillop (1985), using SDS-PAGE techniques, identified three major cytochrome P-450 isozymes in uninduced adult male dogs. Phenobarbital increased the levels of two of these major isozymes, but primarily caused an increase in another (fourth) isozyme. β-Naphthaflavone caused increases in yet another three other isozymes that are only present in very small amounts in naive animals. Hence, as a generality, the beagle dog has at least seven isozymic forms of cytochrome P-450, including a cytochrome P-448 with some homology with that of the rat, but which are differentiated on the basis of molecular weight, substrate specificity, and responses to inducers.

In general, the dog has less ability than the rat to form hydroxylated aromatic metabolites via the MMFO. For example, in the metabolism of amphetamine, the dog produces very little 4-hydroxyamphetamine (as reviewed by Williams, 1972). Cook et al. (1982) reported that the dog, as opposed to the rat, produces no phenoxyl metabolites of disopyramide. Aniline-hydroxylating activity in dogs tends to be less than that of rats. Gregus and colleagues (1983) have reported benzo(a)pyrene-hydroxylating activity in the dog is much less than that of the rat. There are exceptions; for example, the dog has a much higher rate (15 times) of metabolism with 2,2',4,4',5,5-hexachlorobiphenyl than the rat (Duignan et al., 1987). Some care must be taken in interpreting data on aniline hydroxylase in the dog, as this species produces both ortho- and para-aminophenol from aniline at a ratio of 1/2 (p/o) (Williams, 1972). In the rat, this ratio is 6/1. As the common colormetric method (formation of a quinolinidine complex with phenol) of determining aniline hydroxylation is specific for p-aminophenol, the activities reported for aniline hydroxylase in the dog are probably low. With many other typical substrates (dealkylation rather than aromatic hydroxylation), MMFO activity in the dog is often comparable to those of the rat. Microsomal aminopyrine metabolism, for example, is about the same in dogs as in rats (Lan et al., 1983). Gregus, et al. (1983) reported that the rat had about twice the activity with benzphetamine, but four times the activity than with ethylmorphine than dogs. In contrast, dogs have a higher baseline level than rats for 7-ethoxycoumarin (primarily a substrate for P-450–dependent MMFO) and 7-ethoxyresorufin (primarily a substrate for P-448 dependent MMFO) deethylating activities (Gregus et al., 1983; McKillop, 1985), but greater degrees of induction (with either phenobarbital or β-naphthaflavone) occur in the rat than in the dog (McKillop, 1985). Thus, in comparing the rat and the dog (probably the two most common species in toxicity testing), one should not assume that the rat has the more rapid rates of MMFO activity.

There is considerable evidence that the MMFO of rats has stereospecificity. For example, Heimark and Trager (1985) compared the microsomal metabolism of R and S warfarin. The overall rate of oxidation (total product) was much greater with the R entaniomer. There was also a difference in major metabolite from 8-hydroxy-warfarin for the R to 6-hydroxy-warfarin for the S entaniomer. There is some evidence for MMFO stereospecificity in the dog. Cook et al. (1982) examined the disposition of (R) and (S) disopyramide in vivo in dogs. The (R) entaniomer had significantly longer half life than the (S). In addition, a much higher percentage of dose of S-disopyramide was excreted in the urine as the major metabolite. In general, one should expect stereoselective metabolism of racemic mixtures in the dog.

Surprisingly little in-depth work has been reported on the effects of inhibitors on microsomal metabolism in the dog. Golan et al. (1980) compared the effects of three standard inhibitors (metyrapone, tetrahydrofuran, and α-naphthalflavone). Metyrapone proved to be a very potent inhibitor of 7-ethoxycoumarin deethylation in the dog, the IC_{50} being approximately 0.010 mM. This is an order of magnitude lower than the concentration required to achieve comparable inhibition in rat microsomal preparations. In contrast, tetrahydrofuran at 100 mM was more potent in rat rather than dog preparations. As could be expected, α-naphthalflavone, a specific inhibitor for cytochrome P-448–dependent activity, did not inhibit 7-ethoxycoumarin deethylation in either species.

As mentioned, the MMFO is inducible in the dog. McKillop (1985) examined the inducing effect of phenobarbital and β-naphthaflavone in beagle dogs. Phenobarbital (in saline) was administered ip for 7 days; 20 mg/kg for 2 days, 10 mg/kg for 2 days, and 20 mg/kg for the final 3 days. β-Naphthaflavone in arachis oil) was given ip for 6 or 7 days; 10 mg/kg. The phenobarbital treatment increased cytochrome P-450 by approximately 250%, whereas the β-naphthaflavone caused approximately a 100% increase, with a shift from cytochrome P-450 to cytochrome P-488. In contrast, β-naphthaflavone caused a greater increase (175%) in NADPH: cytochrome C reductase than phenobarbital (41%). This latter change contrasts with that of the rat, in which typical P-448 inducers do not cause increases in the reductase activity. The increases were accompanied by the expected increases in enzyme activity: aldrin epoxidase was increased by phenobarbital, 7-ethoxyresorufin deethylase was increased by β-naphthaflavone, and 7-ethoxycoumarin was increased by both. Duignan et al. (1987) used a step-wise regimen (to avoid excessive sedation) to induce beagle dogs with phenobarbital (Na^+ salt): 10 mg/kg (po) for 2 days, followed by 30 mg/kg for 4 days, then 30 mg/kg for a final 8 days. This regimen more than doubled the microsomal concentration of cytochrome P-450 as well as significantly by increasing the activities toward 7-ethoxycoumarin, warfarin, and androstenedione. There were changes in region and site specificity that indicate that induction in the dog, as in the rat, is accompanied by shifts in isozymic character of cytochrome P-450.

Aldrich and Niems (1979) examined the effects of phenobarbital and β-naphthaflavone on the metabolism of caffeine in vivo in the dog. Both phenobarbital (10 mg/kg/day po for 7 days) and β-naphthaflavone (20 mg/kg/day ip for 3 days) decreased the half-life of caffeine, but only β-naphthaflavone caused a qualitative shift in the spectrum of urinary metabolites.

Gascon-Barre et al. (1986) studied the effects of phenobarbital induction of the MMFO on vitamin D metabolism in mongrel dogs. Dogs were given approximately 80 mg/kg/day for 30 days and induction was monitored by following changes *in vivo* [^{14}C]aminopyrine metabolism ($^{14}C\text{-}CO_2$ production). The paper does not mention complications due to the sedative effects of phenobarbital. As might have been expected in an outbred population, some dogs were more inducible than others. In fact, in two dogs, no induction occurred at all. Not surprisingly, induction resulted in increased hepatic catabolism of vitamin D_3. The important points to be stressed here are that variable responses of dogs to inducing agents can be a potential problem and that in vivo clearance of aminopyrine could provide a noninvasive probe for screening of "good" vs "poor" responders to inducing agents of the phenobarbital class.

The inducing effects of drugs and chemicals other than of phenobarbital and β-naphthaflavone (typical experimental tools) have also been studied in the dog. Lan et al. (1983) compared and contrasted the inducing effect of hexahydroindazole (10–250 mg/kg/day for a month) in three species. Increases in relative liver weights occurred in all three species, but increases in microsomal protein only in rats and monkeys. Increases in cytochrome P-450 and aminopyrine metabolism occurred in all three species, but the largest increases (compared to concurrent controls) were observed in dogs.

Abramson et al. (1986) and Abramson and Lutz (1986a,b) have extensively studied the relationship between enzyme induction, in vivo antipyrine metabolism and increases in alpha-1 acid glycoprotein. While the relationship between the latter two parameters is not a simple one, they can be used to monitor the extent of induction by phenobarbital-type agents in the dog. Using these techniques, they demonstrated that phenytoin (Abramson and Lutz, 1986a) and rifampicin (Abramson and Lutz, 1986b) are effective inducing agents in the dog, while medroxyprogesterone was not (Abramson et al., 1986). The latter finding is of interest because medroxyprogesterone has been reported to be an inducing agent in rats. This underscores again the point that there are species-related differences in responses to inducing agents.

Epoxide hydrolase is an important enzyme in the metabolism of reactive arene oxides, but up until 1980 little work had been done to characterize this enzyme in the dog. In 1981, Pacifici et al., reported the activity of hepatic microsomal epoxide hydrolase (with styrene oxide) in the dog to be 9.7 ± 2.0 nmol/min/mg protein, which was intermediate between that of the mouse 1.9 nmol/min/mg) and the baboon (31.3 nmol/min/mg). Gregus et al. (1983) confirmed that the dog has relatively high epoxide hydrolase activity (approx 15 nmol/min/mg protein) compared to many other commonly used laboratory species, including the rat. Little other work has been completed to distinguish, either on structural or substrate specificity basis, epoxide hydrolase of the dog from that of other species. Given its high activity, however, it can be expected to play an important role in xenobiotic metabolism in the dog.

As in other species, conjugative metabolism (other than mercapturic acid formation) has been studied in the dog longer than oxidative metabolism. As reviewed by Hirom et al. (1977), the majority of the conjugative reactions were described in Germany during the latter part of the nineteenth century. The dog, like most mammals, excrete phenols as sulfates and glucuronides. The exceptions to this rule are cats and pigs; the former generally lack the ability to make glucuronides and the latter generally do not make sulfates. In the dog, the ratio of sulfate to glucuronide (at an aromatic hydroxyl group) varies with substrate. For example, with phenolphthalein, the dog will excrete 18% as the glucuronide and 82% as the sulfate (as reviewed by Hirom et al., 1977), whereas with acetaminophen, 75% will be excreted as the glucuronide and 10–20% as the sulfate (Hjelle and Grauer, 1986). With aryl acetates, the dog has a high tendency to form conjugates with amino acids. For example, with benzoic acid, the dog will excrete 82% as the glycine conjugate (hippuric acid) and only 18% as the glucuronide.

Relatively little work has focused on the biochemical and molecular characterization of the enzymes involved in conjugation in the dog. Gregus et al. (1983) examined the in vitro activity of PAPS-sulfontransferase of the dog against four substrates. Activity was noted with all four: the highest with 2-naphthol and the lowest with taurolithocholate. When compared to other species, the sulfotransferase activity of the dog tended to be lower than most.

Gregus et al. 1983 examined the activity of UDP-glucuronosyl transferase against a wide variety of substrates. The dog had somewhat higher activities than the rat with 1-naphthol, p-nitrophenol, estrone, morphine, and digitoxigenin-monodigitoxoside, whereas the opposite was true with diethylstilbestrol and bilirubin. Hence, in terms of relative activity there is little to distinguish the UDP-glucuronosyl transferases of the dog from those of other species. There is evidence, however, of species differences in stereoselectivity. Wilson and Thompson (1984) examined the stereoselectivity of dog hepatic microsomal UDP-glucuronosyl transferase by examining differences in activity toward (R)- and (S)-propranolol. When racemic mixtures were studied, the (S) entaniomer was the preferred substrate, with 3 to 4 times more (S)-propanolol glucuronide produced than that of the (R) entaniomer. Additional experiments with separate entaniomers demonstrated that the K_m and V_{max} of the dog microsomal UDP-glucuronosyl transferase are much higher with the (S) than the (R) entaniomer. In human subjects, plasma levels of (R)-propranolol have been shown to be higher than those of (S)-propranolol (Silbert et al. 1982), whereas the opposite has been shown in dogs (Walle and Walle, 1979), and this difference may be due to the differences in stereospecificity of glucuronidation in the dog vs human (Von Bahr et al., 1982). Stereospecificity of UDP-glucuronosyl transferase with substrates other than propranolol has been reported for other species (Sisenwine et al., 1982). Thus, stereospecificity of UDP-glucuronosyl transferase in not unique to the dog or propranolol.

Schmoldt and colleagues (1987) examined the in vitro glucuronidation rates of dog liver microsomes toward various cardiac glycosides. In contrast to most other species examined, dog UDP-glucuronosyl transferase is capable of conjugating digitoxin; otherwise glucuronidation rates between rats and dogs were similar for all other cardiac glycosides examined. In fact, neither species has detectable activity toward digoxin. As both dog and humans rapidly eliminate (in vivo) administered doses of digoxin, these results suggest that there may be greater similarity between canine and human UDP-glucuronosyl transferase than between the human and rat enzyme with regard to substrate specificity. UDP-Glucuronosyl transferase exits as a family of different isozymes in rats (Knapp et al., 1988). The Schmoldt et al. article (1987) is one of the few to discuss the isozymic character of UDP-glucuronosyl transferase in dogs. By examining a variety of model substrate and various inhibitors, they concluded that while there may be more than one canine isozyme, a single isozyme in the dog was responsible for glucuronidation of all cardiac glycosodise.

The dog has long been recognized to have less active N-acetyl transferase activity than other species (Williams, 1972). This was more recently confirmed by Gregus et al. (1983), who demonstrated that the dog had almost imperceptible activity with five different substrates. This is a qualitative species difference which could result in toxicologically important species-related differences in metabolism. For example, arylamines require acetylation to be activated to mutagens and carcinogens. In an interesting paper, Neis et al. (1985) compared the cytochrome P-450 content, N-acetyltransferase activity, and mutagenic activation activity of canine and human isolated hepatocytes. The mutagenic activation of five different arylamines was examined, and it was found that human hepatocytes had much greater mutagenic "activation" activity; this difference was attributed to the N-acetyltransferase present in human cells. Paroxon, an inhibitor of acetyl transferase, decreased mutagenic activation by human hepatocytes. They noted incidently that dog hepatocytes were approximately the same size as human hepatocytes, but those of the dog had higher concentrations of cytochrome P-450; 210 ± 10 vs 94 ± 2 pmol/10E6 cells. N-Acetylation is thus involved in the activation of arylamines in humans, and therefore the dog may not be the appropriate model in which to study the toxicity (relative to humans) of arylamines.

Arylamines are not only substrates of the MMFO, but they can also be substrates for the flavin-based mixed function oxidase (FMFO). The FMFO of the dog has not been isolated and well characterized like that of the pig or the rat, but differential arylamine metabolism and the use of specific inhibitors has provided a probe for studying the involvement of this enzyme in dog xenobiotic metabolism. 2,[(2,4-Dichloro-6-phenyl)phenoxy]-ethalamine (DPEA) is a specific cytochrome P-450 inhibitor and methimazole is a competitive inhibitor of FMFO. Using these, Hammons et al. (1985) have reported that the FMFO metabolized 2-acetylaminofluorene in pigs and humans, but not in dogs and rats. This group also studied the in vitro metabolism of 1-naphthylamine (1-NA) and 2-naphthylamine (2-NA) in rats, dogs, and humans. N-Hydroxylation is a major pathway in all three species for 2-NA, but not for 1-NA, and this reaction is exclusively mediated by the MMFO. Ring hydroxylation, however, also occurred in all three species, and may be partially mediated by the FMFO as well as the MMFO because it was not completely inhibited by DPEA. For both chemicals, the dog has a higher rate of metabolism than the rat. Interestingly, there were greater individual human-to-human differences in the microsomal metabolism of these chemicals than the differences between rats and dogs.

Like all known and studied mammals, dogs have hepatic cytosolic glutathione S-transferase (GSH-T). Grover and Sims described this enzyme in dogs as early as 1964, and were the first to note the high activity the dog GSH-T has with 1,2-dichloro-4-nitrobenzene. Gregus et al. (1983) examined glutathione S-transferase activity against six different model substrates. Rats and dogs tended to have the equivalent activity with

1-chloro-2,4-dinitrobenzene and 1,2-dichloro-4-nitrobenzene; otherwise rats has much higher activity than dogs with all other substrates examined.

In 1985, Weiner confirmed in mongrel dogs the observation as to GSH-T activity toward 1,2-dichloro-4-nitrobenzene, and further compared the activities of rat and dog cytosolic preparations against seen other substrates and found that activity in the dog ranged from 2.5% (4-nitropyridine N-oxide) to 95% (ethacrynic acid) of those of the rat. Over all, the highest activity in dogs (and rats, for that matter) was obtained with 1-chloro-2,4-dinitrobenzene. Weiner further characterized GSH-T in various cytosolic protein fractions. He found that dog GSH-T exists as four different isozymes composed of three different classes of subunits. In general, this type of isozymic pattern for this enzyme has been seen in other species. The dog enzymes are also not very different with regard to sensitivity to inhibitory ligands, such as bomcresol green or 8-anilino-1-naphthalene (Weiner, 1985). Therefore, except for the expected molecular and quantitative activity differences, GSH-T in the dog is not startlingly different from that of other species. Weiner did observe that dog GSH-T has some activity in the denitrification of organic nitrates, such as isosorbide-2,5-dinitrate, and that this activity was responsible for the rapid in vivo conversion of 2,3-di-O-nitro-adenosine-5'-(N-ethyl-carboxamide) to the mono-nitro chemical in the dog (Wiener et al., 1983). Whether this is a pathway unique to the dog remains to be established.

In general, little in-depth work on extrahepatic metabolism in the dog has been reported, the exception being work done at the Lovelace Inhalation Toxicology Research Institute on the respiratory tract. Halley and Dahl (1983) studied the cytochrome P-450–dependent mono-oxygenase activity in the nasal membrane of several species. The dog tended to have the lowest amount of cytochrome P-450 and the lowest MMFO activities.

Bond et al. (1987) characterized the cellular and regional distribution of xenobiotic-metabolizing enzymes in the respiratory airways of beagles and found detectable cytochrome P-450 dependent activity throughout the airway, from the alar fold to the peripheral lung, but there were regional and substrate differences in specific activities. For example, the ethmoid rubinate had high activities for both benzo(a)pyrene and ethoxy-coumarin metabolism, while higher nasal regions (alar fold, nasoturbinate and maxilloturbinate) had much higher activity with ethoxycoumarin. In general, epoxide hydrolase and glutathione S-transferase activities were present along the entire airway, but tended to be higher in the nasal region and pulmonary airways compared to the major airways. UDP-Glucuronosyl transferase tended to be evenly distributed. These "detoxification" enzymes were present in much greater activity than the MMFO-cytochrome P-450–dependent "activation" system. This work provides an excellent basis for using the dog in the study of site-specific chemical carcinogenesis of the respiratory tract.

For example, Petridou-Fischer and colleagues (1987) studied the in vivo disposition of nasally instilled dihydrosafrole in the dog, and recovered metabolites from the nasopharyngeal mucus, thus confirming the potential importance of the MMFO activities in the upper respiratory tract in the metabolic activation of potential carcinogens.

Other aspects of extrahepatic metabolism in the dog have been partially investigated as part of studies of various species-related differences in target organ toxicity. Garst et al. (1985) examined the pulmonary metabolism of perilla ketone by a variety of species, and concluded that the insensitivity of the dog lung to perilla ketone toxicity resulted from the relatively low amount of cytochrome P-450 with low MMFO activity toward perilla ketone.

Poupko et al. (1983) reported that the dog bladder microsomes had very low activity with both 1- and 2-naphthylamine.

Menard and colleagues (1979) examined both testicular and adrenal cytochrome P-450 in the dog, guinea pig, and rat. The dog and rat had comparable concentrations of adrenal cytochrome P-450 (1.1–1.2 nmol/mg microsome protein), whereas the guinea pig had roughly twice this concentration. In contrast, the dog had the highest concentration of testicular cytochrome P-450 (0.170 nmol/mg microsomal protein) and the rat the lowest (0.067 nmol/mg microsomal protein). Administration of spironolactone, a 7-α-thiosteroid, led to the destruction (40–60%) of the cytochrome P-450s of both tissues in the dog. In contrast, spironolactone had no effect on adrenal cytochrome P-450 in the rat, but caused large decreases (88%) in testicular cytochrome P-450.

Pacifici et al. (1981) reported on species and tissue difference in epoxide hydrolase and glutathione S-transferase. The authors found the epoxide hydrolase activity of the dog kidney to be comparable to that of the guinea pig and rabbit, but less than that of the hamster. Glutathione S-transferase activity of the kidney of the dog (with styrene oxide, the same substrate used to determine epoxide hydrolase activity) tended to be much lower than those of the guinea pig and rat, but higher than those of the human and monkey. Therefore, there are species differences in extrahepatic cytochrome P-450 of which the investigator should be aware, but it does not appear that the dog offers advantages over any other species in the study of specific routes of extrahepatic metabolism.

Very little work has been reported on developmental or age-related changes in drug metabolism in the dog. Tavoloni (1985) examined the age-related development of the cytochrome P-450 MMFO and UDP-glucuronosyl transferase in the beagle dog. Activities were lowest at birth. They increased thereafter, tending to plateau after 6 weeks of age. Increases in the MMFO, but not UDP-glucuronosyl transferase, were induced by phenobarbital.

Baarnhielm et al. (1986) compared and contrasted the in vivo and in vitro metabolism of felodlipne in the rat, dog, and human. Felodipine is a calcium channel blocker which is very lipophilic, well absorbed from the gastrointestinal tract, highly protein bound, and extensively metabolized. Comparative in vitro rates of microsomal metabolism of felodipine were rat>dog>human. There was an excellent correlation between the V_{max}s and the concentrations of cytochrome P-450. The same rank order was observed for in vivo plasma clearance. The authors ran through various pharmacokinetic formulas and concluded that the data obtained in vitro could be used to predict the results in vivo with regard to such parameters as hepatic clearance and extraction ratios. It would appear that with chemicals that are well absorbed and rapidly metabolized, interspecies extrapolations are possible and fairly predictive. In their studies on the disposition of etodolac, Cayen and colleagues (1981) observed that felodlipne also was well absorbed, partially metabolized (different metabolites in dog and rat), and undergoes extensive intrahepatic circulation. There were differences in the serum half-life (human>dog>rat) and clearance (dog>human>rat), but there was greater similarity between the dog and human. In general, the dog appears to be a better pharmacokinetic model (more predictive of behavior in human subjects) for humans than the rat or other rodents for chemicals that are well absorbed and have a high hepatic clearance.

REFERENCES

Abramson, F., and Lutz, M. (1986a) The effects of phenytoin dosage on the induction of alpha-1-acid glycoprotein and antipyrine clearance in the dog. *Eur. J. Drug Metab. Pharmacokin.* 11, 135–143.

Abramson, F., and Lutz, M. (1986b) The kinetics of induction by rifampicin of alpha-1-acid glycoprotein and antipyrine clearance in the dog. *Drug Metab. Dispos.* 14, 46–51.

Abramson, F., Moore, C., and Hill, M. (1986) Medroxyprogesterone acetate does not induce antipyrine clearance and only weekly increases alpha-1-acid glycoprotein in beagle dogs. *Res. Commun. Chem. Pathol. Pharmacol.* 53:65–78.

Adam, W.S., Calhoun, M.L., Smith, E. M., and Stinson, A. W. (1970) *Microscopic Anatomy of the Dog. A Photographic Atlas.* Thomas, Springfield, Illinois, pp. 1–292.

Adams, D. R., and Hotchiss, D. K. (1983) The canine nasal mucosa. *Zbl. Vet. Med. C. Anat. Histol. Embryol.* 12, 109–125.

Al-Bagdadi, F.A., Titkemeyer, C.W., and Lovell, J.E. (1977) Hair follicle cycle and shedding in male beagle dogs. *Am. J. Vet. Res.* 38, 611–616.

Aldridge, A., and Neims, A. (1979) The effects of phenobarbital and β-naphthaflavone on the elimination kinetics and metabolite pattern of caffeine in the beagle dog. *Drug Metab. Dispos.* 7, 378–382.

Amacher, D., and Smith, D. (1987) Differences in the constructive forms of hepatic cytochrome P-450 in male and female adult beagle dogs. *J. Chromatogr.* 419, 61–73.

Amann, R.P. (1982) Use of animal models for detecting specific alterations in reproduction. *Fund. Appl. Toxicol.* 2, 13–26.

Andersen, A.C. (1970) *The Beagle as an Experimental Dog.* Iowa State University Press, Ames, pp. 1–616.

Andersen, A.C., and Goldman, M. (1970) Growth and development, in *The Beagle as an Experimental Dog*, Andersen, A.C., ed. Iowa State University Press, Ames, pp. 43–105.

Andersen, A.C., and Rosenblatt, L.S. (1974) Survival of the beagle under natural and laboratory conditions, in Andersen, A.C., Boyden, E.A., and Dougherty, J.H., eds. *Dogs and other large mammals in aging research.* Vol. 1. MSS Information Corp., New York, pp. 19–25.

Anderson, C., and Danylchuk, K. D. (1978) Bone-remodeling rates of the beagle: A comparison between different sites in the same rib. *Am. J. Vet. Res.* 39, 1763–5.

Anderson, C., and Danylchuk, K.D. (1979a) Studies on bone-remodeling rates in the beagle: a comparison between similar biopsy sites on different ribs. *Am. J. Vet. Res.* 40, 294–6.

Anderson, C., and Danylchuk, K.D. (1979b) Studies on bone-remodeling rates in the beagle: Age-related variations in cortical bone remodeling measurements in male beagles 10 to 26 months of age. *Am. J. Vet. Res.* 40:869–72.

Anderson, C., and Danylchuk, K.D. (1979c) Appositional bone formation rates in beagles. *Am. J. Vet Res.* 40, 907–910.

Armstrong, R.B., Saubert, W., Seeherman, H.J., and Taylor, C.R. (1982) Distribution of fiber types in locomotory muscles in dogs. *Am. J. Anat.* 163, 87–98.

Asbury, A.K. (1973) Renaut bodies. A forgotten structure. *J. Neuropathol. and Exp. Neurol.* 32, 334–343.

Asbury, A.K., and Johnson, P.C. (1978) *Pathology of the Peripheral Nerve.* Saunders, Philadelphia, pp. 1–311.

Baarnhielm, C., Dahlback, H., and Skanberg, I. (1986) *In vivo* pharmacokinetics of felodipine predicted from studies in rat, dog, and man. *Acta Pharmacol. Toxicol.* 59, 113–122.

Baetjier, A.M. (1968) Role of environmental temperature and humidity in susceptibility to disease. *Arch. Environ. Health* 16, 565–579.

Bailey, C.S., and Morgan, J.P., (1983) Diseases of the spinal cord, in *Textbook of Veterinary Internal Medicine. Diseases of the Dog and Cat.* Vol. 1. 2nd ed., Ettinger, S.J., ed. Saunders, Philadelphia, pp. 532–608.

Barker I.K., and Van Dreumel, A.A. (1985) The alimentary system, in *Pathology of Domestic Animals.* Vol. 2. 3rd ed., Jubb, K.V.F., Kennedy, P.C., and Palmer, N., eds. Academic Press, San Diego, pp. 1–237.

Barron, C.N., and Zaunders, L.Z. (1966) Visceral larva migrans in the dog. *Pathol. Vet.* 3, 315–330.

Bartley, M.H., Taylor, G.N., Jee, W.S.S. (1970) Teeth and mandible, in *The Beagle as an Experimental Dog*, Andersen, A.C., ed. The Iowa State University Press, Ames, pp. 189–225.

Bebiak, D.M., Lawler, D.F., and Reutzel, L.F. (1987) Nutrition and management of the dog. *Vet. Clin. North Am. Small Anim. Pract.* 17, 505–533.

Beierwaltes, W.H., and Nishiyama, R.H. (1968) Dog thyroiditis: Occurrence and similarity to Hashimoto's struma. *Endocrinology* 85, 501–508.

Bekaert, D.A. (1982) *Handbook of diseases from dogs and cats to man*. California Veterinary Medical Association, Moraga.

Bellhorn, R.W. (1974) A survey of ocular findings in eight-to-ten-month-old beagles. *J. Am. Vet. Med. Assoc.* 164, 1114–1116.

Besch, E.L., Kadono, H., and Brigman, R.L. (1984) Body temperature changes in dogs exposed to varying effective temperatures. *Lab. Anim. Sci.* 34, 177–180.

Bond, J., Harkema, J., and Russell, V. (1988) Regional distribution of xenobiotic metabolizing enzymes in respiratory airways of dogs. *Drug Metab. Dispos.* 16, 116–124.

Breazile, J.E. (1976) Ear, in *Textbook of veterinary histology*, Dellmann, H.D., and Brown, E.M., eds. Lea & Febiger, Philadelphia, pp. 443–456.

Brewster, R.D., Benjamin, S.A., and Thomassen, R.W. (1983) Spontaneous cor pulmonale in laboratory beagles. *Lab Anim. Sci.* 33, 299–302.

Brown, E.M. (1976) Urinary system, in *Textbook of veterinary histology*, Dellmann, H.D., and Brown, E.M., eds. Lea & Febiger, Philadelphia, pp. 267–318.

Brown, E.M., and Dellman, H.D. (1976) Lymphatic system, in *Textbook of veterinary histology*, Dellman, H.D., and Brown, E.M., eds. Lea & Febiger, Philadelphia, pp. 163–184.

Calhoun, M.I., and Stinson, A.W. (1976) Integument, in *Textbook of veterinary histology*, Dellmann, H.D., and Brown, E.M., eds. Lea & Febiger, Philadelphia, pp. 459–493.

Cameron, A.M., and Faulkin, L.J. Jr. (1971) Hyperplastic and inflammatory nodules in the canine mammary gland. *J. Natl. Cancer Inst.* 47, 1277–1287.

Campbell, S.A., Hughes, H.C., Giffin, H.E., Landi, M.S., and Mallon, F.M. (1988) Some effects of limited exercise on purpose-bred beagles. *Am. J. Vet. Res. (U.S.).* 49, 1298–1301.

Capen, C.C. (1985) The endocrine glands, in *Pathology of domestic animals*, Vol. 3. 3rd ed. Jubb, K.V.F., Kennedy, P.C., and Palmer, N., eds. Academic Press, San Diego, pp. 237–303.

Cayan, M., Kraml, M., Ferdinandi, E., Greselin, E., and Dvornik, D. (1981) The metabolic disposition of etodolac in rats, dogs and man, *Drug Metab. Rev.* 12:339–362.

Christensen, G.C. (1967) The urogenital system and mammary glands, in *Anatomy of the Dog*, Miller, M.E., Christensen, G.C., and Evans, H.E., eds. Saunders Company, Philadelphia, pp. 741–806.

Christie, D.W., and Bell, E.T. (1971) Endocrinology of the oestrus cycle in the bitch. *J. Small Anim. Pract. (Engl.)* 12, 383–389.

Contran, R.S., Kumar, V., and Robbins, S.L. (1989) *Robbins pathologic basis of disease*. 4th ed., Saunders, Philadelphia, pp. 703–754.

Cook, C., Karim, A., and Sollman, (1982) Stereoselectivity in the metabolism of disopyramide enantiomers in rat and dog. *Drug Metab. and Dispos.* 10, 116–121.

Cronkite, E.P. (1973) Blood and lymph, in *Best and Taylor's physiological basis of medical practice*, Brobeck, J.R., ed. Williams & Wilkins, Baltimore, pp. 4–129.

Crow, S.E. (1980) Neoplasms of the preproductive organs and mammary glands of the dog, in *Current therapy in theriogenology: diagnosis, treatment and prevention of reproductive diseases in animals*. Saunders, Philadelphia, pp. 640–646.

Cupps, D.T., Anderson, L.L., and Cole, H.H. (1969) The estrous cycle, in *Reproduction in domestic animals*, Cole, H.H., and Cupps, P.T., eds. Academic Press, New York, pp. 219–250.

De Boer, A.G., Moolenaar, F., De Leede, L.G.J., and Breimer, D.D. (1982) Rectal drug administration: Clinical pharmacokinetic considerations. *Clin. Pharmacokinet.* 7, 285–311.

Dellman, H.D. (1976a) Respiratory system, in *Textbook of veterinary histology*, Dellman, H.D., and Brown, E.M., eds., Lea & Febiger, Philadelphia, pp. 187–203.

Dellman, H.D. (1976b) Endocrine system, in *Textbook of veterinary histology*, Dellman, H.D., Brown, E.M., eds. Lea & Febiger, Philadelphia, pp. 373–399.

Dellman, H.D. (1976c) Eye system, in *Textbook of veterinary histology*, Dellman, H.D., and Brown, E.M., eds. Lea & Febiger, Philadelphia, pp. 423–443.

Dellman, H.D., and Venable, J.H. (1976) Cardiovascular system, in *Textbook of veterinary histology*, Dellman, H.D., and Brown, E.M., eds. Lea & Febiger, Philadelphia, pp. 143–160.

Detweiler, D.K. (1980) The use of electrocardiography in toxicological studies with beagle dogs, in *Cardiac toxicology*. CRC Press, Boca Raton, Florida.

Detweiler, D.K., Patterson, D.F., Buchanan, J.W., and Knight, D.H. (1979) The cardiovascular system, in *Canine medicine. Vol. 2*, Catcott, E.J., ed. American Veterinary Publications, Santa Barbara, California, p. 813.

Doige, C. (1988) Skeletal system, in *Special veterinary pathology*, Thomson, R.G., ed. Decker, Toronto and Philadelphia, pp. 467–507.

Duignan, D., Sipes, G., Leonard, T., and Halpert, J. (1987) Purification and characterization of the dog hepatic cytochrome P-450 isozyme responsible for the metabolism of 2,2',4,4',5,5'-hexachlorobiphenyl. *Arch. Biochem. Biophys.* 255, 290–303.

Duncan, J.R., and Prasse, K.W. (1986) *Veterinary laboratory medicine. Clinical pathology.* Iowa State University Press, Ames, pp. 3–285.

Dungworth, G.L. (1985) The respiratory system, in *Pathology of domestic animals*. Vol. 2. 3rd ed., Jubb, K.V.F., Kennedy, P.C., and Palmer, N.; eds. Academic Press, San Diego, pp. 413–556.

Earl, F.L., Miller, E., and Van Loon, E.J. (1973) Teratogenic research in beagle dogs and miniature swine, in *The laboratory animal in drug testing: 5th symposium internal committee lab animals*, Spiegel, H., ed. pp. 233–247.

Eckenfels, A. (1980) On the variability of the direction of the cardiac vector and of the T-, Q- and S-waves in the normal ECG of the conscious beagle dog. *Arzneimittelforschung 30*(10), 1626–1630.

Eckenfels, A., and Trieb, G. (1979) The normal electrocardiogram of the conscious beagle dog. *Toxicol. Appl. Pharmacol.* 47, 567584.

Eisenbrandt, D.L., and Phemister, R.D. (1977) Radiation injury in the neonatal canine kidney. I. Pathogenesis. *Lab. Invest.* 37, 437–446.

Eisenbrandt, D.L., and Phemister, R.D. (1978) Radiation injury in the neonatal canine kidney. II. Quantitative morphology. *Lab. Invest.* 38, 225–231.

Eisenbrandt, D.L., and Phemister, R.D. (1979) Postnatal development of the canine kidney: Quantitative and qualitative morphology. *Am. J. Anat.* 154, 179–194.

Eisenbrandt, D.L., and Phemister, R.D. (1980) Counting renal corpuscles in tissue sections. *Virchows Arch. B. Cell Pathol.* 32, 177–184.

El Etreby, M.F., and Wrobel, K.H. (1978) Effect of cyproterone acetate, d-norgestrel and progesterone on the canine mammary gland. *Cell Tissue Res.* 194, 245–267.

Engle, E.T. (1946) No seasonal breeding cycle in dogs. *J. Mammals* 27, 79–81.

Ettinger, S.J. (ed.) (1989) Textbook of Veterinary Internal Medicine. 3rd ed. Saunders, Philadelphia.

Fox, M.W. (1965a) Environmental factors influencing stereotyped and Allelomimetic behavior (overt reaction to social stimulation) in animals. *Lab. Anim. Care* 15, 363–370.

Fox, M.W. (1965b) *Canine behav.* Thomas, Springfield, Illinois.

Fritz, T.E., Zeman, R.C., Poole, C.M., and Norris, W.P. (1966) Studies on the spontaneous disease and pathology in the experimental beagle. *Argonne Natl. Lab. Biol. Med. Res. Div. Ann. Rept.* ANL-7278, pp. 114–115.

Fritz, T.E., Zeman, R.C., and Norris, W.P. (1967) Studies on the spontaneous disease and pathology in the experimental beagle colony. *Argonne Natl. Lab. Biol. Med. Res. Div. Ann. Rep.* ANL-7409, pp. 283–284.

Fritz, T.E., Zeman, R.C., and Zelle, A.R. (1970) Pathology and familial incidence of thyroiditis in a closed beagle colony. *Exp. Molec. Pathol.* 12, 14–30.

Fritz, T.E., Lombard, L.S., Tyler, S.A., and Norris, W.P. (1976) Pathology and familial incidence of orchitis and its relation to thyroiditis in a closed beagle colony. *Exp. Mol. Pathol.* 24, 142–158.

Fulper, L.D., Cleary, R.W., Harland, E.C., Hikal, A.H., and Jones, A.B. (1987) Comparison of serum progesterone levels in dogs after administration of progesterone by vaginal tablet and vaginal suppositories. *Am. J. Obstet. Gynecol.* 156, 253–256.

Gaebler, O.H., and Choitz, H.C. (1964) Studies of body water and water turnover determined with deuterium oxide added to food. *Clin. Chem.* 10, 13–18.

Garst, J., Wilson, W., Krstensen, N., Harrison, P., Corbin, J., Simon, J., Philpot, R., and Szabo, R. (1985) Species susceptibility to the pulmonary toxicity of 3-furyl isomyl ketone (perilla ketone): *In vivo* support for the involvement of the lung monooxygenase system. *Anim. Sci.* 60, 248–257.

Gascon-Barre, M., Vallieres, S., and Huet, P. (1986) Influence of phenobarbital on the hepatic handling of [^{3}H]vitamin D_3 in the dog. *Am. J. Physiol.* 251, G627–G635.

Georgi, J.R., and Anderson, R.C. (1975) *Filaroites hirthi* Sp. N. (Nematoda: Metastrongyloidea) from the lung of the dog. *J. Parasitol.* 61, 337–339.

Georgi, J.R., Fleming, W.J., Hirth, R.S., and Cleveland, D.J. (1975) Preliminary investigation of the life history of filaroides hirthi Georgi and Anderson. *Cornell Vet.* 66, 309–323.

Getty, R. (1967) The Eye, orbit and adnexa, in *Anatomy of the dog*, Miller, M.E., Christensen, G.C., and Evans, H.E., eds. Saunders, Philadelphia, pp. 837–847.

Giles, R.C., Kwapien, R.P., Geil, R.G., and Casey, H.W. (1978) Mammary nodules in beagle dogs administered investigational oral contraceptive steroids. *J. Natl. Cancer Inst.* 60, 1351–1364.

Gill, J. (1982) Comparative morphology and ultrastructure of the airways, in *Mechanisms in respiratory toxicology*, Witschi, H., and Netteshein, P., eds., CRC Press, Boca Raton, Florida, pp. 3–25.

Glaister, J.R. (1986) *Principles of toxicological pathology*. Taylor and Francis, London and Philadelphia, pp. 1–223.

Goll, D.E., Stromer, M.H., and Robson, R.M. (1977) Skeletal muscle, nervous system, temperature regulation, and special senses, in *Duke's physiology of domestic animals*, Swenson, M.J., ed. Cornell University Press, Ithaca, New York, and London, pp. 504–651.

Gorton, R.L. (1978) Energy conservation in water heating and HVAC systems, in *Laboratory animal housing. Proceedings of a symposium organized by the ILAR committee on animal housing*, Washington, D.C., pp. 179–183.

Gregus, Z., Watkins, J., Thompson, T., Harvey, M., and Rozman, K., and Klaassen (1983) Hepatic phase I and II biotransformations in quail and trout: Comparison to other species commonly used in toxicity testing. *Toxicol. Appl. Pharmacol.* 67, 430–441.

Green, R.A. (1983) Bleeding Disorders, in *Textbook of veterinary internal medicine. Diseases of the dog and cat.* Vol. 2, Ettinger, S.J., ed., Saunders, Philadelphia, pp. 2076–2098.

Greene, C.E., and Oliver, J.E. (1983) Neurological examination, in *Textbook of veterinary internal medicine. Diseases of the dog and cat.* Vol. 1, Ettinger, S.J., ed. Saunders, Philadelphia, pp. 419–460.

Greve, J.H., and Gaatar, S.M. (1964) Effect of hypothyroidism on canine demodicosis. *Am. J. Vet. Res.* 25, 520–522.

Grover, P., and Sims, P. (1964) Conjugations with glutathione. distribution of glutathione S-aryltransferase in vertebrate species. *Biochem. J.* 90, 603–606.

Gulamhusein, A.P., Harrison-Sage, C., Beck, F., and Al-Alousi, A. (1980) Salicylate-induced teratogenesis in the ferret. *Life Sci.* 27, 1799–1805.

Guttman, P.H. (1970) Renal pathology, in *The beagle as an experimental dog*, Andersen, A.C., ed. The Iowa State University Press, Ames, pp. 546–558.

Guy, R.C. (1989) The effect of overnight water deprivation on pharmacokinetic and clinical chemistry and hematology parameters in the dog. (abstract). Presented at the 10th Annual Meeting of the American College of Toxicology, Williamsburg, Virginia.

Hadley, W., and Dahl, A. (1982) Cytochrome P-450–dependent monooxygenase activity in nasal membranes of six species. *Drug Metab. Dispos.* 11, 275–276.

Hammons, G., Guengerich, F., Weis, C., Beland, F., and Kadlubar, F. (1985) Metabolic oxidation of carcinogenic arylamines by rat, dog and human hepatic microsomes and by purified flavin-containing and cytochrome P-450 monooxygenases. *Cancer Res.* 45, 3578–3585.

Hardy, R.M. (1983) Diseases of the liver, in *Textbook of veterinary internal medicine. Diseases of the dog and cat.* Vol. 2 Ettinger, S.J., ed. Saunders, Philadelphia, pp. 1372–1454.

Hargis, A.M. (1988) Integumentary system, in *Special veterinary pathology,* Thomson, R.G., ed. Decker, Toronto and Philadelphia, pp. 1–68.

Harleman, J.H., Suter, J., and Fischer, M. (1987) Intracytoplasmic eosinophilic inclusion bodies in the liver of beagle dogs. *Lab. Anim. Sci.* 37, 229–31.

Hartman, H.A., Robinson, R.L., and Visscher, G.E. (1975) Naturally occurring intracytoplasmic inclusions in the canine exocrine pancreas. *Vet. Pathol.* 12, 210–219.

Harvey, C.E., O'Brien, J.A., Rossman, L.E., and Stoller, N.H. (1983) Oral, dental, pharyngeal, and salivary gland disorders, in *Textbook of veterinary internal medicine. Diseases of the dog and cat.* Vol. 2, Ettinger, S.J., ed. Saunders, Philadelphia, pp. 1126–1191.

Heimark, L., and Trager, W. (1985) Stereoselective metabolism of conformational analogues of warfarin by β-naphthaflavone-inducible cytochrome P-450. *J. Med. Chem.* 28, 503–506.

Henry, G.A., Long, P.H., Burns, J.L., and Charbonneau, D.L. (1987) Gastric spirillosis in beagles. *Am. J. Vet. Res.* 43, 831–836.

Heywood, R., Hepworth, P.L., and Van Abbe, N.J. (1976) Age changes in the eyes of the beagle dog. *J. Small Anim. Proct.* 17, 171–177.

Hirom, P., Idle, J., and Milburne, P. (1977) Comparative aspects of the biosynthesis and excretion of xenobiotic conjugates by nonprimate mammals, in *Drug metabolism: From microbes to man.* Park, D., and Smith, R., eds. Cranea, Russak, New York, pp. 299–329.

Hirth, R.S., and Hottendorf, G.H. (1973) Lesions produced by a new lungworm in beagle dogs. *Vet. Pathol.* 10, 385–407.

Hite, M., Hanson, H.M., Bohidar, N.R., Conti, P.A., and Mattis, P.A. (1977) Effect of cage size on patterns of activity and health of beagle dogs. *Lab. Anim. Sci.* 27, 60–64.

Hjelle, J., and Grauer, G. (1986) Acetaminophen induced toxicosis in dogs and cats. *J. Am. Vet. Med. Assoc.* 188, 742–746.

Holmes, D.D., and Smith, P.D. (1969) Inclusion bodies in hepatic cytoplasm of dogs and rats after administering endotoxin. *Am. J. Vet. Res.* 30, 811–815.

Holst, P.A., and Phemister, R.D. (1974) Onset of diestrus in the beagle bitch: Definition and significance. *Am. J. Vet. Res.* 35, 401–406.

Hottendorf, G. H., and Hirth, R. S. (1974) Lesions of spontaneous subclinical disease in beagle dogs. *Vet. Pathol.* 11, 240–258.

Hubben, K., Patterson, D. F., and Botts, R. P. (1963) Telangiectasis in canine heart values. *Zbl. Vet. Med.* 10, 195–202.

Hulland, T.J. (1985) Muscles and tendons, in *Pathology of domestic animals.* Vol. 1, Jubb, K.V.F., Kennedy, P.C., and Palmer, N., eds. Academic Press, San Diego, pp. 139–199.

Humason, G.L. (1972) *Animal tissue techniques.* W.H. Freeman, San Francisco, pp. 1–641.

Illanes, O., Morris, R., and Skerritt, G.C. (1988) Myelinated axons in peripheral nerves of adult beagle dogs: Morphometric and electrophysiological measurements. *Res. Vet. Sci.* 45, 181–185.

Innes, J.R.M., and Saunders, L.Z. (1962) *Comparative neuropathology.* Academic Press, New York, p. 665.

Ishmael, J., and Howell, and J. McC. (1967) Siderofibrotic nodules of the spleen of the dog. *J. Small Anim. Pract.* 8, 501–510.

Jaenke, R.S., Phemister, R.D., and Norrdin, R.W. (1980) Progressive glomerulesclerosis and renal failure following perinatal gamma radiation in the beagle. *Lab. Invest.* 42, 643–655.

James, R.W., and Heywood, R. (1979) Age-related variations in the testes and prostate of beagle dogs. *Toxicology* 12, 273–279.

Jee, W.S.S., Bartley, M.H., Cooper, R.R., and Dockum, N.L. (1970) Bone structure, in *The beagle as an experimental dog*, Andersen, A.C., ed. Iowa State University Press, Ames, pp. 162–188.

Jenkins, T.W. (1978) *Functional mammalian neuroanatomy*. Lea & Febiger, Philadelphia, pp. 1–480.

Jochle, W., and Anderson, A. (1977) The estrus cycle in the dog: A review. *Theriogenology* 7, 113–140.

Jorch, U.M., and Anderson, C. (1980) Haversian bond-remodeling measurements in young beagles. *Am. J. Vet. Res.* 41, 1512–5.

Jubb, K.V.F., Kennedy, P.C., and Palmer, N. (1985) Bones and joints, in *Pathology of domestic animals*. Vol. 1, Jubb, K.V.F., Kennedy, P.C., and Palmer, N., eds. Academic Press, San Diego, pp. 1–138.

Katz, L.N., Soskin, S., and Frisch, R. (1934) Variations in contour of the records found in serial electrocardiograms of the dog. *Proc. Soc. Exp. Biol. (N.Y.)* 32, 208–209.

Kirchner, B.K., Port, C.D., Magoc, T.J., Sidor, M.A., and Ruben, Z. (1990) Spontaneous bronchopeumonia in laboratory dogs infected with untyped *Mycoplasma* spp. *Lab Anim. Sci.* 40, 625–628.

Knapp, S., Green, M., Tephly, T., Baron, J. (1988) Immunohistochemical demonstration of isozyme- and strain-specific differences in the intralobular localizations and distributions of UDP-glucuronosyl transferase in livers of untreated rats. *Mol. Pharmacol.* 33, 14–21.

Kunkle, B.N., Norrdin, R.W., Brooks, R.K., and Thomassen, R.W. (1982) Osteopenia with decreased bone formation in beagles with malabsorption syndrome. *Calcif. Tissue Int.* 34, 396–402.

Krantz, J.C., Carr, C.J., Bird, J.G., and Cook, S. (1948) Sugar alcohols. XXVI. Pharmacodynamic studies and polyalkylene derivatives of hexitol anhydride partially fatty esters. *J. Pharmacol. Exp. Ther.* 93, 188–195.

Kuwabara, T., and Cogan, D.G. (1977) The eye, in *Histology*. Weiss, L., and Greep, R.O., eds. McGraw-Hill, New York. pp. 1119–1164.

Kwapien, R.P., Giles, R.C., Geil, R.G., and Casey, H.W. (1980) Malignant mammary tumors in beagle dogs dosed with investigational oral contraceptive steroids. *J. Natl. Cancer Inst.* 65, 137–142.

Lalich, J., Cohen, L., and Walker, G. (1941) The frequency of electrocardiographic variations in normal unanesthetized dogs. *Am. Heart J.* 22, 105–111.

Lan, S., Weinstein, S., Keim, G., and Migdalof, B. (1983) Induction of hepatic drug metabolizing enzymes in rats, dogs, and monkeys after repeated administration of an anti-inflammatory hexahydroindazole. *Xenobiotica* 13, 329–335.

Liversidge, G.G., Nishihata, T., Englel, K.K., Higuchi, T. (1986) Effect of suppository shape on the systemic availability of rectally administered insulin and sodium salicylate. *Intern. J. Pharmacol.* 30, 247–250.

Lovell, J.E., and Getty, R. (1967) The integument, in *Anatomy of the Dog*, Miller, M.E., Christensen, G.C., and Evans, H.E., eds. Saunders, Philadelphia, pp. 875–888.

Lusk, G. (1931) *Elements of the science of nutrition*. Saunders, Philadelphia, pp. 144–169.

Maita, K., Masuda, H., and Suzuki, Y. (1977) Spontaneous lesions detected in the beagles used in toxicity studies. *Exp. Anim.* 26, 161–167.

Martin, R.K., Albright, J.P., Jee, W.S.S., Taylor, G.N., and Clarke, W.R. (1981) Bone loss in the beagle tibia: Influence of age, weight and sex. *Calcif. Tissue Int.* 33, 233–238.

Mawdesley-Thomas, L.E. (1968) Lymphocytic thyroiditis in the dog. *J. Small Animal Pract.* 9, 539–550.

Mawdesley-Thomas, L.E., and Jolly, D.W. (1967) Autoimmune disease in the beagle. *Vet. Rec.* 80, 553–554.

McDonald, L.E. (1969) Reproductive patterns in dogs, in *Veterinary endocrinology and reproduction*. Lea & Febiger, Philadelphia, pp. 377–385.

McEntee, K. (1990) *Reproductive pathology of domestic animals*. Academic Press, San Diego, pp. 1–401.

McGavin, M.D. (1983) Muscle biopsy in veterinary practice. *Vet. Clin. North Am. Small Anim. Pract.* 13, 135–144.

McKillop, D. (1985) Effects of phenobarbitone and β-naphthaflavone on hepatic microsomal drug metabolizing enzymes on the male beagle dog. *Biochem. Pharmacol.* 34, 3137–3142.

Menard, R., Guenthner, T., Kon, H., and Gillette, J. (1979) Studies on the destruction of adrenal and testicular cytochrome P-450 by spironolactone. *J. Biol. Chem.* 254, 1726–1733.

Michaud, L., and Elvenjem, C.A. (1944) Nutritional requirements of the dog. *Nutr. Abstr. Rev.* 13, 321–331.

Miller, M.E., Cristensen, G.S., and Evens, H.E. (1967) *Anatomy of the dog*. Saunders, Philadelphia, pp. 1–941.

Mizejewski, G.J., Baron, J., and Poissant, G. (1971) Immunologic investigations of naturally occurring canine thyroiditis. *J. Immunol.* 107, 1152–1160.

Mosberg, A.T., and Hayes, A.W. (1989) Subchronic toxicity testing, in *Principles and methods of toxicology*. 2nd ed. Hayes, A.W., ed. pp. 221–236.

Moulton, J.E. (1990) *Tumors in domestic animals*. University of California Press, Berkeley, Los Angeles, pp. 1–672.

Muller, G.H., Kirk, R.W., and Scott, D.W. (1983) *Small animal dermatology*. Saunders, Philadelphia, pp. 1–889.

Munkelt, H.F. (1948) Air purification and deodordization by use of activated charcoal. *Refrig. Eng.* 56, 222–229.

Murti, G.S., and Borgmann, R. (1965) Intracytoplasmic periodic-acid-schiff- positive nonglycogenic globules in canine liver: Their histochemical characterization. *Am. J. Vet. Res.* 26, 63–67.

Musser, E., and Graham, W.R. (1968) Familial occurrence of thyroiditis in purebred beagles. *Lab. Anim. Care* 18, 58–68.

Namand, J., Sweeney, W.T., Creame, A.A., and Conti, P.A. (1975) Cage activity in the laboratory beagle: a preliminary study to evaluate a method of comparing cage size to physical activity. *Lab. Anim. Sci.* 25, 180–183.

Nebon, L.W., Weikel, J.H., Jr., and Reno, F.E. (1973) Mammary nodules in dogs during four years' treatment with megestrol acetate or chlormadinene acetate. *J. Natl. Cancer Inst.* 51, 1303–1311.

Neis, J., Yap, S., Van Gamert, P., Roelofs, H., and Henderson, P. (1985) Mutagenicity of five arylamines after metabolic activation with isolated dog and human hepatocytes. *Cancer Lett.* 27, 53–60.

Nelson, L.W., and Kelly, W.A. (1974) Changes in canine mammary gland histology during the estrous cycle. *Toxicol. Appl. Pharmacol.* 27, 113–122.

Nelson, L.W., Weikel, J.H., Jr., and Reno, F.E. (1973) Mammary nodules in dogs during four year's treatment with megestrol acetate or chlormadinone acetate. *J. Natl. Cancer Inst.* 51, 1303–1311.

Newberne, J.W., Robinson, V.B., Estill, L., and Brinkman, D.C. (1960) Granular structures in brains of apparently normal dogs. *Am. J. Vet. Res.* 21, 782–786.

Newton, W.M. (1972) An evaluation of the effects of various degrees of long term confinement on adult beagle dogs. *Lab. Anim. Sci.* 22, 860–864.

NIH (National Institutes of Health) (1985) *Guide for the care and use of laboratory animals*. U.S. Department of Health and Human Services, NIH Publication No. 86-23.

Noel, P.R.B. (1970) The challenge of selecting the suitable animal species in toxicology, in *The problems of species difference and statistics in toxicology*, Vol. XI, Baker, S.B. De C., Tripod, J., and Jacob, J., eds. Excerpta Medica Foundation, Amsterdam, pp. 57–69.

Norrdin, R.W., and Shih, M.S. (1983) Profiles of cortical remodeling sites in longitudinal rib sections of beagles with renal failure and parathyroid hyperplasia. *Metab. Bone Dis. Rel. Res.* 5, 353–359.

Norris, W.P., Poole, C.M., Fry, R.J., and Kretz, N.D. (1968) A study of thermoregulatory capabilities of normal, aged, and irradiated beagles. *Argonne Natl. Lab.* pp. 166–169.

Nutrient Requirements of Dogs (1985) *Subcommittee on Dog Nutrition, National Research Council.* National Academy Press, Washington, D.C.

Oghiso, Y., Fukuda, S., and Hda, H. (1982) Histopathologic studies on distribution of spontaneous lesions and age changes in the beagle. *Jpn. J. Vet. Sci.* 44, 941–950.

Osborne, C.A., Finco, D.R., and Low, D.G. (1983) Pathophysiology of renal disease, renal failure, and uremia, in *Textbook of veterinary internal medicine. Diseases of the dog and cat.* Vol. 2, Ettinger, S.J., ed. Saunders, Philadelphia, pp. 1733–1792.

Pacifici, G., Boobis, A., Brodie, M., McManus, M., and Davies, D. (1981) Tissue and species differences in enzymes of epoxide metabolism. *Xenobiotica* 11, 73–79.

Patridou-Fischer, J., Whaley, S., and Dahl, A. (1987) *In vivo* metabolism of nasally instilled dihydrosafrole [1-(3,4-methylenedioxyphenyl)propane] in dogs and monkeys. *Chem. Biol. Interact.* 64, 1–12.

Payne, B.J., Lewis, H.B., Murchison, T.E., and Hart, E.A. (1976) Hematology of laboratory animals, in *Handbook of laboratory animal science.* Vol. 3, Melby, E.C., and Altman, N.H., eds. CRC Press, Cleveland, Ohio, pp. 383–461.

Phemister, R.D. (1974) Nonneurogenic reproductive failure in the bitch. *Vet. Clin. North Am.* 4, 573–536.

Pick, J.R., and Eubanks, J.W. (1965) A clinicopathologic study of heterogeneous and homeogeneous dog populations in North Carolina. *Lab. Anim. Care* 15, 11–17.

Pickrell, J.A., Dubin, S.E., and Elliott, J.C. (1971) Normal respiratory parameters of un-anesthetized beagle dogs. *Lab. Anim. Sci. (U.S.).* 21, 677–679.

Poupko, J., Radmski, T., Santella, R., and Radomski, J. (1983) Organ, species, and compound specificity in the metabolic activation of primary amines. *J. Natl. Can. Inst.* 70, 1077–1088.

Prasse, K.W. (1983) White blood cell disorders, in *Textbook of veterinary internal medicine. Diseases of the dog and cat.* Vol. 2, Ettinger, S.J., ed. Saunders, Philadelphia, pp. 2001–2045.

Prince, J.H., Diesem, C.D., Eglitis, I., and Ruskell, G.L. (1960) *Anatomy and histology of the eye and orbit in domestic animals.* Thomas, Springfield, Illinois, pp. 65–98.

Ohta, K., Motoya, M., Komori, M., Miura, T., Kitada, M., and Kamataki, T. (1989a) A novel form of cytochrome P-450 in dogs (P-450-D3 is a low spin form of cytochrome P-450 but with catalytic and structural properties similar to P-450d). *Biochem. Phamacol.* 38, 91–96.

Ohta, K., Kitada, M., Ohi, H., Komori, M., Nagashima, K., Sato, N., Kozo, Muroya, K., Kodama, T., Nagao, M., and Kamataki, T. (1989b) Interspecies homology of cytochrome P-450 cross-reactive with anti-rat P-448-H antibodies in liver microsomes from dogs, monkeys, and humans. *Mutat. Res.* 226, 163–167.

Richter, C.P. (1938) Factors determining voluntary ingestion of water in normals and in individuals with maximum diabetes insipidus. *Am. J. Physiol.* 122, 668–675.

Richter, W.R., Stein R.J., Rdzok, E.J., Moize, S.M., and Bischoff, M.B. (1965) Ultrastructural studies of intranuclear crystalline inclusions in the livers of dogs. *Am. J. Pathol.* 47, 587–599.

Robbins, G.R. (1965) Unilateral renal agenesis in the beagle. *Vet. Rec.* 77, 1345–1347.

Rubin, L.F., and Saunders, L.Z. (1965) Intraocular larva migrans in dogs. *Pathol. Vet.* 2, 566–573.

Runkle, R.S., (1964) Laboratory animal housing—Part II. *J. Am. Inst. Arch.* 41, 77–80.

Saville, P.D., and Krook, L. (1969) Gravimetric and isotopic studies in nutritional hyperparathyroidism in beagles. *Clin. Orthop. Rel. Res.* 62, 15–24.

Saunders, L.Z., and Rubin, L.F. (1975) *Ophthalmic pathology of animals.* Karger, Basel, pp. 1–253.

Schiavo, D.M., and Field, W.E. (1974) The incidence of ocular defects in a closed colony of beagle dogs. *Lab. Anim. Sci.* 24, 51–56.

Schmoldt, A., Herzfeldt, B., Von Mayerinick, L., and Benthe, H. (1987) Evidence for a digitoxin conjugating UDP-glucuronosyl transferase in the dog. *Biochem. Pharmacol.* 36, 3951–3955.

Schwartz, L.W. (1987) Pulmonary responses to inhaled irritants and the morphological evaluation of these responses, in *Inhalation toxicology, research methods, applications and evaluation.* Salem, H., ed. pp. 293–348.

Searcy, G.P. (1988) Hemopoietic system, in *Special veterinary pathology.* Thompson, R.G., ed. Decker, Toronto, pp. 269–310.

Sekhri, K.K., and Faulkin, L.J. (1970) Mammary gland, in *The beagle as an experimental dog,* Andersen, A.C., ed. Iowa State University Press, Ames, pp. 327–349.

Sherding, R.C. (1983) Diseases of the small bowel, in *Textbook of veterinary internal medicine. Diseases of the dog and cat* Vol. 2, Ettinger, S.J., ed. Saunders, Philadelphia, pp. 1278–1346.

Shifrine, M., and Wilson, F.D. (1980) *The canine as a biomedical research model: Immunological, hematological, and oncological aspects.* Technical Information Center, U.S. Department of Commerce, Springfield, Virginia.

Shimizu, N., Mori, H., Kato, D., Okamoto, T., Koyama, H., Sako, T., Kawase, K., Uchino, T., Motoyoshi, S., Funabashi, N., and Nakazawa, M. (1986) Electrocardiograms of 1139 beagle dogs recorded by autoanalyzing electrocardiographs: Changes in ECG values with aging. *Bull. Nippon Vet. Zootech. Coll.* 35, 71–76.

Shively, J.N., and Epling, G.P. (1970) Fine structure of the canine eye: Cornea. *Am. J. Vet. Res.* 31, 713–722.

Silber, B., Holford, N., and Riegelman, S. (1982) Stereoselective disposition and glucuronidation of propanolol in humans. *Pharm. Sci.* 711, 699–703.

Simionescu, N., and Simionescu M. (1977) The cardiovascular system, in *Histology,* Weiss, L., and Greep, R.O., eds. McGraw-Hill, New York, pp. 373–431.

Sisenwine, S., Tio, C., Hadley, F., Liu, A., Kimel, H., and Reulius, H. (1982) Species related differences in the stereoselective glucuronidation of oxazepam. *Drug Metab. Dispos.* 10, 605–608.

Snow, G.R., Karambolova, K.K., and Anderson, C. (1986) Bone remodeling in the lumbar vertebrae of young adult beagles. *Am. J. Vet. Res.* 47, 1275–7.

Sokolowski, J.H. (1973) Reproductive features and patterns in the bitch. *J.A.A.H.A.* 9, 71–81.

Sokolowski, J.H. (1977) Reproductive patterns in the bitch. *Vet. Clin. North Am.* 7, 653–666.

Sokolowski, J.H., Zimbelman, R.G., Goyings, L.S. (1973) Canine reproduction: Reproductive organs and related structures of the nonparous, parous and postpartum bitch. *Am. J. Vet. Res.* 34, 1001–1013.

Spencer, P.S., and Bischoff, M.C. (1982) Contemporary neuropathological methods in toxicology, in *Nervous system toxicology,* Mitchell, C.L., ed. Raven Press, New York, pp. 259–275.

Sprague, R.H., and Anisko, J.J. (1973) Elimination patterns in the laboratory beagle. *Behavior (Netherl.)* 47, 257–267.

Stevens, C.E. (1977) Comparative physiology of the digestive system, in *Dukes' Physiology of Domestic Animals,* Swenson, M.J., ed. Cornell University Press, Ithaca, New York, pp. 216–232.

Stinson, A.W., and Calhoun, M.L. (1976) Digestive system, in *Textbook of Veterinary Histology,* Dellman, H.D., and Brown, E.M., eds. Lea & Febiger, Philadelphia, pp. 207–264.

Street, A.E., Chesterman, H., Smith, G.K., and Quinton, R.M. (1968) The effect of diet on blood urea levels in the beagle. *J. Pharmacol. Pharmacol. (Engld).* 20, 325–6.

Strombeck, D.R. (1979) *Small animal gastroenterology.* Stonegate Publishing, Davis, California, pp. 1-564.

Stuart, B.P., Phemister, R.D., and Thomassen, R.W. (1975) Glomerular lesions associated with proteinuria in clinically healthy dogs. *Vet. Pathol.* 12, 125–144.

Sullivan, N.D. (1985) The nervous system, in *Pathology of domestic animals.* Vol. 1, Jubb, K.V.F., Kennedy, P.C., and Palmer, N., eds. Academic Press, San Diego, California, pp. 201–338.

Tabaru, H., Ogawa, H., Otsuka, H., and Ito, K. (1987) Effects of xylazine on arterial blood pressure, heart rate, and electrocardiogram in spinal dogs. *Jpn. J. Vet. Sci.* 49, 391–394.

Tavoloni, N. (1985) Postnatal changes in hepatic microsomal enzyme system in the puppy. *Biol. Neonate* 47, 305–16.

Thompson, S.W., Cook, J.E., and Hoey, H. (1959a) Histochemical studies of acidophilic crystalline intranuclear inclusions in the liver and kidney of dogs. *Am. J. Pathol.* 35, 607–623.

Thompson, S.W., Wiegand, R.G., Thomassen, R.W., Harrison, M., and Turbyfill, C.L. (1959b) The protein nature of acidophilic crystalline intranuclear inclusions in the liver and kidneys of dogs. *Am. J. Pathol.* 35, 1105–1115.

Titkemeyer, C.W., and Calhoun, M.L. (1955) A comparative study of the structure of the small intestine of domestic animals. *Am. J. Vet. Res.* 16, 152–157.

Tilley, L.P. (1985) *Essentials of canine and feline electrocardiography: Interpretation and treatment.* Lea & Febiger, Philadelphia.

Tsutsui, T., Tsuji, J., Kawakami, E., Yamada, Y., Amano, T., and Yamauchi, M. (1986) Studies on the sexual maturity of the male dog: Development of the testis and accessory reproductive organs. *Bull. Nippon Vet. Zootechnical Coll.* 35, 115–123.

Tucker, W.E. (1962) Thyroiditis in a group of laboratory beagles. *Am. J. Comp. Pathol.* 38, 70–74.

Tuffery, A.A. (1987) *Laboratory animals an introduction for new experimenters.* Wiley,

Valli, V.E.O. (1985) The hematopoietic system, in *Pathology of domestic animals.* Vol. 3, Jubb, K.V.F., Kennedy, P.C., and Palmer, N., eds. Academic Press, San Diego, California, pp. 83–236.

Venable, J.H., and Dellmann, H.D. (1976) Muscular tissue, in *Textbook of veterinary histology,* Dellman, H.D., and Brown, E.M., eds. Lea & Febiger, Philadelphia, pp. 111–123.

Von Bahr, C., Hermansson, J., and Lind, M. (1982) Oxidation of (R)- and (S)-propranolol in human and dog liver microsomes. Species differences in stereoselectivity. *J. Pharmacol. Exp. Ther.* 222, 458–462.

Vymetal, F. (1965) Renal aplasia in beagles. *Vet. Rec.* 77, 1344–1345.

Walle, T., and Walle, U. (1979) Stereoselective oral bioavailability ($\pm$) propranolol in the dog. A GC-MS study using a stable isotope technique. *Res. Comm. Chem. Pathol. Pharmacol.* 23, 453–464.

Warner, R.L., and McFarland, L.Z. (1970) Integument, in *The beagle as an experimental dog.* Andersen, A.C., ed. Iowa State University Press, Ames, pp. 126–148.

Wasserman, R.H. (1977) Bones, in *Duke's physiology of domestic animals,* Swenson, M.J., ed. Cornell University Press, Ithaca, New York, pp. 413–432.

Weber, A.F., Hasa, O., and Sautter, J.H. (1958) Some observations concerning the presence of spirilla in the fundic glands of dogs and cats. *Am. J. Vet. Res.* 19, 677–680.

Weiser, M.G., Spanger, W.L., and Gribble, D.H. (1977) Blood pressure measurement in the dog. *J. Am. Vet. Med. Assoc.* 171, 364–368.

Wiener, H. (1986) Heterogeneity of dog-liver glutathione S-transferase evidence of unique temperature dependence of the catalytic process. *Eur. J. Biochem.* 157, 351–363.

Wiener, H., Krivanek, P., and Kolassa, N. (1983) Metabolism and disposition of 2',3'-di-O-nitroadenosine-5'-(N-ethyl-carboxamide) in dogs. *Biochem. Pharmacol.* 12, 1899-1906.

Wilcock, B.P. (1985) The eye and ear, in *Pathology of domestic animals.* Vol. 1, Jubb, K.V.F., Kennedy, P.C., and Palmer, N., eds. Academic Press, San Diego, California, pp. 349–406.

Williams, R.T. (1971) Species variations in drug bio-transformations, in *Fumdamentals of drug metabolism and drug disposition,* LaDu, B., Mandel, H., and Way, E., eds. Williams & Wilkins, Baltimore, pp. 206–252.

Wilson, B., and Thompson, J. (1984) Glucuronidaton of propranolol by dog liver microsomes effects of enamtiomeric inhibition and detergent treatment on stereoselectivity. *Drug. Metab. Dispos.* 12, 161–164.

Wintrobe, M.M., Lee, G.R., and Boggs, D.R., et al. (1981) *Clinical hematology.* Lea & Febiger, Philadelphia, p. 281.

Woods, J.E., and Besch, E.L. (1974) Influence of group size on heat dissipation from dogs in a controlled environment. *Lab. Anim. Sci.* 24, 72–78.

Yager, J.A., and Scott, D.W. (1985) The skin and appendages, in *Pathology of domestic animals,* Vol. 1, Jubb, K.V.F., Kennedy, P.C., and Palmer, N., eds. Academic Press, San Diego, California, pp. 407–549.

Yates, W.D.G. (1988) Respiratory system, in *Special veterinary pathology,* Thompson, R.G., ed. Decker, Toronto and Philadelphia, pp. 69–122.

9

Nonhuman Primates

Toxicology: **Gene B. Fuller and William C. Hobson**
New Mexico Regional Primate Research Laboratory (PRL),
New Mexico State University
Holloman Air Force Base, New Mexico

                             David M. Renquist
University of Tennessee, Memphis
Memphis, Tennessee

Pathology: **Curtis D. Port**
G. D. Searle and Company
Skokie, Illinois

Metabolism: **Christopher P. Chengelis**
WIL Research Laboratories, Inc.
Ashland, Ohio

Toxicology   **Gene B. Fuller, William C. Hobson, and**
                                    David M. Renquist

The phylogenetic and physiological similarity between humans and nonhuman primates has resulted in an increased demand for certain species in safety and efficacy assessments of new drugs and biologics. Only a few of almost 200 primate species are utilized in toxicology studies. These mainly include the most popular New World monkey (squirrel monkey), Old World monkeys (cynomolgus monkey, rhesus monkey, and baboon), and the great apes (chimpanzees).

Because of the genotypic and phenotypic resemblance to humans, nonhuman primates have been used in the study of induced or naturally occurring human diseases such as acquired immunodeficiency syndrome (AIDS), hepatitis, diabetes mellitus, and atherosclerosis. Our understanding of the human brain, vision, aging, reproductive function, and behavior has been enhanced by studies in primates. Efficacy and safety evaluations of drugs, vaccines, and biotechnology products are often conducted in nonhuman primates prior to approval for general use by the public. A failure to investigate the potential teratogenic effects of thalidomide in a primate model prior to exposing pregnant women resulted in tragic consequences in the 1950s and early 1960s (Somers, 1963). Unfortunately, the teratogenicity of thalidomide could not be demonstrated in rodents prior to human exposure, but was subsequently shown to cause fetal abnormalities in primates (Hendrickx et al., 1966; Hendrickx, 1973).

In spite of the obvious predictive value of primates for human responses, they must be utilized conservatively. Where nonprimate models are acceptable and will yield applicable results, they should be the model of choice. This is because of a complex of factors which have both limited primate supply and increased their cost.

Loss of habitat, capture methods, and export restrictions have diminished the supply of wild-caught primates and greatly increased their cost. Domestically bred animals are a major source now, but owing to housing costs, new regulations and special handling procedures resulting from the potential transmission of fatal infectious diseases to humans, costs have increased concurrently. Nevertheless, the humane use of nonhuman primates as a physiological, pharmacological, and toxicological model for safety assessment of new drugs and biotechnology products will increase and will require prudent use of primate inventories.

The intent of this section is to define the utilization of nonhuman primates in toxicology studies and to describe the basic husbandry and technical procedures used in a primate facility. It is not intended to be an exhaustive review of the voluminous primatology literature. (See King et al., 1988, for an excellent summary of the role of nonhuman primates in research.)

HUSBANDRY

Husbandry includes all aspects of housing and adequate care. Primates encompass a variety of species ranging from lower forms such as the tree shrews to the great apes. Much in the literature has generalized the nonhuman primate as one animal when in reality the primate can be as small as several grams (e.g., the shrews) to over 100 kg (e.g., the great apes). The primary genus utilized in toxicological studies has been the Asian macaque with lesser emphasis on the New World monkey and the chimpanzee. The primary thrust of this section will be on the macaque with specific reference when necessary to New World primates and apes. New regulations as promulgated by Congress and enacted through the Animal Welfare Act, Parts I, II, and III further define the need to provide optimal caging; adequate Veterinary care; protocol development through scientific and Animal Care Committee review; and programs geared toward a variety of diverse procedures in assuring the "normality" of a primate during research use. Included in this are requirements for psychological and environmental enrichment programs which are now being defined by a variety of scientific and regulatory bodies.

Institutional Policy and Regulatory Issues

Institutional animal facilities and programs should be operated in accordance with the Animal Welfare Act (PL-89-544) as amended by current regulations (now utilizing the National Institutes of Health's (NIH) *Guide for the care and Use of Laboratory Animals* (1985) and *Public Health Policy on Human Care and Use of Laboratory Animals* (1986) as the standard) and other applicable federal, state and local laws, regulations, and policy. Nothing in the regulations intends to restrict the investigator's freedom to conduct animal experiments in accordance with scientific or humane principles. Any program of husbandry must be developed considering the proper care and humane treatment of the animals used in research or testing. The particular needs of the toxicology program must also consider first the principles noted in the regulations. Aspects of conservation, alternatives to animal use, elimination of experimental duplication, and strong scientific principles must be paramount in experimental design.

The U.S. Department of Agriculture (USDA)/Animal Welfare Regulations (*Federal Register*, 1989) mandate the appointing of an Animal Care and Use Committee (ACUC) to review the humane principles and the total Animal Care and Use Program. Included in this review are semiannual facility and program reviews; protocol review concerning euthanasia, appropriate care, and related issues; and provision of an annual written report to the responsible administrative official on the status of the Institutional Animal Care and Use Program. Special consideration of restraint needs and multiple surgical use as scientifically justified come under the purview of the IACUC.

Facilities

The Physical Plant

A key to a successful research toxicological program is the design of the animal facilities. A good design assures efficiency in animal care and personnel movements and provides managers with the facilities necessary for an economic and sound animal care program. A basic design premise is to accommodate projects involving both small and large numbers of primates.

Briefly, the following functional areas are essential to assure that diverse projects, different primate species, dosing and collection requirements, and husbandry and sanitation needs can be met (*Guide for the Care and Use of Laboratory Animals*, 1985).

1. Separation of primate housing from administrative or human occupancy areas. Areas with animal procedure rooms (as distinguished from laboratories) can be adjacent to basic animal housing areas.
2. Special areas such as quarantine or receiving require isolation from primary study rooms or laboratories to assure project contiguity and disease-free studies.
3. Separate areas for surgery, necropsy, postsurgical care, clinical pathology, radiography, diet preparation, or animal treatment.
4. Office areas for administration and facility support areas, separate from animal areas.
5. Support areas for personnel; e.g., lockers, showers, and toilets.
6. Feed and supply storage and receiving areas.
7. Caging storage, washing facilities, and incinerator or waste disposal.

The size and complexity of the above areas depends on the size of the facility. A facility under 1000 ft^2 has much different requirements from a facility housing numerous primates with areas of thousands of square feet. Efficiency and economy in utilization of research worker's time must be carefully balanced with the need to separate animal and human facilities. Careful consideration of personnel and animal traffic patterns must be utilized in the design of animal facilities. Security has become a key issue in animal facility design. Barriers, entry locks, separate corridors, and/or separate floors all can enhance security.

Building Materials

Economy, maintenance, and sanitation are key in the selection of materials for the research facility. Key features of an animal room are durability, esthetics, and ease of sanitation requirements while providing a humane and comfortable housing area free of pathogens and vermin hiding places.

Construction Criteria

The design of primate housing areas is unique. Basic aspects to consider are:

1. Corridor widths of adequate size to permit easy movement of caging to wash area and bumper guards to prevent wall or corner damage.

2. Animal room doors with self-closures; swinging toward the corridor only when an anteroom is present. Preferable construction is solid or metal doors to eliminate vermin hiding places.
3. Floors of durable, sanitary nonslip construction; e.g., epoxy or sealed concrete.
4. Walls of sealed impervious paints or coatings using coved and sealed junctions at floor and ceiling.
5. Ceilings of nonpermeable construction or sealed with washable coatings. Light fixtures of waterproof sealed construction.

Ventilation, Temperature, and Humidity Control

Nonhuman primates have specific requirements for ventilation, temperature, and humidity. New World primates are specifically affected by humidities less than 50%, causing potential upper respiratory afflictions (*Guide for the Care and Use of Laboratory Animals*, 1985). Ventilation at 10–15 air changes per hour is essential to reduce environmental aerosol contamination as well as to provide odor and ammonia control. Recirculation of air is not advised unless it has been treated to remove particulate or toxic gaseous contaminants (Besch, 1980).

Temperature control is highly recommended to assure appropriate ranges of temperature from 64.4 to 84.2°F (18–29°C) (*Guide for the Care and Use of Laboratory Animals*, 1985). The two most important considerations in the physical environment of primates are humidity and temperature as they closely correlate to metabolism and behavior. Humidity is recommended at between 30–70% for New World species. The toxicological laboratory must be more sensitive to temperature or humidity variations because such finite measurements as cellular parameters and hormonal indices can be affected by environmental variances (Gortan and Besch, 1974).

Power and Lighting

Steady uninterrupted power with backup emergency generators is essential to assure that a drug evaluation can be appropriately tracked free from the influences of power outages on animal physiology. Lighting of sufficient intensity is necessary to provide good husbandry and sanitation practices, observation of animals, security, and safe working conditions. A biphasic or a variable intensity system may be necessary in certain facilities to provide adequate observations, yet provide soft diffused lighting for the majority of the day; thus avoiding eye/retinal damage. Illumination of 75–125 foot-candles (Bellhorn, 1980) has been recommended for observation periods. Time-controlled systems are essential in a research animal facility to assure regular circadian rhythms.

Lights should be sealed and preferably of fluorescent type. Some facilities have gone to the daylight ultraviolet bulb to simulate natural lighting.

Drainage

Adequate waste control is essential to assure that contamination, odor, and waste stoppage of drains do not occur. Many projects have failed because of disease transmission from sewage overflow. All waste fixtures should be of adequate size to permit full flow of waste biscuits, feces, hair, and similar materials. Sizes from 4 to 6 in are recommended (*Guide for the Care and Use of Laboratory Animals*, 1985) with appropriate floor sloping. Cages should be provided with flush pans and troughs to direct and keep waste off of the floors. Facilities using dry paper or bedding systems should have adequate disposal systems for these materials. Lockable drain covers may be necessary to prevent improper materials from being deposited into the drains.

Storage Areas

A variety of storage areas are necessary to permit effective husbandry procedures. These include clean food and bedding storage, refrigerated food storage to prevent vitamin and nutrient deterioration; refuse storage areas for dry bedding or paper; and equipment storage for clean or dirty caging, disinfectants, and personnel items (masks, gloves, etc.).

External Environmental Influences

The animal facility should be free of unusual external influences. Adrenal and immune cellular function can be affected by sudden noise. Cage washing areas should be separate and apart from animal rooms. Sound-proofing materials should also be utilized to prevent unwelcome noise in the animal facility (Fletcher, 1976; Peterson, 1980).

Fire alarm tests should be done with muffled alarms to prevent severe animal distress (which has included abortions in sensitive primate species).

Several recent studies have shown that a simple turning on of a light or sudden personnel intrusion at off hours can have long-lasting effects on primate behavior and hormonal evaluations.

Sanitation Facilities

Critical to the husbandry of any facility is the need for areas for washing and sterilizing animal cages, racks, water bottles, and similar accessories. The USDA/Animal Welfare Regulations mandate the sanitation/washing of cages on a 2-week minimum. Temperatures not lower than 180°F are recommended with use of appropriate disinfectants (*Guide for the Care and Use of Laboratory Animals*, 1985). Key factors to consider in sanitation facilities are:

1. Location related to traffic, animal rooms, elevators, and waste disposal
2. Soundproofing
3. Utilities such as hot and cold water, steam, drainage, and power
4. Proximity to storage
5. Ventilation and employee safety
6. Access and corridor width

The size of the facility dictates whether hand washing using brushes and portable units is satisfactory or whether large mechanical cabinet washers are necessary.

Animal Rooms

Animal rooms for toxicological experiments should be designed with the ability to house either large or small numbers of animals and to provide project segregation. Usually this is best accomplished by having a variety of sizes of animal rooms. Recently the use of laminar flow or bubble-isolette room systems have been designed to permit multiple studies in fairly large rooms.

Generally, animal rooms should have an anteroom provided with a sink and area for outer garments storage; e.g., disposable coveralls, masks, gloves, and foot wear.

The animal room proper should be constructed with all of the parameters noted above to permit an effective sanitary and humane environment. Recent concerns about psychological enrichment may dictate play areas, group housing areas, or special cage constraints to assure animal well-being and to provide the opportunity for exercise. Social needs will probably be paramount as new regulations are being developed, and will certainly influence animal room design, research, and husbandry management techniques.

Support Areas

Personnel support areas, including appropriate break areas, locker rooms, and shower areas, are essential to any husbandry program. These areas should be carefully designed and managed for traffic flow to prevent risks to animals and personnel from contamination and disease.

Special Areas

Most facilities will have special needs for aseptic surgery, involving pre- and postoperative care, surgeon scrub areas, and operating rooms; pathology and necropsy rooms; clinical pathology; radiology support; treatment and procedure areas; etc. The size and complexity of the facility will dictate the size of each of the above areas, but all are necessary parts in the support of the overall facility, husbandry, and management procedures.

Biohazard Areas

The study of drugs for AIDS, hepatitis, and similar diseases dictates the need for special facilities to work with hazardous agents whether chemical, biological, or physical. Each project will dictate the need for the level of contaminant. The Centers for Disease Control (CDC) has listed four levels for dealing with potential biological hazards (from BSL-1 to BSL-4), each with specific criteria. Special hoods, filters, room negative pressures, procedures, and personnel practices are involved. The reader is referred to the CDC (1988) publication on *Biosafety in Microbiological and Biomedical Laboratories* for reference to this vital area.

Caging and Equipment

The well-being and health of the nonhuman primates is critical to the success of a research project. One of the most important factors in this success is the microenvironment of the primate, the caging or housing system. The housing environment should assure that the research objectives can be met through minimizing experimental variables and assuring the "normality" of the animal via the maintenance of health and well-being. The NIH Guide (1985) provides the following factors to consider in any housing system.

1. Provide adequate space to assure freedom of movement and normal postural adjustments with a resting place.
2. Comfortable environment.
3. Escape-proof caging.
4. Easy access to food and water.
5. Adequate ventilation.
6. Meets the biological needs of the animal.
7. Keeps animals dry and clean.
8. Reduces unnecessary physical restraint.
9. Protects animals from known hazards. Added to this is behavioral "normality" through environmental enrichment.

Individual Housing

Cages for nonhuman primates must meet the space recommendations noted in the NIH Guide (1985). Table 1 lists the current space requirements (*Guide for the Care and Use of Laboratory Animals*, 1985). New regulations were promulgated in February 1991, requiring facilities to have programs in environmental enrichment for primates.

Table 1 Individual Housing

Animals	Weight (kg)	Type of housing	Floor area/animal		Height[a]	
			ft^2	m^2	in	cm
Nonhuman primates[b]						
group 1	>1	Cage	1.6	0.15	20	50.80
group 2	1–3	Cage	3.0	0.28	30	76.20
group 3	3–10	Cage	4.3	0.40	30	76.20
group 4	10–15	Cage	6.0	0.56	32	81.28
group 5	15–25	Cage	8.0	0.74	36	91.44
group 6	>25	Cage	25.1	2.33	84	213.36

[a]From the resting floor to the cage top.
[b]The designated groups are based on approximate sizes of various nonhuman primate species used in biomedical research. Examples of species included in each group are:
  Group 1—marmosets, tamarins, and infants of various species
  Group 2—capuchins, squirrel monkeys, and similar species
  Group 3—macaques and African species
  Group 4—male macaques and large African species
  Group 5—baboons and nonbrachiating species larger than 15 kg
  Group 6—great apes and brachiating species
Institutions are encouraged to provide alternatives to individual caging. Infants and juveniles can be housed in group cages, for example. If adults are to be housed in groups, it is essential that only compatible animals be kept together. Newly grouped animals must be closely monitored to detect injuries due to fighting. Space in group cages should be enriched with structures such as resting perches and shelters. The minimum height of pens and runs used to house nonhuman primates should be 6 ft (1.8 m). For chimpanzees and brachiating species (orangutans, gibbons, spider monkeys, and woolly monkeys), the minimum cage height should be such that the animals can, when fully extended, swing from the cage ceiling without having their feet touch the floor.

Historically, cages have been constructed of a variety of materials. Caging must be constructed of sturdy durable materials and designed to reduce the possibility of contamination to adjacent cage units. All surfaces should be smooth and free from sharp edges or broken wires. A minimum of ledges, corners, or angles is recommended to prevent dirt or fecal retention. The squeeze device should be easily operable to avoid primate injury. The cage should facilitate animal observations, and provide feeding access and appropriate watering devices. Cage designs have included wall-mounted, floor, rack (Fig. 1), and permanent installations, all of which are satisfactory depending on species and project needs. The cage requirement for an adult chimpanzee is much different than for the New World monkey, mostly a function of space and strength of design.

Group Housing

The social needs of the nonhuman primate are well known. The majority of toxicological experimentation requires individual housing of primates. The new regulations now being formulated may dictate social housing except for very specific exceptions. Investigators may have to develop procedures using pair housing on specific dosing requirements or use of specialized caging designs to permit pair housing during nonobservation or dosing periods; e.g., nighttime hours. Animals can be housed socially in groups during off-study periods with little difficulty if space and facilities permit. New facility designs should

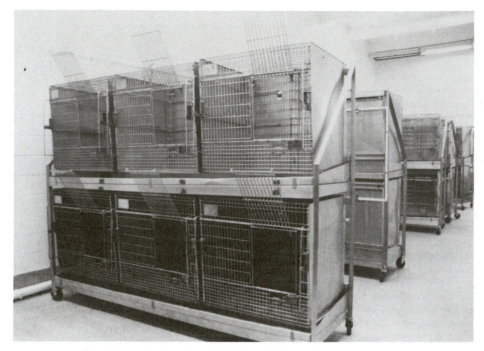

Figure 1 Six-cage rack for mature macaques.

incorporate the ability to group house animals when not required for individually housed projects. Group caging has its own set of requirements which by necessity must consider group dynamics, behavioral needs, usable surface areas, volume vs square footage, escape areas, and management practices.

Equipment Ancillary to the Cage

Equipment necessary to move the cage, handle the animal, and maintain safety to the handler and animal is essential to the husbandry operation. This equipment can include cage lifts, transfer cages, and restraint apparatus (e.g., pole and collar, leather gloves, capture gun, nets).

Systems of Removing Waste

The two primary methods of waste handling are dry and wet methods. Dry methods involve the use of bedding or plastic or paper liners under the cage. This system permits aerosol-free waste removal and cleaning of animal rooms, yet has the disadvantage of excessive waste disposal and high labor. The alternative system is the wet procedure using water under high pressure to move the waste down the trough to the floor drains. The advantage of this system is fast cleanup with the disadvantage of aerosolization and potential contamination of adjacent animals and personnel. A modification of this method using a low-pressure manual or automatic flush system may be the best approach. The use of wall-mounted proportionators allowing dual disinfectant/rinse flushing reduces contamination possibilities.

Cages and Housing for the Great Apes

The most important considerations for housing the ape, specifically the chimpanzee, are strength, environmental and behavioral enrichment, space for adequate movement and exercise, and design simplicity. Group housing of chimps may become the rule. New rules for individual housing will probably require at least two times the current space recommendations for adult chimpanzees of 25 ft^2. This certainly will have a direct impact on housing requirements and protocol design.

Environmental Enrichment and Special Concerns

Congress has coined the term "psychological enrichment" as a housing requirement for nonhuman primates (*Federal Register,* 1991). Essentially this has been meant to include environmental enrichment, social housing, behavioral well-being, and similar terms. Any research primate facility must take measures to assure that programs are in place utilizing and developing techniques to enrich the environment of primates on or off study. Although we have historically been concerned for primates' well-being, we must now specifically state our program for environmental enhancement related to normal behavior. Recent studies have shown long-lasting effects on cellular immune function and steroid levels by the simple movement of a new animal into the room environment. We must definitely concern ourselves with these aspects, not only for public perception, but also for the animals' well-being and the successful conduct of studies.

Nutrition and Water

Fortunately, there are adequate diets available commercially for some nonhuman primates. Unfortunately, the exact nutritional requirements for most species of primates are unknown. Most importantly, concern must be shown with the feeding techniques, feeding frequency, and feeding receptacles used with primates. Careful observation of feeding behavior is essential. An empty feed cup does not signify a primate is eating because most of the biscuits may be on the floor. Nor does a half-empty feed cup indicate an animal is not eating adequately as each animal's metabolic rate is different.

Physical Form and Presentation

The majority of commercial primate feed is produced through an extrusion process resulting, after baking, in a very hard product. A young primate may find the product to be unpalatable unless softened by soaking. (The liquid used for moistening must be provided to the primate, as the vitamin C sprayed on the biscuit will be rinsed off into the liquid if discarded.)

Various projects dealt with in toxicology require oral dosing using a specific vehicle. Careful attention to amount of vehicle, particularly on twice or three times a day dosing regimens, is required to avoid "filling" the primate up with resultant reductions in food intake and potential nutritional deficiency.

The food must be kept palatable to the primate. Feed presented on the bottom of the cage without a feed cup may be contaminated by urine or feces, causing disease or an iatrogenic anorexia.

Available Diets and Analysis

Commercial diets have been developed for the usual species in toxicological research. These diets are usually adequate and can be followed with pre- or postproject analysis. Certified diets are also available. Careful attention to dates of manufacture and rotation of feed stuffs is a necessity. Primate diet should be utilized within 90 days of manufacture to avoid vitamin C deficiency. Analysis of noncertified commercial and noncommercial diets should be made to avoid potential contamination. Commercial diets have been found to have "close to biological effect" levels of various heavy metals.

Food Restriction

Specific projects may require food restriction. Several studies have shown food restrictions lessen tumors and increase the life span (Weindrick and Walford, 1988). These studies may have promise in certain studies to detect carcinogens. Current projects in nonhuman primates by the National Institute on Aging are on the effects of diet restriction on the life span. Food restriction studies require careful analysis to assure that animal well-being is not compromised as related to scientific gain.

Water

Clean fresh water should be available at all times. Modern husbandry systems provide water through filtered automatic water systems. Clean water bottles are also an acceptable method to provide water and have the advantage of quickly determining water consumption. Water can be an important source of potential contaminants which can interfere with a variety of study results. Careful analysis for lead, polychlorinated biphenyls (PCBs), and biological contaminants should be part of quality assurance assays.

Prevention of Disease and Injury

Procurement, Quarantine, and Conditioning

The assurance that the animal model used is of high quality and healthy is essential to any research program. This is particularly critical for nonhuman primates, which for the most part are obtained from wild/feral sources in China, Indonesia, or the Philippines. Only a few primates are bred in the United States under quality conditions.

Inherent then is the need to quarantine the primate for a set period of time to assure the highest quality animal for use. The primary reason for the quarantine length is to detect potential tuberculosis with further emphasis on immunizations and latent or clinical disease control (Renquist, 1975). Recent outbreaks of Ebola-like disease have required the CDC to publish new quarantine guidelines for control of this devastating disease (CDC, 1990).

Procurement Sources.   Nonhuman primates that are usually purchased for laboratory use may be categorized as: wild caught–unconditioned, wild caught–conditioned, or domestically bred. Less frequently, research protocols require that wild-caught monkeys be trapped and delivered under conditions that preclude contact with other primates, and, in some instances, cesarean-delivered or specific pathogen–free monkeys are required. From a strictly economic point of view, wild-caught monkeys are the least expensive to provide for research, whereas domestically bred monkeys are the most expensive. In terms of quality, however, the converse situation occurs. Procurement requirements, quarantine methods, assurance of personnel safety, therapeutic regimens, and husbandry procedures will vary according to the category of monkey used.

Quarantine and Conditioning Procedures.   Because the majority of monkeys used for research are wild caught, quarantine and conditioning procedures that pertain to the macaque will be described. It should be understood, however, that the following procedural descriptions may not be applicable to all institutions which utilize nonhuman primates because of differences in research needs, staffing, and facilities.

Wild-caught macaques (in this case, cynomolgus are described) are trapped by local villagers, collected in holding compounds by primate dealers, and shipped directly to the research facility by an animal importer.

The quarantine facility should consist of standard animal rooms equipped with squeeze-back cages. Prior to receipt of newly arrived monkeys, each cage should be washed in a cage washer and sanitized and the room washed under pressure, disinfected, and rinsed thoroughly. Iodophores and phenolics should be used for their tuberculocidal properties.

Purchased monkeys are delivered in crates containing individually segregated animals. Shipment lots can contain up to 100 animals. Immediately after receipt into the institutional quarantine facility, the monkeys are transferred from their shipping containers to quarantine cages directly and without handling. Drinking water and fruits are offered to assist in adaptation.

The animals are fed a commercial 15% protein monkey chow supplemented with fruit on the afternoon of arrival and allowed to acclimatize for 1 week. After acclimatization, the monkeys are sedated with ketamine HCl (5 mg/kg, im) and examined. Stress to the animals and hazards associated with physical restraint are contraindicated; mild chemical restraint is better for the animal's welfare and personnel safety. An electronic thermometer with an acrylic, rectal probe is used to obtain temperatures. The probe is shielded with a disposable plastic cover, which is changed between animals. Elevated temperature in the sedated primate is an accurate disease indicator unlike in the physically restrained animal. If indicated, fecal cultures are taken prior to taking of temperature. The animals are then examined for respiratory problems, suspicious enlargements, oral herpetic lesions, lacerations, dermatitis, and ectoparasitism. Minor problems, including wounds and dermatitis, are treated at this time and supportive therapy is administered to monkeys with diarrhea or dehydration. Consideration of severe disease problems in individual monkeys which may require extensive workup is reserved until all animals have been examined. Additional fecal cultures and hematological evaluations are performed as indicated.

Following physical examination, monkeys are tested for tuberculosis using 0.1 ml of veterinary mammalian tuberculin, full strength, administered intradermally in the eyelid (National Academy of Sciences [NAS], 1981; *Non-Human Primates—Standard Guidelines for the Breeding Care and Overall Management of Lab Animals*). Each monkey is given an antihelmintic (thiabendazole, 100 mg/kg) prophylactically, using an 8 French pediatric stomach tube. Since the pharyngeal reflex is not abolished by ketamine, the danger of intratracheal intubation is minimal.

Prophylactic injections of benzathine and procaine penicillin G (300,000 U, im) may be indicated dependent on disease status, etc. Vitamins C and B complex (0.25–0.50 ml, im) may also be given.

Monkeys are tattooed consecutively using a combination of letters and numbers per institution policy. Information such as weight, abnormalities, and clinical signs is entered on the animal's individual record. The monkey is then returned to its cage.

The quarantine period procedures are based on recommendations by the National Academy of Sciences (1981). In summary, monkeys are quarantined for 90 days in order to diagnose and eradicate tuberculosis (TB). A total of five consecutive, negative TB tests on each animal (after receipt) in each room must be achieved prior to releasing the group from quarantine. All reactors are examined, radiographed, sacrificed, and necropsied.

All monkeys in the facility are observed twice daily by a veterinarian, who prescribes treatments and institutes diagnostic protocols for sick or debilitated animals. Urgency is paramount in any primate facility. For example, a debilitated animal which exhibits anorexia, nasal discharge, or diarrhea requires prompt attention. Treatment is initiated immediately to alleviate clinical signs; specific therapy is begun after the results of diagnostic tests have been evaluated.

A brief resume of treatment procedures is as follows: Diarrhea is treated with Kaopectate (5 ml/kg, p.o.) after sedation with ketamine. Cultures are made when blood or mucus is seen in the feces and a broad-spectrum bacteriolytic agent is given immediately. This original treatment is continued or changed depending on the results of culture and sensitivity testing. Antidiarrheal agents, which have been used successfully, are amino pentamide hydrogen sulfate (0.1 mg/10 lb, im), chloramphenicol (50 mg/kg/day, im), kanamycin sulfate® (10 mg/kg, im), and sulfa combinations. Because specific animal groups usually harbor bacteria with similar antibiotic sensitivities, one drug can usually be employed for treatment. Bacteriolytic agents are continued for at least 5 days after cessation of clinical signs. Fluid therapy (lactated Ringer's [iv or sc] or oral electrolyte) is essential for all monkeys with diarrhea or dysentery.

Pneumonia is a problem during the winter months owing to shipping delays at airports and inclement weather. Severe epizootics of pneumonia have occurred in rhesus or cynomolgus monkeys which were associated with measles (rubeola) outbreaks the first few weeks of quarantine (Potkay et al., 1971). Vaccination with modified live measles vaccine is indicated. Supportive therapy, including administration of antibiotics such as chloramphenicol, kanamycin, penicillin, or gentamicin is recommended to treat pneumonia caused by secondary bacterial invaders. The selection of antibiotics should be based on the results of culture and sensitivity tests.

Other disease problems include amebiasis, dermatophytosis, and miscellaneous traumatic injuries. Most of these entities become manifest during the first 14–21 days after arrival. Thereafter, the health status of most animals stabilizes considerably.

Blood is obtained from selected animals to further evaluate their health status and for reference serology. Seventeen to 21 days following the receipt into the facility, feces of monkeys selected at random are analyzed for the presence of parasites and pathogenic bacteria. Specific antihelmintics, antiprotozoal agents, and antibiotics are prescribed as indicated to individual monkeys or to groups. Animals are observed and treated for the remaining quarantine period as required.

The foregoing description of quarantine and conditioning procedures is applicable to cynomolgus and other macaques obtained from the wild (Renquist, 1975; NAS, 1981). Domestically bred macaques which have been tested and found to be free of infectious diseases communicable to humans (e.g., shigellosis herpes B virus infection and tuberculosis) do not require such rigid quarantine measures. It is necessary, however, to provide a sufficient period of time for such monkeys to become adapted to a laboratory cage environment, since the majority are born and raised in large harem-type cages or corrals. During the adaptation period, valuable baseline date (hematological, serological, microbiological, and physiological) may be compiled for individual monkeys.

Occupational Health Program

Transmission of disease between primates and humans has been described. Recently, cases of herpes B, latent in the macaque but fatal in humans, have been incriminated in several deaths of animal handlers (CDC Morbidity Mortality Report, 1987). An Occupational Health Program is essential including preemployment screens for tuberculosis and physical examination with complete medical history. Banked reference serum samples and continuous monitoring is necessary with evaluation by the physician to assure employee health. The reader is referred to the NAS (1981) standards for specific information on evaluation criteria (CDC Morbidity Mortality Report, 1987).

The establishment and maintenance of quality standard operating procedures on personnel cleanliness, animal handling, clothing requirements, and personnel operating procedures should be the norm for any facility.

Common Diseases

The information on primate diseases could fill a small volume. The diseases and descriptions noted herein are those most common to the primate toxicology laboratory.

Respiratory Diseases. Pneumonia is seen in primate colonies and is most often due to changes in environment related to stress of shipment, or sudden changes in temperature, humidity, or temperature. In macaques, this is often a complication of rubeola (measles) and specific bacterial pathogens; e.g., *Bordetella* or *Streptococcus*. Appropriate antibiotics and measles vaccination is recommended (Good and May, 1971).

Enteric Diseases. Diarrhea and/or dysentery are probably the most common diseases in nonhuman primates. The major causative organism is *Shigella* with *Salmonella* or *Campylobacter* running a close second (Weil et al., 1971; Renquist, 1987a). Unfortunately, latent infection without clinical signs is common and can be exacerbated by the rigor of the experimental protocol. Clearing protocols may be necessary to reduce the latent carrier state; however, these antibiotic regimens are often costly and time consuming. Appropriate therapy when evidence of clinical disease is seen is often the best approach.

Tuberculosis. The bane of the research laboratory is tuberculosis caused by a variety of mycobacterial organisms (Renquist, 1987a). Appropriate tuberculin testing coupled with rigorous quarantine can eliminate this disease if observed prior to study initiation.

Viral Diseases. Measles (rubeola) is the most common viral disease. Certainly other viral pathogens, e.g., poxviruses, hepatitis, simian hemorrhagic fever, and rabies have also caused problems in a variety of research facilities. Most recently, serious concerns have been caused by herpes B (Renquist, 1987b). Unfortunately, the incidence of herpes B antibody approaches 60% in most colonies. Herpes B is latent in macaques, causing a fever blister–type lesion with no ill effects. When an individual is scratched or bitten by a positive primate, fatal consequences may result. The CDC has developed a set of guidelines for herpes B exposure and Ebola-like disease which should be carefully followed for both liability and employee health aspects (CDC Morbidity Mortality Report, 1987, 1990).

Licensing and Records

Licensing

The Animal Welfare Act (Public Law 89-544), as amended most recently in 1991 (*Federal Register*, 1991), requires the registration and inspection of primate facilities. The USDA Animal Plant Health Inspection Service is involved with enforcement. Direct importers of primates must also be registered with the Centers for Disease Control.

Other regulations and agencies covering primates and their care and use are the Department of the Interior; Federal Wildlife Permit Regulations; Convention on International Trade in Endangered Species of Wild Fauna and Flora (CITES); and the National Academy of Sciences, Institute of Laboratory Animal Resources.

Records

Accurate record keeping is required by law and is essential from the source to the completion of project. This involves source country, date of receipt, importer, age, sex, body weight, and tattoo numbers. This is particularly critical for animals for which a federal wildlife permit is required or when animals are on the threatened or endangered Convention on International Trade in Endangered Species list (e.g., chimpanzees).

STUDY DESIGN

The design of a study protocol is dependent upon the intended indication of the drug or biological product and the population for which it is intended (Hobson and Fuller, 1987). Guidelines issued by regulatory agencies such as the Food and Drug Administration (FDA) or similar agencies of other countries usually provide input into studies designed for safety assessment. Study duration ranges from single-dose acute studies through subchronic multiple dose studies of up to 90 days in length to chronic multiple-dose studies which may be up to 1 year in duration.

Drugs that are intended for the reproductively active population sometimes require a three-segment testing plan (not to be confused with the standard three-segment reproductive evaluation in rodents) (Hendrickx and Cukierski, 1987; Hendrickx and Binkerd, 1990). In segment I, menstrual cycles and hormone levels (estrogen, progesterone, luteinizing hormone, and follicle-stimulating hormone) are monitored for 90–180 days, depending on protocol design, and spermatogenesis and testosterone levels are evaluated in males during a minimum 60-day treatment period. In segment II studies, pregnant females are treated during the period of organogenesis (gestation days 21–89) and a cesarean section usually performed on day 100 for assessment of fetal abnormalities. The late gestational effects of a test material are examined in segment III studies. Pregnant females are administered the drug from gestation days 90–150 for evaluation of any abnormal neonatal neurological or behavioral responses.

Dose levels tested are usually based on a proposed human dose or exposure. The lowest dosage in a safety evaluation study is usually greater than the expected human dose and should define the highest no-effect level. The highest dose is some multiple (e.g., 10–100×) of the proposed clinical human dose and should induce toxicity. The mid-dose is an intermediate level usually with minimal toxicity to provide characterization of a dose response to the test article.

DOSING TECHNIQUES

The dosing technique utilized in safety studies with nonhuman primates approximates as closely as possible the expected route of exposure in humans. Dosing procedures used in research protocols will vary depending upon the experimental objectives or the biochemical characteristics of the compound. Typically, pharmaceuticals are administered orally by gavage and biotechnology-derived proteins are given either intravenously, intramuscularly, or subcutaneously. Other less common routes of dose administration are intranasal, intraperitoneal, and occasionally test materials are given in alternate oral routes such as in fruit slices, sugar cubes, or a fruit drink.

Oral

Oral administration of drugs in safety-evaluation studies has generally been conducted in squirrel monkeys or young macaques and in limited numbers of immature baboons. The reasons for the size limitations in nonhuman primate models is the expense of special handling equipment and the size and aggressive nature of mature monkeys and great apes. Also, an adequate amount of historical data is available only in a limited number of primate species. Procedures must be employed which are nonstressful for the animal, yet protect personnel and animals from injury. Infectious disease agents which may be carried by some of the primate models such as the herpes B virus and Ebola virus may be transmitted to animal handlers with potentially fatal consequences. However, with proper training of personnel in the handling of nonhuman primates, oral toxicity studies may be successfully conducted and the potential risks minimized.

Techniques for oral administration of a test article include stomach or nasogastric intubation, capsule (by gavage), or (when palatable) on a piece of fruit or in a drink such as fruit juice. Oral or nasogastric gavage is the most commonly utilized technique.

Gavage

In the gavage procedure, a tube is introduced into the esophagus either through the mouth or nostril and the test article flushed into the stomach.

Equipment. Commercially available gavage tubes ranging in size from 8 to 12 French (ID) are utilized for most oral gavage of liquids. When specialized tubing is required (e.g., for capsules) tygon or polyethylene tubing of appropriate size is utilized. The end of the tube is beveled, then blunted by heat to prevent esophagal or stomach punctures.

A syringe is attached to the tube for delivery of the test article and/or the flushing solution. An 8 French feeding tube is generally used for nasogastric intubation (Fig. 2) when small volumes or low-viscosity liquids are presented or for stomach tubing of small primates (e.g., squirrel monkeys or infant macaques).

Although large monkeys may be manually restrained for dosing procedures, the risk of

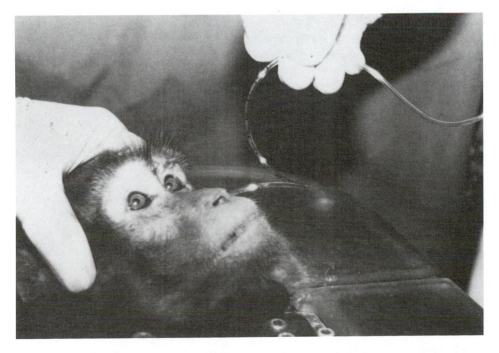

Figure 2 Nasogastric dose administration.

injury to personnel is high, as the head of the animal must be held securely by animal technicians.

A chair restraint system offers the advantage of minimum exposure to the animal's head and limbs, thus less risk for animal handling personnel. In addition, this restraint system is less stressful to the animal than manual restraint, as the animal is not touched by the technician (Anderson and Houghton, 1983).

When using this system an aluminum or hard plastic collar is placed around the neck of an anesthetized animal and remains in place for the duration of the study. Aluminum poles with snap-type hooks are inserted into the cage and attached to the collars. The animal is led from the cage and placed in a chair (Fig. 3) and the collar secured to the chair. In this manner, minimal handling of the animal's head is required for dosing. After dosing, the animal can be led back to the cage and released. Animals adapt to this handling procedure very quickly.

Chimpanzees have been utilized on a limited basis for acute nonterminal toxicity studies. Animals of this size are usually maintained anesthetized for serial bleeds over a

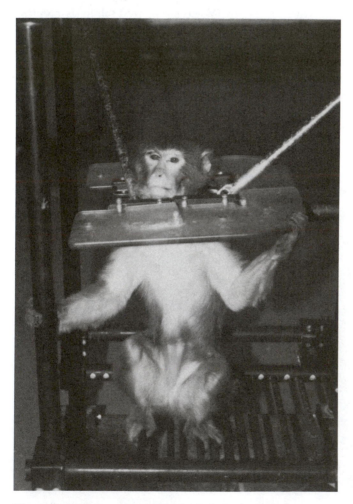

Figure 3   Rhesus monkey held in chair for oral gavage.

maximum of 6 hours after which they can be lightly dosed with ketamine HCl for subsequent bleeds. Some chimpanzees can be trained for alert bleeding, but only experienced personnel should be allowed to handle the animal.

Test Article Preparation. The test article is usually prepared on the day of dosing. When the compound is soluble in an aqueous medium, distilled water may be used as the diluent. Control animals should be administered a volume equivalent to that received by the high-dose animals. The dosing volume for nonhuman primates usually does not exceed 10 ml/kg body weight for oral dosing. If the test article is insoluble, a suspension may be prepared with methylcellulose or equivalent suspending agents with or without the wetting agent Tween 80. If stability testing has been conducted for test compounds under varying laboratory and storage conditions, bulk quantities may be prepared and maintained for longer periods of time; e.g., weekly, every other week, monthly or for the study duration.

Dose Administration. Individual doses are drawn up into graduated syringes in the laboratory. Syringes are labeled with the animal number, the study, and group color code and is verified by a research technician not involved in the dose preparation. Syringes are placed in a rack, also color coded, and transported to the animal room. Three research technicians are utilized for the dosing procedure for large toxicity studies; e.g., 32–48 animals. Monkeys are fasted overnight prior to a morning dosing. Two handlers, each with a pole, are required to capture an animal and place it in the primate chair. The door to the animal's cage is opened slightly, a pole inserted, and the pole attached to a ring on the collar. The animal is restrained within the cage, the door opened and the other pole attached to the ring on the opposite side of the collar. The animal is then led out of the cage and into the chair for restraint. The third technician, meanwhile, has the animal's dosing syringe and tube (nasogastric or oral) available for dose administration. A technician, wearing appropriate gloves and arm covers, restrains the animal's head, the tube is inserted and slight negative pressure is applied to the syringe to check for air bubbles indicating a possible lung intubation. The dose is administered, a flushing syringe containing a small amount of vehicle attached and the remaining contents of the tube flushed into the stomach. The tube is removed and the animal is observed for a moment to observe for vomiting. The poles are reattached to the collar and the animal returned to the cage. The dosing procedure requires approximately 3–5 min per animal.

Risks to the animals are minimal if proper procedure is followed; however, if the dose is inadvertently placed in the lung rather than the stomach chances for animal survival are minimal.

Caustic or irritating compounds or large gavage volumes may induce an emetic response which, if aspirated in the lungs, can result in the death of the animal. When aspiration of a corrosive test substance occurs more than once or twice in a study, consideration must be given to reducing the dose or canceling the study.

Capsule

Plain gelatin or enteric-coated capsules are administered when testing a potential new drug delivery system or when a slower absorption rate is required. The technique for dosing with capsules is similar to oral dosing with a liquid. The plain or coated capsule is slightly wedged into the end of a 8- to 14-in length of tygon tubing of slightly larger inside diameter than the diameter of capsule. A syringe, usually containing 10–15 ml of tap water, is attached to the end of the tube. The capsule-plugged end of the tube is intubated and the capsule flushed into the stomach. Several capsules may be administered simultaneously if a size larger capsule is used to plug the end of the tubing and smaller capsules placed loosely in the bore of the dry tube. Several capsules can, in this way, be administered to one animal without repeated intubations. Several hundred milligrams of test article may be administered in this manner. Commercially prepared capsules or specially coated caplets offer the advantage of minimal chances for a dosing error. Plain gelatin capsules, whether prepared by the toxicology laboratory or a sponsor, have the potential disadvantage of dissolving very rapidly. Saliva from a struggling monkey or one that bites the intubation tube will prematurely dissolve or rupture the capsule prior to flushing into the stomach. Prestudy adaptation training will minimize these problems. For example, once daily intubation of empty gelatin capsules for 1 to 2 weeks prior to study initiation will be sufficient to establish cooperation from most animals.

Diet

Nonhuman primates have a propensity for playing with their food and throwing it from their cage or breaking it up and dropping it through the cage floor, thus making it nearly impossible to quantitate dietary consumption or to deliver a standard dose contained in the diet. On a limited basis, small quantities of test material have been placed on sugar cubes, in small pieces of fruit, or dissolved in a fruit drink such as Tang. Animal technicians will present the test article–treated food item and observe to verify that it is consumed by the animal. Liquid may be administered from a syringe such that the animal voluntarily drinks the dosing solution. Problems encountered with these methods include removal of portions of the sugar cube or fruit from their mouth and refusing to complete the dosing, or losing some of the fruit drink through spillage or refusal to swallow all of their dose solution, making quantitation of the total dose administered difficult. These problems are minimal or nonexistent if the test article/food mixture is highly palatable to the animal. Additionally, the effects of the content of such vehicles on metabolism of the compound must be ascertained as part of the study design.

Intravenous

The intravenous route of drug administration is now the most common for safety or efficacy studies. This has resulted from the large number of recombinant proteins being developed for treatment of various diseases and monoclonal antibodies targeted for certain cancerous tumors. The cephalic and saphenous veins are the most accessible for acute subchronic or chronic venipuncture. All veins, including the femoral and the jugular, can be catheterized for acute or subchronic intravenous infusions, although many veins require a surgical cut-down procedure for catheter introduction. In addition, specialized restraint devices are required for protection of the catheters from the animals (e.g., primate chairs, vascular ports, or jacket-tether systems).

Cephalic and Saphenous

The two largest, most accessible superficial veins for venipuncture are the cephalic and saphenous. The cephalic vein is located on the dorsal arm near the bend of the elbow of the nonhuman primate. The saphenous vein can be found on the ventral side of the leg from the knee to the ankle. Toxicology studies requiring a single daily injection for as long as a year can be performed successfully if proper techniques are utilized.

Alert-Capture Technique.   Study animals are housed singly in squeeze-back cages for the study duration. Wearing appropriate protective apparel (lab-specific clothing, gloves, mask, arm guards), trained technicians capture the animals and administer the test article. Squirrel monkeys are caught by technicians wearing heavy leather gloves with long gauntlets by reaching into the cage, placing a thumb and forefinger firmly around the animal's body, and gently removing it from the cage. The animal is restrained on a table, stomach down, by the technician exposing the back of the leg for a saphenous injection by a second technician.

Macaques and small baboons are usually not removed from their cages for treatment. The animal is pulled to the front of the cage by the squeeze mechanism, which is locked in position. The technician carefully maneuvers an arm or leg near the feeding hole in the lower front of the cage. Once the foot or hand is gripped tightly, the squeeze mechanism is allowed to return approximately one-third of the width of the cage, permitting the animal to lean toward the rear of the cage. The limb can now be extended through the hole for accessibility to the vein (Fig. 4). Prior to injection, a portable clipper is used to remove the hair from 2 to 4 in along the length of the vein. The exposed area is cleaned with an alcohol pad and pressure applied to the vein with the thumb while holding the limb with

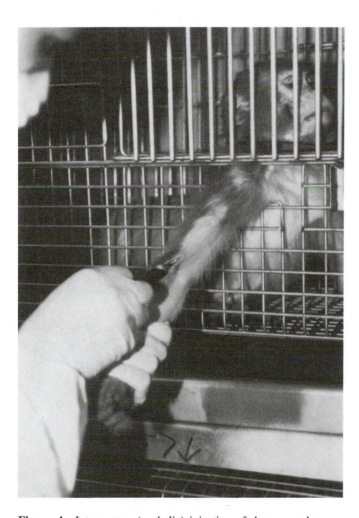

Figure 4 Intravenous (cephalic) injection of rhesus monkey.

the hand. Pressure is applied proximal to the intended injection site. As blood flow is impeded, the vein becomes visible to the technician. The needle, attached to the dosing syringe, is placed bevel up against the skin. Pressure is exerted until there is a slight give, usually indicating entry into the vein. Slight back pressure on the syringe will draw blood into the hub of the needle, verifying venous placement, at which point the test compound may be administered.

Syringe and needle sizes vary with the volume and characteristics of the compound to be injected. Needle sizes usually range from 21 to 25 gauge and syringes from 1 to 10 ml. Total injection volumes range from less than 1 to 10 ml per injection. Injection volumes of greater than 5 ml are more successful when a small butterfly catheter is placed into the vein for dosing. This is best done by two technicians, one to restrain the limb and ensure that the butterfly is not dislodged and the second to administer the dose through the distal end of the catheter and subsequently flush the remaining dose with appropriate vehicle (e.g., saline).

Chair Restraint Technique.   Studies requiring an intravenous infusion for periods of time ranging from 30 min to several hours are conducted using primate restraint chairs (Fig. 5).

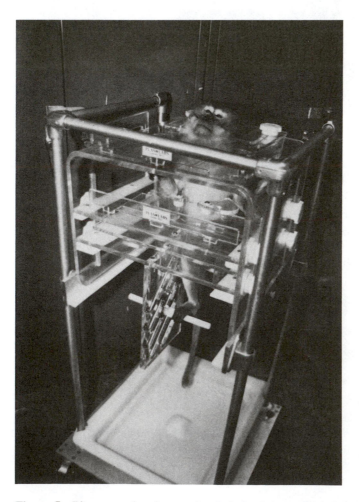

Figure 5   Rhesus monkey in restraint chair for intravenous infusion.

Animals should normally be adapted to chairs prior to study initiation. Two-hour chairing sessions every other day for 2 weeks reduces stress related to the chairing procedure. Animals are first anesthetized with ketamine HCl (approximately 10 mg/kg) and an indwelling catheter introduced (Fig. 6) into the cephalic or saphenous vein (Flynn and Guilboud, 1988). The animal is placed in a restraint chair and allowed to recover from the anesthesia prior to dosing. If the cephalic vein is used for dosing, some provision must be made to secure the opposite hand and arm to prevent the catheter from being pulled from the vein by the animal's free hand. The prepared dose is drawn up in an appropriate-sized syringe and placed on an infusion pump set to deliver the designated dose concentration at a preset rate. An extension tube is attached from the syringe to the catheter for delivery of the dosing solution. The volume of the extension tube must be known so that extra test article can be prepared for total delivery of the dose. Animals can be held in the chairs for up to 12 hr without inducing unacceptable stress to the animal, but a shorter restraint period, e.g. 6 hr, is desirable. At the termination of dosing, the catheter is removed, hemostasis induced, and the animals anesthetized, removed from the chairs, and returned to their cages.

Femoral and Jugular Veins

Jacket-Tether Technique. The femoral and jugular veins are ideal for chronic infusion studies. Placement of an indwelling catheter requires a minor surgical cut-down but offers the advantage of animal inaccessibility to the catheter if it is channeled under the skin to an exit site located on the back of animal and protected by a jacket and tether system (Bryant, 1980). The test article can be delivered via an infusion pump over extended periods of time (i.e., several hours or days). These procedures are applicable for New and Old World monkeys but are not feasible for animals as large as adult chimpanzees.

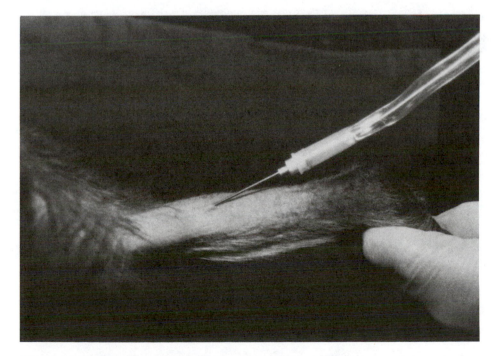

Figure 6 Placement of a saphenous indwelling catheter.

Animals are acclimated to the tethers and jackets for two weeks prior to placement of the catheter. During this period, the jacket is worn by the animal while the tether (flexible steel tube) hangs freely in the cage unattached to the animal. After the acclimatization period, the animal is sedated and taken to the surgery suite. The animal is prepared for surgery and an incision made in the skin above the vein and/or artery to be catheterized. The vessel is located and separated from connective tissue by blunt dissection. The vessel is elevated with suture to impede blood flow and a small cut is made in the vessel with iris scissors. A catheter introducer is inserted into the incision to facilitate introduction of the catheter.

The catheter is inserted into the vein or artery for 5–8 in, depending upon the size of the animal. The most desirable placement of the catheter is in the femoral artery or vein so that the catheter tip extends to either the vena cava or aorta, facilitating infusion and/or blood sampling procedures. The catheter is held in place by ligatures placed around the vessel and on both sides of an elevation (or "donut") located several inches up the catheter. This prevents the catheter from being pulled from the vein or artery by pressure exerted from normal body movement. As an additional precaution, a stress loop is made in the catheter and anchored with suture just under the skin. A trocar is used to tunnel the catheter under the skin to the middle of the back where it is exited. The catheter is then passed through the mounting plate attached to the jacket and through the tether to the appropriate channel on the underside of the swivel. Another length of catheter is attached to the same channel on the top of the swivel and then to an infusion pump. Aseptic technique in handling the exposed end of the catheter is extremely important to the success of this system. Frequent observations for potential problems with jackets and the tethering system are important if study objectives are to be met (Fig. 7). Primates are particularly

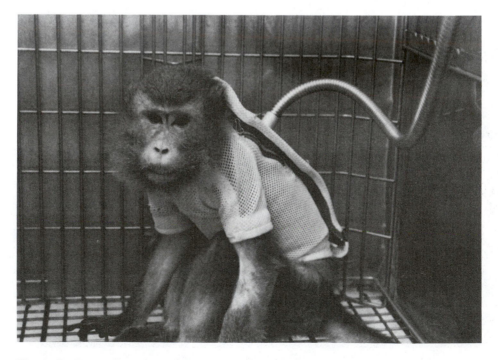

Figure 7 Cynomolgus monkey fitted with a jacket and tether for chronic infusion.

adept at manipulating this system, and thus require frequent monitoring to correct animal attempts to remove the jacket.

Vascular Port Technique. The vascular port is a subcutaneously implanted device which provides chronic vascular access and eliminates multiple venipunctures (Dalton, 1985). The injection port is a silicone rubber septum housed in a rigid elastomeric base that can be anchored with sutures under the skin. The placement of the vascular port is usually in the middle of the back from which the catheter is tunneled under the skin to the femoral vein for catheterization, as described earlier. Catheter patency is maintained with a heparin-saline lock.

Dosing is performed by injecting the test article into the port and the catheterized vein. Animals are lightly sedated for ease of handling and safety concerns. Location of the port and septum is easily accomplished by palpation. The area of the skin above the port is sterilized with alcohol or Betadine, the needle inserted through the septum, and dosing initiated. The heparin-saline solution is used to flush the remaining test article from the catheter and the patency lock restored.

Intramuscular

Intramuscular administration of a test compound provides reasonably quick absorption depending upon the vehicle. Biologicals delivered in oil are released much slower than from an aqueous carrier. In nonhuman primates, the injection site is usually the outer thigh, although the triceps are also utilized in larger animals.

Monkeys and small baboons can be dosed alert, whereas large baboons and chimpanzees should be sedated. The cage squeeze mechanism allows the monkey to be captured and a leg or arm exited through the feeding opening in the front of the cage. Hair is clipped from the injection site and the site disinfected with an alcohol or Betadine pad. Using an appropriate-size needle and syringe, the skin and muscle are penetrated. A slight vacuum is applied to the syringe to check for possible venous puncture. If blood is drawn into the syringe, the needle should be removed and the process repeated. If no blood appears, the plunger is depressed slowly until the dose is administered. The needle is then removed and pressure applied to the injection site for approximately 30 sec with a gauze pad to complete the dosing procedure.

Dosing volume should be limited to less than 1 ml to minimize pain. If larger dosing volumes are required, two injection sites should be utilized.

Subcutaneous

Subcutaneous administration of a test compound is frequently utilized in toxicity studies when a slower absorption rate is required. The dose is delivered between the dermal and muscle layers, usually in the area of the inner thigh. The loose skin at this site allows for volumes up to 3 ml to be administered. Other subcutaneous injection sites commonly utilized are the back and limbs for smaller volumes of dosing material (less than 0.5 ml).

Capture procedures for the animals are as previously described. The injection site is shaved, cleaned, and sterilized with an alcohol or Betadine pad. The skin is grasped between the thumb and forefinger and pulled up and away from the muscle. The skin is penetrated with the needle at approximately a 15-degree angle to the injection site. As the plunger is depressed, a small bubble should appear as the dosing progresses. There should be no resistance to the injection. If resistance is noted and the bubble is firm, close to the surface, and appears white in color, then the injection is being administered intradermally.

The needle should be inserted deeper into the space between the skin and muscle and the dosing completed. One animal technician should restrain the animal while another administers the dose. This ensures complete delivery of the test compound and prevents possible injury to the animal or handler.

Miscellaneous Routes of Exposure

Intranasal

The development of aerosol drug delivery systems for inhalation therapy has resulted in increased intranasal toxicity assessments. Test articles are administered into each nare with the aid of an aerosolizer pump. Discharge from the reservoir can be accurately calibrated, but total delivery into the nasal cavity is not always successful in an alert animal. Dosing of the larger monkeys is best accomplished using the pole and collar chair system as previously described. This technique allows for better control of the head while the delivery tube is placed a short distance into the nostril for dose administration.

Intraperitoneal

Although not a common route for exposure to a test compound in nonhuman primates, intraperitoneal injections or infusions permit rapid absorption into the portal circulation. In humans, this route would place therapeutic agents in close proximity to tumors of the abdominal organs; thus nonhuman primate testing by this route may occur on a limited acute basis.

The jacket-tether system is ideal for continuous intraperitoneal infusions for extended periods of time. This method has been utilized successfully to deliver tumor-specific monoclonal antibodies in safety-evaluation studies. Serial interperitoneal injections (needle or catheter) of nonhuman primates are not recommended because of the high probability of infection as well as the potential for bladder or intestinal puncture. Single injections are usually performed on anesthetized animals. The entire abdomen and inner upper thigh is shaved, cleaned, and sterilized. Using a Betadine swab (or solution) the injection site, which is 1–2 in below and 1–2 in lateral to the navel, is again sterilized.

The skin is pulled slightly to the center of the abdomen with the thumb of one hand while inserting the needle at an angle of approximately 45 degrees into the injection site with the other hand. The purpose for pulling the skin to one side and placing the needle or catheter at an angle ensures that when the needle/catheter is removed an interrupted channel into the body cavity is established. This reduces bleeding and decreases the chances for infection. A short catheter (2 in) or needle reduces the chances of perforating the bladder, intestine, or other organs. The location of the needle/catheter can be checked by injecting 1–2 ml of saline followed by gentle vacuum with a syringe. If blood, fecal material, urine, or fluid other than saline is aspirated into the syringe, the procedure must be reattempted on the opposite side. Health-threatening consequences could result from organ perforation; thus the veterinarian should be notified immediately and appropriate antibiotic therapy begun.

If an organ is not punctured, release thumb pressure on the skin, which will stabilize the needle or catheter for injection. As the plunger of the syringe is depressed, attention must be directed at the injection site for possible swelling, which would indicate a subcutaneous or intramuscular dose. If swelling occurs, dosing is stopped and the procedure repeated. Following completion of the injection, the needle/catheter is removed and pressure applied to the injection site for approximately 30 sec followed by observation for any bleeding or swelling at the site.

Infrequent Routes of Dose Administration

Drug delivery systems designed for special therapeutic applications have been evaluated in safety studies but are not considered "routine" procedures. Such procedures include osmotic mini pumps or other drug-containing implants, topical administration, rectal administration via suppositories or liquids, and sublingual dosing. Many applications require surgical procedures or can only be administered to anesthetized animals or animals physically restrained in primate chairs. Such methods are typically utilized only for acute dosing protocols and are considered unacceptable for subchronic or chronic toxicity assessments. Inhalation toxicology is an unique area requiring specialized equipment and facilities not usually found in general toxicology laboratories and is thus beyond the scope of this review.

DATA AND SAMPLE COLLECTION TECHNIQUES

Almost all Good Laboratory Practice (GLP) primate studies require data collection by observation, physical examination, and body weights; most studies also utilize urine and blood collection for clinical chemistry, hematology, endocrine analyses, and drug level determination. A few studies require measurement of cardiovascular parameters, ophthalmic examination (direct or indirect), body temperature, and body measurements. Occasionally more specialized tests or samples such as menstrual cycle status, pregnancy tests, invasive cardiovascular measurements, nerve conduction velocity, EEGs, and tissue biopsy are required. A declining number of toxicity studies require complete necropsy of the test animals. Rising prices and an increased appreciation of the conservation ethic by regulatory agencies probably mean that the number of terminal studies will decline even further.

Sample collection from great apes is limited to nonterminal and non–life-threatening techniques. Tissues occasionally become available from moribund animals which are humanely sacrificed or from animals dying of natural causes.

Both study design and animal inventory planning have recently been impacted by the requirement that primates can only be subjected to one major experimental surgical procedure during their lifetime (*Federal Register*, 1991). If justified, more than one such procedure within a single experimental protocol is allowed if it is scientifically necessary and is approved by the Institutional Animal Care and Use Committee (IACUC).

Daily Observations

Because primates have complex and highly individualized behavior patterns, obtaining meaningful observation data depends on both the experience of the observer and his or her familiarity with individual animals. The movement toward group caging and placement of environment-enriching devices in the cages make this task even more complex. Ideally, observations should be made at the same time(s) each day and by the same observer each day. Changes in behavior or appearance are most important to note. An experienced observer should be quick to note (Silverman, 1988):

Lethargy
Dehydration
Unusual posture
Condition of hair coat
Brightness or dullness of the eyes
Unusual fluid from body orifices

Unusual motions
Self-mutilation
Panting
Hyperactivity
Startle reactions
Apparent pain or discomfort
"Favoring" of individual limbs
Evidence of changes in appetite or water consumption
Changes in stool consistency
Changes at injection sites (where relevant)
Any other unusual behavior or appearance

Physical Examinations

The physical examination can be one of the most important criteria to determine animal acceptability for study. Protocol requirements vary from a generalized physical, including the majority of organ system, e.g., integument, respiratory, cardiovascular, urogenital, musculoskeletal, and lymphatics, to specialized examinations, which can include endocrinological profiles and ophthalmological and/or neurological examinations (Keeling and Wolf, 1975).

Usually, CBC, SMA, and fecal parasite evaluations are included in the general physical examination. Examples of a prestudy physical examination and/or ophthalmic examination form are included (Appendix). Tables 2 and 3 delineate typical normal ranges for clinical chemistry data on nonhuman primates commonly used in toxicity evaluation studies.

Body Weights

Toxicologists who are not used to data from primate studies are often surprised by the variability of body weights within individual monkeys. It is not uncommon in a short study to encounter weight changes of 10% or more which are totally unrelated to the experimental protocol. These changes can be minimized by weighing and feeding at the same time each day. Weights taken just prior to feeding tend to be less variable. Longer-term acclimatization to the room, the diet, and the other animals in the room is also helpful (Renquist, 1975).

Anesthetized animals can be weighed on conventional scales; however, the use of tared transfer boxes allow weights to be taken without sedating animals. Animals can be readily trained to enter the boxes, particularly if they are housed in cages with squeeze-back mechanisms.

Blood Collection

Trained and experienced technicians can collect blood samples from alert (unanesthetized) macaques in most situations without danger to either the animal or the technician. If the technicians are not experienced, if the macaques are large males, if the cages are not the appropriate type, or if the blood volume needed is large then animals should be anesthetized prior to venipuncture. Some studies have shown physiological and immunological changes caused by behavioral stress with alert bleeds (Mason, 1972). These possibilities must be considered in any study design. In certain instances, macaques and adult chimpanzees and baboons can be trained to submit voluntarily to blood collection procedures by experienced technicians (Hein et al., 1989; Vertein and Reinhardt, 1989);

Table 2 Hematology of Nonhuman Primates, Normal Ranges

Test	Units	Squirrel monkey[b] (*Saimiri sciureus*)	Cynomolgus monkey[a] (*Macaca fascicularis*)	Rhesus monkey[a] (*Macaca mulatta*)	Baboon[c,d] (*Papio* sp.)	Chimpanzee[a] (*Pan troglodytes*)
White blood cells (WBC)	Thsd/mm^3	3.4–14.8	4.5–14.0	5.5–15.4	—	7.2–16.8
Red blood cells (RBC)	mill/mm^3	7.1–10.9	4.6–6.5	4.0–6.6	—	4.8–5.8
Hemoglobin (HGB)	gm%	12.9–17.0	10.0–13.1	10.9–15.5	8.7–13.9	12.0–5.8
Hematocrit (HCT)	percent	—	30–41	35.2–47.6	31–43	36.0–49.5
Mean corpuscular volume (MCV)	μ^3	41.4–62.7	57–68	65–79	63–90	64–102
Mean corpuscular hemoglobin (MCH)	$\mu\mu$g	13.9–20.1	18–22	21–27	18–27	20–34
Mean corpuscular hemoglobin concentration (MCHC)	percent	29.2–34.8	30–33	30–34	28–34	27–36
Platelets (PLT)	thsd/mm^3	—	200–550	230–650	225–544	150–450
Reticulocytes	percent	—	0.1–1.1	0–1.9	0.3–2.3	0.5–1.5
Differential:						
Segmented neutrophils (SEGS)	percent	13.0–79.0	10–50	32–83	23–78	55–80
Lymphocytes (LYMPH)	percent	19.0–82.0	50–80	34–69	14–76	12–45
Monocytes (MONO)	percent	0.0–6.0	0–2	0–2	0–3	0–5
Eosinophils (EOS)	percent	0.0–22.0	2–8	0–6	0–8	0–2
Basophils (BASO)	percent	0.0–4.0	0–2	0–1	0–1	0–1
Coagulation:						
Prothrombin time (PT)	sec	—	8.9–12.9	9.4–13.4	11.5–13.0	10.0–13.4
Activated partial thromboplastin time (APTT)	sec	—	16.9–33.9	19.5–25.3	29.5–38.0	18.9–35.6
Fibrin degradation products (FDP)	μg%	—	<8	<8	—	<8
Fibrinogen (FIBRIN)	mg%	—	150–300	187–411	180–230	139–416

[a]Primate Research Laboratory, NMSU; Colony Historical Data.
[b]Abee, C. R. (1985) Medical care of management of the squirrel monkey, in *Handbook of Squirrel Monkey Research*, Rosenblum, L. A., and Coe, C. L. eds. Plenum Press, New York, pp. 484–485.
[c]Hack, C. A., and Gleiser, C. A. (1982) Hematologic and serum chemistry reference values for adult and juvenile baboons (*Papio* sp). *Lab. Anim. Sci.* 32, 502–505.
[d]Kelly, C. A., and Gleiser, C. A. (1986) Selected coagulation values for adult and juvenile baboons. *Lab. Anim. Sci.* 36, 173–175.

however, routine blood collections in the larger species are almost always done under anesthesia (ketamine HCl) (Muchmore, 1973) because of the danger of injury to technicians by stronger animals and increased activity during blood drawing from alert animals can adversely affect some clinical parameters (e.g., will elevate creatine phosphokinase and corticosteroids) (Coe et al., 1985).

Table 3 Blood Chemistry of Nonhuman Primates, Normal Ranges

Test	Units	Squirrel monkey[b] (*Saimiri sciureus*)	Cynomolgus monkey[a] (*Macaca fascicularis*)	Rhesus monkey[a] (*Macaca mulatta*)	Baboon[c,d] (*Papio* sp.	Chimpanzee[a] (*Pan troglodytes*)
Alanine Aminotransferase (ALT)	U/L	4–1612	5–50	5–61	—	0–40
Albumin (ALB)	mg%	—	3.4–5.0	3.6–5.5	3.6–5.5	2.7–5.3
Alkaline phosphatase (ALP)	U/L	6.0–49.0	150–464	45–661	154–1105	142–624
Aspartate aminotransferase (AST)	U/L	—	5–50	12–63	—	0–40
Bicarbonate (BICARB)	mm1/L	—	20–32	96–116	—	25–32
Bilirubin, total (T BILI)	mg%	0.0–1.9	0.1–0.8	0.1–1.2	0.3–0.7	0.1–1.3
Blood urea nitrogen (BUN)	mg%	11.4–42.2	8–28	8.38	9–25	5–22
Calcium (CA)	mg%	4.2–5.8	8.4–11.1	8.1–13.8	8.0–9.6	8.3–12.9
Chloride (CL)	mm1/L	103.0–118.0	100–118	16–29	104–118	94–110
Cholesterol (CHOL)	mg%	116.0–272.0	70–178	62–238	68–232	144–304
Creatine phosphokinase (CPK)	U/L	—	206–630	22–53	—	9–33
Creatinine (CREAT)	mg%	—	0.5–1.2	0.1–1.5	0.8–1.4	0.1–1.3
Gamma glutamyltransferase (GGT)	U/L	—	11–50	24–645	—	42–366
Globulin (GLOB)	mg%	—	1.5–4.8	1.5–4.8	2.4–4.4	1.9–4.9
Glucose (CLUC)	mg%	35.0–148.0	48–80	27–100	50–129	75–117
Lactic dehydrogenase (LDH)	U/L	230.0–760.0	100–446	43–426	99–488	105–439
Phosphorus (PHOS)	mg%	3.2–9.2	2.1–5.5	2.4–8.7	4.7–7.7	3.0–6.4
Potassium (K)	mm1/L	3.5–9.5	3.5–5.0	2.93–5.45	3.2–4.3	3.5–5.3
Protein, total (T PROT)	mg%	—	6.2–7.6	5.9–8.8	5.7–7.8	5.5–7.2
Sodium (Na)	mm1/L	144.0–173.0	135–158	135–158	143–158	133–148

[a]Primate Research Laboratory, NMSU; Colony Historical Data.
[b]Abee, C. R. (1985) Medical care of management of the squirrel monkey, in *Handbook of Squirrel Monkey Research*, Rosenblum, L. A., and Coe, C. L. eds. Plenum Press, New York, pp. 484–485.
[c]Hack, C. A., and Gleiser, C. A. (1982) Hematologic and serum chemistry reference values for adult and juvenile baboons (*Papio* sp). *Lab. Anim. Sci.* 32, 502–505.
[d]Kelly, C. A., and Gleiser, C. A. (1986) Selected coagulation values for adult and juvenile baboons. *Lab. Anim. Sci.* 36, 173–175.

Usually blood samples are collected by venipuncture. Occasionally, samples are collected through temporary indwelling catheters when frequent collections are required, as in pharmacokinetic studies. Rarely, samples are collected through long-term indwelling catheters. In general, venipuncture is preferred because of less damage caused to the veins, less need for anesthesia or minor surgery, and a reduced chance of infections. In some instances, samples have been collected several times daily for up to a month by venipuncture without adverse effects if sterile techniques are used (shave and alcohol prep the collection site).

Venipuncture samples requiring small amounts (less than 5 ml) are usually collected from the cephalic or saphenous veins. The femoral vein is generally used when large blood volumes are required (greater than 5 ml). For cephalic or saphenous vein collections, animals are restrained as described in the section on intravenous drug administration. The skin over the vein is shaved and swabbed with alcohol or an iodine solution. Either a syringe and needle or an evacuated container can be used. The needle should be the smallest size compatible with the sample volume; i.e., 23 gauge for samples under 1 ml, 22 gauge for 1- to 3-ml samples, etc. Smaller needles cause less damage to the vein and lessen the hazard of hematomas forming. Short-bevel needles are preferred when they are available because they have less chance of slicing the vein wall. After withdrawal of the needle, direct pressure should be maintained on the site for 30 sec. If femoral samples are collected (from anesthetized animals), pressure should be maintained on the site for at least 1 min.

The amount of blood that can safely be removed from a primate during the course of a study depends on the study purpose, the study length, total blood volume (Bender, 1955), and the frequency and amount of samples (Keeling and Wolf, 1975). When in doubt, hematological parameters should be monitored frequently to avoid adverse effects. If an important endpoint of the study is an hematological evaluation, then the maximum recommended volume is reduced in order to avoid influencing these endpoints. As a general guideline, up to 0.5 ml/kg body weight can be removed daily for up to 30 days, since that is the minimal rate at which blood is replaced (Huser, 1970). Up to 5 ml/kg can be removed at one time if no other samples have been or will be collected for several weeks (Schalm, 1975). These amounts are maximum and can be expected to temporarily change some hematological parameters. Other schedules and amounts can be determined from those above.

Sympathetic technicians who work with monkeys on a daily basis find that monkeys quickly adapt to routine blood sample collection. After a time they will offer their arm without being restrained or handled. This learning process can be speeded considerably if rewards are provided to cooperative animals.

Some laboratories return red cells to the animal in an attempt to increase the maximum amount of blood that can be collected. In general, this technique should be avoided unless absolutely necessary. Experience has shown that problems of infection and hematological changes outweigh the benefits gained.

When possible, studies should be designed to avoid the need for chronic catheterization for blood sample collection. Catheters can provide a route for serious infections even when the most careful aseptic techniques are used. Moreover, chronically placed catheters frequently develop fibrin flaps over their distal end, effectively blocking blood withdrawal. When catheters are used, their patency can be maintained by keeping them filled with a normal saline solution containing 1–4 IU/ml sodium heparin for injection. A sterile, saturated sucrose-saline-heparin solution may offer additional advantages. In general, one can expect to maintain patency in a chronic catheter for no more than a week, although in some instances, it has been possible (with exceptionally sterile technique) to use catheters for more than a month.

Temporary catheters placed in restrained or anesthetized animals provide a means for collecting very frequent samples over a short period of time. They are introduced by the technique described earlier for intravenous infusion (also see Bowen and Cummins,

1985). Tables 2 and 3 summarize normal ranges for hematology and blood chemistry laboratory values in the five most common primate species.

Urine Collection

Because almost all monkey species play with their food and water, quantitative long-term collection of uncontaminated urine and feces is a difficult task (Baker and Morris, 1979). By placing a collecting pan (with screens optional) under the cage and removing the food and water source, short-term urine samples of reasonable quality can be obtained from a single void specimen. When setting up urine collection cages for metabolism studies, space is provided under the collection pans to place the collection vessel in ice. This is important when total urine collections for 24 hrs are required. Inexpensive, styrofoam coolers can be cut to size to hold the ice.

  Pharmacokinetic studies usually require quantitative urine collection over a limited period of time. This is frequently accomplished by placing the animal in a chair and catheterizing the bladder of females and placing a condom collection device over the penis of males (catheterization of males' bladders is not practical as a routine procedure). If animals are appropriately adapted to the chair, this technique can be used for up to 12 hr. Longer periods of chairing are best interrupted with an exercise period to prohibit any prolonged stress-related changes. Other methods used under acute conditions are a direct sample collection by suprapubic puncture (Keeling and Wolf, 1975) or indirectly by manual bladder expression. Neither method is recommended for subchronic or chronic toxicology studies.

Physiological Measurements

Physiological endpoint measurements are becoming routine in drug safety evaluations. Requests for such measurements resulted from observations of pyrogenic activity of certain proteins and cardiotoxic or neurotoxic effects of monoclonal antibodies. Indications of untoward physiological responses in the past have necessitated a thorough evaluation of these parameters. Usually measurements (except neurological examinations) are obtained under ketamine anesthesia (10 mg/kg) because most protocols require a battery of tests.

Body Temperature (Rectal)

Rectal temperatures are obtained using a digital thermometer coated with lubricant. The animal is placed in the prone position on a table or gurney for rectal accessibility. The surface of the Table is maintained at approximately room temperature with a warming pad. The probe, covered with a lubricated disposable plastic sheath, is inserted into the rectum until body temperature is attained. Rectal temperatures should be recorded as quickly as possible after anesthesia for the most accurate reading.

Systolic Blood Pressure

Systolic blood pressure is obtained using a blood pressure cuff and a vascular flow probe applied to the femoral artery. Diastolic pressure cannot be determined accurately in monkeys by indirect measurement.

  The animal is positioned supinely on a warmed table. The blood pressure cuff is placed securely around the upper thigh with the cuff-positioning arrow situated over the anterior arterial area. Doppler gel is applied on the skin above the artery (distal to the cuff), which is located with the probe. The unit is set on AUDIO so that the area of the strongest arterial signal is localized. The cuff is inflated until the signal is inaudible. Pressure is slowly released until the first "beat" is heard. The reading on the gauge is recorded. The systolic pressure assessment should be repeated at least two additional times to ensure an accurate estimate.

Heart Rate

The method for recording the heart rate requires only the Doppler and probe. Gel is placed on the skin over the artery and an audible heart beat signal located with the probe. Using a stopwatch, the heart rate is counted over 60 sec and recorded. The heart rate can also be determined from electrocardiographs or by using a stethoscope for the counting procedure.

Neurological Evaluation

Any neuromuscular contraindication can be evaluated by a basic subjective evaluation performed by experienced veterinarians or research personnel. A freely moving animal is initially examined in the cage. An example of a grading system is as follows:

Grade	Sign
0	Absence of purposeful movement—paraplegia
1	Unable to stand to support; slight movement when supported by the tail—severe paraparesis
2	Unable to stand to support; when assisted moves limbs readily but stumbles and falls frequently—moderate paraparesis and ataxia
3	Can stand to support but frequently stumbles and falls—mild paraparesis and ataxia
4	Can stand to support—minimal paraparesis and ataxia
5	Normal strength and coordination

Additional tests require the animal to be squeezed to the front of the cage or properly restrained outside the cage. Pelvic or thoracic limb flexor reflexes are assessed by exerting pressure with a hemostat to the lateral and medial digits. The integrity of the reflex arc following painful stimuli is graded as responsive (+) or nonresponsive (–).

Patellar reflexes (femoral nerves) are evaluated with the animal as relaxed as possible. The patellar tendon is lightly tapped with a reflex hammer and subjectively graded as follows:

Grade	Sign
0	No reflex
1	Hyporeflexic
2	Normal
3	Hyperreflexic
4	Clonic

Tissue Biopsy

The need to conserve primates and the requirement for serial tissue samples has increased interest in obtaining tissue by biopsy in primate toxicology studies. Routine techniques for exterior collection of bone marrow, cerebrospinal fluid, liver, kidney, and fat have been developed (Keeling and Wolf, 1975). Other tissues can be collected through surgical procedures. Protocol designs incorporating tissue biopsy of target organs as an alternative to complete necropsy have recently received favorable regulatory consideration.

The techniques for collecting tissue biopsies are specialized to each tissue and should only be conducted under the supervision of an experienced veterinarian. Detailed descriptions of the techniques are beyond the intent of this chapter.

Specialized Information

Pregnancy Tests

Depending on the species, pregnancy can be diagnosed by palpation, radioimmunoassay for chorionic gonadotropin, commercially available urine and blood test kits, and ultrasound. Human test kits which detect the presence of chorionic gonadotropin work well in the great apes. They are of limited value in macaques because of minimal cross-reaction between the reagents and monkey chorionic gonadotropin. Radioimmunoassays for chorionic gonadotropin in macaques are available (Hobson et al., 1975). In general, however, they are only useful for diagnosing pregnancy during days 17–33 following conception, since chorionic gonadotropin secretion is limited to that time in macaques (Hein et al., 1989).

A urinary chorionic gonadotropin kit is available from NIH at cost (Contraceptive Development Branch, Dr. Gabriel Bialy, Bldg EPN, 600A; telephone (301)496-1661).

Like humans, great apes secrete chorionic gonadotropin throughout pregnancy; however, it is difficult to detect prior to day 13 and after day 90 of pregnancy owing to low levels (Reyes et al., 1975).

Experienced technicians can diagnose pregnancy after day 25 by rectal palpation in macaques. Ultrasonography is probably the ultimate technique for pregnancy diagnosis in all primates because it works early and is accurate throughout pregnancy. It is also valuable for detecting fetal death, twins, and other anomalies of pregnancy.

Menstrual Cycles

The great apes and Old World monkeys (baboons and macaques) exhibit menstrual bleeding at the end of a nonfertile cycle (when the corpus luteum has ceased producing progesterone). New World monkeys do not exhibit menstrual bleeding; thus other endpoints (e.g., serum estrogen, progesterone, FSH, etc.) are necessary to follow the reproductive status of the females. The chorionic gonadotropin urinary kit (NIH Kit) can be utilized for pregnancy determination. In addition to observations of menstrual bleeding, chimpanzee menstrual cycles can be followed by observations of their sex skin. The perineal area swells dramatically in response to estrogen in the early part of the menstrual cycle and regresses rapidly immediately following ovulation (Graham et al., 1972).

Because menstrual bleeding is minimal in macaques, simple observation of the animal or the cage floor is not always sufficient to detect the presence of bleeding. Daily swabbing of the exterior vagina with water-dampened cotton-tipped swabs provides an excellent means of following the menstrual cycle. Most female macaques (particularly rhesus monkeys) rapidly learn to "present" for the swabbing so that data from an entire room can be collected in a few minutes.

Ultrasound and X-Ray

Recently, articles have been written describing the use of ultrasound in pregnancy diagnosis and other procedures (Conrad et al., 1989; Farine et al., 1988). Tabular formats on head size, etc., during gestation provide an excellent method to determine stage of pregnancy.

Accurate dating of pregnancy (within ± 2 days of parturition) is possible at early stages of pregnancy. This process permits dosing at specific gestational ages without more drastic intervention.

Radiology is also useful for determining potential fetal abnormalities, or organ dysfunctions. Both instruments, particularly ultrasound, can be utilized to perform size and function aspects of cardiac flow, rhythm, and other cardiovascular phenomena. The specifics of both instruments are outside the scope of this chapter.

Invasive Cardiovascular Procedures

Direct monitoring of central arterial and venous pressure is the most common cardiovascular measurement requiring an invasive procedure. Normally animals are surgically catheterized in the femoral vein or artery, hooked to a direct recording device, and monitored for up to several hours under general anesthesia. Ketamine is not considered suitable for most of these procedures because it causes fluctuations (most often reductions) in both arterial and venous pressure. Sodium pentobarbital is preferred because of its lack of effect on central pressures. Its use, however, means that the animal's breathing must be maintained on a respirator. The new, pressurized, continuous-infusion devices which allow a constant, slow infusion of heparinized saline (0.5 IU/ml) through the transducer and into the animal reduce clotting problems and improve the quality of the recorded data. The same devices can be used for chronic pressure recording in animals fitted with jackets and tethers (see section on chronic intravenous drug administration).

Measurement of cardiac output is possible with the thermal dilution technique in large macaques using human pediatric catheters. Smaller animals are not suitable for this technique because appropriate catheters are not available at this time. Microspheres can be used to estimate cardiac output in smaller animals (Forsyth et al., 1968). Normal cardiovascular values have been reviewed by Bourne (1975).

NECROPSY

Critical to the majority of toxicological procedures is the determination of the cause of death of an animal or abnormal tissues in dose and control groups. The necropsy findings (both gross and histological) can focus the findings of the antemortem study.

Owing to the potential latent viral problems in primates, it is essential that all safety procedures be utilized in any primate necropsy. These procedures are not limited to gloves, masks, special garments, etc.

It is essential that a prenecropsy meeting be held with prosectors, pathologist, and study director to familiarize all concerned with the protocol, previous antemortem findings, etc. This will enable any recorded masses (palpation), unusual clinical signs, etc., to be noted for focus of the necropsy. The necropsy itself can be done using a variety of methods; however, whichever method is used consistently, check-off and record keeping should be the key. Tissues should be closely followed so a direct record path from gross necropsy to slide reading can be maintained.

ACKNOWLEDGMENT

Photographs by Belinda Burnett, B.S., LATG.

APPENDIX

PHYSICAL AND/OR OPHTHALMIC EXAM FORM (STUDY SUPPORT)

ANIMAL NUMBER: _____ :   VERIFY TATTOO
SEX: _____ :   VERIFY SEX
BODY WIEGHT: _____ KG :   SCALE USED: _____
PRL STUDY:_____   AGE OF ANIMAL: _____ N/A: _____
DATE: _____   EXAMINED BY:_____
ANESTHETIC AGENT: _____   PROCEDURES PERFORMED (X):
  ADMINISTERED BY: _____   1. DIRECT OPHTHALMIC EXAM: _____
  AMOUNT:_____ ML (_____ MG/ML)   (Examine cornea, conjunctiva,
TIME: _____ AM   PM   sclera, iris, fundus,
LOT _____ EXPIR: _____   other: _____)
                                                a) EYES DILATED WITH: _____
                                                b) MFR/LOT/EXPIR: _____
                                            2. OTHER PROCEDURES: _____

	Abnormal	Normal	Not observed	Comments
1. INTEGUMENT				1.
2. RESPIRATION				2.
3. CARDIOVASCULAR				3.
4. GASTROINTESTINAL				4.
5. UROGENITAL				5.
6. NERVOUS SYSTEM				6.
7. MUSCULOSKELETAL				7.
8. LYMPHATICS				8.
9. ENDOCRINE				9.
10 SPECIAL SENSES				10.

BODY TEMP:_____ F   HEART RATE:_____ /MIN   RESP:____/MIN   PULSE:_____
THERMOMETER USED:_____   OTHER EQUIPMENT USED: _____

FOLLOW UP TESTING RECOMMENDED: _____
FOLLOW UP TESTING PEFORMED:_____ (X) COMMENTS: _____

PRESTUDY SAMPLES SUBMITTED OR TO BE SUBMITTED WHICH MAY BE USED TO
DETERMINE ELIGIBILITY: _____ CBC   _____ FECAL PARASITOLOGY
                       _____ SMA   _____ URINALYSIS
                       _____ OTHER: _____

OVERALL ANALYSIS:
Based on this physical exam and review of all applicable clinical data
This animal IS: _____ IS NOT:_____approved for study assignment.

DATE: _____   SIGNATURE: _____
COMMENTS: _____
_____
_____

REASON FOR NON-APPROVAL AND RECOMMENDED TREATMENT, IF ANY: _____
_____

Pathology   **Curtis D. Port**

A number of texts have been written that address the subject of nonhuman primate pathology (Benirschke, 1983; Dunn, 1968; Griesemer, 1976; Karger and Basil, 1972; Ruch, 1959) in a variety of ways; e.g., by organ system or as models of human disease. Most are comprehensive and provide ample background and knowledge of any particular disease. It is, therefore, not the intent of this chapter to provide a review of this information. Rather, the intent is to provide a toxicologist who has little or no knowledge of nonhuman primate pathology with enough information to acquaint him or her with the subject for those species most commonly used in toxicology. Also, the intent is to provide adequate references such that an individual can pursue additional reading as needed. Many of the references at the end of this chapter are themselves heavily referenced, and will provide sufficient information.

In most instances, the nonhuman primates used for toxicological studies will have been screened for certain disease agents before a study can begin. Screening is accomplished by the vendor, before shipment, and by the laboratory animal veterinarian after arrival at the using institution. Screening provides some assurance that the animals will be in good health when the study is started. Should clinical signs of disease be seen, the laboratory animal veterinarian should be consulted and his or her recommendations followed.

This section will outline only the most common diseases in four species: the rhesus (*Macaca mulatta*), the cynomolgus (*Macaca fascicularis*), the squirrel (*Saimiri sciureus*), and the common marmoset (*Callithrix jacchus*). Other species are, of course, used in research but are generally used for studies other than toxicology studies.

NONNEOPLASTIC SPONTANEOUS DISEASES

Bacterial Diseases

Bacterial infections are common in nonhuman primates and can be a significant cause of clinical disease. Most prominent are the enteric organisms followed by the respiratory pathogens. Nonhuman primates must be screened for the common bacterial pathogens prior to placing them on study. This process typically requires 6 weeks or longer and will be done by the laboratory animal veterinarian.

Shigellosis, or Bacillary dysentery
Bacillary dysentery is a common disease of primates living in captivity, but does not occur in wild-living simians. The rhesus macaque is most susceptible, followed next by the cynomolgus. The agents which cause bacillary dysentery are of the same subgroups and serotypes of shigellae as cause dysentery in man. These are *Shigella flexneri, S. sonnei, S. schmitzii*, and *S. dysenteriae*. The sources of infection for nonhuman primates are human carriers, infected food, sick animals, and asymptomatic carriers. Cases are most commonly observed when the animals are captured, or when the animals are shipped to a new facility. While it is evident that primates become infected very quickly, the incidence of disease among primates living in captivity for any length of time is low.

The clinical manifestations are variable, and the course of the disease may be divided into acute and chronic forms. In the mildest form, there are few signs of disease, but the stools are softer and are passed more frequently than normal. In the initial stages, the animals sit bent forward with the head between the hunched hind legs. Progressive weakness and prostration occur quite rapidly and emaciation may become quite pronounced. In the severe form of dysentery, the general state of health deteriorates rapidly, with anorexia and prostration. In this instance, the stools are usually liquid, containing mucus and frequently gross blood. Prolapse of the rectum is common. The body temperature is subnormal and untreated animals die in 2 to 3 days. Sometimes, the acute form passes into the chronic form, manifested as a relapsing or chronic debilitating disease.

Apart from clinically affected animals, many primates become so-called "healthy" carriers. The carrier state takes two forms: (1) a transitional form in which the bacilli are excreted for short periods only, and (2) the chronic form in which the bacilli are excreted indefinitely. In short-term carriers, there are no pathological lesions of the gastrointestinal tract. In chronic carriers, however, pathological lesions are quite evident.

The pathological changes in primate dysentery are quite variable and lesions are quite variable and lesions are predominantly localized to the large intestine. In most instances, the intestine is greatly distended, and its serosal surface characteristically covered with petechial hemorrhages. The mesenteric vessels are usually injected, and the intestinal lymph nodes enlarged, hemorrhagic and often necrotic. When opened, the mucosa of the large intestine is unevenly swollen and pink with occasional hemorrhages. The normal plication of the intestine is frequently obscured and purplish red. Ulcers, varying in size from 3 to 4 mm in diameter, may be present. In more severe cases, the process acquires the character of diphtheritic colitis. The mucous membrane of the large intestine shows scattered islets of dirty gray film adhering to it. The small intestine is not commonly involved. In the spleen there may be moderate edema, hyperemia, and sometimes hemorrhages. The liver and kidneys as well as the heart may show toxic changes.

The shigellae infecting nonhuman primates also can cause dysentery in humans, but fortunately not in the most severe form. Shigellosis among animal technicians is rare, and instances of proven transmission from monkey to adult human are rare. On the other hand, slight contact between a nonhuman primate and a child can result in transmission of the disease with serious consequences. Therefore, excluding children as visitors to animal colonies, and particularly primate colonies, is a necessity.

Salmonellosis, or Paratyphoid

Salmonella species are the next most common causes of dysentery in nonhuman primates. Clinical salmonellosis is uncommon; carrier states, however, are quite common, especially in macaques. The disease may occur as a mixed infection with *Shigella*. The serotypes involved are variable, but belong chiefly to groups B, C, D, and E. In groups B and D, *S. typhimurium*, *S. stanley*, and *S. enteritidis* are the most pathogenic. The usual sources of infections are contaminated food and water, usually with rodent or bird feces, healthy carriers, and sick animals. The occurrence of the disease is usually sporadic, but epidemics sometime occur.

Clinically, the disease has an acute beginning characterized by anorexia, prostration, diarrhea with mucus and blood, watery stools, and hypothermia in the more severe cases. At necropsy, the ileum is frequently involved in addition to the colon. This is in distinct contrast to shigellosis. Grossly, the changes have the character of catarrhal enteritis or gastroenterocolitis with hyperplasia of Peyer's patches, lymph nodes, and mesenteric lymph glands. Ulceration of the intestinal mucosa is not present in salmonellosis as a general rule.

Enterocolitis Caused by Proteus

Proteus group organisms are relatively pathogenic, but clinical infection is rare. *Proteus vulgaris* is often associated with epizootic outbreaks of hemorrhagic gastroenterocolitis in newly arrived animals. *Proteus morgani* is also relatively pathogenic. Clinically, the disease is characterized by anorexia, lethargy, flatulence, vomiting, and diarrhea with rapid deterioration in the overall condition and death within less than 36 hr. At necropsy, there is a gastroenteritis characterized by edema, reddening of the intestine, and hemorrhage in the mucosae of both stomach and small intestine, especially the duodenum. There is excessive quantities of mucus in the stomach and to a lesser extent in the small intestine; the contents of the large intestine are liquid or semiliquid. Splenomegaly is common. Microscopically there is hemorrhage of the mucosa and submucosa with moderate edema, necrosis, desquamation of epithelia, lymphoid hyperplasia of Peyer's patches, and solitary lymphoid nodules. There is minimal to no changes in the colon, but enlarged mesentery lymph nodes show hyperplasia of lymphoid elements.

Campylobacteriosis

Campylobacter species are widespread in laboratory animals, both as pathogens and as normal flora, and are important not only from the disease seen in animals, but also from the zoonotic possibilities. *Campylobacter jejuni* has been recognized as a cause of diarrhea in humans. As with other enteric pathogens, fecal-oral spread appears to be the prinicipal route of infection. Primates may acquire the infection in the wild during holding for export, or during transport. The organism has been isolated from several species of primates, including the macaques, baboons, and marmosets. Clinically, signs vary from none to a severe diarrhea. Apparently, the incubation period is from 2 to 5 days. Symptomatic animals show a fever, diarrhea, and occasional vomiting. The stool may contain mucus and blood.

At necropsy, a mild to severe enteritis may be seen, with mucus and/or blood in the intestinal lumen. Microscopic findings are extremely variable. The pathogenesis of the infection is not understood. Why some animals develop a diarrhea and others remain asymptomatic but continually shed the organism is unknown. The toxicologist must realize that stressful procedures may contribute to clinical campylobacteriosis, and that measures for personal protection should be used. An excellent review of campylobacteriosis has been published by Fox (1982).

Bacterial Pneumonia

Pneumonia is a common disease of all nonhuman primates. Respiratory infections are second only to infectious enteritis as a leading cause of death in captive animals. As one might suspect, different species show different susceptibility. In the great majority of cases, pneumonia develops as a complication of some other disease. It may, however, occur as a primary infection in young monkeys up to 6 months of age. In all groups, the most common cause is one of the types of pneumococci (*Diplococcus pneumoniae*). Other organisms that can be involved are *Haemophilus influenzae*, *Bordetella bronchiseptica*, and *Pasteurella* and/or *Klebsiella pneumoniae*.

Clinically, coughing, sneezing, and rhinitis are some of the symptoms of pneumonia. An elevated temperature is characteristic. On x-ray the affected areas show increased opacity and the appearance of shadows. A majority of pneumonias are bilateral. The affected portions of the lung lobes, typically the dependent or diaphragmatic lobes, are dark red or consolidated. Typically, the affected lobe will not collapse when the chest is opened. Histologically, an alveolar exudate is usually prevalent and consists predominantly of neutrophilic leukocytes mixed with erythrocytes, desquamated epithelial cells, and fibrin. The bronchi usually show an ulcerative bronchitis.

Pneumonias caused by *Klebsiella pneumoniae* are characterized by the development of numerous foci of inflammation which have a tendency to fuse. The result is that many lobes become affected and totally consolidated.

Tuberculosis

The most important pathogen causing disease of the respiratory and gastrointestinal system in nonhuman primates is undoubtedly tuberculosis. Although all three strains of the tubercle bacillus are capable of causing tuberculosis, the human strain is the most common. There are marked differences in species susceptibility. The rhesus monkey is exquisitely sensitive, whereas the squirrel monkey, along with other New World primates, is very resistant. In nonhuman primates, the disease may take either pulmonary or alimentary forms and the course may be prolonged.

As in humans, there is a site of primary infection, called the primary focus. This is most commonly found in respiratory or gastrointestinal tissues. Postprimary infection arises by hematogenous or lymphogenous spread. In nonhuman primates, the disease is usually pulmonary and may run a fulminating course. The disease is characterized by numerous firm or hard, light to gray or yellow tuberculous nodules, bulging from a mucous or serous surface. When the tubercles are numerous, the disease is called miliary tuberculosis. In the nonhuman primate, miliary lesions are frequent and, in contrast to humans, calcification of lesions are rare. Microscopically, the characteristic Langhans' giant cells associated with the tubercles may be numerous or may be absent. A rigid testing program of all nonhuman primates is necessary for adequate diagnosis and control of the disease.

An excellent review on the bacterial infections of nonhuman primates has been published (McClure et al., 1986).

Viral Diseases

Viral diseases are important to the toxicologist from two points of view. First, the expression of primate viruses may interfere with a toxicity study and can, at the very least, make the data questionable or difficult to interpret. And second, they pose a threat to human health. Obviously, the viral status of the primates must be considered before the toxicologist begins his or her work.

Although there are approximately 75 nonhuman primate viruses that are distinctly simian (Kalter, 1983), relatively little is known about them or their impact on their hosts. Indeed, the natural host of several simian viruses is unknown, and their pathogenesis is not understood (Kalter, 1983). Two excellent discussions of the simian viruses, their hosts, and the diseases they cause are provided by (Kalter et al., 1988). This section discusses only those which can be hazardous to the conduct or interpretation of a toxicity study or to the individuals conducting that study. In addition, a few viruses that pose a distinct threat to other primates will be discussed.

Herpesvirus Simiae

Herpesvirus simiae, otherwise known as herpes B virus, or simply B virus, affects only Old World primates, including the rhesus and cynomolgus. New World monkeys have their own herpesviruses, which will be discussed later. The organism obviously belongs to the herpesvirus group, which is one of the largest of the viral groups. In primates the source of infection appears to be contacted either through bites or scratches. The incidence of infection in primates is age related, being highest in adults and lowest in juveniles, with a rapid increase at about the time of puberty. Some evidence indicates that infants may be refractory. *Herpesvirus simiae* is considered a highly pathogenic organism for humans. It was first isolated in 1934 from humans bitten by primates. Until 1973 only 24 human infections had been documented. A very extensive report published in 1987 summarizes the history of the disease in humans and the details of the 24 cases (Palmer, 1987). That same year, however, four additional cases in humans occurred at Pensacola and Gulf Breeze, Florida (Centers for Disease Control, 1987). From this outbreak of the human disease, three things were learned: (1) the virus can be shed from a primate with no visible signs, (2) the virus can be transmitted from human to human, and (3) the disease can be controlled by antiviral drugs.

The clinical manifestation of the disease in macaques is quite variable. The natural, primary infection closely resembles *Herpesvirus simplex* infections in humans and may be so minimal as to escape detection. The 1987 outbreak showed us that the virus can be shed without the evidence of overt pathological change. In this instance, the virus was shed in the tears and the only change noted in the animal was a mild conjunctivitis. In most instances, however, the virus expresses itself as a glossitis, or a stomatitis, with ulceration. Vesicles form which rapidly necrose, leaving ulcers, which may appear singly or in groups. These ulcers heal by granulation without scarring. Most lesions occur on the tongue with some on the lip. Lesions rarely develop in the epidermis and other sites. Occasionally, overt fatal disease may occur in chronically infected animals under stress.

It is important that the toxicologist understand that the administration of compounds to Old World primates could result in an expression of the virus and clinical disease. Thus, the technicians working with the animals are at risk. Once the disease is contracted, it is for all intents and purposes fatal. Preventive measures, for example, the pole and collar method of handling primates, must be relied upon to avoid exposure to infected primates. Additionally, the purchase of only herpes B virus–negative monkeys should be considered.

Herpesvirus Tamarinus

Herpesvirus tamarinus, first isolated from South American Marmosets, infects only New World monkeys. Squirrel monkeys are the most susceptible to the virus and act as a reservoir host. Other monkey species with a positive antibody titer include *Saguinus* species, *Ateles* species, and some *Cebus* species. Transmission of the disease is by contract; antibody levels increase following capture, indicating exposure from the trap to the laboratory. The disease in squirrel monkeys is apparently latent, as they show no signs of infection. Transfer of the virus to marmosets and or owl monkeys, however, causes a systemic fatal disease.

The varied spontaneous lesions occurring in owl monkeys, which also apply to marmosets, have been described in great detail by Hunt and Melendez (1966). The lesions reported include a necrotizing and ulceratives stomatitis, glossitis, and serosal petechiae and ecchymoses at all levels below the duodenum in the intestine. In the lung, uniformly red-brown, numerous, small, slightly raised circular foci were present on the pleural surface. The liver had myriads of pale brown-gray foci on the external surface. Microscopically, there was coagulation necrosis of the epithelium down to the muscularis mucosa in the intestine. The lung showed a mild pneumonitis, and the brown-gray foci in the liver were areas of coagulation necrosis. In the liver, inclusions were prominent and giant cells seen. Both eosinophilic and basophilic intranuclear inclusion bodies were present in this disease.

The clinical course in marmosets and owl monkeys is rapid, with death occurring in

4–5 days. No specific clinical signs are associated with the disease, and there is no treatment. Strict segregation or isolation of susceptible species from squirrel monkeys is the only way to control the disease. It is important to note that no clinically documented infections or serological evidence of infection has been reported in humans.

Monkeypox

Monkeypox is occasionally seen in primate colonies, with the macaque species most commonly affected. The source of the infection is the animals themselves, with transfer of the disease by contact. Clinical disease in macaques is of two types. The first is acute or generalized pox in which the animals show marked facial edema that extends into the cervical region, severe respiratory problems, and papillary eruptions that are present over various parts of the body, but particularly on the head and face.

The second type is cutaneous pox, which is the far more common form. In this manifestation, there is a single crop of discrete papules on the skin, which are 1 to 4 mm in diameter. These lesions become pustular and eventually necrose. Reddish brown crusts form over the lesions and eventually drop off in 7–10 days, leaving a small scar. The most common sites of the papular eruption are the buttocks, hands, feet, face, and hind limbs. Microscopically, there is a focal proliferation of the epidermis followed by necrosis. Intracellular edema causes swelling of both cell bodies and nuclei, but large vesicles are only occasionally seen. An invasion of the dermis by neutrophils results in the formation of the pustules.

Hepatitis

Hepatitis is a common disease in the United States (Frances et al., 1984) as well as in a number of developing nations, and is still being studied extensively with the goal of vaccination as a preventative. Of the three types of hepatitis, i.e., A, B, and non-A/non-B, hepatitis A (HAV) is of greatest interest to the toxicologist because it naturally infects the rhesus, cynomolgus, and the marmoset as well as other species (Lankas and Jensen, 1987; Shevtsova, 1988; Slighter et al., 1988; Mathiesen et al., 1978; Dienhart et al., 1975, and Mao et al., 1981). Hepatitis A virus is a hepatotrophic picornavirus, and it has been generally accepted that nonhuman primates become infected after contact with humans, although antibodies to HAV have been detected in cynomolgus from the wild (Burke and Heisey, 1984). Clearly, however, the disease can be transmitted from nonhuman primate to man (Hillis, 1961; Dienstag et al., 1976).

The disease in rhesus or cynomolgus is not clinically evident; the animals do not stop eating or show any other signs. They do, however, show spontaneous, transient increases in alanine aminotransferase (ALT) and aspartate aminotransferase (AST) levels in the serum. Elevations in these enzymes can cause problems when they occur during a toxicity study (Lankas and Jensen, 1987; Slighter et al., 1988). Toxicologists should be careful in ascribing test article toxicity when there is an increased hepatic enzyme activity associated with periportal inflammation due to HAV. The animals seroconvert to a positive antibody status and have transitory immunoglobulin M (IgM) levels during the convalescent period. There is no obvious way of differentiating this disease-induced change from toxic effects.

The pathological lesions in the liver are minimal. There is generalized activation of sinusoidal lining cells, focal hepatocellular necrosis with occasional acidophilic bodies, and cuffs of mononuclear cells in portal areas. The hepatocellular necrosis is most often minimal, although severe cell necrosis can occasionally be found. Proliferation of bile ductules can also be found when portal inflammation is maximal. During recovery, pigment deposits can be seen in Kupffer cells and they persist for some time. Chronic hepatitis never develops.

The virus is shed in the feces for an indeterminate period. Thus, animal and research technicians should wear protective clothing when working with nonhuman primates. Presently, the only means of prevention is administration of immune serum globulin before or after exposure. An effective vaccine would contribute to prevention, but is not currently available.

Simian Type D Retroviruses

Simian AIDS (SAIDS) or simian acquired immunodeficiency syndrome, due to a type D retrovirus, was first described in California in 1983 (Henrickson et al., 1983). Subsequently, several other outbreaks of SAIDS have occurred involving a variety of species, including the rhesus, and cynomolgus. The type D retroviruses that were isolated in these outbreaks were not alike, as shown by restriction endonuclease mapping and antigen characteristics. Originally, the viruses were named by geographic distribution, e.g. SAIDS/D California. Recently, however, a new nomenclature has been proposed to show a close relationship of the viruses (Marx, 1986). The California and New England type D isolates should be referred to as SRV-1 (SAIDS retrovirus type 1). The Washington and Oregon isolates should be referred to as SRV-2.

The viruses involved in SAIDS are cytopathic retroviruses called lentiviruses. Included in this group are the visna virus, equine infectious anemia virus, human immunodeficiency virus (HIV), and the simian T-cell lymphotropic virus. This cytopathic group is related to a group of transforming retroviruses that include the bovine leukemia virus and the human T-cell leukemia viruses I and II. Much has been learned about human acquired immunodeficiency syndrome (AIDS) and HIV, but little as yet is known about the SAIDS viruses and their pathogenesis.

Nonhuman primates with SAIDS present with a wide range of clinical signs. Affected animals have a generalized lymphadenopathy with diarrhea, apathy, and wasting. In addition, there can be a neutropenia, lymphopenia, anemia, and abnormal peripheral blood monocytes. Chronic infections of the skin or gingiva that are unresponsive to treatment have been noted. Not unlike AIDS, other unusual infections are common. These include fungal (*Candida*), protozoan (*Entamoeba histolytica* and/or Toxoplasmosis and cryptosporidiosis) and bacterial (*Shigella, Staphylococcus Streptococcsis*) infections. The hematological changes occurring in SAIDS have been defined by Mackenzie et al. (1986) in rhesus monkeys.

In 1987, (Lerche et al., 1987) documented the natural history of an endemic type D retrovirus infection in group-housed rhesus. Juvenile rhesus denied physical contact with a SAIDS-affected group remained free of disease. Thus, contact is necessary for transmission of the disease and contaminated saliva is considered to be the most significant route of natural infection (Lerche et al., 1986). Aggressive behavior and biting trauma, part of the normal social behavior, are contributory. Other routes of infection may include blood transfusions, urine, and milk.

Pathologically, SAIDS presents in a variety of ways. It can be acute, subacute, or chronic with minimal evidence of clinical disease. Gross lesions include a mild lymphadenopathy to extensive lymph node hypertrophy, splenomegally, and mild to severe weight loss. A recurrent, nonvesicular rash was also noted in one outbreak. Other opportunistic infections and/or neoplasia complicate the picture. Microscopically, the lymph nodes first exhibit marked follicular hyperplasia. Terminally, the nodes are devoid of follicular and paracortical lymphoid elements and can exhibit marked sinus histiocytosis and erythrophagocytosis. The disease is one of profound immunosuppression and in this regard parallels AIDS in humans.

Screening of suspect animals will generally be done by the laboratory animal veterinarian. Procedures should be in place, however, to minimize exposure if an outbreak does occur. These should include detailed individual health records, screening of all animals on a regular basis, and safety procedures that eliminate virus transfer during toxicology studies.

Miscellaneous Viral Diseases

There are several additional viral diseases that the toxicologist should know about. These are very unique diseases and are important because the viruses do infect humans.

Herpesvirus Hominis, *Type 1*.   *Herpes hominis*, also known as *Herpes simplex*, is one of the most prevalent of human viruses and can infect all simians. The virus is capable of producing a disease of variable intensity. The expression of the disease may range from being inapparent to highly fatal. In severely affected nonhuman primates, the pathological lesions are quite similar to those that appear in human infants with the disease.

Cytomegalic Inclusion Disease.   Cytomegalovirus is another herpesvirus that is known to infect a wide variety of nonhuman primate species. The number of simian cytomegalovirus strains or types in unknown. All of the cytomegaloviruses have characteristics in common and can cause inapparent infections as well as overwhelming fatal disease. These viruses are known to be species specific and have an affinity for the salivary glands and kidneys, where they cause characteristic nuclear inclusions, containing deoxyribonucleic acid (DNA), to give an "owl eye" appearance to the cells. A similar disease in human infants will cause serious illness and death.

Simian Measles (Rubeola).   Probably the most important and common viral disease of primates is measles. It is not commonly seen, however, in the toxicology laboratory, as most primates have an immunity to the disease before they arrive. The number of susceptible species to this paramyxovirus is unknown, but measles antibodies have been demonstrated in macaques species and in *Cercopithecus aethiops*, or the African green monkey. Primates in their native habitat do not have antibodies against measles virus, and the virus is thought to spread to simians from human contact. The disease is usually thought to be aerosol transmitted. The clinical manifestations of the disease are quite similar to those seen in humans, with the development of a maculopapular skin rash occurring on body surfaces. The disease generally lasts approximately 3 weeks, after which time the skin appears normal. Deaths have occurred, however, primarily from pneumonia.

Yaba.   This disease was first reported in a colony of rhesus monkeys being held in Yaba, Nigeria, in 1958, and is clinically characterized by subcutaneous tumors (Frances Hadler et al. 1984). The virus morphologically belongs to the pox group, but is antigenically distinct from vaccinia and monkeypox virus. The disease is apparently spread by contact, and clinically manifests itself as a nonencapsulated tumor that is adherent to underlying structures. The affected animals recover spontaneously, with the growth sloughing away and the area healing by granulation. There are no metastases to visceral organs.

Histopathologically, the tumor is a histiocytoma with prominent intracytoplasmic acidophilic inclusions. Accidental and experimental transmission to humans has occurred, with the tumor being histologically identical to the tumor in primate species.

Marburg Virus.   At least 27 people became ill after handling kidney tissue from African green monkeys. The disease occurred in laboratories and hospitals in Germany and Yugoslavia in 1967, with all the monkeys originating from Uganda. The virus remains unclassified and has not been found in nature, although antibodies to the virus has been demonstrated in simians trapped in different localities in Africa and several species of apes in the United States (Lankas and Jensen, 1987; Shevtsova et al., 1988). Only one outbreak of this disease has occurred, and until the virus appears again the disease will remain a mystery.

An extremely well-referenced chapter on viral diseases, along with the laboratory support for diagnosis, has been published (Slighter et al., 1988).

Simian Hemorrhagic Fever.   Several outbreaks of this disease have occurred, since first described in 1964, the latest being in 1988. Macaques are the only species involved and the only primate to acquire the disease naturally. Several other species have been naturally exposed, but were not affected. In the 1988 outbreaks, it is believed that the disease was introduced, at one facility at least, by contact with African green monkeys (personal communication). The virus causing the disease has not been classified and has no serological relationship to a wide variety of other simian viruses.

Clinically, the disease presents as a high fever of sudden onset. Anorexia and depression, along with facial edema and erythema, follow in 48 to 72 hr. Affected animals progessively deteriorate and show prostration, dehydration, and hemorrhagic diathesis such as purpura, melena, epistaxis, and hematemesis. Death generally occurs 10–15 days after the onset of illness and is for all intensive purposes fatal.

Gross lesions are hemorrhages in the intestines and lungs, pallor of the viscera, and splenomegaly. Two regularly seen features are hemorrhagic necrosis of the proximal duodenum and splenomegally. Microscopically, capillary and venous hemorrhages are seen in a variety of organs, with evidence of venous thrombosis, stasis, and vasodilation. Degenerative changes found in the liver, kidney, brain, and bone marrow are thought to be due to hypoxia of the tissues after blood stasis.

The obvious absence of any serological evidence of infection in any of the primate species tested so far indicates that primates do not, apparently, harbor or come in contact with the virus. The source of the infection is, therefore, unknown; the virus must be, however, quite contagious as numerous macaques were lost during the 1988 outbreaks.

Parasitism

Parasitism is one of the most common disease problems in nonhuman primate colonies. The incidence of parasitism in animals that are wild caught is much higher than those raised in captivity. This point is quite important when purchasing animals, as the detrimental effects of parasitism will often be expressed by the stress of capture and confinement. In many instances, secondary invaders can then establish themselves, leading to debilitation with death.

If one considers metazoan and protozoan parasites along with the species they infect, the number of parasites to consider becomes too large for an adequate treatment in this chapter. Therefore, only the most common infections will be discussed, without regard to classification. An excellent review of the pathoparasitology of nonhuman primates has been published (Toft, 1986). The chapter provides numerous references for those who wish to know of a specific parasite or group of parasites.

Strongyloidiasis

Parasites of the genus *Strongyloides* are found in both old and new world primates. *Strongyloides cebus* has been found in squirrel monkeys and *S. fulleborni* in rhesus and cynomolgus. Only adult parasites and larvae are found in the intestinal tract. Migrating larvae are, however, found in other organs. The life cycle is complex, consisting of free-living and parasitic forms.

Diarrhea is the most common clinical manifestation of the disease, coupled with dehydration, listlessness, vomiting, and emaciation. Gross lesions are a catarrhal to hemorrhagic, necrotizing enterocolitis, which can cause a secondary peritonitis. Pulmonary hemorrhage may be seen as a result of migrating larvae. Microscopically, the small intestine of infected animals shows a multifocal erosive and ulcerative enteritis. The mucosa contains numerous parasites and the intestinal villi are short and blunt. In severe infections, a total loss of villi is apparent. In the lungs, acute multifocal or diffuse hemorrhage is common. Larval granulomas may be seen over pleural surfaces.

This disease is diagnosed by identification of typical larvae in the stool or by demonstration of adult females, eggs, and larvae at necropsy.

Esophagostomiasis

Parasites of the genus *Oesophagostomum* are considered to be the most common nematode parasite in Old World monkeys. *Oesophagostomum apiostomum* is the most common species encountered, although parasites of the genus *Ancylostoma* and *Necator*, also members of this strongylid family, are rare in New World monkeys. The adult parasites are located in the large intestine and the life cycle is direct. Continued reinfection results in the sensitization of the host to the parasite. Infected monkeys are usually asymptomatic and the infection goes unrecognized. Monkeys with severe infection may show a general unthriftiness and a general debilitation.

Lesions at necropsy consist of elevated smooth nodules, 2–4 mm in diameter, which are most frequently seen on the serosal surface of the large intestine and cecum. In the unsensitized animal, nodules are of the same color as the surrounding tissue. The nodules may be black or brown, however, if there is an associated hemorrhage. Older nodules usually are white due to caseation of the contents. Microscopically, the nodules are cystlike structures which invariably contain a worm or worm remnants. Although the soft portions of the worm are enzymatically digested, the cuticle remains as a prolonged irritant. The parasites are usually surrounded by chronic inflammatory cells, mainly macrophages; foreign body giant cells sometimes are present. A fibrous capsule of varying degrees of thickness surrounds the centrally located inflammatory mass.

An infection by *Oesophagostomum* can be diagnosed by identifying the eggs in the feces. A diagnosis of esophagostomiasis based solely on typical eggs in the feces should always be questioned, however, as the eggs of the different hookworm species cannot be differentiated one from another. This parasite has been reported to infect humans, and therefore should be considered as a zoonotic disease.

Pulmonary Nematodiasis

Metastrongylids in the genera *Filaroides* and *Filariopsis* are commonly seen in New World primates, especially in squirrel monkeys. The infection is not as severe or is even absent in animals raised in captivity, as the life cycle of the parasite involves the earthworm. The adults are found in the terminal bronchioles, respiratory bronchioles, and pulmonary alveoli, and gross lesions are subtle. When present in fairly large numbers, the pleural surface of the lung has numerous, random, small, elevated, subpleural nodules. Microscopically, there is atelectasis and foci of chronic inflammatory cells. Most infections are subclinical in nature and a diagnosis can be made by finding and identifying the typical lung worm larvae in the feces of the intact animal.

Filariasis

Filariasis is caused by a wide variety of nematodes that are commonly encountered in New World primates, especially squirrel monkeys. At least 12 different species have been described (Mathiesen et al., 1978) and include four species of *Dipetalonema* and seven species of *Tetrapetalonema*. These parasites live in the abdominal or thoracic cavities, or in the subcutaneous tissues of the host. They also may be found in the mesentery, along the pleural lining of the lung, and inside the pericardium. Typically, those parasites that are found in the serous cavities can cause a fibrinopurulent peritonitis or pleuritis with fibrinous or fibrous adhesions. In most instances, the infection is subclinical, and diagnosis is based on the demonstration and identification of the adult worms in the body cavities or subcutaneous tissues, or by the characteristic microfilaria in the blood.

Pulmonary Acariasis

This is an extremely common condition of wild-caught Old World primates, especially the rhesus. Although at least 10 species of lung mites in the genus *Pneumonyssus* have been reported, the most common member is *Pneumonyssus simicola*. The infection in the rhesus is usually asymptomatic and clinical signs are uncommon, although there have been reports of continued coughing. Gross lesions consist of variably sized pale spots or yellowish gray foci randomly located throughout the pulmonary parenchyma. Those located near the surface of the lungs elevate the pleura. These lesions resemble miliary tubercles, but are soft to the touch. Microscopically, the lung mite lesions are characterized by a bronchiolitis, peribronchiolitis, and focal lobular pneumonitis with alveolar collapse. There is thickening of the bronchial wall and loss of lining epithelium. Macrophages laden with a golden brown pigment are always present around the lesions and throughout the lung tissues. Diagnosis of lung mite infection generally occurs at the necropsy table and at the microscope.

Amebiasis

A number of species of ameba may be found in the intestines of various primate species. The most significant is *Entamoeba histolytica*. There are variations of resistance, the macaques being the more resistant. New World species are very sensitive.

The disease is characterized by frequent passage of feces containing blood and mucus. The signs are very similar to those of bacillary dysentery; thus, differential bacteriological diagnosis is important. Pathological changes are found predominantly in the cecum and colon. The mucous membrane shows catarrhal inflammation with a varying number of different size ulcers. They are covered with a white/yellowish coating, with clear bottoms. The margins are raised. Diagnosis of the disease may be difficult and identification of the organism may require repeated samplings as the trophs are quite delicate.

Other Diseases

It suffices to say that there are numerous diseases from each of the above categories that are uncommon or even rare. They are, therefore, of little consequence to the toxicologist, although it should be understood that they exist. These include such diseases as cryptococ-cosis and histoplasmosis as well as superficial mycoses such as ringworm. In most instances, these will not present a problem as they will have been diagnosed during the quarantine period, and the animals eliminated from those intended for a study.

NEOPLASIA

Neoplasia in captive primates is considered to be uncommon (Chapman, 1968; O'Gara and Adamson, 1972). However, the incidence of neoplasia in zoo populations is increas-ing, possibly because of increased life span (McClure, 1979). Squire et al. (1979) reviewed all the tumors occurring in nonhuman primates, and concluded that hemopoietic tumors constitute the commonest type of neoplasm. Lowenstine (1986) reviewed tumor incidence in the primates from 11 institutions. In New World monkeys, gastrointestinal lesions were most common, of which colonic adenocarcinomas in the cotton-topped tamirin or marmoset (*Sanguinus oedipus*) were the most frequent. In Old World primates, principally the macaques, lymphoreticular and hemopoietic neoplasms accounted for about half (43%) of the reported malignancies in macaques.

As in humans, little is understood about the pathogenesis of neoplasia, or the true incidence. Also, little is known of the role of pathogenic viruses in the tumors of nonhuman primates, although it is known that oncogenic viruses can enhance the in-cidence of neoplasia in some infections. Since most toxicologists will be working with young animals, neoplasms should be of no consequence unless they occur as a result of compound administration.

Metabolism   Christopher P. Chengelis

Monkeys have been widely used in biomedical research for many years, and their xenobiotic metabolism has also been extensively studied, though it is not as well characterized as that of the dog. This was probably because the basic biology of the relevant enzymes could be studied in more convenient, less exotic animals. One could, for example, sacrifice a large number of rats for the sole purpose of isolating cytochrome P-450, but few investigators have been willing to do likewise for the monkey. In addition, monkeys represent a phylogenetic class of animals rather than an individual species. Comparing drug metabolism in rhesus and cynomolgus monkeys is like comparing rats and guinea pigs. There are considerable differences between Old World and New World monkeys (Williams, 1972, 1973; Litterst et al., 1976). One has to be careful of broad generalizations based on study of any one family. This section will concentrate on the more common monkeys used in toxicological research. Where such information exists, differences between members of different phylogenetic families will be high-lighted.

Some key parameters of hepatic xenobiotic metabolism in the monkey are highlighted in Table 4. Concentrations of cytochrome P-450 run between 0.5 and 1.3 nmol/mg protein. There are differences between different species of monkeys. Macaques, such as the rhesus, tend to have the highest concentrations, whereas marmosets tend to have the

Table 4 Summary of Hepatic Xenobiotic Metabolizing Enzymes in Monkeys

Enzyme	Concentration or activity	Comments and references
Cytochrome P-450	0.5–1.3 nmol/mg-m	Amri et al., 1986; Lindstrom and Whitaker, 1987; Lan et al., 1983; Challiner et al., 1980; Litterst et al., 1976; Muller-Eberhart et al., 1983. For old world monkeys, highest in rhesus, lowest in marmoset.
Cytochrome b$_5$	0.31–0.32 nmol/mg-m	Roberts et al., 1977.
NADPH:Cytochrome P-450 Reductase	80–220 nmol-min/mg-m	Wide range due to methodological and age-related differences. Maloney et al., 1986. Leakey et al., 1987; Litterst et al., 1976.
MMFO Activities		Large differences between squirrel and rhesus monkeys. Litterst et al., 1976; Leakey et al., 1987; Iverson et al., 1982; Challiner et al., 1980; Lan et al., 1983.
Aminopyrine	3.3–9.2 nmol/min/mg-m	
Aniline	0.30–0.80 nmol/min/mg-m	
Ethoxycoumarin	0.60–0.90 nmol/min/mg-m	
Ethoxyresorufin	0.03–0.08 nmol/min/mg-m	
Epoxide hydrolase		Pacifici et al., 1981, 1983. Species differences, highest in baboon
styrene oxide	14–32 nmol/min/mg-m	
UDP-Glucuronosyl transferase		Leakey et al., 1983; Litterst et al., 1976
1-naphthol	16–20 nmol/min/mg-m	
4-nitrophenol	7–25 nmol/min/mg-m	
Glutathione S-Transferase		High activity in rhesus monkeys Summer and Grier, 1981.
2,4-dinitro-1-chlorobenzene	2.5–7 μmol/min/mg-c	
1,2-dichloro-4-nitrobenzene ethacrynic acid	7 to 33 nmol/min/mg-c	
Protein estimates		Lan et al., 1983; Lindtrom and Whitaker, 1987.
microsomal	18–36 mg/g liver	
cytosolic		

Abbreviations: mg-m = mg microsomal protein
mg-c = mg cytosolic protein

lowest. Litterst et al. (1976) reported that the amounts of cytochrome P-450 and NAD-PH:cytochrome C reductase, and microsomal mixed function oxidase (MMFO) activities (with ethylmorphine, aminopyrine, aniline, biphenyl, or benzo[a]pyrene) were higher (roughly 2.5-fold) in rhesus than in squirrel monkeys. The molecular nature of cytochrome P-450 from monkeys has not been as well characterized as that of rats. Ohmori et al., 1984) isolated and purified cytochrome P-450 from (Japanese) crab-eating monkeys (macaques). They observed that the monkey MMFO has activity against several typical MMFO substrates, but antibodies against monkey cytochrome P-450 did not inhibit rat MMFO activity, suggesting that there may be little structural homology between the two species. Using SDS-PAGE techniques, Challiner et al., (1982) compared microsomal preparations of marmosets treated with different inducing agents. Their results suggest that there are at least four different cytochrome P-450 isozymes in this species. This was confirmed by Kastner and Schultz (1989) using fast ion-exchange protein chromatography. Thus, cytochrome P-450 in monkeys exists, as in all other animal species examined, as a family of different isozymes with differing substrate specificity and sensitivity to different inducing agents.

Ohta et al., (1989) compared the "activation" of four representative different mutagens in the Ames test using microsomes from rats, dogs, monkeys, and humans. In general, monkey microsomes did not have the highest activity with any of the substrates, and most resembled those of the human with regard to both absolute activity and activity relative to the rat or dog. Interestingly, antibodies against rat cytochrome P-448 had the least inhibitory effect with monkey microsomes. This would suggest that despite the similarity between human and monkeys with regard to activity, the molecular structure of their cytochrome P-450's may be quite different.

A few studies on direct interspecies comparisons of in vitro MMFO activity have been reported. (For a review on species-related differences in MMFO activity, see Kato, 1979.) Dohi et al. (1973) reported that the cytochrome P-450 content and the nicotine-metaboliz-ing capability were higher in rhesus monkeys than in dogs. Amri et al. (1986) compared the MMFO of eight different species, including cynomolgus monkeys, to that of humans. The monkeys had essentially the same amount of cytochrome P-450 (approx. 0.75 nmol/mg microsomal protein) as the guinea pig, and more than twice that of the human subjects (0.31 nmol/min). When the maximal velocities were examined with six different model substrates, the monkey consistently had higher activities than the human. In fact, the similarities between the rat and the rhesus monkey were greater than those between the rhesus and the human. In general, the rhesus monkey tends to have higher amounts of cytochrome P-450 than the rat. For example, Lan et al. (1983) noted that rhesus monkeys had cytochrome P-450 concentrations comparable to that of the rat on a protein basis (approx. 1 nmol/mg), but given that the monkey had higher microsomal protein con-centrations, monkeys had the higher concentrations on a gram liver basis (18.8 nmol/g).

Comparatively little work has been published on the molecular nature of the other components (e.g., NADPH:cytochrome C reductase, cytochrome b_5) of the MMFO of monkeys. Given both the importance of these enzymes, as established by work done with rodents, and the assumed phylogenetic similarities between humans and monkeys, this lack of research is somewhat surprising. Schmucker and Wang (1986) isolated and purified the reductase from rhesus monkeys and found that it exists as a single protein with a molecular weight of approximately 77 kDa, which is similar to that of other species. There is immunological cross-reactivity between the NADPH:cytochrome C reductases of the pig and rhesus monkey. Using the techniques available at the time, Nobrega et al. (1969) compared the molecular properties of cytochrome b_5 from New World monkeys (*Aluoouatta fusca*), pigs, chickens, and humans. The properties of the enzyme isolated from the mammalian species were quite similar with regard to molecular weight (10,600–11,400), amino acid composition, trypsin digestion pattern, and spectrophotometric spectra. Perhaps the reason that there has been so little work on these enzymes in the primate is that the available data do not suggest that they are sufficiently different to warrant the use of primates further study in additional studies.

Definite gender- and age-related (postmaturation or senescent) changes in the MMFO have been identified in rats. Relatively few papers have been published on the subject in monkeys. The data published by Litterst et al. (1976) did not identify any sex-related differences in the MMFO (either in enzyme components or activity), nor for that matter, in glutathione S-transferase, UDP-glucuronosyl transferase, or N-acetyl transferase. Sutter et al. (1985) studied the influence of age on the MMFO in female pig-tail macaques (*Macaca nemstrina*) and identified no age-related (2.5–21.0 year) changes in cytochrome P-450 content, NADPH:cytochrome C reductase, or aryl hydrocarbon hydroxylase activity. Maloney and colleagues (1986) examined adult rhesus monkeys ranging from age 1 to 25 years for age differences in the MMFO. They established that there were no age- or sex-related differences with regard to the amount of cytochrome P-450, MMFO activity with ethylmorphine, or the phospholipid content of endoplasmic reticulum. It would appear, therefore, that age- and sex-related changes in the MMFO are not marked in monkeys. A possible age-related increase in cytochrome C the reductase activity has been identified by Maloney et al. (1986) and confirmed in a follow-up paper (Schmucker and Wang, 1987). There is an age-related increase in the specific activity of this enzyme in rhesus monkeys, which is not accompanied by changes in molecular weight or immunoprecipitability. This is in contrast to the situation in the rat (see Chapter 2) where several investigators have shown that the specific activity of NADPH:cytochrome C reductase declines with age. The paradox of how there can be increases in the reductase activity which are not reflected in increases in MMFO activity remains to be resolved. Developmental (pre- and postnatal) changes of the MMFO in monkeys have been examined in a few publications, but not thoroughly explored. Dvorchik and colleagues (1976, 1979) established that fetal stump-tail macaques had higher concentrations of cytochrome P-450 and MMFO activity than those of comparably aged rats, but still had less activity than the adult animals. This observation was confirmed by Leakey and colleagues (1986). They compared the MMFO of near-term fetal rhesus monkeys to both adult monkeys, and adult and near-term fetal rats. The concentration of cytochrome P-450 and activity of the MMFO of the fetal rhesus monkey is much higher than that of the fetal rat, both in absolute terms and relative to comparable adult levels. That is, in the monkey, the fetal cytochrome P-450 concentration was 17% of that of the adult, whereas in the rat the comparable figure was 8.5%. Differences of similar magnitude were seen with aminopyrine N-demethylase and ethoxycoumarin O-deethylase activities. Interestingly, neither fetal rats or monkeys had measurable activity with ethoxyresorufin deethylation, a specific substrate for cytochrome P-448–mediated activity. This observation would suggest that this particular isozyme develops well after birth in both species.

Treatment of the monkey mothers with dexamethasone induced an increase in the MMFO (enzyme components and activity toward most substrates) in fetal monkeys, but not in fetal rats. This work clearly indicates that while monkeys are born with a MMFO that is better developed than that of the rat, it is considerable less active than that of the adult monkey. The monkey probably more closely resembles the human in this regard than a rodent. The inducibility by dexamethasone may provide a useful tool for studying drug-related toxicities of the newborn.

The specificity of inhibitors of the MMFO in monkeys has not been as well characterized as in rats on other rodents. In fact, few papers, if any, discuss the use of the classic inhibitors of MMFO activity, such as metyrapone and SKF-525A, in monkeys. Anderson et al. (1982) reported that DPEA, 4,6-diphenyl-1,10-2-[2,4-dichloro-6-phenyl)phenoxy]ethylamine hydrobromide, at 0.5 mM, effectively inhibited the in vitro microsomal metabolism of N-phenyl-2-naph-tylamine in Rhesus monkeys. Franklin et al. (1977) reported that treatment of stump-tail macaques with methadone for 1 year will result in reversible decreases in cytochrome P-450 and MMFO activity. Mueller-Eberhart and colleagues (1983) reported that allylisopropylacetamide treatment (300 mg/kd/day sc for four days) will result in substantial decreases in cytochrome P-450 and MMFO activity in rhesus monkeys. Unfortunately, the same treatment also inhibits heme oxygenase and increases δ-aminolevulinic acid synthesis, and, therefore, is porphyrogenic. While interesting, such findings are of limited value to the investigator who wishes to design an experiment involving acute inhibition of the MMFO.

Induction of the MMFO has been examined, but not as exhaustively as in other species. Challiner et al. (1980) reported that phenobarbital (20 mg/kd ip for 3 days) caused the expected increases in cytochrome P-450, and the MMFO (in vitro) activities toward aminopyrine and ethoxycoumarin, but not ethoxyresorufin, in marmosets. In vivo, this induction presented as an increase in the urinary excretion of 6-β-hydroxycortisol. This latter finding suggest a noninvasive method for monitoring for induction in monkeys.

This same group (Challiner et al., 1981) also examined the inducing effect of 3-methylcholanthrene (25 mg/kg ip for 3 days) in marmosets. They observed slight but significant increases in cytochrome P-450 and NADPH:cytochrome C reductase, no change in microsomal aminopyrine N-demethylase, a 2.2-fold increase in ethoxycoumarin O-deethylation, and a 10-fold increase in ethoxyresorufin O-deethylase. This is fairly typical of how other species respond to 3-methylchanthrene. Unlike phenobarbital, induction with 3-methylcholanthrene is not associated with an increase in 6-β-hydroxylation of cortisol.

Iverson et al. (1982) reported that cynomolgus monkeys respond to chronic treatment with both aroclor 1248 and 1254 (2 to 5 mg/kg po, 3 times per week for at least 10 weeks) with an approximately twofold increased in cytochrome P-450 with downward shifts in the absorption maximum. Depending on substrate, increases in activity ranged from 155 (with aminopyrine) to 630% (with ethoxyresorufin) of control. The latter finding is consistent with that seen in other species as ethoxyresorufin is considered to be specifically a substrate for cytochrome P-448–mediated activity.

Thorgerisson et al. (1978) reported that treatment of male rhesus monkeys with 3-methylcholanthrene (a single 80 mg/kg dose 24 hr before sacrifice) caused a 57% increase in cytochrome P-450, with the expected downward shift in the maximum absorbence (450–448) and large increase (five- to eightfold) in benzo(a)pyrene hydroxylation activity.

Despite the fact that monkeys have been shown to respond to the classic inducing agents (phenobarbital, PCBs, etc.), there are some isolated reports in the literature which may suggest that the monkey is not as inducible as other animal species. Lindstrom and Whitaker (1987) compared the action of an aromatase inhibitor (LY 56110) in the rat, dog, and rhesus monkey. The chemical was a potent inhibitor of MMFO in the rat. Two weeks of treatment results in substantial MMFO induction in the rat, but not in the monkey.

Peroxisomal-inducing agents represent a class of chemicals that induce not only increases in MMFO activity, but also increases in peroxisomal number and associated enzyme activity, primarily in rodents. Hawkins et al. (1988) has reviewed species differences in responses to peroxisomal proliferators (typically antilipidemic agents related to clofibrate or phthalate-plasticizing agents such as di(2-ethylhexyl) phthalate, DHEP) and found that monkeys are typically far less sensitive to such agents than rodents.

For example, Rhodes et al. (1986) compared the effects of DHEP in rats and marmosets. Both species were given DHEP 2000 mg/kg/day for 14 days. Rats responded with large significant increases in liver weight accompanied by large increases (sixfold) in peroxisomal number and associated enzyme activity (e.g., fourfold increase in palmitoyl CoA oxidation) that were not seen in marmosets. It would thus appear that in terms of microsomal and peroxisomal proliferation, monkeys are better models for the human responses than are rodents.

Aromatic amines may have three different routes of metabolism in the monkey: aromatic hydroxylation catalyzed by the MMFO, N-hydroxylation catalyzed by the MMFO or the FMFO, and N-acetylation, catalyzed by N-acetyltransferase. These pathways are not mutually exclusive. For example, Thorgerisson et al. (1978) reported that hepatic microsomes isolated from rhesus monkeys produces 3-, 5-, and 7-hydroxylated, as well as N-hydroxylated, metabolites from 2-acetylaminofluorene. Radomski and colleagues (1973) compared the metabolism of primary aromatic amines in dogs and monkeys. These chemicals cause bladder cancer in both species. Both species also produce N-hydroxy metabolites (e.g., N-hydroxy-2-naphthylamine from 2-naphthylamine), but excretion of acetylated N-hydroxy metabolites occured only in monkeys. Thus, the N-hydroxy aromatic metabolite are primary bladder carcinogens, and 2-naphthylamine is carcinogenic in both species despite the differences in metabolism. Perhaps such chemicals cause fewer bladder tumors in monkeys than dogs because of the presence of a competing pathway (acetylation). The FMFO has been reported to be active in N-hydroxylation in other species (Ziegler, 1988), but the involvement of this enzyme in N-oxidation in the monkey remains to be fully characterized.

Primary amines can be acetylated (and then hydroxylated) by monkeys, but the available evidence suggests wide differences in activity with different substrates. Litterst et al. (1976) reported that in vitro cytosolic N-acetyl transferase activity of rhesus monkeys was about 4.9 nmol/min/mg protein with p-aminobenzoic acid, but only 0.01 nmol/min/mg with sulfadiazine. Old World monkeys tend to have higher rates of *n*-acetyltransferase activity than New World monkeys.

The metabolism of secondary aromatic amines differ from that of primary amines in that the former are not acetylated nor N-hydroxylated by monkeys. As reported by Anderson et al. (1982), who examined the metabolism of N-phenyl-2-naphthylamine (P2NA) by seven different species, there is no evidence of N-hydroxylation in any species, including the monkey. All seven species formed the same two major metabolites in vitro, although the ratio of 6-hydroxy-P2NA to 4'-hydroxy-P2NA did vary. This ratio was 0.4 for rat, monkey and mouse, whereas it was 1.0 for the dog and human. This is another example of how the monkey is not always the best model for humans. Anderson et al. (1982), also reported evidence that the cytochrome P-450–dependent MMFO rather than the flavin-dependent FMFO is responsible for the metabolism of P2NA. This is one of the few papers to address FMFO in monkeys.

Epoxide hydrolase has been studied, but not extensively characterized in monkeys. In general, monkeys have higher epoxide hydrolase activity (against styrene oxide) than rodents and more closely resemble that of humans. Activity ranges from 14.8 ± 2.3 nmol/min/mg protein reported for rhesus (Pacifici et al., 1983) to 31.3 ± 1.7 for the baboon (Pacifici et al., 1981). Epoxides are substrates for both epoxide hydrolase and glutathione S-transferase. While broad substrate specificity studies have not been done to confirm this point, the work of Pacifici and colleagues suggests that the preferred route of metabolism of epoxides in primates is through epoxide hydrolase, not glutathione conjugation. In comparing primates to rodents in in vivo disposition of a specific xenobiotic, one should not be surprised to find a greater percentage of diol metabolites in monkeys (assuming equivalent MMFO aromatic oxidation activity).

The important conjugative enzyme, glutathione S-transferase, has received some, but hardly exhaustive, scrutiny in the monkey. Litterst et al. (1974) compared glutathione activity S-transferase with 1,2-dichloro-4-nitrobenzene in rhesus and squirrel monkeys. They found that activity ranged from approximately 15 to 25 nmol/min/mg cytosolic protein with no species-related differences. Asaoka and colleagues (1977a,b) character-ized glutathione S-transferase of the Japanese crab-eating monkey and the rhesus monkey. Using various chromatographic techniques, they tentatively identified five isozymes, with various activities against six typical substrates. Thus, as in other species, glutathione exists as a family of isozymes in other monkeys. The pattern present in rat appears to more closely resemble that of the human as opposed to that of the monkey (Asaoka et al., 1977a). Unlike the situation in rats where there are definite isozymic substrate specifici-ties, one glutathione S-transferase isozyme (iv) in the monkey tended to have the highest activity with all substrates examined (Asaoka et al., 1977a).

This enzyme was further examined by Asaoka and Takahashi (1977). It has a molecu-lar weight of 48,000, is composed of two identical subunits (which is consistent with the isozymic structure of GSH-T of other animals), and is competitively inhibited by hexa-chlorobenzene. Summer and Greim (1981) compared the activity GSH-T from the livers of the rat, rhesus monkey, chimpanzee, and human. The model substrates were 1-chloro-2,4-dinitrobenzene (CDNB) and 1,2-dichloro-4-nitrobenzene (DNCNB). With CDNB, rhesus had the highest activity (about 6.5 μmol/min/mg cytosolic protein) followed by the chimpanzee (3.2), the rat (1.8), and then human (1.6). With DCNB, the rat had the highest activity (about 51 nmol/min/mg), followed by the rhesus monkey (2.9), chimpan-zee (9.2), and then human (4.6). This pattern suggests that (1) compared to the rat, primates have comparable or greater activity of glutathione s-transferase, depending on substrate, and (2) rhesus monkeys tend to have greater activity than humans.

Other conjugative (phase 2) reactions have probably been somewhat better character-ized in monkeys than (phase 1) MMFO-catalyzed reactions with regard to similarities to humans. As reviewed by Caldwell (1981), there are some conjugative reactions that have been shown to occur only in humans or monkeys. These include the N'-glucuronidation of methoxysulfonamides, the glucuronidation of cyproheptadine to yield a quarternary glucuronide, and the conjugation of arylacetic acids with glutamine. Williams (1974) extensively reviewed this last reaction. With phenylacetic acid, for example, humans will excrete almost 95% as the glutamate conjugate. Similar results were obtained with monkeys, where, depending on species, up to 90% is excreted as the glutamate conjugate. Interestingly, this is one metabolic reaction where there are not large differences between Old and New World monkeys. Nonprimates such as the rat will produce 80–100% phenylacetate glycine conjugate and no detectable glutamate conjugates.

Dulik and Fenselau (1987) have examined some of aforementioned primate-specific UDP-glucuronosyl transferase reactions in vitro using immobilized enzyme preparations. Interestingly, while they confirmed in vitro that primates have a much higher activity in the glucuronidation of sulfadimethoxine, the human was still found to have roughly 3 times the activity of the rhesus monkey. Additionally, the activity toward both p-nitrophenol and cyproheptadine was more similar between the monkey and rabbit than between the monkey and human.

Others have studied UDP-glucuronosyl transferase activity in the rhesus monkey. Litterst et al. (1974) compared in vitro microsomal UDP-glucuronosyl transferase activity in the rhesus monkey to that of the squirrel monkey. With 4-nitrophenol as the substrate, activity in both species were comparable (approximately 6–14 nmol/min/mg), whereas the squirrel monkey had considerably higher activity with 2-aminophenol (approximately 0.5 vs 2.9 nmol/min/mg). When compared to the rat, the rhesus monkey had higher activity with p-nitrophenol and comparable activity with o-aminophenol.

Pacifici et al., 1986) established that the rhesus monkey has a relatively high transferase activity toward morphine. Leakey et al. (1983, 1984) established that the monkey has activity against a wide variety of (type 1) substrates, including 4-nitrophenol, and 1-naphthol. Activities in adult females were compared to those of the late-term fetus. With natural (type 2) substrates (e.g., steroid hormones on bilirubin), enzyme activities of the fetus were less than 5% than those of the adult, whereas with synthetic substrates (e.g., 4-nitrophenol) activities ran 40–120% of those of the adult.

These results clearly suggest that UDP-glucuronosyl transferase exists as a family of isozymes with differential development in the rhesus monkey. Also, unlike the rat, intrauterine exposure of rhesus monkeys to dexamethasone (10 mg/kg sc given to the pregnant animals 1, 2, and 3 days prior to near-term cesarean section) greatly enhanced the fetal hepatic UDP-glucuronosyl transferase activity toward the type 2 substrates. For example, activity against bilirubin was increased from 3 to 74 nmol/mg/min. Hence, despite the evidence that UDP-glucuronosyl transferase exists as a family of isozymes in both rodents and primates, the genetic and developmental controls are different. As mentioned elsewhere (Chap. 8), there is stereospecificity in the activity of primate UDP-glucuronosyl transferase. For example, when the activities were examined using either (R) or (S) loraepam as a substrates, the rabbit had no stereospecificity, the monkey exclusively glucuronidated the (R) isomer, and human preparation preferred the (R) to the (S) isomer by approximately 4:1 (Dulik and Fenselau, 1987).

Extrahepatic metabolism has not been extensively or systematically examined in monkeys. There are some isolated reports in the literature. For example, Pacifici et al. (1986) demonstrated that the UDP-glucuronosyl transferase present in the gut plays a major role in the metabolism of morphine in the rhesus monkey. They also discussed extrahepatic styrene oxide metabolism in primates (Pacifici et al., 1981, 1983). Thorgeirsson et al. (1978) reported the presence of aromatic hydrocarbon hydroxylase in monkey lungs. However, the current state of the literature does not permit any integrative generalization. Therefore, the subject will not be discussed further.

There are two processes involved in disposition are mentioned here, even though they are not metabolic processes: plasma protein binding and biliary excretion (also see Chap. 1). While they are not metabolic processes, they can play a major role in disposition of a chemical. A tightly bound drug, for example, will not be as rapidly metabolized. There can be wide species differences in plasma protein binding, as reviewed by Cayen (1987). The rhesus monkey is probably the best model for humans. In general, plasma protein binding is greatest in the human and lowest in the mouse. For example, clofibrate is 97 and 95% protein bound in human and rhesus monkey plasma, respectively, whereas it is only 35% bound in the mouse.

The gut flora often play a role in xenobiotic metabolism and toxicity, as reviewed by Rowland (1988). The gut flora of primates differs considerably from that of rodents, and thus may lead to apparent qualitative differences in metabolism. For example, only human subjects and Old World monkeys have been shown to aromatize quinic acid to benzoic acid. If monkeys are treated with neomycin to suppress gut flora, quinic acid is excreted unchanged (Williams, 1974). It would appear that Old World monkeys would be the better model for humans in studying the involvement of gut flora in xenobiotic metabolism. Gut flora are also important because the interplay between gut metabolism and biliary excretion that govern enterohepatic circulation. As reviewed by Levine (1978), most xenobiotics appear in the bile as metabolites, particularly glucuronides. As reviewed by Cayen (1987), monkeys and humans are relatively inefficient in the process of biliary excretion because the molecular weight cut-off for transportation is much lower in rodents than in primates (Levine, 1978). As reviewed by Calabrese (1988), primates have much lower gut flora. β-glucuronidase activity, so the conjugated chemicals that are excreted in bile are less likely to be hydrolyzed and reabsorbed in primates.

Two generalities can be drawn from this work: (1) enterohepatic circulation of a xenobiotic is more likely to occur in rodents than in primates, and (2) in primates, a greater percentage of metabolites will be excreted in the urine than in the feces; however, once a glucuronide metabolite is excreted into the primate gut, it is less likely to be reabsorbed than in the rat.

Isolated hepatocytes have been used extensively to study xenobiotic metabolism in smaller species. Extensive discussion of this in vitro methodology is outside the scope of this book, but it deserves a mention here because of the opportunity it affords to decrease the use of monkeys. Gee et al. (1983) have described a method of isolating hepatocytes from squirrel monkeys. Cell viability was comparable to that of other species. The in vitro metabolism of tolbutamide, as a model chemical, was studied and both the rates of metabolism and spectrum of metabolites determined. They concluded that isolated hepatocytes from the rat, rabbit, dog, and monkey formed the major metabolites reported to occur in vivo at relative rates similar to intact animals. Interestingly, they also concluded that the rabbit rather than the monkey was the better model for human metabolism of tolbutamide. The important point to be made here is that they were able to come to that conclusion using relatively few animals.

In a classic review, Caldwell (1981) concluded that the monkey was the best model for predicting metabolism in humans. His conclusion was based on the fact that there are fewer biochemical differences between the rhesus monkey and humans than for other species. This was confirmed by review of the literature for 32 different chemicals. Differences in routes of metabolism, however, may or may not be of practical importance. For example, Cayen et al. (1985) examined the pharmacokinetics of tolresat in rats, dogs, and monkeys, and concluded that both the dog and the monkey were equally good models, despite large differences in metabolite profiles, for the pharmacokinetic behavior (AUCs and terminal half-lives) of this drug in human subjects. The dog excreted most of the drug (82%) unchanged in the urine, whereas the monkey excreted mostly conjugated tolrestat (49%) or conjugates of other metabolites (32%). In determining which species may be the best model for humans, one should examine both the routes of metabolism and in vivo pharmacokinetic behavior of the parent chemical. The monkey may not always be the best or only model for humans.

REFERENCES

Abee, C. R. (1985) Medical care of management of the squirrel monkey, in *Handbook of Squirrel Monkey Research*, Rosenblum, L. A., and Coe, C.L., eds., Plenum Press, New York, pp. 484–485.

Amri, H., Batt, A., and Siest, G. (1986) Comparison of cytochrome P-450 content and activities in liver microsomes of seven animal species, including man. *Xenobiotica* 16, 351–358.

Anderson, J. H., and Houghton, P. (1983) The pole and collar system. A technique for handling and training non-human primates. *Lab. Anim.* 12, 47–49.

Anderson, M., Mitchum, R., and Beland, F. (1982) Hepatic microsomal metabolism and macromolecular binding of the antioxidant N-phenyl-2-naphthylamine. *Xenobiotica* 12, 31–43.

Asaoka, K., Ito, H., and Takahashi, K. (1977a) Monkey glutathione S-aryl transferases: 1. Tissue distribution and purification from the liver. *J. Biochem.* 82, 973–981.

Asaoka, K, Ito, H., and Takahashi, K. (1977b) Monkey glutathione S-aryl transferases: 1. Properties of the major enzyme purified from the liver. *J. Biochem.* 82, 973–1323.

Baker, B. A., and Morris, G. F. (1979) A cage liner and feeding system to minimize stress to primates undergoing metabolic balance studies. *Lab. anim.* 13, 249–251.

Bearcroft, W. G. C., and Jameson, M. D. (1958) An outbreak of subcutaneous tumors in Rhesus monkeys. *Nature* 182, 195.

Bellhorn, R. W. (1980) Lighting in the animal environment. *Lab. Anim. Sci.* 30, 440–450.

Bender, M. A. (1955) Blood volume of the rhesus monkey. *Science* 122, 156.

Benirschke, K. (1978) *Pathology of Laboratory Animals*, Vol. I, II, F. M. Garner, and T. C. Jones, eds. Springer-Verlag, New York.

Benirschke, K. (1983) Occurrence of spontaneous diseases, in *Viral and Immunological Diseases in Non-human Primates*, Kalter, S. S. ed. A. R. Liss, Inc., New York, pp. 17–30.

Besch, E. L. (1980) Environmental quality within animal facilities. *Lab. Anim. Sci.* 30, 385–406.

Bourne, G. H. (1975) Collected anatomical and physiological data from the rhesus monkey, in *The Rhesus Monkey*, Vol. I, Bourne, G. H., ed. Academic Press, New York, pp. 1–63

Bowen, J. A., and Cummins, L. B. (1985) Intravenous catheterization of infant chimpanzees, in *Clinical Management of Infant Great Apes*. C. Graham, ed. Liss, New York, pp. 131–140.

Bryant, J. M. (1980) A tethering system to accommodate catheter and a temperature monitor for non-human primates. *Lab. Anim. Sci.* 30, 706–708.

Burke, D. S., and Heisey, G. B. (1984) Wild Malaysian cynomologus monkeys are exposed to hepatitis A virus. *Am. J. Trop. Med. Hyg.* 33:940–944.

Calabrese, E. (1988) Comparative biology of test species. *Environ. Health Perspect.* 77, 55–62.

Caldwell, J. (1981) The current status of attempts to predict species differences in drug metabolism. *Drug Metab. Rev.* 12, 221–237.

Cayen, M. (1987) Retrospective evaluation of appropriate animal models based on metabolism studies in man, in *Human Risk Assessment—The Role of Animal Selection and Extrapolation*, Roloff, M., Wilson, A., Ribelin, W., Ridley, W., and Ruecker, F., eds. Taylor & Francis, New York, pp. 99–112.

Cayen, M., Hicks, D., Ferdinndi, E., Kraml, M., Greselin, E., and Dovrnik, D. (1985) Metabolic disposition and pharmacokinetics of the aldose reductase inhibitor Tolrestat in rats, dogs and monkeys. *Drug. Metab. Dispos.* 13, 412–418.

Centers for Disease Control (1984) *Biosafety in Microbiological and Biomedical Laboratories*, HHS Publications, #84-8395. USDHHS, PHS, March.

Centers for Disease Control (1987) B-virus infection in humans—Pensacola, Florida. *MMWR* 36, 289–290, 295–296.

Centers for Disease Control, Morbidity Mortality Report, 1 Oct. 1987. Guidelines for Prevention of Herpes Virus Simiae (B Virus) Inspection in Monkey Handlers, Vol. 36, 41:680–689.

Centers for Disease Control, Morbidity Mortality Report, 22 June, 1990. Update: Filovirus Infection Associated with Contact with Non-Human Primates of Their Tissues, Vol. 39, 24:404–405.

Challiner, M., Park, B., Odum, J., Orton, T., and Parker, G. L. (1980) The effects of phenobarbitone on urinary 6-b-hydroxycortisol excretion and hepatic enzyme activity in the marmoset monkey (Callithrix jacchus). *Biochem. Pharmacol.* 29, 2219–3324.

Challiner, M., Park, B., Odum, J., and Orton, T. (1981) The effects of 3-methylcholanthrene on urinary 6-b-hydroxycortisol excretion and hepatic enzyme activity in the marmoset monkey (Callithrix jacchus). *Biochem. Pharmacol.* 30, 2131–2134.

Chapman, W. L. Jr. (1968) Neoplasia in non-human primates. *J. Am. Vet. Med. Assoc.* 153, 872–878.

Coe, C. L., Smith, E. R., and Levine, S. (1985) The endocrine system of the squirrel monkey, in *Handbook of Squirrel Monkey Research.* L. A. Rosenblum, and Coe, C. L., eds. Plenum Press, New York, pp. 484–485.

Conrad, S. H., Sackett, G. P., and Burbacher, T. M. (1989) Diagnosis of early pregnancy by ultrasound in *Macaca fascicularis. J. Med. Primatol.* 18, 143–154.

Dalton, M. J. (1985) The vascular port. A subcutaneously implanted drug delivery depot. *Lab. Anim.* 14:21–30.

Deinhart, F., Peterson, D., Cross, G., et al. (1975) Hepatitis in marmosets. *Am. J. Med. Sci.* 270, 73–80.

Dienstag, J. L., Davenport, F. M., McCollum, R. W. et al. (1976) Non-human primate-associated viral hepatitis A. *J.A.M.A.* 236, 462–464.

Dohi, T., Kojima, S., and Tsujimoto, A. (1973) Comparative studies of hepatic nicotine metabolizing enzyme activities in monkeys and dogs. *Jpn. J. Pharmacol.* 13, 748–751.

Dulik, D., and Fenselau, C. (1987) Species-dependent glucuronidation of drugs by immobilized rabbit, rhesus monkey, and human UDP-glucuronyltransferases. *Drug. Metab. Dispos.* 15, 473–477.

Dunn, F. L. (1968) The parasites of *Saimiri*: in the context of platyrrhine parasitism, in *The Squirrel Monkey*, Rosenblum, L. A., and Cooper, R. W., eds. Academic Press, New York, pp. 31–68

Dvorchik, B., Stenger, V., and Quattropani, S. (1976) Drug biotransformation in micromses from fetal stumptail macaque, macaca arctoides: Hepatic N-demethylation. *Drug Metab. Dispos.* 4, 423–429.

Dvorchik, B., Stenger, V., and Hartmen, R. (1979) Drug metabolism by the fetal stumptail macaque, (macaca arctoides): Heptic microsomal N-demethylation and glucuronidation as measured by radiometric assays. *Pharmacology* 18, 241–250.

Farine, D., MacCarter, G. D., Timor-Tritch, I. E., Yeh, M-N, and Stark, R. I. (1988) Real-time ultrasonic evaluation of the baboon pregnancy: biometric measurements. *J. Med. Primatol.* 17, 215–221.

Federal Register, 9 CRF Parts 1, 2, 3, Dept. of Agriculture, APHIS, Vol. 54, #168, August 1989.

Fletcher, J. L. (1976) Influence of noise on animals, in *Control of the Animal House Environment.* Laboratory Animal Handbooks, 7, McSheehy, T., ed. Laboratory Animal, London, pp. 51–62.

Flynn, L. A., and Guilloud, R. B. (1988) Vascular catheterization: Advantages over venipuncture for multiple blood collection. *Lab. Anim.* 17, 29–35.

Forsyth, R. P., Nies, A. S., Wyler, F., Neutize, J., and Melmon, K. (1986) Normal distribution of cardiac output in the unanesthetized restrained rhesus monkey. *J. Appl. Physiol.* 25, 736–741.

Fox, J. G. (1982) Campylobacterosis—a "new" disease in laboratory animals. *Lab. Anim. Sci.* 32, 625–537.

Frances, D. P., Hadler, S. C., Prendergast, T. J. et al. (1984) Occurrence of hepatitis A, B, and non-A/non-B in the United States. CDC Sentinel County Hepatitis Study 1. *Am. J. Med.* 76, 69–74.

Gee, S., Green, C., and Tyson, C. (1984) Comparative metabolism of tolbutamide by isolated hepatocytes from rat, rabbit, dog and squirrel monkey. *Drug Metab. Dispos.* 12, 174–178.

Good, R. C., and May, B. D. (1971) Respiratory pathogens in monkeys. *Infect. Immunol.* 3, 87–93.

Gortan, R. L., and Basch, E. L. (1974) Air temperature and humidity response to cleaning water loads in laboratory animal facilities. *ASHRAE Trans.* 80, 37–52.

Graham, C. E., Collins, D. C., Robinson, H., and Preedy, J. R. F. (1972) Urinary levels of estrogens and pregnanediol and plasma levels of progesterone during the menstrual cycle of the chimpanzee: Relationship to the sexual swelling. *Endocrinology* 91, 13–24.

Griesemer, R. A. (1976) Naturally occurring neoplastic diseases in Non-human primates, in *Handbook of Laboratory Animal Science*, Vol. 3, Melby, E. C., Jr., and Altman, N. H., eds. CRC Press, Cleveland, Ohio, pp. 309–323.

Hack, C. A., and Gleiser, C. A. (1982) Hematologic and serum chemistry reference values for adult and juvenile baboons (*Papio* spp). *Lab. Anim. Sci.* 32, 502–505.

Hawkins, J., Jones, W., Bonner, F., and Gibson, G. (1987) The effect of peroxisome proliferators on microsomal, peroxisomal and mitochondril enzyme activities in liver and kidney. *Drug Metab. Rev.* 18, 441–516.

Hein, P. R., Schatorije, J. S. J. O., Frencken, H. J. A. A. M., Segers, M. F. G., and Thomas, C. M. G. (1989) Serum hormone levels in pregnant cynomolgus monkeys. *J. Med. Primatol.* 18, 133–142.

Heiser, H. J. (1970) *Atlas of Comparative Hematology.* Academic Press, New York.

Henderson, B. E., Kissling, R. E., Williams, M. C., et al. (1971) Epidemiological studies in Uganda relating to the "Marburg" agent, in *Marburg Virus Disease*, Martini, G. A., and Siegert, R., eds. Springer-Verlag, Berlin, p. 166.

Hendrickx, A. G. (1973) The sensitive period and malformation syndrome produced by thalidomide in the crab-eating monkey (*Macaca fascicularis*). *J. Med. Primatol.* 2:267–276.

Hendrickx, A. G., and Binkerd, P. E. (1990) Non-human primates and teratological research. *J. Med. Primatol.* 19, 81–108.

Hendrickx, A. G., and Cukierski, M. A. (1987) Reproductive and developmental toxicology in non-human primates, in *Preclinical Safety of Biotechnology Products Intended for Human Use*, Graham, C., ed. Liss, New York, pp. 73–88.

Hendrickx, A. G., and Aelrod, L. R., and Clayborn, L. D. (1966) Thalidomide syndrome in baboons. *Nature* 210, 958–959.

Hennessen, W. (1971) Epidemiology of Marburg virus disease, in *Marburg Virus Disease*, Martini, G. A., and Siegert, R., Eds. Springer-Verlag, Berlin, p. 161.

Henrickson, R. V., Osborn, K. G., Madden, D. L., Anderson, J. H., Maul, D. H., Sever, J. L., Ellingsworth, L. R., Lowenstein, L. J., & Gardner, M. B. (1983) Epidemic of acquired immunodeficiency in rhesus monkeys. *Lancent* 1, 388–390.

Hillis, W. D. (1961) An outbreak of infectious hepatitis among chimpanzee handlers at a United States Air Force base. *Am. J. Hyg.* 73, 316–328.

Hobson, W. C., and Fuller, G. B. (1987) Species selection for safety evaluation of biotechnology products, in *Preclinical Safety of Biotechnology Products Intended for Human Use*, Graham, C., ed. Liss, New York, pp. 55–71.

Hobson, W. C., Faiman, C., Dougherty, W., Reyes, F. I., and Winter, J. S. D. (1975) Radioimmunoassay of rhesus monkey chorionic gonadotropin. *Fertil. Steril.* 26, 93–97.

Hunt, R. D., and Melendez, L. V. (1966) Spontaneous *Herpes*-T infection in the owl monkey (*Aotus trivirigatus* . *Pathol. Vet.* 3(1), 1–26.

Iverson, F., Truelove, J., and Hierlihy, S. (1982) Hepatic microsomal enzyme induction by aroclors 1248 and 1254 in cynomologus monkeys. *Food Chem. Toxicol.* 20, 307–310.

Kalter, S. S. (1983) Primate Viruses—Their Significance, in *Viral and Immunological Diseases in Non-human Primates*, Vol. 2, Kalter, S. S., eds. Liss, New York, pp. 67–89.

Kalter, S. (1986) Overview of simian viruses and recognized virus diseases and laboratory support for the diagnosis of viral infections, in, *Primates—The Road to Self-Sustaining Populations*, Benirschke, K., ed. Springer-Verlag, Berlin, pp. 571–679.

Karger, S. (1972) *Pathology of Simian Primates*, Part I, R. N. T-W-Fiennes, R. N., ed. Basel.

Kastner, M., and Schultz, T. (1987) Ion-exchange fast proteinliquid chromatography: Optimization of the purification of cytochrome P-450 from marmoset monkeys. *J. Chromatographr.* 397, 153–163.

Kato, R. (1979) Characteristics and differences in the hepatic mixed function oxidases of different species. *Pharmacol. Ther.* 6, 41–98.

Keeling, M. E., and Wolf, R. H. (1975) Medical management of the rhesus monkey, in *The Rhesus Monkey*, Vol. II, Bourne, G. H., ed. Academic Press, New York, pp. 11–96.

Kelly, C. A., and Gleiser, C. A. (1986) Selected coagulation reference values for adult and juvenile baboons. *Lab. Anim. Sci.* 36, 173–175.

King, F. A., Yarbrough, C. J., Anderson, D. C., Gordon, T. P., and Gould, K. G. (1988) Primates. *Science* 240, 1475–1482.

Lan, S., Weinstein, S., Keim, G., and Migdalof, B. (1983) Induction of hepatic drug-metabolizing enzymes in rats, dogs, and monkeys after repeated administration on an anti-inflammatory hexahydroindazole. *Xenobiotica* 13, 329–335.

Lankas, G. R., and Jensen, R. D. (1987) Evidence of hepatitus A infection in immature rhesus monkeys. *Vet. Pathol.* 24, 340–344.

Leakey, J., Althaus, Z., Bailey, J., and Slikker, W. (1983) UDP-Glucuronyltransferase activity exhibits two developmental groups in liver from foetal rhesus monkeys. *Biochem. J.* 214, 1007–1009.

Leakey, J., Althaus, Z., Bailey, J., and Slikker, W. (1985) Dexamethasone increases UDP-glucuronyltransferase activity towards bilirubin, oestradiol and testosterone in foetal liver from rhesus monkeys during late gestation. *Biochem. J.* 214, 1007–1009.

Leakey, J., Althaus, Z., Bailey, J., and Slikker, W. (1986) Dexamethasone induces hepatic cytochrome P-450 content and increases certain monooxygenase activities in rhesus monkey fetuses. *Biochem. Pharmacol.* 35, 1389–1391.

Lerch, N. W., Osborn, K. G., Marx, P. A., Prahalada, S., Maul, D. H., Lowensteine, L. J., Munn, R. J., Bryant, M. L., Henrickson, R. V., Arthur, L. O., Gilden, R. V., Barker, C. S., Hunter, E., and Gardner, M. B. (1986) Inapparent carriers of simian acquired immune deficiency syndrome type D. retrovirus and disease transmission with saliva. *J. Natl. Cancer Inst.* 77, 489–495.

Lerch, N. W., Marx, P. A., Osborn, K. G., Maul, D. H., Lowenstine, L. J., Beviss, M. L., Moody, P., Henrickson, R. V., and Gardner, M. B. (1987) Natural history of endemic Type D retrovirus infection and acquired immune deficiency syndrome in group-housed rhesus monkeys. *J. Natl. Cancer Inst.* 79, 847–854.

Levine, W. (1987) Biliary excretion of drugs and other xenobiotics. *Ann. Rev. Pharmacol. Toxicol.* 18, 81–96.

Lindstrom, T., and Whitaker, G. (1987) Disposition of the aromatase inhibitor LY56110 and associated induction and inhibition studies in rats, dogs and monkeys. *Fund. Appl. Toxicol.* 8:595–604.

Litterst, C., Gram, T., Mimnaugh, Lever, P., Emmerling, D., and Freudenthal, R. (1976) A comprehensive study of in vitro drug metabolism in several laboratory species. *Drug Metab. Dispos.* 4, 203–207.

Lowenstine, L. J. (1986) Neoplasms and proliferative disorders in non-human primates, in *Primates—The Road to Self-Sustaining Populations*, Benirschke, K., ed. Springer-Verlag, Berlin, pp. 781–814.

Mackenzie, M., Lowenstine, L., Lalchandani, R., Lerche, N., Osborn, K., Spinner, A., Bleviss, M., Henrickson, R., and Gardener, M. (1986) Hemotologic abnormalities in SAIDS. *Lab. Anim. Sci.* 36, 14–19.

Maloney, A., Schmucker, D., Vessey, D., and Wang, R. (1986) The effects of aging on the hepatic microsomal mixed function oxidase system of male and female monkeys. *Hepatology* 6, 282–287.

Mao, J. S., Go, Y. Y., Huang, H. Y., et al. (1981) Susceptibility of monkeys to human hepatitis A virus. *J. Infect. Dis.* 144, 55–60.

Marx, P. A. (1986) Overview of Simian AIDS, in *Animal Models of Petrovirus Infection and Their Relationship to AIDS*, Salzman, L. A., ed. Academic Press, Orlando, Florida, pp. 131–144.

Mason, J. W. (1972) Corticosteroid response to chair restraint in the monkey. *Am. J. Physiol.* 222, 1291–1294.

Mathiesen, L. R., Drucker, J., Lorenz, D., et al. (1978) Localization of hepatitis A antigen in marmoset organs during acute infection with hepatitis A virus. *J. Infect. Dis.* 138, 369–377.

McClure, H. M. (1979) Neoplastic diseases of non-human primates: Literature review and observations in an autopsy series of 2176 animals, in *The Comparative Pathology of Zoo Animals*,

Montali, R., and Migaki, G., eds. *Smithsonian Institution Press Washington, D.C.*, pp. 549–565.

McClure, H. M., Brodie, A. R., Anderson, D. C., and Swenson, R. B. (1986) Bacterial infections of non-human primates, in *Primates—The Road to Self-sustaining Populations*, Benirschke, K., ed. Springer-Verlag, Berlin, pp. 531–556.

Muchmore, E. (1973) Clinical care of non-human primates. *J. Med. Primatol.* 2, 341–352.

Muller-Eberhard, U., Eiseman, J., Foidart, M., and Alvares, A. (1983) Effect of heme on allylisopropylacetamide induced changes in heme and drug metabolism in the Rheses monkey (Macaca mulatta). *Biochem. Pharmacol.* 32, 3765–3769.

National Academy of Sciences (1986) *Non-Human Primates—Standard Guidelines for the Breeding Care Overall Management of Lab Animals*, 3rd ed., Revised, Washington, D.C.

National Institutes of Health (1985) *Guide for the Care and Use of Laboratory Animals*. Publication #86-23, ILAR.NRC.

Nobrega, F., Araujo, P., Pasetto, M., and Raw, I. (1969) Some properties of cytochrome b5 from liver microsomes of man, monkey, pig, and chicken. *Biochem. J.* 115, 849–856.

O-Gara, R. W., and Adamson, R. H. (1972) Spontaneous and induced neoplasms in non-human primates, in *Pathology of Simian Primates*, Fiennes, R.N.T.-W., ed. Kerger, Basel, pp. 190–238.

Ohmori, S., Motohashi, K., Misukazu, M., Kanakubo, Y., Igarshi, T., Ueno, K., and Kitagawa, H. (1984) Purification and properties of cytochrome P-450 from untreated monkey liver microsomes. *Biochem. Biophys. Res. Commun.* 125, 1089–1095.

Ohta, K., Kitada, M., Ohi, H., Komori, M., Nagashima, K., Sato, N., Muroya, K., Kodama, T., Nagao, M., and Kamataki, T. (1989) Interspecies homology of cytochrome P-450: Toxicological significance of cytochrome P-450 cross reactive with anti-rat P-448-H antibodies in liver microsomes from dogs, monkeys, and humans. *Mutat. Res.* 226, 163–167.

Orton, T., Adam, H., Bentley, M., Holloway, B., and Tucker, M. (1984) Clobuzarit: Species differences in the morphological and biochemical response of the liver following chronic administration. *Toxicol. Appl. Pharmcol.* 73, 138–151.

Pacifici, G., Boobic, A., Brodie, M., McManus, M., and Davies, D. (1981) Tissue and species differences in enzymes of epoxide metabolism. *Xenobiotica* 11, 73–79.

Pacifici, G., Lindberg, B., Glaumann, H., and Rane, A. (1983) Styrene oxide metabolism in Rhesus monkeys liver: Enzyme activities in subcellular fractins and in isolated hepatocytes. *J. Pharmacol. Exp. Therp.* 226, 869–875.

Palmer, A. E. (1987) B. virus, *Herpesvirus Simiae*: Historical perspective. *J. Med. Primatol.* 16, 99–130.

Peterson, E. A. (1980) Noise and laboratory animals. *Lab. Anim. Sci.* 30, 422–439.

Potkay, S., Ganaway, J. R., Rogers, N. G., and Kirard, (1971) An epizootic of measles in a colony of rhesus monkeys (*Macaca mulatta*). *Am. J. of Vet. Res.* 27, 33–39.

Primate Research Laboratory, New Mexico State University, Colony Historical Data.

Public Health Policy on Humane Care and Use of Laboratory Animals (1986) Office for Protection from Research Risks, National Institutes of Health, September.

Radomski, J., Conzelman, G., Rey, A., and Brill, E. (1973) N-Oxidation of certain aromatic amine, acetamides, and nitro compounds by monkey and dogs. *J. Natl. Cancer Inst.* 50, 989–995.

Renquist, D. M. (1975) Importance of the Source, Proper Procurement and Quarantine Procedures. *Cancer Monograph*, Vol 12. *Proceedings of Symposia on Biohazards and Zoonotic Problems of Primate Quarantine and Research.*

Renquist, D. M. (1987A) Selected biohazards of naturally infected nonhuman primates. *J. Med. Primatol.* 16, 91–97.

Renquist, D. M. (1987B) Zoonoses acquired from pet primates. *Vet. Clin. North Am., Small Anim. Pract.* 17(1), 219–240.

Reyes, F. I., Winter, J. S. D., Faiman, C., and Hobson, W. C. (1975) Serial serum levels of gonadotropins, prolactin and sex steroids in the nonpregnant and pregnant chimpanzee. *Endocrinology* 96, 1447–1455.

Rhodes, C., Orton, T., Pratt, I., Batten, P., Bratt, H., Jackson, S., and Elcombe, C. (1986) Comparative pharmacokinetics and subacute toxicity of di(2-ethylhexyl)phthalate (DEHP) in rats and marmosets: Extrapolation of effects in rodents to man. *Environ. Health Perspec.* 65, 299–308.

Roberts, S., Franklin, M., Snyder, E., and Beck, E. (1977) Effects of chronic oral methadone on hepatic microsomal drug metabolism in monkeys. *Toxicol. Appl. Pharmacol.* 42, 607–612.

Rowland, I. (1988) *Role of the Gut Flora in Toxicity and Cancer*. Academic Press, New York.

Ruch, T. C. (ed.) (1959) *Diseases of Laboratory Primates*. Saunders, Philadelphia.

Schlam, D. W. (1975) Materials and methods for the study of the blood including brief comments on factors to be considered in interpretation, in *Veterinary Hematology*, Jain, N. C., and Carroll, E. J., eds. Lea and Febiger, Philadelphia, p. 24.

Schmidt, S., Au, W., Hill, D., Kadlubar, F., and Slikker, W. (1983) Cytochrome P-450–dependent oxidation of the 17alpha-ethnyl group of synthetic steroids: D-homoannulation or enzyme activation. *Drug Metab. Dispos.* 11, 531–536.

Schmucker, D. and Wang, R. (1986) Effects of aging on the properties of rhesus monkeys in liver microsomal NADPH-cytochrome C (P-450) reductase. *Drug Metab. Dispos.* 15, 225–232.

Shevtsova, Z. V., Lapin, B. A., Doroshenko, N. V., et al. (1988) Spontaneous and experimental hepatitis in old world monkeys. *J. Med. Primatol.* 14, 73–82.

Silverman, J. (1988) How to briefly examine common laboratory animals. *Lab. Anim.* 17, 38–39.

Slighter, R. G., Kimball, J. P., Barbolt, T. A., et al. (1988) Enzootic hepatitis A infection in Cynolmolgus monkeys. *Macaca fascicularis. Am. J. Primatol.* 14, 73–82.

Somers, G. E. (1963) The fetal toxicity of thalidomide. *Proc. Eur. Soc. Study Drug Toxic.* 1, 49–58.

Squire, R. A., Goodman, D. C., Valerio, M. G., et al. (1979) Tumors, in *Pathology of Laboratory Animals*, Bernirschke, K., Graner, F. M., and Jones, T. C., eds. Springer-Verlag, Berlin, pp. 1052–1283.

Summer, K., and Greim, H. (1981) Hepatic glutathione S-transferases: Activities and cellular location in rat, rhesus monkey, chimpanzee and man. *Biochem. Pharmacol.* 30, 1719–1720.

Sutter, M., Wood, G., Williamson, L., Strong, R., Pickham, K., and Richardson, A. (1985) Comparison of the hepatic mixed function oxidase system of young adult, and old nonhuman primates. *Biochem. Pharmacol.* 34, 2983–2987.

Thorgeirsson, S., Sakai, S., and Adamson, R. (1978) Induction of monooxygenases in rhesus monkeys by 3-methylcolanthrene: Metabolism and mutagenic activation of N-2-acetylminofluorene and benzo(a)pyrene. *J. Nat. Canc. Insti.* 60:365–369.

Toft, J. D. (1986) The pathoparasitology of non-human primates: A review, in *Primates—The Road to Self-Sustaining Populations*, K. Benirschke, K., ed. Springer-Verlag, Berlin, pp. 571–679.

Vertein, R., and Reinhardt, V. (1989) Training female rhesus monkeys to cooperate during in-home cage venipuncture. *Lab. Primate Newsletter* 38, 1–3.

Weil, J. D., Ward, M. K., and Spertzel, R. O. (1971) Incidence of shigella in conditioned rhesus monkeys (*Macaca mulatta . Lab. Anim. Sci.* 21:434–437.

Weindruck, R. and Walford, R. L. (1988) *The Retardation of Aging and Disease by Dietary Restriction*, Thomas, Springfield, Illinois

Williams, R. T. (1971) Species variations in drug biotransformations, in *Fundamentals of Drug Matabolism and Drug Disposition*, LaDu, B., Mandel, H., and Way, E., eds. Williams & Wilkins, Baltimore, pp. 206–252.

Williams, T. (1974) Interspecies variations in the metabolism of xenobiotics. *Biochem. Soc. Trans.* 2, 359–377.

Ziegler, D. (1988) Flavin containing monooxygenases: Catalytic mechanism and substrate specificities. *Drug Metab. Rev.* 19, 1–32.

10

Alternative Species

Christopher P. Chengelis
WIL Research Laboratories, Inc.
Ashland, Ohio

This book has concentrated on the eight most commonly used laboratory animals. As illustrated on Table 1, many other different types of species are used in biomedical research and toxicological assessment that have not been discussed. See Chapter 12 for a more complete discussion on animal model selection. For example, the chicken is a common model for organophosphate insecticide-induced neurotoxicity (Murphy, 1986), but we have made no mention of the chicken in this book (nor will we again). Discussing all uses for all species used would have resulted in an encyclopedia, not a convenient source book. These less commonly used species, however, should not be totally ignored. The practice of good science demands that a species be appropriate to the question being pursued. The principle of responsible use of animals demands that we consider the replacement of higher animals with lower species. Here we will discuss some less commonly used species that could be used as replacements for other species in some types of toxicity testing. These will be earthworms, fish, and pigs.

EARTHWORMS

Earthworms are invertebrate, cold-blooded animals which collectively belong to the phylum Annelida, class Oligochaeta, and order Megadrili. Earthworms have been one of the more common species used to test chemicals for potential hazardous impact on the environment. The U.S. Food and Drug Administration (FDA), for example, includes protocols for the study of earthworms in their *Environmental Assessment Handbook*. As recently reviewed elsewhere (Chengelis, 1990), earthworms could also be used for lethality assessment and/or rankings in place of rodents. The more common species of earthworm used, and their sizes, used in such testing are listed in Table 2. There is some debate as to which species is best for testing purposes. Some investigators prefer *Lumbricus terrestris* because of its larger size and relative sensitivity (Dean-Ross, 1983). Others prefer *Eisena foetida* (and the majority of publications mention this species) because of its small size, prevalence in the environment, and relatively low cost (Neuhauser et al., 1986). While there are differences in sensitivity (Neuhauser et al., 1985a), this appears to be more a matter of individual preference. The use of *L. rubellus*

Table 1 Example of Uncommonly used Animal Species

Species	Model or applications
Armadillo	Leprosy
Aplysia	Behavioral studies
Bear	Sleep/hibernation
Bat	Hearing, sonar, microcirculation
Chicken	Insecticide toxicity, renal excretion
Cat	CNS physiology
Crab	Toxicity screen
Fish	Drug metabolism, carcinogenicity, environmental impact
Hydra	Teratogenetic testing
Insects (Cricket, Fly)	Genetic damage
Japanese quail	Environmental studies
Lobster	Peripheral nerves
Nude mouse	Antitumor drug testing
Owl	Sleep physiology
Pigeon	Behavioral problems
Pig	Surgical models, cardiovascular studies, dermal absorption studies
Salamander	Severed limb regeneration
Sheep	ARDS and other pulmonary phenomenon

has advantages in an urban area because it is easier to obtain, it is still the same size as *E. foetida,* and it is free of the objectionable odor that often accompanies *E. foetida.* See Table 3 for a comparison of acute toxicity for various chemicals in *L. rubellus* vs *E. foetida.* In many instances, *L. rubellus* is more sensitive, and therefore may be a more appropriate model for lethality screening.

The basic biology of earthworms has been reviewed by Laird and Kroger (1981) and Roberts and Dorough (1985). Worms differ sufficiently from the mammals with which most toxicologists are familiar that a brief review is necessary here.

Earthworms are highly specialized for life in the soil. The outermost barrier of the body is a thin chitinous cuticle, under which is an epidemral layer which contains mucous secretory glands and nerve receptor cells. Some of these are the light receptors which make earthworms photophobic. Locomotion is affected by contractions of the two layers of muscle cells which are underneath the epidermis; a circular layer and a longitudinal layers. The circular muscle layers are responsible for the segmented appearance of

Table 2 Earthworm (Phylum Annelida, Class Chaetopoda) Species Commonly used in Environmental Impact Testing

Species	Common name	Length (cm)
Allolobphora caliginosa	Field worm	5–20
Eisena foetida	Manure worm	5–12.5
Lumbricus rubellus	Red worm	5–12.5
Lumbricus terrestris	Night crawler	10–30

Table 3 Earthworm Comparative Toxicity

	LC$_{50}$ (μg/cm^2)	
Chemical	*Eisena foetida*	*Lumbricus terrestris*
Carbofuran	0.30	0.31
Aldicarb	3.20	0.02
Carbaryl	9.00	0.28
Malathion	13.5	0.27
Parathion	14.8	1.21
Acephate	851	692

Source: From Roberts and Dorough, 1984.

earthworms. The central nervous system consists of two ganglia per segment interconnected by a double nerve cord. The circulatory system is a closed loop system with five hearts and two primary vessels. Respiration is by passive diffusion across the body walls. Earthworms have a coelom, the fluid-filled cavity situated between the body wall from the digestive tract. It permits the worm to crawl in one direction while food is passing through the digestive tract in the other. Interestingly, while hermaphroditic, earthworms do not self-fertilize. They mate, with two exchanges of sperm and both partners developing cocoons.

Metabolism

Xenobiotic metabolism has been examined but not thoroughly explored in earthworms. The subject has been reviewed by Stenersen (1984). Because of their size, *L. terestris* has been the species best studied. It has been shown to have cytochrome P-450–dependent mono-oxygenase activity, metabolizing aldrin to dieldrin, for example. This highest concentration has been found in the typhosole, the large fold in the earthworm's intestine. Glutathione S-transferase has also been described (Stenersen, 1984). As in mammalian toxicology, it has long been recognized that species differences in toxicity in worms can be due to the differences in metabolism. For example, Gilman and Vardonis (1974) reported that the difference in sensitivity of *L. terrestris* vs *E. foetida* to carbofuran is due to differences in the metabolic distribution of carbofuran.

Husbandry

Caring for earthworms is not difficult (Laird and Kruger, 1981). They literally feed on decaying organic matter found in the soil. One needs only to keep them in moist soil in a cool (15–20°C) dark place. Many papers described supplementing this regimen with animal droppings for *E. foetida* (Roberts and Dorough, 1984). It is important that distilled water be used to moisten the soil, as the earthworm can be quite sensitive to organochlorochemicals. For most studies, husbandry procedures are relatively simple. The worms can be kept in the supplier container in a cool dark place, and used within 48 hr. Prior to use, worms are rinsed off with distilled water, and left in a large Petri dish or beaker on a water-loaded filter paper for a few hours in a darkened room. Worms obtained from domestic bait shops may be of uneven quality and age, and should be sorted. Worms that are obviously smaller, larger, or not as active as the others should not be used.

Dosing Techniques

A variety of dosing techniques have been described in the literature. These include mixing the test article matrices (such as artisol), dipping in aqueous solutions, topical applications, microinjections, and contact on filter paper (Heimbach, 1984; Fisher, 1984; Serda and Furst, 1987).

Microinjection techniques, where the small amounts of test article are injected into the hemocoel or peristrom are quite time consuming and can be quite traumatizing (Roberts and Dorough, 1985). Therefore, these techniques are not generally recommended.

Dips in which the worms are placed in a beaker containing a test article solution for 2 hr and then maintained in soil as usual for 1 week have been described (Dean-Ross, 1983). The main disadvantage of this system is that the worms have to be manipulated several times.

Several papers (Heinbach, 1986, Neuhauser, 1985b) describe experiments in which the test article is mixed with artificial soils of various compositions in which the worms are then left to reside for 2–4 weeks. This is the method of choice for subchronic studies, and is essentially a cross between a dermal application study and a dietary admix study, as the test article will not only be absorbed across the outer cuticle, but also is ingested.

All of these routes have very real disadvantages for use in acute lethality testing. With soilborne tests, for example, dead worms will decay and disappear. Hence, one must be prepared to dig frequently through the soil in order to obtain time-to-death estimates. The technique recommended here for this purpose is the filter paper contact method, and this will be the focus of the remainder of this discussion.

Forty-Eight-Hour Contact Test

The 48-hr contact test has proven to be a fast and resource-effective way of assessing acute toxicity of chemicals in earthworms. The fundamentals of this test are outlined on Table 4. The standardized method, approved by the European community (EEC) is discussed by Neuhauser et al. (1986). This is for environmental impact assessment where cross-laboratory comparisons are important. If, however, one wishes to adopt this technology for the purposes of screening new chemicals, then variants of this method are acceptable, as internal consistency is more important than interlaboratory compar-

Table 4   Earthworm 48-Hour Contact Test Acute Lethality

---

1. Place filter paper of known size (9 cm or 12 × 6.7 cm) in a Petrie dish or standard scintillation vial
2. Take test article up in acetone or some other volatile solvent.
3. Slowly and evenly deposit known amounts of test article solution onto filter paper.
4. Dry thoroughly with air or nitrogen gentle stream.
5. Add 1 ml of distilled water. Let wet filter paper.
6. Add worm *(L. rubellus)*. Keep in 400–500 mg range
7. Ten replicate vials per concentration.
8. Store/incubate in the absence of light at 15–20°C for 48 hours.
9. Examine for lethality (swollen, lack of movement upon warming up to room temp, lack of response to tactile stimulation).
10. Express dose as $\mu g/cm^2$ and mortality as usual. Calculate LC_{50} using standard techniques.
11. Always include negative and positive (benchmark) controls.

---

isons. There are two important considerations. First, because of seasonal variation in the quality of earthworms obtained from suppliers, positive controls or comparator chemicals should be included on every assay run. Second, distilled water must be used, as worms are quite sensitive to contaminants that may occur in chlorinated water. The filter paper should completely cover the sides of the vessel; otherwise, the worms will simply crawl up the sides to escape the adverse stimulus the chemical contact may provide. General fundamental standards for toxicity testing in nonvertebrates are discussed elsewhere (Anonymous, 1980).

Using these techniques, Robert and Dorough (1984, 1985) and Neuhauser et al. (1986) have compared acute toxicity in a variety of organic chemicals in several earthworm species. A comparison of the lethality of selected insecticides in *E. foetida* and *L. rubellus* has been given in Table 3. While there are some obvious quantitative differences between worm species, in general the rank order of toxicity is about the same. All earthworms are very sensitive to carbofuran under the conditions of this test.

Neuhauser et al. (1985) have proposed a toxicity rating scheme based on acute lethality in the earthworms which is similar to the more familiar scheme based on acute lethality in rodents (Table 5). Roberts and Dorough (1985) and Neuhauser et al. (1985) have published extensive compilations of acut lethality in worms and compared these to acute lethality in rats and mice. A selection of these is shown in Table 6. According to the toxicity rating scheme of Neuhauser, most of these chemicals are in the same toxicity category whether based on results from either *E. foetida* or mice. This may suggest that replacing the LD_{50} with the LC_{50} for rating toxicity (for a Department of Transportation shipping permit, for example) deserves serious consideration.

To the extent that the 48-hr contact test is artificial is that earthworms are in direct contact with a chemical in a closed system, it may not be truly reflective of toxicity of a chemical to earthworms in the environment. Van Leemput et al. (1989) compared the LC_{50} for enilconazole (a fungicide) in the 48-hr contact test vs a 14-day artificial soil test (OECD guideline 207; protocol summarized on Table 7). In the contact test, the LC_{50} was 12.8 $\mu g/cm^2$ (filter paper), whereas in the 14-day artificial soil test, the LC_{50} was 541 $\mu g/g$ (soil). Hence, even given the longer exposure period of the artificial soil test, worms were less sensitive to chemical toxicity in this milieu. The same phenomenon is true for other chemicals (Van Leemput et al. 1989) Thus, while the 48-hr contact test has utility as a predictive, screening, or ranking tool, it has limited value in direct environmental assessment. Additionally (as discussed by Van Gestel et al., 1989), lethality is a poor parameter to use in assessing the impact of environmental exposure of earthworms to

Table 5 Earthworm Toxicity Toxicity Rating

Rating	Designation	Rat LD_{50}	*Eisena foetida* LC_{50}
1	Supertoxic	<5	<1.0
2	Extremely toxic	5–50	1.0–10.0
3	Very toxic	50–500	10–100
4	Moderately toxic	500–5000	100–1000
5	Relatively nontoxic	>5000	>1000
		(mg/kg)	($\mu g/cm^2$)

Source: From Neauhausser et al., 1985.

Table 6 Earthworm Acute Lethality Comparative Values

Chemical	*Eisena foetida* (LC_{50})	Mouse (LD_{50})
2,4-Dinitrophenol	0.6 (1)	45 (2)
Carbaryl	14 (3)	438 (3)
Benzene	75 (3)	4700 (4)
1,1,1-Trichloroethane	83 (3)	11,240 (5)
Dimethylphthalate	550 (4)	7200 (5)

Source: From Roberts and Dorough, 1985.

chemicals. Reproductive function is of greater importance for the maintenance of populations. These authors recommended using cocoon production rather than lethality as a more sensitive endpoint in artificial soil tests. Their reasoning appears to be quite sound. In addition, cocoon counts are easily quantifiable, and provide an alternative parameter for assessing toxicity in the artificial soil test where the animals are difficult to see and change in behavior, therefore, is difficult to assess.

Advantages/Disadvantages

The main advantages of the 48-hr contact test are the savings of time and money. The cost savings fall into three categories. First, earthworms are cheap. One hundred *L. rubellus* will cost about $2.00. The 100 mice they could replace in toxicity screens, for example, would cost $125.00–$175.00. Second, earthworms require no vivarium space, and their use could decrease the number of rodents used, resulting in a net decreasing in vivarium use. Third, adapting the 48-hr contact test would require little capital investment other than a dedicated under-the-counter refrigerator set at 15– 20°C. Otherwise, the assay

Table 7 Earthworm 14-Day Toxicity Test in Artificial Soil (OECD Guideline 207)

1. Prepare artificial soil; 10% sphagnum peat, 20% kaolinite clay, 69% construction sand, and 1% calcium carbonate (all % by weight).
2. Obtain worms *(E. foetida)* from supplier. Only adults (400–700 mg) with a well-developed clitellum should be used. Keep for 14 days in shallow trays containing artificial soil before the start of the study.
3. Test article concentrations in test soil are in terms of micrograms per grams of dry weight. Stock solutions in distilled water can be diluted and mixed with soil in a household mixer. Hydrophobic substances can be taken up in a small amount of solvent and mixed with a small amount of test soil. After evaporation of the solvent, the treated soil can be thoroughly mixed with additional soil to obtain appropriate concentrations.
4. For each concentration, four 1-L beakers were filled with 750 g of treated soil. Moisture content was adjusted to 35–40 g H_2O/100 g of soil. Ten worms are added to each beaker. Beakers were covered with perforated plastic.
5. Maintain at 20°C ± 2°C, 12/12 hr light/dark cycle.
6. After 7 and 14 days, earthworms are removed from the test soil, counted, and sorted. Those not responding to mechanical stimuli are sorted as dead.
7. Mortality data can be analyzed by conventional means.

Source: From Van Leemput et al., 1989.

can be easily performed in a standard biochemistry laboratory. With regard to time savings, the standards lethality test with rodents require 7–14 days of postdosing observations. The 48-hr contact test is completed in 48 hr. Not only is the turnaround faster, but the amount of time that technical personnel will have to spend observing animals and recording observations will be decreased. An incidental advantage to earthworms is that they are cold-blooded vertebrates, and thus exempt from the requirements of animal welfare laws.

There are two main disadvantages to the use of earthworms in acut toxicity testing. First, there are a limited number of endpoints. Other than death and a few behavioral abnormalities (Stenersen, 1979; Drewes et al., 1984) the test does not yield much qualitative information. Second, there probably is some institutional bias. Because the test is not cutting-edge technology (no tissue culture) and uses a nonmammalian model, it has been easy to dismiss the utility of the test.

FISH

Fish, like earthworms, have commonly been used to assess potential environmental impact. Some of the more common species of fish used, and their scientific names, are listed on Table 8. Most fish used in toxicity studies belong to the superclass Gnathostoma, class Osteichthyes, subclass Actinoptergii, infraclass Teleostei, division Eutelaosti. They are, of course, cold-blooded vertebrates. In addition to environmental impact studies, the potential use of fish in carcinogenicity testing has been recognized since the early 1970s, when it was reported that some fish develop hepatic neoplasias to many of the same chemicals that rodents do. In fact, the possible use of fish in carcinogenicity testing was the subject of a National Cancer Institute–sponsored symposium in 1981. This practice, however, has not gained wide acceptance. Despite the data suggesting that fish may, in fact, make good models for carcinogenicity testing. Here, the use of the rainbow trout (*Oncorhynchus mykiss*, formerly *Salmo gairdneri*) and the Japanese medaka (*Oryzias latipes*) in carcinogencity testing will be reviewed.

Table 8 Toxicity Testing in Fish Species Studied

Common name	Formal name	Use[a]
Bluegill	*Leopomis macrochirus*	E
Carp	*Cyprinus carpio*	M
Channel catfish	*Ictalurus punctatus*	E
Cobra guppy	*Poecilia reticulata*	C
Cod	*Gadus morhau*	M
Fathead minnow	*Pimphales promelas*	E
Gulf killfish	*Fundulus grandis*	C
Inland silverside	*Menidia berylllina*	C
Japanese medaka (rice fish)	*Oryzias latipes*	C
Rainbow trout	*Oncorhynchus mykiss (Salmo gairdneri)*	E, C, M
Toad fish	*Opsanus tau*	M
Trench	*Tinca tinca*	M
Sheepshead minnow	*Cyprinodon variegatus*	C, E

[a]E = environmental impact; C = carcinogenicity; M = metabolic studies.

Husbandry

Fish obviously require water and need to be kept in either glass aquaria or fiber glass or stainless steel tanks. Water should be of consistent quality from a consistent source. Oxygen content, hardness, and alkalinity should be monitored. So long as water quality is consistently monitored and maintained, both the rainbow trout and Japanese medaka are remarkably free of background diseases. Temperature needs to be maintained at 12–17°C for trout and 22–27°C for medaka. Rates of water turnover in flow-through systems have been described in terms such as 6–10 volume changes per day or 3 L per hr. Published papers describe using aerated well water or dechlorinated tap water. Frequent analysis of potential confounding contaminants should be routine. Lighting can be 12/12 hr cycles. Commercial diets are available for both trout and medaka.

Dosing Techniques

The dosing techniques most often mentioned in the literature include (1) intraperitoneal injection, (2) mixing with water for either static or flow-through exposure, and (3) dietary admix. The intraperitoneal technique is only suitable for treating larger fish and only for single exposures. Exposure in solution under static conditions requires relatively small amounts of material, is much easier to control, and has been shown to be effective for short-term exposure. Flow-through conditions require relatively large amount of material (and generate large amounts of potentially contaminated water) and require extensive engineering safeguards to prevent the exposure of laboratory personnel to potential carcinogens. Flow-through systems allow for longer-term exposure.

A variety of different systems have been described (see Walker et al., 1985, for an example). Water-based delivery requires a certain level of aqueous solubility that may not always be achievable. In that case, dietary admix is the preferred dosing technique. In fact, dietary admix has proven to be a reliable and effective method for dosing large numbers of fish over long dosing periods, and using considerably less test article than flow-through methods. Various methods have been described for preparing the diets, such as dissolving the test article in a highly volatile solvent and applying it by micropipet to individual pellets or mixing it up with salmon oil prior to dressing the basal diet prior to feeding. Exposures are described in terms of parts per million (of test article in the diet). Other dosing techniques have been described in papers in which the emphasis was on studying drug metabolism where relatively small numbers of fish were used in acute preparations. Most of these, such as intra-aortic injection, would be impractical to use for carcinogenicity studies.

Metabolism

Xenobiotic metabolism in medaka has not been extensively examined. This discussion will, therefore, focus on xenobiotic metabolism of the rainbow trout. Some parameters of xenobiotic metabolism are summarized in Table 9. Microsomal mixed function oxidase (MMFO) activity has been studied in the rainbow trout in fairly extensive studies since mid 1970 (see Stegman and Kloepper-Sams, 1987, for a review). Trouts have identifiable activity with most of the substrates that rats do, but the activity tends to be less. No sex- or age-related differences have been discussed in the literature. Gregus et al. (1983) have published comparisons of several of the key enzyme systems in trout to those of the rat (Table 9). In most instances, the trout had comparable or even higher activity.

Table 9 Rainbow Trout Hepatic Xenobiotic
Metabolism

Parameter	Trout	Rat
Liver/body weight ratio (%)	1.1	4.0
Microsomal protein (mg/g)	28.1	25.7
Cytosolic protein	74.5	93.7
Cytochrome P-450	0.34	0.51
MMFO activity		
benzphetamine	0.2	2.2
ethylmorphine	0.1	3.8
ethoxyresorufin	0.4	0.1
Epoxide hydrolase		
styrene oxide	9.0	6.0
UDP-Glucuronosyl transferase		
4-nitrophenol	1.0	5.0
testosterone	0.06	0.01
Glutathione S-transferase		
dichloronitrobenzene	5	75
ethacrynic acid	30	40
N-Acetyl transferase		
2-Aminofluorene	4	0.1
4-Aminobenzoate	0.03	0.06
Temperature	25°C	37°C

Estimated enzyme activities: nmol/min/mg protein.
Source: From Gregus et al., 1983.

The remarkable aspect of the trout MMFO is the high degree with which it responds to 3-methcholanthrene (3-MC)–type inducing agents. For example, Voss et al. (1982) reported that 5 days of treatment, by dietary admix with polychlorinated biphenyl (PCB) (100 ppm), resulted in large increases in cytochrome P-450 content as well as increases in 7-ethoxyresorufin, 7-ethoxycoumarin, and benzo(a)pyrene metabolism in rainbow trout (Table 10).

Further, Erickson et al. (1988) have reported that exposure of trout to as little as 1 ppm piperonyl butoxide for 3 weeks in a continuous flow-through system resulted a three-fold increase in cytochrome P-450, a 17-fold increase in ethoxycoumarin demethylase, and a 36-fold increase in ethoxyresorufin demethylase, the latter considered a marker for cytochrome P-448 or 3-MC–type induction.

In fact, because of the extreme responsiveness of trout to this type of induction, Julkman et al. (1986) have proposed using fish MMFO activity to monitor pollutant levels in a body of water.

Interestingly, trout are not responsive to phenobarbital-type induction (Stegeman and Kloepper-Sams, 1987). For example, Miyauchi (1984) reported that phenobarbital pretreatment did not increase the metabolism or the mutagenicity (in the Ames assay) of 2-acetylaminoflourene, whereas pretreatment with PCBs or 3-MC caused increases in both (Table 11). In addition, α-napthaflavone, an inhibitor of cytochrome P-448 activity, inhibited revertant colony formation, whereas metyrapone, an inhibitor of cytochrome

Table 10 Induction of Hepatic Xenobiotic Metabolism
in Trout with Aroclor

Parameter	Control	+PCB[a]
Cytochrome P-450 (nmol/mg)	0.15 ± 0.04	0.29 ± 0.05
MMFO Activity		
ethoxyresorufin	0.06 ± 0.02	4.07 ± 0.44
ethoxycoumarin	0.04 ± 0.0	0.49 ± 0.02
benzo(a)pyrene	0.004 ± 0.006 (nmole/min/mg)	0.97 ± 0.04

[a]Following dietary exposure to 100 ppm aroclor 1254 (polychlorinated biphenyl) for 5 weeks.
Source: From Voss et al., 1982.

P-450 activity, had no effect on revertant colony formation. Thus, trout differ from
rodents with regard to inducibility in both selectivity and degree of response.

Trout microsomal enzymes are assayed at room temperature (25°C) or even lower. These are temperatures where MMFO activities in the rat would be severely
compromised. The fact that trout have comparable enzyme activities at lower temperature optima than rats is an example of species differences in adaptation. Trout, like
all fish, are poikilothermic. How do trout control MMFO activity at different body temperatures? Would small temperature variations affect carcinogen activation? Egaas
and Varanasi (1981) compared MMFO activity of rainbow trout kept at either 7 or
16°C. When benzo(a)pyrene metabolism was examined in vitro at 29°C, the fish kept at

Table 11 Inuction of Hepatic Xenobiotic
Metabolism in Trout (Using the Ames Assay)

	Mutagenicity	
Treatment group	BENZP[a]	2-AAF[b]
Untreated	20	300
3-Methylcholanthrene	140	600
+α–naphthaflavone	20	90
+metyrapone	130	500
Phenobarbital	20	290
+α–naphthaflavone	20	90
+metyrapone	20	220

Approximate number of revertant colonies (test strain
TA 98) per plate. S-9 Fractions from fish treated with
either 3-methylchoanthrene or phenobarbital. Inhibitors
(α-naphthaflavone or metyrapone) used in vitro (0.1
mM).
[a]BENZP = benzo(a)pyrene.
[b]2-AAF = 2-acetylaminofluorene.
Source: From Miyauchi, 1984.

the lower temperature had significantly higher activity. Similar results were obtained by Blanck et al. (1988). They compared trout held at 5 vs 20°C. They observed that both benzo(a)pyrene and ethoxycoumarin metabolism at 18°C in vitro was more rapid in the preparations from the fish maintained at the lower temperature (Table 12). However, when in vitro incubations were conducted at the same temperatures at which the fish were kept (i.e., microsomes from fish maintained at 5°C were incubated in vitro at 5°C), there were no differences in enzyme activity. Hence, the rainbow trout has a mechanism for responding to changes in environmental temperature in order to maintain constant MMFO activity. As noted also in Table 12, the different ambient temperatures do not alter cytochrome P-450 content, but do change NADPH:cytochrome C reductase activity. Thus, it would appear that trout respond to changes in ambient temperature by varying the ratio of cytochrome P-450 to the reductase in order to maintain constant MMFO activity. Small variations (group to group in temperature) should not effect carcinogen variation.

Most carcinogens, particularly hepatic carcinogens, require metabolic activation. There are two criteria that should be met to support a conclusion that reactive metabolites are being produced. First, irreversible binding to tissue macromolecules must occur. With regard to the trout, Darnerud et al. (1989) have reported that 1,2-dibromoethane and chloroform form irreversibly bound metabolites in trout exposed in vivo. Egaas and Varanasi (1981) demonstrated that trout had the capacity when assayed in vitro (with S-9 or postmitochondrial supernatant fractions) to catalyze the irreversible binding of benzo(a)pyrene to deoxyribonucleic acid (DNA). Loveland et al. (1988) demonstrated that hepatocytes isolated from rainbow trout were capable of producing metabolites of aflatoxin that irreversibly bound to native DNA. With regard to mutagenic activity, Miyauchi demonstrated that trout hepatic preparations could activate mutagens (2-aminoanthracene and 2-acetylaminofluorene) in the Ames *Salmonella* assay. Thus, it would appear that trout are quite capable of the metabolic activation of carcinogens.

Table 12 Hepatic Xenobiotic Metabolism in Trout

	Ambient temp. (°C)	Temperature Effects	
		Kept at 20°C	Kept at 5°C
Cytochrome P-450 (nmole/mg)	18	0.10	0.11
NADPH:Cytochrome C Reductase (nmol/min/mg)	18	24.9	47.7
benzo(a)pyrene (pmol/min/mg)	18	17	57
	20	21	—
	5	—	17
Ethoxycoumarin (pmol/min/mg)	18	27	83
	20	37	
	5	—	31

Microsomal enzyme activities in vivo from mature rainbow trout. Water temperatures were recorded at the time of harvest. N = 15–20.
Source: From Blanck et al., 1989.

Examples of Carcinogenicity in Fish

Numerous reports of chemical carcinogenicity in fish exist and only a few illustrative reports will be presented here. Hendricks et al. (1985) studied the carcinogenicity of benzo(a)pyrene in rainbow trout. The study was initiated with 3-month-old trout fingerlings (3.3 g). They were continuously fed a dietary admixture containing 1000 ppm benzapyrene for 18 months. The results are summarized on Table 13. While there was no difference in mortality, there were decreases in body weight, increases in liver to body weight ratio, and a significant increase in hepatic carcinomas. Thus, benzo(a)pyrene is a positive hepatic carcinogen in rainbow trout. There were no hepatic neoplasias in the control group, which is a common observation (e.g., very low tumor background rate) in carcinogenicity studies in fish.

Shelton et al. (1984) reported that diethylnitrosoamine (100 ppm by dietary admix) produced liver tumors in trout with 12 months of treatment, and that cotreatment with polychlorinated biphenyls (MMFO-inducing agents) greatly enhance the tumor yield (Table 14).

Hawkins and Hinton and their colleagues have reported on the carcinogenicity of methylazoxyethanol (Hinton et al., 1984) and benzo(a)pyrene (Hawkins et al., 1988) in medaka (Table 15). They have also identified tumors in medaka in organs other than the liver. (For a more complete review of carcinogenicity testing with medaka and other aquarium fish, see Hawkins et al., 1985). Benzo(a)pyrene, diethylnitrosamine, and methylazoxymethanol are presumed, if not confirmed, human carcinogens. Thus, it would appear that rainbow trout and Japanese medaka are viable species in which to test suspect human hepatic carcinogens.

Advantages and Disadvantages

There are three main advantages to using fish in carcinogenicity testing. First, they have an extremely low background tumor rate, which enhances the sensitivity of the assays. Second, fish are less expensive to purchase and maintain than rodents. Group sizes of 100 or more (particularly with medaka) become quite manageable. Third, a positive carcinogen will generally show up in fish within 1 year's time. Rodent studies generally last for 18 months (mice) to 30 months (rats). Medaka have certain advantages over trout that magnify the cost savings. For example, they will thrive in waters maintained at room temperature, whereas the cooler temperature optimum of the rainbow trout generally

Table 13 Rainbow Trout Carcinogenicity Study

	Control	BP
N	114	114
Deaths	5	3
Body weights	425 ± 153	364 ± 125 g
Liver/body weight	0.66 ± 0.16	0.70 ± 0.13 %
Liver neoplasia		
Altered hepatic foci	0	4.5%[a]
Carcinoma	0	21%

Study started with 3-month-old trout fingerlings (3.3 g), fed 100 ppm bennzo(a)pyrene (BP) by dietary admixture *ad libitum* for 18 months.
[a]Incidence of animals having the lesion.
Source: From Hendricks et al., 1985.

Table 14   Rainbow Trout Carcinogenicity Study

	Control	DEN	DEN + AC
N	120	120	120
Deaths	1	2	28
Liver row	0.77 ± 0.08	0.65 ± 0.11	0.89 ± 0.13
Liver neoplasia	0	10.2%	40.2%

Trout fingerlings fed 1100 ppm diethylnitrosamine (DEN), or DEN + 100 ppm aroclor (AC) 1242, by dietary admixture for 12 months.
Source: From Shelton et al., 1984.

requires the use of energy-dependent cooling systems. The larger size of the trout requires greater aquarium space. The smaller size of the medaka is an advantage at necropsy, where Medaka are fixed and slide mounted in toto for histological examination, saving both time spent on dissection and other histology laboratory resources.

There are three main disadvantages in using fish for carcinogenicity testing. First, compared to rodents, only relatively few tumors, primarily carcinomas of the liver, have been described in fish. Hence, it would appear to be prudent to use carcinogenicity testing in fish as an adjunct to testing in at least one mammalian species. On the basis of current data, fish would be best used in confirming potential hepatic carcinogens. Second, the assays cannot be adapted without capital changes to the standard vivarium. Third, as with earthworms, there is an ill-defined institutionalized bias against nonmammalian animal models. One could argue, however, that a chemical shown to be carcinogenic across a broad phylogenetic spectrum of species is a stronger candidate to be a human carcinogen than one shown to be positive in only one sex or species.

MINIPIGS

Background

The use of pigs *(Sus scrufa)* in biomedical research is hardly novel. They have been extensively used for surgical (Swindle et al. 1988) and physiological (primarily car-

Table 15   Medaka Carcinogenicity Study

	Incidence of hepatic tumors	
Dosage groups	At 24 weeks	At 36 weeks
Negative control	0/82	1/89 (~1.1%)
Solvent control	1/75	1/97 (~1.0%)
1–4 PPB	1/75	1/94 (~1.1%)
8–34 PPB	0/70	0/96 (0%)
200–220 PPB	8/76	26/73 (~36%)[a]

Initiated with two 6-hr exposure periods to benz(a)pyrene, 6 days apart when fish were 6–10 days of age. Maintained for 36 weeks under standard aquarium conditions.
[a]Twenty had adenomas and six had carcinomas of the liver.
Source: From Hawkins et al., 1988.

diovascular, renal, and digestive) research (Khan, 1984; Clausing et al., 1986) for years. Until relatively recently, their use in toxicity testing was uncommon except in the testing of veterinary or herd-management drugs intended for use in swine. Because of their well-accepted physiological similarities to humans, minipigs are becoming increasingly attractive toxicological models. In fact, they are already more frequently used in nutritional toxicology studies (Clausing et al., 1986). Among the more common experimental animals, pigs are the only one whose use is on the increase (Khan, 1984). Their expense (both in procurement and maintenance) and their relatively large size mitigated against their use in more general toxicity testing. Size differences are summarized on Table 16. The development of minipigs has resulted in a strain of more manageable size. In addition, the increase in expense in the use of dogs, as well as the perceived lay opposition to their uses, make minipigs even more attractive as a nonrodent species for general toxicity studies. The dog is a far more common companion animal and many of the recent developments in animal care and use laws have made specific provisions about the care of dogs. Minipigs have been shown to be more sensitive to a wide variety of drugs and chemicals (e.g., carbaryl, methylmercury) than dogs (Khan, 1984). The FDA has kept its own breeding colony of minipigs since the early 1960s. In short, there are scientific, economic, and sociological reasons that make minipigs good toxicological models. The reader is referred to an excellent short review by Phillips and Tumbleson (1986) that puts the issue of minipigs in biomedical research into the context of modeling in general.

Table 16 Comparison of Typical Weights for Common Laboratory Animals

Species	Age	Weight (males and females)
Mouse (CD-1)	21 DAYS	12 g (male and females)
	30DAYS	23 g (M), 21 g (F)
Rat (Wistar)	25 DAYS	63 g (M), 60 g (F)
	90 DAYS	350 g (M), 240 g (F)
Hamster (Syrian)	26 DAYS	56 g (M), 55 g (F)
	90 DAYS	125 g (M), 115 g (F)
Guinea pig (Hartley)	20 DAYS	235 g (M, F)
	60 DAYS	625 g (M), 525 g (F)
Beagle dog (Hazleton)	8–9 MONTHS	10.5 kg (M), 8.5 kg (F)
Minipig (Hanford)	1 MONTH	4.5 kg (M, F)
	6 MONTHS	37 kg
Minipig (Yucatan)	1 MONTH	3.5 kg
	6 MONTHS	27 kg
Micropig	1 MONTH	3.5 kg
	6 MONTHS	18 kg

Several breeds of miniature swine have been developed. These include in the United States, the Yucatan micro- and minipigs, the Handford, the Sinclair, the Pitman-Moore, and the Hormel. The Yucatan and the Sinclair tend to be the most commonly used. Panepinto and Phillips (1986) have discussed the characteristics, advantages, and disadvantages of the Yucatan minipig in some detail (1986). In Europe, the Gottinger minipig is extensively used. At sexual maturity (4–6 months) the typical minipig weighs 20–40 kg, as compared to 102 kg for the more common pig, 8–15 kg for the dog). Micropigs weigh about 14–20 kg at sexual maturity. The minipig and the dog have comparable life spans; for example, Peggins et al. (1984) reported that the average life span for miniature swine is 15–17 years. The average beagle dog may have a life span of 8–12 years. Most of this discussion will focus on the purpose-bred minipigs, primarily the Yucatan and the Sinclair. Information on regular swine will be used to illustrate further specific examples.

Husbandry

Housing

A general review of handling and husbandry have been described by Panepinto (1986) and Swindle et al. (1988). Young weanling pigs can be kept for short periods of time (up to 1 month) in standard dog cages with the floor modified with narrow mesh to account for the smaller foot of the pig. After that, however, their rapid growth generally makes such caging inappropriate. Larger stainless steel cages would be extremely expensive. Standard dog runs could have enough floor space to be converted for pigs, but smooth flooring does not provide appropriate footing for pigs and needs to be covered with wood chip bedding (Swindle et al., 1986). While pigs are very social, they do not have to be group housed; as discussed by Barnett and Hemsworth (1986), individually housed swine show little evidence of a chronic stress response. Insufficient space, on the other hand, can cause chronic stress in pigs. Hunsaker et al. (1984) have described an inexpensive caging system for miniature swine that is appropriate for toxicology studies. The flooring and walls are constructed of 0.50-cm welded wire coated with polyvinyl chloride polymer. As described, the unit has sufficient room for two pigs, separated by a partition. These units are relatively inexpensive and provide more than sufficient floor space (about 17 ft^2 per pig) to meet the recommendations for pigs.

Water and Feed

Like all animals, pigs should be permitted free access to potable water, preferably from a municipal water supply intended for human consumption. Drinking water intended for pigs does not have to be filtered or deionized. Various diets have been described. Because of their size (i.e., high maintenance charges and test articles demand), pigs have seldom been used for chronic studies where the possibility of waterborne environmental contaminants could influence a study.

For miniature swine, the consistent use of a certified chow from a major manufacturer is recommended (Swindle et al., 1986). Free access to feed is not recommended as pigs will eat to excess. Available feed should be restricted to approximately 4% of body weight per day to prevent the animals from becoming obese.

Restraint and Dosing

In general, minipigs are docile, and easily socialized and trained. Barnett and Harnsworth (1986) recommended a socialization regimen of 2 min of gentle interaction (e.g., stroking, etc.). Pigs, like most experimental animals, are rarely simply kept and fed, but have to be occasionally restrained so samples can be taken and other measurements made. Restraint methods designed for commercial swine should not be used for laboratory swine. Panepinto et al., (1983) have described a sling method that provides restraint with minimal stress. The most frequently mentioned dosing routes in the literature are dietary admix, dermal (topical), gavage, and intravenous injections. Generally, minipigs are restrained in a sling while being dosed by the active route such as gavage. If the experiment requires the implantation of, for example, an indwelling catheter, minipigs can be anesthetized with ketamine (20 mg/kg im) as described by Swindle and co-workers (1986) and by Terris and Simmons (1982).

Clinical Laboratory

Clinical chemical and hematological parameters for minipigs have been studied. Ranges for some of the more commonly examined parameters from Yucatan minipigs are summarized in Tables 17 and 18 (from Radin et al., 1986). Parson and Wells (1986) have published similar data on the Yucatan minipig. Brechbuhler et al. (1984) and Oldigs (1986) have published on the Gottinger minipig. Middleton and co-workers have published extensive lists (organized by age and sex) on the hematological parameters (Burks et al., 1974) and serum electrolytes (Hutcheson et al., 1979) for the Sinclair minipig. In general, the clinical laboratory picture of the various strains are quite similar. No real differences between sexes have been identified, but age can be very much a factor. For example, serum creatinine can be 33% higher in 3-month-old as compared to 18-month-old Sinclair minipigs (based on data reported by Burks et al., 1979). As with other species, health status, feed composition, feeding regimen, fasting state, season, time of day, etc., can affect clinical laboratory results in the minipig. Toxicological experiments should not be run without concurrent controls.

Table 17   Minipig Clinical Chemistry Parameters in Different Strains (mean ± SD)

Parameter	Yucatan	Gottinger
Glucose (mmol/L)	3.75 ± 0.64	5.98 ± 1.01
Urea (mmol/L)	7.84 ± 2.64	3.19 ± 1.15
Creatinine (μmol/L)	115 ± 16	52.2 ± 11.1
Total protein (q/L)	74 ± 9	54.0 ± 4.6
Albumin (q/L)	50 ± 6	26.2 ± 6.0
Bilirubin total (μmol/L)	3.42 ± 1.37	—
Triglycerides (mg/L)	267 ± 134	565 ± 250
Total cholesterol (mmol/L)	1.85 ± 0.38	1.65 ± 0.38
γ-Glutamyl transpeptidase (U/L)	61.6 ± 11.2	—
Alanine aminotransferase (U/L)	72.5 ± 13.6	—
Aspartate aminotransferase (U/L)	40.3 ± 5.9	—
Na^+ (mmol/L)	140.5 ± 4.2	142.3 ± 3.00
K^+ (mmol/L)	4.1 ± 0.3	3.94 ± 0.32
Cl^- (mmol/L)	103.1 ± 4.3	101.3 ± 3.6
Ca^{++} (mmol/L)	2.62 ± 0.18	2.58 ± 0.16
$PO_4^=$ (mmol/L)	2.41 ± 0.26	1.61 ± 0.30

Sources: Parsons and Wells, 1986; Brechbuler et al., 1984; Oldigs, 1986.

Table 18 Minipig Hematological Parameters in Different Strains

Parameter	Sinclair	Yucatan
Red blood cell ($10^6/mm^3$)	7.61 ± 0.15	7.0 ± 0.80
Hemoglobin (g/dL)	14.87 ± 0.18	14.9 ± 1.20
Hematocrit (%)	44 ± 0.5	44.6 ± 4.1
Mean corpuscular, volume (fL)	58.5 ± 0.8	64.4 ± 3.7
Mean corpuscular hemoglobin (pg)	19.8 ± 0.3	21.4 ± 1.3
Mean corpuscular hemoglobin concentration (g/dL)	33.9 ± 0.3	33.2 ± 0.8
White blood cell ($10^3/mm^3$)	12.73 ± 0.41	12.6 ± 3.0
Lymphocytes ($10^3/mm^3$)	7.25 ± 0.24	5.75 ± 1.52
Neutrophil (per mm^3)	4.47 ± 0.24	5.27 ± 1.29
Eosinophils (per mm^3)	534 ± 57	517 ± 31
Monocyte (per mm^3)	422 ± 35	945 ± 71
Basophils (per mm^3)	89 ± 15	63 ± 1.3
Platelets ($10^3/mm^3$)	—	441 ± 119

Sources: Burks et al., 1977 (12-month-old, sexes pooled); Radin et al., 1986.

Xenobiotic Metabolism

Some critical parameters of hepatic microsomal drug metabolism in the minipig, common swine, and rats are given in Table 19. As most investigators tend to use younger minipigs, the values reported in this table are for young (less than 4 years old) minipigs. Relatively few papers have examined the MMFO of minipigs in any detail. Peggins et al. (1984) have examined the MMFO in a broad age range (10 months to 12 years) of Hanford minipigs. They identified definite age-related differences. The amounts of cytochrome P-450, the MMFO activity with aniline and p-chloro-N-methylaniline, and glucuronosyl transferase activity were all significantly higher in middle-age (5–8 years) vs young (less than 4 years) minipigs. Freudenthal et al. (1976) examined Hanford minipigs in the 2- to 8-month age range, and obtained somewhat different cytochrome P-450 (approximately 0.95 nmol/mg) values than did Peggins et al. (1984) (approximately 0.50 nmol). The reported ranges for aniline hydroxylase (about 0.70 nmol/min/mg) and UDP-glucuronosyl transferase (about 50 nmol/min/ mg) were similar in the two papers. Hence, the available data on the MMFO of young Hanford minipigs is fairly consistent.

Little work has been reported on isozymic cytochrome P-450 characteristics, the response to inducers, or the specificity of inhibitors. An exception to this is the work by Muller et al. (1980) comparing the effects of arochlor induction on the subsequent responses in the Ames *Salmonella* mutagenicity test of seven different species with five different known mutagens. Animals were treated with a single dose of arochlor 1254 (500 mg/kg ip in sesame oil) and sacrificed 5 days later. The minipig responded in the same fashion as rats and mice, with large increases (3.9-fold) in ethylmorphine demethylase activity. Liver fractions from untreated minipigs had low activation in the Ames assay with benzo(a)pyrene, cyclophosphamide, and dethylnitrosamine. In contrast, liver preparations from induced animals add greatly increased activity (5 10-fold) in the Ames assay with these mutagens. This is a pattern very similar to that seen in the rat. Thus, the MMFO of the minipig is inducible and the resulting changes in metabolism may not be dissimilar from those produced by the rat.

The flavin adenosine dinucleotide (FAD) containing mono-oxygenase (FMFO) has

Table 19 Comparison of Xenobiotic Metabolism Systems in Rat and Pig

Enzyme	Rat[a]	Minipig[b]	Common swine[a]
Cytochrome P-450[c]	0.59 ± 0.04	0.95 ± 0.02	0.30 ± 0.04
MMFO activity[d]			
ethylmorphine	5.09 ± 0.34	8.53 ± 0.51	1.39 ± 0.16
ethoxyresorufin	0.134 ± 0.022		0.88 ± 0.02
Epoxide hydrolase			
styrene oxide	8.36 ± 2.48	—	11.4 ± 1.67
UDP-Glucuronosyl transferase			
1-naphthol	6.43 ± 1.66	—	5.50 ± 0.89
4-nitrophenol	4.51 ± 0.50	5.5 ± 1.5	9.38 ± 1.07
Glutathione S-transferase			
DNCB	2659 ± 168	—	2746 ± 499
DCNB	118 ± 8.8	—	2.44 ± 0.23
PAPS Sulfotransferase			
2-naphthol	0.785 ± 0.066	—	0.095 ± 0.025
Acetyltransferase			
p-aminobenzoate	0.77 ± 0.23	—	0.621 ± 0.111

[a]From Smith et al., 1984, and Watkins and Klaassen, 1986.
[b]From Fruedenthal et al., 1975, or Peggins et al., 1984.
[c]nmol/mg microsomal protein.
[d]All enzyme activities: nmol/min/mg (either microsomal or cytosolic) protein.

traditionally been studied in hog liver slaughter houses obtained from (Tynes and Hodgeson, 1984; Souhaili El Amri et al., 1987). Interestingly, when FMFO activity is compared between species, substrate specificities are found to be generally very similar (Tynes and Hodgeson, 1984). Recently, Rettie et al. (1990) have isolated and studied the FMFO from Yucatan minipig liver. As with the enzyme studied from other species, the hepatic enzyme exists as a single isozymic species, is active with both dimethylanaline (N-oxide formation) and alkyl p-tolyl sulfides (sulfoxidation), and is enantioselective in metabolite formation. It would thus appear that the minipig does not differ appreciably from regular swine in the presence or activity of FMFO.

Perhaps some aspects of minipig xenobiotic metabolism can be inferred from studies in regular swine. For example, Rendic et al. (1984) demonstrated that cimetadine and ranitidine are excellent inhibitors of the porcine MMFO in vitro, and is probably also inhibitory in microsomal preparations from minipigs. Walker et al. (1978) reported on epoxide hydratase activity in various species, including the pig. Depending on the substrate, the pig had activities equivalent to or greater than that of the rat. This was confirmed by Smith et al. (1984) and Watkins et al. (1986). The MMFO, epoxide hydrolase, UDP-glucoronosyl transferase, N-acetyl transferase, glutathione S-transferase, and sulfotransferase activities in regular swine may be used to help infer the expected activity in minipigs until more complete and specific information appears in the literature on minipigs.

Other aspects of xenobiotic metabolism in minipigs have received even less scrutiny, and can only be inferred from the literature. For example, Kirby et al. (1980) reported that ethylene dibromide (EDB) is rapidly metabolized and cleared by minipigs in a fashion similar to that reported for rats. As EDB is a substrate for the rat liver glutathione S-transferase system that of minipigs must have some characteristics in common with that of the rat.

There are relatively few papers that compare in vivo pharmacokinetic behavior of a specific chemical in the minipig vs another animal. Schneider et al. (1977) reported on the toxicology and pharmacokinetics of cyclotrimethylenetrinitramine in the rat and minipig. Rats convulsed within the first several hours after receiving this chemical, whereas minipigs convulsed at 12–24 hrs later. This is consistent with the observation that at 24 hr postdosing (100 mg/kg po), the plasma levels were 3.0 μg/ml in rats and 4.7 μg/ml in minipigs. Other differences in pharmacokinetics and metabolism between the two species were described. The latent period for convulsion development was more similar between minipigs and humans than between rats and humans. The implication in this paper is that the minipig is a more suitable model for the study of the toxicity and metabolism of the nitramines than rats.

General Toxicity Testing

Are minipigs an appropriate species for the general toxicity testing of new drugs and chemicals? This question is perhaps best addressed by comparing the toxicity of known chemicals in minipigs with that observed in other animals. Unfortunately, relatively few examples of the use of minipigs in a safety assessment package have been published. In one of the few such examples, Van Ryzin et al. (1980) published on the toxicity of proquazone (a nonsteroidal anti-inflammatory drug [NSAID]) in rats, dogs, and minipigs. Rats in general are exquisitely sensitive to NSAIDs, and proquazone was no exception; dosages of 25 mg/kg/day (13 weeks) and above caused evidence of gastrointestinal (GI) toxicity. In dogs, dosages as high as 75 mg/kg were without effect, and higher dosages caused emesis, anorexia, and anemia, but no GI lesions. In a longer-term study, however, evidence of gastric damage was produced in the dog. In minipigs, dosages ranged from 6 to 94 mg/kg/day (26 weeks). Dosage-related mortality, diarrhea, and gastric ulceration was observed at all levels. In this particular example, if the minipig had been used in place of the dog, somewhat different conclusions regarding the safety of proquazone would have been reached. Generalizing from this single case, minipigs may be more similar to rats than to human beings in their response to NSAIDs.

The toxicity of relatively large numbers of chemicals has been investigated in regular swine (summarized in Table 20). These studies did not use minipigs, but still may be used to infer the toxic syndrome in minipigs. After all, if pigs cannot with reasonable certainty predict the toxicity in a different breed of pig, how reliable can they be in predicting the toxicity of chemicals in human beings? In general, these publications suggest that the toxic syndromes produced in pigs reliably predict the toxicity of drugs and chemicals in human beings. There are some notable quantitative and qualitative differences. As mentioned, pigs appear to be more sensitive to the gastrointestinal effects of NSAIDS (a quantitative difference with humans). Pigs primarily develop methemaglobinemia (a qualitative difference with humans) in response to acetaminophen rather than liver damage (Artwhol et al., 1988).

Table 20 Summary of Literature on Toxicity in the Pig

Chemical (References)	Syndrome	Comments
3-Nitro-4-hydroxy-phenyl arsonic acid (Rice et al., 1985)	Subchronic dosing lead to exercise inducible muscle tremors and clonic convulsions.	Controlled lab study, dietary admix, Landrace pigs, 20 kg.
Lead (Lassen, 1979)	Only mild clinical signs despite blood levels of 240 μg/ml and decreases in ALAD, hemoglobin, and HCT.	Controlled lab study, oral administration in solution, crossbred 6-week-old pigs, 17–24 kg.
Polybrominated biphenyls (Howard, 1980)	200 ppm in diet for 12 weeks led to decreases in lymphocyte mitogen response in sow and piglets (4 weeks postpartum). No changes in bactericidal activity. Large increases in pre-β lipoprotein.	Controlled lab study, dietary admix, two-generational study of immunotoxicological effects.
Zearalenone (Jones and Smith, 1982)	10 μg/g feed for 4 weeks caused increases in uterine weight with no effect on growth or feed efficiency.	Controlled lab study, dietary admix Yorkshire gults, included comparisons with rats.
Chlorpyrifos (Scheidt et al., 1987)	Exposure of newborn piglets prior to healing of umbilical and tail wounds led to severe signs of organophosphate insecticide toxicity: lethargy, ataxia, salivation, and diarrhea.	Controlled lab study to follow up a case report, gravid, crossbred sows, aerosol exposure.
Acetaminophen (Artwhol et al., 1988)	Acutely, major clinical sign of toxicity was met-hemolgobin formation. Relatively mild effects on liver—primarily dose related increases in glycogen (500–2000 mg/kg iv over 90 min).	Controlled lab study, intravenous infusion, crossbred male and female swine.
Gossypol (Haschek et al., 1989)	Severe cardiotoxicity: diffuse myofiber atrophy with perinucular vaculation. Liver damage (marked centrilobular congestion and necrosis).	Clinical report, feedlot swine problem traced to cottonseed supplementation of feed.
Fenbendazole (Hayes et al., 1983)	When given at 200 mg/kg for 14 days, caused transient leukopenia and increased serum sorbitol dehydrogenase, but not histopathological lesions.	Controlled lab study, oral gavage, female Yorkshire Pigs 18–24 kg.
Aflatoxin B[1] (Osona and Edds, 1982)	0.2 mg/kg/day for 10 days causes increased serum alkaline phosphatase, sorbitol dehydrogenase, prothrombine time, and partial thromboplastin times. Decreases in total P and β-, γ-globulins.	Controlled lab study, emphasis primarily on clinical pathology parameters.

Table 20   *(continued)*

Chemical (References)	Syndrome	Comments
Tumeric oleoresin (Bille et al., 1985)	60, 296, 1551 mg/kg/day. Dose-related increases in thyroid and liver weights. Pericholangitis, hypoplasia of the thyroid, changes in epitheial cells in kidney and bladder.	Controlled lab study, dietary admix, crossbred swine.
Diacetoxyscirpenol (Weaver et al., 1985)	0, 2, 4, 8, and 16 ppm. Decreases in feed consumption and weight gain at all dosages. Multifocal proliferative, gingival, and lingual lesions. Glandular and mucosal small intestine hyperplasia.	Controlled lab study, dietary admix, crossbred weanling pigs
Lasalocid (Oehme et al., 1984)	3.78 mg/kg/day was a no effect level; 53 mg/kg/day was lethal	Part of literature review
Toxaphene (DiPietro et al., 1979)	Ataxia, lethargy, depression, diarrhea, seizures, increased rectal temperatures	Clinical case report, findings attributed to improper use of a topical preparation.
T-2 Toxin (Lorensona ct al., 1985)	Cyanosis, anorexia, lethargy, pneumonia, necrotic lymph tissue, necrotizing gastroenteritis, and other lesions. Depressed lymphocytes and macrophage function, but no effect on RBCs	Controlled lab study.

Reproductive Toxicity and Teratogenicity

While the rat and the rabbit will probably remain the mainstay of reproductive developmental toxicity testing, the minipig has several attractive features which may make it an appropriate model when one of these other species is not. The estrus cycle is approximately 20 days, which certainly makes the minipig a more convenient nonrodent model than dogs for reproductive toxicity studies. The gestation period is about 114 days and the critical period for organogenesis is days 11 through 35 (Hayama and Kokue, 1985). Average litter size is about six, with weaning in about 5 weeks. The piglets are born quite well developed, and make very good models for behavioral teratogenicity testing. These aspects would make the pig more attractive than the monkey for teratogenicity testing. Other aspects of the porcine reproductive system make pigs good models for other types of research as well. Sows have the epitheliochorial type of placenta, which blocks the transplacental passage of proteins, and therefore the newborn piglet is free of antibodies. The minipig is, therefore, also an excellent model for gnotobiotic research, as discussed by Mandel and Travnicek (1987). For example, Kim et al. (1980) used the gnotobiotic minipig model in their studies of natural killer cells and antibody-dependent cellular toxicity.

Numerous examples of teratogenic studies with minipigs can be found in the literature. Ivankovic (1979) studied the teratogenic effects of N-alkyl-nitorosureas using the Gottingen minipig. He demonstrated, for example, that a single dose of (70 mg/kg ip) ethylnitro-sourea given 13 days postcoitus to the sow causes severe bone malformations in the piglets. This chemical class is also teratogenic to rats and hamsters.

Hayama and Kokue (1987) have published on the natural incidences of various malformations and functional deficits in the Gottinger minipig; many other practical aspects of teratogenicity testing in minipigs are discussed in their review article, which is highly recommended reading. They studied pyrimethamine (a folic acid antagonist, given in the feed at an average of 3.6 mg/kg/day on days 11 through 35 of gestation) and established that it causes a high incidence of major malformations such as cleft palate, clubfoot, and micrognathia.

Dexter et al. (1983) have examined Sinclair minipigs, which will voluntarily consume (i.e., do not avoid) alcohol, as a potential model for the human fetal alcohol syndrome (FAS). They reported that alcohol (20% in drinking water) causes a progressive decrease in litter size and piglet weight, but does not result in the more common FAS-related malformation such as microcephaly and narrowed palpebral fissures.

Dermal Toxicity

While rabbits are commonly used for the assessment of primary dermal irritation, pigs have generally been considered to be better models for the more sophisticated study of dermal permeability and toxicity. As reviewed by Sambuco (1985), human and porcine skin are similar with regard to sparsity of the pelage, thickness and general morphology, epidermal cell turnover time, and size, orientation, and distribution of vessels in the skin. The particularly thin haircoat and lack of pigments of the Yucatan minipig makes it particularly ideal for dermal studies. The size of the animal also provides the additional practical advantage of abundant surface area for multiple site testing.

Sambuco has described the sunburn response of the Yucatan minipig to ultraviolet (UV) light, suggesting that this species would also make a good model in phototoxicity as well as photocontact dermatitis studies. Thirty 12-cm sites were demarcated, permitting the study of 15 different dermal dosages of UV radiation.

Mannisto and co-workers (1984) have published a series of articles on the dermal toxicity of the anthralins in the minipig. In one experiment (Mannisto et al., 1984), 24 sites per minipig were used to assess the acute dermal irritation of various concentrations to four different chemicals per site. The range of concentrations tested permitted them to calculate the median erythema concentration and median irritation concentrations with relatively few animals. They were able to show clear differences between anthralin congeners (antipsoriatic drugs) with regard to irritation. When compared to other species (mouse and guinea pig) the response of the minipig was the most similar to humans in that in both species these chemicals are delayed irritants, and several days postexposure may pass before the maximal irritant response is presented.

In a second experiment (Hanhjarvi et al., 1985), the chronic, cumulative dermal effects of anthralin chemicals were studied in minipigs. Using only 12 animals, they were able, by having 32 sites per animal, to study the effects two different chemicals (dithranol and butanthrone; both anthralins) in three different formulations at three different concentrations each. The protocol also included observations for systemic toxicity, clinical laboratory measurements, plasma drug analyses, and gross and histopathological examinations.

In a third report (very similar to the second), Hanhjarvi et al. (1985) clearly demonstrated that the type of vehicle can greatly influence irritation in that dithranol was clearly more irritating when applied in parafin than when applied in a gel. They were also able to demonstrate that while dithranol was less irritating than butantrone acutely, the cumulative irritations (mean scores at the end of 6 months of six times per week applications) were quite similar (Mannisto et al., 1986). There was no evidence of systemic toxicity nor of test article in plasma with either species.

Cardiovascular Toxicity

In general, the published literature consistently maintains that the cardiovascular systems of swine and humans are very similar. For example, as reviewed by Lee (1986), swine, including minipigs, have a noticeable background incidence of atherosclerotic lesions, and that swine fed high lipid diets will develop even more extensive atherosclerotic lesions. High lipid diets will produce lesions similar to advanced atheromatous lesions seen in humans. While few drugs or chemicals have been shown to cause atherosclerosis, this information has three general applications to toxicology and pharmacology. First, the feeding regimen of minipigs should be carefully controlled in general toxicity studies to minimize the incidence of arterial disease, especially in long-term studies. Second, the pathologist should be aware of the natural background of this disease when preparing a diagnosis. Third, the minipig could provide a convenient model for the study of atherosclerotic disease and the screening of potential therapies.

The minipig has been used to study cardiotoxicity. Van Vleet et al. (1984) reported that minipigs were the only other species studied other than dogs to develop cardiac damage in response to large doses of minoxidil. In both pig and the dog, minoxidil cardiotoxicity is characterized by vascular damage (with hemorrhage in the arterial epicardium) and myocardial necrosis (mostly of the left ventricular papillary muscles). Interestingly, in the dog the atrial lesion is largely restricted to the right atrium, whereas in the pig it is restricted to the left atrium. These lesions can be produced in roughly 50% of the minipigs given 10 mg/kg of minoxidil for 2 days and sacrificed 48 hr after the last dose (Herman et al., 1986, 1988). Herman and colleagues have published extensive descriptions of minoxidil-induced lesions in minipigs in comparison to those produced in dogs (Herman et al., 1988, 1989). The right vs left arterial difference is believed to be due to differences in the anatomical pattern of coronary circulation between two species (Herman et al., 1988).

Minipigs are also sensitive to the cardiotoxic effect of doxorubicin (1986). When given six intravenous injections of either 1.6 or 2.4 mg/kg of doxorubicin at 3-week intervals, minipigs develop cardiac lesions similar to those seen in dogs, rabbits, and other experimental animals (Herman et al., 1986). The lesion is characterized by cytoplasmic vacuolation and varying degrees of myofibrillar degeneration and loss. Thus, the minipig is sensitive to the cardiotoxic effect of two well-known and extensively studied chemicals. Therefore, it is a suitable nonrodent species for the general assessment of the cardiotoxicity.

Advantages and Disadvantages

There are two disadvantages to the use of minipigs. The first is their size. While minipigs are smaller than regular swine, at maturity they are generally larger than beagle dogs. The second is their expense: They are not only larger than dogs, but currently carry higher purchasing costs. Among the advantages are the facts that they are long lived, cooperative animals with well-defined physiological and metabolic characteristics. As they are not either popular companion animals (like dogs) or physically resemble humans (like monkeys), minipigs are not specifically discussed in animal "welfare" laws like the other two species. Depending on their final form, new animal welfare regulations could make the space and maintenance costs for dogs and monkeys very prohibitive. This may make minipigs increasingly more attractive as a nonrodent species for general toxicity testing.

REFERENCES

Anonymous (1980) Standard practice for conducting acute toxicity tests with fishes, macroinvertebrates and amphibians. *Annual Book (1980) of American Society for Testing and Materials Standards* (Designation E729-80), pp. 400–4224.

Artwhol, J., Henne-Bruns, D., Carter, E., and Cera, L. (1988) Acetaminophen toxicosis: A potential model for acute liver failure in swine. *Vet. Hum. Toxicol.* 30, 324–328.

Barnett, J., and Hensworth, P. (1986) The impact of handling and environmental factors on the stress response and its consequences in swine. *Lab. Anim. Sci.* 36, 366–369.

Bille, N., Larsen, J., Hansen, E., and Wurtzen, G. (1985) Subchronic oral toxicity of tumeric oleoresin in pigs. *Food Chem. Toxicol.* X, 967–973, 1985.

Blanck, J., Lindstrom-Seppa, P., Agren, J., Hanninen, O., Rein, H., and Ruckpaul, K. (1989) Temperature Compensation of hepatic microsomal cytochrome P-450 activity in rainbow trout. I. Thermodynamic regulation during water cooling in autumn. *Comp. Biochem. Physiol.* 93C, 55–60.

Brechbuhler, T., Kaeslin, M., and Wyler, F. (1984) Reference values of various blood constituents in young minipigs. *J. Clin. Chem. Clin. Biochem.* 22, 301–304.

Burks, M., Ymbleson, M., Hicklin, K., Hutcheson, D., and Middleton, C. (1977) Age and sex related changes of hematologic parameters in sinclair (S-1) miniature swine. *Growth* 41, 51–62.

Chengelis, C. (1990) Examples of alternative use in toxicology for common species. *J. Am. Coll. Toxicol.* 9, 319–342.

Clausing, P., Beitz, H., Gericke, S., and Solecki (1986) On the usefulness of minipigs in toxicology testing of pesticides. *Arch. Toxicol.* 9 (Suppl.), 225–271.

Cook, W., Osweiller, G., Hyde, W., and Stahr, H. (1985) Levamisole toxicosis in swine. *Vet. Hum. Toxicol.* 27, 388–389.

Darnerud, P., Lund, B., Bittebo, E., and Brandt, I. (1989) 1,2-Dibromoethanc and chloroform in the rainbow trout *(Salmo gairdneri):* Studies on the distribution of the nonvolatile and irreversibly bound metabolites. *J. Toxicol. Environ. Health* 26, 209–221.

Dean-Ross, D. (1983) Methods for the assessment of the toxicity of environmental chemicals to earthworms. *Reg. Toxicol. Pharmacol.* 3, 48–59.

Dexter, J., Tumbleson, M., Decker, J., and Middleton, C. (1983) Comparison of the offspring of three serial pregnancies during voluntary alcohol consumption in sinclair (S-1) miniature swine. *Neurobehav. Toxicol. Teratol.* 5, 229–231.

DiPietro, J., and Haliburton, J. (1979) Toxaphene toxicosis in swine. *J. Am. Vet. Med. Assoc.* 175, 452–453.

Drewes, C., Vining, E., and Callahan, C. (1984) Non-invasive electrophysiological monitoring: A sensitive method for detecting sublethal neurotoxicity in earthworms. *Environ. Toxicol. Chem.* 3, 559–607.

Egaas, E., and Varanasi, U. (1981) Effects of polychlorinated biphenyls and environmental temperature on in vitro formation of benzo(a)pyrene metabolites by liver of trout *(Salmo gairdneri). Biochem. Pharmacol.* 31, 561–566.

Erickson, D., Goodrich, M., and Lech, J. (1988) The effect of piperonyl butoxide on hepatic cytochrome P-450–dependent monooxygenase activities in rainbow trout *(Salmo gaidneri)*. *Toxicol. Appl. Pharmacol.* 94, 1–10.

Fisher, S. (1984) A comparison of standardized methods for measuring the biological activity of pesticides to the earthworms. *Lumbricus terrestris. Ecotoxicol. Environ. Safety* 8, 564–571.

Freudenthal, R., Leber, P., Emmerling, D., Kerchner, G., and Campbell, D. (1976) Characterization of the hepatic microsomal mixed-function oxidase system in miniature pigs. *Drug Metab. Dispos.* 4, 25–27.

Gad, S. (1990) Recent developments in replacing, reducing and refining animal use in toxicologic research and testing *Fund. Appl. Toxicol.* 15, 8–16.

Galitzer, S., and Oehme, F. (1984) A literature review of the toxicity of lasalocid, a polyether antibiotic. *Vet. Hum. Toxicol.* 26, 322–326.

Gilman, A., and Vardanis, A. (1974). Carbofuran. Comparative toxicity and metabolism in the worms *Lumbricas terrestris* and *Eisenia foetida. J. Agric. Food Chem.* 22, 625–628.

Gregus, Z., Watkins, J., Thompson, T., Harvey, M., and Rozman, K., an Klaassen (1983) Hepatic phase I and II biotransformations in quail and trout: Comparison to other species commonly used in toxicity testing. *Toxicol. Appl. Pharmacol.* 67, 430–441.

Hanhijarvi, H., Nevalainen, T., and Mannisto, P. (1985) A six month dermal irritation test with anthralins in the gottingen miniature swine. *Arch. Toxicol.* 8 (Suppl.), 463–468.

Haschek, W., Beasley, V., Buck, W., and Finnell, J. (1989) Cottonseed meal (gossypol) toxicosis in a swine herd. *J. Am. Vet. Med. Assoc.* 195, 613–615.

Hawkins, W., Overstreet, R., Fournie, J., and Walker, W. (1985) Development of aquarium fish models for environmental carcinogenesis: Tumor induction in seven species. *J. Appl. Toxicol.* 5, 261–264.

Hawkins, W., Walker, W., Overstreet, R., Lytle, T., and Lytle, J. (1988) Dose-related carcinogenic effects of water-born benzo(a)pyrene on liver in two small fish species. *Ecotoxicol. Envir. Safety* 16, 219–231.

Hayama, T., and Kokue, E. (1985) Use of the Goettingen miniature pig for studying pyrimethamine teratogenesis. *CRC Crit. Rev. Tox.* 14, 403–421.

Hayes, R., Oehme, F., and Leipold, H. (1983) Toxicity investigation of fenbendazole, and antithelminitic of swine. *Am. J. Vet. Res.* 44, 1108–1111.

Heimbach, F. (1984) Correlation between three methods for determining the toxicity of chemicals to earthworms. *Prestic. Sci.* 15, 605–611.

Hendricks, J., Meyers, T., Shelton, D., Casteel, J., and Bailey, G., (1985). Hepatocarcinogenicity of benzo(a)pyrene to rainbow trout by dietary exposure and intraperitoneal injection. *J. Nat. Cancer Inst.* 74, 839–851.

Herman, E., Young, R., Balazs, T. and Ferrans, V. (1986). The evaluation of acute and chronic cardiotoxicity in miniature swine. *Swine Biomed. Res.* 3, 1659–1670.

Herman, E., Ferrans, V., and Young, R. (1988). Examination of Minoxidil-induced acute cardiotoxicity in miniature swine. *Toxicology* 48, 41–51.

Herman, E., Ferrans, V., Young, R., and Balazs, T. (1989). A comparative study in minoxidil-induced myocardial lesions in Beagle dogs and miniature swine. *Toxicol. Pathol.* 17, 189–191.

Hinton, D., Lantz, R., and Hampton, J. (1984). Effect of age and exposure to a carcinogen on the structure of the Medaka liver: A morphometric study. *Natl. Cancer Inst. Monogr.* 65, 239–249.

Howard, S., Werner, P., and Sleight, S. (1980). Polybrominated biphenyl toxicosis in swine: Effects of some aspects of the immune system in lactating sows and their offsprings. *Toxicol. Appl. Pharmacol.* 55, 146–153.

Hunsaker, H., Norden, S., and Allen, K. (1984). An inexpensive caging method for miniature swine suitable for trace-element studies. *Lab. Animal. Sci.* 2, 386–387.

Hutcheson, D., Tumbleson, M., and Middleton, C. (1979). Serum electrolyte concentrations in sinclair (S-1) miniature swine from 1 through 36 months of age. *Growth* 43, 62–70.

Ikeda, G., Miller, E., Sapienza, P., Michel, T. and Sager, A. (1985) Maternal-Foetal distribution studies in late pregnancy. I. Distribution of [N-methyl-^{14}C]Betaine in tissues of Beagle dogs and miniature pigs. *Food Chem. Toxicol.* 23, 609–614.

Ivankovic, S. (1979). Teratogenic and carcinogenic effects of some chemicals during prenatal life in rats, Syrian hamsters and minipigs. Natl. Can. Inst. *Monograph* Vol. 1979 M51, 103–115.

James, L., and Smith, T. (1982) Effect of dietary alfalfa on zearalenone toxicity and metabolism in rats and swine. *J. Anim. Sci.* 55, 10–118.

Julkunen, Schiller, Muller, D., Klinger, W., and Hanninen, O. (1986) Monooxygenase activity of fish liver in biomonitoring aquatic environment. *Arch. Toxicol.* 9(Suppl.), 378–381.

Kahn, M. (1984) Minipig: Advantages and disadvantages as a model in toxicity testing. *J. Am. Coll. Toxicol.* 3, 337–342.

Kim, Y., Huh, N., Koren, H., and Amos, B. (1980) Natural killing (NK) and antibody-dependent cellular cytotoxicity (ADCC) in specific pathogen-free (SPF) miniature swine and germfree piglets. I. Comparison of NK and ADCC. *J. Immunol.* 125, 755–762.

Kirby, K., and Tremmel, H., and Keisert, J. (1980) Determination and metabolism of ethylene dibromide in minipigs. *Bull. Environ. Contam. Toxicol.* 24, 774–777.

Laird, J., and Kroger, M. (1981) Earthworms *CRC Crit. Rev. Environ. Control* 11, 189–218.

Lassen, E., and Buck, W. (1979) Experimental lead toxicosis in Swine. *Am. J. Vet. Res.* 40, 1359–1364.

Lee, K. (1986) Swine as animal models in cardiovascular research. *Swine Biomed. Res.* 3, 1481–1496.

Lorenzana, R., Beasely, V., Buck, W., and Ghent, A. (1985) Experimental T-2 toxicosis on serum enzymes and biochemistry, blood coagulation and hematology. *Fund. Appl. Toxicol.* 5, 893–901.

Loveland, P., Wilcox, J., Hendricks, J., and Bailey, G. (1988) Comparative metabolism and DNA binding of aflatoxin B1, Aflatoxin M1, aflatoxicol, and aflatoxicol-M1 in hepatocytes from rainbow trout. *Carcinogen* 9, 441–446.

Mandel, L., and Travnicek, J. (1987) The minipig as a model in gnotobiology. *Die Nahrung.* 31, 613–618.

Mannisto, P., Havas, A., Haasio, K., Hanhijarvi, H., and Mustakallio, K. (1984) Skin irritation by dithranol (anthralin) and its 10-aceyl analogues in 3 animal models. *Contact Dermatitis* 10, 140–145.

Mannisto, P., Hanhijarvi, H., Kosma, V., and Collan, Y. (1986) A 6-month dermal toxicity test with dithranol and butantrone in miniature swine. *Contact Dermatitis* 15, 1–9.

Miyauchi, M. (1984) Conversion of procarcinogens to mutagens by the S-9 fraction from the liver of rainbow trout (Salmo gairdneri): Inducibility with PCB, 3-methylcholanthrene and pheno-barbital and inhibition by metyrapone and alpha-naphthaflavone. *Comp. Biochem. Physiol.* 79C, 363–367.

Mueller, D., Nelles, J., Deparade, E., and Arni, P. (1980) The activity of S-9 liver fractions from seven species in salmonella/mammalian-microsome mutagenicity tests. *Mut. Res.* 70, 279–300.

Murphy, S. (1986) Toxic effects of insecticides in *Casurett and Doull's Toxicology: The Basic Science of Poisons*, Klaassen, C. Amdur, M., and Doull, J., eds. Macmillan, New York, pp. 519–581.

Neuhauser, E., Durkin, P., Malecki, M., and Antara, M. (1985a) Comparative toxicity of ten organic chemicals to four earthworm species. *Comp. Biochem. Physiol.* 83C, 197–200.

Neuhauser, E., Loehr, C., Malecki, M., Milligan, D., and Durkin, P. (1985b) The toxicity of selected organic chemicals to the earthworm *Eisenia fetida. J. Environ. Qual.* 14, 383–388.

Neuhauser, E., Loehr, C., and Malecki, M., (1986) Contact and artificial soil tests using earth-worms to evaluate the impact of wastes in soil, in *Hazardous and Industrial Solid Waste Testing: Fourth Symposium, ASTM STP 886.* Petros, J., Lacy, W., and Conway, R., eds. American Society for Testing and Materials. Philadelphia, pp. 192–202.

Oldigs, B. (1986) Effects of internal factors upon hematological and clinical chemical parameters in the Gottinger miniature pig. *Swine Biomed. Res.* 2, 809–813.

Osuna, O., and Edds, G. (1980) Toxicology of aflatoxin B1, warfarin, and cadmium in young pigs: Clinical chemistry and blood coagulation. *Am. J. Vet. Res.* 43, 1387–1394.

Panepinto, L. (1986) Laboratory methodlogy and management of swine in biomedical research. *Swine Biomed. Res.* 1, 97–109.

Panepinto, L., and Phillips (1986) The Yucatan miniature pig: Characterization and utilization in biomedical research. *Lab. Animal Sci.* 36, 344–347.

Panepinto, L., Phillips, R., Norden, S., Pryor, P., and Cox, R. (1983) A comfortable, minimum stress method of restraint for yucutan miniature swine. *Lab. Anim. Sci.* 33, 95–97.

Pang, V., Lambert, R., Felsberg, P., Beasley, V., Buck, W., and Haschek, W. (1987) Experimental T-2 toxicosis in swine following inhalation exposure. Effects on pulmonary and systemic immunity, and morphologic changes. *Toxicol. Pathol.* 15, 308–319.

Parsons, A., and Wells, R. (1986) Serum biochemistry of healthy Yucatan miniature pigs. *Lab. Anim. Sci.* 36, 428–430.

Peggins, J., Shipley, L. and Weiner, M. (1984) Characterization of age related changes in hepatic drug metabolism in miniature swine. *Drug Metab. Dispos.* 12, 379–381.

Pesonen, M., Celander, M., Forlin, L., Anderson, T. (1987) Comparison of xenobiotic biotransformation enzymes in kidney and liver of rainbow trout *(Salmo gairdneri). Toxicol. Appl. Pharmacol.* 91, 75–84.

Phillips, R., and Tumbleson, M. (1986) Models. *Swine Biomed. Res.* 1, 437–440.

Radin, M., Weiser, M., and Frettman, M. (1986) Hematologic and serum biochemical values for Yucatan miniature swine. *Lab. Anim. Sci.* 36, 425–427.

Rendic, S., Ruf, S., Weber, P., and Kajfez, F. (1984) Cimetidine and ranitidine: Their interaction with human and pig liver microsomes and with purified cytochrome P-450. *Eur. J. Drug. Metab. Pharmacokinet.* 9, 195–200.

Rettie, A., Bogucki, B., Lim, I., and Meier, P., (1990) Stereoselective sulfoxidation of a series of alkyl P-tolyl sulfides by microsomal and purified flavin containing monooxygenases. *Mol. Pharmacol.* 37, 643–651.

Rice, D., Kennedy, S., McMurray, C., and Branchflower, W. (1985) Experimental 3-nitro-4-hydroxyphenylarsonic acid toxicosis in pigs. *Res. Vet. Sci.* 39, 47–51.

Roberts, R., and Dorough, H. (1984) Relative toxicities of chemicals to the earthworm *Eisenia foetida. Environ. Toxicol. Chem.* 3, 67–78.

Roberts, B., and Dorough, H. (1985) Hazards of chemicals to earthworms. *Environ. Toxicol. Chem.* 4, 307–323.

Romert, P., and Matthiessen, M. (1984) Fine structure of hepatocytes from mini-pigs and mini-pig fetuses exposed to alcohol (ethanol) in vivo. *Acta Anat.* 120, 190–195.

Sambuco, P. (1985) Miniature swine as an animal model in photodermatology: Factors influencing sunburn cell formation. *Photodermatology* 2, 144–150.

Scheidt, A., Long, G., Knox, K., and Hubbard, S. (1987) Toxicosis in new born pigs associated with cutaneous application of an aerosal spray containing chloropyrifos. *J. Am. Vet. Med. Assoc.* 191, 1410–1412.

Schneider, N., Bradley, S., Andersen, M. (1977) Toxicology of cyclomethylenetrinitramine: Distribution and metabolism in the rat and the miniature swine. *Toxicol. Appl. Pharmacol.* 39, 531–541.

Serda, S., and Furst, A. (1987) Acute toxicity of selenium to earthworms. *Proc. West. Pharmacol. Soc.* 30, 127–228.

Shelton, D., Hendricks, J., and Bailey, G. (1984) The hepatocarcinogenicity of diethylnitrosamine to rainbow trout and its enhancement by aroclors 1242 and 1254. *Toxicol. Lett.* 22, 27–31.

Smith, G., Watkins, J., Thompson, T., Rozman, K., and Klassen, C. (1984) Oxidative and conjugative metabolism of xenobiotics by livers of cattle, sheep, swine and rats. *J. Anim. Sci.* 58, 386–395.

Stegman, J., and Kloepper-Sams, P. (1987) Cytochrome P-450. Isozymes and monooxygenase activity in aquatic animals. *Environ. Health Perspec.* 71, 87–95.

Stenersen, J. (1979) Action of pesticides on earthworms. Part I: toxicity of cholinesterase-inhibiting insecticides to earthworms as evaluated by laboratory tests. *Prestic. Sci.* 10, 66–74.

Stenersen, J. (1984) Detoxication of xenobiotics by earthworms. *Comp. Biochem. Physiol.* 78C, 249–252.

Swindle, M., Smith, A., and Hepburn, B. (1988) Swine as models in experimental surgery. *J. Invest. Surg.* 1, 65–79.

Tynes, R., and Hodgson, E. (1984) The measurement of FAD-containing-oxygenase activity in microsomes containing cytochrome P-450. *Xenobiotica* 14, 515–520.

Van Gestel, C., Van Dis, W., Van Breeman, E., and Sparenburg, P. (1989) Development of a standardized reproduction toxicity test with the earthworm species *Eisenia-fetida-andrei* using copper, pentachlorophenol, and 2,4-dichloroaniline. *Ecotoxicol. Environ. Safety* 18, 305–312.

Van Leemput, L., Swysen, E., Woesternborghs, R., Michielsen, Meulderman, W., and Heykants, J. (1989) On the terrestrial toxicity of the fungicide imasalil (enilconazole) to the earthworm species *Eisenia-foetida*. *Ecotoxicol. Environ. Safety* 18, 313–320.

Van Ryzin, R., and Trapold, J. (1980) The toxicology profile of the anti-inflammatory drug proquazone in animals. *Drug Chem. Toxicol.* 3, 361–379.

Van Vleet J., Herman, E., and Ferrans, V. (1984) Cardiac morphologic alterations in acute Minoxidil cardiotoxicity in miniature Swine. *Exp. Mol. Pathol.* 41, 10–25.

Voss, S., Shelton, D., and Hendricks, J. (1982) Effects of dietary aroclor 1254 and cyclopropane fatty acids on hepatic enzymes in rainbow trout. *Arch. Environ. Contam. Toxicol.* 11, 87–91.

Walker, C., Bentley, P., and Oesch, F. (1978) Phylogenetic distribution of epoxide hydratase indifferent vertebrate species, strains and tissues measured using three substrates. *Biochem. Biophys. Acta* 539, 427–434.

Walker, W., Manning, C., Overstreet, R., and Hawkins, W. (1985) Development of aquarium fish models for environmental carcinogenesis: An intermittent-flow exposure system for volatile, hydrophobic chemicals. *J. Appl. Toxicol.* 5, 255–260.

Watkins, J., and Klassen, C. (1986) Xenobiotic biotransformation in livestock: Comparison to other species commonly used in toxicity testing. *J. Anim. Sci.* 63, 933–942.

Weaver, G., Kurtz, H., Bates, F., Mirocha, C., Behrens, J., and Hagler, W. (1981) Diacetoxyscirpenol toxicity in pigs. *Res. Vet. Sci.* 31, 131–135.

11

Clinical Pathology of Laboratory Animals

Robert L. Hall
Hazleton Wisconsin, Inc.
Madison, Wisconsin

In the context of conventional toxicology studies, clinical pathology usually encompasses routine hematology, clinical chemistry, and urinalysis tests. The majority of tests are the same as those used in human medicine to establish a minimum database. There are, of course, species differences for reference ranges, interpretation of changes, methodology, and the value or appropriateness of individual tests. The choice of tests for a given study depends upon a number of factors, including objective of the study, test species, test material(s) or conditions, duration of the study, and regulatory requirements.

The results of clinical pathology tests are used to identify general metabolic and pathological processes. Although specific "diagnoses" or toxicological mechanisms are infrequently identified, test results help to direct further study by narrowing the possibilities. Alterations in test results are rarely the only evidence of biologically important *adverse* toxicological effects. Clinical observations and/or anatomical pathology findings usually corroborate pathologically meaningful laboratory findings. On the other hand, it is relatively common to observe minor effects of a test material only in the clinical pathology results. For example, changes in homeostatic mechanisms to maintain normal fluid, electrolyte, and acid-base balance secondary to a test material that alters water consumption or acid load may be reflected only in urinalysis results.

The ability to identify subtle changes in a group of treated animals that are compared directly with a control group is much greater than in an individual animal compared with historical reference ranges. In safety assessment studies, this fact inevitably leads to important decisions concerning the nature of a subtle change. Is it simply an alteration in normal homeostatic mechanisms, or is it an early indication of a more significant adverse effect? This question can be difficult to answer. It is clearly not as simple as referring to a table of historical reference ranges.

Accurate interpretation of laboratory results requires not only an understanding of the tests themselves, it also requires knowledge of species differences, study design, the test material(s) or conditions, clinical observations, and anatomical pathology findings. The interpretation of one test result, e.g., high serum urea nitrogen, is dependent on the results of another, i.e., urine specific gravity. The urine specific gravity result is the difference between an interpretation of prerenal azotemia, as with dehydration, and renal azotemia, as with chronic renal failure.

With respect to regulated safety assessment studies, required or recommended clinical pathology tests have important limitations in their ability to demonstrate toxicological effects. Some of the limitations are due to timing of sample collection and analysis during the study, and some are related more to the actual tests. In fact, some of the recommended tests are outdated or inappropriate and should either be eliminated or used only in specific circumstances. To add to the confusion, recommended test lists vary among regulatory agencies, both inside and outside of the United States.

This chapter will address (1) the use and potential misuse of clinical pathology reference ranges, (2) sources of variation in laboratory test results and their potential impact on data interpretation, (3) the characteristics and interpretation of routine hematology, clinical chemistry, and urinalysis tests used in toxicology studies, and (4) aspects of laboratory test results that are unique to individual laboratory animal species. For more in-depth discussions of the laboratory tests and their interpretation, the reader is referred to Sanderson and Phillips (1981), Duncan and Prasse (1986), Jain (1986), Kaneko (1989), and Loeb and Quimby (1989).

REFERENCE RANGES

The term *normal range* has been replaced by the more appropriate terms *reference range* or *reference interval*. The word *normal* occasionally caused confusion because it implied that values outside of the range were, by definition, abnormal. However, because most laboratory test reference intervals are statistically constructed to include the range of values found in 95% of a population of healthy, or "normal," individuals, it should not be surprising that approximately 1 out of 20 results for a specific test (e.g., serum glucose concentration) from a group of "normal" animals is outside of the historical reference range. Taking this idea a step further, and because of the fact that a minimum hematology and clinical chemistry database consists of approximately 30 individual test results, it should also not be surprising that a "normal" animal will often have at least 1 test result that falls outside of the historical reference ranges. In this light, it is easy to see that study designs requiring all animals have "normal" clinical pathology test results as a prerequisite for inclusion in the study are too restrictive if taken literally.

Another potentially confusing aspect of the term *normal range* is that it seems to imply that a test result within the range is, by definition, normal, and therefore the organ system or metabolic process being assessed by that test is also normal. Unfortunately, severely abnormal animals may have laboratory values well within the reference range. For example, a dog with advanced liver cirrhosis often has serum liver enzyme activities within the established reference ranges for those tests. An animal with leukemia may have a "normal" white blood cell count. Certain aspects of a disease condition may mask abnormalities in a laboratory test. Dehydration may mask anemia or hypoproteinemia. The decrease in plasma volume due to fluid loss will spuriously increase red blood cell count and serum protein concentration. Acidosis may mask total body potassium depletion as intracellular potassium ions exchange with extracellular hydrogen ions, resulting in a "normal" serum potassium concentration.

Reference ranges are influenced by many variables, and a number of these will be discussed in the following section. Of particular importance is the individual laboratory performing the tests and the specific methodology employed. For instance, the temperature at which enzyme assays are conducted will greatly influence results; the higher the temperature, the higher the reference range. It is difficult and potentially misleading to use reference ranges found in the literature for the interpretation of study data. Whenever possible, investigators should establish in-house reference ranges. Because of a number of limitations, not the least of which is economic, this is not always feasible. For this reason, reference ranges for common hematology and clinical chemistry tests in the eight principal laboratory animal species described in this book have been included with this chapter (Tables 1–8). These ranges are presented to serve as general guidelines and to show differences among the species. They represent a composite of ranges found in the literature and at Hazleton Wisconsin, Inc. When reference ranges are established in-house, it is important that they be periodically updated. Changes in test methodology, animal supplier, and animal husbandry or handling practices are examples of variables that will cause "old" reference ranges to become obsolete.

Reference ranges do not replace the need for control animals in large studies designed to assess the toxic potential of a test material. Because it is not possible to repeatedly duplicate a standard set of study conditions, there is no substitute for age- and sex-matched control animals from the same supplier undergoing the same procedures as the test animals. For instance, test results from animals receiving a purified diet cannot be compared directly with reference ranges established on animals fed a conventional diet. In small investigational studies with few or no control animals, however, reference ranges are necessary for identifying potential toxic effects.

Reference ranges should never be relied upon as the sole means of making judgments concerning the biological importance of a test material–related effect. As previously mentioned, values outside of the reference range do not necessarily indicate an abnormal condition and values within the reference range do not necessarily signify a normal condition. Wild-caught monkeys tend to have wide reference ranges for most parameters. The finding that the mean serum alanine aminotransferase activity of a treated group is significantly higher than that of the control group should not be dismissed as toxicologically unimportant simply because the mean activity of the treated group falls within the upper reference limit. On the other hand, reference ranges for serum urea nitrogen concentration in rats are generally very narrow. If addition of test material to the drinking water of rats caused reduced water consumption, it is quite possible that the mean serum urea nitrogen concentration for these rats would be significantly higher than for the control animals and would exceed the upper reference limit without a meaningful toxic effect on the kidney.

Given the variety of caveats described for the use of reference ranges, it is necessary to emphasize their value. Proper assessment of the significance of laboratory findings is only possible with a firm understanding of what is typical for healthy animals under similar conditions. Reference ranges serve as the starting point, a point of reference, from which one can move toward an appropriate conclusion based on all of the variables that may have impacted a particular study.

SOURCES OF VARIATION IN LABORATORY MEASUREMENTS

As previously mentioned, the need for developing in-house reference ranges is based on the fact that many variables, such as methodology, affect test results, and that controlling these variables is best accomplished within one's own laboratory. In addition, however, there are sources of variation that can affect the results of individual animals within a group and thereby complicate data interpretation. Most variables can be categorized as either physiological, procedural, or artifact. Examples of these are discussed in the following paragraphs.

Age-Related Changes

Age-related changes must always be considered, and reference ranges should be established in accordance with the age of animals used most often by the individual laboratory. As young animals mature, typical changes in most species include decreasing reticulocyte count, mean corpuscular volume, serum alkaline phosphatase activity, and serum inorganic phosphorus concentration and increasing red blood cell count, hematocrit, hemoglobin concentration, total serum protein concentration, and serum globulin concentration. In many species, neutrophil count will increase and lymphocyte count will decrease with age. As a population of animals becomes older, test results exhibit greater variability because of subclinical disease conditions such as progressive nephropathy in rats. Reference ranges therefore become wider.

Strain and Gender Differences

Strain differences can be important, especially in mice and rats, just as species differences in nonhuman primates. Gender-related differences also occur, but they are often subtle. Depending on the laboratory's need, it may be desirable to combine the data from both sexes into a single reference range. On the other hand, the effects of estrus may be extremely important, as in ferrets with estrus-induced bone marrow hypoplasia. Axenic animals may have significant differences from others of their species, especially with respect to leukocyte counts and serum globulins. Hibernation in hamsters affects a variety of laboratory tests.

Effect of Diet

Diet has an effect on laboratory data. Changes in cholesterol are obvious in some species fed atherogenic diets, but less obvious changes can occur in tests such as serum urea nitrogen concentration in animals fed diets containing different types or amounts of protein. Data from animals fed purified diets should always be carefully examined. Small errors in the formulation of these diets can have a significant effect on health. For most species, fasting is a generally accepted practice designed to help stabilize the test results. However, fasting may actually be a detriment in rabbits and mice.

Excitement and Stress

Excitement and stress can have pronounced effects on laboratory data. Excitement is associated with endogenous catecholamine release and stress with endogenous corticosteroid release. The effects of catecholamines on test results are immediate, whereas those of corticosteroids take longer. The most obvious changes observed in excited or frightened animals (e.g., untrained, unanesthetized monkeys) affect leukocytes and serum glucose concentration. Endogenous corticosteroid release also affects these parameters, but somewhat differently. If possible, clinical pathology testing should be delayed for at least a week following shipping to avoid stress-related changes.

Choice of Collection Site and Use of Anesthesia

The most familiar procedural influences on laboratory test results are those associated with sample collection site and the use of anesthesia. Many investigators have analyzed the differences in data resulting from choice of collection site and anesthesia. This is especially true for the rat in which a variety of bleeding techniques have been used (Neptun et al., 1985; Suber and Kodell, 1985). The principal message of these works is that one should use the technique with which they have had good success and with which they are comfortable. While specific study objectives may occasionally dictate which bleeding technique is most appropriate, it is very difficult to consistently obtain high-quality specimens if the techniques are not used routinely. Furthermore, very few research facilities have the resources to establish reference ranges for more than one or two bleeding techniques. Choice of bleeding site and anesthesia appear to have their greatest effect on peripheral blood cell counts. Serum enzyme activities, especially for enzymes derived from muscle, are also notably affected by bleeding site.

Artifacts

Due to Hemolysis

One of the most common causes of variation due to artifact is in vitro hemolysis. Free hemoglobin may interfere with a variety of assays depending upon the method and instrumentation used. In addition, lysis of erythrocytes releases intracellular constituents such as aspartate aminotransferase, lactate dehydrogenase, inorganic phosphorus, and potassium that cause spuriously high serum activities and concentrations. There are species differences for erythrocyte intracellular potassium concentration that are discussed later in the chapter.

While hemolysis is generally obvious and can, therefore, be considered when interpreting data, poor laboratory procedures can have effects that are not grossly evident. Intracellular erythrocyte constituents will leach into serum if clotted blood samples are not centrifuged and separated quickly. In addition, serum glucose concentration will decrease at a rate of about 7–10 mg/dl each hour. These changes, along with the potential of analytical drift by laboratory instrumentation, are some of the reasons why randomization of animals for blood collection is extremely important. For example, if control animals in a large study are bled first and high-dose animals last, and the serum is not separated from the clotted blood until after the last animal is bled, then serum lactate dehydrogenase activity and inorganic phosphorus concentration may be statistically lower in the high-dose group simply because their blood did not sit as long before separation.

Due to Multiple Bleeding Intervals

Sometimes overlooked are the effects of multiple bleeding intervals. It is relatively easy to create iatrogenic, blood-loss anemia in animals that are bled frequently for pharmacokinetic studies or for serial test determinations such as plasma cholinesterase activity. In the absence of control animals undergoing the same procedures, it may be difficult to separate test material effects from those of the multiple blood collections.

Due to Urine Collection Procedures

Timed urine collection procedures, as currently practiced in most toxicology laboratories, cannot avoid a number of artifacts in the urinalysis results. It is virtually impossible to make a long-term collection (16–24 hr) in such a way as to prevent bacterial contamination and proliferation. Preservatives have disadvantages, and it is very difficult to keep the samples constantly chilled. Because of these problems, the list of artifacts is long: bacteria proliferate; urine pH increases because urease-producing bacteria result in ammonia formation; highly alkaline urine can cause false-positive proteinuria with reagent strip methods; glucose is consumed by proliferating bacteria; volatile ketones leave solution;

bilirubin is oxidized by light to biliverdin, which does not react with reagent strips; cells and casts disintegrate over time; and crystals form, especially those that occur in alkaline urine.

Well-conceived standard operating procedures and careful study design can help to eliminate or reduce many potential sources of variation. However, it is always necessary to consider their impact when interpreting clinical pathology data.

CLINICAL PATHOLOGY TESTS AND INTERPRETATIONS

Hematology

The hematology tests routinely performed during toxicology studies evaluate erythrocytes, leukocytes, platelets, and coagulation. Many automated cell counters can determine red blood cell (RBC) count, hemoglobin, hematocrit, mean corpuscular volume (MCV), mean corpuscular hemoglobin (MCH), mean corpuscular hemoglobin concentration (MCHC), white blood cell (WBC) count, and platelet count from as little as 100 μl of anticoagulated whole blood. Because erythrocytes of the common laboratory species are smaller than human erythrocytes, the cell counters must be adjusted to ensure accuracy. In addition, platelet counts from rodents are often higher than the upper limit for some analyzers (1 million/μl) and adjustments are sometimes necessary for the instrument to report the high counts. At this time, cell counters that perform WBC differential counts on human blood are generally unable to determine accurate differential counts on blood from multiple species. The differential count done by microscopic examination of a stained blood film is still the method of choice, although it is fairly time consuming and labor intensive. If an automated cell counter is unavailable, a considerable amount of information can be acquired from a packed cell volume (PCV; essentially the same as hematocrit) obtained by microhematocrit tube centrifugation, a WBC count performed on a hemocytometer, and examination of the blood film for cell morphology, estimation of platelet count, and WBC differential count. The common coagulation tests, prothrombin time (PT) and activated partial thromboplastin time (APTT), can be done manually or using one of the newer automated coagulation analyzers. Like the cell counters, some of the newer light-impedance analyzers must be specifically set up for animal specimens.

Erythrocytes
Anemia. Perhaps the most common clinical pathology findings in toxicology studies are mild decreases in RBC count, hemoglobin concentration, and hematocrit (the percentage of whole blood made up of erythrocytes). When values for these tests are below their lower reference limits, the condition is called anemia. Considering the fact that a healthy human produces about 100 billion new erythrocytes per day, it is not surprising that test materials causing effects such as lower body weight will also affect erythrocyte mass. The RBC count, hemoglobin concentration, and hematocrit will parallel each other as long as cell size and hemoglobin content do not change. The erythrocyte indices, MCV and MCHC, measure individual cell size and hemoglobin concentration. Reticulocyte count and erythrocyte morphology are critical pieces of information for determining the potential causes of anemia.

The general diagnostic approach to anemia is simple. The first step is to determine whether the anemia is regenerative or nonregenerative.

Regenerative Anemia. In regenerative anemia, the hematopoietic tissues are actively trying to replenish the lost erythrocytes by increasing production and release of new ones into circulation. Following acute blood loss or hemolysis, it takes approximately 3–4 days for the new erythrocytes, or reticulocytes, to appear in peripheral blood. Reticulocytes can be counted as a percentage of erythrocytes on a peripheral blood film stained with a vital stain such as new methylene blue. It is best to determine the absolute reticulocyte count by multiplying the reticulocyte percentage (relative reticulocyte count) times the RBC count. A severely anemic animal can have a high relative reticulocyte count and yet have an absolute reticulocyte count that is no greater than a normal animal. In this case, the animal would not be showing an appropriate regenerative response for its degree of anemia. With the typical Romanowsky stains used for WBC differential counts, reticulocytes are larger and stain slightly more basophilic than the other erythrocytes. During a regenerative response, the erythrocyte morphology would be described by the terms anisocytosis (variable size) and polychromasia (variable color). Nucleated red blood cells and Howell-Jolly bodies are often more numerous in peripheral blood films of animals with regenerative anemia, but they also occur in some forms of nonregenerative anemia. Basophilic stippling of erythrocytes is a seldom seen change that may occur during regeneration; it is primarily associated with lead toxicity, however. During a regenerative response, the erythrocyte indices usually show a higher MCV because of the influx of larger young cells and a lower MCHC because these large cells have a lower hemoglobin concentration.

The two primary causes of regenerative anemias are blood loss and hemolysis. In addition to the erythrocyte changes, blood loss is usually characterized by lower serum protein concentrations. The source of the blood loss may be identified by clinical observations, necropsy findings, or tests such as fecal and urine occult blood. Hemolytic conditions do not generally cause changes in serum protein concentrations. Hepatosplenomegaly, icterus, bilirubinemia, and bilirubinuria may be associated findings. When hemolysis is suspected, careful examination of the peripheral blood films can sometimes identify the mechanism.

Heinz Body Anemia: Oxidizing agents may cause Heinz bodies; irreversibly precipitated hemoglobin attached to the internal surface of the erythrocyte membrane. Affected cells are removed from circulation by the mononuclear phagocyte system; the process is called extravascular hemolysis. Although Heinz bodies can usually be seen with Romanowsky stains, they are much more readily identified with vital stains such as those used to count reticulocytes. The size and number of Heinz bodies are dependent on the causative agent, the dose, and the time after exposure. Heinz bodies observed in chronic, low-level exposures may be small and difficult to see. Acute, high-dose exposures cause large, prominent Heinz bodies and a variety of other morphological changes such as ghost cells (remnants of cell membrane without associated hemoglobin). Agents that produce Heinz bodies have the potential to cause methemoglobinemia and vice versa. Whenever one is observed, the other should be evaluated.

Immune-Mediated Hemolytic Anemia: Many agents can induce immune-mediated hemolytic anemia, although this tends to be an idiosyncratic reaction. There are three general mechanisms by which this occurs: the agent acts as a hapten bound to the erythrocyte membrane; the agent elicits an antibody response and the antigen-antibody complex binds to the erythrocyte membrane; or the agent causes the immune system to mistakenly recognize normal erythrocyte antigens as foreign. Immune-mediated hemolysis is also extravascular. Macrophages of the mononuclear phagocyte system may phagocytize entire erythrocytes or just portions of the membrane coated with immunoglobulin. In the latter case, spherocytes are formed which can be identified microscopically on a peripheral blood film. Animals with immune-mediated hemolytic anemia may be severely anemic, but they usually exhibit a pronounced reticulocytosis. The erythrocytes are less osmotically resistant, and the osmotic fragility test has been performed to support the diagnosis. Unfortunately, this test is nonspecific and labor intensive. Antiglobulin, or Coombs' tests may help to confirm the diagnosis by identifying immunoglobulin and/or complement on the cell surfaces. This test requires species-specific anti-immunoglobulin or anticomplement. Agglutination indicates a positive test. Occasionally, an animal's fresh whole blood will exhibit autoagglutination in the test tube or on a wet mount of the blood; this is provisional evidence that the animal may have immune-mediated disease.

Hemolytic Anemia Due to Parasites: Hemotropic parasites can cause hemolytic anemia, but with the exception of malaria, caused by *Plasmodium* organisms in nonhuman primates, this is an infrequent cause of anemia. Malarial organisms are intracellular and cause hemolysis via multiplication and rupture of the cell. They are readily observed during microscopic examination of blood films, but their appearance in blood fluctuates and it may be necessary to examine blood specimens at multiple intervals. Extracellular organisms that attach to the surface of the cell, such as *Eperythrozoon coccoides* in mice and *Hemobartonella* species in rodents and dogs, are rarely a problem with today's laboratory-reared animals. The infections are generally subclinical, but manifestations of hemolytic anemia can be induced by splenectomy or immunosuppression. Interestingly, subclinical infections in mice may alter certain responses in immune function tests and lead to erroneous conclusions.

Fragmentation Anemia: An unusual form of hemolysis that is rarely observed in toxicology studies is fragmentation anemia. Injury to highly vascular tissue such as the lung, liver, or intestine with the formation of fibrin strands across small vessels can lead to intravascular lysis of erythrocytes as they are "clotheslined" by the fibrin during passage through the vessels. The observation of schistocytes (helmet cells) on peripheral blood films is evidence of the process. Fragmentation anemia may also occur with vascular neoplasms such as hemangiosarcoma. Disseminated intravascular coagulation (DIC) is characterized by, among other things, schistocyte formation. Unfortunately, this condition is usually so severe that the animals bleed to death or die from major organ dysfunction before regeneration is possible.

Nonregenerative Anemia. This type of anemia is characterized by the absence of polychromasia and reticulocytosis. In toxicology studies, nonregenerative anemia is far more common than regenerative anemia. In most cases, it is associated with overall poor health of the treated animals (e.g., poor weight gain or food consumption, poor grooming habits, dull haircoat), and an exact mechanism for the finding is not clear. The erythrocytes appear normal in color (normochromic) and size (normocytic). These animals are only mildly anemic, just enough so that their values can be distinguished from the control animals. Other types of nonregenerative anemia are distinguished by their severity, the presence of morphologically distinct cells, or additional findings that identify the etiology.

Aplastic Anemia: If hematopoietic pluripotent stem cells are injured, as in irradiation or benzene toxicity, the anemia becomes progressively worse because senescent cells are not replaced. This form of anemia is called aplastic anemia. Typically, however, the animal will die from the consequences of severely decreased WBC count (infections) or platelet count (hemorrhage) long before it becomes severely anemic. This is because the circulating survival time of erythrocytes is several weeks, whereas it is only about a week for platelets and about a day for most leukocytes. Agents that damage the microenvironment necessary for hematopoiesis can have a similar effect. In addition, it is possible for a single cell line to be severely depleted without an effect on the others.

Anemia of Chronic Disease and Iron Deficiency Anemia: Chronic inflammatory lesions are associated with mild to moderate nonregenerative anemia. This is not unusual in chronic studies. The putative mechanism is a decrease in the transfer of iron to developing erythrocytes. The cells are normochromic and normocytic. In contrast, iron deficiency, most commonly associated with chronic blood loss or inadequate dietary iron, is characterized by cells that are hypochromic (inadequate hemoglobin) and microcytic. Animals with long-standing iron deficiency anemia have a low MCV and MCHC.

Megaloblastic Anemia: Humans that have folate or vitamin B_{12} deficiency have macrocytic erythrocytes because these nutrients are necessary for deoxyribonucleic acid (DNA) synthesis and developing erythrocytes undergo fewer divisions before maturation. The anemias that result are referred to as megaloblastic, and asynchronous development of erythrocyte precursors is observed in bone marrow smears. Although folate and vitamin B_{12} deficiency are not a problem in animals, agents such as methotrexate that block folate synthesis, or cyclophosphamide, an alkylating agent that inhibits DNA synthesis, can cause megaloblastic anemia in animals.

Nonregenerative Anemia Associated with Chronic Renal or Liver Failure: Chronic renal failure is associated with a moderate to severe nonregenerative, normochromic, normocytic anemia. Although the mechanism sometimes involves decreased erythropoietin, this hormone is often increased during renal failure. There are a number of "uremic toxins" that have been implicated in the anemia of chronic renal disease, and it is undoubtedly a combination of factors that cause decreased hematopoiesis. Chronic liver failure is also associated with moderate anemia. Acanthocytosis, an erythrocyte morphological abnormality characterized by several blunt cytoplasmic projections resembling pseudopodia, is sometimes a feature of this anemia. The mechanism is believed to be an imbalance in the cholesterol:phospholipid ratio in the cell membrane. As with the anemia of renal failure, the anemia of liver failure is not nearly as significant to the animal as the primary organ dysfunction. Endocrine disorders such as hypothyroidism and hypoadrenocorticism may also have mild nonregenerative anemia as part of the disease syndrome.

Nonregenerative Anemia Associated with Leukemia: Finally, nonregenerative anemia is typically a feature of leukemia. The cells are generally normochromic, normocytic unless it is the erythrocytic line that is neoplastic. The principal mechanism of the anemia is the "crowding out" of normal hematopoietic tissue by the neoplastic cell proliferation which competes for nutrients. An interesting exception is large granular lymphocyte leukemia of Fischer-344 rats. By an unknown mechanism, this form of leukemia is associated with a predictable immune-mediated hemolytic anemia that is regenerative.

Polycythemia. Increased RBC count, polycythemia, is fairly unusual in toxicology studies. The most common cause of relative polycythemia is simple dehydration. Relative polycythemia may also be observed secondary to lung disease which causes systemic hypoxia and triggers erythropoietin production. A similar mechanism occurs with systemic alkalosis. By increasing the affinity of hemoglobin for oxygen, alkalosis causes the renal tissue sensors to detect hypoxia, triggering erythropoietin production.

Leukocytes

The examination of leukocytes is part of the minimum hematological database. It includes the quantitative determination of total and differential WBC counts and the qualitative assessment of cellular morphological abnormalities. The differential WBC count enumerates granulocytes (neutrophils, eosinophils, and basophils), lymphocytes, and monocytes. Increased numbers of these cells are called neutrophilia, eosinophilia, basophilia, lymphocytosis, and monocytosis, respectively. Neutropenia, eosinopenia, and lymphopenia refer to decreases. The normal cell counts for basophils and monocytes are so low that decreases are difficult to recognize. Relative counts (percentages) for the different types of leukocytes, obtained by doing the differential count, are of little or no value without knowledge of the total WBC count. A dog with 70% neutrophils could be normal or have neutrophilia or neutropenia depending on the total WBC count. Unfortunately, some of the regulatory guidelines for carcinogenicity studies require differential counts but do not require total WBC counts. By looking only at the relative count data, a 90% lymphocyte count with 100,000 lymphocytes/μl cannot be distinguished from a 90% lymphocyte count with 5000 lymphocytes/μl. Because it is not always possible to microscopically distinguish neoplastic lymphocytes from normal lymphocytes, nothing in the reported data would indicate the possibility of lymphocytic leukemia in the first case. Differential WBC counts should always be reported as absolute numbers.

Neutrophils and lymphocytes are the principal cell types found in peripheral blood, and toxicological effects on leukocytes usually involve these two cell lines. While primary effects occur, the changes observed are most commonly secondary changes in response to primary toxicity of other tissues or organ systems.

Excited or frightened animals may have a physiological leukocytosis (increased WBC count) due to endogenous catecholamine release. Increased heart rate, blood pressure, or muscular activity mobilizes cells that normally marginate along the endothelium of smaller vessels. The addition of these cells may more than double the number flowing freely in circulation and consequently increase the WBC count proportionately. Neutrophilia and lymphocytosis can both occur.

A steroid or stress-induced leukocyte response refers to a combination of changes observed in animals receiving corticosteroids or producing increased endogenous corticosteroids because of some stressful condition. It generally consists of a mature neutrophilia (no immature neutrophils such as bands or metamyelocytes), lymphopenia, eosinopenia, and sometimes monocytosis depending on the animal species. The mature neutrophilia develops as a consequence of increased release of segmented cells from the bone marrow storage pool, decreased margination of cells, decreased movement of cells into tissues, and increased stability of lysosomal membranes. Lymphopenia results from steroid-induced lysis and cell redistribution. Eosinopenia develops as a result of decreased production and release from the bone marrow. And monocytosis, when it occurs, is thought to result from mobilization of marginated cells. It is interesting that the stress-induced leukocyte response is a relatively infrequent finding in toxicology studies even though the study design or the test material often create physical conditions that would appear to be quite stressful.

Neutrophils.   The primary function of the neutrophil is phagocytosis of small particulate matter (e.g., bacteria). The neutrophil is also an integral cellular component of inflammation. It is therefore not unusual to observe neutrophilia secondary to nearly any inflammatory lesion caused by a test material. Unless moderately severe, however, dermal inflammation may not induce increases in neutrophil count. The term *left shift* indicates an increased number of immature neutrophils in circulation. A left shift can occur whenever an inflammatory lesion has a significant demand for neutrophils and immature cells are released from the bone marrow. Lesions that cause a left shift are almost always easily identified, if not by physical examination and the evaluation of other laboratory data, then certainly at necropsy. They frequently involve infectious organisms that have invaded tissue damaged by the test material. A "degenerative" left shift describes the situation of a normal or decreased neutrophil count with more immature than mature neutrophils. It generally indicates a severe infection such as might occur with aspiration pneumonia or during a study using indwelling intravenous catheters that become contaminated, leading to systemic bacterial infection. In severe conditions such as these, when the demand for neutrophils is extreme, so-called toxic neutrophils may be observed. These are neutrophils with morphological changes such as cytoplasmic basophilia, vacuolation, or granulation and Döhle bodies (small, bluish-gray cytoplasmic inclusions that represent aggregated rough endoplasmic reticulum).

Neutropenia occurs for three primary reasons. There may be extreme demand for and consumption of neutrophils as described above. There may be sequestration of neutrophils along the endothelium in capillary beds as occurs in endotoxic shock. And there may be decreased production of neutrophils. Irradiation, chemotherapeutic drugs, inorganic solvents, and estrogens are examples of agents that cause damage to myeloid precursors. It is very common for these agents to also affect erythrocyte and platelet production, but neutropenia and increased susceptibility to bacterial infection will be the hematological problem first encountered. On rare occasion, drugs have been known to induce immune-mediated neutropenia.

Lymphocytes. These are responsible for a wide variety of immune system functions. Although there are many lymphocyte subpopulations, it is not possible to distinguish them by light microscopic examination. Lymphocytes are unique among leukocytes in that they recirculate. That is, lymphocytes leave the vascular system through venules in lymph nodes and ultimately return to the blood through the thoracic duct. They are long-lived cells compared with other leukocytes. The most common cause of lymphocytosis is the physiological lymphocytosis associated with excitement, as previously described. Occasionally increased lymphocyte counts are observed with chronic infections (especially in rodents), and much less frequently with hypersensitivity syndromes and immune-mediated diseases.

Much more common than lymphocytosis is the presence of morphologically distinct lymphocytes sometimes called "reactive" lymphocytes, or immunocytes. They can be seen in low numbers secondary to any type of antigenic stimulation and are so common that no mention is usually made of their presence.

Lymphopenia occurs most frequently as a part of the steroid or stress-induced leukocyte response. Agents that cause neutropenia, such as chemotherapeutic agents, will usually cause lymphopenia as well. Because of the many subpopulations of lymphocytes, it is difficult to know the biological significance of a small change in lymphocyte number. It is possible that a small change could represent an effect on a specific subpopulation of cells. This is the case with HIV infection in humans, but this author is not aware of examples of chemical agents having such a specific effect.

Eosinophils, Basophils, and Monocytes. Absolute eosinophil, basophil, and monocyte counts are normally very low (usually $<1000/\mu l$) and quite variable. It is very unusual, therefore, to be able to detect toxicological effects on these cell types. Eosinophilia may occur secondary to some hypersensitivity syndromes. Eosinopenia may occasionally result from the steroid or stress-induced leukocyte response. The primary function of the monocyte is phagocytosis and digestion of large particulate matter such as senescent cells, necrotic cellular debris, and large microorganisms. Monocytes process antigens and present them to lymphocytes in a more antigenic form. Monocytosis may occur secondary to lesions involving extensive tissue destruction such as neoplasms with associated necrosis or hemolytic anemia.

Leukemia. It is not unusual for a small percentage of rodents (control and treated animals) to develop leukemia in a carcinogenicity study. Animals with leukemia do not always have elevated WBC counts, and neoplastic cells may be difficult to find on peripheral blood films. Unfortunately, when neoplastic cells are present it large numbers, it is often difficult to identify the specific cell type using routine staining procedures and light microscopic examination. The likelihood of diagnosing leukemia is greater during the histopathological examination of animals that died on test or are sacrificed in a moribund condition than by doing periodic examinations of the blood as required by regulatory guidelines.

Platelets

Almost immediately following vascular injury, platelets adhere to exposed collagen and begin to aggregate, forming a primary platelet plug that is sufficient to control bleeding from minor injuries of very small vessels. The aggregated platelets release a variety of substances that stimulate vasoconstriction and fibrin formation. The fibrin acts to cement the mass of platelets into a stable hemostatic plug. Signs of thrombocytopenia (decreased platelet count) include petechial and ecchymotic hemorrhages (most easily observed in mucous membranes), melena, and prolonged bleeding from small wounds such as venipuncture sites. Signs are generally not apparent until the count is less than $50,000/\mu$l. Platelet function defects, such as that caused by aspirin, may cause identical signs, but the tendency to do so is much less. In addition to platelet count, platelet function studies measuring adhesion and aggregation are available but impractical except for investigational studies. Bleeding time is an in vivo test that measures the functional ability of platelets to stop the bleeding from a controlled superficial wound. Although commonly used in human medicine, this test is difficult to standardize in animals. It should also be reserved for investigational purposes.

Thrombocytopenia. This occurs as a result of either decreased production or increased consumption of platelets. Toxins that affect erythroid and myeloid progenitor cells often cause injury to megakaryocytes (platelet precursors). Because the circulating lifespan of platelets is about 7–10 days, acute toxicity of megakaryocytes would lead to decreased platelet count in about a week. Increased consumption of platelets may be caused by immune-mediated phenomena or disseminated intravascular coagulation. In the latter, prolonged coagulation times, decreased plasma fibrinogen concentration, and increased fibrin/fibrinogen degradation products (FDPs) are associated findings. One clue for differentiating decreased production from increased consumption is the presence of large macroplatelets in peripheral blood. These generally indicate that there is increased production of young platelets that are larger than normal.

Thrombocytosis. Increased platelet count, thrombocytosis, is rarely a primary effect of a test material. It may be observed as a secondary effect in conjunction with generalized bone marrow stimulation as in hemolytic anemia or some types of inflammatory diseases. Thrombocytosis is also associated with iron deficiency. The increases in platelet numbers that occur in toxicology studies are generally small and not likely to have any biological significance. If platelet counts were markedly elevated, however, the potential for thromboembolic events would be increased.

Coagulation

The coagulation mechanism is traditionally divided into two pathways. The intrinsic pathway, routinely evaluated by the activated partial thromboplastin time (APTT) or the activated coagulation time (ACT), begins with exposure of factor XII to subendothelial collagen or other abnormal surfaces. The extrinsic pathway, evaluated by the one-stage prothrombin time (PT), is initiated by exposure of factor VII to tissue thromboplastin. Both mechanisms share the terminal sequence of events, including conversion of pro-thrombin to thrombin, which in turn converts fibrinogen to fibrin. The coagulation assays can be difficult to perform in smaller laboratory animal species because of sample collection problems.

The assays are not particularly sensitive to small changes in the concentration of clotting factors. In general, the activity of a single factor must be reduced below approximately 30% of normal before coagulation times are prolonged. Given the conditions in most toxicology studies, where animals are exposed to the test material for a prolonged period of time, if there were an effect on the production of a clotting factor, it is likely that the animals would exhibit some form of bleeding diathesis. These include severe hemorrhage externally (e.g., epistaxis or hematochezia) or internally (e.g., subcutaneous hematoma, hemothorax, or hemarthrosis). In most cases, reliance on the coagulation assays to detect a test material effect is probably unnecessary. However, in those situations when there is a known effect or an effect is likely, carefully planned coagulation assays may help to define the clinical picture.

The majority of clotting factors are synthesized by the liver. Liver injury and dysfunction must be quite severe in order to cause depletion of clotting factors sufficient to prolong the coagulation assays. The liver requires vitamin K for the production of functional forms of factors II, VII, IX, and X. Vitamin K antagonists, such as warfarin and diphacinone, cause prolongation of both the intrinsic and extrinsic mechanism assays. Because factor VII has the shortest half-life and is part of the extrinsic mechanism, prolonged PT occurs before prolonged APTT. Since vitamin K is a fat-soluble vitamin, coagulation assays are indicated when test materials are administered that have the potential of depleting fat-soluble vitamins. This is true of some of the recently developed synthetic fats that are not absorbed by the intestine.

Depletion of all clotting factors with subsequently prolonged coagulation times is a feature of DIC. Fibrinogen concentrations and FDP assays are used to help confirm the diagnosis.

Small, statistically significant differences in mean PT or APTT between control and treated animals (e.g., 2 sec) are occasionally observed in toxicology studies. This degree of change has little or no biological impact on the individual animals. However, it should not be casually dismissed because it may be an early indication of a potential problem. Depending on the test material, it may be necessary to design longer studies or increase the dose levels to see if the effect is repeatable and meaningful.

Clinical Chemistry

The clinical chemistry tests routinely performed during toxicology studies generate information concerning carbohydrate, lipid, and protein metabolism, renal function, liver function, hepatocyte injury, and electrolyte balance. Advances in clinical chemistry instrumentation have greatly reduced sample volume requirements and have therefore enabled the laboratory to produce complete biochemical profiles on animals as small as rats without compromising the study because of excessive blood collection. Many newer instruments can use 250 μl of serum or less to run a 17–18 test panel. The vast majority of common tests do not require modification of the methods that are used for testing human samples. There are, however, many differences in the expected ranges of results for individual species. When purchasing an instrument and reagents for work with animal specimens, volume requirements (including dead space) and ranges of linearity are very important considerations.

Carbohydrate, Lipids, and Proteins

Glucose. Serum glucose concentration depends upon intestinal absorption, hepatic production, and tissue uptake of glucose. The balance between hepatic production and tissue uptake is influenced by a variety of hormones, including insulin, glucagon, corticosteroids, adrenocorticotropic hormone (ACTH), growth hormone, and catecholamines. Insulin is the primary factor responsible for the uptake of glucose by tissues. Corticosteroids, catecholamines, and growth hormone are called insulin antagonists because they interfere with insulin's action on cells. Furthermore, hepatic gluconeogenesis is stimulated by glucagon and glucocorticoids, and glycogenolysis is stimulated by glucagon and catecholamines. These actions tend to increase serum glucose concentration. The practice of fasting animals prior to blood collection is primarily intended to avoid the variability that accompanies postprandial intestinal absorption of glucose. Another procedural consideration for glucose analysis is prompt separation of the serum from the clotted blood. As mentioned previously, erythrocyte, and to a lesser degree leukocyte, glycolysis will spuriously reduce serum glucose concentration by approximately 7–10 mg/dl every hour that the blood cells remain in contact with the serum at room temperature.

Hyperglycemia and Hypoglycemia: The most frequently encountered causes of hyperglycemia are failure to fast an animal and catecholamine release secondary to excitement or fear. Animals that become moribund occasionally develop hyperglycemia. Less frequently encountered causes, especially in toxicology studies, include insufficient insulin (diabetes mellitus and pancreatitis) and increased glucocorticoids (hyperadrenocorticism and steroid therapy). Hypoglycemia may result from improper handling of the specimen, malnutrition, malabsorption, severe hepatic disease, endotoxemia, and some tumors, in particular, insulinomas and hepatomas. Occasionally in toxicology studies, treated animals that fail to thrive and gain body weight will also have mildly lower serum glucose concentration (e.g., 10–15 mg/dl) than the control animals even though there are no differences in food consumption. Although the mechanism for this phenomenon is not clear, two possibilities are poor assimilation of the food and alteration of the body's "set-point" for serum glucose. Regardless of the cause, the reduction is probably of little biological importance and is simply a reflection of the overall process that has caused the animals to do poorly.

Cholesterol and Triglycerides. Cholesterol is required for the biosynthesis of bile acids, corticosteroids, and sex steroids. Triglycerides serve as an important source of energy. Serum cholesterol and triglycerides are derived from dietary intake and endogenous synthesis, primarily by the liver. The liver, via the biliary system, is the major excretory pathway for cholesterol. In circulation, cholesterol and triglycerides are components of chylomicrons and the lipoproteins: very low-density lipoprotein (VLDL), low-density lipoprotein (LDL), and high-density lipoprotein (HDL). Chylomicrons, which cause serum to appear lipemic, are produced by intestinal cells after a fatty meal and are rich in triglycerides. Hepatocytes synthesize VLDL, which has less triglyceride than chylomicrons but more cholesterol. The triglycerides in chylomicrons and VLDLs are broken down to free fatty acids and monoglycerides by lipoprotein lipase attached to the surface of endothelial cells, especially in the capillaries of adipose tissue and muscle. Adipocytes tend to reesterify the fatty acids for storage as triglycerides. Muscle tends to oxidize the fatty acids for energy. The loss of triglyceride causes VLDL to become LDL. In humans, about two-thirds of serum cholesterol is transported by LDL. In contrast, HDL, generated by the liver and other tissues, is the principal lipoprotein responsible for cholesterol transport in several animal species. Species differences in lipid metabolism make it quite difficult to correlate effects in animal models with those in humans.

Serum triglyceride concentration is elevated postprandially, while serum cholesterol concentration is relatively stable. Both are elevated in hypothyroidism and diabetes mellitus. Cholesterol is the predominant lipid in hypothyroidism, and triglycerides predominate in diabetes mellitus. In both cases, lipoprotein lipase activity is reduced.

Biliary stasis, whether intrahepatic or extrahepatic, and other forms of liver disease can increase serum cholesterol concentration, but severe liver disease is associated with hypocholesterolemia.

The nephrotic syndrome, which is almost always the result of glomerular injury, is characterized by increased urinary protein excretion, hypoalbuminemia, and hypercholesterolemia. Steroid therapy, and perhaps hyperadrenocorticism, are also associated with increased serum cholesterol concentration. As might be expected, nutrient deficiency and malassimilation can cause decreased serum cholesterol concentration.

Effects on serum cholesterol concentration are relatively frequent findings in toxicology studies. Both increases and decreases are observed. While the changes are usually small and generally believed to represent minor alterations in lipid metabolism, the exact mechanisms involved are rarely identified. Many factors are probably involved, including food consumption and assimilation, body weight and composition, activity, and hormone balance.

Protein.   Total serum protein concentration is a measure of all of the different proteins in plasma with the exception of those that are consumed in clot formation such as fibrinogen and the clotting factors. For this reason, plasma protein concentration is generally about 0.3–0.5 g/dl higher than serum protein concentration.

Albumin: Albumin is the most abundant individual protein and is largely responsible for maintaining intravascular oncotic pressure. Albumin also serves as a storage reservoir of amino acids and as a transport protein, binding most plasma constituents that do not have a specific transport protein.

Globulins: The globulins constitute a heterogeneous population of proteins, including specific transport proteins (e.g., transferrin for iron, lipoproteins for lipids, haptoglobin for hemoglobin, and thyroxine-binding globulin for thyroxine), mediators of inflammation (e.g., complement and C-reactive protein), clotting factors (e.g., fibrinogen, thrombin, and factor VIII), catalysts and inhibitors of biochemical reactions (e.g., enzymes), and immunoglobulins (e.g., IgG, IgM, and IgA). Globulins are nonspecifically categorized by their electrophoretic migration pattern as α-, β-, and γ-globulins. Depending on the animal species, these regions may be further subdivided; most species have two α regions, alpha$_1$ and alpha$_2$. Immunoglobulins are generally found in the γ regions of the electrophoretogram but some, IgM in particular, also extend into the β regions. The liver synthesizes albumin and most of the globulins, with the major exception of immunoglobulins.

Serum Protein Electrophoresis: In most laboratories, total serum protein and albumin concentrations are measured directly, and serum globulin concentration is calculated by subtraction. Serum protein electrophoresis is sometimes valuable for determining the cause of increased or decreased globulin concentration, and its use should be reserved for that purpose. A broad-based increase in γ-globulins, generally the result of antigenic stimulation, is termed a polyclonal gammopathy because plasma cells have produced a heterogeneous population of immunoglobulins in response to the antigenic challenge. A narrow-based increase in γ-globulins in termed a monoclonal gammopathy and is usually the result of a single immunoglobulin class being produced in excess by a single clone of lymphocytes or plasma cells. Most frequently, but not always, the clone of cells is neoplastic (e.g., multiple myeloma). An increase of the α-globulin regions, especially alpha$_2$, frequently occurs secondary to inflammation and the production of acute-phase reactant proteins. These acute-phase proteins (e.g., alpha$_2$-macroglobulin, haptoglobin, and ceruloplasmin) are part of the general response to inflammation.

In general, the cost: benefit ratio of serum protein electrophoresis would indicate that it not be routinely run as part of the minimum database. Unfortunately, some regulatory guidelines recommend routine serum protein electrophoresis in safety assessment studies. If the production of a single, specific protein in the α or β regions were affected by a test material, the absence of change in the other proteins of the same region would probably be sufficient to mask any effect on the electrophoretogram. On the other hand, if the test material does affect a particular region, further identification procedures are necessary because electrophoresis does not identify specific globulin proteins.

Hyperproteinemia: The most frequent causes of hyperproteinemia are dehydration and polyclonal gammopathy secondary to antigenic stimulation. Monoclonal gammopathies are rare in toxicology studies. When uncomplicated dehydration is the cause of hyperproteinemia, both serum albumin and serum globulin concentrations will be increased proportionately.

Hypoproteinemia: This results from either decreased production or increased loss of protein. In dietary toxicity studies, decreased protein production may result from effects on food consumption, digestion, or absorption. Because of the reserve capacity of the liver, hepatic injury must be fairly severe before protein synthesis is notably diminished. However, in large studies, small differences between the control and treated groups may be apparent with mild-to-moderate hepatotoxicity. Loss of protein, both albumin and globulin, occurs with hemorrhage and exudative lesions such as burns. Albumin is the principal protein lost as a result of enteropathies and glomerulopathies. The half-life of albumin is shorter in smaller species; approximately 2 days for mice and approximately 8 days for dogs (Kaneko, 1989). Theoretically, impaired albumin synthesis or albumin loss could be detected earlier in the smaller species. Hydration status of the animal is always an important factor for proper interpretation of changes in serum protein concentrations. Hypoproteinemia, like anemia, can be masked by dehydration. A small, statistically significant decrease in serum albumin concentration is one of the most frequent findings in toxicology studies. The exact mechanism is usually not apparent but a combination of factors, similar to those causing mildly lower glucose, are probably responsible.

Renal Function

Serum urea nitrogen concentration and serum creatinine concentration are used in conjunction with urine specific gravity or osmolality to evaluate renal function. These tests are relatively insensitive to small effects on the kidney, and there are a number of nonrenal causes for serum elevations that must be considered.

Urea Nitrogen.   Urea is synthesized by the liver from ammonia that is absorbed from the intestine or generated by endogenous protein catabolism. It is freely filtered through the glomerulus and excreted in urine. Some urea is passively reabsorbed with water in the proximal tubule; the amount that is reabsorbed is inversely related to rate of urine flow through the tubules. Decreased glomerular filtration rate (GFR) causes serum urea nitrogen concentration to increase. However, because urea production can vary with diet or protein catabolism, serum urea nitrogen elevations do not necessarily indicate kidney disease. Increased serum urea nitrogen concentration, termed azotemia, can be categorized as prerenal, renal, or postrenal.

Prerenal Azotemia: This type of azotemia develops as a result of increased hepatic urea synthesis or decreased renal blood flow. The former may result from high protein diets or conditions that increase protein catabolism such as starvation, fever, infection, tissue necrosis, and high gastrointestinal hemorrhage. Decreased renal blood flow, with subsequently decreased GFR, may result from dehydration, shock (hemorrhagic or circulatory), or cardiovascular disease. The changes in serum urea nitrogen concentration caused by increased urea synthesis are typically small, but those caused by decreased renal perfusion are dependent on the degree of GFR reduction and can be quite large. The concentrating ability of the kidney is not affected by these conditions. In the case of prerenal azotemia due to dehydration, the kidneys will attempt to conserve body water and urine specific gravity will be elevated.

Renal Azotemia: This type of azotemia develops as a result of primary renal disease or toxicity. The renal lesions can be acute or chronic. Unfortunately, because of the sizable reserve capacity of the kidney, serum urea nitrogen concentration does not increase until approximately 75% of the kidneys' nephrons are nonfunctional. By this time, renal concentrating ability is usually impaired and urine specific gravity is isosthenuric (i.e., the same as the glomerular filtrate: 1.008–1.012). An indication of the chronicity of the renal lesions may be gleaned from the hematology data. Concurrent nonregenerative anemia suggests that the lesions are chronic.

Postrenal Azotemia: This type of azotemia results from obstruction of the urinary outflow tract. This is rarely observed in toxicology studies, but test materials that promote urinary calculi formation might cause this condition.

Creatinine.   This is a nonprotein nitrogenous waste material that is freely filtered by the glomerulus and, unlike urea, is not reabsorbed by the tubules. It is formed at a fairly constant rate by the breakdown of creatine, a molecule that stores energy in muscle as phosphocreatine. Serum creatinine concentration is influenced by muscle mass and conditioning but is relatively independent of dietary influences and protein catabolism. Although it tends to rise and fall more slowly, serum creatinine concentration parallels changes in serum urea nitrogen concentration caused by alterations in renal blood flow, renal function, or urinary outflow.

Endogenous creatinine clearance is sometimes used as a measure of GFR because blood levels of creatinine are relatively stable over short intervals, creatinine is freely filtered, and creatinine is not significantly secreted or reabsorbed. Endogenous creatinine clearance may underestimate the true GFR because of the presence of noncreatinine chromagens that spuriously increase the measure of serum creatinine concentration but not urinary creatinine concentration.

Liver Function and Hepatocyte Injury

The critical metabolic, synthetic, and excretory roles of the liver and the abundant enzymatic machinery needed to perform these functions result in a large number of biochemical parameters that may be altered due to toxicity. On the other hand, the large functional reserve of the liver makes possible a significant loss of tissue with minimal or no detectable change in routine laboratory tests. While no single test is superior for detecting liver toxicity, the pattern of abnormal findings in a battery of tests may help to determine the location and severity of liver lesions.

Many enzymes have been identified that have increased serum activity when hepatocellular damage is present. Although these enzyme activities are not measures of liver function, they can detect cellular degeneration or necrosis. The utility of a particular enzyme depends on a number of factors, including relative specificity to liver, intrahepatic location, intracellular location, concentration gradient between cell and serum, serum half-life, in vitro stability, and the ease, accuracy, and economy of measurement. Alanine aminotransferase (ALT), aspartate aminotransferase (AST), sorbitol dehydrogenase (SDH), lactate dehydrogenase (LDH), and glutamate dehydrogenase (GDH) are some of the enzymes that have been used to evaluate hepatocellular damage. Each has advantages and disadvantages, some of which depend on the laboratory animal species being tested.

Serum ALT Activity. In general, serum ALT activity, formerly known as serum glutamic pyruvic transaminase (SGPT), is the most useful enzyme activity for identifying the presence of hepatocellular damage. The enzyme is found in many tissues, but its greatest concentration in most species is within hepatocytes. For practical purposes, significant elevations of serum activity result only from hepatocyte ALT. The enzyme is primarily cytosolic, and its concentration within the cell is up to 10,000 times greater than that in the serum. Therefore, ALT may leak into serum in any condition that alters membrane permeability to a sufficient degree. Leakage does not require cell death; elevated activity does not imply necrosis. The magnitude of serum activity elevation is proportional to the number of affected hepatocytes and is not indicative of the reversibility of the lesion. For example, it is possible to have higher serum ALT activity following reversible cellular hypoxia secondary to hypovolemic shock than might occur with focal necrosis caused by a localized hepatic abscess. Of course, the greatest elevations result from severe lesions that affect a large portion of the liver tissue.

Following an acute hepatotoxic episode, serum ALT activity will rise within 12 hr. Depending upon the injury, the activity will peak in 1–2 days and then decline. Prolonged elevations may reflect increased production of ALT in regenerative liver tissue or continued leakage from cells whose close proximity to the primary lesion has resulted in degenerative changes secondary to the altered microenvironment. However, acute studies designed so that clinical pathology tests are run 14 days after a single administration of the test material are likely to miss changes in serum ALT activity even if the test material causes marked hepatotoxicity (e.g., carbon tetrachloride).

Increased serum ALT activity is not specific for primary hepatocellular disease. Bile duct obstruction also causes increased activity. The probable mechanism is that retained bile salts physically damage the cell membranes of surrounding hepatocytes. Drugs such as corticosteroids and anticonvulsants appear to induce ALT production. These drugs can also cause pathological changes that result in enzyme leakage, however, and without histopathological examination, it is difficult to determine whether an elevation is due to enzyme induction or drug-induced disease.

Serum AST and LDH Activities. Serum AST (formerly serum glutamic oxaloacetic transaminase; SGOT) and LDH activities tends to parallel serum ALT activity with respect to liver damage. Unfortunately, they are not liver-specific because of high concentrations in other tissues, especially muscle. In small species, blood collection techniques sometimes cause increased variability among animals, reflected in wider reference ranges. There appears to be no advantage in determining both of these enzyme activities, and AST is generally preferred. In most species, elevations in serum AST activity due to hepatotoxicity are not as pronounced as the elevations in serum ALT activity; this may occur because a portion of AST is mitochondrial. Corticosteroids and anticonvulsants affect AST in a similar manner as ALT. Decreased serum activities of AST and/or ALT are occasionally observed in toxicology studies and may indicate decreased hepatocellular production or release, inhibition of the enzymes' activity, interference with the enzyme assay, or an effect on the coenzyme, pyroidoxal 5'-phosphate (vitamin B_6). Decreased serum activity of these enzymes has not been shown to be a pathologically important phenomenon.

Serum SDH and GDH Activities. Serum SDH and GDH activities, neither of which are used in human medicine in the United States, have occasionally been recommended as good indicators of hepatic toxicity in laboratory animal species. Increased serum activity of each enzyme is liver specific; SDH is a cytosolic enzyme and GDH is mitochondrial. Theoretically, in order for serum GDH activity to increase, the cell damage must be relatively severe. Elevations in serum SDH activity return to baseline levels faster than for other liver enzymes because of a short serum half-life. The major drawback for both of these enzymes is the assay. Their lack of popularity in human medicine is responsible for the absence of standard automated procedures.

There are a few serum enzymes, originating from hepatocytes and biliary epithelial cells, that increase as a result of increased production secondary to intrahepatic or extrahepatic cholestasis and biliary proliferation. These include serum alkaline phosphatase (AP), γ-glutamyl transferase (GGT), leucine aminopeptidase (LAP), and 5'-nucleotidase (5'N). The most commonly used are AP and GGT. Both are bound to cytoplasmic and microsomal membranes. The mechanism for the cholestasis-induced production is uncertain, but bile acids are thought to stimulate enzyme synthesis.

Serum AP Activity. In the dog, serum AP activity is the most sensitive test for detecting cholestasis. It lacks specificity, however. Isoenzymes of AP are produced by cells of the intestine, kidney cortex, liver, bone, placenta, and myeloid series. Techniques for isoenzyme separation are available, but they are not easily used. Regardless, there are some guidelines that aid in the interpretation of increased serum AP activity. Normal serum AP activity in most adult animals is primarily the liver isoenzyme. Young, growing animals have an increased amount of the bone isoenzyme in serum secondary to increased osteoblast activity. In humans, but not dogs, placental isoenzyme is increased during pregnancy. The isoenzymes of liver and bone have half-lives of about 3 days in the dog, whereas those of intestine, kidney, and placenta are only 3–6 min. It is very unlikely that any of the latter three isoenzymes will produce serum elevations. Elevations in the bone isoenzyme rarely exceed three to five times the normal adult levels, even in young animals and animals with metabolic bone diseases. Corticosteroids and anticonvulsants can induce liver isoenzyme production. Knowledge of the test material characteristics may help to identify probable drug-induced increases. In some dogs, a unique steroid-induced isoenzyme can cause extremely high serum AP activity.

Because of cell swelling and pressure obstruction of small bile ductules, primary hepatocellular toxicities can and do cause enough intrahepatic cholestasis to elevate serum AP activity. Periportal lesions induce greater increases than do centrilobular lesions. Extrahepatic cholestasis, as might be seen with pancreatitis or biliary calculi, stimulates higher serum AP activity than intrahepatic cholestasis. Unfortunately, the degree of elevation is rarely sufficient for differentiating primary hepatocellular toxicity from primary biliary toxicity.

Serum GGT Activity.   In the last decade, serum GGT activity became popular because it purportedly had fewer interpretation problems than serum AP activity. Although its highest tissue concentrations are in the kidney and pancreas, serum elevations are reported to occur only with hepatobiliary lesions and certain drug therapies. Like AP, it can be induced by steroids and other drugs. Unlike AP, it is not affected by bone growth or disease. Furthermore, its serum activity is less likely to increase secondary to primary hepatocellular toxicity or intrahepatic cholestasis due to hepatocellular swelling. In laboratory animal species, GGT appears somewhat less sensitive to hepatobiliary disease than AP; however, there are some exceptions (Leonard et al., 1984; Ghys et al., 1975).

Serum LAP and 5'N activities have been investigated as alternatives to serum AP activity but have not found general acceptance. In some models of liver toxicity, 5'N appears to be more sensitive than AP. Further investigation is warranted.

The absence of change in serum hepatic enzyme activities does not signify an absence of hepatic toxicity. As previously mentioned, elevations can be missed by poor timing of clinical pathology testing. Furthermore, serum enzyme activities do not constitute hepatic function tests. The liver can be severely dysfunctional and yet have little or no ongoing cellular degeneration.

Bilirubin.   Heme breakdown by cells of the mononuclear phagocyte system produces bilirubin. Hemoglobin from senescent erythrocytes provides about 85% of all bilirubin; hemoglobin from ineffective erythropoiesis provides another major source. Macrophage enzymes split hemoglobin into heme and globin, and heme is broken down into biliverdin and iron. Biliverdin reductase converts biliverdin to bilirubin, which is then released into circulation. At this point, the bilirubin is known as free, unconjugated, prehepatic, or indirect-reacting bilirubin. It is not water soluble and circulates bound to albumin. Hepatocytes remove unconjugated bilirubin from plasma and prepare it for removal from the body by a 4-step process that includes uptake, conjugation, secretion, and excretion. Secretion of conjugated bilirubin across the canalicular membrane is the rate-limiting step in the process, and small amounts of conjugated or direct-reacting bilirubin escape into plasma, not bound to albumin. Conjugated bilirubin is freely filtered through the glomerulus. In most species, it is reabsorbed by the renal tubular epithelium, but in the dog the renal threshold is low and traces of bilirubin are normal in concentrated urine.

The van den Bergh test differentiates unconjugated (or indirect) bilirubin from conjugated (or direct) bilirubin. The test is not very sensitive and should not be run unless the total bilirubin concentration is greater than 2 to 3 mg/dl. It was designed to help distinguish prehepatic causes of hyperbilirubinemia from hepatic or posthepatic causes in clinical cases. In toxicology studies, however, the combination of clinical observations, other laboratory data (e.g., hematocrit and liver enzyme activities), and anatomical pathology findings are usually more than sufficient to determine the mechanism of hyperbilirubinemia. Laboratory determination of direct and indirect bilirubin is generally of little value.

Hyperbilirubinemia: Prehepatic or unconjugated hyperbilirubinemia is a very uncommon finding in toxicology studies. It occurs almost exclusively as a result of acute, moderate to severe hemolysis. If hepatocytes are unable to process the large amount of unconjugated bilirubin produced by the mononuclear phagocyte system during a hemolytic episode, there will be an increase in total serum bilirubin concentration consisting primarily of the free form. It has been estimated that the healthy liver has the capacity to metabolize up to 30 times more free bilirubin than normal before hyperbilirubinemia results. A hemolytic event sufficient to overload a normal liver and cause unconjugated hyperbilirubinemia can be expected to exhibit other evidence of hemolysis. Unconjugated hyperbilirubinemia may occur with less severe hemolysis if diminished hepatic function already exists. There are a number of nonhemolytic unconjugated hyperbilirubinemia syndromes in humans that result from biochemical defects in the uptake and conjugation of free bilirubin. The Gunn rat is an animal model of defective conjugation.

Conjugated hyperbilirubinemia occurs as a result of impaired secretion of bilirubin, obstruction of bile outflow, or both. Because bilirubin secretion is the rate-limited step, any disease that damages the hepatocyte can potentially increase serum conjugated bilirubin concentration. Obstruction to bile flow may be either intrahepatic or extrahepatic in origin. As with serum AP activity, periportal lesions will induce greater hyperbilirubinemia than will centrilobular lesions and extrahepatic obstructions cause higher serum bilirubin concentration than do intrahepatic obstructions. In the dog, when hyperbilirubinemia is the result of a cholestatic process, serum AP activity will always be elevated.

Hyperbilirubinemia is most commonly due to increases in both conjugated and unconjugated bilirubin. For instance, hemolytic diseases can cause secondary hepatocyte dysfunction due to hypoxia. The result is swollen hepatocytes that have impaired ability to secrete conjugated bilirubin. Alternately, biliary obstruction can cause secondary hepatocyte damage that may decrease the uptake and conjugation of free bilirubin.

Unlike hepatic enzyme activities, serum bilirubin concentration is a measure of liver function. In the absence of hemolysis, hyperbilirubinemia is an indication that the liver is not functioning properly. In most examples of hepatotoxicity, however, there is normal total serum bilirubin because of the tremendous functional reserve of the liver. In the dog, where some conjugated bilirubin is excreted in urine, a 70% hepatectomy will not elevate serum bilirubin concentration.

It is interesting to note that human patients receiving anticonvulsant therapy have lower serum bilirubin levels than the population as a whole. Enzyme induction apparently enhances the metabolism and excretion of bilirubin and could potentially mask an otherwise elevated bilirubin level.

Bile Acids. These are synthesized from cholesterol by hepatocytes, conjugated to an amino acid, secreted into the biliary system, and eventually excreted into the intestine. Bacteria transform some of the primary bile acids to secondary bile acids in the intestine. There is a very efficient enterohepatic circulation of bile acids, with the greatest part of the reabsorption occurring from the ileum. Portal blood returns the bile acids to the liver for uptake, reconjugation, and resecretion. Any toxicity that affects the liver can potentially alter one of the steps in the metabolism of bile acids and cause increased levels in serum. While not commonly used in toxicology studies at this time, total serum bile acid concentration is sensitive and specific for hepatobiliary toxicity. By itself, however, total serum bile acid concentration does not provide enough information to discriminate between different types of hepatic lesions. Like serum bilirubin concentration, bile acids are a measure of a hepatic function.

The synthetic role of the liver has been previously mentioned concerning glucose, cholesterol, urea nitrogen, and a variety of proteins. Severe hepatocellular dysfunction may cause decreased serum urea nitrogen concentration, hypoglycemia, hypocholesterolemia, hypoproteinemia (especially hypoalbuminemia), and prolonged coagulation times. On the other hand, liver disease may result in hypercholesterolemia and hyperglobulinemia. The pattern of changes elicited by liver toxicity is complex and multifaceted. Examination of the entire biochemical profile, along with hematological and urinalysis findings, is necessary to properly evaluate liver toxicity.

Calcium and Inorganic Phosphorus

Calcium.   Serum calcium concentration is affected by parathyroid hormone, calcitonin, and vitamin D and represents a balance between intestinal absorption, bone formation and reabsorption, and urinary excretion. Serum inorganic phosphorus concentration is affected by the same hormones, but is more sensitive to dietary intake and urinary excretion. In order to interpret the changes in either of these parameters, it is helpful to know the results of the other. Unfortunately, one of the regulatory agencies does not have inorganic phosphorus on its list of recommended tests for safety assessment studies.

Approximately 50% of serum calcium is ionized. As such, it is biologically active and participates in neuromuscular activity, bone formation, coagulation, and other biochemical mechanisms. Approximately 40% of serum calcium is bound to albumin in an inactive, unionized state. The remaining serum calcium is complexed to anions such as phosphate and citrate.

Hypercalcemia.   This is relatively uncommon in toxicology studies unless the test material, like some plant toxins, has properties of vitamin D. Miscellaneous causes of hypercalcemia include hypervitaminosis D, primary hyperparathyroidism, pseudohyperparathyroidism (i.e., secondary to some types of neoplasia), and occasionally renal disease.

Hypocalcemia.   Mildly decreased serum calcium concentration, secondary to hypoalbuminemia, is a frequent finding in toxicology studies. In these studies, signs of hypocalcemia do not occur because ionized calcium is relatively unaffected. Other miscellaneous and much less frequent causes of hypocalcemia include hypoparathyroidism, nutritional hyperparathyroidism, acute pancreatitis, puerpural tetany in the bitch, and renal disease.

Hyperphosphatemia and Hypophosphatemia.   Increased serum inorganic phosphorus concentration is a normal finding in young animals. It may be as high or higher than serum calcium concentration. Serum inorganic phosphorus concentration is very sensitive to GFR and may be increased with prerenal, renal, or postrenal azotemia. Other less frequent causes of hyperphosphatemia include hypervitaminosis D, hypoparathyroidism, and nutritional hyperparathyroidism due to excess dietary phosphorus. Greatly decreased food consumption may cause hypophosphatemia, and this is sometimes observed in dietary toxicity studies if the animals refuse to eat.

Sodium, Potassium, and Chloride

Sodium is the major cation in serum and is the principal determinant of extracellular fluid volume (i.e., hydration status). Potassium is the major intracellular cation. Serum potassium concentration is maintained within narrow limits because of its critical role in neuromuscular and cardiac excitability. Chloride is the major anion in serum and serves to support fluid homeostasis and balance cation secretion.

While reference ranges for these parameters may appear fairly wide, the range of results in a well-controlled study is often quite narrow. Occasionally, very small statistically significant differences occur between control and treated groups in toxicology studies. Unfortunately, the mechanism for the difference is usually not apparent.

In most instances, serum sodium and chloride concentrations tend to parallel each other. Hypernatremia is relatively rare, but hyperchloremia may sometimes occur secondary to secretory diarrhea with metabolic acidosis. In this condition, renal tubular reabsorption of chloride is increased because of decreased availability of bicarbonate. Decreased serum sodium and chloride concentrations can occur with gastrointestinal losses (e.g., vomiting or diarrhea), polyuric renal losses (e.g., chronic renal failure or diabetes mellitus), diuretics, and hypoadrenocorticism (a rare finding in toxicology studies). Vomiting may cause hypochloremia and normonatremia because chloride, as hydrochloric acid, may be lost in excess of sodium.

Serum potassium concentration is a relatively poor indicator of total body potassium because of shifts between intracellular and extracellular compartments. Increased serum potassium concentration occurs with acidosis due to the exchange of extracellular hydrogen ions for intracellular potassium ions. Severe tissue necrosis and anuric or oliguric renal disease are infrequent causes of hyperkalemia. Decreased serum potassium concentration, like the changes in sodium and chloride, is associated with gastrointestinal losses and polyuric renal losses. Potassium is also sensitive to decreased dietary intake and serum concentrations may be decreased along with inorganic phosphorus in animals that refuse to eat. Finally, an infrequent cause of hypokalemia is alkalosis.

Urinalysis

Urinalysis is part of the minimum laboratory database for clinically ill patients. It provides a specific evaluation of the urogenital tract as well as information concerning more generalized conditions. As a general observation, however, urinalysis is utilized improperly in many toxicology studies. For the most part, this is due to the technical difficulties associated with collecting a large number of urine specimens from small laboratory animals. The method by which urine is collected greatly influences the value and interpretation of the data obtained. If a toxin is known or suspected to affect the urinary system, measures can be taken to provide appropriate specimens for urinalysis (i.e., by catheterization, cystocentesis, or carefully collected voided samples). Usually, however, when a large number of animals are being tested with a test material of unknown toxic potential, and regulatory guidelines require urinalysis, the most efficient method of urine collection (i.e., in a collection vessel at the bottom of a metabolic cage) produces a multitude of artifacts that diminish the value of the test results and may make interpretation impossible. Voided urine traverses the urethra, vagina or prepuce, and perineum or preputial hairs where it can acquire both cells and bacteria. Added to the environmental contaminants in the bottom of a cage (e.g., cleaning chemicals, feces, bacteria, food, and hair) and given time (16–24 hrs) to incubate, it is little wonder that urinalysis data from timed collections in a metabolic cage are less than desirable. Furthermore, it is nearly impossible to keep the collection vessel chilled during a prolonged collection and preservatives such as toluene have disadvantages that preclude their use. The following discussion of the various parts of the urinalysis addresses the major issues of interpretation with respect to potential false-positive and false-negative results.

The urinalysis consists of two parts: physicochemical properties and sediment evaluation. The physicochemical properties include color, clarity, volume (for timed collections), specific gravity, and the reagent strip tests (pH, protein, glucose, ketones, bilirubin, urobilinogen, and occult blood). Some reagent strips have additional tests for nitrite (indicates presence of nitrite-producing bacteria) and leukocyte esterase, but these are not particularly valuable for animal specimens. Urinary enzyme activities, for the identification of renal tubule toxicity, are sometimes determined in investigational studies on test materials that are known or potential renal toxins.

Urinary sediment evaluation is a semiquantitative microscopic measure of the presence of cells, casts, bacteria, and crystals. In order to properly evaluate changes in the physicochemical properties of urine, it is important to know the urine sediment results. The reverse is also true.

Urine Volume and Specific Gravity

Timed urine volume and urine specific gravity are the only measures of renal function in the urinalysis. They demonstrate the ability of the kidneys to perform work. The loss of urine concentrating ability generally precedes the development of azotemia as a consequence of primary renal disease. Urine specific gravity, as determined by refractometry, is an approximation of the solute concentration, but it is dependent on molecular size and weight as well as the total number of solute molecules. Urine specific gravity usually varies inversely with urine volume. Animals that have lost the ability to concentrate their urine will have decreased urine specific gravity and increased urine volume. However, since urine specific gravity is a function of fluid intake, solute intake, glomerular filtration, renal tubular cell health, and other factors, the range of values that can be considered physiologically normal (e.g., 1.001–1.075) is quite large.

Hyposthenuria (i.e., urine specific gravity = 1.001–1.007) is sometimes observed in toxicology studies. Perhaps the most common cause is a leaky water bottle or automatic water system. More importantly, however, some nonhuman primates develop psychogenic polydipsia which results in excretion of very dilute urine. Because of high urine flow through the kidney, these animals may develop medullary washout and lose the ability to concentrate urine even if water is withheld. If water is unavailable, they can rapidly become dangerously dehydrated. For this and other reasons, it is probably inappropriate to withhold water from nonhuman primates. Unfortunately, some monkeys play with their water source habitually and make urinalysis results from cage-bottom specimens meaningless. There are many diseases that cause hyposthenuria, but these rarely occur in toxicology studies.

Isosthenuria (i.e., urine specific gravity = 1.008–1.012), also referred to as "fixed" specific gravity, occurs with advanced renal disease. Isosthenuria and hyposthenia are particularly meaningful when serum urea nitrogen concentration is elevated or the animal is dehydrated. If the urine sample is free of water contamination, this combination of findings indicates primary renal disease. Isosthenuria and hyposthenuria may also occur if the test material has diuretic activity.

When an animal is dehydrated and its kidneys are functioning properly, urine should be more concentrated than plasma. In toxicology studies, urine specific gravity is sometimes higher in treated groups than in controls because the treated groups are not eating and drinking normally. Occasionally, test materials cause excessive gastrointestinal fluid losses that result in relative dehydration.

If water contamination of the urine sample is avoided, timed urine volume (e.g., 16 or 24 hrs) and urine specific gravity are probably the most valuable urinalysis tests routinely performed. The other tests have too many complicating factors given the typical procedure for urine collection.

Reagent Strip Tests

Urine pH varies with diet; high-protein meat diets usually produce acid urine and cereal or vegetable diets usually produce alkaline urine. While test materials may alter urine pH, it is not a good indicator of acid-base balance. As urease-producing bacteria multiply in a standing urine sample, ammonia is produced and urine pH becomes more alkaline. Loss of carbon dioxide from specimens in open containers will also cause urine pH to rise.

A small amount of urine protein, as measured with reagent strips, is a normal finding in most animals, especially if the urine is concentrated. A large amount of protein, especially in dilute urine, is abnormal. Increased protein excretion may be due to glomerular injury, defective tubular reabsorption, hemorrhage, inflammation, or the presence of proteinaceous material from the lower urogenital tract in voided specimens. The sediment findings may help to interpret the cause of proteinuria. The reagent strip reactions measure albumin better than globulin so a false negative is possible in rare instances. The most common spurious findings are false positives owing to the effect of highly alkaline urine on the reagent strip reaction or contamination of the urine with quaternary ammonium compounds commonly used as disinfectants. Alternative methods of urine protein determination are sometimes used if these problems are suspected or if the urine protein result is expected to be an important piece of information.

Urine glucose is normally negative. Glucosuria is most commonly observed as a result of hyperglycemia, greater than 180 mg/dl in the dog, and the failure of the renal tubules to reabsorb the increased glucose load entering the glomerular filtrate. Diabetes mellitus is the most frequent disease associated with glucosuria. In toxicology studies, glucosuria is very rare, but it could possibly occur with test materials that affect proximal tubular cells, decreasing their ability to reabsorb filtered glucose. False-negative findings for urine glucose can occur as a result of bacterial proliferation and consumption of glucose.

Ketonuria is occasionally observed in debilitated, anorectic animals and animals that have been fasted for a prolonged period of time. Ketonuria indicates that energy metabolism has shifted to incomplete oxidation of fatty acids. As might be expected, diabetic animals often have ketonuria. False-negative findings for urine ketones can occur as a result of bacterial degradation and the loss of volatile ketones from open containers.

Bilirubinuria, especially in concentrated urine, is a normal finding in the dog, but an abnormal finding in other species. Increased urine bilirubin occurs as a result of the same conditions that cause hyperbilirubinemia, but it often precedes the change in blood. False-negative findings for urine bilirubin can occur from prolonged exposure of the urine specimen to light which will oxidize the bilirubin to biliverdin.

Theoretically, urine urobilinogen tests the patency of the bile duct. Once conjugated bilirubin reaches the intestine, bacterial action converts some of it to urobilinogen, a portion of which is reabsorbed by the intestine. Most of the reabsorbed urobilinogen is removed by the liver, but a small amount is normally excreted in the urine. Therefore, a negative urine urobilinogen is supposed to indicate an obstructed bile duct. There are a multitude of problems with this test, and its value is questionable in any circumstance. It generally is determined simply because it exists on the same reagent strip as the other tests.

Positive findings for urine occult blood frequently occur in normal animals. The origin of the blood is generally not known, but estrus in females is a common source. The reagent strips do not discriminate between erythrocytes, hemoglobin, and myoglobin. Results of this test must be correlated with the microscopic findings for proper interpretation. Hematuria occurs secondary to inflammation, trauma, or neoplasia of the urogenital tract and bleeding disorders.

Urine Sediment Evaluation

Small numbers of erythrocytes, leukocytes, and epithelial cells are normal findings in urine sediment. Large numbers, however, are abnormal. A variety of lesions can be responsible for hematuria and pyuria, at any level of the urogenital tract. Large epithelial cells (i.e., squamous and transitional cells) generally do not indicate serious abnormalities, but the presence of many small epithelial cells (i.e., renal tubular cells) is indicative of renal tubular lesions. Unfortunately, unless associated with granular or cellular casts, it is often difficult to distinguish renal tubular cells from other cells. Furthermore, prolonged exposure of all cells to the somewhat hostile environment of urine leads to degenerative changes or cell lysis. This is one of the major problems with prolonged, timed urine collections. If sediment detail is important, other means of urine collection should be used.

Casts are cylindrical molds of protein and/or cells that form within the lumens of renal tubules. An occasional hyaline (i.e., proteinaceous) or granular cast can be a normal finding. An increased number of these casts or the presence of any cellular casts is an abnormal finding. Increased hyaline cast formation occurs when there is increased protein loss from the kidney. Cellular casts (erythrocyte, leukocyte, or epithelial) are rarely observed in animal urine, but if found, would indicate a severe renal lesion. Cellular casts become granular casts as the cells within the cast degenerate. Granular casts, therefore, are also an indication of a renal lesion. Waxy casts are occasionally seen. They represent the final stage of degeneration of the cellular cast and indicate prolonged, local or diffuse, intrarenal urine stasis. Broad casts are identified by their width and represent casts formed in collecting ducts or pathologically dilated portions of the nephron. As with waxy casts, broad casts indicate intrarenal urine stasis. While cells can originate all along the urogenital tract, cylinduria (increased number of casts) identifies renal involvement. As with cells, casts will degenerate when exposed to urine too long.

Because of the urine collection methods normally used, bacteria are a consistent finding in laboratory animal urine. In order for true bacteriuria to be confirmed, other collection methods must be used.

Crystals are also common findings in the urine of laboratory animals. The type of crystal is dependent on the urine pH. Triple phosphate, amorphous phosphate, calcium carbonate, and ammonium urate crystals are frequently seen in alkaline urine, and urate, oxalate, and hippurate crystals are associated with acid urine. Other types of crystals may be observed. A test material will occasionally form crystals in urine; the significance of this depends on the presence of these crystals in renal tubules or the development of calculi. Ammonium biurate crystals are associated with liver failure, and hippurate crystals are associated with ethylene glycol toxicity.

SPECIES DIFFERENCES

Rat (Table 1)

Hematology

Rats have relatively small erythrocytes; MCV is generally between 50 and 60 femtoliters (fl) in adults. Central pallor is usually observed, and mild-to-moderate anisocytosis and polychromasia are normal findings that correspond to reticulocyte counts of 1–3%. Howell-Jolly bodies and nucleated red blood cells are occasionally observed. Crenation, fragmentation, and poikilocytosis of erythrocytes are commonly observed but are usually artifacts of slide preparation. Erythrocyte survival time is approximately 45–68 days (Jain, 1986). Hematocrits are generally between 40 and 50% and are slightly higher for males than for females.

Table 1 Clinical Pathology Reference Ranges Rat—Young Adult, CD

Test	Units	Male	Female
Red blood cell count	x10^6/μl	6.7–9.0	5.7–9.0
Hemoglobin	g/dl	13.0–17.0	11.0–17.0
Hematocrit	%	44–55	39–55
Mean corpuscular volume	fl	55–65	55–65
Mean corpuscular hemoglobin	pg	16–22	17–22
Mean corpuscular hemoglobin concentration	%	28–34	28–34
Platelet count	x10^3/μl	700–1500	700–1500
Prothrombin time	sec	12–17	12–18
Partial thromboplastin time	sec	17–27	17–27
White blood cell count	x10^3/μl	3.0–14.5	2.0–11.5
Segmented neutrophils	x10^3/μl	0.3–3.0	0.1–2.0
Band neutrophils	x10^3/μl	0.0–0.0	0.0–0.0
Lymphocytes	x10^3/μl	3.0–12.0	1.0–10.0
Monocytes	x10^3/μl	0.0–0.5	0.0–0.3
Eosinophils	x10^3/μl	0.0–0.3	0.0–0.3
Basophils	x10^3/μl	0.0–0.0	0.0–0.0
Nucleated red blood cell count	/100 WBC	0–2	0–2
Glucose	mg/dl	70–125	70–120
Total protein	g/dl	5.6–7.1	5.5–7.3
Albumin	g/dl	3.9–4.9	4.0–5.2
Globulin	g/dl	1.5–2.3	1.4–2.0
Cholesterol	mg/dl	42–90	45–100
Triglyceride	mg/dl	30–90	15–40
Urea nitrogen	mg/dl	10–16	10–19
Creatinine	mg/dl	0.5–0.8	0.5–0.8
Total bilirubin	mg/dl	0.0–0.2	0.0–0.2
Aspartate aminotransferase	IU/L	60–300	80–250
Alanine aminotransferase	IU/L	25–55	25–50
Alkaline phosphatase	IU/L	85–245	60–110
γ-Glutamyl transferase	IU/L	0–1	0–1
Creatine kinase	IU/L		
Calcium	mg/dl	8.5–10.5	8.5–10.2
Inorganic phosphorus	mg/dl	6.0–9.5	6.0–9.0
Sodium	mmol/L	139–155	139–155
Potassium	mmol/L	4.4–5.7	4.0–5.5
Chloride	mmol/L	100–115	100–113

White blood cell counts range from about 3000–12,000/μl; counts for males tend to be slightly higher than for females. In young rats, lymphocytes comprise as many as 90% of the total cell count. With age, however, the neutrophil:lymphocyte ratio is closer to 40:60. Rat granulocytes sometimes have lobulated, ring-shaped nuclei. Immature granulocytes, such as band and metamyelocyte neutrophils, appear as distinctive "doughnut" ring forms with a smooth nuclear membrane. Primary granules of the rat neutrophil are small and faint.

Inflammatory lesions in the rat cause a neutrophilic leukocytosis, often accompanied by a lymphocytosis. Older rats with chronic lesions such as cage sores or tumors with ulcerated, infected surfaces can have very high WBC counts (e.g., >50,000/μl) that must be distinguished from leukemia. A high percentage of Fischer-344 rats develop large granular lymphocyte leukemia after a year of age (Stromberg, 1985). In addition to high numbers of neoplastic cells in peripheral blood, the hematologic findings are also characterized by the development of an acute, immune-mediated hemolytic anemia exhibiting spherocytosis and reticulocytosis.

The rat spleen exhibits active hematopoiesis throughout life. In the bone marrow, the M:E ratio is usually between 1:1 and 1.5:1.0. Megakaryocytes are abundant, and lymphocytes are common, comprising up to 20% of the nucleated cell population. Mast cells are more prominent in rat bone marrow than in bone marrow from other laboratory animal species.

Platelet counts in rats are very high; averaging about 1,000,000/μl. Lower counts are frequently due to sampling-induced platelet aggregation, and platelet clumps are often observed on peripheral blood films. Prothrombin time and partial thromboplastin time in the rat are similar to other species.

Clinical Chemistry

In most respects, clinical chemistry findings and interpretations for the rat are not unusual. Because of the rat's prominence in biomedical research, however, there are numerous references in the literature covering a wide range of subjects relating to clinical chemistry. A high percentage of these report on the sources of variation such as the time of day when bled, method of handling, blood collection site, or anesthetic used. Several other references compare the merits of different tests for identifying lesions caused by various models of toxicity. For example, which of several liver enzymes is the best for identifying a specific model of liver toxicity? Rather than list the details of these reports, some generalizations will be made.

As with most species, serum glucose concentration is one of the most sensitive parameters to variations in handling and sample collection. Increased concentration due to experimental manipulations other than food consumption are often attributed to the effect of endogenous catecholamines and corticosteroids on glycogenolysis, gluconeogenesis, and insulin antagonism. While total serum cholesterol in the rat is relatively resistant to atherogenic diets, a variety of disease conditions in older animals are associated with hypercholesterolemia. The reference range for cholesterol in aged rats is quite wide. In contrast to humans, high-density lipoprotein is the predominant lipoprotein in the rat; the same is true of many other laboratory animal species. The γ-globulin fraction of serum protein determined by electrophoresis is remarkably low in the young adult rat, but as in most species, it increases with the age of the animal and with exposure to antigenic stimulation.

In young adults, serum urea nitrogen and creatinine concentrations have narrow reference ranges. With age, however, the common occurrence of chronic progressive nephropathy, especially in males, affects the ranges.

Numerous liver enzymes have been studied and variously advocated for the study of hepatic toxicity in the rat. In general, serum ALT, SDH, and GDH activities have been the best indicators of hepatocellular injury. Because ALT activity is the simplest to determine, it has generally been adopted by most laboratories as the standard liver enzyme.

There has been considerable discussion concerning the relative merits of serum AP, GGT, and 5'N activities for the evaluation of hepatobiliary or cholestatic disease. It has been argued that serum AP activity is not specific or sensitive in the rat and that changes in serum activity are due to changes in the intestinal isoenzyme. The experience of this author is that serum AP activity will increase in the rat in association with some hepatobiliary lesions and in the absence of visible histological gastrointestinal involvement. However, serum AP activity does not appear to be as sensitive to cholestasis in the rat as it is in the dog. Furthermore, depending on the conditions of the experiment, serum AP activity has been shown to either increase or decrease secondary to food restriction (Oishi et al., 1979; Schwartz et al., 1973). In either case, the changes are small. Serum GGT activity is essentially nonexistent in normal rats, but a few studies have shown increased activity secondary to hepatobiliary toxins (Leonard et al., 1984; Ghys et al., 1975). This author has rarely observed increased serum GGT activity in the rat. It is possible that the hepatobiliary damage must be severe before an increase occurs. Serum 5'N has been used infrequently in the rat but has been shown, in certain disease models, to parallel increases in serum AP and GGT activity (Kryszewski et al., 1973).

Electrolyte findings are not notably different in the rat. Like the erythrocytes of mice and humans, however, rat erythrocytes have high potassium concentration and hemolysis will yield spuriously high serum potassium values (Meeks, 1989).

The rat is commonly used as a test animal for organophosphate and carbamate products. It is interesting to note that plasma cholinesterase activity in females is approximately three to four times higher than in males. While this difference is absent in very young animals, it becomes noticeable around 6–8 weeks of age. Red blood cell cholinesterase activity is similar in males and females.

The primary adrenocorticosteroid in the rat is corticosterone.

Urinalysis

Proteinuria is a common finding in rats, especially males, increasing with age and the development of chronic progressive nephropathy. Males begin to excrete low molecular weight sex-dependent proteins around 8 weeks of age (Alt et al., 1980). Larger proteins, including albumin, are excreted with the development of the nephropathy.

Mouse (Table 2)

Hematology

Mice have the smallest erythrocytes of the common laboratory animal species; MCV is generally between 45 and 55 fl. Central pallor is usually observed, but because of the cell's small size, it is inconsistent. Moderate anisocytosis and polychromasia are normal findings and correspond to reticulocyte counts of 2–5%. Mice have the highest reticulocyte counts among adult laboratory animals. Howell-Jolly bodies are a frequent normal finding, and nucleated red blood cells are occasionally observed. Fragmentation and crenation of erythrocytes are commonly observed, but these are usually artifacts of slide preparation. Erythrocyte survival time is the shortest among common laboratory animals, approximately 40–50 days (Bannerman, 1983). Hematocrit is relatively high, especially if mice are fasted before sample collection. Although generally between 40 and 50%, hematocrits above 50% are frequently observed. Considering the small erythrocyte size, it is not surprising that mouse RBC counts are the highest encountered, ranging 8–11 million/ml.

Mice generally have WBC counts ranging from 2000–10,000/μl; counts for males tend to be slightly higher than for females. Lymphocytes normally comprise about 70–80% of

Table 2   Clinical Pathology Reference Ranges Mouse—Young Adult, CD-1

Test	Units	Male	Female
Red blood cell count	$\times 10^6/\mu l$	9.0–11.3	9.0–11.5
Hemoglobin	g/dl	13.5–17.0	14.5–17.5
Hematocrit	%	45–55	45–57
Mean corpuscular volume	fl	47–55	45–55
Mean corpuscular hemoglobin	pg	13–16	13–16
Mean corpuscular hemoglobin concentration	%	29–34	29–34
Platelet count	$\times 10^3/\mu l$	900–1900	900–1800
Prothrombin time	sec	7–20	7–20
Partial thromboplastin time	sec		
White blood cell count	$\times 10^3/\mu l$	2.0–10.0	1.0–12.0
Segmented neutrophils	$\times 10^3/\mu l$	0.3–2.0	0.3–2.5
Band neutrophils	$\times 10^3/\mu l$	0.0–0.0	0.0–0.0
Lymphocytes	$\times 10^3/\mu l$	1.0–7.0	1.0–9.0
Monocytes	$\times 10^3/\mu l$	0.0–0.3	0.0–0.3
Eosinophils	$\times 10^3/\mu l$	0.0–0.5	0.0–0.5
Basophils	$\times 10^3/\mu l$	0.0–0.0	0.0–0.0
Nucleated red blood cell count	/100 WBC	0–2	0–2
Glucose	mg/dl	80–160	80–150
Total protein	g/dl	5.0–7.4	4.8–7.0
Albumin	g/dl	3.5–5.0	3.4–5.0
Globulin	g/dl	1.5–3.5	1.0–2.5
Cholesterol	mg/dl	90–170	50–130
Triglyceride	mg/dl	60–160	40–130
Urea nitrogen	mg/dl	15–45	15–40
Creatinine	mg/dl	0.3–0.8	0.2–0.6
Total bilirubin	mg/dl	0.1–1.0	0.1–0.9
Aspartate aminotransferase	IU/L	70–400	70–400
Alanine aminotransferase	IU/L	25–200	25–100
Alkaline phosphatase	IU/L	30–80	40–100
γ-Glutamyl transferase	IU/L	0–3	0–3
Creatine kinase	IU/L		
Calcium	mg/dl	8.5–11.5	8.5–11.5
Inorganic phosphorus	mg/dl	7.0–11.5	7.0–11.5
Sodium	mmol/L	145–167	145–165
Potassium	mmol/L	5.0–8.5	5.0–8.5
Chloride	mmol/L	110–125	110–125

the total cell count, but the percentage of neutrophils increases with age. Like the rat, mouse granulocytes often have lobulated, ring-shaped nuclei. Sometimes the ring is broken, and the nucleus appears similar to those of most mammals. As in the rat, immature granulocytes appear as distinctive "doughnut" ring forms with a smooth nuclear membrane. In the mouse, neutrophil primary granules are small and very faint.

As with most species, inflammatory lesions in the mouse result in an increased absolute neutrophil count. Similar to the rat, however, this is often accompanied by an increase in absolute lymphocyte count. Older mice with chronic lesions also get remarkably high WBC counts, easily greater than 50,000/μl. Similar to rabbits, and in contrast to dogs, corticosteroids cause decreased absolute monocyte count in the mouse (Jain, 1986).

In addition to bone marrow, the mouse spleen exhibits active hematopoiesis throughout life. Erythropoiesis appears greater than granulopoiesis in the spleen, and the reverse is true in marrow where the average myeloid-to-erythroid ratio is usually around 1.5:1.0. Megakaryocytes are abundant in both locations. Lymphocytes are commonly found in bone marrow preparations from mice and may comprise up to 25% of the nucleated cell population.

Mice have the highest platelet counts encountered among laboratory animals. Counts normally range between 1 and 2 million/ml. Because sample collection is often problematic, it is not unusual to have lower counts due to platelet aggregation and observe platelet clumps on peripheral blood films. Prothrombin time in the mouse appears to be similar to other species, but reported partial thromboplastin times (55–110 sec) are longer than for most other laboratory animals (Allen, 1962). This could easily be due to methodology differences.

Clinical Chemistry

The limited volume of available serum (or plasma) has a great impact on clinical chemistry procedures in mice. Even with the many advances in biomedical technology, it remains very difficult to complete a moderately full biochemical profile. It is impossible if hematology tests are also desired. Evaporation during handling and testing can have a major effect when the total sample is only a few hundred microliters. Study design must accommodate these limitations. Tests should be individually selected on the basis of expected effects or areas of concern. The number of tests measuring similar effects, such as urea nitrogen and creatinine for kidney dysfunction or multiple liver enzymes for hepatocellular injury, should be reduced to a single choice. Tests that exhibit large variation among individuals, such as electrolytes, may be of little value. If both hematology and a full biochemical profile are deemed necessary, then the number of animals tested should be increased so that individuals can be designated for one or the other test procedure. Pooling of samples for clinical chemistry analysis is not recommended.

In general, clinical chemistry reference ranges for mice are quite wide. This is probably indicative of some of the difficulties associated with sample collection and analysis. Because precollection fasting is not generally practiced, values for serum glucose and triglyceride concentrations are moderately higher than those normally observed with other species that have been fasted. Serum urea nitrogen values also tend to be higher, and concentrations as high as 40 mg/dl are common in normal mice.

Serum ALT and SDH activities are both useful for the detection of hepatocellular injury. Because serum AST and LDH activities are more easily influenced by muscle injury, such as occurs with handling or blood collection, these enzymes are less desirable if sample volume limitations are a concern. It is important to note, however, that serum ALT activity is also affected by handling. When compared with control mice that were either not handled or tail-handled one hour prior to blood collection, mice that were grasped by the body had serum ALT activity nearly four times greater (Swaim et al., 1985). An interesting enzyme activity phenomenon is associated with lactic dehydrogenase virus in mice. This viral infection induces decreased clearance of serum enzymes resulting in elevations of LDH and AST activity, among others (Riley, 1978). In contrast to most laboratory animal species, salivary amylase is responsible for most of the serum amylase activity in the mouse and may increase with salivary gland injury.

The most notable electrolyte findings in the mouse are the reported reference ranges which are high and wide (e.g., 112–193 mEq/l for sodium; Everett and Harrison, 1983). It is likely that evaporation of the small samples has had some impact on the high end of these ranges. With respect to potassium, mouse erythrocytes have a high intracellular concentration (similar to humans but in contrast to dogs), and hemolysis will cause spuriously high serum potassium concentration.

The primary adrenocorticosteroid in the mouse is corticosterone.

Hamster (Table 3)

Hematology

Many hematological characteristics of hamsters are similar to other rodents, but there are a few differences. Their erythrocytes are morphologically similar to those of rats. The

Table 3 Clinical Pathology Reference Ranges Syrian Hamster—Adult

Test	Units	Male	Female
Red blood cell count	x10^6/μl	6.0–8.5	6.0–8.0
Hemoglobin	g/dl	12.5–16.5	12.0–16.0
Hematocrit	%	35–50	35–45
Mean corpuscular volume	fl	52–65	52–65
Mean corpuscular hemoglobin	pg	19–23	19–23
Mean corpuscular hemoglobin concentration	%	32–36	32–36
Platelet count	x10^3/μl	300–900	300–900
Prothrombin time	sec		
Partial thromboplastin time	sec		
White blood cell count	x10^3/μl	4.0–10.0	4.0–10.0
Segmented neutrophils	x10^3/μl	0.5–3.5	0.5–3.5
Band neutrophils	x10^3/μl	0.0–0.0	0.0–0.0
Lymphocytes	x10^3/μl	2.5–8.0	2.5–8.0
Monocytes	x10^3/μl	0.0–0.5	0.0–0.5
Eosinophils	x10^3/μl	0.0–0.3	0.0–0.3
Basophils	x10^3/μl	0.0–0.0	0.0–0.0
Nucleated red blood cell count	/100 WBC	0–2	0–2
Glucose	mg/dl	50–100	50–100
Total protein	g/dl	5.3–7.0	5.3–7.0
Albumin	g/dl	3.5–4.5	3.5–4.5
Globulin	g/dl		
Cholesterol	mg/dl	50–200	50–200
Triglyceride	mg/dl		
Urea nitrogen	mg/dl	12–25	12–25
Creatinine	mg/dl	0.3–0.7	0.3–0.7
Total bilirubin	mg/dl	0.1–0.5	0.1–0.5
Aspartate aminotransferase	IU/L	20–100	20–100
Alanine aminotransferase	IU/L	20–50	20–50
Alkaline phosphatase	IU/L	50–200	50–200
γ-Glutamyl transferase	IU/L		
Creatine kinase	IU/L		
Calcium	mg/dl	10.0–13.5	10.0–13.5
Inorganic phosphorus	mg/dl	4.5–9.0	4.5–9.0
Sodium	mmol/L	145–155	145–155
Potassium	mmol/L	4.0–7.0	4.0–7.0
Chloride	mmol/L	98–110	98–110

cells are approximately 50–60 fl in volume, and most exhibit some central pallor. Mild-to-moderate anisocytosis and polychromasia corresponds to a reticulocyte count of about 1–3% in the adult. Howell-Jolly bodies and nucleated red blood cells are occasionally observed on blood films from normal adults. Erythrocyte survival time is approximately 60 to 70 days, but it increases greatly during hibernation and may reach as high as 160 days (Brock, 1960). Hematocrit is generally in the range of 35–45%, and it also increases during hibernation. At the end of hibernation, reticulocyte production increases. Unlike mice and rats, the spleen does not contribute to normal erythropoiesis.

The normal WBC count is approximately 5000–10,000/μl, and lymphocytes are the predominant nucleated cell, making up about 75% of the total. In contrast to RBC count, WBC count decreases during hibernation. Hamster neutrophils are similar to those of mice and rats and frequently appear in peripheral blood as lobulated ring-forms with fine, faintly eosinophilic primary granules. Band neutrophils and metamyelocytes have a distinctive ring or "doughnut" appearance with a smooth nuclear membrane. They are readily identified in bone marrow smear preparations. Although the normal myeloid-to-erythroid ratio has been reported as high as 10:1 in hamsters (Desai, 1968), it is probably closer to 2:1. Lymphocytes, a prominent finding in the bone marrow of other rodents and guinea pigs, do not represent more than a few percent of the marrow cell population.

While the clotting time for hamster whole blood is fairly rapid, prothrombin time and partial thromboplastin time are similar to those of most laboratory species (Desai, 1968; Dodds, 1977). Platelet counts in hamsters are not quite as high as in mice and rats, and the platelets are more difficult to see on peripheral blood films.

Clinical Chemistry

Serum glucose concentration in the hamster is similar to other species but is said to increase during hibernation (Lyman and Leduc, 1953) as do total serum protein and albumin concentration (South, 1958). Chinese hamster lines have been developed as models of insulin-dependent diabetes mellitus and as expected exhibit hyperglycemia, hypercholesterolemia, and hypoinsulinemia (Gerritsen, 1982). Of the small laboratory animals, hamsters appear to have the highest total serum cholesterol concentration (Carroll and Feldman, 1987). Amyloidosis is a common disease affecting older hamsters and similar to other species, hamsters with renal amyloidosis develop azotemia, hypoproteinemia, hypoalbuminemia, and hypercholesterolemia (Murphy et al., 1984).

Serum AP and ALT activities appear to be valuable as markers for liver injury, and serum LDH and creatine kinase activities increase in hereditary myopathy in Syrian hamsters (Homburger et al., 1966).

The primary adrenocorticosteroid in hamsters is corticosterone, but cortisol is also present and will increase under the influence of ACTH (Albers et al., 1985; Ottenweller et al., 1985).

Guinea Pig (Table 4)

Hematology

Guinea pig erythrocytes are the largest among common laboratory animals. Their MCV is generally between 75 and 90 fl; similar in size to human erythrocytes. The cells have central pallor and exhibit mild anisocytosis and polychromasia that corresponds to a reticulocyte count of 1–2.5%. Howell-Jolly bodies and nucleated red blood cells are rarely observed. The erythrocytes have a survival time of approximately 80–90 days. Hematocrit is generally in the range of 40–50%. An interesting phenomenon, unique to the guinea

Table 4 Clinical Pathology Reference Ranges Guinea Pig—Adult

Test	Units	Male	Female
Red blood cell count	x10^6/μl	4.8–6.8	4.5–6.5
Hemoglobin	g/dl	12.0–16.0	12.0–15.5
Hematocrit	%	38–52	36–50
Mean corpuscular volume	fl	70–88	75–90
Mean corpuscular hemoglobin	pg		
Mean corpuscular hemoglobin concentration	%	28–33	28–33
Platelet count	x10^3/μl	300–800	300–900
Prothrombin time	sec		
Partial thromboplastin time	sec		
White blood cell count	x10^3/μl	2.0–12.0	2.0–12.0
Segmented neutrophils	x10^3/μl	0.5–3.5	0.5–4.5
Band neutrophils	x10^3/μl	0.0–0.0	0.0–0.0
Lymphocytes	x10^3/μl	1.5–10.0	1.5–9.0
Monocytes	x10^3/μl	0.0–0.5	0.0–0.5
Eosinophils	x10^3/μl	0.0–0.5	0.0–0.5
Basophils	x10^3/μl	0.0–0.0	0.0–0.0
Nucleated red blood cell count	/100 WBC	0–1	0–1
Glucose	mg/dl	75–110	75–110
Total protein	g/dl	5.0–6.3	4.5–6.0
Albumin	g/dl	2.5–4.0	2.2–3.5
Globulin	g/dl		
Cholesterol	mg/dl	25–80	30–80
Triglyceride	mg/dl	10–70	10–70
Urea nitrogen	mg/dl	15–30	15–25
Creatinine	mg/dl	0.5–0.8	0.5–0.8
Total bilirubin	mg/dl	0.0–0.3	0.0–0.3
Aspartate aminotransferase	IU/L	30–80	30–75
Alanine aminotransferase	IU/L	30–70	25–65
Alkaline phosphatase	IU/L	60–100	50–100
γ-Glutamyl transferase	IU/L	5–15	5–15
Creatine kinase	IU/L	200–500	150–500
Calcium	mg/dl	9.5–11.5	9.5–11.5
Inorganic phosphorus	mg/dl	4.0–8.5	4.0–8.5
Sodium	mmol/L	130–142	130–142
Potassium	mmol/L	4.0–6.0	4.0–6.0
Chloride	mmol/L	103–112	103–112

pig, is the development of an acute hemolytic anemia in response to high dietary cholesterol (Yamanaka et al., 1967). The belief is that alterations in membrane lipid content may render the erythrocytes more susceptible to lysis.

The most unique feature of guinea pig leukocytes is the Kurloff body, a cytoplasmic inclusion observed in a small number of mononuclear cells believed to be T lymphocytes because of their ability to form rosettes of rabbit erythrocytes (Jain, 1986). Kurloff bodies are a glycoprotein complex that generally appear as a single, large, round-to-oval, purplish red, homogeneous inclusion. On occasion, a cell will have multiple smaller inclusions. Although the function of the Kurloff body is not known, they are observed more frequently in females than males, especially during the first 3 months of life, and appear to increase during pregnancy or with exogenous estrogen administration (Ledingham, 1940). In general, Kurloff bodies occur in less than 5% of circulating leukocytes.

Guinea pig neutrophils appear similar to those of humans in that the nuclei are distinctly segmented and the cytoplasm contains conspicuous reddish primary granules. The granules are not as large or prominent as those of the rabbit heterophil, but some authors refer to the guinea pig neutrophil as a heterophil. The cells are easily distinguished from eosinophils. In contrast to other species, guinea pig lymphocytes exhibit alkaline phosphatase activity (Kaplow, 1969). This has significance because alkaline phosphatase activity is sometimes used to cytochemically differentiate neutrophils which exhibit activity in most species, from monocytes and lymphocytes, which normally do not.

The normal WBC count in the guinea pig ranges from approximately 5000 to 10,000/ μl and will increase slightly with age. Regardless of age, the neutrophil:lymphocyte ratio remains approximately 1:2. Similar to mice and rats, as many as 25% of the cells in normal bone marrow of guinea pigs are lymphocytes. The typical myeloid:erythroid ratio is about 1.5:1.0.

With respect to coagulation, guinea pigs are unique among laboratory animals because of their relatively low concentration of the factor VII clotting protein. Consequently, one-stage prothrombin times for the evaluation of the extrinsic clotting system are longer in the guinea pig; as long as 50–100 sec in one study (Kaspareit, 1988). Automated coagulation analyzers that automatically stop if an assay has not begun to form fibrin within 50 sec would be inappropriate for use on guinea pig samples. Thrombin time also appears to be relatively prolonged in guinea pigs. On the other hand, activated partial thromboplastin time is similar to other species.

Clinical Chemistry

There is not much information available concerning the clinical chemistry of guinea pigs. One of the most noteworthy items is that serum ALT activity is said to be insensitive and nonspecific as a marker for hepatocellular injury. Part of this stems from the finding that the activity of ALT in other tissues such as muscle is as high as it is in the liver. In addition, liver ALT activity in the guinea pig is localized primarily within mitochondria, and theoretically would be less likely than cytoplasmic enzyme to enter circulation secondary to hepatocellular damage. Regardless of these considerations, however, liver toxicity should remain the most likely interpretation for elevated serum ALT activity in the guinea pig. The rabbit is another example of a species for which ALT activity is not specific for the liver, but when treated with CCl_4, serum ALT activity is rapidly and markedly elevated. Normal serum ALT activity in the guinea pig is similar to that of other species.

Total serum cholesterol concentration will increase when guinea pigs are fed cholesterol-rich diets, but contrary to most species, the amount of HDL cholesterol also increases. Normally, the guinea pig has a smaller amount of HDL cholesterol than other laboratory animals or humans. Its predominant lipoprotein is LDL.

The primary adrenocorticosteroid in the guinea pig is cortisol. While there is considerable homology among species with respect to the structure of insulin, guinea pig insulin is substantially different and is associated with differences in activity and receptor concentration (Zimmerman et al., 1974).

Rabbit (Table 5)

Hematology

Normal rabbit erythrocytes are slightly smaller than those of the dog; MCV is generally between 55 and 70 fl. The cells have central pallor and exhibit moderate anisocytosis and

Table 5 Clinical Pathology Reference Ranges New Zealand White Rabbit—Young Adult[a]

Test	Units	Male	Female
Red blood cell count	$\times 10^6/\mu l$	5.0–7.2	5.0–7.2
Hemoglobin	g/dl	10.5–15.0	10.5–15.0
Hematocrit	%	32–45	32–45
Mean corpuscular volume	fl	55–65	55–70
Mean corpuscular hemoglobin	pg	19–23	19–23
Mean corpuscular hemoglobin concentration	%	30–35	30–35
Platelet count	$\times 10^3/\mu l$	300–750	300–750
Prothrombin time	sec		
Partial thromboplastin time	sec		
White blood cell count	$\times 10^3/\mu l$	4.0–13.0	4.0–13.0
Segmented neutrophils	$\times 10^3/\mu l$	1.0–6.0	1.0–6.0
Band neutrophils	$\times 10^3/\mu l$	0.0–0.0	0.0–0.0
Lymphocytes	$\times 10^3/\mu l$	2.0–9.0	2.0–9.0
Monocytes	$\times 10^3/\mu l$	0.0–0.5	0.0–0.5
Eosinophils	$\times 10^3/\mu l$	0.0–0.4	0.0–0.4
Basophils	$\times 10^3/\mu l$	0.0–1.0	0.0–1.0
Nucleated red blood cell count	/100 WBC	0–1	0–1
Glucose	mg/dl	105–190	100–190
Total protein	g/dl	5.2–7.5	5.2–7.5
Albumin	g/dl	4.0–5.5	3.5–5.5
Globulin	g/dl	1.0–2.5	1.0–2.5
Cholesterol	mg/dl	25–70	30–100
Triglyceride	mg/dl	50–180	30–180
Urea nitrogen	mg/dl	11–25	11–25
Creatinine	mg/dl	0.9–1.7	0.9–1.7
Total bilirubin	mg/dl	0.1–0.5	0.1–0.5
Aspartate aminotransferase	IU/L	15–45	15–45
Alanine aminotransferase	IU/L	15–50	15–50
Alkaline phosphatase	IU/L	40–140	40–140
γ-Glutamyl transferase	IU/L	0–10	0–10
Creatine kinase	IU/L		
Calcium	mg/dl	13.0–15.5	12.5–15.5
Inorganic phosphorus	mg/dl	3.0–9.0	2.0–9.0
Sodium	mmol/L	133–152	133–150
Potassium	mmol/L	3.5–6.0	3.5–6.0
Chloride	mmol/L	96–106	96–106

[a]Not fasted.

mild polychromasia that corresponds to a reticulocyte count of 1–4%. Howell-Jolly bodies and nucleated red blood cells are rarely observed on blood films from normal rabbits. The erythrocytes have a survival time of approximately 45–70 days. Hematocrit is generally in the range of 35–45%.

Rabbit leukocytes have some unique features. The rabbit neutrophil, commonly referred to as a heterophil, is morphologically distinct from neutrophils of other mammals. Although the term *heterophil* has been used to describe the neutrophil of other laboratory animal species, the rabbit's heterophil is clearly unique. The cytoplasm contains many primary granules that are large, irregularly shaped, and darkly eosinophilic. Unless the cells are viewed in the same microscopic field, it may be difficult for the inexperienced observer to distinguish rabbit heterophils from eosinophils. Rabbit eosinophils have larger primary granules that are round and stain dull orange. The granules may partially obscure the eosinophil's bilobed or segmented nucleus. Rabbits are the only laboratory animal species to normally have circulating basophils counted during a standard differential white blood cell count. These cells have many dark purplish granules that obscure the nucleus. As many as 10% of the leukocytes in normal animals may be basophils.

The normal white blood cell count in the rabbit, approximately 5000–12,000/μl, is similar to the dog. The heterophil:lymphocyte ratio is approximately 1:2 in young adult animals and 1:1 in older animals. In response to acute inflammation, the rabbit's heterophil:lymphocyte ratio will increase, but in contrast to the dog, its white blood cell count generally will not (Toth and Krueger, 1989). Similar to most species, rabbits develop lymphopenia secondary to stress or exogenous corticosteroid administration. In addition, corticosteroids induce monocytopenia in the rabbit.

A rare condition of rabbit leukocytes is Pelger-Hüet anomaly. Observed in several species, including humans, this hereditary trait is characterized by failure of granulocyte nuclei to develop normal segmentation. In the heterozygous state, neutrophil morphology gives the appearance of a permanent left shift (i.e., the neutrophils always appear to be band forms), but the cells are not dysfunctional. Selective breeding in the rabbit can produce a homozygous state which is invariably lethal.

Because normal serum calcium concentration is much higher in the rabbit than other species, there is a potential for technical difficulties when performing coagulation tests. Calcium chelators such as citrate or oxalate are used for sample collection, and it is possible that overfilling collection tubes that have been prepared using the recommended anticoagulant to blood ratios may allow some fibrin formation to take place. If problems with tests such as prothrombin time, activated partial thromboplastin time, or thrombin time are encountered, consideration should be given to the sample collection method.

Clinical Chemistry

Fasting is recommended prior to blood collection for most species in order to standardize sampling conditions for the generation of, and comparison to, reference range values. For most experimental purposes, fasting rabbits for sample collection may be unnecessary because it appears to have less effect on serum concentrations of parameters such as glucose and triglycerides than in other species. This may be due in part to the practice of coprophagy. Furthermore, the notable effect of fasting on rabbit body weight data may necessitate bleeding nonfasted animals in order to maintain proper conditions for other study objectives.

The most conspicuous biochemical differences between rabbits and other laboratory animals involve serum albumin and calcium concentrations. Unmodified, routine chemistry methods (e.g., bromcresol green or bromcresol purple) for determination of serum albumin concentration will yield falsely elevated values. In fact, albumin concentration will often exceed total serum protein concentration. Serum protein electrophoresis results indicate that albumin actually comprises about 60–70% of serum protein. The cause of the spuriously high values determined with routine methods is not known. Results may be improved, however, by using a rabbit albumin standard for calibration.

Rabbits have higher total serum calcium than any other laboratory animal. While values as high as 16 mg/dl are not uncommon in normal rabbits, they would clearly indicate severe hypercalcemia in other species. The reason for the difference is not known. Despite its relatively high serum calcium, mineralization of soft tissue lesions is not a prominent histological finding in the rabbit. The VX_2 carcinoma of the rabbit is a model of tumor-associated hypercalcemia (Wolfe et al., 1978).

Serum cholesterol concentration varies more due to strain and gender than other parameters. As with many species, serum cholesterol concentration increases with age and is greater in females. Rabbits are more sensitive to dietary induction of hyper-cholesterolemia than most species and serve as a model to study atherosclerosis (Clarkson et al., 1974). Diet-induced hypercholesterolemia in rabbits is remarkable in that serum levels can reach as high as 3000 mg/dl. The serum in these animals is extremely lipemic and complicates serum biochemical analysis. Ultracentrifugation may be necessary to clear the serum samples.

The primary adrenocorticosteroid in the rabbit is corticosterone. Rabbits are very sensitive to exogenous corticosteroids and develop typical signs and laboratory results for hyperadrenocorticism including hyperglycemia and increased serum aminotransferase activities. The latter is associated with diffuse vacuolization of hepatocytes.

Urinalysis

Because of its physical characteristics, rabbit urine is not routinely examined. The thick, turbid appearance is due to mucin and abundant calcium carbonate and triple phosphate crystals. The crystals may cause falsely elevated urine specific gravity if refractometric readings are made on samples that have not been centrifuged. Furthermore, the crystals make it difficult to visualize other formed elements in the urine sediment. In general, urinalysis is not recommended as part of the routine laboratory database in this species.

Ferret (Table 6)

Hematology

Compared with dogs, ferrets have relatively small erythrocytes; MCV is generally between 50 and 60 fl. Central pallor is usually observed. The cells exhibit only slight anisocytosis and polychromasia, even though reticulocyte counts have been reported as high as 12–14% in normal ferrets (Thornton et al., 1979). Others report much lower reticulocyte counts, 0–1%, which correlate better with the erythrocyte morphology (Sherrill and Gorham, 1985). Howell-Jolly bodies and nucleated red blood cells are occasionally observed as might be expected since the spleen retains some hematopoietic capacity. Hematocrits tend to be slightly higher than those of the dog and generally range from 45 to 55%.

The WBC counts of the ferret range from about 5000 to 15,000/μl. The neutrophil: lymphocyte ratio ranges from about 40:60–60:40. Leukocyte counts, morphology, and response to inflammation are similar to those of the dog.

Ferret platelet counts average approximately 500,000/μl, and platelet morphology is similar to other laboratory animal species. Prothrombin time in ferrets is slightly longer than in dogs but is similar to rats.

The most unusual feature of ferret hematology is estrus-induced bone marrow hypoplasia (Kociba and Caputo, 1981; Bernard et al., 1983; Sherrill and Gorham, 1985). Because the ferret is an induced ovulator, estrus may be prolonged if the female is not bred. Under the influence of endogenous estrogen, bone marrow hypoplasia develops in as many as 50% of the females with protracted estrus. The hematological signs are characterized by an initial increase in platelet count and WBC count at the beginning of estrus followed

Table 6   Clinical Pathology Reference Ranges Ferret—Young Adult

Test	Units	Male	Female
Red blood cell count	x10^6/μl	7.0–11.0	6.5–10.0
Hemoglobin	g/dl	14.0–18.0	14.0–17.5
Hematocrit	%	45–55	40–50
Mean corpuscular volume	fl	50–60	50–60
Mean corpuscular hemoglobin	pg	18–20	18–20
Mean corpuscular hemoglobin concentration	%	32–36	32–36
Platelet count	x10^3/μl	300–700	300–900
Prothrombin time	sec	14–17	14–17
Partial thromboplastin time	sec		
White blood cell count	x10^3/μl	4.0–15.0	4.0–15.0
Segmented neutrophils	x10^3/μl	2.0–11.0	2.0–11.0
Band neutrophils	x10^3/μl	0.0–0.0	0.0–0.0
Lymphocytes	x10^3/μl	2.0–7.0	2.0–7.0
Monocytes	x10^3/μl	0.0–0.8	0.0–0.8
Eosinophils	x10^3/μl	0.0–0.8	0.0–0.8
Basophils	x10^3/μl	0.0–0.2	0.0–0.2
Nucleated red blood cell count	/100 WBC	0–1	0–1
Glucose	mg/dl	90–150	90–150
Total protein	g/dl	5.3–7.5	5.3–7.5
Albumin	g/dl	2.5–4.0	2.5–4.0
Globulin	g/dl		
Cholesterol	mg/dl	100–250	100–250
Triglyceride	mg/dl		
Urea nitrogen	mg/dl	15–30	15–30
Creatinine	mg/dl	0.3–0.9	0.3–0.9
Total bilirubin	mg/dl	0.1–0.7	0.1–0.7
Aspartate aminotransferase	IU/L	30–120	30–120
Alanine aminotransferase	IU/L	50–200	50–200
Alkaline phosphatase	IU/L	20–100	20–100
γ-Glutamyl transferase	IU/L		
Creatine kinase	IU/L		
Calcium	mg/dl	8.5–10.5	8.5–10.5
Inorganic phosphorus	mg/dl	4.0–8.5	4.0–8.5
Sodium	mmol/L	145–160	145–155
Potassium	mmol/L	4.3–6.0	4.3–6.0
Chloride	mmol/L	110–125	110–125

later by pancytopenia (e.g., platelet count <50,000/μl; hematocrit <30%; WBC count <2,500/μl). The thrombocytopenia may be responsible for hemorrhaging that further lowers the hematocrit and leads to severe, fatal anemia. Systemic bacterial infections are sometimes associated with the leukopenia. Examination of bone marrow from severely affected animals reveals depletion of all hematopoietic cell precursors.

Clinical Chemistry

In general, clinical chemistry test results from normal ferrets more closely resemble those of the dog than any other common laboratory animal. Serum glucose, protein, and lipid concentrations are similar. For example, total serum cholesterol in the ferret and dog is relatively high for most laboratory animals, but comparable to humans. Serum urea nitrogen and creatinine concentrations are similar to the dog. Serum ALT activity tends to be slightly higher than in the dog, but serum AP activity is somewhat lower. As with all other species, serum AP activity decreases with age. In contrast to mice, rats, hamsters, and monkeys, hemolysis does not spuriously increase serum potassium concentration. Like the dog, it is thought that ferret erythrocytes have a low concentration of intracellular potassium (Lee et al., 1982).

Thyroid and adrenocortical hormone levels and their response to stimulation or suppression tests have been investigated (Garibaldi et al., 1988a,b; Heard et al., 1990). Resting values for serum thyroxine (T_4), triiodothyronine (T_3), and cortisol concentrations are similar to dogs. Stimulation with thyroid-stimulating hormone (TSH) causes increased T_4 but not T_3. Stimulation with adrenocorticotropic hormone (ACTH), intravenously or intramuscularly, increases serum cortisol. Intravenous dexamethasone suppression (0.2 mg/animal) appears to decrease cortisol by greater than 50% at 3 and 5 hr postdose (Heard et al., 1990), whereas intramuscular dexamethasone (0.1 mg/kg) had little effect at 6 hr postdose (Garibaldi et al., 1988b). These findings seem to support the belief that the ferret is a relatively steroid-resistant species.

Urinalysis
Like the dog, bilirubinuria is a common finding. The threshold for bilirubin excretion is apparently lower in these species than in most others.

Dog (Table 7)

Hematology
Dog erythrocytes are smaller than those of humans (MCV is generally between 60 and 75 fl), but the cells have the classic biconcave disc shape with an obvious area of central pallor. Because the normal reticulocyte count is less than 1%, anisocytosis and polychromasia are minimal. Howell-Jolly bodies and nucleated red blood cells are rarely observed in normal adults. Sampling and slide preparation artifacts such as crenation, fragmentation, and poikilocytosis are less frequently observed in dogs than in smaller laboratory animals, especially rodents. Erythrocyte survival time is the longest of the common laboratory animals, approximately 100–120 days (Jain, 1986). Hematocrits are generally between 40 and 50% and are slightly higher for males than for females. Compared with most species, dog erythrocytes are relatively resistant to osmotic lysis as measured by osmotic fragility tests.

White blood cell counts range from about 5000 to 15,000/μl. Laboratory-reared beagles tend to have lower and less variable counts than the general dog population. In contrast to the other species, neutrophils normally outnumber lymphocytes. The neutrophil:lymphocyte ratio is typically about 60:40–70:30. Dog neutrophils have segmented nuclei, and their primary granules are much fainter than those in human neutrophils.

Typical inflammatory lesions in the dog generally cause a neutrophilic leukocytosis. The presence of a left shift, as in all species, depends upon the severity of the lesion and the inciting agent. Lymphopenia, secondary to stress-induced endogenous corticosteroid, often occurs with serious inflammatory diseases. In the dog, leukocyte counts greater than 50,000/μl occur with closed infections such as pyometra or prostatic abscess. Dogs typically respond to exogenous corticosteroid treatment with a mature neutrophilia, lymphopenia, eosinopenia, and monocytosis.

Table 7   Clinical Pathology Reference Ranges Beagle Dog—Young Adult

Test	Units	Male	Female
Red blood cell count	x10^6/μl	5.5–7.7	5.5–7.6
Hemoglobin	g/dl	12.5–17.0	12.3–17.0
Hematocrit	%	38–51	36–50
Mean corpuscular volume	fl	60–71	62–72
Mean corpuscular hemoglobin	pg	20–24	20–24
Mean corpuscular hemoglobin concentration	%	32–35	31–35
Platelet count	x10^3/μl	240–550	270–550
Prothrombin time	sec	5.8–8.2	6.0–8.0
Partial thromboplastin time	sec	9.0–13.0	9.5–13.5
White blood cell count	x10^3/μl	6.4–14.6	5.6–15.2
Segmented neutrophils	x10^3/μl	3.0–9.5	3.0–10.5
Band neutrophils	x10^3/μl	0.0–0.0	0.0–0.0
Lymphocytes	x10^3/μl	1.0–6.0	1.5–5.5
Monocytes	x10^3/μl	0.0–0.9	0.0–0.8
Eosinophils	x10^3/μl	0.0–0.8	0.0–0.7
Basophils	x10^3/μl	0.0–0.1	0.0–0.1
Nucleated red blood cell count	/100 WBC	0–1	0–1
Glucose	mg/dl	82–120	85–125
Total protein	g/dl	5.0–6.5	5.0–6.3
Albumin	g/dl	3.0–3.9	3.1–4.0
Globulin	g/dl		
Cholesterol	mg/dl	120–220	120–230
Triglyceride	mg/dl		
Urea nitrogen	mg/dl	7–18	7–22
Creatinine	mg/dl	0.5–0.8	0.5–0.8
Total bilirubin	mg/dl	0.0–0.2	0.0–0.2
Aspartate aminotransferase	IU/L	15–45	15–45
Alanine aminotransferase	IU/L	22–48	20–50
Alkaline phosphatase	IU/L	68–190	65–200
γ-Glutamyl transferase	IU/L		
Creatine kinase	IU/L	35–580	40–540
Calcium	mg/dl	10.2–12.0	9.8–12.1
Inorganic phosphorus	mg/dl	6.6–8.4	6.0–8.2
Sodium	mmol/L	143–158	142–156
Potassium	mmol/L	4.4–6.5	4.3–6.5
Chloride	mmol/L	108–118	109–120

Hematopoiesis is confined to the bone marrow in normal dogs. Extramedullary hematopoiesis, usually in the spleen, may be observed in moderate-to-severe anemia with marked regeneration. The M:E ratio in the bone marrow is usually from 1:1 to 2:1. In contrast to rodents, lymphocytes generally comprise less than 5% of the nucleated cell population.

Platelet counts in dogs are generally in the range of 200,000/μl–500,000/μl. Inherited factor VII deficiency, an autosomal recessive trait, affects many beagle dogs from commercial breeding colonies. The disease is mild, causing no obvious bleeding problems with the exception of increased tendency to bruise. The dogs may also have increased susceptibility to systemic demodecosis. The disease is usually detected when prothrombin times are measured in a group of dogs and one or more have notably longer times. The difference, however, may only be 2 or 3 sec.

Clinical Chemistry

The popularity of the dog as a pet is primarily responsible for the extensive database that has been accumulated concerning its clinical pathology findings in health and disease. The relative ease of sample collection eliminates many variables, such as collection site and anesthesia, that influence the interpretation of data from smaller animals. It is rather natural, therefore, to think of the dog as the "norm" and to compare other species with it. In this respect, clinical chemistry findings appear fairly straightforward. A few notable features of clinical chemistry in the dog will be discussed here.

When compared with the "street" population of dogs, laboratory-reared beagle dogs have very narrow ranges for several parameters, especially total protein, albumin, globulin, urea nitrogen, creatinine, ALT, and AST. Carbohydrate metabolism in dogs is similar to that in humans, and glucose tolerance tests have been well documented (Kaneko, 1989). The range for total serum cholesterol concentration is higher and wider than for smaller laboratory species; values over 200 mg/dl are relatively common. Like many laboratory animals, but unlike humans, HDL is the most abundant lipoprotein.

Serum ALT activity is both sensitive and specific for hepatocellular injury, but as in other species, certain compounds may stimulate enzyme production and cause small increases in the absence of pathological change. Serum AP activity in the dog is very sensitive to intrahepatic or extrahepatic cholestasis but will increase with a variety of hepatic lesions. In addition, the dog has a unique steroid-induced AP isoenzyme that can be markedly elevated after administration of exogenous corticosteroids or secondary to hyperadrenocorticism. In these conditions, the hepatic isoenzyme activity will also increase. Serum GGT and 5'N activities parallel serum AP activity during cholestasis and are more specific for biliary diseases. The degree of change for GGT, however, is not as great as for AP. Decreasing activity of the osteoblastic isoenzyme of AP is responsible for the gradual lowering of serum AP activity with age. Serum GGT and 5'N activities are unaffected by changes in bone metabolism.

Total serum bilirubin concentration is slow to increase in cholestatic diseases in the dog because the renal threshold for bilirubin is low. Bilirubinuria is a common finding, even for normal dogs.

Findings for electrolytes are similar to those in humans. However, because dog erythrocytes have a low intracellular potassium concentration, hemolysis does not cause spuriously high serum potassium values.

Thyroid and adrenocortical hormone tests are well documented (Kaneko, 1989). The size of the dog makes it a very suitable species for stimulation and suppression studies. Cortisol is the primary adrenocorticosteroid in the dog.

Urinalysis

As mentioned previously, bilirubinuria is a normal finding in the dog, especially in concentrated urine.

Nonhuman Primates (Table 8)

Hematology

Although the size of nonhuman primate erythrocytes is somewhat species dependent, they are generally smaller than those of humans. The MCV for cynomolgus monkeys (approx-

Table 8 Clinical Pathology Reference Ranges Cynomolgus Monkey—Adult, Wild-Caught

Test	Units	Male	Female
Red blood cell count	$\times 10^6/\mu l$	5.2–7.8	5.5–7.6
Hemoglobin	g/dl	10.5–14.0	10.0–13.5
Hematocrit	%	36–49	34–48
Mean corpuscular volume	fl	57–75	57–73
Mean corpuscular hemoglobin	pg	16–22	16–22
Mean corpuscular hemoglobin concentration	%	27–32	27–32
Platelet count	$\times 10^3/\mu l$	180–650	175–750
Prothrombin time	sec	9.0–12.5	9.0–12.0
Partial thromboplastin time	sec	16.0–29.0	16.0–29.0
White blood cell count	$\times 10^3/\mu l$	5.0–18.0	3.5–18.0
Segmented neutrophils	$\times 10^3/\mu l$	0.5–7.5	0.5–9.0
Band neutrophils	$\times 10^3/\mu l$	0.0–0.0	0.0–0.0
Lymphocytes	$\times 10^3/\mu l$	2.0–12.0	1.0–10.0
Monocytes	$\times 10^3/\mu l$	0.0–0.5	0.0–0.5
Eosinophils	$\times 10^3/\mu l$	0.0–0.7	0.0–0.7
Basophils	$\times 10^3/\mu l$	0.0–0.2	0.0–0.2
Nucleated red blood cell count	/100 WBC	0–1	0–1
Glucose	mg/dl	45–100	40–100
Total protein	g/dl	7.3–9.8	7.1–9.8
Albumin	g/dl	3.7–5.0	3.5–5.0
Globulin	g/dl	3.2–5.0	3.2–5.4
Cholesterol	mg/dl	110–190	100–200
Triglyceride	mg/dl	20–100	30–80
Urea nitrogen	mg/dl	15–26	12–30
Creatinine	mg/dl	0.8–1.2	0.7–1.1
Total bilirubin	mg/dl	0.1–0.8	0.1–0.8
Aspartate aminotransferase	IU/L	20–100	15–105
Alanine aminotransferase	IU/L	15–200	20–230
Alkaline phosphatase	IU/L	100–1100	150–600
γ-Glutamyl transferase	IU/L	40–170	30–160
Creatine kinase	IU/L	150–1100	150–1000
Calcium	mg/dl	8.9–11.3	8.6–11.0
Inorganic phosphorus	mg/dl	5.1–8.9	4.1–8.1
Sodium	mmol/L	148–169	148–172
Potassium	mmol/L	4.0–6.0	4.0–6.5
Chloride	mmol/L	101–116	102–117

imately 58–72 fl) is less than that for rhesus monkeys (approximately 70–80 fl). Among laboratory animals, monkey erythrocytes tend to have the largest, most obvious area of central pallor. The cells often appear somewhat hypochromic, and MCHC is generally lower in monkeys than in other species. Values less 30% for MCHC are frequently observed. Because of these findings, there is a concern that low-grade iron deficiency may be a subclinical problem affecting laboratory primates. The normal reticulocyte count is less than 1%; anisocytosis and polychromasia are minimal. Howell-Jolly bodies and nucleated red blood cells are rarely observed in normal adults. Erythrocyte survival time is

approximately 85–100 days (Jain, 1986; Kreier, 1970). Hematocrits are generally between 35 and 45% and tend to be higher for males than for females.

Subclinical malarial infection, recognized by the presence of intracellular *Plasmodium* trophozoites and schizonts, is relatively common in wild-caught, imported cynomolgus and rhesus monkeys (Donovan et al., 1983; Stokes et al., 1983; Schofield et al., 1985). Clinical disease is unusual without complicating factors such as disease-induced or drug-induced immunosuppression and splenectomy. Most frequently noted as an incidental finding on peripheral blood films of healthy animals, infections will occasionally cause an acute hemolytic anemia in animals secondary to experimental manipulations.

White blood cell counts range from about 5,000 to 20,000/μl. The extended reference range is mostly due to a physiological leukocytosis observed in "untrained" animals bled without chemical restraint. The release of catecholamines may double the WBC count by mobilizing cells, both neutrophils and lymphocytes, from the marginal pool to the circulating pool. While this "alarm" or "fright" reaction can probably occur in any laboratory species, it appears to have the greatest effect on nonhuman primates. In nonhuman primates, lymphocytes are increased more than neutrophils during this reaction. The upper limit of reference ranges for anesthetized or trained animals is closer to 12,000/μl. The neutrophil:lymphocyte ratio is generally around 40:60 or 50:50 but may reach 30:70 in excited animals. Neutrophil morphology is similar to that in humans; primary granules are prominent.

As in the dog, hematopoiesis is confined to the bone marrow. The M:E ratio is usually from 1:1 to 1.5:1. Lymphocytes generally comprise less than 5% of the nucleated cell population.

Platelet counts are generally in the range of 300,000–600,000/μl. Coagulation times, PT and APTT, are slightly longer than for dogs but similar to man.

Clinical Chemistry

As might be expected, clinical chemistry results for wild-caught monkeys are quite variable; the reference ranges for most parameters are broad. Although fasting serum glucose concentration is lower in the monkey than in other laboratory species, the "alarm" reaction can cause glucose values high enough to be confused with diabetes mellitus. High serum glucose concentrations (e.g., >150 mg/dl) should be checked with repeated serum glucose tests and urinalysis for glucose and ketones. Monkeys with diabetes mellitus frequently have high serum cholesterol and triglyceride concentrations. Atherogenic diets also cause increased serum cholesterol and triglyceride concentrations.

Wild-caught monkeys often have surprisingly high total serum protein and globulin concentrations; values over 9.0 and 5.0 g/dl, respectively, are not uncommon. The etiology is thought to be subclinical inflammatory or infectious disease with chronic antigenic stimulation causing a polyclonal gammopathy. Serum urea nitrogen and creatinine concentrations are higher and much more variable than in dogs.

Serum enzyme activities also tend to be highly variable. Increased serum activity of muscle enzymes (e.g., creatine kinase, AST, and LDH) may be observed secondary to iatrogenic muscle injury associated with handling or intramuscular injections of anesthetic. Alanine aminotransferase, although present in muscle tissue in the monkey, is relatively specific and sensitive for hepatocellular injury. A fairly common cause of increased serum ALT activity in cynomolgus and rhesus monkeys is subclinical, enzootic hepatitis A infection (Slighter et al., 1988). Increased activity correlates with seroconversion to the virus and periportal inflammation. Because a percentage of animals entering a facility for use in toxicology studies are not already infected, exposure and infection may take place during the actual study period causing sporadic, high serum ALT activities in a few individuals. These results often confound the interpretation of the enzyme data.

Serum AP activity is much higher in cynomolgus monkeys than in any other laboratory animal species, and GGT may be of more value in the diagnosis of hepatobiliary disease in the monkey than in other species.

Values for serum electrolytes are extremely variable in unanesthetized monkeys. Serum sodium and chloride concentrations may range up to 170 and 125 mmol/L, respectively. The reason for these extremely high results is not known, but in the anesthetized animal, values over 155 and 115 mmol/L are unusual. In the monkey, serum potassium concentration may be spuriously elevated due to hemolysis since erythrocyte intracellular potassium concentration is high.

Cortisol is the primary adrenocorticosteroid in the monkey. Values in marmosets are higher than in macaques (Loeb, 1989). The same is true of T_3 and T_4 (Kaack et al., 1979).

REFERENCES

Albers, H. E., Yogev, L., Todd, R. B., and Goldman, B. D. (1985) Adrenal corticoids in hamsters: Role in circadian timing. *Am. J. Physiol.* 248, R434–R438.

Allen, R. C., Meier, H., and Hoeg, W. G. (1962) Distribution of coagulation proteins in normal mouse plasma. *Science* 135, 103.

Alt, J. M., Hackbarth, H., Deerberg, F., and Stolte, H. (1980) Proteinuria in rats in relation to age-dependent renal changes. *Lab. Anim.* 14, 95–101.

Bannerman, R. M. (1983) Hematology, in *The Mouse in Biomedical Research*, Vol. III, *Normative Biology, Immunology, and Husbandry*, Foster, H. L., Small, J. D., and Fox, J. G., eds. Academic Press, New York, pp. 293–312.

Bernard, S. L., Leathers, C. W., Brobst, D. F., and Gorham, J. R. (1983) Estrogen-induced bone marrow depression in ferrets. *Am. J. Vet. Res.* 44, 657.

Brock, M. A. (1960) Production and life span of erythrocytes during hibernation in the golden hamster. *Am. J. Physiol.* 198, 1181.

Carroll, R. M., and Feldman, E. B. (1989) Lipids and lipoproteins, in *The Clinical Chemistry of Laboratory Animals*, Loeb, W. F., and Quimby, F. W., eds. Pergamon Press, New York, pp. 95–116.

Clarkson, T. B., Lehner, N. D. M., and Bullock, B. C. (1974) Specialized research applications. I. Arteriosclerosis research, in *The Biology of the Rabbit*, Weisbroth, S. H., Flatt, R. E., and Kraus, A. L., eds. Academic Press, New York, pp. 155–166.

Desai, R. G. (1968) Hematology and microcirculation, in *The Golden Hamster—Its Biology and Use in Medical Research*, Hoffman, R. A., Robinson, P. F., and Magalhaes, H., eds. Iowa State University Press, Ames, pp. 185–191.

Dodds, W. J., Raymond, S. L., Moynihan, A. C., and McMartin, D. N. (1977) Spontaneous atrial thrombosis in aged Syrian hamsters. II. Hemostasis. *Thromb. Haemos.* 38, 457–464.

Donovan, J. C., Stokes, W. S., Montrey, R. D., and Rozmiarek, H. (1983) Hematologic characterization of naturally occurring malaria *(Plasmodium inui)* in cynomolgus monkeys *(Macaca fascicularis)*. *Lab. Anim. Sci.* 33, 86–89.

Duncan, J. R., and Prasse, K. W. (1986) *Veterinary Laboratory Medicine*, 2nd ed., Iowa State University Press, Ames.

Everett, R. M., and Harrison Jr., S. D. (1983) Clinical biochemistry, in *The Mouse in Biomedical Research*, Vol. III, *Normative Biology, Immunology, and Husbandry*, Foster, H. L., Small, J. D., and Fox, J. G., eds. Academic Press, New York, pp. 313–326.

Garibaldi, B. A., Pecquet Goad, M. E., Fox, J. G., and Murray, R. (1988a) Serum thyroxine and triiodothyronine radioimmunoassay values in the normal ferret. *Lab. Anim. Sci.* 38, 455–458.

Garibaldi, B. A., Pecquet Goad, M. E., Fox, J. G., Sylvina, T. J., and Murray, R. (1988b). Serum cortisol radioimmunoassay values in the normal ferret and response to ACTH stimulation and dexamethasone suppression tests. *Lab. Anim. Sci.* 38, 452–454.

Gerritsen, G. C. (1982). The Chinese hamster as a model for the study of diabetes mellitus. *Diabetes* 31, 14–25.

Ghys, A., Thys, O., Hildebrand, J., and Georges, A. (1975). Relation between hepatic and renal function tests and ultrastructural changes induced by 2-N-methylpiperazinomethyl-1,3-diazafluoranthen 1-oxide (AD-3579), a new experimental antileukemic drug. *Toxicol. Appl. Pharmacol.* 31, 13–20.

Heard, D. J., Collins, B., Chen, D. L., and Coniglario, J. (1990). Thyroid and adrenal function tests in adult male ferrets. *Am. J. Vet. Res.* 51, 32–35.

Homburger, F., Nixon, C. W., Eppenberger, M., and Baker, J. R. (1966). Hereditary myopathy in the Syrian hamster: Studies on pathogenesis. *Ann. N. Y. Acad. Sci.* 138, 14–27.

Jain, N. C. (1986). *Schalm's Veterinary Hematology*, 4th ed., Lea & Febiger, Philadelphia.

Kaack, B., Walker, L., Brizzee, K. R., and Wolf, R. H. (1979). Comparative normal levels of serum triiodothyronine and thyroxine in nonhuman primates. *Lab. Anim. Sci.* 29, 191–199.

Kaneko, J. J. (1989). *Clinical Biochemistry of Domestic Animals*, 4th ed., Academic Press, San Diego.

Kaplow, L. S. (1969). Alkaline phosphatase activity in peripheral blood lymphocytes. *Arch. Pathol.* 82, 69–72.

Kaspareit, J., Messow, C., and Edel, J. (1988). Blood coagulation studies in guineapigs *(Cavia porcellus)*. *Lab. Anim.* 22, 206–211.

Kociba, G., and Caputo, C. A. (1981). Aplastic anemia associated with estrus in pet ferrets. *J. Am. Vet. Med. Assoc.* 178, 1293.

Kreier, J. P. (1970). Erythrocyte life span and label elution in monkeys *(Macaca mulatta)* and cats *(Felis catus)* determined with chromium-51 and diisopropyl fluorophosphate-32. *Am. J. Vet. Res.* 31, 1429.

Kryszewski, A. J., Neale, G., Whitefield, J. B., and Moss, D. W. (1973). Enzyme changes in experimental biliary obstruction. *Clin. Chem. Acta* 47, 175–182.

Ledingham, J. C. G. (1940). Sex hormones and the Foa-Kurloff cell. *J. Pathol. Bacteriol.* 50, 201–219.

Lee, E. J., Moore, W. E., Fryer, H. C., and Minocha, H. C. (1982). Haematological and serum chemistry profiles of ferrets *(Mustela putorius furo)*. *Lab. Anim.* 16, 133–137.

Leonard, T. B., Neptun, D. A., and Popp, J. A. (1984). Serum gamma glutamyl transferase as a specific indicator of bile duct lesions in the rat liver. *Am. J. Pathol.* 116, 262–269.

Loeb, W. F., and Quimby, F. W., (1989). *The Clinical Chemistry of Laboratory Animals*, Pergamon Press, New York.

Lyman, C. P., and Leduc, E. H. (1953). Changes in blood sugar and tissue glycogen in the hamster during arousal from hibernation. *J. Cell. Comp. Physiol.* 41, 471–492.

Meeks, R. G. (1989). The rat, in *The Clinical Chemistry of Laboratory Animals*, Loeb, W. F., and Quimby, F. W., eds. Pergamon Press, New York, pp. 19–25.

Murphy, J. C., Fox, J. G., and Niemi, S. M. (1984). Nephrotic syndrome associated with renal amyloidosis in a colony of Syrian hamsters. *J. Am. Vet. Med. Assoc.* 185, 1359–1362.

Neptun, D. A., Smith, C. N., and Irons, R. D. (1985). Effect of sampling site and collection method on variations in baseline clinical pathology parameters in Fischer-344 rats. 1. Clinical chemistry. *Fund. Appl. Toxicol.* 5, 1180–1185.

Oishi, S., Oishi, H., and Hiraga, K. (1979). The effect of food restriction for 4 weeks on common toxicity parameters in male rats. *Toxicol. Appl. Pharmacol.* 47, 15–22.

Ottenweller, J. E., Tapp, W. N., Burke, J. M., and Natelson, B. H. (1985). Plasma cortisol and corticosterone concentrations in the golden hamster *(Mesocricetus auratus)*. *Life Sci.* 37, 1551–1557.

Riley, V., Spackman, D. H., Santisteban, G. A., Dalldorf, G., and Hellstrom, I. (1978). The LDH virus: An interfering biological contaminant. *Science* 200, 124–126.

Sanderson, J. H., and Phillips, C. E. (1981). *An Atlas of Laboratory Animal Haematology*, Oxford University Press, Oxford, England.

Scholfield, L. D., Bennett, B. T., Collins, W. E., and Beluhan, F. Z. (1985). An outbreak of *Plasmodium inui* malaria in a colony of diabetic rhesus monkeys. *Lab. Anim. Sci.* 35, 167–168.

Schwartz, E., Tornaben, J. A., and Boxill, G. C. (1973). The effects of food restriction on hematology, clinical chemistry, and pathology in the albino rat. *Toxicol. Appl. Pharmacol.* 25, 515–524.

Sherrill, A., and Gorham, J. (1985). Bone marrow hypoplasia associated with estrus in ferrets. *Lab. Anim. Sci.* 35, 280–286.

Slighter, R. G., Kimball, J. P., Barbolt, T. A., Sherer, A. D., and Drobeck, H. P. (1988). Enzootic Hepatitis A infection in cynomolgus monkeys *(Macaca fascicularis)*. *Am. J. Primatol.* 14, 73–81.

South, F. E., and Jeffay, H. (1958). Alterations in serum proteins of hibernating hamsters. *Proc. Soc. Exp. Biol. Med.* 98, 885–887.

Stokes, W. S., Donovan, J. C., Montrey, R. D., Thompson, W. L., Wannemacher Jr, R. W., and Rozmiarek, H. (1983). Acute clinical malaria *(Plasmodium inui)* in a cynomolgus monkey *(Macaca fascicularis)*. *Lab. Anim. Sci.* 33, 81–85.

Stromberg, P. C. (1985). Large granular lymphocyte leukemia in F344 rats. *Am. J. Pathol.* 119, 517–519.

Suber, R. L., and Kodell, R. L. (1985). The effect of three phlebotomy techniques on hematological and clinical chemical evaluation in Sprague-Dawley rats. *Vet. Clin. Pathol.* 14, 23–30.

Swaim, L. D., Taylor, H. W., and Jersey, G. C. (1985). The effect of handling techniques on serum ALT activity in mice. *J. Appl. Toxicol.* 5, 160–162.

Thornton, P. C., Wright, P. A., Sacra, P. J., and Goodier, T. E. W. (1979). The ferret, *Mustela putorius furo*, as a new species in toxicology. *Lab. Anim.* 13, 119–124.

Toth, L. A., and Krueger, J. M. (1989). Hematologic effects of exposure to three infective agents in rabbits. *J. Am. Vet. Med. Assoc.* 195, 981–986.

Wolfe, H. J., Bitman, W. R., Voelkel, E. F., Griffiths, H. J., and Tashjian, A. H. (1978). Systemic effects of the VX$_2$ carcinoma on the osseous skeleton. *Lab. Invest.* 38, 208–215.

Yamanaka, W., Ostwald, R., and French, S. (1967). Histopathology of guinea pigs with cholesterol induced anemia. *Proc. Soc. Exp. Biol. Med.* 125, 303–306.

Zimmerman, A., Moule, M., and Yip, C. (1974). Guinea pig insulin. II. Biological activity. *J. Biol. Chem.* 249, 4026–4029.

12

Model Selection and Scaling

Shayne Cox Gad
Becton Dickinson and Company
Research Triangle Park, North Carolina

This entire book is directed at the premises that (1) animals can serve as accurate predictive models of toxicity in humans (or other species), (2) the selection of an appropriate species to use is key to accurate prediction in man, and (3) understanding the strengths and weaknesses of any particular model is essential to understanding the relevance of specific target organ toxicities to what would be expected in humans. Each of these premises requires some examination.

It is a fundamental hypothesis of toxicology that adverse effects caused by chemical entities in animals are generally the same as those induced by those entities in humans. There are many who point to individual exceptions to this and conclude that the general principle is false. Yet, as our understanding of molecular biology advances and we learn more about the similarities of structure and function of higher organisms at the molecular level, the more it becomes clear that the mechanisms of chemical toxicity are largely identical in humans and animals. This increased understanding has caused some of the same people who question the general principle of predictive value to in turn suggest that our state of knowledge is such that mathematical models or simple cell culture systems could be used just as well as intact animals to predict toxicities in man. This last also misses the point that the final expressions of toxicity in humans or animals is frequently the summation of extensive and complex interactions on cellular and biochemical levels. Zbinden (1987) has published extensively in this area, including a very advanced defense of the value of animal models. Lijinsky (1988) has reviewed the specific issues about the predictive value and importance of animals in carcinogenicity testing and research. Though it was once widely believed (and still is believed by many animal rights activists) that in vitro mutagenicity tests would replace animal bioassays for carcinogenicity, this is clearly not the case on either scientific or regulatory grounds. Though there are differences in the responses of various species (including humans) to carcinogens (Gregory, 1988), the overall predictive value of such results (when tempered by judgment) is clear. Additionally, though, many propose that there is little data to support that findings of toxicity in animals have been predictive of adverse effects in humans (because agents found toxic in animals are generally not knowingly given to humans). This is not the case—see Zbinden (1987) or refer to recent events surrounding azidothymidine (AZT) or retionines.

The principal problem in using animal models as predictions of toxicity in humans lies in the second major premise cited at the beginning of this chapter. As will be addressed in the first major section of this chapter, the theoretical basis for selection of the appropriate animal model is well established and often quoted (Plaa, 1976) but rarely adhered to. As the core chapters in this book should have established, each commonly used model species has both strengths and weaknesses. Probably the greater weakness in the current practice of toxicity testing is a lack of care in selection of the appropriate model. Our third premise is this very point: Each model species has strengths and weakness, and an understanding of these in evaluating findings in the species we actually use in essential to establishing the relevance (or lack of relevance) of findings.

This is, of course, one reason that toxicity is generally evaluated in at least two species. As Plaa (1976) and Litchfield, (1962) have pointed out, adverse effects found in two separate and diverse model species have a much higher predictive power for the outcome of exposure in humans. A subset of this consideration (susceptibility factors) is addressed in the next chapter. Susceptibility factors are differences in either the animal model or human population (such as age, sex, disease, diet, physiological state, or strain) which can markedly influence the toxicity of a chemical entity and the course of an induced pathogenesis. Many times the predictive value of our animal studies could be improved by altering elements of protocol or experimental design to allow for the existence of susceptibility factors in a target populations. Another corollary of this third premise is that there are times when adverse effects have nothing to do with what will happen in humans. Clayson (1988) has reviewed the case for this in terms of carcinogenicity, but the argument is not limited to that.

MODEL SELECTION

The key points in selecting the most appropriate animal species as a model are to start by clearly identifying the objective of the studies to be performed and then to utilize all available information on both available model species and the mode of action and pharmacokinetics of the compound to be studied.

If the objective of a study is limited to acting for a screen or a "single endpoint"–type assay (Gad and Chengelis, 1988), then a much wider range of species will be appropriate than if greater discrimination is required.

Given all that has been presented in the core chapters on test systems, the characteristics of different species and how one extrapolates from one species to another, the next obvious question is how are test species actually selected?

The obvious theoretical best choice would be the species considered at risk, which would leave us with no difficulty in extrapolating from one species to another.* For some applications (veterinary agents or where the concern is for the effects of potential exposures to domesticated animals or wildlife), it is possible to take this approach. But for most cases, where the real life concern is potential toxicity to humans, a laboratory animal species must be selected as although chemical are still occasionally administered to people for experimental purposes, there are legal and ethical issues which make this a rare case indeed before at least some acute toxicity data has been gathered in a species other than humans (National Academy of Science 1975). Even then, initial toxicity tests carried out

---

*Though, as will be seen later in this chapter under "Limitations of Models", not all members of the same species (even disregarding sex and strain differences) respond the same.

in humans are generally at low dose levels compared to the toxic doses predicted from animal experiments. The design of acute toxicity studies in which humans are used is commonly directed at the evaluation of alterations in blood chemistry, measurable physiological variables, and the analysis of the agent and its metabolites in the blood, urine, feces, and tissues (Nosal and Hladka, 1968; Rider et al., 1969). With pesticides and a few other environmental agents, useful human acute toxicity data has been obtained by the study of accidentally exposed individuals (Brown, 1980).

What then would constitute the best choice of models? There is a set of characteristics that most would agree constitute the "ideal" animals on scientific grounds. These include (1) similarity of absorption, distribution, metabolism, and excretion to humans; (2) sensitivity of the species to the agent closely resembling that of humans; (3) evolutionary level of the animal; (4) ability of the species to express the full range of responses that humans would (such as emesis); (5) ability to make all pertinent measurements in a meaningful way; and (6) stages of the life span should correlate directly to those of humans.

However, there is also a set of desired characteristics for an ideal species to possess from a technical management point of view. These criteria are:

1. Have a low body weight. The weight of the experimental animal is so important because during the early stages of development of new commercial chemicals only small quantities of the test material may be available.
2. Be easy to bleed and large enough to supply a reasonable amount of blood.
3. Be easy to obtain or breed and maintain in the laboratory.
4. Be easy to handle and to administer test agents to by the various desired routes.
5. Should have a short life span.
6. Physiology and metabolism should approximate those of humans.
7. Should not pose a disease threat to handlers.

Each of these ideal features is secondary to the desire to have a model that responds exactly as our target species. However, there is no animal species that mimics humans in all respects, so that the ultimate choice depends on the balance of conflicting factors. For example, consider the case of the selecting a model to predict the effects of agents on the gastrointestinal tract of humans (Fara et al., 1988). There is not single best model, with the common species (rat, mouse, and dog) generally being more sensitive than humans to such agents as nonsteroid anti-inflammatory drugs (NSAIDs). It is all too easy to suggest that the animal of choice should fit the criteria enumerated above, but in actuality these are empty words. Actual selections are made generally on practical and "political" criteria rather than these logical points.

The data necessary to make decisions based on practical considerations has largely been incorporated into the tables in the core chapters of this book. Economic considerations turn out to be among the most important. These include the cost of the animal and its upkeep, availability of test animals, housing requirements, and a host of other factors that tend to push selection toward smaller, established test animal species.

The possibilities for selection are, of course, much wider. The subkingdom of vertebrate animals alone contains a great number of species, which can be classified into distinct categories, as shown in Table 1.

But only a few of this multitude of possible species has actually been employed at any time. And the eight species that are discussed in-depth in this chapter represent virtually all (99.9%) of the animals currently used in acute toxicology. Why is this?

Table 1 Approximate Distribution
of the Vertebrate Animal Species

Category	No. of distinct species
Fish	23,000
Amphibians	2,000
Reptiles	8,500
Mammals	4,500
All vertebrates	43,000

Source: Rothschild, 1961.

How Species Are Actually Selected

There are two major sets of factors which actually drive the process of model selection in acute toxicology, with rare exceptions.

First, economic considerations such as ease of commercial production and availability, housing, life span, etc., have, as was pointed out above, favored the use of small laboratory animals. In the resulting enthusiasm for establishing rodents as the satisfactory test models, toxicologists have conveniently overlooked the fact that there have been few studies correlating the toxicity of specific compounds in humans and these animal species. The available information suggests a moderate-to-fair direct correlation (Litchfield 1961, 1962). Difficulties in validating alternative or new test systems have tended to preclude any improvement of the model systems that are employed. There is an urgent need for a nonrodent species with a life span of up to 5 years that does not have the problems inherent in the dog or primate. Ferrets, marmosets, miniature pigs, and a number of other species have been investigated during the last 15 years, but only now have people begun to use one of these (the ferret) to any extent. There is clearly an opportunity for the commercial animal breeder here, but it may be that the essential criteria are impossible to meet and the underlying societal inertia is too great. Stevenson (1979) has discussed these aspects in the wider context of general toxicology.

The second major set of factors can only be classified generally as custom or habit. What the scientists and technicians are used to using, and what the regulators are used to interpreting data from, is generally what we tend to continue doing. The resulting inertia is the greatest impediment not only to proper model selection, but also to adaptation of new or improved study designs and to the development and use of in vitro models. The frequently raised issue of "validation" for any proposed change in what the science of toxicology does is all too often more accurately stated as, "Show us that it gives us the same answers—we know how to deal with those, even if they are wrong."

To fulfill these two sets of factors, animals are then actually selected for acute testing based on the following steps.

1. Which species will meet test design needs?
2. What is species availability?
3. How much test compound is available? If the amount is limited, the smallest (body weight) species that will meet other needs will be selected.

4. What species is the least expensive, both in terms of costs directly associated with the animals and indirect costs (the easier an animal is to handle, for example, the lower are the labor costs associated with the study). There are some special cases of species selection being based on expense. The most common of these is where the compound (usually a drug) being studied is very expensive or in extremely short supply. As a result, using the smallest possible animals reduces compound use. In this sense, small primates are often "less" expensive than dogs.

5. Will the species selected meet regulatory guidelines (usually easy, as these either dictate a species for a particular test or simply specify rodent or nonrodent) and have regulatory "acceptance" (not so easy)?

6. What have we used in the past? This question usually actually comes first, generating a list of candidate species.

Special Cases in Species Selection

There are a number of the routes of exposure which have a particular species which is by habit (frequently based on a form of folklore) especially favored.

In inhalation, there are several special considerations of anatomy and physiology which dictate model selection. The following three factors should be strongly considered in species selection for inhalation studies.

1. Mouth (10 μ filtration) vs nose (3 μ filtration) breathers. A human versus rodent comparison, with considerable resulting differences in both particular/droplet filtration and regional absorption.

2. Number of "daughter" generations of air passages. These are the number of successive times that air passages in the respiratory tree branches. There are 35 in the human.

3. Distribution of major compartments in the respiratory tract. Humans have:

Nasopharyngeal (NP)
    Nasal cavity
    Mouth
Tracheobronchial (TB)
    Larynx
    Trachea
    Bronchials
Alveolar sacs
    Pulmonary (P)

The rat is far and away the most common species used in inhalation, even though it is an obligatory nose breather and its respiratory morphophysiology is much different than that of humans (it has five lung lobes and a total lung surface area of 7.5 m^2—10% of that of humans).

Folklore says that primates are the best inhalation model for humans. However, the closest similarity in respiratory structure and function is probably found in the horse or donkey. Besides the rat, commonly used species include none of these, however. Rather, the mouse and dog are the only other commonly used species in inhalation.

Likewise, dermal studies are by custom performed on the rabbit because its dermal absorption is "greater" than that of humans, making it the most sensitive model. As has been presented in a review by Gad and Chengelis (1988), this in fact is not the case.

Neither is it true that in the general case the dermal absorption and skin morphology of the pig most resemble humans (as originally reported by Bartek et al., 1972). Rather, the answers as to which species is either most sensitive or most resembles humans depend very much on the structural characteristics of compounds in question. Recent efforts and suggestions by some that all toxicity tests be performed on a common species, such as the rat, merit wider consideration. If we as scientists are not willing or able to select models on a scientific basis of what will provide us with the best prediction of what would happen in humans, then the argument of at least using a single common model that we understand the weaknesses of becomes a compelling one.

Caution

Having considered the general process of model selection, one should next be aware of the limitations and peculiarities of the common models, and of some of the variations that occur within a species due to differences between strains of animals.

LIMITATIONS OF MODELS

Despite our best efforts, when human exposures to a chemical entity (such as a drug) occur, the results do not always come near what was expected based on animal studies. For the population as a whole, there are a number of possible explanations. Some of these are presented in Table 2.

An example of these types of problems in the extrapolation of toxicity data from one species to another can be found in published studies on fenclozic acid, which was a potential new anti-inflammatory drug (Alcock, 1971). No adverse effects were observed

Table 2 Some Reasons Why Data Obtained in Animal Studies Does Not Always Match Human Experience

1. The animal species selected differ in response from humans. The same measurement or experiments in a different animal species may have been more predictive.
2. Differences in absorption, distribution, and/or metabolism may be present.
3. The anatomy involved in the model may differ from that in people.
4. Different animal strains of the same species may generate different results.
5. The pathological nature of any lesions produced may differ at either a macroscopic or microscopic level.
6. There may be critical differences between the species at subcellular, cellular, receptor or physiological levels that lead to different responses. This is particularly true in terms of our current use of clinical chemistry findings to identify "target organs" in animals when these enzymes may not have the same relationship to pathogenesis in animals as in humans. Consider, for example, the animal clinical chemistry associations review of hepatic function and damage indicators in animals species "correct."
7. Experimental conditions in the animal model may yield qualitatively different data over the course of several experiments, and it may be unclear which set is.
8. The "dose" required to produce the observed results in animals is never achieved in humans.
9. The target dose in humans cannot be achieved in test animals.
10. The human population we are concerned about may differ from the population in general, and in so doing may have special characteristics which were not adequately represented in our animal model population.

to occur in the mouse, rat, dog, rhesus monkey, patas monkey, rabbit, guinea pig, ferret, cat, pig, cow, or horse, but the drug caused acute cholestatic jaundice in humans.

Beyond the difficulties in extrapolating from one or more test animals populations to the overall human population, there are a number limitations to the standard model populations which are imposed by two forms of "good scientific practice" that is employed in conducting toxicity studies. Both of these practices have as their rationale the maximization of the sensitivity of the test system, with the underlying good intention of therefore providing the greatest possible protection to people. This is not actually the effect, however.

The first of these practices is that toxicity testing has traditionally been performed at high doses. Even in acute toxicity studies which have the objective of predicting potential target organs and mechanisms of toxicity for humans at much lower doses, the study is considered suspect if all (or for some people, any) animals survive at the highest dose level tested. This use of a maximum administrable dose and large fractions thereof is a spillover from carcinogenesis testing and times when our ability to detect effects was crude. It can frequently produce errors or difficulties in prediction of effects in people, such as those in Table 3.

The second practice is that of using test animal populations which are as homogeneous as possible. This current strategy for quantifying toxicity for the most part evaluates toxicity in homogeneous populations, whether in animals or in humans, whether in vitro or in vivo. Such an approach minimizes the expression of background biological variability and, therefore, generates the most readily quantifiable and "sensitive" estimates of predicted toxicity. In actual target populations which are more heterogeneous than the model population with respect to, among other things, susceptibility and resistance to the compound in question, this may not be the case. The rationale may not be truly applicable to effects on humans, where a toxicity in even a relatively small susceptible population would not be acceptable. Adjustments for this wider range of susceptibility in the population of potentially exposed humans is most commonly accounted for as being part of what is involved in the use of safety factors in setting allowable limits for human exposure. This may not be either accurate or adequate.

The underlying view is that a potentially toxic exposure occurs with the interaction of the chemical and a model population in a particular space and time. This experimental

Table 3 Reasons Why High Dose Toxicity Testing Is Usually Not Predictive of Human Effects

1. Solubility of the compound may be limiting.
2. Kinetics may be nonlinear (e.g., an enzyme may be saturated) and absorption may be decreased.
3. Michaelis-Menten kinetics may be applicable, and the blood levels may be greater than predicted in animals.
4. Metabolites formed in the animal studies may cause toxicity that would not occur with lower doses (high doses of phenacetin are one of many examples).
5. Detoxification mechanisms in the liver or elsewhere may be depleted or saturated (examples are high doses of acetaminophen in the liver or of hexavalent chromium in the lungs).
6. Bioavailability of the dose form may be entirely different at lower doses due to local physiological effects (such as irritation) in the high dose animal studies.
7. High dose levels in animals may overwhelm organ systems which would not be affected at lower doses, causing effects which serve to mask those seen at lower blood levels.

event of exposure must be characterized by the range of "dose"; type of exposure; characteristics of the exposed population (weight, sex, strain, etc.); the biological characteristics of the effect at the molecular, cellular, tissue, organ, individual, and population levels; and over a spectrum of effects from physiological through pathological and behavioral. The toxicity of the exposure must be characterized in terms of the severity of the effect—for example, clinical signs, disability, and/or death. Later, someone must consider the relevance and acceptability of an observed effect to human society. As a corollary of the principles of experimental design, each variable in a protocol is rigidly fixed within a narrow range. And we use a "high-class" test population—the healthiest, most nutritionally adequately fed young adult animal population possible. These laboratory animals have been carefully bred to make them as genetically defined as possible, and are maintained in clean cages under narrowly controlled environmental conditions. Thus, toxicologists traditionally utilized a very robust and (at best) narrowly representative population of animals under the best of environmental conditions.

How then do we predict for the real-life susceptibility human populations we are most concerned about, or at least allow for them in our predictions? In many cases, perhaps one should utilize special "at-risk" model populations in such tests. For example, if older individuals or those with compromised cardiovascular function are known to constitute a significant part of the potentially exposed human population, study designs should incorporate groups of animals that can serve to determine if such conditions render the animals (and therefore potentially people) more susceptible to toxic effects or if it changes the nature of the expression of the toxic effect.

Susceptibility to an effect at any particular moment in a biological organism is determined by three sets of variables affecting the biological state of the organism at the time of exposure that are largely "invisible" to the outside world: genetic constitution, previous life experience, and momentary physiological state. Genetic constitution is determined by factors of strain, species, family, congenital abnormalities, and any acquired alterations. Species factors are the result of the selection of major genetic components over the course of evolution, and have already been discussed. Strain factors have largely been determined by selective breeding for concentration of genetic characteristics by the laboratory animal breeder, and considerations of strain will be presented later in this chapter.

But there are a number of factors which are part of the other two variables above (life experience and momentary physiological state) which are not generally characteristically represented or considered in our test animal population and yet do exist in humans and do contribute to the biological outcome of a chemical exposure. These can be considered "susceptibility factors." Chapter 13 will explore the problem of susceptibility in detail.

CROSS-SPECIES EXTRAPOLATION

For all the other words in this volume about the relevance of the test systems that are described, one should never forget that none of the animal species we use is other than a model for the human being. And ultimately the continued use of animals in predictive testing must depend on how well we can use the data from these animal models to predict the outcome in people. The activity of transforming results in members of one animal species (say rats) to one or more populations of another species (such as people) is called cross-species extrapolation, or scaling (though technically scaling is actually limited to the act of making adjustments for differences in sizes or rates).

Each step in the scaling process adds an additional degree of uncertainty to the final product. Wise and prudent scientific practice calls for at least three courses of action in seeking to give the best quality (i.e., least uncertain) final product in the form of what does this mean to humans. These courses of action are: (1) have as few steps in the prediction process as possible; (2) have as little uncertainty as possible associated with each step; and (3) understand the places and ways in which the selected model fails as a predictor. Each of these courses of action is not only an integral part of the extrapolation process, but also contributes heavily to proper model (test species) selection.

All the efforts so far in this book have focused primarily on step 2 and part of step 3 above—performing various tests in a manner that gives us the least imprecise and most relevant data possible, and understanding the associated weaknesses of the model systems we employ. As such, our efforts and resulting extrapolations to this point have generally been for the animal species that data were being developed in. Ultimately it is necessary to predict what these data would mean in humans. With the wide range of effects we are concerned about here, what conversion factor (or factors) can we derive that would allow us to equate "x" dose or exposure in rats or "y" effect in dogs with what would be seen in humans at the same or different doses? The tools at hand for the effort consist of a collection of mathematical methods (generally based on either body weight or body surface area as a means of quantitatively bridging the gap) and a set of logical and empirical rules that have been developed over the years.

The mathematical aspects will be addressed primarily in this section of the chapter, whereas the "rules" will appear in the sections that follow. Though there is some scientific basis for these mathematical conversions, it is not on a point-for-point basis and from one to two orders of magnitude of uncertainty are generally involved. Such extrapolations clearly have both quantitative and qualitative aspects, and the rules seek to limit the uncertainty about the qualitative aspects. Some form of pharmacokinetic and metabolic study would provide us with active agent concentrations at target organ sites as well as other information of value in safety assessments (Hawkins and Chasseaud, 1985). While this would be the best approach to such qualitative modeling, even these methods have both difficulties and limitations of their own accompanying their clear advantages (Gillette, 1979), and are expensive and generally not available for support of most cases of data interpretation. An extension of this approach is that of physiological modeling (Gibson and Starr, 1988), which seeks to develop a quantitative compartmental model for each identified organ or organ system.

The qualitative aspects of species-to-species extrapolations are best addressed by a form of classification analysis tailored to the exact problem at hand. This approach identifies the known physiological, metabolic, and other factors which may be involved in the risk-producing process in the model species (for example, the skin sensitization process in the guinea pig), establishes the similarities and differences between these factors and those in humans, and comes up with means to bridge the gaps between these two (or at least identifies the fact that there is no possible bridge).

Table 4 presents an overview of the classes of factors which should be considered in the initial step of a cross-species extrapolation. Examples of such actual differences which can be classified as one of these factor are almost endless.

The absorption of compound from the gastrointestinal tract and from the lungs is generally comparable among vertebrate and mammalian species. There are, however, differences between herbivorous animals and omnivorous animals due to the differences

Table 4 Classes of Factors to Be Considered in Species-to-Species Extrapolations of Toxicity

I. Relative sensitivity of model (compared to humans)
    A. Pharmacological
    B. Receptor
    C. Life span
    D. Size
    E. Metabolic function
    F. Physiological
    G. Anatomical
    H. Nutritional requirements
    I. Reproductive and developmental processes
    J. Diet
    K. Critical reflex and behavioral responses (such as emetic reflex)
    L. Behavioral
    M. Rate of cell division
    N. Other systemic defense mechanisms
    O. Can endpoint of interest be expressed in both species?
II. Relative population differences
    A. Size
    B. Heterogeneity
    C. Selected nature of test population (model populations are "high class" compared to the human population)
III. Differences between test and real world environment
    A. Physical (temperature, humidity, etc.)
    B. Chemical
    C. Nutritional

in stomach structure. The problem of distribution within the body probably relates less to species than to size, and will be discussed a little later. Primarily endogenous metabolism, xenobiotic metabolism of foreign compounds, metabolic activation, or toxicantion/detoxification mechanisms (by whatever name) is perhaps the critical factor, and this can differ widely from species to species. The increasing realization that the original administered compound is not necessarily the ultimate toxicant makes the further study of these metabolic patterns critical.

In terms of excretory rates, the differences between the species are not great: small animals tend to excrete compounds more rapidly than large animals in a rather systematic manner. Boxenbaum (1982) has generalized this to the concept of "pharmacokinetic time," which is related to relative body size.

The various cellular and intracellular barriers seem to be surprisingly constant throughout the vertebrate phylum. In addition, it is becoming increasingly clear that the various receptors, such as DNA and the neurotransmitters, are comparable throughout the mammalian species.

There are life-span (or temporal) differences that are not considered adequately, nor have they been in the past. It takes time to develop (for example) a cellular immune response and at least some of this time may be taken up by actual cell division processes. Cell division rates appear to be significantly higher in smaller animals. Mouse and rat cells turn over appreciably faster than do human cells—perhaps at twice the rate. On the other hand, the latent period for expression of many effects is also much shorter in small animals than in large ones.

Another difficulty is that the life span of humans is from 4.4 to 66.0 times (Gad and Chengelis, 1988) that of common test species. Thus, there is generally a much longer time available for many toxicities to be expressed or developed in people than in test animals. These sorts of temporal considerations are of considerable importance, and this area of chronotoxicology has not yet begun to really be explored.

Body size, irrespective of species, seems to be important in the rate of distribution of foreign compounds throughout the body. A simple example of this is that the cardiac output of the mouse is on the order 1 ml/min, and the mouse has a blood volume of about 1 ml. The mouse is, therefore, turning its blood volume over every minute. In humans, the cardiac output per minute is only 1/20th of the blood volume. So the mouse turns its blood over 20 times faster than the human, which has clear implications for the comparative rates at which xenobiotics are systemically distributed in these two species.

Another aspect of the size difference which should be considered is that the large animal has a much greater number of susceptible cells that may interact with potential toxic agents, though there is also a proportionately increased number of "dummy" (hyporesponding) cells.

Rall (1979), Oser (1981), and Borzelleca (1984) have published articles reviewing such factors, and Calabrese (1983) had published an excellent book on the subject.

Having delineated and quantified species differences (even if only having factored in comparative body weights or relative body surface areas), one can now proceed to some form of quantitative extrapolation (or scaling).

There are currently two major approaches to scaling for use with general toxicities. These are by body weight and by body surface area (Calabrese, 1983; Schmidt-Nielsen, 1984). Both of these are single variable or two dimensional models, and represent alternate simple forms of what are called allometric equations. Davidson et al. (1986) have presented the generalized form of such equations as

$$Y = aW^n$$

where W is body weight, n is the slope of the derived line, and a is a scaling factor. Certain authors (e.g., Yates and Kugler, 1986 for example) have proposed that a multidimensional model would be more accurate. Such a form of allometric equation is probably too complicated for use in most cases in toxicology, however, and its use would be inappropriate considering the relatively imprecise nature of the data generated.

The body weight approach is the most common general approach to scaling in toxicology—particularly in regulatory toxicology testing. There are several ways to perform a scaling operation on a body weight basis, the most often employed being to simply calculate a conversion factor (K) as

$$K = \frac{\text{Weight of human (70 kg ``standard'')}}{\text{Weight of average test animal}}$$

More exotic methods for doing this, such as that based on a form of linear regression, are reviewed by Calabrese (1983), who believes that the body weight method is preferable.

A difficulty with this approach is that the body weights of any population of animals or people change throughout life, and in fact even at a common age will present considerable variation. Custom is, therefore, to use an "ideal person" (70 kg for men and 50 kg for women) or "ideal" animal weight (for which there is considerable less consensus).

The alternatives are the body surface area methods, which attempt to factor in differences in metabolic rates based on the principle that these changes are in proportion to body surface area (since as the ratio of body surface area to body weight increases, relatively more energy is required to maintain a constant body temperature). As long ago as 1938, Benedict published a comparison of body weight vs basal metabolic rates for species from mice to elephants which showed a linear relationship between the two variables. Pinkell (1958) and Freireich et al. (1966) later found a similar relationship for effective/tolerated doses of cancer chemotherapeutics, and most recently Otterness and Gans (1988) have reported that the effective dose of (NSAIDs) could be scaled between species and models by surface area. There are several methods for making such conversions, each having a ratio of dose to the animal's body weight (in mg/kg) as a starting point, resulting in a conversion factor with mg/M^2 as the units for the product of the calculations.

The Environmental Protection Agency (EPA) version of the surface area scaling equation is generally calculated as

$$(M_{human}/M_{animal})^{1/3} = \text{Surface area}$$

where M = mass in kilograms. Another form is calculated based on constants that have been developed for a multitude of species of animals by actual surface area measurements (Spector, 1956). The resulting formula for this approach is

$$A = KW^{2/3}$$

where A = surface area in square centimeters, K = a constant, specific for each species, and W = body weight in grams. A scaling factor is then simply calculated as a ratio of the surface area of a human over that of the model species.

Most recently, direct measurements of indicators of damage (much as tissue DNA damage; Visek, 1988 and Slaga, 1988) has been proposed as the ultimate means of cross-species scaling of exposures.

The best scaling factor is not generally agreed upon. Though the majority opinion is that surface area is preferable where a metabolic activation or deactivation is known to be both critical to the adverse effect–causing process and present in both humans and the model species, these assumptions may not always be valid. And for the conditions under which most toxicity testing is performed, these facts are generally unknown. Table 5 presents a comparison of the weight and surface area extrapolation methods for the eight common laboratory animal species and humans. Brown et al. (1988), on reviewing the currently available data, likewise have concluded that though "correlations exist among risk levels in various species, many factors appear to influence toxicity that are not captured in a simple scaling rule." These factors are commonly those pointed out in Table 4.

Schneiderman et al. (1975) and Dixon (1976) have published comparisons of these methods, but Schmidit-Nielsen (1984) should be considered the primary source on scaling in interspecies comparisons.

When one is concerned about specific target organ effects, frequently the earliest indicator of such an effect is an alteration in organ weight out of proportion to what is to be expected due to changes in overall body weight (Gad et al., 1984) or to changes in a

Table 5 Extrapolation of a Dose of 100 mg/kg in the Mouse to Other Species

Species	Weight (g)	Surface[a] area (cm.^{2})	Extrapolated dose based on (mg) body weight (A)	Extrapolated dose based on (mg) body surface area (B)	ratio A/B
Mouse	20	46.4	2	2	1.0
Rat	400	516.7	40	22.3	1.80
Hamster	50	126.5	5	5.4	1.08
Guinea pig	400	564.5	40	24.3	1.65
Ferret	500	753.9	50	32.5	1.54
Rabbit	1500	1272.0	150	54.8	2.74
Dog	12000	5766.0	1200	248.5	4.82
Monkey	4000	2975.0	400	128.2	3.12
Man	70000	18000.0	7000	775.8	9.8

[a]Surface area (except in the case of man) values calculated from the formula:

Surface area $(cm^2) = KW^{2/3}$

Where K is a constant for each species and W is the body weight (values of K and the surface area for man are taken from Spector, 1956).

standard such as brain weight. It should be pointed out that a form of scaling is involved in detecting such effects, as adjustments to organ weight to account for alterations in overall body weight can take several forms. Either simple ratios (Angervall and Carlstrom, 1963; Weil and Gad, 1980; Gad and Weil, 1981), or analysis of covariance, or species or organ specific allometric methods (Trieb et al., 1976; Lutzen et al., 1976) may be employed.

An alternative approach to achieving society's objective for the entire risk assessment process (that is, protecting the human population from unacceptable levels of voluntary risk) is the classic approach of using safety factors. This is still the methodology used in determining what are acceptable risks, given the uncertainties involved, in phase I human clinical trials of a new drug would be based on animal safety data. The presumed degree of uncertainty in these cases is instructive. In 1972, Weil summarized this approach as,

> In summary, for the evaluation of safety for man, it is necessary to: (1) design and conduct appropriate toxicologically tests, (2) statistically compare the data from treated and control animals, (3) delineate the minimum effect and maximum no ill-effect levels (NIEL) for these animals, and (4) if the material is to be used, apply an appropriate safety factor, e.g., (a) 1/100 (NIEL) or 1/50 (NIEL) for some effects or (b) 1/500 (NIEL), if the effect was a significant increase in cancer in an appropriate test.

This approach has served society reasonably well over the years, once the experimental work has identified the potential hazards and quantitated the observable dose-response relationships. The safety factor approach has not generally been accepted or seriously entertained by regulatory agencies for carcinogens, mutagens, or teratogen, but is well established for other toxic effects of drugs and chemicals (Weil, 1972), and Johnson has recently (1988), after reviewing a broad range of developmental and maternal toxicity data proposed that "where the effect in the embryo is only seen at maternally toxic doses and exposure is below the adult toxic doses, relatively modest safety factors are sufficient for safe cross species extrapolation." Until such time as the more elegant risk assessment procedures can instill greater public and scientific confidence, the use of the safety factor approach to bridge our collective uncertainty about the difference between species responses should perhaps not be abandoned so readily for more "mathematically precise and elegant" procedures, but rather should be reviewed and perhaps revised for some areas of greater uncertainty (Dawson and Stara, 1983).

As a final sanity check to any multistep process of hazard assessment, the data points generated by any other studies (particularly any human exposures) of the endpoint of interest should be evaluated to determine if they fall within the range expected based upon the assessment. If we find that the available real-world data does not fit our extrapolation model at this point, then as scientists we have no choice but to reject such a model or assessment and start anew.

Embodied in the safety factor approach are two of the "rules" for cross-species extrapolation, which are actually general comparative statements of relationships between species.

In general, as animal species become larger, they also become more sensitive to short-term toxicities. This effect may be credited to a number of mechanisms (such as increases of available target tissues and decreases of metabolic rate as size increases), but it is true even for nonmammalian species such as fish (Anderson and Weber, 1975) and birds (Hudson et al., 1979). The rule even applies somewhat to differences in body size within the same age class of the same sex of the same species.

What this rule means is that as a rule of thumb, the sensitivity of a larger species (such as a dog or human) to a short-term toxicity will be greater than that of a smaller species (such as a mouse or rat). There are, of course, exceptions and wide variations from linearity in this relationship (such as hamsters being much less sensitive to the neurotoxicity of DDT than are mice, as reported by Gingell and Wallcave in 1974). And those toxicities which are mediated or modulated by structurally different features (such as those toxicities associated with the skin, where general rules fall completely apart across broad ranges of structual classes; Nixon et al., 1975; Campbell and Bruce, 1981) are subject to even less certainty under this rule.

There are also those who believe that humans are more sensitive than any test species, even if that species is larger than humans (such as a cow or horse). Lehman (1959) published, for example, the relationships shown in Table 6.

It should be noted that much data on effects in humans are biased by humans being better (or at least more sensitive and louder) indicators of adverse effects. Differences in sensitivity between the sexes are, in the majority, such that females are more sensitive than males. Data to support this will be reviewed later in this chapter.

SPECIAL CASES: MATCHING CHARACTERISTICS FOR SPECIAL POPULATIONS

There are many factors which can alter the physiological state an individual (or the fraction of available chemical moiety in an individual—see Table 7), and in so doing make them more (or, in some few cases, less) susceptible to the adverse effects of a chemical. These include (but are not limited to) immunological experience, physiological factors such as stress, age, illness, conditioning factors (such as obesity and malnutrition), and sex. Proper model selection and experimental design require that these factors be

Table 6 Some Relations of Drug Toxicity in Experimental Animals Compared to Humans

Species	Weight (kg)	Weight ratio animal/human	Drug dose ratio	Sensitivity: drug dose ratio/weight ratio
Man	60	1	1	1
Cow	500	8	24	Human 3× as sensitive
Horse	500	8	16	Human 2× as sensitive
Sheep	60	1	3	Human 3× as sensitive
Goat	60	1	3	Human 3× as sensitive
Swine	60	1	2	Human 2× as sensitive
Dog	10	1/6	1	Human 6× as sensitive
Cat	3	1/20	1/2	Human 10× as sensitive
Rat	0.4	1/150	1/15	Human 10× as sensitive

The value in this table are averages and their validity can not be checked against original data as Lehman (1959) only reported them as being from numerous sources.

identified and considered. Chapter 13 (susceptibility factors) will consider these and related factors on a theoretical basis in more detail.

Sex

Sex hormones may be the target or sex hormones may modify a particular toxic response which then may account for differential responses between the sexes to toxic materials. The current consensus is that (as was pointed out earlier) females are more susceptible than males to the acute toxic effects of many chemicals, though males and females of the same strain, age, and general condition will react in a qualitatively similar manner.

As a result of reviewing the acute oral and dermal toxicities of 98 pesticides to rats, Gaines (1969) concluded that by the oral route the majority were more toxic to females than to males. He found the reverse true for only 9 out of the 98 pesticides tested: aldrin, chlordane, heptachlor, abate, imidan, methyl parathion, fenchlorphos, schradan, and metepa. Pallotta et al. (1962) found the same pattern for the antibiotic acetoxycyclohex-imide in rats but not in dogs (where there was no sex difference).

Indeed, a review of the published literature on pesticides by Kato and Gillete (1965) found that such sex differences are common in rodents but less so in other mammals, though the information on these other species is not as definitive. Even with rodents and pesticides, however, it should be remembered that this is a general rule and not a universal

Table 7 Factors Which May Increase the Fraction of Available Chemical Moiety in the Systemic Circulation

1. Renal impairment
2. Liver impairment
3. Hypoalbuminea
4. Presence of other moieties that displace test agent from proteins in circulation.
5. Pregnancy

truth. Steen et al. (1976) found mevinphos to be more toxic to male Mongolian gerbils than to females, whereas Gaines (1960) found the reverse to be the case for this compound in rats. These observations were in accord with published data on hexabarbitone sleeping times, as shown in Table 8. In general, most barbiturates cause longer sleeping times in females than in males. Likewise, as a class organophosphates are lethal in lower doses in female rats than in males.

Shanor et al. (1961) found that in humans there is a statistically significant difference between the plasma cholinesterase levels of healthy young males and females (activity levels in females are from 64 to 74% of males), but that this difference disappeared in older people. There was no significant variation between the sexes in erythrocyte cholinesterase—a finding confirmed by Eben and Pilz (1967). Naik et al. (1970) likewise found there to be no significant difference between males and females in either total brain cholinesterase or in brain acetylcholine. These findings suggest that the distribution characteristics of toxicants working by cholinesterase inhibition mechanisms may be critical to their acute toxicity and that these distribution characteristics may be altered by the sex of the animal.

Krasovskij (1975) reviewed data on the acute toxicities of 149 chemicals and compared the results for males versus those for females. For both rats and mice, he found that the females tended to be more sensitive than the males, though not by large amounts (generally the differences were on the order of from 8 to 12%, being a little greater in rats than in mice).

Depass et al. (1984) looked at oral and dermal lethality of a number of previously studied compound on which the results had largely been published. To assess the effect of sex, they calculated the correlation coefficient (r) between the LD_{50} results for the two sexes. For 91 oral studies, r was found to be 0.93, whereas for 17 dermal studies with skin abrasion and 28 without, the r values were 0.73 and 0.96, respectively. The LD_{50} values between the two sexes were, in other words, strongly associated. However, when the values were compared using paired t-tests, there was a statistically significant trend towards higher LD_{50}'s in the males.

Similarly, Bruce (1985) reviewed studies from files on 48 chemicals and found that for only three of these there was evidence of lower LD_{50} values among the males than the females, and that none of these differences approached statistical significance. In 13 cases, however, the males had significantly higher LD_{50} values than the females. For these 13 studies, male LD_{50} values averaged 29% higher than those for females.

Table 8 Relative Hexobarbitone Sleeping Times for Each Sex in Two Different Rodent Species

Sex	Mean sleeping time (min)		
	Mongolian gerbil[a]	rat[b]	mouse[c]
Male	105 + 9.6	22 + 4	34 + 5
Female	70 + 6.9	67 + 15	31 + 5

The reported sex difference did not occur in rats less than 4 weeks old.
[a]Maines and Westfall, 1971.
[b]Quinn et al., 1958.
[c]Vessell, 1968.

Imbalances of hormones other than those related to sexual function have also been shown to alter the susceptibility of animals to the toxic effects of chemicals. Hyperthyroidism, hyperinsulinism, adrenalectomy, and stimulation of the pituitary have all been demonstrated to be capable of modifying the effects of selected toxicants (Dauterman, 1980; Doull, 1980).

Stress

Stress and the variability of animals underlying biological rhythms (the complex interactions of physiological responses to chronologically ordered external factors) are among the least accounted for valuables in toxicology. Though they have both been studied and identified as important determinants of sensitivity to toxicity, standard practice does not evaluate these effects or seek to factor them in predicting human effects.

Stress is a broad term for specific morphological, biochemical, physiological, and/or behavioral changes experienced by an organism in response to a stressful event or "stressor" (Vogel, 1987). Such changes can be quite drastic. Plasma levels of epinephrine in resting rats are approximately 100 pg/ml, but in a stressed rat can approach 2000 pg/ml. Cessation of the stressful event usually terminates the stress response and the organism returns to its baseline homeostasis. However, if the stress response is very intense or long lasting, a return to the original homeostasis may not occur and a new biological equilibrium may be established. The consequences of this new condition can be either beneficially (such as exercise induced stress strengthening the heart) or detrimental (such as job-induced stress causing ulcers or hypertension) to the organism.

The typical behavioral stress responses are fear, tension, apprehension, and anxiety. Physiological stress responses can include changes in gastric secretion and motility and increases in blood pressure and heart rate. Biochemical changes are widespread during stress and include significant increases in the levels of plasma catecholamine and corticosteroids or marked changes in brain neurotransmitter concentrations. Although these are only typical response examples, most biochemical and physiological systems are probably affected during stress. Thus, potential toxicants interact with quite different physiological and/or biochemical systems during stress and the resulting outcomes of such interactions are bound to be quite different under these altered conditions.

In experimental toxicology, it is customary to use nonstressed animals to evaluate the extent and modes of action of chemicals. However, animals and humans are seldom nonstressed, but rather are frequently challenged by stressful events in the real world, responding with stress manifested as some of the previously mentioned responses. Thus, agents acting at specific biochemical sites or on physiological processes will encounter different conditions during rest and stress, resulting in differences in their effects. In addition, the true action of some agents may only be revealed during stress. Thus, the variable of stress should probably be included during experimentation to better approximate (or model) various real-life situations and to predict more accurately the actions of chemicals under all types of environmental conditions.

The literature does very clearly reflect that the actions of biologically active substances can be altered during stress. Toxic effects can be increased or decreased, and the results must be interpreted in this context before they can be generalized or extrapolated to the human population. Guinea pigs show an increased susceptibility to the lethal effects of ouabain during stress. Natelson et al. (1979) report that only 9% of nonstressed animals die, whereas 50% succumb to the same dose of ouabain if the animals are stressed.

Similarly, the delayed neuropathology to triorthotolyl phosphate in hens is almost tripled by stress (Enrich et al., 1983), and Stokinger (1959) indicated the considerable influence that stress can have on the dose-dependent distribution of some of the elements in the body.

It has also been demonstrated that injections of adrenocorticotropic hormone (Vaccarezza and Wilson, 1964a,b) caused increases both in plasma and cell cholinesterase in rats, but that adrenalectomy caused a progressive decline in the circulating RBC cholinesterase but had no effect on plasma cholinesterase in rats. In people, injections of adrenocorticotropic hormone also gave rise to increases in plasma and circulating cell cholinesterases (Vaccarezza and Pelts, 1960).

In reporting investigations of parathion in rats, Kling and Long (1969) demonstrated the influence that dietary stress could have on the time course of the response of cellular cholinesterase, while not altering the overall quantitative outcome. In fact, much of life (for at least the laboratory animals species) consists of a habitat that exhibits a recurrence of a sequence of events in an ordered manner relative to time. The effect of many biologically active agents, particularly toxicants, must interfere with these normal patterns and resulting biological cybernetics. Though Scheving et al. (1974) have held that there was little evidence that acute toxicity displayed significant differences relative to circadian rhythms, this conclusion seems suspect. There are clear relationships between biorhythms, stress, and the endocrine functions.

Circadian differences in response to a range of chemicals such as nikethamide, ethanol, chlordiazepoxide (Librium), methopyrapone, and ouabain have been observed in the mouse. Halberg et al. (1960) demonstrated that there was a potency ratio alteration of from 3.2 to 1.0 for the bioassay of *Escherichia coli* endotoxin carried out at 12-hr time intervals. And working with rats, Lenox and Frazier (1972) demonstrated that the mortality due to methadone was influenced by a circadian cycle.

Stress due to fasting has been shown to alter the permeability of the blood-brain barrier to some chemicals (Angel, 1969). Indeed, selective starvation can also influence sensitivity—Boyd et al. (1970) demonstrated that feeding protein-deficient or protein-rich diets to rats could markedly alter the LD_{50} values for many pesticides.

Likewise, for some toxicants the influence of single or multiple housing can also significantly alter the results of a range of outcomes in acute toxicity tests, with marked variations in sensitivity (and the direction even of the influence) to this housing variable between different species.

Age

Age is an endogenous factor which alters an organism's response to exposure to a test chemical. Very young or old animals may be either more or less sensitive to toxic effects than fully developed young or mature animals, and indeed may even have qualitatively different responses. Older rats, for example, are almost immune to the carcinogenic actions of most chemicals. Neonates are more susceptible to the actions of opiates.

Traditionally, what is used to perform tests in our studies are young adult animals. However, much of our human population is either very young or old, and clearly not physiologically comparable to young adults.

Age variation may give rise to differences in susceptibility to acute intoxication by different chemicals and there is not a simple rule for relating age to the sensitivity or nature of the toxic response. Goldenthal (1971) published an extensive review of the comparative acute toxicity of agents to newborn and adult animals. During the early stages of life, anatomical, physiological, metabolic, and immunological capabilities are not fully developed.

Substantial differences in susceptibility can sometimes even be related to small age differences. With rodents, a few months difference in age can markedly alter the response to chemicals that influence either the central nervous or immunological systems.

Biological aging is both time and species dependent (Mann, 1965). For the purposes of acute toxicity, it is generally convenient to consider the stages of biological age as being neonatal, infant, young adult, and old. There is no clear dividing line between these stages in any species, though their length was loosely defined at the beginning of this chapter. Rather, development and aging are a continuum on which there is both species and individual variation. For some laboratory-bred species, however, such as the rat, there is a fairly linear relationship between the logarithm of body weight and the reciprocal of the animal's age (Gray and Addis, 1948), which can be expressed as:

$$\log_{10}[W] = \frac{-K}{d} + \log_{10}A$$

where W = weight in grams, K = slope, d = age in days, and A = the estimated asymptote or limit for W.

There are in fact an entire family of statistical methods for adjusting different structural and functional characteristics for age. Mattfeldt and Mall (1987) give an excellent overview of these allometric methods.

The toxicological response to both exogenous and endogenous physiological chemicals (such as epinephrine and acetylcholine) can vary with age. Bus and Herman (1971) demonstrated that newborn mice were significantly less sensitive to epinephrine and norepinephrine than were adults, but that the reverse held true for acetylcholine. Naik et al. (1970) found that brain acetylcholine concentrations increased with body weight/age until maturity, whereas brain cholinesterase activities was variable at lower weight/age and became less variable as weight/age increased. Shanor et al. (1961), using a large population sample of young adults (ages 18–35 years) and older people (ages 70–80 years) found that the plasma cholinesterase activity was approximately 24% higher in the young males than in the old males, but that no such difference existed for females or for RBC cholinesterase.

Older animals also show a large number of alterations in their response to potential toxicants when compared to young adults.

Disease

Disease states can modify a variety of kinetic and physiological parameters, altering the baseline homeostatic condition. Earlier, it was pointed out that a number of conditions (such as liver or renal disease) could increase the amount of available drug moiety in the systemic circulation. The ability to understand how pathological conditions can modify the kinetics and effect of exogenous chemicals requires an understanding of the interrelationships between these various parameters.

Stress due to infection can alter the responses of animals to biologically active chemicals. In 1972, Safarov and Aleskerov found that the dipping of sheep in an ectoparasiticide depressed antibody production and reduced the ability of the sheep to survive infections. It has been shown that some chemicals adversely affect the natural immunological defense systems, although this appears to be associated more with persistent agents retained in the organism than with those agents which are rapidly cleared. Liver (by decreasing biotransformation) and renal (by disrupting both excretory and metabolic functions) diseases associated with a preexisting condition or old age may contribute to a greater sensitivity to a toxicant. Hyperthyroid states also have been shown to increase sensitivity to the toxic effects of several classes of drug, particularly selected psychoactive agents (Zbinden, 1963).

Physiological State

The influence of diet on the response of animals and humans to toxins is well established. The toxicity of specific agents can be increased or decreased by alterations of dietary protein or the various micronutrients (an example being the decreased sensitivity of protein-deficient animals to CCl_4). Two conditions which occur in humans and are not generally recognized as diseases (obesity and subclinical malnutrition or marginal nutrition) can also alter the biological affects of chemicals and serve to increase the susceptibility of individuals to toxic actions.

Obesity may well alter the distribution and storage of a xenobiotic, especially when it is markedly lipophilic. Obesity is also generally accompanied in humans and test animals by reduced or impaired respiratory, cardiovascular, and renal function, all of which will also alter the manner and degree to which an agent may be toxic.

Subclinical malnutrition or marginal nutrition is the other end of the scale from obesity usually, but not always or absolutely. An individual person's or animal's diet may be calorically adequate (or even oversupplied), but nutritionally marginal in terms of vitamins, proteins, minerals, and other nutrients. Any such marginal nutrient state clearly presents the possibility of an increased susceptibility to a toxic or adverse outcome of exposure to a xenobiotic, particularly if said nutritional state means limited or deficient metabolic and/or enzymatic defense mechanisms. Or if the potential toxicant acts to reduce the available limiting nutrient. The principal biotransformation of toxicants is performed by the microsomal mixed function oxidase system (or MMFO), which is depressed by a deficiency of essential fatty acids, vitamin A, or proteins.

Boyd et al. (1970) and Boyd (1972) reviewed the effects of nutritional status on acute toxicity, showing alteration in the responses of rodents. Mehrle et al. (1973) demonstrated that the LC_{50}s of chlordane in rainbow trout were altered by the brand of commercial diet the fish were maintained on beforehand. Furthermore, the nutritional status of animals used to prepare or provide tissues for in vitro studies can change the microsomal metabolism and other aspects of responsiveness of the tissue (Kato and Gillette, 1965).

Toxins also have the potential to induce nutritional deficiencies, but these are generally of concern only in cases of longer-term exposure.

MODELS

This entire volume has focused on animal models in toxicology and is based on the premise that these models are not only a valid approach to predicting the adverse effects of chemicals in humans, but are the primary model for such predictions.

In vivo models are not the only means, however, and a brief review of the status of alternatives to them is called for. Classes of in vitro alternatives are in vitro models (which do not use intact higher organisms but do use some form of test system) and mathematical or SAR approaches (which construct theoretical analogies but require no actual generation or interpretation of new data).

In Vitro Models

In vitro models, at least as screening tests, have been with us in toxicology for some 20 years now. The last 5–10 years have seen a great upsurge in interest in such models. The increased interest is due to economic and animal welfare pressures and technological improvements.

In vitro systems per se have a number of limitations which can contribute to their not being acceptable models. Some of these reasons are detailed in Table 9.

At the same time there are substantial potential advantages in using in vitro systems. The scientific advantages of using cell or tissue culture in toxicological testing are isolation of test cells or organ fragments from homeostatic and hormonal control, accurate dosing, and quantitation of results. It is important to devise a suitable model system which is related to the mode of toxicity of the compound. Tissue and cell culture have been used in two very different ways in screening studies. First, they have been used to examine a particular aspect of the toxicity of a compound in relation to its toxicity in vivo. Second, they have been used as a form of rapid screening to compare the toxicity of a group of

Table 9 Possible Interpretations When In Vitro Data Do Not Predict Results of In Vivo Studies

1. Chemical is not absorbed at all or is poorly absorbed in in vivo studies.
2. Chemical is well absorbed but is subject to first-pass effect in liver.
3. Chemical is distributed so that less (or more) reaches the receptors than would be predicted on the basis of its absorption.
4. Chemical is rapidly metabolized to an active or inactive metabolite that has a different profile of activity and/or different duration of action than the parent drug.
5. Chemical is rapidly eliminated (e.g., through secretory mechanisms).
6. Species of the two test systems used are different.
7. Experimental conditions of the in vitro and in vivo experiments differed and may have led to different effects than expected. These conditions include factors such as temperature or age, sex, and strain of animal.
8. Effects elicited in vitro and in vivo differ in characteristics.
9. Tests used to measure responses will probably differ greatly for in vitro and in vivo studies, and the types of data obtained may not be comparable.
10. The in vitro study did not use adequate controls (e.g., pH, vehicle used, volume of test agent given, samples taken from sham-operated animals).
11. In vitro data cannot predict the volume of distribution in central or in peripheral compartments.
12. In vitro data cannot predict the rate constants for chemical movement between compartments.
13. In vitro data cannot predict whether linear nonlinear kinetics will occur with specific chemical in vivo.
14. In vitro data cannot predict whether linear or nonlinear kinetics will occur with specific dose of a chemical in vivo.
15. Pharmacokinetic parameters (e.g., bioavailability, peak plasma concentration, half-life) cannot be predicted based solely on in vitro studies.
16. In vivo effects of chemical are due to an alteration in the higher order integration of an intact animal system, which cannot be reflected in a less complex system.

compounds. Additionally, target organ–specific in vitro models offer a powerful means of explaining the mechanisms behind toxicities observed in intact organisms.

SUMMARY

If the human population we are concerned about is such that one or more of these susceptibility factors is present in a substantial portion of the members, steps should be taken to design studies so that such individuals are adequately represented ("i.e., matched") by an appropriate model in the test animal population. Barring that, or in the face of having existing data on studies performed in a standard manner, consideration should be given to these factors when attempting to predict outcome of exposures in people.

Individual Biological Variation

There are also individual animal-to-animal variations in temperature, health, and sensitivity to toxicities which are recognized and expected by experienced animal researchers, but are only broadly understood. The resulting differences in response are generally accredited to "individual biological variation." This same phenomenon has been widely studied and observed among humans, and is expected by any experienced clinician. Examples of such individual variations in humans include isoniazid, succinylcholine, and glucose-6-phosphate levels and/or activities. In the first of these, "slow inactivators" who are deficient in acetyltransferase, and therefore acetylate agents such as isoniazid only slowly, and are thus more liable to suffer from the peripheral neuropathy caused by an accumulation of isoniazid. At the same time, people with more effective acetyltransferase require larger doses of isoniazid to benefit from its therapeutic effects, but in so doing are more likely to suffer liver damage.

Likewise, individuals with atypical or low levels of serum cholinesterase may exhibit prolonged muscle relaxation and apnea following an injection of a standard dose of the muscle relaxant succinylcholine. And glucose-6-phosphate dehydrogenase deficiency is responsible for the increased probability of some individuals given primaquine or antipyrine to suffer from a hemolytic anemia.

Species Variation

Though anyone who has had to work in biological research with intact animals should be aware of the existence of wide variability between species, examples which are specific to toxicology should be presented here along with some degree of comparison of relative species sensitivity for a number of specific agents. Table 10 presents an enumeration of target organ toxicities which are specific to several model-specific species commonly used in toxicology.

The rodenticide zinc phosphide is dependent on the release of phosphine by hydrochloric acid in the stomach for its activation and efficacy (Johnson and Voss, 1952). As a result, dogs, and cats are considerable less sensitive than rats and rabbits since the former species secrete gastric hydrochloric acid intermittently while the latter secrete it almost continuously.

That this case is not a rare one can be quickly established by examining some data sets where we have comparative oral lethality data on several species (including humans), such as those presented in Table 11.

Hottendorf has published a review of the predictive value of seven animal model

Table 10 Species-Specific Toxic Effects

Type of Toxicity	Structure	Sensitive species	Mechanism of toxicity
Ocular	Retina	Dog	Zinc chelation
Ocular	Retina	Any with pigmented retinas	Melanin binding
Stimulated basal metabolism	Thyroid	Dog	Competition for plasma binding
Ocular	Retina and optic nerve	Primates	Formic acid formation
Porphyria	Liver	Human, rat, guinea pig, mouse, and rabbit	Estrogen enhanced sensitivity
Tubular necrosis	Kidney	Rats (males)	Androgen enhanced sensitivity[a]
Urolithiasis	Kidney and bladder	Rats and mice	Uricase inhibition
Teratogenesis; mortality	Fetus	Rats and mice	Uricase inhibition
Cardiovascular	Heart	Rabbits	Sensitivity to microvascular constriction

[a]More sensitive than humans for many agents (such as caprolactam and halogenated solvents).
Source: Adapted from Gralla, 1986, with modification.

Table 11 Comparative Human Acute Lethal Doses and Animal LD_{50}s (mg/kg via oral route)

Chemical	Human LD_{LO}[a]	LD_{50} values			
		mouse	rat	rabbit	dog
Aminopyrine	220	358	685	160	150
Aniline	350	300	440		195
Amytal	43	345	560	575	
Boric acid	640	3450	2660		
Caffeine	192	620	192	224	140
Carbofuran	11	2	5		19
Carbon tetrachloride	43	12800	2800	6380	
Cycloheximide		133	3		
Lindane	840		125	130	120
Fenoflurazole		1600	283	28	50

[a]LD_{LO} = lowest observed lethal dose.

species across a range of compounds with different target organs, finding the rat, mouse, and monkey to be generally the best individual predictors while the guinea pig and hamster were the least accurate predictors.

REFERENCES

Alcock, S. J. (1971) An anti-inflammatory compound: Non-toxic to animals, but with an adverse action in man. *Proc. Eur. Soc. Stud. Drug Tox.* 12, 184–190.

Anderson, P. D., and Weber, L. J. (1975) Toxic response as a quantitative function of body size. *Toxicol. Appl. Pharmacol.* 33, 471–481.

Angel, G. (1969) Starvation, stress and the blood brain barrier. *Dis. Nerv. Syst.* 30, 94–97.

Angervall, L., and Carlstrom, E. (1963) Theoretical criteria for the use of relative organ weights and similar ratios in biology. *J. Theoret. Biol.* 4, 254–259.

Animal Clinical Chemistry Association (1988) Assessment of hepatic function and damage in animal species. *J. Appl. Toxicol.* 8, 249–254.

Animal Welfare Act of 1987, PL 99-198, CFR 9 (Vol. 52, No. 61, 10292–10322).

Baker, H. J., Lindsey, J. R., and Weisbroth, S. H. (1979) *The Laboratory Rat.* Vol. I. Academic Press, New York, pp. 411–412.

Bartek, M. J., LaBudde, J. A., and Maibach, H. I. (1972) Skin permeability in vivo. Comparison in rat, rabbit, pig and man. *J. Invest. Dermatol.* 58, 114–123.

Belehradek, J. (1957) A unified theory of cellular rate processes based upon an analysis of temperature action. *Protoplasma* 48, 53–71.

Benedict, F. C. (1938) *Vita Energetics: A Study in Comparative Basal Metabolism.* Carnegie Institute, 503, 1–215.

Borzelleca, J. F. (1984) Extrapolation of animal data to man, in *Concepts in Toxicology*, Vol. I, Tegeris, A. S., ed. Krager, New York, pp. 294–304.

Boxenbaum, H. (1982) Interspecies scaling, allometry, physiological time and the ground plan of pharmacokinetics. *J. Pharmacokinet. Biopharmacol.* 10, 201–227.

Boyd, E. M., Dodos, I., and Krijnen, C. J. (1970) Endosulfan toxicity and dietary protein. *Arch. Environ. Health* 21, 15–19.

Brown, A. M. (1961) Sleeping time response of time-random bred, inbred and F_1-hybrids to pentobarbitone sodium. *J Pharmacol. Pharmacol.* 13, 679–687.

Brown, V. K. (1980) *Acute Toxicity in Theory and Practice.* Wiley, New York.

Brown, S. L., Brett, S. M., Gough M., Radricks, J. V., Tardiff, R. C., and Turnball, D. (1988) *Reg. Toxicol. Pharmacol.* 8, 191–206.

Bruce, R. D. (1985) An up-and-down procedure for acute toxicity testing. *Fund. Appl. Toxicol.* 5, 151–157.

Brus, R., and Herman, Z. S. (1971) Acute toxicities of adrenaline, noradrenaline and acetylcholine in adult and neo-natal mice. *Dissert. Pharm. Pharmacol.* 23, 435–437.

Burrell, G. A. (1912) The use of mice and birds for detecting carbon monoxide after mine fire and explosions. Technical Paper 11, Department of Interior, Bureau of Mines, Washington, D.C., pp. 3–16.

Calabese, E. J. (1983) *Principles of Animal Extrapolation.* Wiley, New York.

Campbell, R. L., and Bruce, R. D. (1981) Comparative dermatotoxicology. *Toxicol. Appl. Pharmacol.* 59, 555–563.

Clayson, D. B. (1988) Needs for biological risks assessment in interspecies extrapolation. *Environ. Health Perspect.* 77, 93–97.

Dauterman, W. C. (1980) Physiological factors affecting metabolism of xenobiotics, in *Introduction to Biochemical Toxicology*, Hodgeson, E., Guthrie, F. E., eds. Elsevier, New York.

Davidson, I. W. F., Parker, J. C., and Beliles, R. P. (1986) Biological basis for extrapolation across animal species.

Depass, L. R., Myers, R. C., Weaver, E. V., and Weil, C. S. (1984) *Alternative Methods in Toxicology*, Vol. 2. *Acute Toxicity Testing*, Mary Ann Liebert, New York, 141–153.

Dixon, R. L. (1976) Problems in extrapolating toxicity data from laboratory animals to man. *Environ. Health Perspect.* 13, 43–50.

Doull, J. (1980) Factors influencing toxicology, in *Casarett and Doull's Toxicology*, Doull, J., Klaassen, C. D., and Amdur, M. O., eds. Macmillan, New York.

Dubois, K. P., and Geiling, E. M. K. (1959) *Textbook Toxicology*. Oxford University Press, New York, pp. 11–12.

Dawson, M. L., and Stara, J. F. (1983) Regulatory history and experimental support of uncertainly (safety) factors *Reg. Toxicol. Pharmacol.* 3, 224–238.

Eben, A., and Pilz, W. (1967) Abhangigbeit der Acetylcholinesterase-acktivata in Plasma and Erythrocyten von der alter and geschlecht der Ratte. *Arch. Toxicol.* 23, 27–34.

Ehrich, M., and Gross, W. B. (1983) Modification of triorthotolyl phosphate toxicity in chickens by stress. *Toxicol. Appl. Pharmacol.* 70, 249–254.

Ensminger, M. E., and Olentine, C. J. (1978) Mink nutrition, in *Feeds and Nutrition-Complete*. Ensminger Publishing, Cloves, California, pp. 997–1017.

Evans, R. H. (1982) Ralston Purina Co., St. Louis, Missouri.

Fara, J. W., Anderson, L. D., Casper, A. C. T., and Myrback, R. E. (1988) Assessment and validation of animal models to evaluate topical effects of substances on gastrointestinal mucosa. *Pharmaceut. Res.* 5, 165–170.

Freireich, E. J., Gehan, E. A., Rall, D. P., Schmidt, L. H., and Skipper, H. E. (1966) Quantitative comparison of toxicity of anticancer agents in mouse, rat, hamster, dog, monkey and man. *Cancer Chemother. Rep.* 50, 219–244.

Gad, S. C., and Chengelis, C. P. (1988) *Acute Toxicology: Principles and Methods*. Telford Press, Caldwell, New Jersey.

Gad, S. C., and Weil, C. S. (1980) Statistical analysis of body weight—a reply. *Toxicol. Appl. Pharmacol.* 57, 335–337.

Gad, S. C., Smith, A. C., Cramp, A. L., Gavigan, F. A., and Derelanko, M. J. (1984) Innovative designs and practices for acute systemic toxicity studies, *Drug Chem. Toxicol.* 7, 423–434.

Gaines, T. B. (1960) The acute toxicology of pesticides to rats. *Toxicol. Appl. Pharmacol.* 2, 88–99.

Gaines, T. B. (1969) Acute toxicology of pesticides. *Toxicol. Appl. Pharmacol.* 14, 515–534.

Garattini, S. (1985) Toxic effects of chemicals: Difficulties in extrapolating data from animals to man. *Crit. Rev. Toxicol.* 16, 1–29.

Gibson, J. E., and Starr, T. B. (1988) Opportunities for improving techniques for interspecies extrapolation in the risk assessment process. *Environ. Health Perspect.* 77, 99–105.

Gillette, J. R. (1979) Extrapolating from microsomes to mice to men. *Drug Metab. Dispos.* 7, 121–123.

Gingell, R., and Wallcave, L. (1974) Species differences in the acute toxicity and tissue distribution of DDT in mice and hamsters. *Toxicol. Appl. Pharmacol.* 28, 385–394.

Goldenthal, E. I. (1971) A compilation of LD_{50} values in newborn and adult animals. *Toxicol. Appl. Pharmacol.* 18, 185–207.

Gralla, E. J. (1986) Species specific toxicoses with some underlying mechanisms, in *Safety Evaluation of Drugs and Chemicals*, Lloyd, W. E., ed. Hemisphere, New York, pp. 55–81.

Gray, H., and Addis, T. (1948) Rat colony testing by Zucker's weight-age relation. *Am. J. Physiol.* 153, 35–40.

Gregory, A. R. (1988) Species comparison in evaluating carcinogenicity in humans. *Reg. Toxicol. Pharmacol.* 8, 160–190.

Halberg, F., Johnson, E. A., Brown, B. W., and Bittner, J. J. (1960) Susceptibility rhythm to *E. coli* endotoxin and bioassay. *Proc. Soc. Exp. Biol. Med.* 103, 142–144.

Haley, T. J., Dooley, K. L., and Harmon, J. R. (1973) Acute oral toxicity of N-2-fluorenlyacet-amide (2FAA) in several strains of mice. *Proc. Soc. Exp. Biol. Med.* 143, 1117–1119.

Hawkins, D. R., and Chasseaud, C. F. (1985) Reasons for monitoring kinetics in safety evaluation studies. *Arch. Toxicol.* 8 (Suppl.), 165–172.

Holmes, D. D. (1984) *Clinical Laboratory Animal Medicine*. Iowa State University Press, Ames.

Hottendorf, G. H. (1987) Species differences in toxic lesions, in *Human Risk Assessment*, Roloff, M. V., ed. Taylor & Francis, Philadelphia, pp. 87–95.

Hudson, R. H., Haegele, M. A., and Tucker, R. K. (1979) Acute oral and percutaneous toxicity of pesticides to mallards: Correlations with mammalian toxicity data. *Toxicol. Appl. Pharmacol.* 47, 451–460.

Johnson, E. M. (1988) Cross-species extrapolations and the biologic basis for safety factor determinations in developmental toxicology. *Reg. Toxicol. Pharmacol.* 8, 22–36.

Johnson, H. D., and Voss, E. (1952) Toxicological studies of zinc phosphide. *J. Am. Pharm. Assoc. (Sci. Ed.)* 41, 468–472.

Kato, R., and Gillette, J. R. (1965) Sex difference in the effects of abnormal physiological states on the metabolism of drugs by rat liver microsomes. *J. Pharmacol. Exp. Ther.* 150, 2285–291.

Krasovskij, G. N. (1975) Species and sex differences in sensitivity to toxic substances, in *Methods Used in the USSR for Establishing Biologically Safe Levels of Toxic Substances* World Health Organization, Geneva.

Lehman, A. J. (1959) Some relations of drug toxicities in experimental animals compared to man, in *Appraisal of Safety of Chemicals in Foods, Drugs and Cosmetics*. Association of Food and Drug Officials of the United States.

Lenox, R. H., and Frazier, T. W. (1972) Methadone induced mortality as a function of the circadian cycle. *Nature* 239, 397–398.

Lijinshy, W. (1988) Importance of animal experiments in carcinogenesis research. *Environ. Mol. Mutagen.* 11, 307–314.

Litchfield, J. T. (1961) Forecasting drug effects in man from studies in laboratory animals. *J. Am. Med. Soc.* 177, 34.

Litchfield, J. T. (1962) Symposium on clinical drug evaluation and human pharmacology. *Clin. Pharmacol. Ther.* 3, 665–672.

Lutzen, L., Trieb, G., and Pappritz, G. (1976) Allometric analysis of organ weights: II. Beagle dogs. *Toxicol. Appl. Pharmacol.* 35, 543–551.

Maines, M. D., and Westfall, B. A. (1971) Sex difference in the metabolism of hexobarbital in the Mongolian gerbil. *Proc. Soc. Exp. Biol. Med.* 138, 820–822.

Mattfeldt, T., and Mall, G. (1987) Statistical methods for growth allometric studies. *Growth* 51, 86–102.

Mitruka, B. M., Rawnsley, H. M., and Durham, V. V. (1976) *Animals for Medical Research*. Wiley, New York.

Naik, S. R., Anjaria, R. J., and Sheth, U. K. (1970) Studies on rat brain acetylcholine and cholinesterase. Part 1. Effect of body weight, sex, stress and CNS depressant drugs. *Ind. J. Med. Res.* 58, 473–479.

National Academy Sciences (1975) *Experiments and Research with Humans: Values in Conflict*, Academy Forum, 3rd in series. Washington, D.C.

Natelson, B. H., Hoffman, S. L., and Cagin, N. A. (1979) A role for environmental factors in the production of digitalis toxicity. *Pharmacol. Biochem. Behav.* 12, 235–237.

National Institutes of Health (1985) *Guide for the Care and Use of Laboratory Animals*, HHS, Publication No. 85-23.

Nixon, G. A., Tyson, C. A., and Wertz, W. C. (1975) Interspecies comparisons of skin irritancy. *Toxicol. Appl. Pharmacol.* 31, 481–490.

Nosal, M., and Hladka, A. (1968) Determination of the exposure to fenitrothion on the basis of the excretion of p-nitro-m-cresol by the urine of persons tested. *Arch. Gewerbepath. Gewerbehyg.* 25, 28–38.

Otterness, I. G., and Gans, D. J. (1988) Nonsteroidal anti-inflammatory drugs: An analysis of the relationship between laboratory animals and clinical doses, including species scaling. *J. Pharm. Sci.* 77, 790–795.

Pallotta, A. J., Kelly, M. J., Rall, D. P., and Ward, J. W. (1962) Toxicology of acetoxycyclohex-imide as a function of sex and body weight. *J. Pharmacol.* 136, 400–405.

Pinkel, D. (1958) The use of body surface area as a criterion of drug dosage in cancer chemother-apy. *Cancer Res.* 18, 853–856.

Plaa, G. L. (1976) Animal models in the safety evaluation process. *Austral. J. Pharm. Sci.* NSS: 57–63.

Priestly, J. (1772) On different kinds of air. *Philosophical Transactions.*

Pyle, N. J. (1940) Use of ferrets in laboratory work and research investigations. *Am. J. Pub. Health* 30, 787–796.

Quinn, G. P., Axelrod, J., and Brodie, B. B. (1958) Species, strain and sex differences in metabolism of hexobarbitone aminopyrine antipyrine and aniline. *Biochem. Pharmacol.* 1, 152–159.

Rall, D. P. (1979) Relevance of animal experiments to humans. *Environ. Health Perspect.* 32, 297–300.

Rider, J. A., Moeller, H. C., Puletti, E. J., and Swader, J. I. (1969) Toxicity of parathion, systox, octamethyl pyrophosphoramide and methyl parathion in man. *Toxicol. Appl. Pharmacol.* 14, 603–611.

Rothschild, Lord (1961). *A Classification of Living Animals.* Longmans, London.

Rozman, K. (1988) Disposition of xenobioties: Species differences. *Toxicol. Pathol.* 16, 123–129.

Safarov, Y. B. and Aleskerov, S. A. (1972) Effects of pesticides in producing relapses in animals recovering from bacterial infections. *Probl. Vet. Sanit.* 43, 213–218.

Scheving, L. E., Mayerbach, H. V., and Pauly, J. E. (1974) An overview of chronopharmacology. *J. Eur. Toxicol.* 7, 203–227.

Schmidt-Nielsen, K. (1984) *Scaling: Why Is Animal Size So Important?* Cambridge University Press, New York.

Schneiderman, M. A., Mantel, N., and Brown, C. C. (1975) *Ann. N.Y. Acad. Sci.* 246, 237–248.

Schwenk, M. (1988) Mucosal biotransformation. *Toxicol. Pathol.* 16, 138–146.

Shanor, S. P., van Hees, G. R., Baart, N., Erdos, E. G., and Foldes, E. F. (1961) The influence of age and sex on human plasma and red cell cholinesterase. *Am. J. Med. Sci.* 242, 357–361.

Slaga, J. J. (1988) Interspecies comparisons of tissue DNA damage, repair, fixation, and replica-tion. *Environ. Health Perspect.* 77, 73–82.

Smith, R. L. (1974) The problem of species variations. *Ann. Nutr. Alimen.* 28, 335.

Spector, W. S. (1956) *Handbook of Biological Data.* Saunders, Philadelphia.

Steen, J. A., Hanneman, G. D., Nelson, P. L., and Folk, E. D. (1976) Acute toxicity of mevinophos to gerbils. *Toxicol. Appl. Pharmacol.* 35, 195–198.

Stevenson, D. E. (1979) Current problems in the choice of animals for toxicity studies. *J. Toxicol. Environ. Health* 5, 9–15.

Stockinger, H. E. (1953) Size of dose: Its effect on distribution in the body. *Nucleonics* 11, 24–27.

Trieb, G., Pappritz, G., and Lutzen, L. (1976) Allometric analysis of organ weights. I. Rats. *Toxicol. Appl. Pharmacol.* 35, 531–542.

Vaccarezza, J. R., and Peltz, L. (1960) Effect of ACTH on blood cholinesterase activity in normal subjects and respiratory-allergy patients. *Presse Med.* 68, 723–724.

Vaccarezza, J. R., and Willson, J. A. (1964a) The effect of ACTH on cholinesterase activity in plasma, whole blood and blood cells of rats. *Experientia* 20, 23.

Vaccarezza, J. R., and Willson, J. A. (1964b) The relationship between corticosterone administra-tion and cholinesterase activity in rats. *Experientia* 21, 205.

Vessell, E. S. (1968) Genetic and environmental factors affecting hexobarbital metabolism in mice. *Ann N.Y. Acad. Sci.* 151, 900–912.

Visek, W. J. (1988) Issues and current applications of interspecies extrapolation of carcinogenic potency as a component of risk assessment. *Environ. Health Perspect.* 77, 49–54.

Vogel, W. H. (1987) Stress-the neglected variable in experimental pharmacology and toxicology. *Trends Pharmacol. Sci.* 7, 35–37.

Weil, C. S. (1972) Guidelines for experiments of predict the degree of safety of a material for man. *Toxicol. Appl. Pharmacol.* 21, 194–199.

Weil, C. S., and Gad, S. C. (1980) Applications of methods of statistical analysis to efficient repeated dose toxicology tests. 2. Powerful methods for analysis of body liver and kidney weight data. *Toxicol. Appl. Pharmacol.* 52, 214–226.

Wills, J. H. (1968) Pharmacology, in *The Golden Hamster—Its Biology and Use in Medical Research*, Hoffman, R. A., Robinson, P. F., Magalhaes, H., eds. Iowa State University Press, Ames.

Yates, F. E., and Kugler, P. N. (1986) Similarity principles and intrinsic geometries: Contrasting approaches to interspecies scaling, *J. Pharm. Sci.* 75, 1019–1027.

Zbinden, G. (1963) Experimental and clinical aspects of drug toxicity, in *Advances in Pharmacology*, Garratini, S., and Shore, P. A., eds. Academic Press, New York, pp. 1–112.

Zbinden, G. (1987) *Predictive Value of Animal Studies in Toxicology.* Centre for Medicines Research, Carshalton, U.K.

13

Susceptibility Factors

Shayne Cox Gad
Becton Dickinson and Company
Research Triangle Park, North Carolina

Susceptibility factors are conditions or characteristics which make individual animals or discrete groups of animals (or people) differentially more sensitive to the toxicity of an agent. Or to expression of manifestations of the toxicity. Such factors should be considered from two different perspectives. First, if undesired they may serve to either confound the results of experiments, or by increasing the variability of response in text populations, decrease the sensitivity of test systems. Second, if our concern is the health and safety of more sensitive individuals in the population (as opposed to the young, healthy adult population whom our usual test animal pool represents), then incorporation of such factors in selecting model populations is essential.

There are many factors which can alter the physiological state of an individual (or the fraction of available chemical moiety—see Table 1), and in so doing make them more (or, in some few cases, less) susceptible to the adverse effects of a chemical. These include (but are not limited to) immunological experience; psychological factors such as stress, age, illness; conditioning factors (such as obesity and malnutrition); and sex. There are also environmental factors such as temperature, humidity and time of day which can serve as susceptibility factors.

As a starting place for examining the influence (and possible uses) of susceptibility factors, we should first consider the "base case." That is, what is the nature of the commonly used animal model?

THE DEFINED ANIMAL MODEL

Over the last 15–20 years, it has become accepted practice in toxicology to use bred-to-purpose, genetically defined (usually inbred) and specific pathogen–free (SPF) experimental animals. Such animals are most commonly obtained fom commercial vendors and put on study while they are young adults in the log phase of growth.

Festing (1979a) in his review of the development of these animal stocks has called them "defined" animals in terms of their microbiological flora, genetic background, and environmental and nutritional care.

Table 1 Factors Which May Increase the Fraction of Available Chemical Moiety in the Systemic Circulation

1. Renal impairment
2. Liver impairment
3. Hypoalbumineia
4. Presence of other moieties that displace test agent from proteins in circulation
5. Pregnancy

Microbiological Definition

Animals, like humans, suffer from infectious diseases ranging from those causing only mild symptoms to acute disease outbreaks with high mortality. Although some of these diseases may be partially controlled by medication, both the disease and the medication may seriously interfere with experimental work. Fortunately, most of the infectious disease of laboratory animals may be controlled simultaneously by the use of SPF techniques (Bleby, 1976).

Stocks of SPF animals were initially developed by hysterectomy of the pregnant females just prior to parturition using aseptic surgical techniques. The young were resuscitated in a building designed to prevent the entry of disease-causing organisms, or in closed isolators, and then hand-reared using a sterile milk substitute. This procedure immediately eliminates a wide range of pathogenic organisms which are normally trans-mitted from mother to offspring because young within the uterus are usually microbially sterile. Such SPF animals are normally free of all parasites, many viruses, and most pathogenic bacteria. Once established, such colonies breed well and can be used to supply high-quality breeding stock which does not carry the risk of introducing disease when introduced into an existing colony. Commercial breeders supply SPF mice, rats, guinea pigs, rabbits, and cats. Although some other species have been derived into SPF con-ditions, they are not freely available at present. Such SPF animals have (or offer) the following advantages:

A colony of animals carrying infectious pathogenic organisms is likely to be more variable than a group of SPF animals, and therefore more animals will be needed to achieve the same degree of statistical precision. For example, it has been shown that underweight mice carried five times as many parasitic nematodes as their normal-weight littermates (Eaton, 1972). Although in this case cause and effect cannot be separated, it seems reasonable to assume that such an uneven parasite burden will lead to increased variability among the experimental animals. This means that for the same statistical precision, more "parasitized" animals may be needed than if the animal were free of such parasites.

In conventional animals, there is the danger that the effects of disease may be mistaken for the actions of the experimental treatment. Vitamin A deficiency, for example, has been recorded as causing pneumonia and lung abscesses in rats, when in fact all that the deficiency is doing is to increase the severity of the infectious chronic respiratory disease found in all non-SPF rats (Lindsey et al., 1971). Pneumonia does not occur in SPF rats which are vitamin A deficient. The activation of latent disease through the experimental treatment can be extremely misleading as the control animals not subjected to the same degree of stress may be unaffected (Baker et al., 1971).

In some cases, mild infections may mask the results of an experimental treatment. For example, rats are widely used in inhalation toxicology, yet the lesions of chronic respiratory disease may completely obscure the effects of the experimental treatment. In one case, chlorine gas caused lung lesions, but as the animals grew older the differences between the treated and control groups were completely obscured by the chronic respiratory disease, so that the two groups became histologically indistinguishable (Elmes and Bell, 1963).

Many long-term studies require a substantial number of animals to reach old age. As fewer SPF animals die as a result of infectious disease, fewer animals need to be started in each experimental group (Lindsey et al., 1971). Thus, for long-term studies SPF animals may be substantially more economical than conventional ones. A sidelight of this is that the use of SPF animals has advanced survivability to the point that consideration has been given to lengthening some study types (such as carcinogenicity).

Genetic Definition

Laboratory animals should also be genetically defined. Behavior, response to drugs, size, weight, and shape of many organs, numbers, and types of spontaneous tumors, and response to antigens depends not only on the species, but also on the strain of animal (Festing, 1979a). Inbred strains of mice, rats, hamsters, and guinea pigs produced as a result of at least 20 generations of brother:sister mating are readily available. They are much better experimental subjects than the more widely used outbred "white" mice and rats for most studies. As early as 1942, Strong wrote that:

> It is the conviction of many geneticists that the use of the inbred mouse in cancer research has made possible many contributions of a fundamental nature that would not have been otherwise. Perhaps it would not be out of place to make the suggestion that within the near future all research on mice should be carried out on inbred animals or on hybrid mice of known (genetically controlled) origin where the degree of biological variability has been carefully controlled.

Gruneberg (1952) even went so far as to state that, "The introduction of inbred strains into biology is probably comparable with that of the analytical balance into chemistry."

The main characteristics of genetically defined inbred strains are:

1. All individuals of a strain are genetically identical (isogenic). The genetic uniformity of inbred strains means that each strain can be genetically typed for characters such as their blood group in the knowledge that all animals within that strain will be the same. Such data are essential in many immunological and cancer research studies, and cannot be gathered in outbred stocks, where each individual is genetically unique. Isogenicity also leads to phenotypic uniformity for all highly inherited characters, and this means that the statistical precision of an experiment using these animals is increased.
2. Inbred strains are genetically stable. Once a strain has been developed it stays genetically constant for many years. Non-inbred strains may change as a result of selective forces, but such forces cannot act on inbred strains, which can only change as a result of the accumulation of mutations—a slow process. This stability means that background data on strain characteristics remains constant for long periods— allowing for the use of such information in planning experiments.
3. Inbred strains are internationally distributed. This means that experiments conducted

on some of the commoner inbred strains, which are maintained in laboratories throughout the world, may easily be confirmed at laboratories in entirely different parts of the world. Moreover, if many laboratories are working with the same strain, background data on the strain are accumulated much faster.

4. Each strain has a unique set of characteristics which may be of value in research. In some cases, a strain may have a disease which in some way models a similar condition in humans. The best known of such models are the strains with a high incidence of a particular type of cancer. The inbred mouse strain C3H develops a very high incidence of breast tumor, strains AKR and C58 develop leukemia, SJL develop reticulum-cell sarcoma (Hodgkin's disease), and some sublines of strain 129 develop teratomas. Other strains develop autoimmune anemia (NZB), amyloidosis (YBR and SJL), congenital cleft palate (A and CL), hypertension and heart defects (BALB/c and DBA/2 mice, and SHR and GH rats), obesity and diabetes (NZO, PBB and KK mice), and even a preference for alcohol when given a free choice of 10% alcohol or plain water (strain C57BL mice).

Each of these strains may be studied in order to obtain a better understanding of the disease in the mouse or rat. Once it is understood in the animal, it will be easier to understand in the human, even though it is unlikely that the conditions are exactly comparable in animals and humans. In fact, it is clear from a study of a disease such as hypertension in the rat that the cause of the hypertension in SHR and GH is entirely different (Simpson et al., 1973), emphasizing that diseases of this sort in humans can have several different causes. Obviously, in such cases, some animal models may mimic a human disease relatively closely, whereas in other cases there is little resemblance. Table 2 lists some examples of the models of disease that can be found among inbred strains of mice.

Inbred stains do not neet to model any human disease in order to be of value in research. Strains can usually be found to differ for almost every characteristic studied, including many aspects of behavior, response to a wide range of drugs and chemicals, response to antigens, response to infectious agents, incidence of spontaneous diseases, and even anatomical features. These differences can be of great value in research in a number of different ways. At the most trivial level, if a scientist is studying a response to some treatment effect, it is often possible for him to find, by surveying a number of inbred strains, a strain which is highly sensitive to his experimental treatment. In some cases this will mean that fewer animals are needed to achieve the same degree of statistical precision in future experiments. In other cases, the more sensitive strain may well show the effect sooner than resistant strains, and this may reduce the time and facilities needed to complete the experiment.

At a slightly more sophisticated level, a comparison of sensitive and resistant strains may give extremely valuable information about the mechanism of some treatment effect. For example, if two strains differ in sensitivity to a drug, it would be of great interest to know whether this is because of differences in absorption, metabolism, excretion, or target organ sensitivity. Such a study could give information that would be extremely useful in evaluating the likely effect of the drug in humans. Preferably, such studies should be carried out on two or more sensitive and two or more resistant strains in order to show whether the results are uniquely strain dependent, or can be generalized.

Any two inbred strains will normally differ from each other at several thousand

Table 2 Examples of Disease Models and Characteristics of Interest in Inbred Strains of Mice

Character	Strain(s)
Alcohol (10%) preference	C57BL, C57BL, C57BR/cd
Aggression/fighting	SJL, NZW
Audiogenic seizures	DBA/2
Autoimmune anaemia	NZB
Amyloidosis	YBR, SJL
Cleft palate	CL, A
Chediak-Higashi syndrome	SB
Hypertension and/or heart defects	BALB/c, DBA/1, DBA/2
Hyperprolinaemia and prolinuria	PRO
Obesity and/or diabetes	NZO, PBB, KK, AY
Osteoarthropathy of knee joints	STR/1
Polydipsia	SWR, SWV
Resistance to myxovirus infection	A2G
Tumors	
leukaemia	AKR, C58, PL, RF
reticulum-cell sarcoma (Hodgkin's disease)	SJL
lung tumors	A
hepatomas	C3Hf
mammary tumors	C2H, C3HA-A^{vy}, GRS/A, RIII
ovarian teratomas	LT
induced plasmacytomas	BALB/c, NZB
testicular texatomas	B129/terSV
complete absence of spontaneous tumors	X/Gf
Whisker eating	A2G

Source: From Festing, 1978.

different genetic loci. However, sets of inbred strains which differ from one another at only one or a few loci have been developed in order to study in greater detail those loci which are of particular importance in biomedical research. These are known as sets of congenic strains, and most of them have been developed in order to study the major histocompatibility complex (MHC). This complex locus is responsible for a range of immunological reactions, including immune responses and graft rejection. Obviously, if two strains can be developed which are genetically identical apart from the MHC, it becomes possible to study the MHC in detail simply by comparing the two strains. Such strains can be developed either as a result of a fortuitous mutation within an inbred strain, or by deliberate breeding using conventual genetic back-crossing techniques. Several hundred strains of this type have been developed, and they are not widely used in immunology and cancer research. They have undoubtedly given much insight into the biology of the mouse MHC, which in many respects is very similar to the MHC in humans. There are more than 500 known mutants and variants in the mouse, and a further 100 in the rat, though in the rat many of these have now been lost. Some of these mutants appear to mimic similar mutants in several species, including humans, and may therefore be regarded as "models" of human disease. Other mutants lack an organ such as the

Table 3 Examples of Mouse Mutants of Medical Interest and of Biochemical and Immunological Polymorphisms

Models of disease	Mouse mutants of biomedical interest	
	gene	name
Anemia	sla	Sex-linked anemia
	Sl	Steel
	W	Dominant spotting
Chediak-Higashi syndrome	bg	Beige
Diabetes and/or obesity	A^y	Yellow
	A^{vy}	Viable yellow
	db	Diabetes
	db^{ad}	Adipose
	ob	Obese
Inborn errors of metabolism	his	Histidinaemia
	pro	Prolinemia
Kidney disease	kd	Kidney disease
Muscular dystrophy	dy	Dystrophia-muscularis
	dy^{2j}	Dystrophia-muscularis-2J
Neuromuscular mutants	jp	Jimpy
	med	Motor and plate disease
	qk	Quaking
	Swl	Sprawling
	Tr	Trembling
Genetic alterations or deficiencies		
Embryonic defects	t-allets	Tailless alleles
Hair absent	hr	Hairless
	hr^{rh}	Rhino
	N	Naked
Hair and thymus absent	nu	Nude
Growth hormone absent	dw	Dwarf
Resistance to androgen	Tfm	Testicular feminization
Sex reversal	Sxr	Sex reversal
Spleen absent	Dh	Dominant hemimelia
	Biomedical and immunological polymorphisms	

Polymorphism	Gene locus
Aromatic hydrocarbon	Ahh
Pancreatic	Amy-2
β-D-Galactosidase activity	Bgs
Liver catalase	Ce-1
Erythrocyte antigens	Ea-1 to Ea-7
Esterases (serum and kidney)	Es-1 to Ds-7
Friend virus susceptibility	Fv-1, Fv-2
G-6-PD regulators	Gdr-1, Gdr-2
Haemoglobin alpha chain	Hba
Haemolytic complement	He
Histocompatibility	H-1 to H-38
Immunoglobulin	Ig-1 to Ig-4
Macrophage antigen-1	Mph-1

Table 3 *(continued)*

Polymorphism	Gene locus
Major urinary protein	Mup-1
Phosphoglucomutase	Pgm-1, Pgm-2
Sex-limited protein	Slp
Thymus cell antigen-1	Thy-1
Thymus leukemia antigen	Tla

Source: From Festing, 1978.

thymus, spleen, tail, or eyes, or they suffer from some hormone deficiency or a developmental defect. Such mutants can be extremely valuable for certain types of research even though they may not resemble any human condition. A list of some of these mutants, classified into models of disease, a genetic alterations and deficiencies, and biochemical and immunological polymorphisms is given in Table 3. There are, for example, a number of types of genetically determined obesity and diabetes which have been extremely useful as models of similar conditions in humans (Festing, 1979b). Such animals help to show up the immense complexity of the regulation of body fat via the hormonal control of a range of metabolic interactions, each of which may be controlled by regulatory mechanisms which interact with one another. Thus, the finding of a particular biochemical abnormality is no guarantee that it is the cause of the observed obesity. It is much more likely that it is a secondary effect of the primary genetic defect. However, although many of these models of obesity may have no exact counterpart in humans, they may still be useful in screening drugs with a potential for reducing obesity (Cawthorne, 1979).

One of the most important mutants causing genetic alterations or deficiencies is the athymic nude mutation in the mouse. A similar mutation has now been described in the rat (Festing et al., 1978). The thymus is essential for the full development of the immune system, and homozygous nude mice or rats are deficient in the cell-mediated type of immune response. They are of value in fundamental studies of immune mechanisms as well as in applied cancer research. This is because, lacking the cell-mediated immune response, they are unable to reject transplanted foreign tissue, including transplants of human tumors. Such transplanted human tumors usually grow, but they retain all the characteristics of human tissue. Therefore, it is possible not only to study human tumors when growing in an animal, but it is also possible to study the effect of drugs on such tumors. This is obviously of more value than having to rely simply on the study of animal tumors in animals.

Recently, there has been a great increase in interest in mutants. This probably follows the successful development of the nude mouse as a research model.

ENVIRONMENTAL AND NUTRITIONAL CONDITION

The need to house the defined laboratory animal in defined and stabilized environmental conditions, with a nutritionally adequate and controlled diet, is now becoming recognized. Both diet and environment can drastically alter the physiology of the animal and its response to drugs and other experimental treatments. Moreover, animals obtained from a commercial breeder may well take 2 or more weeks to acclimatize to their new environment. During this period their physiological responses may be unpredictable, depending on the difference between the two environments (Grant et al., 1971).

SUSCEPTIBILITY FACTORS

With all the effort (and reasons behind it) that goes into obtaining a "defined" test animal with a relatively narrow range of variation in responses, what then are the components or factors which lead some animals to be more sensitive to the toxicity of agents than others?

Consideration of the problem shows that susceptibility factors fall into two large groups—intrinsic and external. The intrinsic factors include sex, stress, age, disease, physiological state (all of which were discussed in detail in the previous chapter), species variations, and strain and animal variations ("biological variation"). External or environmental factors, meanwhile, include temperature, humidity, light, and time of day.

Summary

If the human population we are concerned about is such that one or more of these susceptibility factors is present in a substantial portion of the members, steps should be taken to design studies so that such individuals are adequately represented by an appropriate model in the test animal population. Barring that, or in the face of having existing data on studies performed in a standard manner, consideration should be given to these factors when attempting to predict outcome of exposures in people.

Species Peculiarities

There are a number of quirks associated with various of the common species of laboratory animals used in toxicology. Many of these are not well presented in the toxicology literature, though Oser (1981) has done his best to overview problems specific to the rat and Gralla (1986) has published a review of eight species-specific responses to toxicants (a modified form of which is presented in Table 5). Most of these peculiarities hold at least the potential to impact on study design and interpretation. Presented here are those that the authors believe should be considered in model selection for acute studies.

Species Variation

Though anyone who has had to work in biological research with intact animals should be aware of the existence of wide variability between species, examples which are specific to toxicology should be pointed out along with a comparison of species sensitivities for a number of specific agents.

The rodenticide zinc phosphide is dependent on the release of phosphine by hydrochloric acid in the stomach for its activation and efficacy (Johnson and Voss, 1952). As a result, dogs and cats are considerably less sensitive than rats and rabbits, since the former species secrete gastric hydrochloric acid intermittently, whereas the latter secrete it almost continuously. That this case is not a rare one can be quickly established by examining some data sets where we have comparative oral lethality data on several species (including humans), such as those presented in Table 6.

There are numerous additional examples of such differences in pharmacology (Tedeschi and Tedeschi, 1968). But just as important as these variations in general patterns or effect are the species-specific responses that are associated with the commonly employed animal models.

Rat. The rat is commonly accepted as the best animal model in toxicology, the closest to

Table 5 Species-Specific Toxic Effects

Type of toxicity	Structure	Sensitive species	Mechanism of toxicity
Ocular	Retina	Dog	Zinc chelation
Ocular	Retina	Any with pigmented retinas	Melanin binding
Stimulated basal metabolism	Thyroid	Dog	Competition or binding
Porphyria	Liver	Human, rat, guinea pig, mouse, and rabbit	Estrogen enhanced sensitivity
Tubular necrosis	Kidney	Rats (male)	Androgen enhanced sensitivity[a]
Urolithiasis	Kidney & bladder	Rats and mice	Uricase inhibition
Teratogenesis; fetal mortality	Fetus	Rats and mice	Uricase inhibition
Cardiovascular	Heart	Rabbits	Sensitivity to microvascular constriction

[a]More sensitive than humans for many agents (such as caprolactam and halogenated solvents).
Source: Adapted from Gralla, 1986, with modification.

our ideal (Oser, 1981). Table 7 presents a list of some of the commonly known advantages and disadvantages of the rat as a model for humans.

Calabrese (1983) has published a good comparative review of the rat as a model for humans across a wide range of toxicological and biological parameters, and should be consulted for details on these

Mice. Mice share many advantages and disadvantages of the rats as a model for humans, such as an inability to vomit (i.e., no emetic response). Additionally, their small size and high metabolic rate cause the extent of many toxic effects to be exaggerated as homeostatic mechanisms are "overshot."

Table 6 Comparative Human Acute Lethal Doses and Animals LD_{50}s (mg/kg via oral route)

Chemical	Human LD_{LO}[a]	LD$_{50}$ values Mouse	Rat	Rabbit	Dog
Aminopyrine	220	358	685	160	150
Aniline	360	300	440		195
Amytal	43	345	560	575	
Boric acid	640	3450	2660		
Caffeine	192	620	192	224	140
Carbofuran	11	2	5		19
Carbon tetrachloride	43	12800	2800	6380	
Cycloheximide		133	3		
Lindane	840		125	130	120
Fenoflurazole		1600	283	28	50

[a]LD_{LO} = lowest observed lethal dose.

Table 7 Advantages and Disadvantages of the Rat as an Experimental
Model for Humans

Advantages	Disadvantages
Commonly used	Anatomic
Small size	lack of gallbladder
Minimal housing space	yolk-sac placenta
Prolific	multiple mammae over body surface
Short gestation	no emetic reflex
Short lactation	fur covered
Omnivorous	thinner stratum corneum
Dry diet acceptable	no bronchial glands
Dosing by multiple routes	Physiological
Inexpensive	estrus and menstrual cycles
Low maintenance cost	multiparous
Docile	hematology
Intelligence	obligatory nose breather
	concentrated urine
	limited hypersensitivity response
	Metabolic
	purines to allantoin
	clinical chemistry
	enzymatic biotransformation
	high β-glucuronidase activity
	Nutritional
	mineral requirements
	vitamin requirements
	ascorbic acid biosynthesis
	histidine biosynthesis
	Behavior
	nocturnal
	coprophagy
	cannibalism
	Maintenance requirements
	temperature and humidity control
	noise control

Guinea Pigs. The systemic immune response in the guinea pig is exaggerated. As a result, though for many immune parameters, it is the best common model for humans, the animal is subject to exaggerated respiratory and cardiovascular expressions of immunologically evoked events.

Rabbits. There are no specific pathogen-free rabbits currently commercially available. Rather, the animals tend not to be as homogeneous nor of as high quality as the other common laboratory animal species. Indeed, they tend to harbor a wider range of subclinical infections which show a seasonal variation in their degree of expression (animals with a visible disease problem are more common in the spring and fall), and the stress of experimentation can cause these subclinical infections to be expressed.

Also, the alterations in dermal vascular flow which accompany the changes in phases of hair growth cause marked alterations in percutaneous absorption and in so doing may alter many dermally related responses to chemicals.

Dog. The dog is currently the first-choice nonrodent model for toxicity studies. It is generally very cooperative. The major physiological peculiarity it has that affects toxicity testing is the ease with which it is provoked to vomit. This makes oral dosing at best impractical, and at worst impossible in the case of many compounds, even if the material is encapsulated or given in diet.

Considerations of Strain

Thus far we have focused on the differences between the different species of common laboratory animals and on how this should influence our choice of a model. But for each of the two species that are used the most in toxicology (the rat and mouse), there is the additional level of complexity caused by differences between strains.

There are three different genetic categories of strains of rodents used in toxicological research: random bred, inbred and F_1 hybrids (or outbred). Random bred animals are produced in large colonies where mating occurs randomly among males and females from unrelated litters. Commercially performed random breeding should not be unplanned, but rather occur in such a manner as to minimize inbreeding. Inbred animals are the result of sister-brother or parent-offspring matings. Twenty or more generations of sister-brother and/or parent offspring mating are necessary to establish an inbred strain. Outbred animals are the results of matings between two inbred strains and are usually more vigorous than either of the parental strains. Animals within an inbred or outbred strain are essentially identical genetically, serving to remove a significant source of biological variability.

Strains also exist of the other laboratory animal species, but are generally neither as rigorously defined or of as great a concern, and have been less studied as a source of variation within toxicity studies.

That stain differences within species are a source of significant and broad differences in results has now been well established, in many cases with varying degrees of knowledge of the underlying mechanistic basis. The resistance of some strains of rabbits to atropine is believed to be due to the hydrolysis of the drug by atropine sterase, controlled by the gene A_8, belonging to the group containing the gene which governs black pigmentation. As a result, resistance to atropine and black pigmentation are often associated (Sawin and Glick, 1943). Likewise, some strains of rabbits possess a pseudococaine esterase that makes their insensitivity to this drug extreme.

There are also varieties within strains. These result from various factors which in total are labeled genetic drift, and can lead to significant differences in response to toxicants. An example is the resistance that some wild rats have developed to the anticoagulant rodenticides (Gratz, 1973; Zimmermann and Matschiner, 1974), requiring that new forms of rodenticides be developed.

Strain variations in response to biologically active agents arise from the same general mechanistic differences as do species differences. Although these (Hilado and Furst, 1978) pharmacogenetics have been the subject of numerous reviews (Kalow, 1962, 1965; Meier, 1963a,b; Vessel, 1969; Hathway, 1970; Moore, 1972; Lange and Vessel, 1976), it is still the case that few investigators have studied the mechanisms of variation in higher animals (Becker, 1962). And the differences in handling characteristics have generally not appeared in the literature before.

Biological Variation

There are also individual animal-to-animal variations in temperature, health, and sensitivity to toxicities which are recognized and expected by experienced animal researchers, but are only broadly understood. The resulting differences in response are generally accredited to "individual biological variation." This same phenomenon has been widely studied and observed among humans, and is expected by an experienced clinician. Examples of such individual variations in human include isoniazid, succinylcholine, and glucose-6-phosphate levels and/or activities. In the first of these, "slow inactivators" who are deficient in acetyltransferase, and therefore acetylate agents such as isoniazid only slowly, and are thus more liable to suffer from the peripheral neuropathy caused by an accumulation of isoniazid. At the same time, people with more effective acetyltransferase require larger doses of isoniazid to benefit from its therapeutic effects, but in so doing are more likely to suffer liver damage.

Likewise, individuals with low levels of serum cholinesterase may exhibit prolonged muscle relaxation and apnea following an injection of a standard dose of the muscle relaxant succinylcholine, and glucose-6-phosphate dehydrogenase deficiency is responsible for the increased probability of some individuals given primaquine or antipyrine to suffer from a hemolytic anemia. Some of these as seen in mice are listed in Table 2.

ENVIRONMENTAL FACTORS

Temperature

Changes in temperature may alter the toxicity of a compound. As examples, at ambient temperatures colchicine and digitalis are more lethal to the rat than to the frog. But the sensitivity of the frog can be increased by raising the environmental temperature of the two species. The duration of response also decreases as the temperature is raised, suggesting that a temperature-dependent biotransformation of these compounds is involved.

Temperature may include both the background environmental temperature and the internal, physiologically regulated temperature of the animal itself. Many chemicals can profoundly alter body temperature to the acceleration of reaction rates, but rather were due to alterations in the rates of physical factors, such as the absorption rate.

Keplinger et al. (1959) investigated the toxicity of 58 chemicals under different ambient conditions, including temperature. He found that many of the patterns of acute toxicity response were biphasic relative to ambient temperature, with some temperature in the ambient range being associated with a peak sensitivity in many cases.

Humidity

Selisko et al. (1963) investigated the effects of a number of environmental factors on the acute IP toxicity of nicotine to mice and found only humidity to have a significant influence. Humidity does not have a marked influence on absorption through the skin except at the extreme limits of its range (Neely et al., 1967), and the relationship between humidity and transdermal water loss in sweating animal species in not linear (Grice et al., 1972). The relationships in nonsweating species (which include all of our common laboratory species) is even more complex (Neely et al., 1967).

The physiological status of the test animal in terms of hydration can markedly influence its response to toxicants. Muller and Vernikos-Danelis (1968) showed that the LD_{50}s of caffeine and dextroamphetamine in mice were markedly affected by both ambient temperature and the animals' hydration, with caffeine showing a large potentiation of toxicity at 30°C, whereas dextroamphetamine showed much less change. At lower temperatures (22 and 15°C) the acute toxicity of both compounds was much less influenced by hydration (Cremer and Bligh, 1969).

Environmental temperature and humidity are generally closely related and as such have frequently been considered together (Lange and Vessel, 1976). Understanding the basis for the temperature dependence of many of the actions of biologically active compounds has been an area of significant progress over the last 20 years. Belehradek (1957) successfully combined his own and other investigators' research to produce unified theory of cellular rate processes based on an analysis of the actions of temperature. He concluded that the rate processes based on an analysis of the actions of temperature. He concluded that the rate of biological processes is primarily dependent on the resistance of cellular matter to the free movement of molecules within the cells rather than the rate of actual chemical reactions themselves. He was enthusiastic about the relationship between the rate responses of cellular systems and Slotte's temperature-viscosity relationship formula. Brody (1964) has, however, reviewed the applicability of this last to vertebrate animals and pointed out its shortcomings.

The relationship between responses to toxicants and ambient temperature in animals is sometimes paradoxical. Unsinger (1957) investigated this in mice and found a series of biphasic relationships with "optimal," or peak, ranges. Mean oxygen consumption per unit body weight diminishes as temperature increases further. Likewise, he measured the rectal temperatures occurring when the ambient temperature was 25°C, increasing on either side of this temperature.

Ahdaya et al. (1976) investigated thermoregulation in mice exposed to parathion, carbaryl, and DDT at temperatures of 1, 27, and 38°C. All three of the pesticides were found to be least toxic at 27°C. Doull (1972) has reviewed these temperature-dependent responses for many chemicals and presented the hypothesis that temperature is directly correlated with the magnitude and inversely correlated with the duration of the biological response to biologically active xenobiotics in many organisms. Though this temperature dependence stands as a general rule, there are a number of special case exceptions. And it is clear that the effect of temperature on one response variable may not necessarily be predictive of effects on other biological response variables.

Baetjer and Smith (1956) found that the onset of death, rate of dying, and rate of recovery due to parathion in mice were more rapid, whereas the mortality was higher at 35.6°C than at 22.8°C. At 15.5°C, the onset of death was delayed and the total mortality was greater than at 22.8°C. They also investigated the influence of both pre- and postexposure temperatures on the response of the mice and determined that mortality varied directly with the pre- and inversely with the postexposure ambient temperatures. Their conclusion was the results could not be attributed.

Barometric Pressure

Interest in the effect of atmospheric pressure on the toxicity of chemicals is fairly recent, arising from human activities in space and deep sea diving vessels. At high altitudes, the toxicity of digitalis and strychnine are decreased, whereas that of amphetamine is increased. The influence of atmospheric pressure seems to be mainly (but not entirely) attributable to altered physiological oxygen tension rather than a direct pressure effect (Brown, 1980). Recently this interest has taken a new turn as concern as to the possible hazard of fires and atmospheric contaminants on submarines has surfaced.

Light

Whole body irradiation with electromagnetic radiation, including light, increases the toxicity of central nervous system (CNS) stimulants and decreases that of CNS depressants. The toxicity of analgesics such as morphine does not seem to be altered. Many toxicants to exhibit a diurnal pattern of response in animals that is generally related to the light pattern. In rats and mice, P-450 enzyme activity is at its greatest at the beginning of the dark phase of the cycle.

Social Factors

A variety of social factors (interactions between individual animals and between animals and research workers) can modify the toxicities of chemicals in animals and undoubtedly also in humans. Animal handling, housing (singly or in groups), types of cages, and laboratory routine are all important components of such considerations.

Edward (1982) should be consulted for a good overview of the factors to be considered in the design and operation of a laboratory in terms of both good science and economic and regulatory considerations.

Temporal Factors

Most biological organisms are influenced, directly and/or indirectly, by a stream of daily and annual variations in their environment. These variations include light, temperature, social interactions, and food, and have resulted in a notable cyclical variations in function. Table 8 presents some of the better established of these.

Many of these cycles can be considerably amplified and/or modified. Liver function, for example, includes liver glycogen (which is also seasonally variable), glycogen phosphorylase, tyrosine transaminase, tryptophan pyrrolase, and esterase; some of these rhythmic changes are reflected in hepatic cell ultrastructure. Renal function includes urine volume and pH, and excretion of sodium, potassium, chloride, phosphate, uric acid, adrenal cortex, and probably other tissues as well. Blood leukocytes other than eosinophils show daily variation, although the eosinophilic changes have probably been the most studied. Reviews of these topics are to be found in Reinberg and Ghata, 1964; Aschoff, 1965; Brunning, 1967; Conroy and Mills, 1970; Mills, 1973, and Gall, 1977.

Many unicellular organisms also show cyclically varying functions; for example, cell generation time, photosynthetic capacity, phototaxis, and luminescence. In higher plants, growth, leaf and petal movement and CO_2 fixation are rhythmic functions, and in fungi, spore discharge (Wilkins, 1973).

Table 8 Physiological functions showing time based cyclic variations

Activity/sleep
Body temperature
Pain threshold
Adrenocortical function
Skin histamine sensitivity
Liver function
Renal function
Eosinophil count
Mitotic rates
Food consumption
Body weight

An interesting feature of these rhythms is that they continue when rhythmic external stimuli are removed. If the daily light/dark cycle is turned into continuous light and if temperature variation is suppressed, and if, in humans, clues like watches and clocks and fixed meal times are removed, the rhythmic variation in function continues, but with a period which may differ slightly from the original 24 hr. This is the so-called "free-running" period. A 24-hr rhythm may become, for example, 25.0 or 22.9 hr (usually, however, between 20 and 28 hr), and settles to this new period indefinitely until external clues are restored. This phenomenon is the origin of the expression "circadian," meaning about a day's length.

Considerable work has gone into trying to identify the biological clock which maintains these rhythms, so far without clear-cut success. Does the clock reside in an organ, (for example, the CNS or the adrenal cortex), or is it a celluar function? The answer is probably both: that the cell has mechanisms which allow it to entrain to environmental rhythms, and that in higher organisms these become systematized in regulatory organs to coordinate the functioning of the body as a whole in response to environmental changes (Mills, 1966, 1973).

Both unicellular organisms and avian and mammalian cells in culture show circadian rhythms in the absence of exogenous influences (Bruce, 1965). Present arguments center around whether the cellular clock is based on sequential DNA transcription or to biochemical networks with natural oscillatory periods. A more recent hypothesis suggests that the cell membrane, with its stable lipids and mobile protein ionic gates, may serve as an oscillator with the underlying slow periodically (Njus et al., 1974).

The majority of the laboratory animals used in toxicology are nocturnal, and they do not change while in the laboratory. Our procedures rarely take the fact and implication of this underlying biological activity rhythm into account.

Diurnal rhythms (more correctly nychthemeral; diurnal refers to daytime, nocturnal to the night) are probably the most important, but there are almost certainly other cyclical changes in physiological function, connected to season or to sexual function, which for the most part we disregard, and which may occasionally be important.

The significance of circadian variation for drug action and toxicology will depend very much on the nature of the drug, its absorption characteristics, and on the way in which it is administered. Toxicity from continuous atmospheric exposure is not likely to show much circadian dependence, nor from a drug only slowly absorbed or slowly metabolized to an active component. But these are perhaps the exceptions, and with the increasing range of drugs showing some clinical effectiveness, many of which also carry undesirable side effects, it would seem sensible to administer these in a regimen which allows them to exert their maximum desired effect with a minimum of side effects. While drugs acting on the CNS, the cardiovascular system, and the kidney and the steroids are obvious candidates for such consideration, there is evidence that susceptibility to infection is also circadian dependent, and chemotherapeutic agents and the antibiotics may not be outside such an inquiry.

In addition, a sizeable proportion of the population has its biological clock thrown into potential disarray. Besides the pilots and aircrew of long-distance flights and the jet-set traveler, the night-shift work force is numerous enough, and includes not only the factory workers and truck drivers, but hospital staffs, police, airport control tower staff, and watchkeepers at sea, all carrying considerable responsibility. If there is a relationship between drug action and the circadian cycle. it deserves proper evaluation.

REFERENCES

Ahdaya, S. M., Shah, P. V., and Guthrie, F. E. (1976) Thermoregulation in mice treated with parathin, carbaryl or DDT. *Toxicol. Pharmacol.* 35, 575–580.

Angel, G. (1969) Starvation, stress and the blood brain barrier. *Dis. Nerv. Syst.* 30, 94–97.

Aschoff, J. (ed.) (1965) *Circadian Clocks.* North-Holland, Amsterdam.

Baetjer, A. M., and Smith, R. (1956) Effect of environmental temperature on reaction of mice to parathion, an anticholinesterase agent. *Am. J. Physiol.* 186, 39–46.

Baker, H. J., Cassell, G. H., and Lindsey, J. R. (1971) Research complicants due to Haemobartonella and Eperythrozoon infection in experimental animals. *Am. J. Pathol.* 64, 625–656.

Becker, W. A. (1962) Choice of animals and sensitivity of experiments *Nature* 193, 1264–1266.

Belehradek, J. (1957) A unified theory of cellular rate process based upon an analysis of temperature action. *Protoplasma* 48, 53–71.

Bleby, J. (1976) "Disease-free (SPFE) animals,' in *The UFAE handbook on the Care and Management of Laboratory Animals*, 5th ed., Churchill Livingstone, Edinburgh.

Boyd, E. M., Dodos, I., and Krijnen, C. J. (1970) Endosulfan toxicity and dietary protein. *Arch. Environ. Health* 21, 15–19.

Brody, S. (1964) *Bioenergetics and Growth.* Hafner, New York.

Brown, V. K. (1980) *Acute Toxicity in Theory and Practice.* Wiley, New York.

Bruce, V. G. (1965) Cell division and the circadian clock, in Aschoff, J., ed., *Circadian Clocks.* North-Holland, Amsterdam, pp. 125–138.

Bruce, R. D. (1985) An up-and-down procedure for acute toxicity testing. *Fund. Appl. Toxicol.* 5, 151–157.

Brus, R., and Herman, Z. S. (1971) Acute toxicities of adrenaline, noradrenaline and acetylcholine in adult and neo-natal mice *Dissert. Pharm. Pharmacol.* 23, 435–437.

Bunning, E. (1967) *The Physiological Clock.* Longmans, New York.

Calabese, E. J. (1983) *Principles of Animal Extrapolation.* Wiley, New York.

Cawthorne, M. A. (1979). The use of animal models in the detection and evaluation of compounds for the treatment of obesity, in *Animal models of obsesity*, Festing, M. F. W., ed. Macmillan, London, pp. 79–90.

Conroy, R. T. W. L., and Mills, J. N. (1970) *Human Rhythms.* Churchill, London.

Corcharan, G. B., and Wong, B. K. (1987). Obesity as a risk factor in drug-induced organ injury: Increased liver and kidney damage by acetaminophen in the obese overfed rat. *JET* 241, 921–927.

Corcoran, G. B., and Salazar, D. E. (1988) Obesity as a risk factor in drug induced organ injury. II. Increased renal cytochrome P-450 in the obese overfed rat. *Drug Metab. Dispos.* 16, 898–900.

Cremer, J. E., and Bligh, J. (1969) Body temperature and responses to drugs. *Br. Med. Bull.* 23, 299–306.

Dauterman, W. C. (1980) Physiological factors affecting metabolism of xenobiotics, in *Introduction to Biochemical Toxicology*, Hodgson, E., and Guthrie, F. E., eds. Elseivier, New York.

Depass, L. R., Myers, R. C. Weaver, E. V., and Weil, C. S. (1984) *Alternative Methods in Toxicology*, Vol 2. *Acute Toxicity Testing.* Mary Ann Liebert, New York, pp. 141–153.

Doull, J. (1972) The effect of physical environmental factors on drug response, in *Essays in Toxicology*, Vol. 3. Hayes, W. J., ed. Academic Press, New York.

Doull, J. (1980) Factors influencing toxicology, in *Casarett and Doull's Toxicology*, Doull, J., Klaassen, C. D., and Amdur, M. O., eds. Macmillan, New York.

Eaton, G. J. (1972) Intestinal helminths in inbred strains of mice. *Lab. Anim. Sci.* 22, 850–853.

Eben, A., and Pilz, W. (1967) Abhangigbeit der acetylcholinesterase-acktivatat in plasma and erythrocyten von der alter und geschlecht der ratte. *Arch. Toxicol.* 22, 27–34.

Edwards, A. G. (1982) Animal care and maintenance, in *Principles and Methods of Toxicology*, Hayes A. W., ed. Raven Press, New York, pp. 321–345.

Ehrich, M., and Gross, W. B. (1983) Modification of triorthotolyl phosphate toxicity in chickens by stress. *Toxicol. Appl. Pharmacol.* 70, 249–254.

Elmes, P. C., and Bell, D. P. (1963) The effects of chlorine gas on the lungs of rats with spontaneous pulmonary disease. *J. Pathol. Bacteriol.* 86, 317–326.

Festing, M. F. W. (1978) Genetic variation and adaptation in laboratory animals, in *Das Tier in Experiment*, Weihe, W. H. ed. Hans Huber, Bern, pp. 16–32.

Festing, M. F. W. (1979a) *Inbred Strains in Biomedical Research*. Macmillan, London.

Festing, M. F. W. ed. (1979b). *Animal Models of Obesity*. Macmillan, London.

Festing, M. F. W. (1981) The "defined" animal and the reduction of animal use, in *Animals in Research*, Sperlinger, D., ed. Wiley, New York.

Gaines, T. B. (1960) The acute toxicity of pesticides to rats. *Toxicol. Appl. Pharmacol.* 2, 88–99.

Gaines, T. B. (1969) Acute toxicology of pesticides *Toxicol. Appl. Pharmacol.* 14, 515–534.

Gall, D. (1977) Temporal variations in toxicity, in *Current Approaches in Toxicology*, Ballantyne, B., ed. John Wright, Bristol, England.

Gillete, J. R. (1979) Extrapolating from microsomes to mice to men, *Drug Metab. Dispos.* 7, 121–123.

Goldenthal, E. I. (1971) A compilation of LD_{50} values in newborn and adult animals. *Toxicol. Appl. Pharmacol.* 18, 185–207.

Grant, L., Hopkins, P., Jennings, G., and Jenner, F. A. (1971). Period of adjustment of rats used for experimental studies. *Nature* 232, 135.

Gray, H., and Addis, T. (1948) Rat colony testing by Zucker's weight-age relation. *Am. J. Physiol.* 153, 35–40.

Grice, K., Sattar, H., and Baker, H. (1972) The effect of ambient humidity on transepidermal water loss. *J. Invest. Dermatol.* 58, 343–346.

Gruneberg, H. (1952). *The Genetics of the Mouse*, 2nd ed. Nijhoff, The Hague.

Halberg, F., Johnson, E. A., Brown, B. W., and Bittner, J. J. (1960) Susceptibility rhythm to E. coli endotoxin and bioassay *Proc. Soc. Exp. Biol. Med.* 103, 142–144.

Hathway, D. E. (1970) Species, strain and sex differences in metabolism, in *Foreign Compound Metabolism and Mammals*, Hathway, D. E., ed. Chemical Society, London.

Heston, W. E. (1975) Testing for possible effects of cedar wood shavings and diet on the occurrence of mammary gland tumours and hepatomas in C3H-A^{vy} and C3H-A^{vy} fB mice *J. Natl. Cancer Instit.* 54, 1011–1014.

Hilado, C. J., and Furst, A. (1978) Reproducibility of toxicity data as a function of mouse strain, animal lot and operator *J. Combust. Tox.* 5, 75–80.

Johnson, H. D., and Voss, E. (1952) Toxicological studies of zinc phosphide. *J. Am. Pharm. Assoc.* (Sci. Ed.) 41, 468–472.

Kalow, W. (1962) *Pharmacogenetics—Heredity and the Response to Drugs*. Saunders, Philadelphia.

Kalow, W. (1965) Dose-response relationship and genetic variation. *Ann N.Y. Acad. Sci.* 123, 212–218.

Kato, R., and Gillette, J. R. (1965) Sex difference in the effects of abnormal physiological states on the metabolism of drugs by rat liver microsomes *J. Pharmacol. Exp. Ther.* 150, 2285–291.

Keplinger, M. L., Lanier, G. E., and Deichmann, W. B. (1959) Effects of environmental temperature on the acute toxicity of a number of compounds in the rat, *Toxicol. Appl. Pharmacol.* 1, 156–161.

Krasovskij, G. N. (1975) Species and sex differences in sensitivity to toxic substances, in *Methods Used in the USSR for Establishing Biologically Safe Levels of Toxic Substances*. World Health Organization, Geneva.

Lang, C. M., and Vessell, E. S. (1976) Environmental and genetic factors affecting laboratory animals: Impact on biomedical research. *Fed. Proc.* 35, 1123–1124.

Lenox, R. H., and Frazier, T. W. (1972) Methadone induced mortality as a function of the circadian cycle. *Nature* 239, 397–398.

Leonard, B. E. (1988) Stress, the immune system and psychiatric illness. *Stress Med.* 4, 207–213.

Lindsey, J. R., Baker, H. J., Overcash, R. G., Cassell, G. H., and Hunt, C. E. (1971) Murine chronic respiratory disease. *Am. J. Pathol.* 64, 675–716.

Meier, H. (1963a) Potentialities for and present status of pharmacological research in genetically controlled mice, in *Advances in Pharmacology*, Vol. 2, Garattini, S., and Shore, P. A. eds. Academic Press, New York.

Meier, H. (1963b) *Experimental Pharmacogenetics: Physiopathology of Heredity and Pharmacologic Responses.* Academic Press, New York.

Mills, J. N. (1966) Human circadian rhythms. *Physiol. Rev.* 46, 128–171.

Mills, J. N. (ed.) (1973) *Biological Aspects of Circadian Rhythms.* Plenum Press, London.

Moore, D. H. (1972) Species, Sex and Strain Differences in Metabolism, in *Foreign Compound Metabolism in Mammals* Hathway, D. E., ed. Chemical Society, London.

Muller, P. J., and Vernikos-Danellis, J. (1968) Alteration in drug toxicity by environmental variables. *Proc. West. Pharmacol. Soc.* 11, 52–53.

Naik, S. R., Anjaria, R. J., and Sheth, U. K. (1970) Studies on rat brain acetylcholine and cholinesterase, pt 1. Effect of body weight, sex, stress and CNS depressant drugs. *Ind. J. Med. Res.* 58, 473–479.

Natelson, B. H., Hoffman, S. L., and Cagin, N. A. (1979) A role for environmental factors in the production of digitalis toxicity. *Pharmacol. Biochem. Behav.* 12, 235–237.

Neely, W. A., Turner, M. D., and Taylor, A. E. (1967) Bidirectional movement of water through the skin of a non-sweating animal. *J. Surg. Res.* 7, 323–328.

Njus, D., Sulzman, E. M., and Hastings, J. W. (1974) Membrane model for the circadian clock. *Nature* 248, 116–120.

Oser, B. L. (1981) The rat as a model for human toxicology evaluation, *J. Toxicol. Environ. Health* 8, 521–542.

Palotta, A. J., Kelly, M. J., Rall, D. P., and Ward, J. W. (1962) Toxicology of acetoxycyclohex-imide as a function of sex and body weight. *J. Pharmacol.* 136, 400–405.

Reinberg, A., Cervais, P., and Pollack, E. (1973) Circadian rhythms during drug-induced coma. *Int. J. Chronobiol.* 1, 157–162.

Sabine, J. R., Horton, B. J., and Wicks, M. B. (1973) Spontaneous tumours in C3H-A^{vy} and C3H-A^{vy} fB mice: High incidence in the United States and low incidence in Australia. *J. Natl. Cancer Instit.* 50, 1237–1242.

Safarov, Y. B. and Aleskerov, S. A. (1972) Effects of pesticides in producing relapses in animals recovering from bacterial infections *Probl. Vet. Sanit.* 43, 213–218.

Sawin, P. B., and Glick, D. (1943) Atropinesterase, a genetically determined enzyme in the rabbit. *Proc. Natl. Acad. Sci.* 29, 55–59.

Scheving, L. E., Mayerback, H. V., and Pauly, J. E. (1974) An overview of chronopharmacology *J. Eur. Toxicol.* 7, 203–227.

Selisko, O., Hentschel, G., and Ackermann, H. (1963) Uber die abhangigkeit her mittleren todlichen dosis (LD$_{50}$) von exogenen Faktoren. *Arch. Int. Pharmacodyn. Ther.* 45, 51–69.

Shanor, S. P., van Hees, G. R. Baart, N., Erdo, E. G., and Foldes, E. F. (1961) The influence of age and sex on human plasma and red cell cholinesterase. *Am. J. Mws. Axi.* 242, 357–361.

Simpson, F. O., Phelan, E. L., Clark, D. W. J., Jones, D. R., Gresson, C. R., Lee, D. R., and Bird, D. L. (1973) Studies on the New Zealand strain of genetically hypertensive rats. *Clin. Sci. Mol. Med.* 45, 15s–21s.

Steen, J. A., Hanneman, G. D., Nelson, P. L., and Folk, E. D. (1976) Acute toxicity of mevinophos to gerbils. *Toxicol. Appl. Pharmacol.* 35, 195–198.

Strong, L. C. (1942) The origin of some inbred mice. *Cancer Res.* 2, 531–539.

Stockinger, H. E. (1953) Size of dose; its effect on distribution in the body. *Nucleonics* 11, 24–27.

Tedeschi, D. H., and Tedeschi, R. E. (1968) *Importance of Fundamental Principles in Drug Evaluation*, Raven Press, New York.

Usinger, W. (1957) Respiratorischer stoffweschel und korpetemperature der weissen mans in thermoindefferenter umgebung. *Pfugers Arch.* 264, 520–535.

Vaccarezza, J. R., and Peltz, L. (1960) Effect of ACTH on blood cholinesterase activity in normal subjects and respiratory-allergy patients. *Presse Med.* 68, 723–724.

Vaccarezza, J. R., and Willson, J. A. (1964a) The effect of ACTH on cholinesterase activity in plasma, whole blood and blood cells of rats. *Experientia* 20, 23.

Vaccarezza, J. R., and Willson, J. A. (1964b) The relationship between corticosterone administration and cholinesterase activity in rats. *Experientia* 21, 205.

Vessell, E. S. (1969) Recent progress in pharmacogenetics, in *Advances in Pharmacology and Chemotherapy*, Vol. 7, Garattini, S., Goldin, A., Hawking, F., and Koplin, I. J., eds. Academic Press, New York.

Vogel, W. H. (1987) Stress—The neglected variable experimenta pharmacology and toxicology. *Trends Pharmacol. Sci.* 7, 35–37.

Wilkins, M. B. (1973) Circadian rhythms in plants, in Mills, J. N., ed. *Biological Aspects of Circadian Rhythms*. Plenum Press, London, pp. 235–279.

Zbinden, G. (1963) Experimental and clinical aspects of drug toxicity, in *Advances in Pharmacology*, Garratini, S., and Shore, P. A., eds. Academic Press, New York.

14

Laws and Regulations Governing Animal Care and Use in Research

Curtis D. Port
G. D. Searle and Company
Skokie, Illinois

Laws governing the care and use of animals in research are not new, and have their beginnings in nineteenth century England as a result of the antivivisection movement (French, 1975). The first law governing research on animals was passed in 1822 and was amended in 1835 and 1849. The British Cruelty to Animals Act of 1876 was passed in the hope it would frustrate or hinder antivivisectionist activity; it was amended in 1912. Several proposals for reform of the 1876 amended law were made during the 1970s, all of which were unsatisfactory and included the Halsbury and Fry Bills (Hampson, 1979). In 1979, the animal welfare movement put its proposals into a document prepared by the Committee for Reform of Animal Experimentation (CRAE), which was submitted to Parliament. Proposals for reform are continuing to be submitted to Parliament; these proposals constantly change the balance between the interests of scientists and animal welfare groups. Two articles offer a detailed discussion of the Cruelty to Animals Act and a summary and discussion of recent British laboratory animal legislation (Heath, 1986; Hollands, 1986).

England's concern for the welfare of animals used in research spread to Europe. Proposals to regulate experimentation have been introduced in many countries, including the countries of Scandinavia, West Germany, the Netherlands, Belgium, France, and Italy (Springier, 1981). Austria and Switzerland have very detailed laws governing animal research. In December of 1987, a Swiss national referendum prohibiting the use of all animals in research was defeated. An article discussing Swiss animal welfare legislation and a proposed ban on experiments using vertebrate as well as invertebrate animals was published in 1985. The article also compares Swiss, French, and West German animal welfare legislation (Freudiger, 1985).

In 1969, a resolution limiting animal research was presented to the Consultative Assembly of the Council of Europe and was adopted in 1971 as Recommendation #621. The previously mentioned CRAE paper contained proposals that were cross-referenced with the Council of Europe Convention (Heath, 1986). Subsequently, a committee of experts was gathered together and called the Ad Hoc Committee of Experts on the

Protection of Animals. This Committee founded the European Convention on the use of live animals for experimental purposes. It is clear that the issues of animal protection and animal research will probably be addressed through international discussions, possibly through the Council of Europe. Guiding principles for biomedical research involving animals have been developed and proposed by the Council for International Organizations of Medical Sciences (CIOMS) (Howard-Jones, 1985).

In the United States, animal welfare and animal rights activists have sought the adoption of Federal laws and regulations to establish standards for the current treatment of animals used in experiments, and they have been largely successful. In general, animal research is regulated by three acts: (1) the Animal Welfare Act, (2) the Public Health Service Act, and (3) the Food and Drug Administration's Good Laboratory Practice Act. In addition, a number of state, county and municipal laws may apply. A brief summary of the three federal laws follow.

1. The Animal Welfare Act was passed on August 24, 1966, was amended on December 24, 1970, on April 22, 1976, and December 23, 1985. These laws require that all institutions doing animal experimentation with warm-blooded animals (except rodents and birds) must be registered and licensed by the U.S. Department of Agriculture (USDA). In addition, these laws establish standards of humane care, housing, handling, transportation, exercise, and veterinary medical care with the appropriate use of anesthetics, analgesics, tranquilizing drugs, or euthanasia. The USDA enforces these laws by unannounced inspections. Violations of the standards are punishable by fine or imprisonment or both.

2. The Public Health Service (PHS) has issued an act on humane care and use of laboratory animals which regulates the use of animals for research in federal grants awarded by the National Institutes of Health (NIH) and National Science Foundation (NSF) (Public Health Service, Department of Health and Human Services, November 20, 1985). The PHS act requires that each awarding institution establish an Institutional Animal Care Committee (IACC) which must review and approve all animal protocols, inspect and report semiannually their findings, and submit an assurance that the requirements of the policy have been met, to be accepted by the NIH. For guidance throughout these compliance requirements, the IACC refers to the *Guide for the Care and Use of Laboratory Animals* (Guide), published by the Department of Health and Human Services of the NIH (1985). The Office for Protection from Research Risks (OPRR) of the NIH enforces the act, with unannounced inspections, if they deem an irregularity has occurred. Violations of any PHS policy are punishable by withdrawal of all federal funds from the investigator, department, and/or institution along with other punitive actions.

3. The Good Laboratory Practice (GLP) regulations prescribe good laboratory practices for conducting nonclinical laboratory studies that support, or are intended to support, applications for research or marketing permits for products regulated by the FDA (Food and drug Adinistration, Department of Health and Human Services, December 22, 1978). The legislation and regulations apply to nonclinical safety studies but not to nonclinical efficacy studies, and cover: (a) food and color additives, (b) animal food additives, (c) human and animal drugs, (d) medical devices for human use, (e) biological products, and (f) electronic products. A nonclinical laboratory study means any in vivo or in vitro experiment in which a test article is studied prospectively, in a test system, under laboratory conditions to determine its safety. The GLP regulations have specific requirements for animal facilities and animal care as well as the collection, storage, and retrieval of the records of the study.

DISCUSSION OF UNITED STATES LAWS AND REGULATIONS

The Animal Welfare Act

President Lyndon B. Johnson signed this act into law on August 24, 1966, authorizing, for the first time, legal requirements for the humane care and treatment of dogs, cats, rabbits, hamsters, guinea pigs, and nonhuman primates used for research, testing, teaching, or experimentation. Responsibility for caring out the legislative intent for this humane care and treatment law was given to the United States Department of Agriculture (USDA).

The authority of this first piece of legislation was very limited, and its main thrust was preventing the illegal transfer of family pets (dogs and cats) to research institutions. The only persons affected by this law were the researchers and the dealers supplying the regulated animals. If a laboratory did not use dogs or cats, that laboratory was not regulated, regardless of what other animals were used. Once a facility was licensed or registered because they used dogs or cats, the other species, i.e., rabbits, hamsters, guinea pigs, and nonhuman primates, were also regulated. In addition, only those dealers supplying dogs or cats to research laboratories were regulated.

The Animal Welfare Act had other limitations. Jurisdiction of the regulating agency was limited to the care and treatment of research animals only while they were in the institution's holding facility. This jurisdiction ceased once an animal was assigned to an investigator. Also, the original legislation provided for the regulation of animals while they were transported by the supplier, but not when moved by common carrier.

The Animal Welfare Act was amended on December 24, 1970, and greatly expanded the responsibility and the influence of the USDA in several ways. The list of animals covered under the act was enlarged from six species to include all warm-blooded animals whether dead or alive. Domestic livestock and poultry used for food or fiber, however, were excluded. Marine mammals, birds, and laboratory rats and mice were also excluded from regulation, at the discretion of the Secretary of Agriculture. Regulated businesses now included exhibitors such as zoos and circuses, operators of auction sales handling domestic dogs and cats, and dealers or brokers selling regulated animals as pets.

The 1970 amendments required every research facility to submit an annual report showing that the facility followed professionally accepted standards governing the care, treatment, and use of animals during actual research or experimentation. Included were the appropriate use of anesthetics, analgesics, and tranquilizing drugs. The act prohibited the Secretary of Agriculture, however, from promulgating rules, regulations, or orders circumscribing the design, outlines, or performance of actual research.

The Animal Welfare Act was again amended on April 22, 1976. The authority of the Act was expanded to cover transportation, including common carriers and intermediate handlers which transported regulated animals. The Act also specifically included any dogs for hunting, security, or breeding, and prohibited animal fighting ventures. In addition, on September 20, 1979, Standards for Marine Mammals were adopted with input from the Marine Mammal Commission, the National Marine Fisheries Service, the U.S. Fish and Wildlife Service, and the marine mammal industry. This 1979 amendment governed the humane handling, care, treatment, and transportation of warm-blooded aquatic animals or marine mammals.

The authority for the development of standards governing the care and use of laboratory animals is contained in Section 13 of the Animal Welfare Act. This section delineates the responsibility of the Secretary of Agriculture to develop standards to govern the humane handling, care, treatment, and transportation of animals by dealers, research facilities, and exhibitors. Such standards include minimum requirements regarding handling, housing, feeding, and watering of animals. Standards for sanitation, ventilation, shelter from extremes of weather and temperatures as well as adequate veterinary care are specified. This section also states that the Secretary shall promulgate standards to govern the commercial transportation of animals and the handling, care, and treatment of animals by intermediate handlers, air carriers, or other carriers consigned by any dealer, research facility, exhibitor, operator of an auction sale, other person, or governmental body.

It should also be noted that this section empowers the Secretary of Agriculture to revise, delete, or add regulations or standards without the consent of Congress as long as the changes are within the confines of Act's wording. These regulations state the requirements by which the Act will be implemented and the standards specify the minimum conditions of care and treatment which are required.

The legal framework through which the Animal Welfare Act is administered consists of three parts: (1) Definitions, (2) Regulations, and (3) Standards, collectively all called regulations. These can be found in Title 9 of the Code of Federal Regulations (CFR). The prescribed rule-making method consists of first publishing any proposal in the *Federal Register* (FR), a daily listing of regulatory actions by the Government. After the public has an opportunity to comment, usually after a period of 60 to 90 days, a revised version of the regulation is published in the FR as well as in the CFR, at which time the publication has the force of law.

Part 1 of 9-CFR, Subchapter A, concerns a definition of terms. In this section, the meanings and definitions of the terms used throughout the Act are specified. Part 2 of 9-CFR, Subchapter A, concerns animal welfare regulations. These regulations address matters such as record keeping, animal identification, holding periods, license fees, confiscation of animals, and other miscellaneous procedures and rules. This section specifies that an institution engaged in research must be registered with the USDA at the lowest level of legal entity. The research institution must permit unannounced inspections of its laboratories by USDA veterinarians to determine if it is complying with requirements of the Animal Welfare Act. Also, the research facility must contract or employ, either full or part time, an attending veterinarian who establishes and maintains programs of disease control and prevention, euthanasia, and veterinary care. The institution must file an annual report with the USDA showing that animals are being treated and cared for in accordance with professionally accepted standards. This report must be signed by a facility official and the attending veterinarian.

Part 3 of 9-CRF, Subchapter A, sets forth animal welfare standards. As written, these standards represent the legal minimum specification for the humane care, handling, treatment, and transportation of animals. The standards are divided into three general categories: Facilities and Operating Standards, Animal, Health and Husbandry Standards, and Transportation Requirements.

Facilities and Operating Standards consists of requirements for facilities in general, indoor facilities, outdoor facilities and primary enclosures. Primary enclosures generally refer to a room, pen, run or cage. Minimum space requirements for the different species have been specified (Table 1). The general facility requirements describe structural strength, availability of water and electric power, storage facilities for food and bedding, disposal of waste, and provisions for washrooms and sinks to maintain cleanliness. Standards for an indoor facility require sufficient heating, adequate ventilation, ample lighting, interior surfaces which are impervious to moisture, and suitable drainage.

Table 1 Minimum Space Recommendations for Laboratory Animals

Animals	Weight	Housing	Floor area/animal		Heights[a]	
Mice	<10 g	Cage	6.0 in^2	38.71 cm^2	5 in	12.70 cm
	10–15 g	Cage	8.0 in^2	51.62 cm^2	5 in	12.70 cm
	15–25 g	Cage	12.0 in^2	77.42 cm^2	5 in	12.70 cm
	>25 g	Cage	15.0 in^2	96.78 cm^2	5 in	12.70 cm
Rats	<100 g	Cage	17.0 in^2	109.68 cm^2	7 in	17.78 cm
	100–200 g	Cage	23.0 in^2	148.40 cm^2	7 in	17.78 cm
	200–300 g	Cage	29.0 in^2	187.11 cm^2	7 in	17.78 cm
	300–400 g	Cage	40.0 in^2	258.08 cm^2	7 in	17.78 cm
	400–500 g	Cage	60.0 in^2	387.12 cm^2	7 in	17.78 cm
	>500 g	Cage	70.0 in^2	451.64 cm^2	7 in	17.78 cm
Hamsters	>60 g	Cage	10.0 in^2	64.52 cm^2	6 in	15.24 cm
	60–80 g	Cage	13.0 in^2	83.88 cm^2	6 in	15.24 cm
	80–100 g	Cage	16.0 in^2	103.23 cm^2	6 in	15.24 cm
	>100 g	Cage	19.0 in^2	122.59 cm^2	6 in	15.24 cm
Guinea pigs	≤350 g	Cage	60.0 in^2	387.12 cm^2	7 in	17.78 cm
	>350 g	Cage	101.0 in^2	651.65 cm^2	7 in	17.78 cm
Rabbits	<2 kg	Cage	1.5 ft^2	0.14 m^2	14 in	35.56 cm
	2–4 kg	Cage	3.0 ft^2	0.28 m^2	14 in	35.56 cm
	4–5.4 kg	Cage	4.0 ft^2	0.37 m^2	14 in	35.56 cm
	>5.4 kg	Cage	5.0 ft^2	0.46 m^2	14 in	35.56 cm
Dogs[b]	<15 kg	Pen/run	8.0 ft^2	0.74 m^2	—	—
	15–30 kg	Pen/run	12.1 ft^2	1.12 m^2	—	—
	>30 kg	Pen/run	24.0 ft^2	2.23 m^2	—	—
	<15 kg	Cage	8.0 ft^2	0.74 m^2	32 in	81.28 cm
	15–30 kg	Cage	12.1 ft^2	1.12 m^2	36 in	91.44 cm
	>30 kg	Cage	b	b	—	—
Nonhuman primates[c]						
group 1	<1 kg	Cage	1.6 ft^2	0.15 m^2	20 in	50.80 cm
group 2	1–3 kg	Cage	3.0 ft^2	0.28 m^2	30 in	76.20 cm
group 3	3–10 kg	Cage	4.3 ft^2	0.40 m^2	30 in	76.20 cm
group 4	10–15 kg	Cage	6.0 ft^2	0.56 m^2	32 in	81.28 cm
group 5	15–25 kg	Cage	8.0 ft^2	0.74 m^2	36 in	91.44 cm
group 6	>25–40 kg	Cage	25.1 ft^2	2.33 m^2	84 in	213.36 cm
group 7	>40	Cage	50.0 ft^2	4.65 m^2	84 in	213.36 cm

[a]Height measured from the floor to top of cage.
[b]These recommendations may vary according to breed and conformation of dogs.
[c]Primates vary in size and are divided into groups as follows:

1. Prosimian primates
2. Marmosets and tamarins
3. Other New World monkeys
4. Langurs and colobines
5. Other Old World monkeys
6. Lesser apes
7. Great apes

Likewise, standards for an outdoor facility require shelter from sunlight, shelter from rain or snow, shelter from cold weather, and drainage. Under primary enclosures, general requirements and space requirements for laboratory animals are specified.

Animal Health and Husbandry Standards covers such topics as feeding, watering, sanitation, number of employees, classification and separation of animals, and veterinary care. Food is of particular importance as food contaminants can have substantial effects of biochemical and physiological processes. Assay of food for contaminants is desirable and maximum concentrations of food contaminants have been set for toxicological studies (Table 2).

Transportation Requirements cover assignments to carriers and intermediate handlers, the time of delivery to carriers, temperature limits for transportation, crate construction, size of primary enclosures used to transport animals, primary conveyances (motor vehicle, rail, air, and boat), food and water, care in transit, terminal facilities, identification and records, health certificates, and handling of animals so that they are not subjected to unsafe or uncomfortable conditions. This section also regulates the number of animals per container.

The Animal and Plant Health Inspection Service (APHIS) is the agency within the USDA that has the responsibility for enforcing the Animal Welfare Act. Inspections are unannounced, and every site must be inspected. Federal facilities are not inspected by APHIS, but they are required to obey the law in the same manner as nonfederal facilities.

Deficiencies in meeting standards are cited as either "major" or "minor" during the inspection. A deadline is set by which time the deficiencies must be corrected. If they have not been corrected, and if there is not justifiable reason, the inspector prepares an "alleged violation" against the facility. This report is submitted to the Interstate Inspection Compliance Staff for review; if the complaint is justified, the case is submitted to the Office of the General Council with a recommendation for prosecution.

Table 2 Maximum Concentrations of Feed Contaminants Considered Acceptable for Natural-Ingredient Rations

Agents	Maximum concentration ($\mu g/g$)
Cadmium	0.05
Selenium	0.50
Polychlorinated biphenyls	0.50
Total DDT (DDE, DDT, TDE)	0.05
Mercury	0.05
Arsenic	0.25
Lead	1.00
Dieldrin	0.01
Lindane	0.01
Heplachlor	0.01
Malathion	0.50
Estrogenic activity	2.00
Total aflatoxins (B_1, B_2, G_1, G_2)	1.00

The Animal Welfare Act was again amended on December 23, 1985, and was now known as Public Law 99-198. On March 31, 1987, the United States Department of Agriculture published Parts 1 and 2, but not 3, of the proposed regulations, allowing 60 days for the Public to comment. Approximately 8000 comments were received by the United States Department of Agriculture on Parts 1 and 2.

On March 15, 1989, the USDA republished Parts 1 and 2 of the proposed rules and added Part 3. The agency allowed 60 days for comment on Parts 1 and 2, only as they relate to Part 3, and 120 days on Part 3.

According to the USDA, over 7500 comments on Parts 1 and 2 of the proposed regulations were submitted to the Department for consideration. Over 8000 on Part 3 were submitted. Most of the comments were received from the research community, which had numerous concerns about the proposed regulations. Chief among there were:

1. The animal welfare standards were being changed arbitrarily; i.e., there was no scientific data provided in support of enclosure size, exercise, lighting, etc.
2. The total economic impact of all three parts of the proposal was prohibitive. The APHIS estimated the cost to be just over $1 billion. The National Association for Biomedical Research estimated the cost to exceed $2 billion. The Pharmaceutical Manufacturers Association estimated that the cost for Part 3 to be at least $630 million for capital expenditures and $105 million in recurring annual expenses.
3. The proposed standards were inconsistent with U.S. Public Health Service requirements. The PHS guidelines were written as performance specifications, not like the strict, inflexible regulations proposed by the USDA.
4. The standards exceeded the statutory authority and intent of Congress. The department intended to impose new standards which lacked scientific validity and will, of necessity, require numerous exceptions or variances.

The USDA, to address these concerns and others, consulted with the U.S. Department of Health and Human Services and with members of the Interagency Research Animal Committee, and republished the regulations as a final rule on August 31, 1989, effective as of October 30, 1989. (Animal and Plant Health Inspection Service, United States Department of Agriculture (8/31/89), FR, Vol. 54, No. 168, 36112.) Parts 1 and 2 of these Animal Welfare regulations have been significantly rewritten and reorganized, but major provisions are really unchanged. The publication also indicates that Part 3, the standards by animal species, is also final, but this refers to the existing Part 3 standards only. Part 3 will be published as a final rule at a later date.

Part 1 contains several new or expanded definitions. Part 2, the regulations, has undergone extensive revisions, such that all the requirements pertaining to research facilities have been placed in one subpart. The text that follows is a brief summary of important points.

I will first address the new or extended definitions in Part 1 and then briefly summarize the important issues in Part 2.

Part 1

The first definition indicates an organizatonal change within the United States Department of Agriculture, Animal and Plant Health Inspection Service (APHIS). This reorganization creates a Regulatory Enforcement Animal Care (REAC) organization unit charged with responsibility for administering the Animal Welfare Act and Regulations for APHIS. This reorganization means that there will be one APHIS veterinarian inspecting only animal facilities within each area or district.

There has been a great deal of controversy over the fact that the USDA as the authority to regulate rats and mice, though they have never included laboratory rats and mice in the regulations. Therefore, in the final rule, the definition of animal excludes rats of the genus *Rattus* and mice of the genus *Mus* that have been bred for use in research. Rodents of other genera, such as kangaroo rats, are included within the definition. The agency has also clarified when farm animals are covered by the regulations. They indicate that the agency has the authority to regulate farm animals when used for biomedical research or testing purposes. Those farm animals used or intended for use as food or fiber, or used in agricultural research to improve the quality of food and fiber, are not covered. It is interesting to note that research involving animals that are studied in their natural habitat without any invasive procedure and without harming or materially altering their behavior are exempt.

In the definitions published on March 15, 1989, the USDA added the term *animal care and use procedure* in lieu of "protocol," to avoid any misunderstanding or implication that the USDA intended to become involved in the evaluation of the design, outlines, guidelines, and scientific merit of proposed research. In this final rule they have replaced the term *animal care and use procedure* with the Public Health Service Policy term *activity*. The term *activity* is defined to mean those elements of research, testing, or teaching procedures that involve the care and use of animals. Since this term is used throughout the regulations, it is important to understand this change.

The definition of euthanasia has been revised. Previously the definition included the term *immediate death* without evidence of pain or distress. The new definition states euthanasia to mean the humane destruction of an animal accomplished by a method that produces rapid unconsciousness and subsequent death without evidence of pain or distress. The numerous methods of euthanasia, listed by the AVMA Panel on Euthanasia, are consistent with this definition.

To make the distinction between research that is conducted under captive conditions vs that which is conducted in the wild, a new definition of the term *study area* has been added. This term is defined as any building, room, area, enclosure, or other containment outside of a core facility or centrally designated or managed area in which animals are housed for more than 12 hr.

In the previously published regulations, the USDA refers to the Chief Executive Officer of a research facility as a responsible institutional official with authority to bind that facility. This phrase is being replaced with the single term *institutional official*, which means the individual at a research facility who is authorized to legally commit on behalf of the research facility.

Since there was such confusion about the definition of a major operative experiment, that definition has been revised. It means any surgical intervention that penetrates and exposes a body cavity, or any procedure which produces permanent impairment of physical or physiological functions. Thus, the USDA is leaving it up to the principal investigator and the Institutional Animal Care Committee to determine whether a major operative procedure has produced a permanent impairment of the animal's physical or physiological function. If it has, the animal cannot be used again for survival surgical procedures.

The definition of a principal investigator has been revised. It now includes any person associated with the research facility who uses or intends to use live animals in research, testing, or experiments. This includes individuals who are not necessarily an employee of that facility.

There has been considerable controversy about when a procedure is painful. Although the definition has not been changed, the new regulations do note that a procedure in which pain is relieved is still considered to be a painful procedure, and the provisions of the Act which address the conduct of a painful procedure apply. This fact is good to know when assigning pain categories for a particular procedure in the USDA annual report.

Part 2

As previously stated, Part 2, the regulations, has been expensively rewritten. A new Subpart, Subpart C, has been added that consolidates all of the regulations in Part 2 applicable to research facilities.

In the regulations published on March 15, 1989, there was a great deal of concern that the Institutional Animal Care Committee and attending veterinarian were allocated too much responsibility and authority such that they functioned, in effect, as enforcement agents for the APHIS. The language of the regulations has been changed to make it clear that the committee and the veterinarian shall perform as agents of the research facility and that compliance with regulations are ultimately the responsibility of the research facility. Further, the language of the Act has been changed to conform more closely with that of the Public Health Service Act. Accordingly, the following requirements have been removed:

1. The final rule does not contain a requirement that the research facility maintain an up-to-date list of Committee Members indicating their degrees, position, and qualifications.
2. The requirement that the committee must file an inspection report within 10 business days after completing its inspection of all animal areas.
3. The proposed requirement for deficient notification reports and the 30-day correction period have been removed from the final rule.
4. The requirement that each research facility establish a written policy which assures that no animal is used in more than one major operative experiment from which it is allowed to recover is removed.
5. The requirement for documentation of personnel training has been removed.
6. The requirement that a copy of all written reports, detailing and explaining exceptions to the regulations, be attached to the research facility annual report has been removed.
7. No written program of adequate veterinarian care is required if a full-time veterinarian is on the staff at a facility.
8. There is no reference to an established reporting procedure whereby laboratory or research facility employees can report suspected violations of the Act.

Several new requirements pertaining to the role of the Institutional Animal Care Committee have been added.

The first is that the committee review and evaluate, at least once every 6 months, all activities involving animals to include a review of the programs for humane care and use of animals.

Second, the revised proposal would allow subcommittees to perform these inspections, and would also permit ad hoc consultants to assist in conducting evaluations.

The inspection report must be reviewed and signed by a majority of committee members, and must include any minority views. In its report, the committee shall set forth a specific plan and schedule, with dates, for correcting deficiencies. Deficiencies must be identified as minor or significant and uncorrected significant deficiencies must be reported, in writing, to the APHIS within 15 days.

As in the previously published rule, the committee is authorized to review and approve, require modifications in, or withhold approval of those components of proposed activities involving animals used in research. This review includes justification for a departure from acceptable procedures, in writing, presented by the principal investigator.

There are two major requirements involved in the presentation of a proposed activity. First, the principal investigator must supply a narrative description, in writing, of the methods and the *sources* that were used to determined that alternatives were not available. The sources consulted could be *Biological Abstracts*, *Index Medicus*, *Current Research Information Service*, and the Animal Welfare Information Center, operated by the National Agricultural Library. Second, the principal investigator must provide written assurance that the proposed activities do not *unnecessarily* duplicate previous experiments. It should be noted that Committee meeting minutes must be made available to the APHIS to determine whether alternatives were in fact discussed, and the written narrative of information and sources consulted made part of the Committee record. Research facilities will be held responsible if it is subsequently determined that an alternative procedure was available to accomplish the objectives of the proposed experiment, or that an experiment is unnecessarily duplicative.

Previously, a copy of all written reports detailing and explaining exceptions to the regulations had to be attached to the research facility annual report. The law now prescribes that only a summary of all departures from the regulations, including a brief explanation of the departure and identification of the species and the number of animals affected by the exception, must be attached to the annual report. This requirement could amount to a considerable amount of work for the principal investigator, but does not completely reveal departures from the regulations as previously required.

The final rule also requires written notification of the Committees disposition of each proposed activity involving the care and use of animals. If the Committee decides to withhold approval or suspend the activity, it must provide the principal investigator and the research facility with a written statement explaining its decision. The principal investigator can then respond appropriately. If the activity is suspended, the law also requires that the institutional official be appraised that the facility had not been operating in compliance with the regulations, by virtue of the suspended disapproved activity. The institutional official must then review the reasons for the suspension with the committee and take appropriate corrective action in order to bring the facility back into compliance. The institutional official must report the corrective actions to the APHIS

As previously stated, there is no requirement that training be documented. The final rule only requires that training and instruction be made available and that the qualifications of personnel be reviewed with sufficient frequency to fulfill the facilities responsibilities to insure its personnel are qualified, and that it is in compliance with the regulations. The law does list, however, those areas in which training must be make available.

Last, the law allows the APHIS representatives to enter facilities during business hours for inspection purposes, and to take photographs to document their findings. It is interesting to note that these findings must be in noncompliance with the law, although the APHIS does not define noncompliance.

In conclusion, Parts 1 and 2 of the new regulations have been written as performance specifications rather than engineering specifications. Thus, they are in close agreement with the Public Health Service *Guide for the Care and Use of Laboratory Animals*. The regulations clearly place the burden of compliance on the facility, but at the same time allow that facility a good deal more flexibility for compliance. The anticipated date for republication of the Part 3 proposals to implement the exercise for dogs and psychological well-being of primate requirements is not known at this time.

Health Research Extension Act

The Public Health Service (PHS) has had a long-standing policy requiring institutions to establish and maintain proper measures to ensure the appropriate care and use of all animals involved in research, research training, and biological testing activities conducted or supported the PHS. This policy was originally entitled Public Health Service Policy on Humane Care and Use of Laboratory Animals by Awarding Institutions. Under this policy, no activity involving animals could be conducted or supported by the PHS until the institution conducting the activity provided a written assurance acceptable to the PHS, setting forth compliance with this policy. The *Guide for the Care and Use of Laboratory Animals*, published by the Institute of Laboratory Animal Resources (ILAR), was used to assist scientific institutions in using and caring for laboratory animals in a way judged to be professionally appropriate, and was used as the working document to implement the policy.

The Health Research Extension Act of 1985, P.L. 99-158, gave a statutory foundation to the long-standing Public Health Service Policy on Humane Care and Use of Laboratory Animals. The PHS Policy is now entitled Public Health Service Policy on Humane Care and Use of Laboratory Animals and incorporates several new changes into the old policy.

The first major change is that the Chief Executive Officer shall appoint an Institutional Animal Care Committee, qualified through the experience and expertise of its members to oversee the institution's animal program, facilities, and procedures. This Committee shall consist of not less than five members, and shall include at least: (1) a Doctor of Veterinary Medicine, with training or experience in laboratory animal science or medicine, who has direct or delegated program responsibility for activities involving animals at the institution, (2) one practicing scientist experienced in research involving animals, (3) one member whose primary concerns are in a nonscientific area, and (4) one individual who is not affiliated with the institution in any way other than as a member of the IACC and is not a member of the immediate family or a person who is affiliated with the institution.

The new policy enumerates the responsibilities of the Institutional Animal Care Committee. These responsibilities include: (1) the inspection of the institutional animal facilities at least once every 6 months and a review of the institution's program for humane care of animals at least once every 6 months, using the *Guide for the Care and Use of Laboratory Animals* as a basis for evaluation. (2) Review concerns involving the care and use of animals at the institution, and make recommendations to the institutional official regarding any aspects of the institution's program, facilities, or personnel training. (3) Review and approve, require modifications to secure approval, or withhold approval of those sections of grant applications pertaining to animals, and will have the authority to suspend an activity not conducted in accordance with Animal Welfare Act, the *Guide for the Care and Use of Laboratory Animals*, the institution's assurance, or the PHS Policy.

The reporting requirements of the Institutional Animal Care Committee are also spelled out. At least once every 12 months, the IACC, through the institutional official, shall report in writing any change in the institutions programs or facilities, any change in the description of the institution's program for animal care and use, any changes in the IACC membership, and notice of the dates the IACC conducted its semiannual evaluations of the institutions programs and facilities. Alternatively, when there are no changes to report, the IACC shall submit a letter to the Office of Protection and Research Risks (OPRR) stating that there are no changes. Also, the IACC through the institutional official, shall promptly provide the OPRR with a full explanation of the circumstances and action taken with the respect to any serious or continuing noncompliance with the policy, any serious deviation from the provisions of the NIH Guide, or any suspension of an activity by the IACC. It is also stipulated that reports filed under this policy shall include any minority views filed by members of the IACC.

Per the amended PHS Policy, institutions must maintain on file, for at least 3 years, its approved PHS assurance, minutes, attendance and activities of the IACC, records of applications and proposed significant changes in animal care and use, records of IACC semiannual reports and recommendations, and records of accrediting body determinations. All records must be accessible for inspection and copying by authorized personnel.

Each awarding institution is subject to review at any time by PHS staff and advisors, which may include a site visit, in order to review compliance with PHS policy and the NIH Guide. The Director of the NIH can suspend or revoke a grant or contract if (1) the conditions of animal care, treatment, or use in an entity which is receiving a grant, a contract, or cooperative agreement involving research on animals do not meet established applicable guidelines, (2) the entity has been notified by the Director of NIH of such determination and has been given a reasonable opportunity to take corrective action, and/or, (3) no action has been taken by the entity to correct such conditions.

The second major change in the new PHS policy is that the policy now requires that applicants now assure the NIH of the availability of instruction at their institution in humane practices of animal care and in research methods that minimize the use of animals and limit animal distress. The Guide encourages special training programs to ensure research is conducted in a humane and scientifically accepted manner. The Act also requires that the NIH Director take appropriate action to convey to scientists and others, involved with research or experimentation involving animals, information respecting the methods found to be valid and reliable.

Many laboratories using animals in research, such as pharmaceutical laboratories, do not receive grants from the federal government. As such, they are not subject to the rules and regulations of the Health Research Extension Act. These laboratories do, however, have a high regard for animal welfare and the quality of scientific research that uses experimental animals. Accordingly, they have chosen to be accredited by the American Association for Accreditation of Laboratory Animal Care (AAALAC). The AAALAC is a nonprofit corporation directed by representatives of 31 scientific and professional organizations that are members of the corporation. It was organized in 1965 to conduct a voluntary program for the accreditation of laboratory animal care facilities and programs. The accreditation program is concerned with encouraging high standards for the care and use of laboratory animals, including appropriate veterinary care, controlling variables that might adversely affect animal research, and protecting the health of animal research workers. For those facilities not receiving federal grants, accreditation is extremely important. Accreditation tends to improve morale in the facility and to continue the emphasis on quality. In addition to providing the accredited institution and animal care staff with internal pride, AAALAC accreditation assures prospective investigators and clients that high-quality animal care is being provided. The Institute of Laboratory Animal

Resources, National Research Council's *Guide for the Care and Use of Laboratory Animals* is used as a basis for evaluation of these institutions. Currently there are 521 accredited institutions in the United States and throughout the world.

The Good Laboratory Practices Act

Many researchers outside of the pharmaceutical industry are not aware that portions of their work may place their institutions under the Food & Drug Administration's (FDA) Good Laboratory Practice (GLP) regulations. The GLP regulations (43FR, p. 60013, December 22, 1978) prescribed Good Laboratory Practices for conducting nonclinical laboratory studies that support, or are intended to support, applications for research or marketing permits for products regulated by the FDA. The legislation and regulations apply to nonclinical safety studies, but not to nonclinical efficacy studies, and cover: (1) food and color additives, (2) animal food additives, (3) human and animal drugs, (4) medical devices for human use, (5) biological products, and (6) electronic products. A nonclinical laboratory study means any in vivo or in vitro experiment in which a test article is studied prospectively in a test system, under laboratory conditions, to determine its safety. In the opinion of the legal staff of the FDA, any laboratory work that supports the safety of a product placed before the FDA or an investigational permit for licensing must be conducted in accordance with the GLPs.

For all facilities that are subject to FDA inspection, Section 58.15 of the GLP regulations state:

> a testing facility shall permit and authorize employees of the Food & Drug Administration, at reasonable time, and in a reasonable manner, to inspect the facility and to inspect all records (and copy them) and specimens required to be maintained regarding studies within the scope of this part.

The organization and personnel of testing facilities are also examined under the GLP regulations and must meet the following requirements:

1. Personnel shall have the education, training, and experience necessary to perform their assigned duties.
2. Each testing facility shall maintain current summaries of the training, experience, and job descriptions of each individual engaged in or supervising the study.
3. A sufficient number of personnel for proper conduct of the study, according to the protocol, shall be employed.
4. Standard Operating Procedures (SOPs) shall be in writing and available to FDA personnel. These shall cover all phases of the study.
5. Personnel shall take the personal sanitary and health precautions necessary to avoid contamination of the test and control articles as well as the test systems.
6. Personnel shall wear clothing appropriate for the duties they perform.
7. An individual with an illness that may affect the results of the study shall be excluded from contact with the test system (and test and/or control articles).

Physical facilities, including those for animals, are covered in several paragraphs of the Regulations. The Regulations state that each testing facility shall be of a suitable size and construction and in a location to facilitate the proper conduct of nonclinical laboratory studies. In addition, the facility shall be designed to allow a degree of separation sufficient to prevent any other function or activity from having an adverse effect on the study.

The Regulations also state that the animal care facility shall have a sufficient number of rooms to ensure: (1) separation of species or test systems; (2) isolation of individual projects; (3) quarantine of animals, and (4) routine and specialized housing of animals. Rooms or areas separate from those just mentioned shall provide: (1) isolation of studies being conducted with hazardous materials; (2) separate areas for the diagnosis, treatment, and control of laboratory animal diseases, (3) facilities for the collection and disposable of all animal waste and refuse or for its safe and sanitary storage. Disposal facilities shall minimize vermin infestation, odors, disease hazards and environmental contamination; and (4) animal facilities shall be designed, constructed and located in such a way as to minimize disturbances that interfere with the study.

The Regulations require that documentation of care and maintenance of the facility will be available. This documentation must be initialed by the Study Director and may not have any erasures. Only those facilities or rooms used by the investigator in performing the reportable study are subject to FDA review, or compliance with the GLPs, not the entire institution and all of its animal facilities.

Animal care is specifically covered by the GLPs, and includes written SOPs, quarantine of animals, diagnosis of disease and authorization for treatment, proper identification of animals, animal housing (see Table 1), feed (see Table 2), water and bedding as well as documentation of the use of pest control materials.

The collection, storage, and retrievable of data and records is essential for the support and documentation of information submitted to the FDA for the testing and licensing of products. All raw data, experiment documentation, SOPs, protocols, and special and final reports shall be retained and are subject to FDA review. Records must be retained for at least 2 years following the date on which an application for a research or marketing permit is approved by the FDA. Records must be retained for 5 years following the date on which the results of nonclinical laboratory studies are submitted to the FDA in support of an application for a research or marketing permit. Summaries of training, experience, and job descriptions in each of these situations should be retained, along with other testing facility employee records, for the same lengths of time.

In 1987, the FDA issued a final rule that amends the regulations specifying Good Laboratory Practice procedures for nonclinical laboratory studies (Food and Drug Administration, Department of Health and Human Services, September 4, 1987). The amendments clarify, delete, or amend several provisions of the GLP regulations to reduce the regulatory burden on testing facilities. Significant changes were made in the provisions respecting quality assurance, protocol preparation, test and control article characterization, and retention of specimens and samples. These changes will not compromise the objective of the GLP regulations, which is to assure that the quality and integrity of the safety data submitted in support of approval of regulated products. Also, in 1988, FDA issued an LD_{50} Test Policy (Food and Drug Administration, Department of Health and Human Services, October 11, 1988).

Other Federal Regulatory Acts

In addition to the Good Laboratory Practice standards for conducting nonclinical research studies, as published by the Federal Food and Drug Administration, other federal statutes also contain standards for animal care and use. These are the Toxic Substances Control Act (TSCA) (U.S. Environmental Protection Agency, 1976) and the Federal Insecticide, Fungicide, and Rodenticide Act (FIFRA) (U.S. Environmental Protection Agency, 1970), both promulgated by the Environmental Protection Agency (EPA). Test guidelines for hazard evaluation of pesticides and for health effects have also been published by the EPA (U.S. Environmental Protection Agency, 1976, 1978, 1985).

There is little difference in the requirements for animal care and use between the FDA and the TSCA and FIFRA Acts. In fact, the wording of these acts is, in most instances, the same. There is considerable difference, however, between the requirements of these Acts and those of the Animal Welfare Act and the Health Research Extension Act. Most notable is that the FDA, FIFRA, and TSCA Acts do not require an Animal Care Committee, nor specific training requirements for personnel conducting the studies. The EPA does require, however, the submission of a statement of compliance with good laboratory practice standards when a test is submitted to the agency. In this respect, it is similar to the Health Research Extension Act. Further, if there is noncompliance with Good Laboratory Practice standards, the EPA will not consider any data toward demonstrating that the substance is safe for the purposes of TSCA or for applications for research or marketing permits under FIFRA. Persons violating these provisions are subject to civil and criminal penalties. Last, the TSCA and RIFRA Acts do not have words preventing the rules, regulations, or standards from being construed as dictating research methodology, such as found in the Animal Welfare Act or the Health Research Extension Act.

STATE AND MUNICIPAL LAWS AND ORDINANCES

Following through on the ultimate objective of prohibiting all animal research, animal rights activists have introduced bills or ordinances into state legislatures and municipalities restricting or prohibiting the use of animals. Most notable are the pound laws. All 50 states and many municipalities had laws or regulations releasing pound animal to research laboratories. Many, however, were repealed and currently there are 12 states that prohibit the use of pound animals for research (National Association for Biomedical Research, 1988). Similarly, some municipal ordinances ban the release of pound animals, most notable among them being the Los Angeles, California, and Cambridge, Massachusetts, ordinances.

In addition, bills prohibiting eye irritancy tests, including the Draize test, have been introduced into state legislatures. Some are limited only to acute toxicity tests for the purpose of testing cosmetics and household products. Others, in addition, prohibit the LD_{50} acute toxicity test. Some of these bills have passed; others have been defeated.

It is clear that animal welfare proponents have directed, and will continue to direct, their efforts toward the passage of state laws and municipal ordinances. In 1985, legislation affecting the availability or use of animals in research was introduced in 21 state legislatures (O'Connor, 1986).

NOTE ADDED IN PROOF

After the chapter on laws and regulations governing animal research was completed, the last subparts (9 CFR, Part 3, Subparts A and D) of the amendments to the Animal Welfare Act were published in the February 15, 1991 *Federal Register,* effective on March 18, 1991. These subparts require research facilities to develop plans for the exercise of dogs and the care of nonhuman primates to assure their psychological well-being. Written documents describing the plans must be developed, made available to APHIS for inspection, and implemented by August 14, 1991. To minimize the amendment's economic impact, major capital improvements may be phased in over 3 years, with complete compliance delayed until February 15, 1994.

REFERENCES

Animal and Plant Health Inspection Service, United States Department of Agriculture. (August 31, 1989) *Fed. Reg.* 54, (168), 36112–36163.

Department of Health and Human Services, Public Health Service, National Institutes of Health. (1985) *Guide for the Care and Use of Laboratory Animals.* NIH Publication no. 85-23.

Food and Drug Administration, Department of Health and Human Services. (December 22, 1978) 43FR, p. 60013.

Food and Drug Administration, Department of Health and Human Service. (September 4, 1987) 21 FR, Vol. 2, No. 172, p. 33768.

Food and Drug Administration, Department of Health and Human Services. (October 11, 1988) 53FR, p. 39650.

French, R. D. (1975) *Antivivisection and Medical Science in Victorian Society.* (Princeton University Press, Princeton, NJ).

Freudiger, U. (1985) Public initiative for the abolition of vivisection, called the "Weber Initiative." (English translation). *Schweiz Arch. Tierheilkd.,* 127, 635–649. (In German with English summary.)

Hampson, J. (1979) Animal welfare—A century of conflict. *New Scientist,* 84, 280–282.

Heath, M. (1986) British law relating to experimental animals—Its provisions and restriction. *Anim. Technol.* 37, 131–136.

Hollands, C. (1986) The animals (Scientific Procedures Act, 1986). *Lancet* 2, 32–33.

Howard-Jones, N. (1985) A CIOMS ethical code for animal experimentation. *WHO Chron.* 39, 51–56.

National Association for Biomedical Research (personal communication). (1988).

O'Connor, K. (1986) Laws, regulation, and legislation affecting the use of animals in research. *Public Affairs: Fed. Am. Soc. Exp. Biol. Proc.* 45, 9a.

Public Health Service, Department of Health and Human Services. (November 20, 1985) Health Research Extension Act. *Public Law* 99-158.

Springier, D. (1981) *Animals in Research. New Perspectives in Animal Experimentation.* (Wiley, Chichester, England), p. 865.

U.S. Environmental Protection Agency. (1970) Federal Insecticide, Fungicide, and Rodenticide Act. (FIFRA). 7 U.S.C., 136 et. seq.

U.S. Environmental Protection Agency. (1976a) Toxic Substances Control Act (TSCA) 15. U.S.C., 160.1 et. seq.

U.S. Environmental Protection Agency. (1976b) Proposed health effects test standards for Toxic Substances Control Act: Test rules and proposed good laboratory practice standards for health effects. *Fed. Reg.* 44, 44054–44059, 44066–44067.

U.S. Environmental Protection Agency. (1978) Proposed guidelines for registering pesticides in the U.S. Hazard evaluation: Humans and domestic animals. *Fed. Reg.,* 43, 37336–37345, 37351–37356.

U.S. Environmental Protection Agency. (1985) Health effects testing guidelines. *Fed. Reg.* 50, 39397–39398.

APPENDIX

Commercial Sources of Laboratory Animals

Shayne Cox Gad
Becton Dickinson and Company
Research Triangle Park, North Carolina

Source	Rat	Mouse	Hamster	Ferret	Beagle Dog	Rabbit	Guinea Pig	Primate
Camm	X					X	X	
Charles River	X	X	X			X	X	X
Davidson Mill							X	
Elm Hill							X	
Hare						X		
Hazleton					X	X		X
Hilltop	X	X					X	
Holtzman	X							
Marshall Farms				X	X			
Millbrook Farm						X		
Sasco	X	X	X				X	
Taconic	X	X						
White Eagle					X			

[a]This list is representative, and not meant to be exhaustive. The reader is referred to *Lab Animal* Vol. 16, No. 7 (Oct. 1987) for a more complete listing.

ADDRESSES AND PHONE NUMBERS

CAMM RESEARCH LAB ANIMALS
414 Black Oak Ridge Road
Wayne, N.J. 07470
201/694-0703

CHARLES RIVER LABORATORIES,
    INC.
251 Ballardvale Street
Wilmington, MA 01887-0630
800-522-7287

DAVIDSON MILL BREEDING LABS
231 Fresh Pond Road
Jamesburg, N.J. 08831
201/821-9094

ELM HILL BREEDING LABS
71 Elm Street
Chelmsford, MA 01824
508/256-2322

HARE MARLAND
P.O. Box X
Hewitt, N.J. 07421
201/728-3745

HAZLETON RESEARCH PRODUCTS,
    INC.
P.O. Box 7200
Denver, PA 17517
800/345-4114

HILLTOP LAB ANIMALS, INC.
P.O. Box 183
Scottdale, PA 15683
800-245-6921 or 412/887-8480

HOLTZMAN LABORATORY
ANIMALS
P.O. Box 4220
Madison, WI 53711
608/271-6441

MARSHALL FARMS
R.D. 1, Box 91
North Rose, N.Y. 14516
315/587-2295

MILLBROOK FARM RABBITS
Box 513
Amherst, MA 01004
413/253-5083

SASCO, INC.
319 S. 17th St., Suite 340
P.O. Box 66 DTS
Omaha, NE 68101
402/346-3300

SIMONSEN LABORATORIES, INC.
1180C Day Road
Gilroy, CA 95020
408/847-2002

TACONIC
33 Hover Ave.
Germantown, N.Y. 12526
518/537-6208

WHITE EAGLE LABORATORIES, INC.
2003 Lower State Road
Doylestown, PA 18901
215/398-3868

REFERENCES

Animal and Plant Health Inspection Service, USDA, (11/2/79) 44FR, No. 214, 63488.
Animal and Plant Health Inspection Service, USDA, (3/31/87) 9CFR, no. 61, 10292.
Animal and Plant Health Inspection Service, USDA, (3/15/89) *Fed. Reg.* Vol. 54, No. 49.
Animal and Plant Health Inspection Service, USDA, (8/31/89) 9CFR, Vol. 54, No. 168, 36112.
Department of Health and Human Services, Public Health Service, National Institutes of Health
    (1985) *Guide for the Care and Use of Laboratory Animals.* National Institutes of Health
    Publication No. 85–23.

Food and Drug Administration, Department of Health and Human Services (December 22, 1978) 43FR 60013.

Food and Drug Administration, Department of Health and Human Services (September/4/1987) 21 CFR, Vol. 2, No. 172, 33768.

Food and Drug Administration, Department of Health and Human Services (October 11, 1988) 53FR, 39650.

French, R. D. (1975). *Antivivisection and Medical Science in Victorian Society*. Princeton University Press, Princeton, New Jersey.

Freudiger, U. (1985). Public initiative for the abolition of vivisection, called the "Weber Initiative." (English Translation). *Schweiz Arch. Tierheilkd.* 127, 635–49. (In German with English summary).

Hampson, J. (1979) Animal welfare—A century of conflict. *New Scientist* 84, 280–282.

Heath, M. (1986) British law relating to experimental animals—its provisions and restrictions. *Anim. Technol.* 37, 131–6.

Hollands, C. (1986). The animals (Scientific Procedures Act, 1986). *Lancet* 2, 32–3.

Howard-Jones, N. (1985). A CIOMS ethical code for animal experimentation. *W.H.O. Chron.* 39, 51–6.

National Association for Biomedical Research (personal communication) (1988).

O'Connor, K. (1986) Laws, regulation, and legislation affecting the use of animals in research. *Public Affairs: Federation of American Societies for Experimental Biology Proceedings*, 45:9a.

Public Health Service, Department of Health and Human Services (1985) Health Research Extension Act, *Public Law*, pp. 99–158.

Sperlinger, D. (1981) *Animals in Research. New Perspectives in Animal Experimentation*. Wiley, Chichester, England.

U.S. Environmental Protection Agency (1970) Federal Insecticide, Fungicide, and Rodenticide Act (FIFRA). 7 U.S.C., 136 et seq.

U.S. Environmental Protection Agency (1976) Toxic Substances Control Act (TSCA) 15. U.S.C., 160.1 et seq.

U.S. Governmental Protection Agency (1978) Proposed guidelines for registering pesticides in the U.S. hazard evaluation: Humans and domestic animals. *Fed. Reg.* 43, pp. 37336–37345; 37351–37356.

U.S. Government Protection Agency (1976) Proposed health effects test standards for toxic substances control act test rules and proposed good laboratory practice standards for health effects. *Fed. Reg.* 44, pp. 44054–44059; 44066–44067.

U.S. Environmental Protection Agency (1985) Health effects testing guidelines. *Fed. Red. 50*, pp. 39397–39398.

Index

Absorption, 9
Accutane, 4
Acute toxicity studies, 193–195, 546–547
ADME, 10
Age-related differences, 115
AIDS, 675
Amebiasis, 720
Amyloidosis, 301
Analgesia and anesthesia, 307–308, 367–368, 371, 457, 507–510
Angiectasis, 236
Animal identification, 180–183
Animal rights, 2
Animal Welfare Act, 676
Atrial thrombosis, 239
AZT, 8, 813

Biliary proliferations, 94
Biohazard, 680
Biotechnology, 497
Blood collection, 62–73, 306–308, 365, 454–456, 593, 700–704
Blood pressure, 66–67, 312, 704–705
Buehler procedure, 371–375

Campylobacteriosis, 712
Capsule administration, 48–49, 691–692

Carcinogenicity, 40–41, 197–199, 320, 548, 749
Cardiovascular parameters, 63–67, 521, 588–593
  toxicity, 759
Cataractogenesis, 353
Chinese hamsters, 297
Chronic toxicity, 197
Clinical chemistry values, 80, 313, 355–356, 525, 702, 752, 790–801
Clinical pathology, 78–79, 230–231, 312–317, 355, 522–530, 701, 753, 765–811
Congenital defects, 86
Conjugation reactions, 122–129
Contaminants (diet), 35–36
Cross-species extrapolation, 820–826

Dermal carcinogenicity, 205–208
Dermal dosing, 452
Dermal irritation and toxicity, 4–59, 305–306, 461–462, 758–759, 817–818
Dietary admix, 44–45, 209–211, 692
Disease models, 318–320, 738
Diseases, 415–416, 831–832
Distribution, 9–10
Dosing, 6, 41–61, 206–229, 362–365, 451–454, 513–517, 582–587, 691–699, 740, 744

Draize scale, 373
Drinking water, 211–213

Ear notching, 181–182
Earthworms, 737–743
ECG, 63–65, 312, 590–593
Elixir of sulfanilamide, 3
Enterotoxemia, 471
Epoxide hydrolase, 120–122
European hamster, 297
Excretion, 16
Extrahepatic metabolism, 130–133, 341–
    342

Femoral vein, 53–54
Filariasis, 720
First systematic use of animals, 1
FISN, 243–249
Five Freedoms, 357
Foci of cellular alterations, 94
Food restriction, 36
Footpad injection, 364
Functional observational battery (FOB), 62–
    63

Gavage, 45–48, 206–209, 365
Genetic definition, 843–847
Genetic tox studies, 200–203
Glomerulonephropathy, 91–92
GLPs, 873–874
Guinea pig maximization test, 375–
    380
Gut flora metabolism, 342

Hamster enteritis, 327–328
Hamster species, 296–299
Hemangioma, 238
Hemangiosarcoma, 238
Hepatitis, 715–716
Heritable translocation assay, 201–
    202
Herpes virus tamarinus, 714
Host resistance test, 389–390

Ideal species, 815
Identification (animal), 180–183
Induction (metabolic), 108
Inhalation, 59–61, 227–229, 320–321,
    516, 817
Intradermal, 223–224, 306, 364, 453–
    454
Intramuscular, 55–56, 220–221, 306, 364,
    453, 516, 584, 697
Intranasal, 698
Intraperitoneal, 54–55, 217–220, 306, 454,
    584–585, 698
Intravenous, 49–54, 213–217, 306, 364–
    365, 453, 514–516, 585–586, 692–
    697
In vitro models, 832–834

Jugular vein, 52–53

Keratoconjunctivitis, 37–38

Lash lure, 3
LD_{50}, 26
Legal restrictions, 500
Limitations of models, 818–820
Lungs, 132

Marburg disease (virus), 718
MEST, 203–204
Metabolism, 8, 10–16, 103–134
Microbial host-mediated assay, 202–
    203
Microbiological definition, 842–843
Mites, 461
MMFO, 103–113, 331–333, 419–425,
    480–489, 722–729, 753–755
Morbidity and mortality (rats), 85
Mouse ear swelling, 203–204
Mouse micronucleus assay, 201
Murine lymphomas, 249–251
Mutagenicity test, 813
Mycoplasmosis, 82–83
Mycotic diseases, 416

Necropsy, 74–75, 76–78, 231–232, 603–604, 608–610
Neoplasia, 97–102, 396–397, 478, 721
Neurobehavioral examinations, 62–63
Neurological examination, 705
Nonneoplastic lesions, 325
Normal physiological values:
  mouse, 167–168
  rabbit, 443–444
  rats, 22–23
NSAIDs, 4, 815

Ocular administration, 4–53
Ocular irritation, 459–460
Oraflex, 4
Oral route, 41–42, 206–216, 305, 513, 582–583, 451–452
Orfila, 1
Organ weights, 266–272, 357, 362, 397, 537
Ototoxicity, 353

Peroxisomal proliferation, 118–119
Pigs, 749–760
Pharmaceuticals, 371
Photosensitization, 383
Physical examinations, 61–62, 229–230, 587–588, 700
Pinworms, 82, 241
Pneumocystis carinii, 552
Polyarteritis, 236
Pregnancy tests, 706–707
Probability criteria, 97
Proliferative colitis, 554
Pyrogen test, 463

Radiculoneuropathy, 92
Recommended dietary content, rat, 34–35
Rectal route, 58, 586–587
  renal hyaline droplets, 86
  renal tubular degeneration, 86
Reproductive data:
  dogs, 571
  ferrets, 520
  guinea pig, 354

  hamster, 311
  mouse, 167
  rabbit, 443–444
  rat, 23
Retinenes, 813

Salmonellosis, 711
Scurvy, 361
Segment II studies, 43
Sendai virus infection, 81, 303, 329
Sensitization severity, 379
Shaving, 365–367
Shigellosis, 710
Short-term toxicity studies, 195–196
Sialodacryoadenitis, 37–38, 80–81
Simian hemorrhagic fever, 718
Skin painting studies, 204–205
Sources of variation, 767–769
Special populations, 826
Species differences, 16, 22, 24, 168, 317, 391–393, 598–599, 790–809, 834–836
Split adjuvant test, 380–383
Strain differences, 113–115, 169–170, 247, 275, 317–318
Strains, 165, 392
Stress, 829–830
Study designs, 24, 39–41, 458–462
Subcutaneous route, 56–57, 221–223, 305–306, 362–363, 453, 583, 697–698
Sulfanilamide, 3
Syrian hamster, 296–297

Teratology study, 43, 200, 321, 353, 369–370, 466, 548–549, 757–758
Test article preparation, 45–46, 691
Testicular atrophy, 87
Thalidomide, 3, 4, 675
Tissue biopsy, 705
Toe clipping, 182
Topical route, 57–58, 225–227
Treponematosis, 468
Tuberculosis, 687
Tumor incidences:
  hamsters, 305, 330
  mice, 171, 235–236, 237
  rats, 25, 98
Tyzzer's disease, 302–303, 328, 468, 472

Urine collection, 73–74, 307, 456, 594, 704

Vaginal route, 586–587, 454
Viral diseases, 687

Yaba, 717

Zomax, 4